Contents in Brief

Each update, each change has been made in hopes of providing a premier text to guide the nursing student in their quest for a quality education toward the entry into what I believe to be one of the most satisfying career choices. With each topic I have read and each page written I am in awe of nursing and all it encompasses. None of this would have been possible without the unwavering support of my family, friends, and colleagues.

To my husband Anthony and my daughter Jaelyn Elizabeth, whose love and cheers have encouraged me in this process, I appreciate your support and understanding of the long hours and hard work needed to bring this book to publication. I love you both.

To my writing partner, Kelly Gosnell, words cannot express my respect for your hard work and dedication to our dream to produce a work we are infinitely proud of. You have been a source of strength and friendship in this endeavor. I look forward to many future chapters of writing adventures. Finally to the Elsevier team, I thank you for the continued belief in this title and the partnership striving to produce it.

Kim Cooper

To my husband Ed and my daughters Katelyn and Kinsey, I thank you for your love, patience, and understanding during the time it took to complete this endeavor starting with the seventh edition. Your acceptance of the demands on my time made it all possible. In the last edition I expressed my gratitude to the newest family members, Jared and Miles. Since that time, we have added three new family members to the life of a nursing textbook author. Taj, Ivory, and Owen have now become a part of our textbook! I appreciate all you have done to support and brighten the road along the way.

To all my wonderful family, friends, and colleagues, your constant support and belief in me while completing this project mean more to me than I can express.

To my writing partner, Kim Cooper, without you getting me into the crazy world of ancillary writing years ago, I would not have had the opportunity to tackle this fantastic opportunity of nursing textbook authorship with you. It has been, and hopefully will continue to be, an awesome ride.

Kelly Gosnell

Adult Health Nursing

A tailored education experience —

Sherpath book-organized collections

Sherpath book-organized collections offer:

Objective-based, digital lessons, mapped chapter-by-chapter to the textbook, that make it easy to find applicable digital assignment content.

Adaptive quizzing with personalized questions that correlate directly to textbook content.

Teaching materials that align to the text and are organized by chapter for quick and easy access to invaluable class activities and resources.

Elsevier ebooks that provide convenient access to textbook content, even offline.

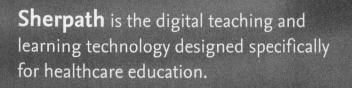

Sherpath is the digital teaching and learning technology designed specifically for healthcare education.

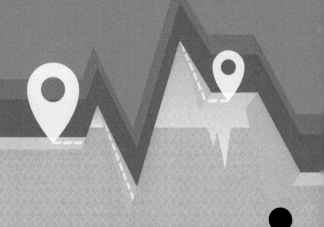

VISIT
myevolve.us/sherpath
today to learn more!

21-CS-0280 TM/AF 6/21

Adult Health Nursing

EDITION

9

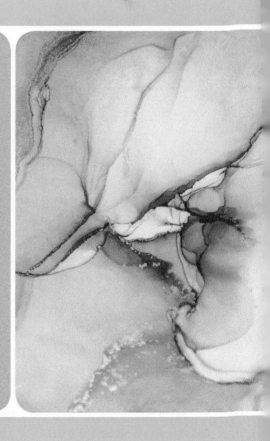

Kim Cooper, RN, MSN
Associate Professor and Dean
School of Nursing
Ivy Tech Community College
Terre Haute, Indiana
President, Indiana State Board of Nursing

Kelly Gosnell, RN, MSN
Associate Professor and Department Chair
School of Nursing
Ivy Tech Community College
Terre Haute, Indiana

ELSEVIER

Elsevier
3251 Riverport Lane
St. Louis, Missouri 63043

ADULT HEALTH NURSING, NINTH EDITION   ISBN: 978-0-323-81161-3
Copyright © 2023 by Elsevier, Inc. All rights reserved.

No part of this publication may be reproduced or transmitted in any form or by any means, electronic or
mechanical, including photocopying, recording, or any information storage and retrieval system, without
permission in writing from the publisher. Details on how to seek permission, further information about the
Publisher's permissions policies and our arrangements with organizations such as the Copyright Clearance
Center and the Copyright Licensing Agency, can be found at our website: www.elsevier.com/permissions.

This book and the individual contributions contained in it are protected under copyright by the Publisher
(other than as may be noted herein).

Notice

Practitioners and researchers must always rely on their own experience and knowledge in evaluating
and using any information, methods, compounds or experiments described herein. Because of rapid
advances in the medical sciences, in particular, independent verification of diagnoses and drug dosages
should be made. To the fullest extent of the law, no responsibility is assumed by Elsevier, authors, editors
or contributors for any injury and/or damage to persons or property as a matter of products liability,
negligence or otherwise, or from any use or operation of any methods, products, instructions, or ideas
contained in the material herein.

Previous editions copyrighted 2019, 2015, 2011, 2006, 2003, 1999, 1995, and 1991.

Library of Congress Control Number: 2021945618

Senior Content Strategist: Brandi Graham
Senior Content Development Specialist: Laura Goodrich
Publishing Services Manager: Julie Eddy
Senior Project Manager: Cindy Thoms
Senior Book Designer: Renee Duenow

Printed in the United States of America

Last digit is the print number: 9 8 7 6 5 4 3 2 1

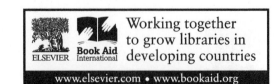

Working together
to grow libraries in
developing countries

www.elsevier.com • www.bookaid.org

Acknowledgments

The ninth edition of this textbook has seen progression geared toward the NCLEX® Next Generation case studies and alternative format questions have been added. At the same time, this edition has maintained the strong foundation that it has historically been recognized for. Special thanks to our photographer, Dr. Katelyn Gosnell Richey, for her hard work in adding more than 100 new photographs between *Foundations of Nursing* and *Adult Health Nursing*; to our many family, friends, and colleagues for volunteering to be our models; and to Ivy Tech Community College, Terre Haute, Indiana, for their willingness to share their facility setting for many of the updated photographs.

The work on the ninth edition kicked off under the direction of Nancy O'Brien, Content Strategist. She was a returning team member from the eighth edition. Shortly after work began she transitioned to a much deserved retirement. We are thankful for Laura Goodrich, Senior Development Specialist, and Cindy Thoms, Senior Project Manager. Their unwavering support and continued belief in our vision were invaluable in the completion of the works. The tireless work behind the scenes has been immeasurable in the quest to bring this edition to fruition.

The role of the practical nurse is to be a key member of the health care team. The education of these dedicated men and women is needed to prepare them for entry to practice. Those contributors, reviewers, and dedicated colleagues have shared invaluable expertise in this journey in bringing this work to life, and we are forever indebted.

Contributors and Reviewers

CONTRIBUTORS

Mary Brown, RN, MEd, MSN CNE
Program Director (Retired)
Nursing
Yavapai College
Prescott, Arizona

Emily Cannon, DNP, RN
Assistant Professor
School of Nursing
Indiana State University
Terre Haute, Indiana

Jeffrey Coto, DNP, MS-CNS, RN
Valparaiso University
CONHP
Valparaiso University
Valparaiso, Indiana

Farzana Dalal, RN, MSN
Instructor
Nursing
Ivy Tech Community College
Terre Haute, Indiana

Michele Gonser, RN, MSN
Director of Quality Improvement
Nursing
Ivy Tech Community College
Fort Wayne, Indiana

Catherine (Cathy) S. Moe, BSN, MS, EdD
Associate Professor-Dean (Retired)
Nursing
Lakeview College of Nursing
Danville, Illinois
Visiting Faculty
Nursing
University of Illinois
Champaign, Illinois
Assistant Professor
Nursing
Lakeview College of Nursing
Charleston, Illinois

REVIEWERS

Amanda Churchman, RN, MSN
PN Program Director
Red River Technology Center
Duncan, Oklahoma

Heather L. Clark, DNP, RN
Practical Nursing Program Director
Penn State University
Center Valley, Pennsylvania

Linda Cline, RN, MSN/Ed
Practical Nursing Program Director
Assistant Professor
Southwest Virginia Community College
Cedar Bluff, Virginia

Odelia Garcia, MS, MSN, BSN, RN
Vocational Nursing Instructor
Texas State Technical College – Harlingen
Harlingen, Texas

Alice M. Hupp, BS, RN
Lead Instructor
North Central Texas College
Gainesville, Texas

Lorraine Kelley, BSHA, RN
Faculty
Pensacola State College
Pensacola, Florida

Molly M. Showalter, MSN Ed, RN
Interim Director Vocational Nursing Program
Texas Southmost College
Brownsville, Texas

Elaine Kay Strouss, MSN, BSN, RN
Dean of the School of Health Sciences
Community College of Beaver County
Monaca, Pennsylvania

LPN/LVN Advisory Board

Nancy Bohnarczyk, MA
Adjunct Instructor
College of Mount St. Vincent
New York, New York

Nicola Contreras, BN, RN
Faculty
Galen College
San Antonio, Texas

Dolores Cotton, MSN, RN
Practical Nursing Coordinator
Meridian Technology Center
Stillwater, Oklahoma

Patricia Donovan, MSN, RN
Director of Practical Nursing and Curriculum Chair
Porter and Chester Institute
Rocky Hill, Connecticut

Nancy Haughton, MSN, RN
Practical Nursing Program Faculty
Chester County Intermediate Unit
Downingtown, Pennsylvania

Dawn Johnson, DNP, RN, Ed
Practical Nurse Educator
Reno, Nevada

Mary E. Johnson, RN, MSN
Director of Nursing
Dorsey Schools
Roseville, Michigan

Bonnie Kehm, PhD, RN
Faculty Program Director
Excelsior College
Albany, New York

Tawnya S. Lawson, MS, RN
Dean, Practical Nursing Program
Hondros College
Westerville, Ohio

Kristin Madigan, MS, RN
Nursing Faculty
Pine Technical and Community College
Pine City, Minnesota

Hana Malik, DNP, FNP-BC
Academic Director
Illinois College of Nursing
Lombard, Illinois

Mary Lee Pollard, PhD, RN, CNE
Dean, School of Nursing
Excelsior College
Albany, New York

Barbara Ratliff, MSN, RN
Nursing Program Chair
Cincinnati State Great Oaks School of Practical Nursing
Cincinnati, Ohio

Mary Ruiz-Nuve, RN, MSN
Director of Practical Nursing Program
St. Louis College of Health Careers
St. Louis, Missouri

Renee Sheehan, RN, MSN/Ed
Director of Nursing, Vocational Nursing
Nursing Assistant Programs
Summit College
Colton, California

Fleur de Liza S. Tobias-Cuyco, BSc, CPhT
Dean, Director of Student Affairs, and Instructor
Preferred College of Nursing
Los Angeles, California

To the Instructor

The ninth edition of *Adult Health Nursing* was developed to educate the practical/vocational nursing student in the fundamentals of nursing required to care competently and safely for a wide variety of patients in various settings. As the level of knowledge and responsibility increases for LPN/LVNs in all health care settings from acute to community-based care, it is essential that a text such as *Adult Health Nursing* be available to educate the student for the growing demands of this profession.

This full-color companion text to *Foundations of Nursing* provides the knowledge base necessary for the expanding role of the LPN/LVN while remaining accessible, clearly written, user-friendly, and portable. This new edition was revised to incorporate the most current and clinically relevant information available.

Finally, it is our belief that nursing will always be both an art and a science. This philosophy is reflected throughout the text.

ORGANIZATION AND STANDARD FEATURES

The organization of the ninth edition continues to follow the strengths of the previous edition, based on positive comments from educators and students. An overview of anatomy and physiology and a separate chapter on care of the surgical patient from the preoperative phase, through surgery, and care during the postoperative phase. Several chapters have received extensive revisions in order to provide the most current information for the student. These chapters include Chapter 8, *Care of the Patient With a Cardiovascular or a Peripheral Vascular Disorder*; Chapter 9, *Care of the Patient With a Respiratory Disorder*; Chapter 11, *Care of the Patient With an Endocrine Disorder*; and Chapter 12, *Care of the Patient With a Reproductive Disorder*.

TABLE OF CONTENTS

The text begins with an introductory chapter on anatomy and physiology to give students the basis for comprehension of the disorders content to follow. A chapter devoted to care of the surgical patient comes next, followed by chapters covering major disorders by body system. Systems disorders chapters are arranged in an orderly flow but can be studied in any order. New and additional content has been added to ensure that students have access to the most current information. Chapter Organization

Disorders chapters typically are organized in the following format for more effective learning:
- Etiology and Pathophysiology
- Clinical Manifestations
- Assessment (with subjective and objective data)
- Diagnostic Tests
- Medical Management
- Nursing Interventions (including relevant medications)
- Nursing Diagnoses
- Patient Teaching
- Prognosis

NURSING PROCESS

The nursing process as applied to specific disorders is integrated throughout. A special nursing process summary section appears at the end of appropriate chapters, enabling the reader to see more clearly its application to the chapter content as a whole. For this text the authors have replaced nursing diagnoses with a patient problem list to better describe health problems the patient experiences. These statements provide a problem-centered approach to nursing care. We have emphasized the role of the LPN/LVN in the nursing process as follows:
- The LPN/LVN will participate in planning care for the patient based on the patient's needs.
- The LPN/LVN will review the patient's plan of care and recommend revisions as needed.
- The LPN/LVN will follow defined prioritization for patient care.
- The LPN/LVN will use clinical pathways, care maps, or care plans to guide and review patient care.

REFERENCES AND SUGGESTED READINGS

References and Suggested Readings are grouped by chapter and listed at the end of the book for easy access. *Additional Resources* such as websites and agencies are included where applicable.

In the appendixes, *Common Abbreviations* are listed along with The Joint Commission's *Lists of Dangerous Abbreviations, Acronyms, and Symbols* to promote safety in clinical practice in such areas as avoiding dosage errors, and *Laboratory Reference Values* provide quick access to important information.

LPN THREADS

The ninth edition of *Adult Health Nursing* shares some features and design elements with other Elsevier LPN/LVN textbooks. The purpose of these *LPN Threads* is to make it easier for students and instructors to use the variety of books required by the relatively brief and demanding LPN/LVN curriculum. *LPN Threads* include the following:

- Efforts are continually made to keep the *reading level* of our LPN texts around 10th grade to increase the consistency among chapters and ensure the text is easy to understand.
- *Full-color design, cover, photos,* and *illustrations* are visually appealing and pedagogically useful.
- *Objectives* (numbered) begin each chapter. Chapter objectives provide a framework for content and are especially important in providing the structure for the TEACH Lesson Plans for the textbook.
- *Key Terms* with phonetic pronunciations and page number references are listed at the beginning of each chapter. Key terms appear in color in the chapter and are defined briefly, with full definitions in the *Glossary*. Simple phonetic pronunciations accompany difficult medical, nursing, or scientific terms or other words that may be difficult for students to pronounce.
- A wide variety of *special features* related to critical thinking, clinical practice, care of the older adult, health promotion, safety, patient teaching, complementary and alternative therapies, communication, home health care, delegation and assignment, and more. Refer to the To the Student section of this introduction on page xiv for descriptions of each of these features.
- *Critical Thinking Questions* with each Nursing Care Plan give students opportunities to practice critical thinking and clinical decision-making skills with realistic patient scenarios. Answers are provided in the Instructor Resources section on the Evolve website.
- *Key Points,* located at the end of chapters, follow the chapter objectives and serve as a useful chapter review.
- A full suite of *Instructor Resources* including TEACH Lesson Plans and Lecture Outlines, PowerPoint Lecture Slides, Test Bank, and Image Collection. Each of these teaching resources is described in detail below.
- In addition to consistent content, design, and support resources, these textbooks benefit from the advice and input of the *Elsevier LPN/LVN Advisory Board.*

TEACHING AND LEARNING PACKAGE

FOR STUDENTS

- An *Evolve website* provides free student resources, including additional review questions for the NCLEX Examination for every chapter, calculators, and animations and video clips.
- The *Study Guide for Adult Health Nursing* is designed to promote learning, understanding, and application of the content in the textbook. Each chapter ties specific activities to specific objectives rather than simply listing objectives and activities separately. Activities include hundreds of labeling, matching, and fill-in-the-blank questions, each with textbook page references; critical thinking questions with clinical scenarios; and multiple-choice and alternate-format questions for NCLEX review. The complete answer key is provided to instructors in the Instructor Resources section of the Evolve website. *Sold separately.*
- *Virtual Clinical Excursions* is an interactive workbook/online package that guides the student through a multifloor virtual hospital in a hands-on clinical learning experience. Students can assess and analyze information, diagnose, set priorities, and implement and evaluate care. NCLEX-style review questions provide immediate testing of clinical knowledge. *Sold separately.*

FOR INSTRUCTORS

The comprehensive *Evolve Resources With TEACH Instructor Resource* provides a rich array of teaching tools and includes the following:

- *TEACH Lesson Plans With Lecture Outlines,* based on the textbook learning objectives, provide ready-to-use lesson plans that tie together all the text and ancillary components provided for *Adult Health Nursing.*
- A collection of more than 200 *PowerPoint Lecture Slides* are specific to the text.
- A *Test Bank,* delivered in ExamView, provides approximately 1500 multiple-choice and alternate-format NCLEX-style questions. Each question includes the correct answer, rationale, topic, objective, cognitive level, step of the nursing process, and NCLEX category of patient needs, as well as corresponding textbook page references.
- An *Image Collection* contains nearly 500 images from the textbook. Images are suitable for incorporation into classroom lectures, PowerPoint presentations, or distance-learning applications.
- *Answer Keys* are provided for the Critical Thinking Questions in Nursing Care Plans and for the activities in the Study Guide.

To the Student

Designed with you in mind, *Adult Health Nursing* presents fundamental nursing concepts in a visually appealing and easy-to-use format. Here are some of the numerous special features that will help you understand and apply the material.

READING AND REVIEW TOOLS

Objectives introduce the chapter topics, *Key Terms* are listed with page number references, and difficult medical, nursing, or scientific terms are accompanied by simple phonetic pronunciations. Key terms are in color where they are briefly defined in the text, and complete definitions are provided in the Glossary.

Each chapter ends with a *Get Ready for the NCLEX® Examination!* section. *Key Points* follow the chapter objectives and serve as a chapter review. An extensive set of *Review Questions for the NCLEX® Examination* provides immediate opportunity for testing your understanding of the chapter content. Next Generation case studies and alternative format questions have been added to this section in order to aid in preparing for the changes that will be occurring with the NCLEX-PN® examination.

ADDITIONAL LEARNING RESOURCES

The online *Evolve Resources* at http://evolve.elsevier.com/Cooper/adulthealth give you access to even more Review Questions for the NCLEX Examination, animations, and much more.

CHAPTER FEATURES

Skills are presented in a logical step-by-step format with accompanying full-color illustrations. Clearly defined *nursing actions* followed by *rationales* in italicized type show you how and why skills are performed. Each skill includes icons that serve as a reminder to perform the basic steps applicable to *all* nursing interventions:

Check orders.

 Gather necessary equipment and supplies.

 Introduce yourself.

 Check patient's identification.

 Provide privacy.

 Explain the procedure/intervention.

 Perform hand hygiene.

 Don gloves (if applicable).

Nursing Care Plans, developed around specific case studies, include patient problem statements in place of nursing diagnoses. These patient problem statements better describe health problems the patient experiences. These statements provide a problem-centered approach to nursing care. An emphasis is placed on patient goals and outcomes and questions to promote *critical thinking.* These sample care plans are valuable tools that can be used as a guideline in the clinical setting. The critical thinking aspect empowers you to develop sound clinical decision-making skills.

Patient problem statements and interventions are screened and set apart in the text in a clear, easy-to-understand format to help you learn to participate in the development of a nursing care plan.

Evidence-Based Practice boxes summarize the latest research findings and highlight how they apply to LPN/LVN practice.

Medication tables developed for specific disorders provide quick access to action, side effects, and nursing considerations for commonly used medications.

Safety Alert! boxes emphasize the importance of maintaining safety in patient and resident care to protect patients, residents, family, health care providers, and the public from accidents and the spread of disease.

Health Promotion boxes emphasize a healthy lifestyle, preventive behaviors, and screening tests to assist in the prevention of accidents and disease.

Patient Teaching boxes appear frequently in the text to help develop awareness of the vital role of patient/family teaching in health care today.

Coordinated Care boxes throughout the text promote comprehensive patient care with other members of the health care team, focusing on prioritization, assignment, supervision, collaboration, and leadership topics.

Complementary and Alternative Therapies boxes in nearly every chapter give a breakdown of specific nontraditional therapies, along with precautions and possible side effects.

Cultural Considerations boxes explore broad cultural beliefs and how to address the needs of a culturally diverse patient and resident population when planning nursing care.

Communication boxes focus on communication strategies with real-life examples of nurse-patient dialogue.

Life Span Considerations for the Older Adult boxes bring a gerontologic perspective to nursing care, focusing on the nursing interventions unique to the older adult patient or resident.

Home Care Considerations boxes discuss the issues facing patients and caregivers in the home setting.

Contents

Adult Health Nursing

Introduction to Anatomy and Physiology

1

Objectives

1. Identify the difference between anatomy and physiology.
2. Define the term *anatomical position*.
3. List and define the principal directional terms and sections (planes) used in describing the body and the relationship of body parts to one another.
4. Use each word from a given list of anatomical terms in a sentence.
5. List the nine abdominopelvic regions and the abdominopelvic quadrants.
6. List and discuss, in order of increasing complexity, the levels of organization of the body.
7. Differentiate among tissues, organs, and systems.
8. Identify and define three major components of the cell.
9. Discuss the stages of mitosis and explain the importance of cellular reproduction.
10. Differentiate between active and passive transport processes that move substances through cell membranes, and give two examples of each.
11. Describe the four types of body tissues.
12. Discuss the two types of epithelial membranes.
13. List the 11 major organ systems of the body and briefly describe the major functions of each.

Key Terms

active transport (p. 7)
anatomy (p. 1)
cell (p. 4)
cytoplasm (SĪ-tō-plăzm, p. 5)
diffusion (dĭ-FŪ-zhŭn, p. 8)
dorsal (p. 3)
filtration (p. 8)
homeostasis (hō-mē-ō-STĀ-sĭs, p. 4)
membrane (p. 5)
mitosis (mĭ-TŌ-sĭs, p. 6)
nucleus (p. 5)

organ (p. 4)
osmosis (ŏz-MŌ-sĭs, p. 8)
passive transport (p. 7)
phagocytosis (făg-ŏ-sī-TŌ-sĭs, p. 7)
physiology (fĭz-ē-ŎL-ō-jē, p. 1)
pinocytosis (pī-nō-sī-TŌ-sĭs, p. 7)
quarks (p. 4)
system (p. 4)
tissue (p. 4)
ventral (p. 2)

Caring for a person who is sick or injured requires understanding how the human body normally functions, so nurses must be familiar with basic human anatomy and physiology principles. **Anatomy** is the study, classification, and description of structures and organs of the body. **Physiology** explains the processes and functions of the various structures and how they interrelate. The normal, healthy human body is like a finely tuned machine; each part performs a special function. Like a machine, when the body malfunctions, the repairer must understand how to make the necessary repairs to return the body to homeostasis; otherwise, illness, disease, or death may result.

ANATOMICAL TERMINOLOGY

Study of the human body first requires mastery of terms that aid in locating specific structures. To understand the following terms, consider the body in a normal anatomical position, that is, standing erect with the face and palms facing forward (Fig. 1.1):

- *Anterior (or ventral):* To face forward; the front of the body. The chest is located anterior to the spine.
- *Posterior (or dorsal):* Toward the back. The kidneys are posterior to the peritoneum.
- *Cranial:* Toward the head. The brain is located in the cranial portion of the body.
- *Caudal:* Toward the distal end of the body (trunk). A caudal anesthetic may be given.
- *Superior:* Toward the head, or above. The neck is superior to the shoulders.
- *Inferior:* Lower, toward the feet, or below another. The foot is inferior to the ankle.
- *Medial:* Toward the midline. The sternum (breastbone) is located in the medial portion of the chest.
- *Lateral:* Toward the side. The outer area of the leg, the area located on the side, is called lateral.
- *Proximal:* Nearest the origin of the structure; nearest the trunk. The elbow is proximal to the forearm.

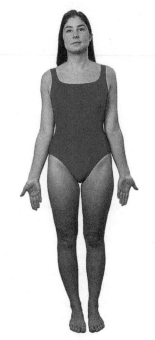

Fig. 1.1 Anatomical position. The body is in an erect or standing posture with the arms at the sides and palms forward. The head and feet also point forward. The right and left sides of the body are mirror images of each other. (From Frank ED, Long BW, Smith BJ: *Merrill's atlas of radiographic positioning and procedures,* ed 1, St. Louis, 2012, Mosby.)

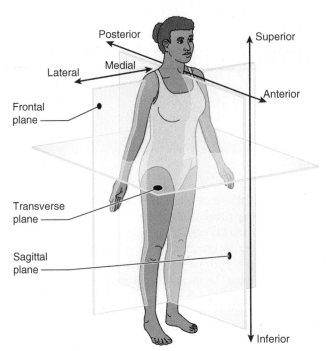

Fig. 1.2 Directions and planes of the body.

- *Distal:* Farthest from the origin of the structure; farthest from the trunk. The fingers are distal to the palm of the hand.
- *Superficial:* Nearer the surface. The skin of the arm is superficial to the muscles below it.
- *Deep:* Farther away from the body surface. The bone of the upper arm is deep to the muscles that surround and cover it.

BODY PLANES

To make it easier to study individual organs or the body as a whole, divide the body into three imaginary planes: sagittal, coronal (frontal), and transverse (Fig. 1.2):

1. The sagittal plane runs lengthwise from the front to the back. A sagittal cut gives a right and a left portion of the body. A midsagittal cut gives two equal halves.
2. The coronal (frontal) plane divides the body into a ventral (front) section and a dorsal (back) section.
3. The transverse plane cuts the body horizontal to the sagittal and frontal planes, dividing the body into caudal and cranial portions.

BODY CAVITIES

Although the body appears to be a solid structure, it is not. It is made up of open spaces, or cavities, that contain compact, well-ordered arrangements of internal organs. The body has two major cavities that are subdivided and contain compact, well-ordered arrangements of internal organs. The two major cavities are

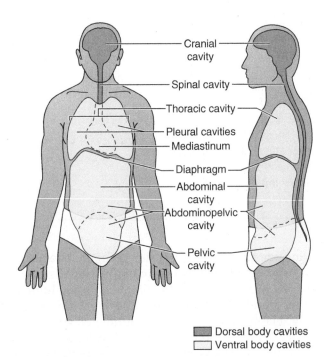

Fig. 1.3 Location and subdivisions of the dorsal and ventral body cavities as viewed from the front (anterior) and the side (lateral).

the ventral and the dorsal body cavities (Fig. 1.3 and Table 1.1).

Ventral Cavity

The **ventral** cavity consists of the thoracic (or chest) cavity and the abdominopelvic cavity (see Fig. 1.3), which are separated by the diaphragm (a muscle directly beneath the lungs).

The thoracic cavity contains the heart and the lungs. Its mid-portion is a subdivision of the thoracic cavity,

Table 1.1	Body Cavities
BODY CAVITY	**ORGAN(S)**
Ventral Body Cavity	
Thoracic Cavity	
Mediastinum	Trachea, heart, blood vessels
Pleural cavities	Lungs
Abdominopelvic Cavity	
Abdominal cavity	Liver, gallbladder, stomach, spleen, pancreas, small intestine, parts of the large intestine
Pelvic cavity	Lower (sigmoid) colon, rectum, urinary bladder, reproductive organs
Dorsal Body Cavity	
Cranial cavity	Brain
Spinal cavity	Spinal cord

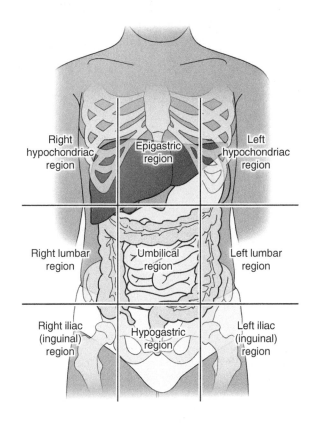

Fig. 1.4 The nine regions of the abdominopelvic cavity. The most superficial organs are shown. Can you identify the deeper structures in each region?

the mediastinum, which contains the trachea, the heart, and the blood vessels. Its other subdivisions are the right and left pleural cavities, which contain the lungs.

The abdominal cavity contains the stomach, the liver, the gallbladder, the spleen, the pancreas, the small intestine, and parts of the large intestine. The pelvic cavity is a subdivision of the abdominal cavity and contains the lower portion of the large intestine (lower sigmoid colon, rectum), urinary bladder, and internal structures of the reproductive system. Because the abdominal and pelvic cavities are not separated by any structure, they are referred to collectively as the abdominopelvic cavity (see Table 1.1).

Dorsal Cavity

The dorsal cavity is composed of the cranial and spinal body cavities. The cranial body cavity houses the brain, whereas the spinal cavity contains the spinal cord. The dorsal body cavity is smaller than the ventral cavity (see Table 1.1).

ABDOMINAL REGIONS

For convenience in locating abdominal organs, anatomists divide the abdomen into nine imaginary regions. The nine regions are identified from right to left and from top to bottom (Fig. 1.4).

The most superficial organs located in each of the nine abdominal regions are shown in Fig. 1.4. The visible organs in each region are as follows: (1) right hypochondriac region, the right lobe of the liver and the gallbladder; (2) epigastric region, parts of the right and left lobes of the liver, and a large portion of the stomach; (3) left hypochondriac region, a small portion of the stomach, and large intestine; (4) right lumbar region, parts of the large and small intestine; (5) umbilical region, a portion of the transverse colon, and loops of the small intestine; (6) left lumbar region, additional loops of the small intestine, and a part of the colon; (7) right iliac region, the cecum, and parts of the small intestine; (8) hypogastric region, loops of the small intestine, the urinary bladder, and the appendix; and (9) left iliac region, portions of the colon, and the small intestine (Patton, 2019).

ABDOMINOPELVIC QUADRANTS

Health professionals frequently divide the abdomen into four quadrants to describe the site of abdominopelvic pain or to locate an internal pathologic condition such as a tumor or abscess (Fig. 1.5). Horizontal and vertical lines passing through the umbilicus (navel) divide the abdomen into right and left upper quadrants and right and left lower quadrants.

STRUCTURAL LEVELS OF ORGANIZATION

Before studying the structure and function of the human body and its many parts, think about how those parts are organized and how they may fit together into a functioning whole. Fig. 1.6 illustrates the different levels of organization that influence body structure and function. The levels of organization progress from the least complex (chemical level) to the most complex

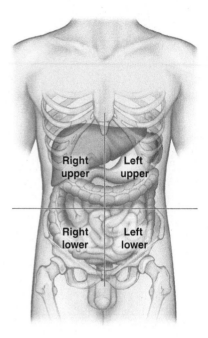

Fig. 1.5 Horizontal and vertical line passing through the umbilicus (navel) divides the abdomen into right and left upper quadrants and right and left lower quadrants. (From Patton KT, Thibodeau GA: *The human body in health and disease,* ed 7, St. Louis, 2018, Elsevier.)

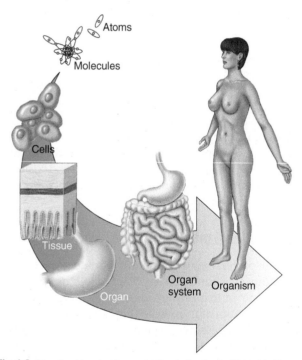

Fig. 1.6 Structural levels of organization in the body. (From Herlihy B: *The human body in health and illness,* ed 5, St. Louis, 2014, Saunders.)

(body as a whole). The structural levels of organization in the body are cells, tissues, organs, and systems.

Although the body is a single structure, it is made up of billions of smaller structures. Atoms and molecules often are referred to as the chemical level of organization (see Fig. 1.6). Atoms are small particles that form the building blocks of matter, once thought to be the smallest complete units of which all matter was made. More recent research has identified the quark. Atoms contain protons, neurons, and electrons; quarks are the building blocks of protons and neutrons that make up the atom (Moskowitz, 2012). Since this discovery, there has been much discussion of whether there is a structure smaller than a quark. Presently, there are many theories, but there is not sufficient evidence to determine that there is any smaller structure (Lincoln, 2014). When two or more atoms unite through their electron structures, they form a molecule. A molecule can be made of atoms that are alike (e.g., the oxygen molecule is made of two identical atoms), but more often a molecule is made of two or more different atoms (e.g., a molecule of water [H_2O] contains one atom of oxygen [O] and two atoms of hydrogen [H]) (see Fig. 1.6).

The existence of life depends on the proper levels and proportions of many chemical substances in the cytoplasm of cells. The cell is considered the smallest living unit of structure and function in our bodies. Although cells are considered the simplest units of living matter, they are extremely complex units.

Tissues are even more complex than cells. A tissue is an organization of many similar cells that act together to perform a common function. Cells are held together and are surrounded by varying amounts and types of gluelike, nonliving intercellular substances.

Organs are more complex than tissues. An organ is a group of several different kinds of tissues arranged to perform a special function. The stomach and intestines shown in Fig. 1.6 are an example of organization at the organ level.

Systems are the most complex units that make up the body. A system is an organization of varying numbers and kinds of organs arranged to perform complex functions for the body. The organs of the gastrointestinal system, shown in Fig. 1.6, permit digestion of ingested food and excretion of waste products. Major organs of the digestive tract include the mouth, esophagus, stomach, and small and large intestines.

CELLS

In the mid-1660s, scientist Robert Hooke discovered the first cell while examining plant fragments under the microscope. The structures reminded him of the cells in a monastery, so he coined the term cell (the fundamental unit of all living tissue) (Fig. 1.7; famousscientists.org, 2014). Many living things are so simple that they consist of just one cell. Conversely, the human body is so complex that it has trillions of cells.

All cells are microscopic but differ greatly in size and shape. Despite their differences, all cells exhibit five unique characteristics of life: growth, metabolism, responsiveness, reproduction, and homeostasis. Homeostasis is achieved when the body's internal environment is relatively constant; this state is maintained naturally by adaptive responses that promote healthy survival.

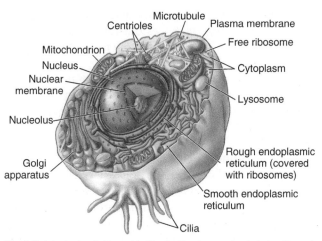

Fig. 1.7 A typical cell. (From Herlihy B: *The human body in health and illness*, ed 6, St. Louis, 2018, Elsevier.)

Structural Parts of Cells

The three main parts of a cell are the plasma membrane, cytoplasm, and nucleus (see Fig. 1.7).

Plasma membrane. The plasma membrane encloses the cytoplasm and forms the outer boundary of the cell. The plasma membrane is a thin and extremely delicate structure. Despite its size and delicacy, it has a precise, orderly structure.

Even though it seems fragile, the plasma membrane is strong enough to keep the cell whole and intact. It also performs other life-preserving functions for the cell, serving as a gateway between the fluid inside the cell and the fluid around it. The plasma membrane is selectively permeable. This means the membrane permits certain substances to enter and leave while not allowing other substances to cross. This membrane separates the cell contents from the dilute saltwater solution called interstitial fluid, or tissue fluid, which surrounds every cell in the body. The plasma membrane also has distinct surface proteins that identify a cell as coming from one individual. This fact is the basis of tissue typing, a procedure performed to determine compatibility before an organ transplantation can occur. Carbohydrate chains attached to the surface of cells often help identify cell types.

Cytoplasm. Cytoplasm, found only within cells, is the internal living material of cells. Also known as protoplasm, it is a sticky, gel-like substance that contains approximately 70% water, as well as food, minerals, enzymes, and other specialized materials. Lying between the plasma membrane and the nucleus of the cell, cytoplasm contains numerous organelles (tiny functioning structures) that help with the processes of the cell. Because organelles are so small, they were not discovered until the development of the powerful electron microscope. (Table 1.2 lists major cell structures and their functions.)

Nucleus. The nucleus is the largest organelle within the cell. It is responsible for cell reproduction and control of

Table 1.2	Some Major Cells and Their Functions
CELL STRUCTURE	**FUNCTION(S)**
Plasma membrane	Serves as the cell's boundary; protein and carbohydrate molecules on the outer surface of the plasma membrane perform various functions (e.g., serve as markers that identify cells of each individual or as receptor molecules for certain hormones)
Endoplasmic reticulum (ER)	Ribosomes attach to rough ER to synthesize proteins; smooth ER synthesizes lipids and certain carbohydrates
Ribosomes	Synthesize proteins; the cell's "protein factories"
Mitochondria	Synthesize adenosine triphosphate; the cell's "powerhouses"
Lysosomes	Serve as cell's "digestive system"
Golgi apparatus	Synthesizes carbohydrates, combines it with protein, and packages the product as globules of glycoprotein
Centrioles	Function in cell reproduction
Cilia	Short, hairlike extensions on the free surfaces of some cells capable of movement; often have specialized functions such as propelling mucus upward over cells that line the respiratory tract
Flagella	Single projections of cell surfaces, much larger than cilia; an example in humans is the "tail" of a sperm cell; propulsive movement makes it possible for sperm to "swim" or move toward the ovum once they are deposited in the female reproductive tract
Nucleus	Dictates protein synthesis, thereby playing an essential role in other cell activities, namely active transport, metabolism, growth, and heredity
Nucleoli	Play an essential role in the formation of ribosomes

the other organelles. The nucleus is surrounded by the nuclear membrane. It contains nucleoplasm, a refined form of cytoplasm, and the nucleolus, the largest structure in the nucleus. The nucleolus is critical in the formation of ribonucleic acid (RNA).

Endoplasmic reticulum. Throughout the cytoplasm lies a system of membranes, or canals, called the endoplasmic reticulum (ER). ER functions as a miniature circulating system for the cell by carrying substances from one part of the cell to another. There are two types of ER: (1) smooth, which is found in cells that deal with fatty substances; and (2) rough, which is found in cells that manufacture proteins (Patton, 2019).

Ribosomes. Ribosomes are tiny structures floating free in the cytoplasm or attached to the rough ER. They are called protein factories because they produce enzymes and other proteins.

Mitochondria. The mitochondria are the powerhouses of the cells. They are bean-shaped with a folded interior membrane. They take food and convert it to a complex energy form, adenosine triphosphate (ATP), for use by the cell. ATP supplies the energy for all activities.

Lysosomes. Lysosomes are small saclike structures containing enzymes that digest food compounds and microbes that have invaded the cell.

Golgi apparatus. The Golgi apparatus usually is located near the nucleus. It is the "packaging plant" of the cell.

It packages certain carbohydrate and protein compounds into globules. Then, it moves outward through the cell membrane, where it breaks open and releases its contents.

Centrioles. The centrioles are paired, rod-shaped organelles. During cell division (mitosis), they aid in the formation of the spindle, a structure necessary for cell reproduction.

Protein Synthesis

Protein is a vital component of every cell in the body. Protein production relies on nucleic acids in the cell's cytoplasm and nucleus. Two important nucleic acids are (1) DNA (Fig. 1.8), which is located only in the nucleus; and (2) RNA, which is located in the nucleus and cytoplasm. The DNA encodes a message for protein synthesis as RNA and sends the RNA to ribosomes in the cytoplasm, where the protein is produced. For this reason, DNA is called the chemical blueprint, and RNA is called the chemical messenger.

Cell Division

All cells in the body, except sex cells, reproduce by **mitosis**, which is a type of somatic (pertaining to nonreproductive cells) cell division in which the original cell divides to form two daughter cells. Each daughter cell has the same characteristics (including the nucleus and cytoplasm) as the original cell. Each daughter cell contains the same number of chromosomes as the parent cell. Each chromosome in the daughter cells contains the complete genetic information of the original chromosome because of duplication of the DNA molecule during interphase (Fig. 1.9).

The chromosomes (spindle-shaped rods) in the cell's nucleus carry the genes that are responsible for the organism's traits, including such hereditary factors as hair and eye color. These chromosomes are composed of DNA. Each body cell in humans contains 46 chromosomes, which exist in pairs. At the time of fertilization, one member of each pair is received from the father, and one is received from the mother to form a total of 23 pairs of chromosomes. These paired chromosomes, except for the pair that determines sex, are alike in size and appearance and carry genes for the same traits.

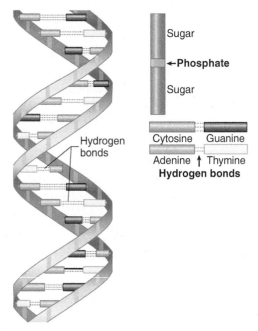

Fig. 1.8 Deoxyribonucleic acid (DNA) molecule. Note that each side of the DNA molecule consists of alternating sugar and phosphate groups. Each sugar group is united to the sugar group opposite it by a pair of nitrogenous bases (adenine-thymine or cytosine-guanine). The sequence of these pairs constitutes a genetic code that determines the structure and function of a cell. (From Patton KT, Thibodeau GA: *Anatomy & physiology,* ed 10, St. Louis, 2019, Elsevier.)

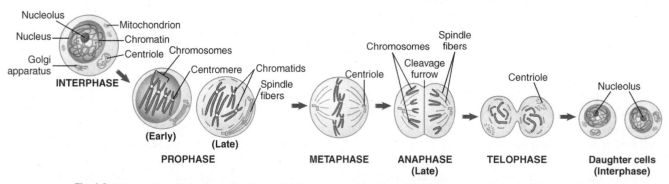

Fig. 1.9 Mitosis. (From Thibodeau GA, Patton KT: *Structure and function of the body,* ed 14, St. Louis, 2012, Mosby.)

During mitosis, the cell goes through four phases: prophase, metaphase, anaphase, and telophase:

1. *Prophase:* In the nucleus, the chromosomes form two strands called chromatids. In the cytoplasm, the centrioles form a network of spindle fibers.
2. *Metaphase:* The nuclear membrane and nucleolus disappear, and the chromosomes are aligned across the center of the cell. The centrioles are at the opposite ends of the cell, and spindle fibers are attached to each chromatid.
3. *Anaphase:* The chromosomes are pulled to the opposite ends of the cell, and cell division begins.
4. *Telophase:* During this final phase of cell division, the two nuclei appear and the chromosomes disperse. At the end of the phase, two new daughter cells appear.

Movement of Materials Across Cell Membranes

For a cell to survive, it must receive food and oxygen and secrete its waste products. A number of processes allow for the mass movement of substances into and out of the cells. These transport processes are classified under two general headings: passive transport and active transport.

The difference between active and passive transport is based on whether energy is required. **Active transport** involves chemical activity that allows the cell to admit larger molecules than would otherwise be possible. Active processes require the cell to expend energy. **Passive transport** processes, on the other hand, do not require energy expenditure. The cell obtains energy for active transport from an important chemical substance called ATP. ATP is produced in the cell from nutrients and releases energy so that the cell can work.

Active transport processes. Active transport is an extremely important process. It allows cells to move certain ions or other water-soluble particles to specific areas. Certain enzymes play a role in active transport, providing a chemical "pump" that helps move substances through the cell membrane. For example, insulin binds with glucose and transports the glucose into the cell. Other active transport processes (Table 1.3) include the following:

- **Phagocytosis** (Greek for "cell-eating"): The process that permits a cell to engulf (or surround) any foreign material and to digest it. The white blood cells in the human body often perform this function.
- **Pinocytosis** (Greek for "cell-drinking"): The process by which extracellular fluid is taken into the cell. The cell membrane develops a saclike indentation filled with extracellular fluid and then closes around it and digests it.
- *Sodium-potassium pump:* The process of actively transporting sodium ions (Na^+) out of cells and potassium ions (K^+) into cells. The sodium-potassium pump maintains a lower sodium concentration in intracellular fluid than in the surrounding extracellular fluid. At the same time, this pump maintains a higher potassium concentration in the intracellular fluid than in the surrounding extracellular fluid. This active transport pump operates in the plasma membrane of all human cells and is essential for healthy cell survival.

Table 1.3   Active Transport Processes

DESCRIPTION		EXAMPLE(S)
Ion Pump		
Movement of solute particles from an area of low concentration to an area of high concentration (up the concentration gradient) by means of a carrier protein structure	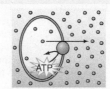	In muscle cells, pumping of nearly all calcium ions to special compartments or out of the cell
Phagocytosis		
Process that permits a cell to engulf or to surround any foreign material and to digest it	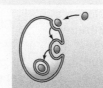	Trapping of bacterial cells by phagocytic white blood cells
Pinocytosis		
Movement of fluid and dissolved molecules into a cell by trapping them in a section of the plasma membrane that pinches off to form an intracellular vesicle; type of endocytosis	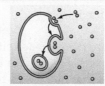	Trapping of large protein molecules by some body cells

The energy required for active transport processes is obtained from ATP (adenosine triphosphate). ATP is involved in all active transport processes.
From Patton KT, Thibodeau GA: *The human body in health and disease,* ed 7, St. Louis, 2018, Elsevier.

Table 1.4 Passive Transport Processes

DESCRIPTION		EXAMPLE(S)
Diffusion		
Movement of solute particles through a membrane from an area of high concentration to an area of low concentration (down the concentration gradient)		Movement of carbon dioxide out of all cells; movement of sodium ions into nerve cells as they conduct an impulse
Osmosis		
Diffusion of water through a selectively permeable membrane in the presence of at least one impermeable solute		Diffusion of water molecules into and out of cells to correct imbalances in water concentration
Filtration		
Movement of water and small solute particles, but not larger particles, through a filtration membrane; movement occurs from an area of high pressure to an area of low pressure		In the kidney, movement of water and small solutes from blood vessels but lack of movement by blood proteins and blood cells; begins the formation of urine

From Patton KT, Thibodeau GA: *The human body in health and disease,* ed 7, St. Louis, 2018, Elsevier.

- *Calcium pump:* Active calcium carriers in the membranes of muscle cells (for example) that allow the cells to force nearly all the intracellular calcium ions (Ca^{2+}) into special compartments or out of the cell entirely. This is important because a muscle cell cannot operate properly unless the intracellular Ca^{2+} concentration is kept low during rest.

Active transport processes require cellular energy to move substances from a low concentration to a high concentration. In contrast, passive transport processes—the movement of small molecules across the membrane of a cell by diffusion—do not require cellular energy and move substances from a high concentration to a lower concentration.

Passive transport processes. The primary passive transport processes (Table 1.4) include the following:

- **Diffusion:** A process in which solid particles in a fluid move from an area of higher concentration to an area of lower concentration, resulting in an even distribution of the particles in the fluid (Fig. 1.10).
- **Osmosis:** The passage of water across a selectively permeable membrane, with the water molecules going from the less concentrated solution to the more concentrated solution (Fig. 1.11).
- **Filtration:** The movement of water and particles through a membrane by force from either pressure or gravity. This membrane contains spaces that allow liquid to pass but are too small to be permeated by solid particles. Movement is from areas of greater pressure to areas of lesser pressure.

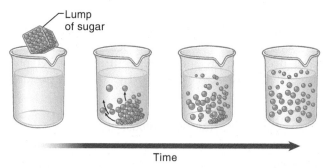

Fig. 1.10 Diffusion. The molecules of a lump of sugar are very densely packed when they enter the water. As sugar molecules collide frequently in the area of high concentration, they gradually move away from each other toward the area of lower concentration. Eventually, the sugar molecules are distributed evenly. (From Patton KT, Thibodeau GA: *The human body in health and disease,* ed 7, St. Louis, 2018, Elsevier.)

TISSUES

Tissues are groups of similar cells that work together to perform a specific function. The body and its organs are composed of the following four main types of tissues: epithelial, connective, muscle, and nervous (Table 1.5).

Epithelial Tissue

Epithelial cells are packed closely together and contain no blood vessels. Epithelial tissue covers the outside of the body and some of the internal structures. The four types of epithelial tissue are (1) simple squamous, (2) stratified squamous, (3) simple columnar, and (4) stratified transitional (see Table 1.5).

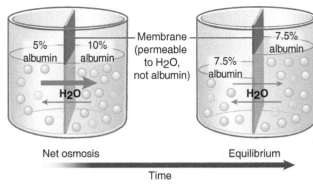

Fig. 1.11 Osmosis. Osmosis is the diffusion of water through a selectively permeable membrane. The membrane shown in this diagram is permeable to water but not to albumin. Because there are relatively more water molecules in 5% albumin than in 10% albumin, more water molecules osmose from the more dilute into the more concentrated solution (as indicated by the *large arrow* in the diagram on the left) than osmose in the opposite direction. The overall direction of osmosis, in other words, is toward the more concentrated solution. Movement across the membrane continues until the concentrations of the solutions equalize. (From Patton KT, Thibodeau GA: *The human body in health and disease*, ed 7, St. Louis, 2018, Elsevier.)

Epithelial tissue serves several important functions in the body, including the following:

- *Protection:* By covering the body and many of its organs, epithelial tissue is a protective barrier against invasion.
- *Absorption:* Certain specialized epithelial cells can absorb material in the body (e.g., the lining of the small intestine can absorb digested nutrients).
- *Secretion:* Mucus is secreted in areas such as the respiratory and digestive tracts.

Connective Tissue

As the name suggests, connective tissue "connects," or joins, tissues or structures of the body, and it supports and protects them. Connective tissue is the most abundant and widely distributed tissue in the body. It exists in various forms: thin and delicate, tough and cordlike, or liquid (blood). Mast cells, plasma cells, and white blood cells are found in connective tissue; red blood cells are not, unless blood vessels have been injured. Unlike the closely packed epithelial tissue, the connective tissue cells are spaced out and surrounded by intercellular fluid, which is composed of protein complexes and tissue fluid.

Some of the most important forms of connective tissue are loose fibrous (areolar) connective tissue, adipose (fat) tissue, fibrous connective tissue, bone, cartilage, blood, and hematopoietic tissue (see Table 1.5).

Muscle Tissue

Muscle tissue is composed of cells that contract in response to a message from the brain or the spinal cord. The three types of muscle cells are (1) skeletal (striated, voluntary), (2) cardiac (striated, involuntary), and (3) visceral (smooth, involuntary) (Fig. 1.12).

Skeletal muscle cells are striated (have a striped appearance) and attach to bones to produce voluntary movement. Skeletal muscle is also known as voluntary muscle because a person has voluntary control over skeletal muscle contractions (see Fig. 1.12A).

Cardiac muscle cells are striated with fibers that branch to form many networks, or webs. These networks are found only in the walls of the heart, and the regular contractions of cardiac muscle produce the heartbeat. In general, cardiac muscle cells are involuntary; that is, a person cannot contract them at will (see Fig. 1.12B).

Smooth (visceral) muscle cells are nonstriated and appear in the viscera, or internal organs, such as the stomach and the intestines as well as in the walls of blood vessels and the uterus. Contractions of smooth muscle propel food and fluid through the digestive tract and help regulate the diameter of blood vessels. Contraction of smooth muscle in the tubes of the respiratory system, such as the bronchioles in the lungs, can impair breathing and result in asthma attacks and labored respiration. In general, smooth muscles are involuntary, but some control can be exerted with biofeedback techniques (see Fig. 1.12C).

Nervous Tissue

Nervous tissue allows rapid communication between the brain or spinal cord and body structures and allows control of body functions. Nervous tissue is composed of two types of cells: neurons and glial cells. The neurons are the nerve cells and transmit impulses or messages. They are the system's functional or conducting units. The glial cells are connecting and supporting cells; they support and nourish the neurons.

Each neuron has three parts: (1) dendrites, which carry impulses toward the cell body; (2) a cell body; and (3) an axon, which carries impulses away from the cell body (see Chapter 14, Fig. 14.1).

MEMBRANES

Membranes are thin sheets of tissue that serve many functions in the body. They cover body surfaces, line and lubricate hollow organs, and protect and anchor organs and bones. The two major types of membranes are epithelial and connective tissue membranes.

Epithelial Membranes

Epithelial membranes usually are composed of a thin layer of epithelial cells with an underlying layer of connective tissue for strength. Epithelial membranes are divided into two subgroups: mucous membranes and serous membranes.

Mucous membranes. Mucous membranes secrete mucus (a thick, slippery material), which keeps the membranes moist and soft and protects against bacterial invasion. Mucous membranes line the body surfaces that open to the outside environment. Examples include the nose; the mouth; and urinary, respiratory, gastrointestinal, and reproductive tracts. The type of epithelium in the mucous membrane varies, depending on its location and function. The esophagus, for example, contains a tough,

Table 1.5   Tissues

TISSUE	LOCATION	FUNCTION
Epithelial		
Simple squamous	Alveoli of lungs	Absorption by diffusion of respiratory gases between alveolar air and blood
	Lining of blood and lymphatic vessels	Absorption by diffusion, filtration, and osmosis
Stratified squamous	Surface of the lining of mouth and esophagus	Protection
	Surface of skin (epidermis)	Protection
Simple columnar	Surface layer of the lining of stomach, intestines, and parts of the respiratory tract	Protection; secretion; absorption
Stratified transitional	Urinary bladder	Protection
Connective[a]		
Areolar	Between other tissues and organs	Connection
Adipose (fat)	Under skin	Protection
	Padding at various points	Insulation; support; reserve food
Dense fibrous	Tendons; ligaments	Flexible but strong connection
Bone	Skeleton	Support; protection
Cartilage	Part of the nasal septum; covering articular surfaces of bones; larynx; rings in trachea and bronchi Disks between vertebrae External ear	Firm but flexible support
Blood	Blood vessels	Transportation
Hematopoietic	Liquid matrix with a dense arrangement of blood cell–producing cells located in red bone marrow	Blood cell formation
Muscle		
Skeletal (striated voluntary); see Fig. 1.12A	Muscles that attach to bones	Maintenance of posture, movement of bones
	Eyeball muscles	Eye movements
	Upper third of the esophagus	First part of swallowing
Cardiac (striated involuntary); see Fig. 1.12B	Wall of heart	Contraction of heart
Smooth (nonstriated involuntary or visceral); see Fig. 1.12C	In walls of tubular viscera of digestive, respiratory, and genitourinary tracts	Movement of substances along respective tracts
	In walls of blood vessels and large lymphatic vessels	Changing the diameter of blood vessels
	In ducts of glands	Movement of substances along ducts
	Intrinsic eye muscles (iris and ciliary body)	Changing the diameter of pupils and shape of the lens
	Arrector muscles of hair follicles	Erection of hairs (gooseflesh)
Nervous	Brain; spinal cord; nerves	Irritability; conduction

[a]Connective tissues are the most widely distributed of all tissues.

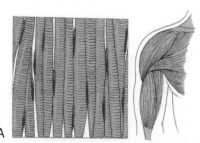 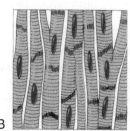 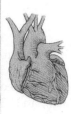 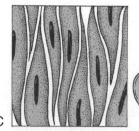 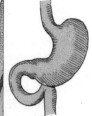

Fig. 1.12 Types of muscle. (A) Skeletal muscle. (B) Cardiac muscle. (C) Smooth muscle.

abrasion-resistant, stratified squamous epithelium. A thin layer of simple columnar epithelium covers the walls of the lower segments of the digestive tract.

In addition to protection, the mucus produced by mucous membranes also serves other purposes. For example, mucus in the digestive tract lubricates food as it moves through the digestive tract, and mucus secreted in the respiratory tract acts as a defense mechanism by trapping microorganisms and preventing their invasion into the respiratory system.

Serous membranes. Serous membranes secrete a thin, watery fluid that prevents friction when organs rub against one another. These membranes line the body surfaces that do not open to the outside environment. Examples include the lungs (pleura), the intestines (peritoneum), and the heart (pericardium). Like epithelial membranes, serous membranes are composed of two distinct layers of tissue: (1) the epithelial sheet, a thin layer of simple squamous epithelium; and (2) the connective tissue layer, a very thin sheet that holds and supports the epithelial cells.

The serous membrane that lines body cavities and covers the surfaces of organs in those cavities is a single, continuous sheet covering two different surfaces.

The parietal membrane lines the wall of the cavity, whereas the visceral membrane covers the surface of the viscera (organs within the cavity).

Connective Tissue Membranes (Synovial Membranes)

Connective tissue (or synovial) membranes are smooth and slick and secrete synovial fluid (a thick, colorless lubricating fluid). Synovial membranes line the joint spaces and prevent friction between the ends of the bones, allowing free movement of the joints. Synovial membranes also line small, cushion-like sacs called bursae, which are found between some moving body parts. Unlike serous and mucous membranes, connective tissue membranes do not contain epithelial components.

ORGANS AND SYSTEMS

When several kinds of tissues are united to perform a more complex function than any tissue alone, they are called organs. Examples are the heart, stomach, and kidneys. These organs working together for the same general purpose make up organ systems, which maintain the whole body. Systems perform a more complex function than any one organ can perform alone (Table 1.6).

Table 1.6   Organ Systems and Their Functions

STRUCTURE	FUNCTION	STRUCTURE	FUNCTION
Integumentary System		**Endocrine System**	
Hair Nails Oil glands Sense receptors Skin Sweat glands	• Protection • Regulation of body temperature • Sense organ • Synthesis of chemicals	Adrenal glands Hypothalamus Ovaries (female) Pancreas Parathyroid glands Pineal gland Pituitary gland Testes (male) Thymus gland Thyroid gland	• Control is slow and of long duration • Examples of hormone regulation: growth, metabolism, reproduction, and fluid and electrolyte balance • Same as nervous system—communication, integration, control • Secretion of special substances (hormones) directly into the blood (e.g., insulin from the pancreas)
Skeletal System		**Cardiovascular (Circulatory) System**	
Bones Joints	• Blood cell formation • Movement (with joints and muscles) • Storage of minerals • Support	Blood vessels Heart	• Immunity (body defense) • Regulation of body temperature • Transportation for nutrition, water, oxygen, and wastes
Muscular System		**Lymphatic System**	
Involuntary or smooth muscles Voluntary or striated muscles	• Maintenance of body posture • Movement • Production of heat	Lymph nodes Lymphatic vessels Spleen Thymus Tonsils	• Maintains body's internal fluid environment by producing, filtering, and conveying lymph • Production of various blood cells • Protection • Transportation
Nervous System		**Respiratory System**	
Brain Nerves Sense organs Spinal cord	• Communication • Contains body's control center • Control • Control is fast acting and of short duration • Integration • Recognition of sensory stimuli • Responsible for all the coordination of body's activities • System functions by production of nerve impulses caused by stimuli of various types	Nose Larynx Pharynx Trachea Lungs Bronchi	• Area of gas exchange in the lungs called alveoli • Exchange of waste gas (carbon dioxide) for oxygen in the lungs • Filtration of irritants from inspired air • Regulation of acid-base balance

Continued

Table 1.6   Organ Systems and Their Functions—cont'd

STRUCTURE	FUNCTION	STRUCTURE	FUNCTION
Digestive System		**Reproductive System**	
Primary Organs		**Male**	

Mouth
Pharynx
Esophagus
Stomach
Small intestine
  (duodenum,
  jejunum, ileum)
Large intestine
  (ascending,
  transverse,
  descending,
  sigmoid)
Rectum
Anal canal
	• Absorption of nutrients
	• Mechanical and chemical
	  breakdown (digestion) of food
	• Undigested waste product that is
	  eliminated is called feces
		Gonads (testes)
		Genital ducts
		  (epididymis,
		  vas deferens,
		  ejaculatory duct,
		  urethra)
		Accessory
		  glands (prostate,
		  seminal vesicles,
		  Cowper
		  glands)
		Supporting
		  structures (penis,
		  scrotum)
			• Fertilization of female sex cells
			• Production of sex cells (sperm)
			• Production of sex hormones
			• Survival of species
			• Transfer of sperm to female sex
			  cells

Accessory Organs		**Female**	

Teeth
Salivary glands
Tongue
Liver
Gallbladder
Pancreas
Appendix
	• Appendix is a structural but not a
	  functional part of the digestive system
	• Function of other structures can
	  be found in the digestive system
	  chapters (see Chapters 5 and 6)
		Gonads (ovaries)
		Accessory organs
		  (uterus, fallopian
		  tubes [oviducts],
		  vagina)
		External genitalia
		  (vulva)
		• Mons pubis
		• Labia majora
		• Labia minora
		• Clitoris
			• Development and birth of offspring
			• Nourishment of offspring
			• Production of sex cells (ova)
			• Production of sex hormones
			• Survival of species

Urinary System			

Kidneys
Ureters
Urinary bladder
Urethra
	• Acid-base balance
	• Clearing or cleaning the blood of
	  waste products; waste product
	  excreted from the body is called urine
	• Electrolyte balance
	• Urethra has urinary and reproductive
	  functions (in male)
	• Water balance
		Accessory glands
		  (Skene glands,
		  Bartholin glands)
		Mammary glands
		  (breasts)	

Get Ready for the NCLEX® Examination!

Key Points

- Anatomy is the study, classification, and description of structures and organs of the body. Physiology explains the function of the various structures and how they interrelate.
- The normal anatomical position of the body is standing erect with the face and the palms of the hands forward.
- For the purposes of study, the body is divided into three imaginary planes: sagittal, coronal (frontal), and transverse.
- The body is divided into two large cavities: the dorsal and the ventral. The dorsal cavity contains the cranial and spinal cavities. The ventral cavity contains the thoracic, abdominal, and pelvic cavities.
- For the purposes of study, the abdominal region is divided into nine regions: right hypochondriac region, epigastric region, left hypochondriac region, right lumbar region, umbilical region, left lumbar region, right inguinal region, hypogastric region, and left inguinal region.
- The cell's major structures are the cytoplasm, nucleus, endoplasmic reticulum, ribosomes, mitochondria, lysosomes, Golgi apparatus, and centrioles.
- Organization is a fundamental characteristic of body structure.
- Cells are considered the smallest living units of structure and function in the body. Although long recognized as the simplest units of living matter, cells are extremely complex.
- Tissues are groups of similar cells that work together to perform a specific function.
- Organs are structures made up of two or more kinds of tissues organized so that they can perform a more complex function than they could alone.
- Systems are groups of organs arranged so that they can perform a more complex function than they could alone.

- To receive nutrition and oxygen and to rid itself of wastes, the cell performs passive transport (diffusion, osmosis, filtration) and active transport (phagocytosis and pinocytosis, as well as the sodium-potassium pump and the calcium pump).
- The body is composed of four main types of tissues: epithelial, connective, muscle, and nervous tissues.
- The major systems of the body are integumentary, skeletal, muscular, nervous, endocrine, cardiovascular (circulatory), lymphatic, respiratory, digestive, urinary, and reproductive.

Additional Learning Resources

SG Go to your Study Guide for additional learning activities to help you master this chapter content.

Be sure to visit the Evolve site at http://evolve.elsevier.com/Cooper/adult/ for additional online resources.

Review Questions for the NCLEX-PN® Examination

1. The nurse is caring for a patient who is experiencing back pain located in the lower portion of the spine. The nurse is correct in documenting this as what area?

   1. Medial
   2. Caudal
   3. Proximal
   4. Dorsal

2. The nurse correctly identifies which organs as being found in the abdominopelvic cavity? *(Select all that apply.)*

   1. Spleen
   2. Urinary bladder
   3. Pancreas
   4. Gallbladder
   5. Rectum

3. The student nurse correctly identifies _____ as when a person's body is maintaining a balanced state within its internal environment.

   1. Homeostasis
   2. Mitosis
   3. Lysosomes
   4. Protein synthesis

4. What process has occurred when the patient inhales oxygen and it passes through the lungs and into the bloodstream (area of higher concentration to an area of lower concentration)?

   1. Phagocytosis
   2. Pinocytosis
   3. Osmosis
   4. Diffusion

5. The nurse correctly identifies which mechanism as the movement of materials across the membrane of a cell by means of chemical activity requiring the expenditure of energy by the cell?

   1. Passive transport
   2. Active transport
   3. Telophase
   4. Transcription

6. What type of tissue is composed of cells that contract in response to a message from the brain or spinal cord?

   1. Epithelial
   2. Connective
   3. Membrane
   4. Muscle

7. The student nurse demonstrates knowledge of basic human anatomy and physiology with which statement?

   1. "Mucous membranes line many organs, open to the outside environment, and are part of the body's defense mechanism against invasion of microorganisms."
   2. "Serous membranes line many organs, open to the outside environment, and are part of the body's defense mechanism against invasion of microorganisms."
   3. "Striated smooth muscle lines many organs, open to the outside environment, and are part of the body's defense mechanism against invasion of microorganisms."
   4. "Visceral, involuntary smooth muscle lines many organs, open to the outside environment, and are part of the body's defense mechanism against invasion of microorganisms."

8. When the body recognizes a foreign body invasion and responds by engulfing or surrounding the foreign material and digesting it, the nurse is accurate in identifying this process as what?

   1. Mitosis
   2. Pinocytosis
   3. Phagocytosis
   4. Filtration

9. A type of cell division of somatic cells in which each daughter cell contains the same number of chromosomes as the parent cell is called what?

   1. Flagella
   2. Mitosis
   3. ER synthesis
   4. Mitochondria

10. When a group of several different kinds of tissues is arranged to perform a special function, the nurse correctly uses which term to describe it?

    1. Cell
    2. Organ
    3. Tissue
    4. System

11. The hypogastric region of the abdominopelvic cavity is located where? *(Select all that apply.)*

    1. Inferior to the umbilical region
    2. Lateral to the left iliac region
    3. Medial to the right iliac region
    4. Lateral to the epigastric region
    5. Superior to the right lumbar region

12. A patient is being admitted to the intensive care unit following a motor vehicle accident that resulted in serious injury to organs in the dorsal cavity. Which organs does the nurse suspect are involved?

    1. Right kidney
    2. Spinal cord
    3. Liver
    4. Gallbladder
    5. Brain

13. The patient had a gunshot wound that damaged the structure that divides the thoracic cavity from the abdominal cavity. The nurse is aware that what structure has been affected?

    1. Mediastinum
    2. Diaphragm
    3. Lungs
    4. Stomach

14. The nurse is caring for a patient with a disease of the endocrine system. Which organs does the nurse identify as possibly not functioning correctly based on this patient's disease? *(Select all that apply.)*

    1. Pituitary gland
    2. Pancreas
    3. Thyroid gland
    4. Spleen
    5. Adrenal glands

Matching

Match each directional term in Column B with its opposite term in Column A.

COLUMN A	COLUMN B
15. _____ Superior	a. Posterior
16. _____ Distal	b. Superficial
17. _____ Anterior	c. Medial
18. _____ Lateral	d. Proximal
19. _____ Deep	e. Inferior

Match the function in Column B with the correct system in Column A.

COLUMN A	COLUMN B
20. _____ Integumentary	a. Provides movement, body posture, and heat
21. _____ Skeletal	b. Uses hormones to regulate body functions
22. _____ Muscular	c. Transports fatty nutrients from the digestive system to the blood
23. _____ Nervous	d. Makes physical and chemical changes in nutrients and absorbs nutrients
24. _____ Endocrine	e. Cleans the blood of metabolic wastes and regulates electrolyte balance
25. _____ Cardiovascular	f. Protects underlying structures, provides for sensory reception, and regulates body temperature
26. _____ Lymphatic	g. Transports substances from one part of the body to another
27. _____ Respiratory	h. Ensures the survival of the species rather than the individual
28. _____ Digestive	i. Uses electrochemical signals to integrate and control body functions
29. _____ Urinary	j. Exchanges oxygen and carbon dioxide and regulates acid-base balance
30. _____ Reproductive	k. Provides a rigid framework for the body and stores minerals

Care of the Surgical Patient

Objectives

1. Identify the purposes of surgery.
2. Distinguish among elective, urgent, and emergency surgery.
3. Explain the concept of perioperative nursing.
4. Discuss the factors that influence an individual's ability to tolerate surgery.
5. Discuss considerations for the older adult surgical patient.
6. Describe the preoperative checklist.
7. Explain the importance of informed consent for surgery.
8. Explain the procedure for turning, deep breathing, coughing, and leg exercises for postoperative patients.
9. Differentiate among general, regional, and local anesthesia.
10. Explain conscious (moderate) sedation.
11. Describe the roles of the circulating nurse and the scrub nurse during surgery.
12. Discuss the initial nursing assessment and management immediately after transfer from the postanesthesia care unit.
13. Identify the rationale for nursing interventions designed to prevent postoperative complications.
14. List the assessment data for the surgical patient.
15. Identify the information needed for the postoperative patient in preparation for discharge.
16. Discuss the nursing process as it pertains to the surgical patient.

Key Terms

ablative (ăb-LĀ-tĭv, p. 16)
anesthesia (ăn-ĕs-THĒ-zē-ă, p. 35)
atelectasis (ă-tĕ-LĔK-tă-sĭs, p. 27)
cachexia (kă-KĔK-sē-ă, p. 45)
catabolism (kă-TĂB-ō-lĭsm, p. 49)
conscious moderate sedation (sĕ-DĀ-shŭn, p. 37)
dehiscence (dē-HĬS-ĕns, p. 44)
drainage (p. 41)
embolus (ĔM-bō-lŭs, p. 27)
evisceration (ĕ-vĭs-ĕr-Ā-shŭn, p. 45)
extubate (ĕks-TŪ-bāt, Table 2.7, p. 42)
exudate (ĔKS-yū-dāt, p. 33)
incentive spirometer (ĭn-SĔN-tĭv spĭ-RŎM-ĕ-tĕr, p. 25)
incisions (ĭn-SĬZH-ŭnz, p. 33)

infarct (ĬN-făhrkt, p. 27)
informed consent (p. 22)
intraoperative (ĭn-tră-ŎP-ĕr-ă-tĭv, p. 17)
palliative (PĂL-ē-ă-tĭv, p. 16)
paralytic ileus (păr-ă-LĬT-ĭk ĬL-ē-ŭs, p. 48)
perioperative (pĕr-ē-ŎP-ĕr-ă-tĭv, p. 17)
postoperative (pōst-ŎP-ĕr-ă-tĭv, p. 17)
preoperative (prē-ŎP-ĕr-ă-tĭv, p. 17)
prosthesis (prŏs-THĒ-sĭs, p. 38)
singultus (SĬNG-gŭl-tŭs, p. 48)
surgery (p. 15)
surgical asepsis (ā-SĔP-sĭs, p. 40)
thrombus (THRŎM-bŭs, p. 27)

Surgery is the area of medicine that addresses diseases, conditions, and traumatic injuries that are difficult or impossible to treat only with medicine. Although the vast majority of surgical procedures are safe and have successful outcomes, patients are frequently fearful of surgery. Nurses can help alleviate much of this fear by providing support and educating patients about their procedures.

Surgery is classified as elective, urgent, or emergent. Elective surgery is not necessary to preserve life and may be performed at a time the patient chooses. Urgent surgery is required to keep additional health problems from occurring. Emergent surgery is performed immediately to save the individual's life or to preserve the

function of a body part or system. Surgical procedures also may be categorized as either major or minor, although all surgeries have an element of risk.

Surgery is performed for various purposes, including diagnostic, ablative, palliative, reconstructive, curative, preventive, transplant, constructive, and cosmetic (Table 2.1). Table 2.2 presents frequently used surgical terminology.

Traditionally, surgical procedures were performed in hospitals. With the current emphasis on decreasing health care costs, the surgical suite may now be in a variety of settings. Although facilities use different terms for surgical settings and processes, some common variations are listed in Box 2.1.

Table 2.1   Classification of Surgical Procedures

TYPE	DESCRIPTION AND EXAMPLES
ADMISSION STATUS	
Ambulatory (outpatient)	Patient enters setting, has surgical procedure, and is discharged on the same day (e.g., breast biopsy, cataract extraction, hemorrhoidectomy, scar revision).
Same-day admit	Patient enters hospital, undergoes surgery on the same day, and remains for convalescence (e.g., carotid endarterectomy, cholecystectomy, mastectomy, vaginal hysterectomy).
Inpatient	Patient is admitted to hospital, undergoes surgery (surgery may occur on a day other than the day of admission), and remains in hospital for convalescence (e.g., amputation, heart transplant, laryngectomy, resection of aortic aneurysm).
SERIOUSNESS	
Major	Involves extensive reconstruction or alteration in body parts; poses great risks to well-being (e.g., coronary artery bypass, colon resection, gastric resection).
Minor	Involves minimal alteration in body parts; often designed to correct deformities; involves minimal risks compared with those of major procedures (e.g., cataract extraction, skin graft, tooth extraction).
URGENCY	
Elective	Performed on basis of patient's choice (e.g., bunionectomy, plastic surgery).
Urgent	Necessary for patient's health (e.g., excision of cancerous tumor, removal of gallbladder for stones, vascular repair for obstructed artery [e.g., coronary artery bypass]).
Emergency or Emergent	Must be done immediately to save life or preserve function of body part (e.g., removal of perforated appendix, repair of traumatic amputation, control of internal hemorrhaging).
PURPOSE	
Diagnostic	Surgical exploration that allows physician to confirm diagnosis; may involve removal of tissue for further diagnostic testing (e.g., exploratory laparotomy [incision into peritoneal cavity to inspect abdominal organs], breast mass biopsy).
Ablative	Excision or removal of diseased body part (e.g., amputation, removal of appendix, cholecystectomy).
Palliative	Surgery for relief or reduction of intensity of disease symptoms; will not produce cure (e.g., colostomy, debridement of necrotic tissue).
Reconstructive	Restoration of function or appearance to traumatized or malfunctioning tissue (e.g., internal fixation of fractures, scar revision, breast reconstruction).
Curative	Surgery that cures the problem or condition.
Preventative	Surgical procedure that prevents any problems or damage from occurring.
Transplant	Replacement of malfunctioning organs (e.g., cornea, heart, joints, kidney).
Constructive	Restoration of function lost or reduced as result of congenital anomalies (e.g., repair of cleft palate, closure of atrial-septal defect in heart).
Cosmetic	Alteration of personal appearance (e.g., rhinoplasty to reshape nose).

Table 2.2   Surgical Terminology

TERM/SUFFIX	INTERPRETATION WITH EXAMPLE
Anastomosis	Surgical joining of two ducts or blood vessels to allow flow from one to another; to bypass an area (e.g., Billroth I, joins stomach and duodenum).
-ectomy	Surgical removal of (e.g., cholecystectomy, removal of the gallbladder).
Lysis	Destruction or dissolution of (e.g., lysis of adhesions, removal of adhesions).
-orrhaphy	Surgical repair of (e.g., herniorrhaphy, repair of a hernia).
-oscopy	Direct visualization with a scope (e.g., cystoscopy, direct visualization of the bladder and urethra by means of a cystoscope).
-ostomy	Opening made to allow the passage of drainage (e.g., ileostomy, formation of an opening of the ileum onto the surface of the abdomen for passage of feces).
-otomy	Opening into (e.g., thoracotomy, surgical opening into the thoracic cavity).
-pexy	Fixation of (e.g., cecopexy, fixation or suspension of the cecum to correct its excessive mobility).
-plasty	Plastic surgery (e.g., mammoplasty, reshaping of the breasts to reduce, lift, reconstruct).

Box 2.1	Common Surgical Settings

Inpatient: Patient hospitalized for surgery.

One-day (same-day surgery): Patient is admitted the day surgery is scheduled and discharged the same day.

Outpatient: Patient (not hospitalized) is admitted either to a short-stay unit or directly to the surgical suite (sometimes referred to as ambulatory surgery).

Short-stay surgical center: Independently owned agency; surgery is performed when overnight hospitalization is not required (also called an ambulatory surgical center or 1-day surgery center).

Short-stay unit: Department or floor where a patient's stay does not exceed 24 hours (sometimes referred to as an outpatient/observation unit).

Mobile surgery unit: A unit that moves from place to place; it moves to the patient instead of the patient traveling to the unit.

PERIOPERATIVE NURSING

The **perioperative** period encompasses the **preoperative** phase (before surgery), **intraoperative** phase (during surgery), and **postoperative** phase (after surgery). Perioperative nursing stresses the importance of providing continuity of care for the surgical patient by using the nursing process. In many hospitals, perioperative nurses assess a patient's health status preoperatively, identify specific patient needs, teach and counsel, attend to the patient's needs in the operating room (OR), and then monitor the patient's recovery. In other facilities, different nurses care for the patient during each phase. Nurses also may delegate certain aspects of perioperative care to appropriate personnel (Box 2.2). It is the nurse's responsibility to ensure that safe, consistent, and effective nursing care is provided during each phase of surgery.

INFLUENCING FACTORS

Every surgical procedure is stressful for the patient. Observing the patient's nonverbal communication and listening to questions help identify the patient's feelings and concerns. By helping the patient to express the concerns, the nurse can offer support, reassurance, and information to address fear of the unknown. Numerous factors (1) affect the individual's ability to tolerate surgery and (2) influence the development of intraoperative and postoperative complications.

Age

Young and old patients do not tolerate major surgical procedures as well as patients in other age groups. Because of their metabolism, patients in these extreme age groups may have a slower response to physiologic changes such as temperature variations, cardiovascular shifts, respiratory needs, and renal function. Nursing assessments and appropriate interventions must be ongoing (see the Lifespan Considerations box).

 Lifespan Considerations

Older Adults

Undergoing Surgery

- Older adults undergoing surgery have higher morbidity and mortality rates than younger people.
- Surgery places a greater stress on older people than on younger people. The patient's physiologic status and coexisting conditions, such as diabetes mellitus or cardiac disease, should be evaluated carefully. The individual's current health status is a more important factor than age when considering the benefits and risks of surgery. Consequently, increasing numbers of older patients are undergoing surgery, and nurses need to know the age-related factors that affect their response to surgical procedures.
- Older patients tend to recover from surgery more slowly than younger patients. Recovery is affected by the level of mental functioning, individual coping ability, and the availability of support systems.
- Older adults have an increased risk of aspiration, atelectasis (collapsed lung), pneumonia, thrombus formation, infection, and altered tissue perfusion because of age-related changes to various body systems.
- Older adults are more likely to experience disorientation or toxic reactions after the administration of anesthetics, sedatives, or analgesics. These reactions result from age-related changes in the hepatic and renal systems and may persist for days after receiving the medication. However, the health care staff should be cautioned to avoid undermedicating an older adult solely based on age, remembering that many elders are in very good physiologic health.
- Preoperative and postoperative teaching may require extra time. The nurse should allow time for the patient to process any information presented. Repeating and reinforcing directions is sometimes necessary.
- When communicating with older adult patients, the nurse should be aware of any auditory, visual, or cognitive impairments.

Physical Condition

Patients in good overall general health have smoother and faster recovery periods than patients with coexisting health problems. The nurse should assess each body system to identify actual and potential problems and determine measures to prevent postoperative complications (Box 2.3).

Nutritional Factors

The body uses carbohydrates, proteins, and fats to supply energy-producing glucose to its cells. Carbohydrates and fats are the primary energy producers, and protein is essential to build and repair body tissue. Under stressful conditions such as recovering from surgery, the body's need for energy and repair increases. Nutritional needs are affected by a patient's age and physical requirements; patients who maintain a sound nutritional diet tend to recover more quickly.

Box 2.2	Delegation Considerations in Perioperative Nursing

- The skills of assessment that are part of preparing a patient for surgery require the critical thinking ability and knowledge application unique to a nurse. For these skills, delegation is inappropriate. However, unlicensed assistive personnel (UAP) may obtain vital signs and weight and height measurements. Instruct UAP on proper precautions for these delegated procedures as needed.
- The skills of preoperative teaching require the critical thinking and knowledge application unique to a nurse. For these skills, delegation is inappropriate. However, UAP may reinforce and assist patients in performing postoperative exercises.
- Review with UAP any precautions for a particular patient (e.g., turning method).
- Be certain staff members know when to inform the nurse if the patient is unable to perform the exercises correctly.
- Coordinating the patient's preparation for surgery requires the critical thinking and knowledge application unique to a nurse. However, UAP may administer an enema or douche in some settings; obtain vital signs; apply antiembolitic stockings; and assist patient in removing clothing, jewelry, and prostheses.
- Instruct UAP in proper precautions when preparing a patient for surgery.
- Instruct UAP in proper observations and precautions if the patient has an intravenous (IV) catheter in place.
- The skills of sterile gowning and gloving can be delegated to a surgical technologist or a nurse who has acquired the proper skills.
- The skill of initiating and managing postoperative care of a patient requires the critical thinking and knowledge application unique to a nurse. However, UAP may obtain vital signs, remove and replace a nasal cannula or oxygen mask during transfers, and provide basic comfort and hygiene measures.

Box 2.3	ABCDEF Mnemonic Device to Ascertain Serious Illness or Trauma in the Preoperative Patient

A *Allergy* to medications, chemicals, and other environmental products such as latex. All allergies are reported to anesthesia and surgical personnel before the beginning of surgery. Place an allergy band on the patient's arm immediately.

B *Bleeding* tendencies or the use of medications that deter clotting, such as aspirin or products containing aspirin, heparin, or warfarin sodium. Herbal medications also may increase bleeding times or mask potential blood-related problems.

C *Cortisone* or steroid use.

D *Diabetes mellitus,* a condition that not only requires strict control of blood glucose levels but also is known to delay wound healing. Patients with diabetes also may have elevated blood glucose levels even after being placed on NPO (nothing by mouth) status because of the body's stress response.

E *Emboli.* Previous embolic events (such as lower leg blood clots) may recur because of prolonged immobility.

F *Fighting ability.* Patients whose immune systems are suppressed are at a much higher risk for development of postoperative infection and are less capable of fighting that infection.

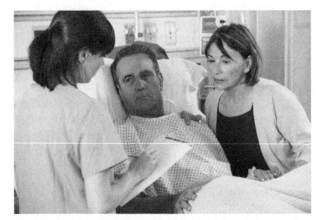

Fig. 2.1 Knowledge deficits often occur when a patient is undergoing his or her first surgical experience.

A complete diet history identifies the patient's usual eating habits, nutritional patterns, and food preferences. Dietary practices are influenced by a patient's ethnic, cultural, religious, and socioeconomic background. Consider this information when offering the patient appropriate foods that are high in energy-producing nutrients. Surgery may decrease a patient's appetite and alter metabolic functions, so observe the patient for signs of malnutrition. If malnutrition is identified promptly, tube feedings, intravenous (IV) therapy, or total parenteral nutrition can be initiated (see Chapters 15 and 18 in *Foundations of Nursing*).

PSYCHOSOCIAL NEEDS

As the patient and family plan for surgery, they frequently express concern and fears about possible outcomes (Box 2.4). Preoperative fear has been linked to intraoperative and postoperative behavior. The preoperative anxiety level influences the amount of anesthesia required, the amount of postoperative pain medication needed, and the speed of recovery from surgery. Each patient's perceptions, emotions, behavior, and support systems should be evaluated to identify factors that may influence the individual's progress through the perioperative period. Patiently and actively listening to the patient, the family, and significant others allows the nurse to address fears and help reduce anxiety (Fig. 2.1).

While the patient prepares for the upcoming surgery, family members and support people are also trying to cope. Families may have additional burdens, such as financial obligations, living changes, and added personal responsibilities. In addition to nursing and medical personnel, social workers, clergy, or patient advocates can provide support for patients and families during this stressful time (see the Patient Teaching box on preoperative care).

Box 2.4   Common Fears Associated With Surgery

- Fear of loss of control is associated primarily with anesthesia. The patient becomes almost totally dependent on the health care team during the surgical experience—even for basic needs such as breathing and life support—while under the influence of anesthesia.
- Fear of the unknown may result from uncertainty about the surgical outcome or a lack of knowledge regarding the surgical experience.
- Fear of anesthesia may include fears of unpleasant induction of or emergence from anesthesia. The patient may fear waking up during the operation and feeling pain while under anesthesia. This fear often is related to loss of control and fear of the unknown.
- Fear of pain or inadequate postoperative analgesia is common. Reassure the patient and significant others that the pain will be controlled.
- Fear of death is a legitimate fear. Even with the great strides in surgery and anesthesia, no anesthetic or operation is perfectly safe for all patients.
- Fear of separation from the usual support group may arise because the patient is separated from spouse, family, or significant others, as well as other support groups, and is cared for by strangers during this highly stressful period.
- Fear of disruption of life patterns relates to surgery and recovery interfering in varying degrees with activities of daily living, social activities, work, and professional activities.
- Fear of change in body image and mutilation is not unusual. Surgery disrupts body integrity and threatens body image.
- Fear of detection of cancer produces a high anxiety level.

Patient Teaching

Preoperative Care

The nurse may assist preoperative patients and their families by providing information about the following:
- Preoperative tests: Reason, preparation
- Preoperative routines: Sequence of events
- Special equipment needed, especially if the patient is undergoing same-day surgery and being discharged home. Items that may be necessary include crutches, orthopedic boots or splints, wheelchair, walker, bedside commode, and shower chair
- Transfer to operating room: Time, checking procedures
- Medications that may be prescribed at discharge: Addressing how the patient will obtain prescribed medication is especially important for the patient who does not have insurance
- Recovery room or postanesthesia care unit
- Place where the patient will awaken
- Frequent monitoring of vital signs
- Return to room when vital signs are stable
- Probable postoperative therapies
- Need for increased mobility as soon as possible
- Need to keep respiratory passages clear
- Anticipated treatments such as an intravenous line, dressing changes, and incentive spirometry
- Pain medication routines (timing sequence, "as needed" [prn] status), other modalities of management such as patient-controlled analgesia and patient-controlled epidural analgesia

SOCIOECONOMIC AND CULTURAL NEEDS

The United States is a nation of diverse individuals of various social, economic, religious, ethnic, and cultural origins. Even regional factors affect the way a patient responds to surgery. It is important to allow patients and families to express themselves openly.

A multicultural perspective (see Chapter 6 in *Foundations of Nursing*) helps nurses to approach patients with respect and individually tailor care to promote recovery (see the Cultural Considerations box).

Cultural Considerations

The Surgical Patient

- Use of the patient's language helps to put an anxious patient at ease. Use an interpreter when possible. Learn some key phrases in foreign languages. Use references such as medical dictionaries, which usually have key phrases listed in an appendix.
- Because some cultures may avoid eye contact and consider it disrespectful, consider limiting eye contact when dealing with these patients.
- Some cultures may not ask for pain medication and may need teaching to help understand how comfort and relief from pain promote healing and a quicker recovery.
- Some cultures are often stoic when ill. Complaints of pain to the nurse may be in general terms such as, "I am uncomfortable." Undertreatment of pain is common.
- With some cultures, verbal consent often has more meaning than written consent because it is based on trust. Fully explain the need for written consent. The patient may be expressive regarding pain. Pain may cause intense fear. Prepare the patient for painful procedures, and develop a care plan to prevent pain. Assistance with toileting or other intimate care also may be an area of concern in which the nurse must consider male/female roles.
- For some cultures, having an interpreter is important, depending on the sensitivity of the subject under discussion, because of modesty. A female family member is expected to be at the bedside to provide care and comfort. Men are the decision makers and support the family; therefore speaking with the male head of the family may be necessary. Eye contact and touch should be avoided in some instances.

MEDICATIONS

Review of the patient's current medication regimen is essential. Polypharmacy (concurrent use of multiple medications) occurs in all age groups but is more common with older adults. The Kaiser Family Foundation (KFF) reported that approximately 89% of people older than age 65 take some kind of prescription medication. Fifty-four percent of those older than 65 years of age report taking four or more prescription medications. The use of multiple medications can lead to adverse drug reactions and interactions with other medications in the perioperative setting.

During the perioperative period, health care providers use medications and agents from several pharmacologic categories, including anesthetics, antimicrobials, anticoagulants, hemostatic agents, steroids, diagnostic imaging dyes, diuretics, central nervous system agents, and emergency protocol medications. An acutely ill patient may receive several drugs at one time. The larger the number of medications, the greater the chance of an adverse interaction.

People also frequently use herbal remedies as alternative or complementary therapy. It is essential to ask the patient about the use of herbal preparations, either as dietary supplements or as medicines, because most patients do not think of them as medications. Even though herbs are natural products, they act like drugs and may interact with or potentiate other medications or interfere with surgical procedures (Table 2.3). Vitamin use also must be addressed because of vitamins' physiologic actions (e.g., vitamin E may prolong bleeding times).

Some medications may be stopped before the patient goes to surgery. The nurse needs to know the purposes and actions of drugs because they may be critical for a patient with coexisting conditions. For example, if a patient with diabetes has the insulin dose withheld before surgery, the nurse must closely monitor the patient's blood glucose level preoperatively and postoperatively. The anesthesiologist, in collaboration with the patient's health care provider and surgeon, determines whether such medications should be taken the day of surgery and postoperatively. Common medications that are not stopped and are given with a sip of water the morning of surgery include antiseizure and cardiac drugs.

Assess the patient for allergies to drugs that may be given during any phase of the perioperative period. If the patient is allergic to a drug, ask him or her to

Table 2.3 Preoperative Considerations for Commonly Ingested Herbs

HERB	COMMON USES	PREOPERATIVE CONSIDERATIONS
Echinacea	Treat cold symptoms	Possible negative impact on the liver. Subsequent interference with hepatic metabolism of certain anesthesia medications.
Ephedra sinica	Decongestant Weight loss	Increased risk of cardiac dysrhythmias. May reduce effectiveness of medications used to treat hypotension.
Feverfew	Migraine prevention	Has anticoagulation factors; potential for increased bleeding. Preoperative assessment should include clotting studies. Discontinue before surgery.
Garlic	Improved immunity High blood pressure and cholesterol	Potential for increased bleeding.
Ginger	Motion sickness Cough Menstrual cramps Intestinal gas	Risk of prolonged clotting times. Preoperative assessment should include clotting studies. Discontinue before surgery.
Ginkgo biloba	Brain function and alertness Tension Erectile dysfunction	Potential for increased bleeding.
Ginseng	Overall well-being Diabetes	May increase anesthetic agent requirements. Potential for hypoglycemia in patients taking insulin or oral diabetes agents.
Guarana	Mental alertness Fatigue	May reduce the efficacy of warfarin. May potentiate sympathetic nervous system stimulants, leading to cardiac complications. May decrease cerebral blood flow.
Kava	Sleep aid Anxiety, tension	May potentiate muscle relaxants. May increase effects of certain antiemetics. Potential for serious liver damage and subsequent decreased hepatic metabolism of certain anesthetic agents.
Licorice	Asthma, eczema, rheumatoid arthritis Expectorant Gastritis	May cause hypertension. Potential for hypokalemia and associated cardiac dysrhythmias.
St. John's wort	Antidepressant Antiviral properties Antiinflammatory action	Should not be used with other psychoactive drugs, monoamine oxidase inhibitors, or serotonin reuptake inhibitors. Discontinue before surgery because of possible drug interactions.
Valerian root	Sedative or tranquilizer effect Sleep aid	Should not be used with sedatives or anxiolytics. May increase effects of central nervous system depressants.

describe specifically the type of reaction. Determine nondrug allergies, including allergies to foods, chemicals, pollen, antiseptics used to prepare the skin for surgery, and latex products. A patient with a history of allergic responsiveness is more likely to have a hypersensitivity reaction to anesthesia agents. Many facilities require such patients to wear an allergy identification band during surgery. Follow facility policy for posting allergy alerts in the patient's medical record.

EDUCATION AND EXPERIENCE

When teaching patients, consider the patient's age, educational level, and communication abilities. Communicate at a level that patients understand. The care plan should include provisions to ensure the patient has understood any new information presented. For example, ask the patient to summarize the information given or to perform a return demonstration.

PREOPERATIVE PHASE

Before surgery, patients require a thorough health assessment. Acute or chronic diseases hinder the body's ability to repair or to adjust to surgical treatment. Disorders of the systems identified in Table 2.4 present high-risk conditions for surgery. Each system is affected further by the patient's age, health, nutritional status, and mental state. Assessment questions

Table 2.4 Surgical Effects on Body Systems

DISEASE OR DISORDER	SURGICAL EFFECTS
CARDIOVASCULAR (See Chapter 8)	
Recent myocardial infarction, dysrhythmias, and heart failure Hypertension	Hypotension and cardiac dysrhythmias are the most common cardiovascular complications of the surgical patient. Early recognition and management before these complications become serious enough to diminish cardiac output depend on frequent assessment of the patient's vital signs.
ENDOCRINE (See Chapter 11)	
Type 1 and type 2 diabetes	Diabetes increases susceptibility to infection and may impair wound healing because of altered glucose metabolism and associated circulatory impairment. Fluctuating blood glucose levels may cause central nervous system malfunction during anesthesia.
GASTROINTESTINAL (See Chapter 5)	
Hiatal hernia	
Ulcers	Preoperative and postoperative medication may be necessary to control gastric acidity.
Esophageal varices	Risk of hemorrhage may increase because of intubation.
Liver disease	Liver disease alters metabolism and elimination of drugs administered during surgery and impairs wound healing because of alterations in protein metabolism.
IMMUNE (See Chapter 15)	
Acquired immunodeficiency syndrome; allergies; immunodeficiency	Disease slows the body's ability to fight infection. Immunologic disorders increase risk of infection and delay wound healing after surgery. Hypothermia during surgery decreases immune function.
MUSCULOSKELETAL (See Chapter 4)	
	Osteoporosis and increased risk for fractures in the older adult place patient at increased risk for injury during surgery.
NEUROLOGIC (See Chapter 14)	
Seizures	Ensure antiseizure medications are at therapeutic levels to prevent postoperative seizures.
Myasthenia gravis	Muscle relaxants may need to be excluded because of patient's decreased ability to reverse their effects.
Cerebrovascular accident	Impaired verbal communication, defective perception of the body, paralysis, and visual disturbances place patient at high risk for injury.
Peripheral vascular disease	Patient has a decreased threshold for peripheral pain.
RESPIRATORY (See Chapter 9)	
Tumors Chronic obstructive pulmonary disease Emphysema Asthma	Lung capacity is decreased and gas exchange slowed. Anesthetic agents reduce respiratory function, increasing risk for severe hypoventilation.
URINARY (See Chapter 10)	
Renal failure	Impaired kidney function decreases excretion of anesthesia and alters acid-base balance.
Tumors	Prostate enlargement may increase risk of urinary tract infection.

regarding the patient's use of chemicals, alcohol, and recreational substances help the health team to select medications. When possible, postoperative care also is adjusted to prevent potential complications. For example, a patient who smokes cigarettes may have impaired alveoli and reduced lung capacity. Mucus and anesthesia by-products may become trapped in the lungs, causing atelectasis and pneumonia. After surgery, breathing exercises and treatments for smokers aid in lung expansion and decrease the risk of respiratory complications.

Additional preoperative questions identify allergies, past surgeries, and infection and disease history. The patient should be asked for a complete list of prescription drugs and over-the-counter medications, as well as vitamins, minerals, and herbal products taken, including home remedies. The patient's vital signs, height, and weight should be measured before surgery to have a baseline for postoperative comparison.

PREOPERATIVE TEACHING

Patient teaching before surgery helps reduce (1) the patient's anxiety associated with fear of the unknown, (2) the amount of anesthesia needed, (3) postsurgical pain, and (4) corticosteroid production. Decreasing postsurgical complications through preoperative teaching speeds wound healing.

Include the patient and family when providing preoperative teaching, and remember that basic terminology and information are easier for them to understand than complex explanations. Frequently verify the patient's understanding of information, ask questions, and encourage responses. Avoid asking questions that can be answered "yes" or "no." Instead of saying, "Do you have any questions?" try asking, "What questions do you have?" If using printed material for preoperative teaching, make sure that the patient is able to read and that the printed material is within the patient's reading level. Printed or video material used in preoperative teaching sessions should be documented. Older adults may have difficulty reading small print or hearing audio material. If the patient does not understand English, an interpreter should explain the information presented. In addition, patients should understand that a nurse will be with them throughout the entire surgical experience.

For surgical procedures that have potential long-term effects, support groups can offer assistance preoperatively. Cancer organizations, amputation support groups, and enterostomal associations are examples of large national organizations that offer peer support.

Ideally the patient is seen in the surgeon's office and preoperative teaching is provided when the surgery is scheduled, when anxiety is not as high. The surgeon provides information regarding the actual surgical procedure, as well as the risks, benefits, and possible outcomes. The surgeon's nursing staff typically provides teaching regarding preoperative instructions,

such as any gastrointestinal (GI) cleansing preparation, or the need for assistive devices to be obtained for use immediately after surgery (e.g., crutches or orthopedic boots). The nurse clarifies what the physician has explained to the patient, reviews the time of the surgery, and witnesses the patient signing the informed consent. If the patient is already in the hospital and a surgery is scheduled, the nurse on the unit provides similar information that the office staff provides, as well as information about the recovery area (e.g., previously assigned units, intensive care, specialty units, or outpatient area). Facilities often have an established teaching program, which includes a systematic preoperative teaching plan and checklist. If a transfer is planned after surgery, it is helpful to take the patient and family on a tour of the new unit. The nurse also should explain that vital signs, dressings, and tubes are assessed every 15 to 30 minutes until the patient is awake and stable.

PREOPERATIVE PREPARATION

Preparation for surgery depends on the patient's age and physical and nutritional status, the type of surgery, and the surgeon's preference. For surgery in a short-stay or ambulatory setting, the workup normally occurs a few days in advance. If the patient is admitted to the hospital, testing may be conducted to assess for potential problems. Preparation frequently includes in-facility testing and evaluation of test results that were completed before admission.

Laboratory Tests and Diagnostic Imaging

Testing before surgery depends on the institution's policies, the health care provider's directives, and the patient's condition. Laboratory tests commonly reviewed before surgery include a urinalysis; a complete blood count; and a blood chemistry profile to assess endocrine, hepatic, renal, and cardiovascular functions. Serum electrolytes are evaluated if extensive surgery is planned or if the patient has associated problems. One essential electrolyte assessed is potassium; abnormal serum potassium levels can lead to dysrhythmias during and after surgery, and the patient's recovery may be delayed by general muscle weakness. A chest x-ray evaluation and electrocardiogram are used to identify disease processes or existing respiratory or cardiac damage. Additional tests are conducted to assess the organ involved in surgery. A blood chemistry profile tests several blood levels, including lipids, blood urea nitrogen (BUN), and creatinine (kidney function), proteins, and electrolytes, as well as liver function.

Informed Consent

The Patient's Bill of Rights affirms that patients must give informed consent (i.e., permission to perform a specific test or procedure) before any procedure is begun. In signing the consent form, the patient must be competent and agree to have the procedure that is stated on the form. The surgeon must explain the risks involved, identify expected benefits, and describe consequences or alternatives for the presenting problem. The nurse frequently is a witness when a patient signs the consent form. A witness verifies only that this is the person who signed the consent and that it was a voluntary consent; the witness cannot verify that the patient understood the procedure. Ideally, the surgeon discusses the surgical procedure with the patient in advance. In some institutions, the surgical consent is completed in the physician's office or in the admissions department before the patient is admitted to the unit. Informed consent should not be obtained if the patient is disoriented, unconscious, mentally incompetent, or, in some agencies, under the influence of sedatives. The nurse must follow agency policy (see Chapter 2, Fig. 2.1 in *Foundations of Nursing*).

If the patient has vision or hearing impairment, additional time may be necessary to explain and obtain the patient's signature on the consent form. For patients who do not understand English, an interpreter may be necessary. A patient should never be coerced into signing a consent that he or she does not understand or that contains information different from that originally given. If necessary, inform the physician that the patient does not understand the procedure. (Refer to Chapter 2 in *Foundations of Nursing* for discussion of informed consent.)

In an emergency, the patient may not be able to give consent for surgery. Every effort is made to locate family members to assume this responsibility. In many cases, consent will be provided by the spouse. In the absence of a spouse, this role may be passed to another legally identified individual (e.g., advance directive). On occasion, telephone permission may be obtained. Hospitals have standard guidelines for obtaining verbal consent. If the patient's life is in danger and family members cannot be located, the surgeon may legally perform surgery. If the patient is deemed incompetent to provide consent, there is a legal process for identifying a legal guardian eligible to provide the consent. If family members object to surgery that the physician believes is essential, a court order may be obtained for the procedure. This practice is used only in extreme circumstances (e.g., when a child's life is in danger). The nurse must follow agency policy in any of these circumstances.

Gastrointestinal Preparation

In the past, the standard GI preparation included placing the patient on nothing by mouth (NPO) status at midnight the night before surgery to decrease the risk of intraoperative and postoperative vomiting and aspiration. Several studies have shown that being NPO for extended periods of time before surgery does not significantly decrease the risk for aspiration and actually increases the patient's risk for dehydration, insulin resistance, and muscle wasting and places a strain on the immune system. In addition, prolonged NPO status increases the patient's anxiety level, thirst, dizziness, and hunger. The American Society of Anesthesiologists (2017) recommendations suggest allowing the patient to have clear liquids up to 2 hours before surgery and a light meal without human milk up to 6 hours before surgery unless the patient has a condition that delays gastric emptying. Fatty meals, meats, and fried foods should be avoided for 8 hours prior to surgery. Regardless of studies, many health care providers continue to place patients on NPO status at midnight before surgery. The nurse must follow any preoperative orders issued by the health care provider.

The patient can have oral care while NPO but should be cautioned not to swallow any fluids used. A wet cloth on the lips helps to relieve dryness. If the patient needs to be hydrated or requires special IV medications, the health care provider may order parenteral fluids or medication. Depending on the procedure, many patients resume eating and drinking on the same day following the surgery.

Because anesthesia relaxes the bowel, a bowel cleanser may be ordered to evacuate fecal material and lessen postoperative GI problems (nausea and vomiting). A cleansing enema or a general laxative may be used. If a bowel preparation is given, chart the type of preparation used, the patient's tolerance to the procedure, and the results. Bowel preps are generally reserved for surgeries involving the small and large intestines. Follow the order of the health care provider. Before bowel surgery, medication (neomycin, sulfonamides, erythromycin) may be given over a period of days to detoxify and sterilize the GI tract. This lessens the chance of infection if fecal contamination occurs during surgery.

Skin Preparation

Before surgery the surgeon may order hair removal at the surgical site. Typically, hair removal is ordered only if it may interfere with exposure, closure, or dressing of the surgical site. During hair removal, the operative site must be treated carefully to remove the hair without injuring the skin (Skill 2.1).

Studies indicate no significant difference in surgical site infection (SSI) rates when comparing the results of no hair removal with hair removal by shaving, clipping, and depilatory cream (Kowalski et al, 2016). Shaving the hair before surgery can create microscopic cuts that increase the risk of SSI. The Centers for Disease Control and Prevention (CDC) strongly recommend not removing hair unless it would interfere with the surgery and if removing hair is necessary, a depilatory agent is suggested (CDC, n.d.). Debate also continues regarding when to perform hair removal if it is indicated. Some surgeons prefer patient hair removal close to the time of the surgical procedure to decrease the time for growth of bacteria and lower the potential for infection. Some surgical departments prepare the patient either in a surgical holding room or in the OR. Each facility should have policies and protocols regarding

Skill 2.1   Performing a Surgical Skin Preparation

CHECK   GATHER   HELLO   ID   PRIVACY   EXPLAIN   WASH   GLOVES

NURSING ACTION (RATIONALE)

1. Refer to medical record, care plan, or Kardex for special interventions. (*Provides basis for care.*)
2. Obtain equipment. (*Organizes procedure.*)
   a. Appropriate light
   b. Operating room prep kit:
   Basin
   Razor
   Sponge with soap
   Waterproof pad
   Cotton-tipped applicators
   c. Clean gloves
3. Introduce self. (*Decreases patient's anxiety.*)
4. Identify patient. (*Identifies correct patient for procedure.*)
5. Explain procedure to patient. (*Improves cooperation and decreases anxiety.*)
6. Perform hand hygiene and, if appropriate, don clean gloves. Know agency policy and guidelines from the Centers for Disease Control and Prevention (CDC) and the Occupational Safety and Health Administration (OSHA). (*Reduces spread of microorganisms.*)
7. Prepare patient for intervention:
   a. Close door to room or pull curtain. (*Provides privacy.*)
   b. Drape for procedure if necessary and position patient. (*Promotes proper body mechanics.*)
8. Raise bed to comfortable working level. (*Promotes proper body mechanics.*)
9. Place towel or waterproof pad under area to be shaved. (*Protects bed and linen from soiling.*)
10. Fill basin with warm water. (*Allows nurse to lather soap and rinse skin.*)
11. Place bath blanket over patient. (*Exposes only area to be shaved.*)
12. Adjust lighting. (*Allows thorough assessment of skin and helps decrease chance of skin impairment.*)
13. Lather skin with antiseptic soap and warm water. (*Cleanses skin, softens hair, and reduces friction from razor.*)
14. If using a razor, hold razor at a 30- to 45-degree angle to skin. (*Minimizes chances of cutting or nicking skin.*)
    a. Shave small areas while holding skin taut.
    b. Use short, smooth strokes. (*Prevents pulling skin.*)
    c. Shave hair in same direction it grows. (*Removes hair close to skin surface.*)
15. Rinse razor frequently. (*Removes accumulation of hair from razor and prevents contamination from dirty water.*)
16. After entire area is shaved, cleanse it with a washcloth and clean, warm water. Dry skin. (*Removes excess shaved hair, body oils, and soil on skin. Reduces number of microorganisms. Promotes patient comfort.*)
17. Reassess skin for cuts, nicks, or hair. (*Prevents growth of microorganisms and possible infections from skin impairment.*)
18. Return patient to appropriate position. (*Provides patient comfort and safety.*)
19. Clean and dispose of equipment. (*Reduces spread of microorganisms.*)
20. Remove and dispose of soiled gloves and wash hands. (*Reduces spread of microorganisms.*)
21. Document. (*Verifies procedure.*)

Special concerns for patients undergoing a surgical skin preparation are as follows:

- Small children may be easily frightened by this procedure, and it may have to be done in the operating room (OR).
- Older adults need a detailed explanation to relieve their anxiety.
- Older adults have less subcutaneous tissue, less skin elasticity, and more delicate skin tissue. Take extreme care when shaving the older adult.
- Older adults are usually more susceptible to infections.

the timing, the method, and the staff responsible for the preoperative skin preparation of surgical patients.

Facility policy or specific surgeon order dictates preoperative skin preparation. The nurse reviews agency policy and the patient chart to determine the area to be prepared. Before the skin preparation, the surgical site is assessed carefully for the presence of any skin impairment (e.g., infection, irritation, bruises, lesions).

The patient also is assessed for any skin allergies. Any abnormal assessment findings must be recorded and reported to the surgeon. Some surgeons require patients shower with an antimicrobial solution the night before or the day of surgery, or both.

Once the patient is in the OR, an antiseptic solution to kill adherent and deeper-residing bacteria is used. Common surgical antiseptic solutions include povidone-iodine (Betadine) and chlorhexidine. The surgeon may place a transparent sterile drape directly over the skin before making an incision.

Latex Allergy Considerations

A focused assessment helps identify patients who may be at risk for latex allergy response. Assessing the patient's experience helps identify those at risk for a systemic reaction (e.g., the patient may relate stories of complicated anesthesia events, hives from blowing up a balloon, or severe swelling of the labia with a urinary catheterization).

With the advent of universal precautions (now called standard precautions) in the late 1980s, the use of latex gloves dramatically increased, and latex allergies were detected much more often. Gloves are worn by all staff members providing health care to patients. Most gloves are powdered to make them easier to put on. The powder absorbs protein allergens from the latex and deposits them on skin and into surgical wounds; it also aerosolizes the protein allergens. Aerosolized latex allergens are carried in ventilation systems, requiring further preventive measures.

Latex allergy occurs in three ways: (1) as irritant contact dermatitis, (2) as type IV allergic reactions, and (3) as type I allergic reactions. The irritant reaction, which is seen most commonly, is actually a nonallergic reaction and results in itchy, dry, and irritated hands. The type IV allergic reaction to latex is a cell-mediated response to the chemical irritants found in latex products. The true latex allergy is the type I allergic reaction, and it occurs shortly after exposure to the proteins in latex rubber. The type I reaction is an immunoglobulin E–mediated systemic reaction that occurs when latex proteins are touched, inhaled, or ingested (Asthma and Allergy Foundation of America, n.d.).

Factors influencing the risk for latex allergy response are the individual's susceptibility and the route, duration, and frequency of latex exposure. Risk factors (Mayo Clinic Staff, n.d.) include the following:
- A job with daily exposure to latex (health care, food handlers, rubber industry workers)
- Children with spina bifida (approximately 50% with disorder) due to early and repeated exposure to latex products through necessary health care provided frequently, beginning at birth
- Food allergies (specifically kiwi, bananas, avocados, chestnuts)
- History of allergies and asthma
- History of reactions to latex (balloons, condoms, gloves)
- Multiple surgical procedures (especially from infancy)

To provide a latex-safe environment for susceptible patients, all surgical patients should be screened for the risk for latex allergy response before admission. Identification of patients at risk is the first step in preventing a reaction.

When a patient with a suspected or known latex allergy is scheduled for surgery, all latex use is avoided, and the patient is admitted directly to the OR as the first

| Box 2.5 | Responding to a Patient's Risk for Latex Allergy |

LATEX ALERT PATIENT (HIGH RISK FOR ALLERGIC RESPONSE)
- Recognize the problem.
- Avoid exposing the patient to latex.
- Notify surgeons and operating room nurses and staff.
- Be prepared to treat anaphylaxis should it occur.
- Be alert to signs and symptoms of a reaction postoperatively.

LATEX ALLERGY PATIENT (SUSPECTED OR KNOWN ALLERGIC RESPONSE)
- Administer prophylactic treatment with steroids and antihistamines preoperatively.
- Prepare a latex-safe environment, include latex-safe supply cart and crash cart.
- Apply cloth barrier to patient's arm under a blood pressure cuff.
- Use medications from glass ampules.
- Do not puncture rubber stoppers with needles.
- Wear synthetic gloves.
- Use latex-free syringes.
- Use latex-safe (polyvinyl chloride) intravenous (IV) tubing.
- Do not use latex equipment (i.e., tubing and spikes on tubing) on IV bags.

case of the day, if possible. Many facilities have converted isolation rooms into latex-safe environments for patients with latex allergy. Nurses must ensure that everyone on the health care team is aware that a patient is, or may be, allergic to latex. A medical alert or allergy band must be placed around the patient's wrist and clearly flagged on the patient's medical record. All natural rubber latex products are removed from the area, and latex-free measures are used for medication preparation. The crash cart must be stocked with latex-free equipment, supplies, and drugs for treating anaphylaxis. Some surgeons order preoperative prophylactic treatment with glucocorticoid steroids and antihistamines. Box 2.5 lists interventions based on Nursing Interventions Classifications (NICs) for the perioperative care of the patient at risk for a latex allergy response (Nursing Interventions and Rationales, 2013).

Respiratory Preparation

If a general anesthetic is administered, it is essential to ventilate the lungs postoperatively to prevent or treat atelectasis, improve lung expansion, improve oxygenation, and prevent postoperative pneumonia. Because the lungs do not expand fully during surgery, mucus and gases remain in the lungs until expelled. Pulmonary exercises can help to expand the lungs and remove these by-products. Preoperative introduction to incentive spirometry has proven helpful.

The nurse usually instructs the patient about the incentive spirometer (IS). The patient should use the IS at the bedside at regular intervals to promote deep breathing (Skill 2.2 and the Patient Teaching box on incentive spirometry). A chart included inside the IS package helps to predict IS capacity based on gender, height, and age.

CHECK

GATHER

HELLO

ID

PRIVACY

EXPLAIN

WASH

GLOVES

NURSING ACTION *(RATIONALE)*

1. Refer to physician's orders, care plan, or Kardex. (Health care facilities frequently require a medical order for incentive spirometry.)
2. Assess patient's respiratory status and lung sounds. Indications for spirometry are (a) asymmetric chest wall movement, (b) increased respiratory rate, (c) increased production of sputum, and (d) diminished lung expansion postoperatively. *(Alerts health care personnel to those patients at risk for respiratory complications during illness or after surgery.)*
3. Explain procedure, and instruct patient in the correct use of the spirometer. Frequently the respiratory therapist will do this. However, it may be the nurse's responsibility to follow up and promote proper technique. *(Understanding improves compliance with use.)*
4. Obtain supplies and equipment. *(Organizes procedure.)*
   a. Incentive spirometer or positive expiratory pressure (PEP) therapy device
   b. Emesis basin
   c. Tissues
   d. Bedside trash bag
   e. Clean gloves (if soiling is likely)
5. Wash hands and don gloves (if soiling is likely). Know agency policy and guidelines from the Centers for Disease Control and Prevention and the Occupational Safety and Health Administration. *(Reduces spread of microorganisms.)*
6. Place prescribed incentive spirometer at the bedside. *(Prepares equipment for procedure.)*
7. Place patient in semi-Fowler or high Fowler position. *(Promotes optimal lung expansion.)*
8. Place tissues, emesis basin, and bedside trash bag within easy reach. *(Enables sanitary disposal of respiratory secretions expectorated during procedure.)*
9. Incentive spirometry
   a. Instruct patient to completely cover mouthpiece with lips (use a nose clip if patient is unable to breathe through the mouthpiece) and to (a) inhale slowly until maximum inspiration is reached, (b) hold breath 2–3 s, and (c) slowly exhale (see Fig. 2.2). *(Promotes maximum inspiration.)*
   b. Instruct patient to relax and breathe normally for a short time. *(Prevents patient from hyperventilating and prevents fatigue.)*
   c. Instruct and encourage patient to gradually increase depth of inspiration. *(Promotes maximum lung expansion.)*
   d. Offer oral hygiene after spirometry is completed. *(Patients often find this refreshing.)*
   e. Store spirometer in an appropriate place, such as the bedside table, until next scheduled time. *(Provides a convenient place for repeated use.)*

10. PEP therapy and "huff" coughing
    a. Wash hands. (Reduces transmission of microorganisms.)
    b. Set PEP device for setting ordered. (The higher the setting, the more effort required.)
    c. Instruct patient to assume a semi-Fowler or high Fowler position, and place nose clip on patient's nose. (Promotes optimum lung expansion and expectoration of mucus.)
    d. Instruct patient to place lips around mouthpiece and (1) take a full breath and exhale two or three times longer than inhalation and (2) repeat this pattern for 10–20 breaths. (Ensures that all breathing is done through the mouth and that the device is used properly.)

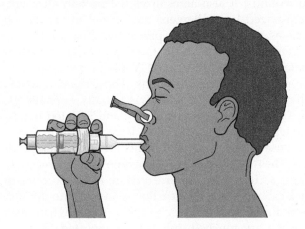

    e. Remove device from mouth, and have patient take a slow, deep breath and hold for 3 s. (Promotes lung expansion before coughing.)
    f. Instruct patient to exhale in quick, short, forced "huffs." ("Huff" coughing, or forced expiratory technique, promotes bronchial hygiene by increasing expectoration of secretions.)
11. Position patient as desired or as ordered. (Helps maintain patient comfort and promotes maximum chest expansion.)
12. Place call light within easy reach. (Maintains patient safety.)
13. Remove and dispose of soiled gloves and wash hands. (Reduces spread of microorganisms.)
14. Assess respiratory status and evaluate patient's response to spirometry. (Provides a basis for repeated use.)
15. Document in nurse's notes patient's respiratory status before and after incentive spirometry, type of spirometry, and any adverse effects from the procedure. (Verifies patient care. Some agencies require such documentation for third-party reimbursements.)
16. Carry out patient teaching (see the Patient Teaching box on incentive spirometry).

The initial postoperative goal is one-third of the predicted value. The amount of air inspired is measured, and the patient is encouraged to attain the established goal. When the patient is able to reach that goal on a regular basis, the goal should be increased. A respiratory therapist may provide preoperative teaching of IS use if the patient is considered at high risk for atelectasis (an abnormal condition characterized by the collapse of lung tissue). Conditions such as chronic respiratory disease and thoracic or abdominal surgery increase the risk for atelectasis.

Patient Teaching

Incentive Spirometry

- After performing incentive spirometry exercises, the patient should practice controlled coughing techniques.
- Teach the patient to examine his or her sputum for consistency, amount, and color changes.
- Before discharge, ask the patient to demonstrate the correct procedure for use of incentive spirometer.
- Administer breathing treatments before the patient's meals to prevent nausea and vomiting.
- To encourage patient use, place the spirometer close by, on the bedside stand. The usual rate of use is 10 breaths hourly during waking hours.

There are two general types of incentive spirometer:
1. *Flow-oriented inspiratory spirometer:* This type of incentive spirometer is inexpensive and measures inspiration. It contains one or more clear plastic cylinder chambers that contain freely movable, colored, lightweight plastic balls or a disk. Instruct the patient to place the mouthpiece in the mouth and inhale slowly and deeply; this raises the balls or disk in the cylinders. Encourage the patient to keep the colored balls or disk floating or raised for at least 2 to 3 seconds. The degree of elevation is marked on the cylinders so that this, plus the length of time the patient maintains elevation, can be recorded (Fig. 2.2).
2. *Volume-oriented spirometer:* This form of incentive spirometer maintains a known volume of inspiration. Encourage the patient to breathe with normal inspired capacity.

Before surgery, help the patient practice coughing (Skill 2.3 and the Patient Teaching box on controlled coughing technique), turning, and deep breathing (Skill 2.4). Because coughing increases intracranial pressure, it usually is contraindicated in cranial and spine-related surgeries. Coughing also is contraindicated after most types of eye surgery (Box 2.6). Patients frequently ambulate within a few hours of surgery or sooner to return cardiovascular and respiratory functions to normal more quickly.

Cardiovascular Considerations

Accompanying the need to turn, cough, and deep-breathe is the need to practice leg exercises (see Skill 2.4). Because blood stasis occurs when the body lies flat, encourage the patient to do leg exercises to assist venous blood flow. Slow venous blood flow can lead to the formation of a thrombus (an accumulation

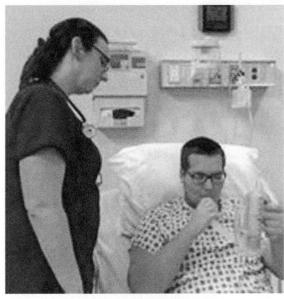

Fig. 2.2 Flow-oriented spirometer.

Patient Teaching

Controlled Coughing Technique

- For the patient entering the hospital for same-day surgery, controlled coughing can be taught in the physician's office, in the preoperative area, or postoperatively.
- The home health nurse may need to reinforce the importance of coughing once or twice an hour during waking hours for the patient receiving home care services.
- Young children or older adults may not understand fully the importance of controlled coughing, and continual reinforcement of teaching and assistance may be needed.
- Teach family members of a young child the procedure so that they may assist the child.
- After brain, spinal, head, neck, or eye surgery, coughing often is contraindicated because of a potential increase in intracranial pressure.
- Instruct the patient to cough instead of just clearing the throat.
- Teach the patient how to splint the incision with a small pillow or blanket, that controlled coughing will not injure the incision, and that there will be less discomfort with splinting.
- Teach the patient to examine the sputum for odor, consistency, amount, and color changes.

of platelets, fibrin, and cellular elements of the blood attached to the interior wall of a vessel, sometimes occluding the lumen). If a thrombus is dislodged, it can travel as an embolus (a traveling or mobilized clot) to the lungs, heart, or brain, where the vessel can be occluded. Without an adequate blood supply, an infarct (localized area of necrosis) can occur. Antiembolism stockings (thromboembolic deterrent stockings) and/or sequential compression devices (SCDs) with an intermittent external pneumonic compression system may be ordered to provide support and to prevent venous thrombus in the lower extremities. Newer models of SCDs are battery operated so that the patient does not have to be tethered to a motor, allowing for use at any time (Skill 2.5 and the Patient Teaching

CHECK GATHER HELLO ID PRIVACY EXPLAIN WASH GLOVES

NURSING ACTION *(RATIONALE)*

1. Refer to medical record, care plan, or Kardex for special interventions. *(Provides basis for care.)*
2. Obtain equipment. *(Organizes procedure.)*
   a. Pillow or bath blanket
   b. Gloves
   c. Emesis basin
   d. Facial tissues
   e. Chair or bed
3. Introduce self. *(Decreases patient's anxiety.)*
4. Identify patient. *(Ensures correct patient for procedure.)*
5. Explain procedure. *(Improves cooperation and decreases anxiety.)*
6. Wash hands and don clean gloves according to agency policy and guidelines from the Centers for Disease Control and Prevention and the Occupational Safety and Health Administration. *(Reduces spread of microorganisms.)*
7. Assist patient to upright position. Place pillow between bed or chair and patient. *(Facilitates deep breathing and optimum chest expansion.)*
8. Demonstrate coughing exercise for patient (see illustration). *(Allows patient to observe nurse and to ask questions.)*
   a. Take several deep breaths. *(Deep breaths expand lungs fully so that air moves behind mucus and facilitates effect of coughing.)*

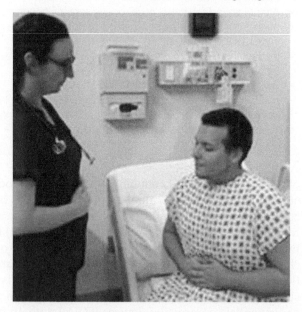

   b. Inhale through nose.
   c. Exhale through mouth with pursed lips.
   d. Inhale deeply again and hold breath for count of three.
   e. Cough two or three consecutive times without inhaling between coughs. *(Consecutive coughs remove mucus more effectively and completely than one forceful cough.)*
9. Caution patient against just clearing the throat instead of coughing. *(Clearing the throat does not remove mucus from deep in airways.)*
10. Before the patient coughs, abdominal or thoracic incision can be splinted with hands, pillow, towel, or rolled bath blanket (see illustration). *(Surgical incision cuts through muscles, tissues, and nerve endings. Deep breathing and coughing place additional stress on suture line and cause discomfort. Splinting incision provides firm support and reduces incisional pulling.)*

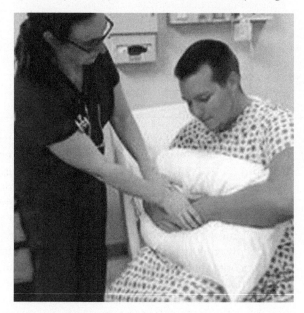

11. Encourage patient to practice coughing once or twice an hour during waking hours, while splinting incisional area. Assist patient as indicated. *(Helps to effectively expectorate mucus with minimal discomfort.)*
12. Remind patient to use tissues and emesis basin for any mucus expectorated. *(Reduces spread of microorganisms.)*
13. Teach patient to examine sputum for consistency, amount, and color changes. *(Changes could indicate respiratory complications such as pneumonia.)*
14. Provide wash cloth and warm water for washing hands and face, provide for oral hygiene, and return patient to comfortable position. *(Provides for patient comfort.)*
15. Remove and dispose of soiled gloves and wash hands. *(Reduces spread of microorganisms.)*
16. Document exercises performed and patient's ability to perform them independently. *(Verifies care given and patient teaching.)*
17. Carry out patient teaching (see the Patient Teaching box on controlled coughing technique).

Skill 2.4   Teaching Postoperative Breathing Techniques, Leg Exercises, and Turning Exercises

NURSING ACTION (RATIONALE)

1. Refer to medical record, care plan, or Kardex for special interventions. (*Provides basis for care.*)
2. Obtain equipment. (*Helps organize procedure.*)
   a. Support pillow, towel, or folded bath blanket
   b. Gloves
   c. Emesis basin
   d. Facial tissues
3. Introduce self. (Decreases patient's anxiety.)
4. Identify patient. (Verifies correct patient for procedure.)
5. Explain procedure to patient. (Improves cooperation and decreases anxiety.)
6. Perform hand hygiene and don clean gloves. Know agency policy and guidelines from the Centers for Disease Control and Prevention and the Occupational Safety and Health Administration. (Reduces spread of microorganisms.)
7. Prepare patient for intervention.
   a. Close door to room or pull curtain. (*Provides privacy.*)
   b. Drape for procedure if necessary.
8. Raise bed to comfortable working level. (*Promotes proper body mechanics.*)
9. Premedicate with pain medication, if indicated. (*Elicits patient compliance.*)

Postoperative Breathing Techniques

10. Place pillow between patient and bed or chair. (Allows for fuller chest expansion [bed or chair is too firm to provide expansion].)
11. Sit or stand, facing patient. (Allows patient to observe nurse.)
12. Demonstrate taking slow, deep breaths. Avoid moving shoulders and chest while inhaling. Inhale through nose. (Prevents panting and hyperventilation. Moistens, filters, and warms inhaled air.)
13. Hold breath for a count of three, and slowly exhale through pursed lips. (Allows for gradual expulsion of air.)
14. Repeat exercise three to five times. Have patient practice exercise. (Allows patient to observe appropriate technique. Allows nurse to assess patient's technique and correct errors.)
15. Instruct patient to take 10 slow, deep breaths q 2 h until ambulatory. (Helps prevent postoperative complications.)

16. If there is an abdominal or chest incision, instruct patient to splint incisional area, using pillow or bath blanket, if desired, during breathing exercises. (Provides support and additional security for patient.)

Leg Exercises

17. Lifting one leg at a time and supporting joints, gently flex and extend leg 5–10 times. (*Stimulates circulation and helps prevent thrombus formation.*)

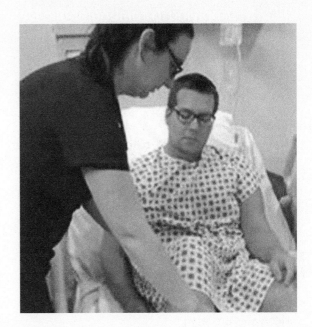

18. Repeat exercise with opposite extremity. Lifting leg while supporting joints, gently flex leg 5–10 times. (*Stimulates circulation and helps prevent thrombus formation.*)
19. Flex ankle with toes pointed toward head, then extend ankle with toes pointed toward foot of bed. (*Uses additional muscle flexion and contraction to stimulate circulation.*)
20. Make circle with ankles of both feet four or five times to the left and four or five times to the right. (*Further stimulates circulation through muscle contraction and flexion.*)
21. Assess pulse, respiration, and blood pressure. (*Aids in determining complications from exercise.*)

Continued

Skill 2.4   Teaching Postoperative Breathing Techniques, Leg Exercises, and Turning Exercises—cont'd

Turning Exercises

22. Instruct patient to assume supine position on right side of bed. Have side rails on both sides of bed in up position. (Positioning begins on right side of bed so that turning to left side will not cause patient to roll toward bed's edge. Side rails in the raised position promote patient safety.)

23. Instruct patient to place left hand over incisional area to splint it. (Supports and minimizes pulling on suture line during turning.)

24. Instruct patient to keep left leg straight and to flex right knee up and over left leg. (Straight leg stabilizes patient's position. Flexed right leg shifts weight for easier turning.)

25. Instruct patient to turn q 2 h while awake. (Reduces risk of vascular and pulmonary complications.)

26. Remove and dispose of soiled gloves and wash hands. (Reduces spread of microorganisms.)

27. Document. (Records patient education and verifies procedure.)

Skill 2.5   Applying Thromboembolic Deterrent Stockings and Sequential Compression Devices

CHECK   GATHER   HELLO   ID   PRIVACY   EXPLAIN   WASH   GLOVES

NURSING ACTION (RATIONALE)

1. Refer to medical record, care plan, or Kardex for special interventions. (*Provides basis for care.*)
2. Obtain equipment. (*Organizes procedure.*)
   a. Thromboembolic deterrent stockings (TEDs) or sequential compression devices (SCDs)
   b. Clean gloves (when appropriate)
   c. Tape measure
3. Introduce self. (*Decreases patient's anxiety.*)
4. Identify patient. (*Identifies correct patient for procedure.*)
5. Explain procedure. (*Improves cooperation and decreases anxiety.*)
6. Perform hand hygiene and, if appropriate, don clean gloves. Know agency policy and guidelines from the Centers for Disease Control and Prevention and the Occupational Safety and Health Administration. (*Reduces spread of microorganisms.*)
7. Prepare patient.
   a. Close door to room, pull curtain, and drape for procedure, if necessary. (*Provides privacy.*)
8. Raise bed to comfortable working level. (*Promotes proper body mechanics.*)
9. Examine legs and assess risk for conditions. (*Helps nurse to determine presence of pigmentation around ankles, pitting edema, or peripheral cyanosis, which may indicate inadequate circulation.*)
10. Assess patient for calf pain, redness, tenderness, warmth, and/or swelling. (*May indicate presence of thrombophlebitis.*)

11. Measure legs for stockings according to agency policy, and order stockings. (*Promotes the correct size to accomplish purpose of stockings.*)

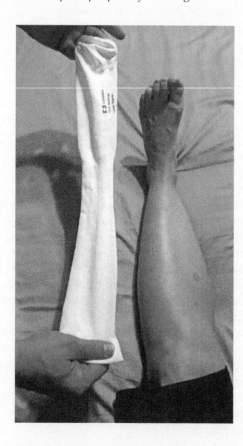

Skill 2.5 Applying Thromboembolic Deterrent Stockings and Sequential Compression Devices—cont'd

Thromboembolic Deterrent Stockings

12. Assist patient to supine position to apply stockings before patient rises. Patient should be recumbent for at least 30 min before application. (*Prevents veins from becoming distended or edema from occurring.*)

13. Turn stockings inside out as far as heel. Place thumbs inside foot part, and slip stocking on until heel is correctly aligned. (*Positions stocking for appropriate application.*)

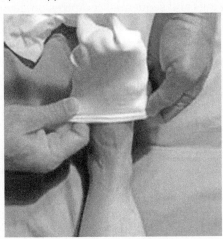

14. Gather fabric and ease it over ankle and up the leg. (Prevents bunching of stocking, which can cause local pooling of blood.)

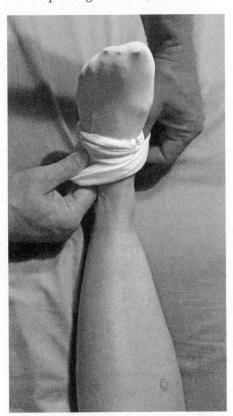

15. Pull leg portion of stocking over foot and up as far as it will go, making certain that gusset lies over femoral artery. Adjust stocking to fit evenly and smoothly with no wrinkles. (*Allows appropriate fit and application, which are vital for maintaining even pressure. Prevents irritation and impediments to circulation.*)

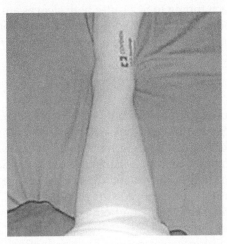

16. Repeat steps 12–15 for opposite extremity. (*Ensures appropriate application.*)

Sequential Compression Devices

17. Place sleeve under patient's leg, with fuller portion at top of thigh or just below knee, depending on ordered length. (*Ensures correct fit.*)

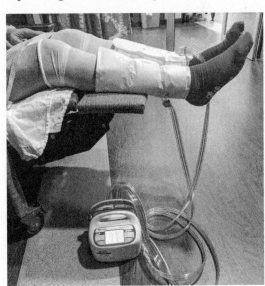

Continued

Skill 2.5 Applying Thromboembolic Deterrent Stockings and Sequential Compression Devices—cont'd

18. Apply sleeve with opening at front of knee and closed portion behind knee. (*Ensures appropriate placement and desired effect.*)
19. When the SCD is in place, make sure there are no wrinkles or creases in stockings. Fold Velcro strips over to secure stockings. (*Allows proper functioning of stockings and prevents irritation.*)
20. Attach tubing to SCD after both sleeves are applied. Align arrows for correct connection and appropriate effect. Plug in unit. (*Allows air to inflate stockings in sequential order.*)

21. Assess patient periodically. (*Determines presence of edema or cyanosis.*)
22. Assess stocking at regular intervals. (*Ensures that top has not rolled down or loosened and that no wrinkles are present.*)
23. Remove and dispose of soiled gloves and wash hands. (*Reduces spread of microorganisms.*)
24. Document. (*Verifies patient care.*)
25. Carry out patient teaching (see the Patient Teaching box on use of thromboembolic deterrent stockings and sequential compression devices).

box on use of thromboembolic deterrent stockings and SCDs). Some surgeons and facilities are no longer using thromboembolic deterrent stockings due to the complications they may cause. These complications include skin breakdown and the stocking rolling at the top, causing increased pressure on vessels.

Consider the following points when applying antiembolism stockings:

- The postoperative patient with abdominal or thoracic incisions will not be able to bend and pull on his or her own stockings.
- Measurements should be taken according to the manufacturer's guidelines to ensure proper size and fit.
- Stockings may be difficult to apply for some patients; the nurse or family members will need to assist.

Patient Teaching

Use of Thromboembolic Deterrent Stockings and Sequential Compression Devices

- Teach the patient how to correctly apply antiembolism stockings.
- Teach the patient appropriate care of the stockings. (Hand wash in warm water and mild soap, do not wring dry, and lay over flat surface to dry.)
- Instruct the patient not to massage legs because of the risk of dislodging a thrombus.
- Teach the patient the signs of possible complications. (If stockings or devices are too restrictive, edema and pain could result.)

Vital Signs

Vital signs mirror the body's response to anesthesia and surgery. Explain to the patient before surgery that it is normal for blood pressure, temperature, pulse, and respiration to be monitored before and after surgery, until the patient stabilizes. The schedule for monitoring vital signs depends on the facility's protocol and

Box 2.6	Surgeries for Which Coughing Is Contraindicated or Modified

Intracranial: Coughing increases intracranial pressure (ICP), leading to cerebrospinal fluid leakage.
Eye: Coughing increases ICP, which then increases intraocular pressure, causing pressure on suture line.
Ear: If patient must cough, mouth must be kept open to prevent pressure backup through eustachian tube to middle ear, causing pressure on suture line.
Nose: If patient must cough, mouth must be kept open to prevent dislodgment of a clot with subsequent bleeding.
Throat: Vigorous coughing may dislodge a clot with subsequent bleeding.
Spinal: Coughing increases spinal canal pressure.

the patient. Preoperative vital signs provide a baseline for determining postoperative stability or identifying related problems. Postoperative vital signs are discussed later in this chapter.

Genitourinary Considerations

After general anesthesia, the urinary bladder's tone is decreased, leading to urinary retention. Assess the patient's normal bladder habits preoperatively and identify when the bladder is full and distended postoperatively. If the patient does not urinate within 8 hours after surgery, assess the patient by palpating above the symphysis pubis to determine if the bladder is distended (Fig. 2.3). Once the patient is awake and tolerating fluids, encourage an adequate fluid intake. Occasionally a urinary catheter is inserted to monitor urinary output. This procedure normally is reserved for a patient undergoing urinary surgery or who may have difficulty voiding or needs the output closely monitored postoperatively. The catheter is removed as soon as possible, based on the patient's condition, either at the conclusion of the surgery or 1 or 2 days postoperatively, to reduce the chance of bladder infection. Once it is removed, encourage the patient to drink

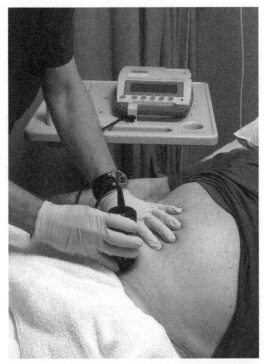

Fig. 2.3 Assess the bladder by palpating the lower abdomen for distention. (From Williams P: *deWit's fundamental concepts and skills for nursing*, ed 5, St. Louis, 2018, Elsevier.)

8 ounces of fluids per hour while awake unless contraindicated. In addition, monitor intake and output (I&O) values until the patient's normal voiding pattern returns. Urinary retention is a common postoperative complication.

Surgical Wounds

Incisions (cuts produced surgically by a sharp instrument to create an opening into an organ or body space) are closed in a variety of ways: with sutures, staples, Steri-Strips, transparent strips, or tissue adhesives. Knowing the type of closure enables the nurse to explain its appearance to the patient. Some surgeries require the removal of exudate, often with a drain. The purpose of the drain should be explained to the patient and monitored and cared for appropriately. Wound care, dressing changes, and drainage systems are described in more detail in Chapter 22 of *Foundations of Nursing*.

Pain

Many individuals undergoing surgical procedures fear the prospect of postoperative pain. Discussion of various pain relief measures should be included in the preoperative teaching. If the patient is considering nonpharmacologic analgesia (e.g., imagery, biofeedback, relaxation techniques), these techniques should be reviewed with the patient, and practice time should be planned. Most patients choose traditional analgesia. Some patients fear that addiction to pain medications may occur, so it is important to reassure patients that

addiction to analgesics rarely occurs in the time frame needed for comfort. For the patient who is apprehensive about intermittent injections, patient-controlled analgesia (PCA) and opioids injected into the epidural space (patient-controlled epidural) offer safe and effective relief for postoperative pain. When the patient can resume oral intake, oral analgesics coupled with nontraditional methods are often effective (see Chapter 21 in *Foundations of Nursing*). Nurses must listen to patient complaints of postoperative pain.

Tubes

Depending on the surgery, patient teaching includes information about nasogastric (NG) tubes, wound drainage units, and IV and oxygen therapy. Allowing patients to view related equipment and understand their purpose lessens the fear associated with them. (See Chapters 14 and 15 in *Foundations of Nursing* for more detailed discussion of the tubes and drains used in the postoperative patient.)

Preoperative Medication

Preoperative medication reduces the patient's anxiety, decreases the amount of anesthetic needed, and reduces respiratory tract secretions. The patient should be told what to expect from preoperative medications. Barbiturates and tranquilizers (e.g., phenobarbital and diazepam [Valium]) sometimes are given for sedation to reduce the amount of anesthetic required. Opioid analgesics (meperidine and morphine) may be administered by intermittent injection or PCA if the patient has pain before surgery; this also reduces the amount of anesthetic required. An introduction to PCA preoperatively helps the patient to understand the concept and how the equipment works. Anticholinergics such as atropine reduce spasms of smooth muscles and decrease gastric, bronchial, and salivary secretions (Table 2.5).

The patient frequently becomes drowsy, notices a dry mouth, and experiences vertigo after receiving a preoperative medication. If the preoperative medication is given on the nursing unit, the patient should be encouraged to void before receiving the medication and must remain in bed after administration of the medication to prevent falls. Safety measures should be instituted, such as placing the bed in a low position and raising side rails and monitoring the patient every 15 to 30 minutes until the patient leaves for surgery. Reassurance and support should be given to the patient, as well as providing a quiet environment on the nursing unit while waiting for transport to the surgical suite. In many institutions, the preoperative medication is given by the anesthesiologist or anesthesia provider, such as a certified registered nurse anesthetist (CRNA), in the preoperative holding area.

For the patient scheduled for surgery, all medications ordered before surgery usually are stopped preoperatively except for those prescribed for long-term conditions,

Table 2.5   Medications for the Perioperative Period

GENERIC NAME	ACTION	NURSING IMPLICATIONS
Benzodiazepines		
midazolam diazepam lorazepam	• Decrease anxiety and produce sedation • Induce amnesia	Monitor for respiratory depression, hypotension, drowsiness, and lack of coordination.
Opioid Analgesics		
morphine fentanyl citrate	• Decrease anxiety • Allow decreased anesthetics	Monitor for respiratory depression, nausea, vomiting, orthostatic hypotension, and pruritus.
H₂ Receptor Antagonists		
famotidine ranitidine	• Reduce gastric acid volume and concentration	Monitor for confusion and dizziness in older adults.
Antiemetics		
metoclopramide droperidol ondansetron HCl (5-HT3 receptor antagonist)	• Enhance gastric emptying • Tranquilizing effect • Prevent postoperative nausea and vomiting	Monitor for sedation and extrapyramidal reaction (involuntary movement, muscle tone changes, and abnormal posture). Instruct patient to report any difficulty in breathing.
Anticholinergics		
atropine sulfate glycopyrrolate	• Reduce oral and respiratory secretions to decrease risk of aspiration • Decrease vomiting and laryngospasm	Monitor for confusion, restlessness, and tachycardia. Prepare patient to expect dry mouth.
Antibiotics		
cefazolin sodium cefotaxime sodium ceftriaxone	• Bactericidal • Minimizes risk of wound infection • Bactericidal • Used for perioperative prophylaxis • Bactericidal • Used for perioperative prophylaxis	If large doses are given, therapy is prolonged, or patient is at high risk, monitor for signs and symptoms of superinfection, including abdominal pain, moderate to severe diarrhea, severe anal or genital pruritus, and severe mouth soreness. Determine patient's history of allergies. If dosing continues, space drug evenly around the clock. Advise patient to complete therapy.
Adrenocortical Steroid		
methylprednisolone	• Decreases inflammation	Determine whether patient has hypersensitivity to drug. Determine whether patient has diabetes mellitus, and anticipate an increase in antidiabetic drug regimen because of raised blood glucose level.
Nonsteroidal Antiinflammatory Drug (NSAID)		
ketorolac	• Reduces intensity of pain • Reduces inflammation	Assess the duration, location, onset, and type of pain the patient is having. Evaluate patient for therapeutic response.
Anticoagulants		
enoxaparin sodium	• Produces anticoagulation • Prevents new clot formation or secondary embolic complications	Do not give IM, but give subQ. Tell the patient not to take aspirin or similar over-the-counter drugs.
heparin sodium		Cross-check heparin dose with another nurse before administering. Use constant rate IV infusion pump. Monitor the patient's partial thromboplastin time diligently. Assess patient's gums for erythema and gingival bleeding; skin for bruises or petechiae; and urine for hematuria.
warfarin sodium		Observe patient for evidence of hemorrhage such as abdominal or back pain, decreased blood pressure, increased pulse rate, and severe headache. Urge patient not to ingest alcohol or make drastic dietary changes. If administration continues, urge patient to notify the physician if he or she experiences black stools; bleeding; brown, dark, or red urine; coffee-ground vomitus; or red-speckled mucus from a cough.

IM, Intramuscular; *IV*, intravenous; *mcg*, microgram; *PO*, per os (by mouth); *q 4–6h*, every 4–6 h; *subQ*, subcutaneously.
Data from *Mosby's 2021 nursing drug reference*, St. Louis, 2021, Elsevier.

DRUG CLASS	IMPLICATIONS FOR THE SURGICAL PATIENT
Anticoagulants	Anticoagulants such as warfarin and aspirin are stopped several days before surgery. Anticoagulants prolong clotting times, which may lead to hemorrhage.
Antihypertensives	Antihypertensives may cause hypotension when combined with anesthetic agents and narcotics used for pain control.
Antiseizure drugs	Long-term use of certain antiseizure drugs (e.g., phenytoin [Dilantin], phenobarbital) can interact with anesthetic agents.
Corticosteroids	If used for an extended period, corticosteroids may prolong bleeding and hamper the body's ability to heal. These drugs also may decrease the body's ability to deal with the stress of surgery as a result of suppression of the adrenal glands.
Diuretics	Because of fluid loss during surgery, diuretics may cause hypotension after surgery and decreased serum potassium level.
Herbal therapies	Several herbal therapies can affect clotting times. Ginseng may increase hypoglycemia with insulin therapy (see Chapter 20 in *Foundations of Nursing*, Complementary and Alternative Therapies boxes for potential complications that may occur when herbal therapies are combined with traditional medications).
Insulin	Blood glucose levels fluctuate, so insulin levels may require adjustment. A patient with diabetes may have reduced need for insulin after surgery because nutritional intake is decreased; conversely, stress response and intravenous administration of glucose solutions can increase dosage requirements after surgery.
Nonsteroidal antiinflammatory drugs (NSAIDs)	NSAIDs inhibit platelet function and may prolong bleeding, leading to possible hemorrhage.

Table 2.6 Medications With Special Implications for the Surgical Patient

such as phenytoin for seizure control (Table 2.6). After surgery, the surgeon prescribes or reorders the necessary medication, as does the primary health care provider.

Anesthesia

Anesthesia means the absence of all sensation, including pain (*an*, meaning "without," plus *esthesia*, meaning "awareness of feeling"). Anesthesia is divided into four categories: general, regional, local, and conscious (moderate) sedation.

General anesthesia. General anesthesia produces amnesia, analgesia, muscle paralysis, and sedation. The patient is in a state of unconsciousness that is reversible. General anesthesia is used for major surgery requiring extensive tissue manipulation. Modern anesthetics are much easier to reverse, and they allow the patient to recover with fewer unwanted effects than in the past.

An anesthesiologist or a CRNA administers general anesthetics through the four stages of anesthesia. Common anesthetic agents include propofol (a nonbarbiturate IV anesthetic), nitrous oxide gas, and desflurane and sevoflurane vapors; muscle relaxants also may be used as an adjunct.

In the induction phase, the patient is awake and the anesthetic often is given intravenously. This phase is complete when the patient loses consciousness. Intubation with an endotracheal tube or use of a laryngeal mask airway (Fig. 2.4) is done at this time to establish an airway.

During the maintenance phase, the patient is kept anesthetized at appropriate levels throughout the

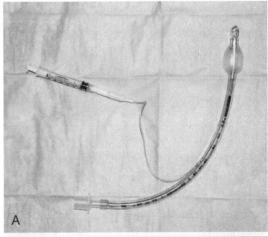

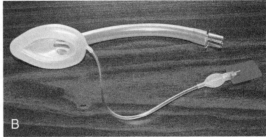

Fig. 2.4 (A) Endotracheal tube. (B) Laryngeal mask airway.

surgical procedure. Anesthesia may be maintained using a combination of inhalation of gases and vapors and IV medications. The patient also receives a continuous supply of oxygen and adjunct medications such as opioid analgesics and muscle relaxants. A combination of small amounts of several medications can mean

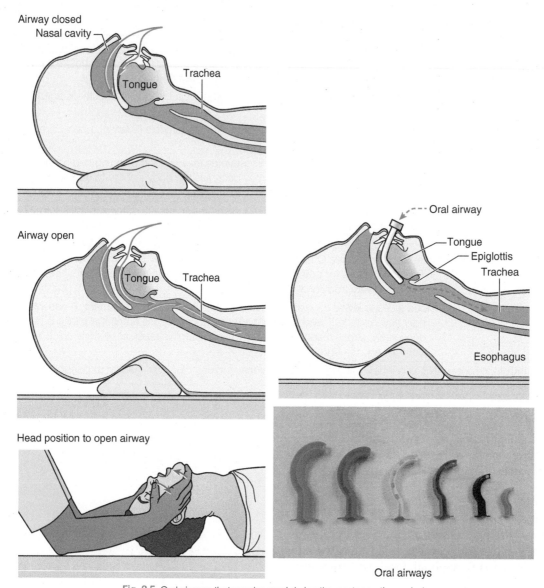

Fig. 2.5 Oral airways that may be used during the postoperative period.

a significant reduction in dose compared with using a single drug.

The duration of anesthesia depends on the length of surgery. Surgical risks influence the duration of surgery. The greatest risks from general anesthesia are the adverse effects of anesthetic agents, including cardiovascular depression or irritability, respiratory depression, and liver and kidney damage.

Patients emerge from anesthesia when procedures are complete and reversal agents are given. Because of the short half-life of the anesthetic agents currently used, emergence often occurs in the OR. The oropharynx is suctioned to decrease the risk of aspiration and laryngeal spasm after extubation. Extubation or removal of the laryngeal airway mask may occur before transfer to the postanesthesia care unit (PACU), depending on the patient's ability to maintain a patent airway. If the patient is having difficulty maintaining a patent airway after extubation, an oral airway may be used to maintain an open airway until the patient is fully conscious (Fig. 2.5).

Regional anesthesia. Regional anesthesia causes loss of sensation in an area of the body and is used for some surgical procedures and pain management. The patient does not lose consciousness with regional anesthesia but usually is sedated. The anesthesiologist or CRNA administers regional anesthetics by infiltration and local application. Fig. 2.6 shows common sites where spinal or epidural anesthetics are administered to achieve a regional block. The sensory pathway that is anesthetized depends on the method of induction.

Infiltration of anesthetic agents may involve one of the following induction methods:
- *Epidural anesthesia:* This procedure is safer than spinal anesthesia because the anesthetic agent is injected into the epidural space outside the dura mater and the depth of anesthesia is lighter.

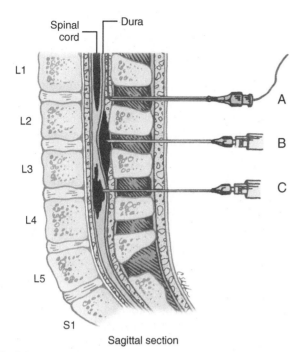

Spinal cord — Dura

L1
L2
L3
L4
L5
S1

A
B
C

Sagittal section

Fig. 2.6 Spinal column—side view with spinal and epidural anesthesia needle placement. (A) Epidural catheter. (B) Single injection epidural. (C) Spinal anesthesia. (Interspaces most commonly used are L4–L5, L3–L4, and L2–L3.) (From Rothrock JC: *Alexander's care of the patient in surgery,* ed 16, St. Louis, 2019, Elsevier.)

Epidural anesthesia blocks sensation in the vaginal and perineal areas and thus often is used for obstetric procedures. The epidural catheter may be left in so that the patient can receive medication via continuous epidural infusion after surgery.

- *Nerve block:* Local anesthetic is injected into a nerve (e.g., brachial plexus in the arm), blocking the nerve supply to the operative site. This type of anesthesia is used commonly for orthopedic surgery involving extremities.
- *Spinal anesthesia:* The anesthesiologist or CRNA performs a lumbar puncture and introduces local anesthetic into the cerebrospinal fluid in the subarachnoid space. Anesthetic effects can extend from the tip of the xiphoid process down to the feet. The position of the patient influences the movement of the anesthetic agent up or down the spinal cord. Spinal anesthesia often is used for lower abdominal, pelvic, and lower extremity procedures; urologic procedures; and surgical obstetrics.

Infiltrative anesthesia involves risks, particularly with spinal anesthesia, because the anesthetic agent may move upward in the spinal cord and affect breathing. This migration of anesthetic depends on the drug type and amount and on patient position. The patient's blood pressure may drop suddenly because of extensive vasodilation caused by the anesthetic block to sympathetic vasomotor nerves and pain and motor nerve fibers. If the level of anesthesia rises, respiratory paralysis may develop, requiring resuscitation by the anesthesiologist. Elevation of the upper body prevents respiratory paralysis. The patient must be monitored carefully during and immediately after surgery.

The patient under regional anesthesia is awake throughout the procedure unless the physician orders a tranquilizer that promotes sleep and/or amnesia. Because the patient is responsive and capable of breathing voluntarily, the anesthesiologist or CRNA does not need to insert an endotracheal tube.

Local anesthesia. Local anesthesia involves loss of sensation at the desired site (e.g., a growth on the skin or the cornea of the eye). The anesthetic agent (e.g., lidocaine) inhibits nerve conduction until the drug is diffused into the circulation. Local anesthetics usually are injected or applied topically. The patient loses sensation of pain and touch, and control over motor and autonomic activities (e.g., bladder emptying). Local anesthesia is used commonly for minor surgical procedures, such as a biopsy of a tumor or removal of a growth. Physicians also may infiltrate the operative area with a local anesthetic to promote postoperative pain relief.

Conscious sedation (moderate sedation). In **conscious sedation**, more recently referred to as *moderate sedation,* the patient is given drugs that depress the central nervous system or provide analgesia to relieve anxiety or provide amnesia during surgical diagnostic procedures. Combinations of sedatives, tranquilizers, anesthetics, or anesthetic gases commonly are used for conscious (moderate) sedation. It is used routinely for procedures that do not require complete anesthesia but rather a depressed level of consciousness. A patient under conscious (moderate) sedation must retain independently a patent airway and airway reflexes and be able to respond appropriately to physical and verbal stimuli.

Advantages of conscious (moderate) sedation include adequate sedation and reduced fear and anxiety as well as minimal risk, amnesia, relief of pain and noxious stimuli, mood alteration, elevation of pain threshold, enhanced patient cooperation, stable vital signs, and rapid recovery. Conscious (moderate) sedation is appropriate for a variety of diagnostic and therapeutic procedures, such as burn dressing changes, endoscopic procedures, certain biopsy procedures, and dental surgeries.

Nurses assisting with the administration of conscious (moderate) sedation must be knowledgeable about anatomy, physiology, cardiac dysrhythmias, procedural complications, and pharmacologic principles related to the particular sedation agents. Nurses also must be able to assess, diagnose, and intervene if an adverse reaction occurs and provide airway management and oxygen delivery. Resuscitation equipment must be readily available.

Positioning the patient for surgery. During general anesthesia the nursing personnel and surgeon often wait to position the patient until he or she is relaxed completely. The choice of position usually is determined by the surgical approach (Fig. 2.7). Ideally the patient's position provides good access to the operative site and sustains

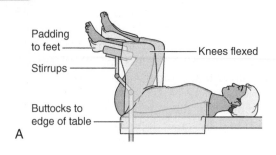

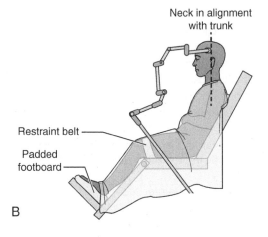

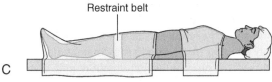

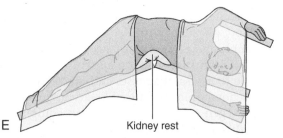

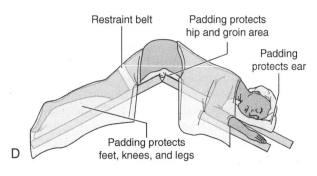

Fig. 2.7 Common perioperative positions and the padding provided to relieve pressure in each position. (A) Lithotomy position, used for vaginal and perineal procedures. (B) Sitting position, used for neurologic procedures. (C) Supine position (the most common position). Potential pressure points are the occiput, scapula, olecranon, thoracic vertebrae, sacrum, coccyx, and calcaneus. (D) Jackknife position, used for gluteal and anorectal surgeries. (E) Lateral kidney position, used for procedures requiring a retroperitoneal approach.

adequate circulatory and respiratory function, but it should not impair neuromuscular structures. The surgical team must consider the patient's comfort and safety, including such issues as age, weight, height, nutritional status, physical limitations, and preexisting conditions. These then are documented for staff members who care for the patient postoperatively. Nurses in postoperative divisions must recognize the discomfort a patient may feel after surgery (e.g., discomfort of the left arm or side of a patient whose right kidney was removed).

An alert person maintains normal range of joint motion by pain and pressure receptors. If a joint is extended too far, pain reminds the person that the muscle joint strain is too great. In a patient who is anesthetized, normal defense mechanisms cannot guard against joint damage, muscle stretch, and strain. The muscles are so relaxed that it is relatively easy to place the patient in a position he or she could not assume while awake. The patient often remains in a given position for several hours. Although it may be necessary to place a patient in an unusual position, it is important that the surgical team attempt to maintain correct alignment and protect the patient from pressure, abrasion, and other injuries (e.g., corneal abrasion). Attachments to the OR table allow protection and padding of extremities and bony prominences. Positioning should not interfere with normal movement of the diaphragm or circulation to body parts. If restraints are necessary, the surgical team should pad the area to be restrained to prevent skin trauma (see Chapter 10 in *Foundations of Nursing*).

Preoperative Checklist

A preoperative checklist often is used by facilities to ensure that all required care has been performed and that the patient is prepared properly for surgery. This form is completed before the patient leaves the nursing unit (Fig. 2.8). Signing the preoperative checklist means that the nurse assumes responsibility for all areas of care included on the list. If the preoperative medication is to be given on the nursing unit, the preoperative checklist must be completed before the medication is administered. Any prosthesis (an artificial replacement for a missing part of the body), contact lenses, dentures, and jewelry and other valuables are removed and either given to family members or placed in a secure area. Some facilities allow patients to wear dentures while in surgery and remove them later. If the patient wears rings and does not want them removed, they should be secured with tape and noted in the chart. The patient should void before the preoperative medication is administered or 1 hour before surgery is scheduled. Although most patients become drowsy after administration of a preoperative medication, a few either become hyperactive or demonstrate no side effects. The nurse should remind the patient to remain in bed, and side rails should be raised and the call light within reach to ensure patient safety.

Kell-Russell Memorial Hospital		Patient name: Jeri Schank		
		Date of Birth (DOB):	05/20/1952	
		Medical ID number:	57982310	

Check the appropriate box and initial	Surgery/Procedure Checklist			
Items Assessed	Check for yes and initial	Non-applicable (N/A) and initial	Comments	Date
1. Informed consent witnessed and signed				
2. ID band on				
3. Blood transfusion consent signed and ID band on				
4. Allergies identified and allergy band on				
5. Allergies, list				
6. Surgical site identified and marked				
7. Height and weight documented in chart				
8. Prosthetic devices removed (eyeglasses, contacts, dentures-full or partial, artificial eye, etc.)				
9. Nail polish, artificial nails, makeup, jewelry, hairpins removed				
10. Skin prep, list				
11. Hospital gown				
12. Anti-embolism stockings				
13. Time of NPO				
14. Lab results in chart				
15. ECG, scans, x-rays, etc. in chart				
16. History and physical in chart				
17. Pre-op vital signs				
18. Voided or catheterized				
19. Pre-op medications administered				
20. Mode of transfer to OR				
Signature of Nurse: *Kate Nicoli, LPN*	Initials of Nurse: *KN*	Signature of Nurse:	Initials of Nurse:	

Fig. 2.8 Preoperative assessment form. *ECG*, Electrocardiogram; *NPO*, Nothing by mouth; *OR*, Operating room.

Eliminating Wrong Site and Wrong Procedure Surgery

The Joint Commission (TJC) established Universal Protocol guidelines to prevent surgeons from performing surgery at the wrong site or performing the wrong procedure. If an invasive surgical procedure is planned, this protocol must be implemented regardless of location (ambulatory surgery centers, hospital, or health care provider's office). The protocol consists of three main steps:

1. Conduct a preoperative verification process that guarantees all relevant documents and test results are available and that they meet the patient's expectations.
2. Mark the operative site with indelible ink, including marking left or right, multiple structures (e.g., toes), and vertebral level(s) of the spine.

3. Just before the start of the procedure, all members of the surgical and procedure team have a timeout (everyone stops what they are doing) to verify they have the correct patient, procedure, site, and any implants.

A legally designated representative or an active patient must be included in all the protocol steps. If the representative or patient refuses to allow marking of the operative site, this must be noted on the procedure checklist (TJC, n.d.).

Transport to the Operating Room

Personnel in the OR notify the nursing unit when it is time for surgery. The transporter checks the patient's identification bracelet against the patient's medical record to be sure the correct person is going to surgery. For transportation on a gurney, the nurses and transporter help the patient to safely transfer from bed to gurney. The ambulatory surgery patient may walk to the OR, allowing more control over the event. The trip to surgery should be as smooth as possible so that the sedated patient does not experience nausea or dizziness.

Family should be allowed to visit before the patient is transported to the OR and then directed to the appropriate waiting area. If family members plan on leaving the facility during the procedure, the nurse should ensure there is a way to contact them.

Preparing for the Postoperative Patient

If the patient was hospitalized before surgery and will return to the same nursing unit, the bed and room should be prepared for the patient's return. The bed is placed in the high position with the bed rails down on the receiving side and up on the other side. A postoperative bedside unit should include the following items:
- Bed pads to protect bed linen from drainage
- Clean gown
- Emesis basin
- Extra pillows for positioning
- IV pole and pump
- Oxygen equipment
- PCA pump, if ordered
- Sphygmomanometer, stethoscope, and thermometer
- Suction equipment
- Wash cloth, towel, and facial tissues

INTRAOPERATIVE PHASE

Intraoperative (within the surgical suite) care focuses on care and protection of the patient. When the patient enters the OR (Fig. 2.9), the patient is identified verbally and by the identification band and medical records. Nursing interventions include warm, personal contact with the patient to humanize the OR's cold, aseptic, and highly technical environment. During surgery and particularly while anesthetized, patients cannot protect themselves from sources of possible harm. Essential

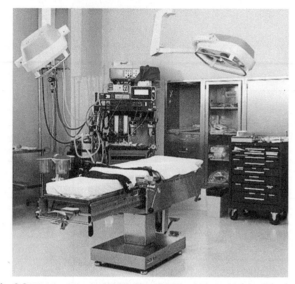

Fig. 2.9 Traditional operating room. (From Lewis SL, Heitkemper MM, Dirksen SR, et al: *Medical-surgical nursing: Assessment and management of clinical problems,* ed 10, St. Louis, 2017, Elsevier.)

elements for monitoring and promoting patient safety include being aware of the potential for harm, recognizing body areas most susceptible to injury, strictly adhering to principles of positioning and asepsis, and monitoring sites for impairment or early signs of injury. The nurse must ensure that small or potentially dangerous objects such as needles and syringes are not placed near the patient. Side rails and safety straps are used, even for the fully conscious patient, to protect the patient from injury. Safety reminder devices may be necessary to protect the delirious, semicomatose, or disoriented patient from injury.

HOLDING AREA

In many facilities the patient enters a surgical care unit called a preanesthesia care unit (or holding area) outside the OR, where the nurse completes the preoperative preparations. Nurses in this unit are usually part of the OR staff and wear surgical scrub suits.

The nurse, anesthesiologist, or CRNA inserts an IV catheter into the patient's vein to establish a route for fluid replacement and IV medications. A large-bore IV catheter is used for optimal infusion of all fluids and possible blood products.

The temperature in the OR is usually cool to aid in hindering the growth of bacteria, so the patient should be offered an extra blanket for warmth and relaxation. This blanket often is placed in a warmer before covering the patient with it. The patient's stay in the holding area is generally brief.

NURSE'S ROLE

In the intraoperative phase, the nurse assumes one of two roles during the surgical procedure: scrub nurse or circulating nurse (Box 2.7). Everyone (nurses, physicians, anesthesia providers) in the OR must practice surgical asepsis (using sterile technique to protect

Box 2.7 Responsibilities of the Circulating Nurse and the Scrub Nurse

RESPONSIBILITIES OF THE CIRCULATING NURSE

- Prepares operating room with necessary equipment and supplies and ensures that equipment is functional.
- Arranges sterile and unsterile supplies; opens sterile supplies for scrub nurse.
- Sends for patient at proper time.
- Visits with patient preoperatively; explains role, identifies patient, verifies operative permit, and answers any questions.
- Performs patient assessment.
- Confirms patient assessment.
- Checks medical record for completeness.
- Assists in safe transfer of patient to operating room table.
- Positions patient on operating room table in accordance with type of procedure and surgeon's preference.
- Places conductive pad on patient if electrocautery is to be used.
- Counts sponges, needles, and instruments with scrub nurse before surgery.
- Assists scrub nurse and surgeons by tying gowns.
- May prepare patient's skin.
- Assists scrub nurse in arranging tables to create sterile field.
- Maintains continuous astute observations during surgery to anticipate needs of patient, scrub nurse, surgeons, and anesthesiologist.
- Provides supplies to scrub nurse as needed.
- Observes sterile field closely for any breaks in aseptic technique and reports accordingly.
- Cares for surgical specimens according to institutional policy.
- Documents operative record and nurse's notes.
- Counts sponges, needles, and instruments when closure of wound begins.
- Transfers patient to gurney for transport to recovery area.
- Accompanies patient to the recovery room and provides a report.

RESPONSIBILITIES OF THE SCRUB NURSE

- Performs surgical hand scrub.
- Dons sterile gown and gloves aseptically.
- Arranges sterile supplies and instruments in manner prescribed for procedure.
- Checks instruments for proper functioning.
- Counts sponges, needles, and instruments with circulating nurse.
- Gowns and gloves surgeons as they enter operating room.
- Assists with surgical draping of patient.
- Maintains neat and orderly sterile field.
- Corrects breaks in aseptic technique.
- Observes progress of surgical procedure.
- Hands surgeon instruments, sponges, and necessary supplies during procedure.
- Identifies and handles surgical specimens correctly.
- Maintains count of sponges, needles, and instruments so that none will be misplaced or lost in wounds.

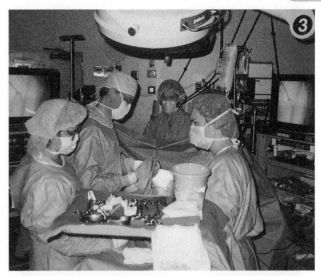

Fig. 2.10 Safe, effective intraoperative care requires team effort. (From Harkreader H, Hogan MA: *Fundamentals of nursing: Caring and clinical judgment,* ed 3, Philadelphia, 2007, Saunders.)

against infection before, during, or after surgery) to prevent microbial contamination of the operative site. The patient is at risk for introduction of infecting organisms through catheters, drains, and the surgical wound. Standards and guidelines for surgical scrubs and skin preparation should be followed strictly. The operation's success and ease greatly depend on group dynamics as professionals work to achieve common goals (Fig. 2.10).

POSTOPERATIVE PHASE

IMMEDIATE POSTOPERATIVE PHASE

During the postoperative phase the OR nurse assists in transferring the patient to the PACU (Fig. 2.11), the recovery room, or the intensive care area. The staff reviews information about the patient's status, including IV fluids, medications, and blood products administered; the surgical dressing; any complications in the OR; and unusual risks for hemorrhage or cardiac irregularities. The OR nurse is an important resource in planning the patient's postoperative care.

Immediate postoperative observation and interventions are focused on maintaining and monitoring the patient's airway, breathing, consciousness, circulation, and system review (Table 2.7). Vital signs are assessed every 15 minutes during the recovery period, and respiratory and GI functions are monitored. The wound is evaluated for any drainage or exudate (fluids from a body cavity, wound, or other source of discharge that slowly seeps from cells, tissue, or blood vessels through small pores or breaks in cell membranes). Once the patient has a patent airway and stable vital signs, is conscious, and responds to stimuli, the anesthesia provider or surgeon approves transfer to the nursing unit. As the patient regains consciousness, relief from pain is often the first need expressed. Frequently, medication is given in the recovery area. Staff members on the nursing unit review documentation from the surgical suite and recovery room to assess how well the patient tolerated the surgery.

The patient's body temperature must be monitored closely. Hypothermia—a rectal temperature of less than 96°F (35.6°C) or an oral temperature of less than 95°F (35°C)—frequently occurs because of body exposure in a cold OR, the effects of cold solutions, or as a possible consequence of some anesthetics. The heat loss in

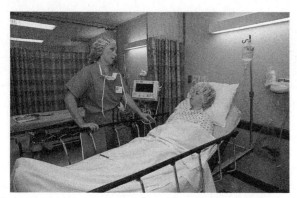

Fig. 2.11 Nurse in a postanesthesia care unit. (From Remmert LA, Sorrentino SA: *Mosby's textbook for nursing assistants*, ed 10, St. Louis, 2021, Elsevier.)

the OR can continue in the PACU, so warmed blankets may be used to increase the patient's body temperature. Another therapy may be used to provide warmth to the patient, convective warming. This therapy uses a disposable cover inflated with warm air from a heating unit placed over the patient; warm air passes out through the underside, so the warm air is moving constantly. In the PACU, the patient's temperature and vital signs are monitored every 15 minutes until vital signs are stable, or more frequently if they are unstable. The frequency and duration of monitoring are dictated by facility PACU policy. Patients are monitored until they are discharged from the PACU, usually at least 1 hour. Before discharge from the PACU, the patient must meet minimum criteria as established by the facility. This often is scored using a system based on assessment of the patient. Assessment variables that determine when the patient may be discharged include the patient's pain level, the presence of nausea or vomiting, ability to urinate, vital signs, cognitive level, and the amount bleeding from the surgical site.

The PACU nurse must be aware that malignant hyperthermia also can occur in the PACU and repeatedly assess the patient for signs of this condition. Malignant hyperthermia is a rare genetic disorder characterized by uncontrolled skeletal muscle contractions leading

Table 2.7	Interventions Associated With Immediate Postoperative Recovery Phase
ASSESSMENT MODE	**INTERVENTION**
A: Airway	• Maintain patency: keep head tilted up and back; may position on side with the face down and the neck slightly extended. • Note presence or absence of gag or swallowing reflex; stay at bedside until gag reflex returns. • Suction until awake and alert. • Provide oxygen if necessary.
B: Breathing	• Evaluate depth, rate, sounds, rhythm, and chest movement. • Assess color of mucous membranes. • Place hand above patient's nose to detect respirations if shallow. • Initiate coughing and deep breathing exercises as soon as patient is able to respond. • Chart time oxygen is discontinued. • Monitor oxygen saturation levels (SaO_2) by pulse oximetry checks.
C: Consciousness	• **Extubate** patient (remove endotracheal tube from airway). • Confirm that patient responds to commands. • Confirm that patient verbalizes responses. • Confirm that patient reacts to stimuli.
C: Circulation	• Monitor temperature, pulse, respirations, and blood pressure q 10–15 min; take axillary, tympanic, or rectal temperature if warranted. • Assess rate, rhythm, and quality of pulse. • Evaluate color and warmth of skin and color of nail beds. • Check peripheral pulses as indicated. • Assess incision and dressing (monitor wound drainage output). • Monitor intravenous lines: solution, rate, site. • Cardiac monitors are usually in place for patients who had general anesthesia.
S: System review	• Assess neurologic functions, muscle strength, and response. • Monitor drains, tubes, and color and amount of output. • Check for pressure, type, and condition of dressings. • Evaluate pain response; may need to give analgesic and monitor patient response. • Observe for allergic reactions. • Assess urinary output if Foley catheter is in place.

to cardiac dysrhythmia and potentially fatal hyperthermia. It occurs when patients predisposed to the disorder are given a combination of certain anesthetic agents. Unless the triggering event is stopped and the body is cooled, death results.

LATER POSTOPERATIVE PHASE

Immediate Assessments

When the patient returns to the nursing unit, the nurse performs a thorough postsurgical assessment. Common initial assessment criteria include a review of vital signs, the IV and incisional sites, any tubes, and postoperative orders. A review of each body system identifies when body functions return and provides a guideline for further assessments. Unless otherwise indicated, it is standard practice in most facilities to monitor vital signs and make general assessments using the "times 4" factor—every 15 minutes times 4 (for 4 times); every 30 minutes times 4; every hour times 4; then every 4 hours, or until assessments are within expected ranges. Table 2.8 details body temperature responses to surgery. A postoperative flow sheet (Fig. 2.12) is used frequently to document the patient's

progress. This is often a computerized form. Significant observations are critical for the patient after surgery.

Although the patient may respond, the level of consciousness is altered; it is important to keep the side rails up and the call light within reach for safety. Until the patient is fully conscious, a pillow should not be placed under the patient's head because this may cause the tongue to obstruct the airway. The patient should be positioned on the side, depending on the type of surgery, or the head of the bed should be raised to a 45-degree angle. Positioning the head higher than the chest reduces the chance of the patient aspirating vomitus. Because nausea and vomiting are normal in the first 12 to 24 hours, an emesis basin should be kept at the bedside. If the patient vomits, the amount should be measured and carefully described in the documentation. Any red or coffee-ground emesis must be reported immediately because this is an indication of GI bleeding. Frequently the patient remains on NPO status for the first few hours after surgery; fluids are introduced gradually. The surgeon may order ice chips followed by clear or full liquids.

Postoperative complications can occur suddenly, making ongoing assessments critical. Vital signs, coupled with the patient's behavior, are an early indication of postoperative complications. A pulse that increases and becomes thready, a declining blood pressure, cool and clammy skin, reduced urinary output, narrowing pulse pressure, and restlessness are usually indicative of hypovolemic shock. Hypovolemic shock in the postoperative period can be a life-threatening emergency and frequently is caused by internal hemorrhage or excessive loss of blood or fluids during surgery (Box 2.8). A drop in blood pressure slightly below a patient's preoperative baseline reading is common after surgery. However, a significant drop in blood pressure, accompanied by an increased heart rate, may indicate hemorrhage, circulatory failure, or fluid shifts. Impending hypovolemic shock cannot be based on one low blood pressure reading. If the patient's blood pressure is showing a trend of dropping, measurements of the pressure should be taken every 5 minutes for 15 minutes to determine the variability. Fluctuations in blood pressure also can mean that the anesthetic is wearing off or that the patient is experiencing severe pain.

In addition to hypotension, manifestations of shock include tachycardia (rapid heartbeat), restlessness, apprehension, and cold, moist, pale, or cyanotic skin. When a patient appears to be going into shock, standard protocol in most facilities includes the following steps: (1) administer oxygen per facility protocol or increase its rate of delivery, unless contraindicated by a respiratory disease or disorder such as chronic obstructive pulmonary disease (COPD); (2) raise the patient's legs above the level of the heart; (3) increase the rate of IV fluid administration as per facility protocol, unless contraindicated because of fluid excretion problems

CAUSE	ASSESSMENT AND INTERVENTION
Table 2.8 Temperature Assessment and Intervention	
HYPOTHERMIA	
Within First 12 h	
Response to surgery, anesthesia, and body exposure	• Monitor temperature readings. • Assess for warmth. • Provide warm blankets. • Do not expose for long periods. • Assess orientation.
HYPERTHERMIA	
24–48 h	
Dehydration Decreased lung activity Inflammatory response to surgery	• Monitor temperature readings. • Monitor intravenous rate. • Encourage fluids. • Assess intake and output (I&O). • Have patient turn, cough, and breathe deeply. • Provide incentive spirometer. • Assess lung sounds. • Observe incision.
After Day 2	
Infection: Respiratory, wound, urinary, or circulatory	• Monitor temperature readings. • Assess lung sounds and expectoration of sputum. • Evaluate incision and drainage. • Monitor I&O. • Encourage fluids (6–8 oz/h) unless contraindicated. • Note urine color, odor, amount, and consistency, and patient's complaints of burning on micturition. • Perform leg exercises q 2 h, and ambulate q 4 h.

Kell-Russell Memorial Hospital	Post-operative Assessment			Patient name: Jeri Schank	
				Date of Birth (DOB):	05/20/1952
				Medical ID number:	57982310
Surgeon:	Operative Procedure:	Date and Time patient received:	Anesthetic Type:	Allergies:	
Time	B/P, P, R, T	Pain Level (0-10 scale)	O₂ Saturation	Assessment	
1300	90/60, 100, 32, 98.4	1	95% on O₂ @2L N/C	Pt. received from PACU via stretcher. Drowsy but able to answer questions. Surgical dressing clean, dry, and intact. See flow sheet for remainder of assessment.	
1315	96/62, 98, 28, 98.2	1	96% on O₂ @2L N/C	Remains drowsy but continues to answer questions. Dressing remains clean, dry, and intact.	
1330	98/62, 94, 26, 98.3	2	93% on O₂ @2L N/C	Drowsy. Encouraged to take deep breaths. Pinpoint shadowed area of sanguineous drainage on dressing. Area marked with time.	
1345	110/70, 94, 28, 98.7	4	96% on O₂ @2L N/C	Less drowsy, reports incisional pain at a 4/10. Encouraged to press PCA for bolus. Patient complied. No increase in drainage on dressing.	
Signature of Nurse: Kate Nicoli, LPN	Initials of Nurse: KN		Signature of Nurse:	Initials of Nurse:	

Fig. 2.12 Postoperative assessment form. *BP, P, R,* Blood pressure–pulse rate–respiratory rate; *PACU,* postanesthesia care unit; *PCA,* patient-controlled analgesia; *O₂ saturation,* arterial oxygen saturation.

or other existing conditions; (4) notify the anesthesia provider and the surgeon; (5) provide medications as ordered; and (6) continue to assess the patient and the patient's response to interventions.

Incision

The incisional dressing must be monitored to assess for bleeding or excessive drainage (e.g., dressings saturated with bright red drainage, or bright red drainage occurring 24 to 48 hours after surgery warrants notifying the surgeon). Normally dressings are not changed but are reinforced during the first 24 hours. To accurately measure the amount of drainage, circle the shadowed drainage markings on the dressing and write the time and date; this technique makes evident any increased bleeding or drainage over time. Dehiscence (the separation of a surgical incision or rupture of a wound

Box 2.8	Possible Causes of Postoperative Shock

- Cardiac dysrhythmias
- Cardiac failure
- Inadequate ventilation
- Loss of blood and other body fluids
- Movement of patient from operating table to gurney
- Pain
- Patient (gurney) being jarred during transport
- Reactions to drugs and anesthesia

closure) may occur 3 days to more than 2 weeks postoperatively. Wound separation in the first 3 days usually is related to technical factors, such as the sutures. Separation within 3 to 14 days postoperatively usually is associated with postoperative complications such as distention, vomiting, excessive coughing, dehydration,

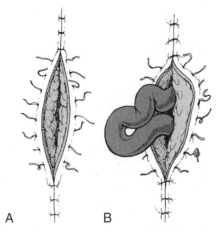

Fig. 2.13 (A) Wound dehiscence. (B) Evisceration.

or infection. Wound separation after 2 weeks usually is associated with metabolic factors, such as cachexia (ill health, malnutrition, and wasting as a result of chronic disease), hypoproteinemia, increased age, malignancy, radiation therapy, and obesity. Wound evisceration (protrusion of an internal organ through a wound or surgical incision, especially in the abdominal wall) also may occur. Wound dehiscence and evisceration require prompt attention (Fig. 2.13). If the patient feels a sudden "give," sutures or staples may have broken. Cover the wound immediately with a sterile dressing moistened with sterile normal saline and notify the surgeon. Tension on the abdomen may be decreased by placing the patient in a semi-Fowler position with the knees slightly flexed. Reassure the patient regarding the situation and inform him or her that surgery will be required. Begin preparing the patient for surgery by placing him or her on NPO status as well as following other facility protocol. Sterile technique procedures—including dressing change and care of the surgical incision with phases of wound healing—are discussed in Chapter 22 in *Foundations of Nursing*.

Ventilation

Immediate postoperative hypoventilation can result from drugs (anesthetics, narcotics, tranquilizers, sedatives), incisional pain, obesity, chronic lung disease, or pressure on the diaphragm. Inadequate ventilation leads to hypoxemia. Arterial oxygen saturation (SaO_2) is monitored either by arterial blood gas measurements or by pulse oximetry.

Because lung ventilation is vital, the patient should be helped to turn, cough, and breathe deeply every 1 to 2 hours until the chest is clear. Having practiced this combination preoperatively, the patient is usually able to remove adequately trapped mucus and surgical gases. To ease the pressure on the incision, help the patient to support the surgical site with a pillow or rolled bath blanket. The hand can be used to splint the incision, but it is not the ideal method. Administration of analgesics, as prescribed, to control pain before

coughing and deep-breathing exercises will increase the effectiveness of these activities. Early mobility and frequent position changes facilitate secretion clearance and improve the ventilation and perfusion in the lungs. Respiratory infections frequently are caused by shallow breathing and poor coughing. The licensed practical nurse/licensed vocational nurse (LPN/LVN) should auscultate (i.e., listen to) the lungs at least every 2 hours to determine the presence of any adventitious (i.e., unusual or abnormal) breath sounds as an early indication of postoperative complications.

If the patient feels chest pain or has a fever, productive cough, or dyspnea (difficulty breathing), atelectasis or pneumonia may be developing. Sudden chest pain along with dyspnea, tachycardia, cyanosis (i.e., a slightly bluish, gray, or dark purple discoloration of the skin), diaphoresis (excessive sweating), and hypotension is a sign of a pulmonary embolism. Raise the head of the bed immediately to decrease dyspnea, and immediately report signs and symptoms to the health care provider because this is a medical emergency. Frequently oxygen therapy is instituted to assist with breathing.

Whenever air exchange is reduced, postoperative recovery slows. Medication, suctioning, and oxygen therapy may be needed to assist the patient in respiratory distress. Mechanical devices, such as the IS, are used to stimulate deep breathing (see Skill 2.2). Patients are encouraged to take 10 deep breaths every hour while awake.

If respiratory complications develop, the health care provider may order nebulizer treatments to deliver bronchodilators and/or steroids or antiinflammatory medications, or intermittent positive pressure breathing (IPPB) treatments to deliver a mixture of air and oxygen; medication can be added to enhance respirations. IPPB treatments use positive pressure to expand the lungs for better distribution of medication. Chest percussion and postural drainage constitute a form of chest physiotherapy that combines positioning and percussion movements to lung areas to help dislodge and move secretions; this also may be ordered by the health care provider. This treatment, as well as IPPB, usually is delivered by a respiratory therapist.

Pain

Because postoperative pain is to be expected, it is important for the nurse to monitor and assess the patient for pain postoperatively. Effective pain management allows for early ambulation, promotion of adequate rest, and fewer postoperative complications. Depending on the type of surgery, acute pain usually begins to subside within 24 to 48 hours, and pain medication is adjusted as necessary. In the early stages of recovery, comfort interventions may help to ease pain. After the acute phase, comfort measures may be the only interventions required (Box 2.9).

A patient's level of pain can be difficult to evaluate. If the patient is able to communicate verbally, ask the patient to rate the pain on a scale of 0 to 10 or 0 to 5, depending on facility policy. There are standard pain indexes (restlessness, moaning, grimacing, diaphoresis), but some patients may not exhibit signs outwardly. Objective pain factors are signs that the body is responding to "pain"; these include vital sign changes (blood pressure lowers in the immediate postoperative period and elevates in response to pain after about 12 hours, and pulse increases), restlessness, diaphoresis, and pallor. The patient's description of discomfort represents subjective pain factors. Pain behaviors are influenced by the patient's culture and past experiences. Behaviors include moaning, grimacing, and favoring a body area.

The effectiveness of analgesic measures differs with each person; if relief is not obtained, changing the medication or administration schedule may provide effective pain control. Many patients wait to request or accept analgesics until pain is at its worst. Explain that pain medication is more effective if

Box 2.9   Postoperative Comfort Measures for Pain

DECREASE EXTERNAL STIMULI
- Darken room; close drapes.
- Keep TV and radio off or low.
- Monitor hall traffic and noise.
- Assess staff interruptions.
- Check room for noise—dripping water, buzzing lights, constant intercom messages.

REDUCE INTERRUPTIONS
- Plan care to allow rest.
- Post "Do Not Disturb" sign.
- Unplug telephone, if acceptable to patient.
- Restrict visitors.
- Pull curtains around bed.

ELIMINATE ODORS
- Discuss offending odors and assess elimination.
- Remove from room all dressings that are soiled with exudate.
- Remove food trays immediately after meals.

NURSING INTERVENTIONS
- Ask patient about normal relaxation patterns and practices.
- Have patient practice deep-breathing and relaxation techniques.
- Plan rest periods.
- Provide back rub.
- Engage patient in conversation; ask about concerns and fears.
- Encourage diversional activities.
- Reposition and support with pillows, bed rolls.
- Check tube placement.
- Offer warm fluids if indicated.
- Reduce room clutter.
- Provide restful environment.

taken at the onset of pain. Remember that each patient interprets pain differently and has a personal pain tolerance level; pain is whatever the patient says it is.

The success of pain management depends on the surgery, the patient's emotional state, and postoperative complications. Patients experiencing chronic pain may have more difficulty obtaining relief than individuals with acute episodes. Commonly used analgesic measures are nurse-administered narcotics, patient-controlled IV medications (see Chapter 21 in *Foundations of Nursing*), and pain control via a transcutaneous electrical nerve stimulation (TENS) unit (Fig. 2.14). When attached to the skin, the TENS unit applies electrical impulses to the nerve endings and blocks transmission of pain signals to the brain. The PCA system is a pump that is programmed to dispense only a given amount of medication. The patient can self-administer an analgesic by pressing a control button. The PCA system must be monitored by the nurse at least every 3 to 4 hours or as directed by facility policy. Nonpharmacologic pain control measures such as repositioning and diversional activities may be effective in treating pain. (Refer to Chapter 21 in *Foundations of Nursing* for pain management.)

Urinary Function
Anesthesia depresses urinary function, so it is important for the nurse to assess the bladder area for distention and changes in renal function. It routinely takes 6 to 8 hours for voiding to occur after surgery. If patients do not void within 8 hours, catheterization may be necessary, but it should be used only if necessary. Before use of catheterization to treat urinary retention, try noninvasive measures such as having the patient listen to running water, placing the hands in warm water, or ambulating to the bathroom or bedside commode, if able, to facilitate voiding. Helping male patients to stand often encourages voiding. Usually I&O is measured while a Foley catheter is in place, while the patient is receiving IV therapy, and immediately after a Foley catheter has been removed. The urine measurement should continue until the

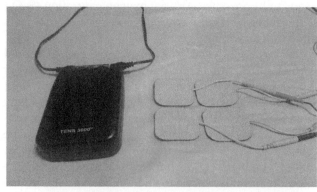
Fig. 2.14 Transcutaneous electrical nerve stimulation (TENS) unit.

patient is voiding without difficulty. Determination of serum blood urea nitrogen (BUN) may be ordered by the health care provider daily until the patient has recovered.

Fluid deficit may result from inadequate replacement of body fluids lost during surgery or from continued fluid losses. Fluid excess may occur from large amounts of IV fluids when kidney function is inadequate. A urinary output of 30 mL/h is considered acceptable postoperatively. Unless the patient has had urinary tract surgery, urine should be clear and yellow and smell like ammonia.

Venous Stasis

Venous stasis (a disorder in which the normal flow of fluid through a vessel of the body is slowed or halted) is the underlying cause of thrombus formation. Performing leg exercises every 2 hours and using intermittent pneumatic compression devices and compression stockings aid the circulatory system and help prevent deep vein thrombosis. Assessment of the feet and legs includes palpating for pedal pulse (i.e., pulse on upper surface of foot) and noting the skin's color and temperature. If edema, aching or cramping, sensitivity, redness, inflammation, warmth, or pain occurs in the calf or leg, thrombophlebitis should be suspected. The patient is to remain in bed until the health care provider can perform an evaluation. The patient should be instructed not to cross the legs when in bed and be encouraged to be out of bed as much as possible (if not contraindicated) to prevent venous stasis. If the bed has a knee gatch (i.e., a bed jointed to allow knee flexion), it should not be used with the postoperative patient, because this promotes venous stasis in the lower legs.

Surgical patients are at increased risk of developing life-threatening deep vein thrombosis and pulmonary embolism. Not only does surgery injure blood vessels, but anesthesia and inactivity also cause venous stasis. Surgery, however, is not the only risk factor. Others include pregnancy, myocardial infarction, heart failure, stroke (cerebrovascular accident or brain attack), cancer, sepsis, and immobility. Effective methods to prevent deep vein thrombosis include early and frequent ambulation and leg exercises. Antiembolism stockings and pneumatic compression devices are also useful preventive measures.

The external SCD (see Skill 2.5) is used on many postoperative patients, especially those patients who are at increased risk of developing deep vein thrombosis and pulmonary embolism. Many surgeons require that the device be placed on the patient preoperatively so that therapy can be initiated during surgery or in the immediate postoperative period without delay. This device includes an air pressure pump and cuffs, one for each entire leg, calf, or foot. Continuous inflation and deflation of the cuffs decrease pooling of venous blood in the legs and improve venous return to the heart. The pressure cuffs automatically inflate to the prescribed setting and deflate in cycles, with inflation lasting approximately 10 to 15 seconds and deflation lasting approximately 45 seconds. This system is contraindicated for any patient with acute thrombophlebitis or deep vein thrombosis. Their use in these patients could lead to an embolism.

When ambulating the patient, turn the pump off and remove the cuffs. The SCD should not be disconnected for more than 30 minutes. If the patient is scheduled for diagnostic examinations that require leaving the nursing unit for longer than 30 minutes, the compression pump, the cuffs or sleeves, and the instructions on operation should travel with the patient if traditional SCDs are used. If battery-operated SCDs are used, ensure that the batteries are charged fully.

The treatment usually continues for 72 hours postoperatively or until the patient is ambulating well. Orthopedic patients may be instructed to use the SCDs for longer periods because mobility is often more impaired. The cuffs should be removed daily to assess skin integrity and to provide skin care. Documentation of the use of the intermittent external pneumatic compression system and any abnormal reaction, such as numbness or tingling, should be included in the patient's record.

Activity

Early ambulation is a significant factor in hastening postoperative recovery and preventing postoperative complications. The exercise of getting in and out of bed and walking during the early postoperative period has numerous benefits (Box 2.10). Ambulation usually is contraindicated for patients with severe infection or thrombophlebitis.

Box 2.10 Effects of Early Postoperative Ambulation

- Increased circulation
- Increased kidney function
- Increased mental alertness from increased oxygenation to brain
- Increased metabolism
- Increased micturition (urinary elimination)
- Increased peristalsis
- Increased rate and depth of breathing
- Nutrients required for healing are more available to wound
- Prevention of abdominal distention and gas pain
- Prevention of atelectasis and hypostatic pneumonia
- Prevention of constipation
- Prevention of loss of muscle tone
- Prevention of paralytic ileus
- Prevention of thrombophlebitis
- Prevention of urinary retention
- Promotion of expulsion of flatus
- Restoration of nitrogen balance

Assessment. Before helping the patient to ambulate for the first few times after major surgery, assess the following:

1. Level of alertness: Ask the patient simple questions or to follow simple commands
2. Cardiovascular status (orthostatic hypotension, i.e., a drop of 25 mm Hg in systolic pressure and a drop of 10 mm Hg in diastolic pressure when moving from a lying to sitting position)
   a. Assess pulse and respiratory rate and depth while patient is supine and then after sitting.
   b. Observe skin color for pallor while patient is sitting.
   c. Note complaints of vertigo while patient is sitting.
3. Motor status
   a. Assess muscle strength of patient's legs.
   b. Assess sitting ability.

It is also important to consider any preoperative limitations to ambulation. The patient with arthritis or arteriosclerosis may take longer to move and to adjust to standing and walking. The patient who used a walker preoperatively needs assistance for a longer time before using the walker again. Family members are important in assisting patients with any physical limitation and in providing emotional support during postoperative recovery.

Nursing interventions. Nursing interventions are as follows:

1. Encourage muscle-strengthening exercises before ambulation.
   a. Have patient bend knees, lower knees, press back of knees hard against bed.
   b. Have patient alternately contract and relax calf and thigh muscles 10 times, using the following cycle: contract, relax, rest.
2. Obtain vital signs, and if within normal limits, have patient sit on side of bed (legs dangling) to adapt to the upright position before ambulating for the first time. Be certain that the pulse has stabilized (returned to baseline) before patient attempts ambulation.
3. If the patient has an NG tube, clamp it while the patient ambulates and then reconnect it.
4. Keep urinary tube connected to drainage bag, and keep the drainage receptacle below the level of bladder to prevent reflux of urine.
5. Attach IV bag to a movable pole.
6. Make sure two people assist in ambulating an unsteady patient receiving IV fluids.
7. Encourage the patient to walk farther at each ambulation.

The word *ambulate* means to move from place to place or to walk. Sitting in a chair is not ambulation. After ambulating, the patient may sit in a chair but should be advised to stand and walk at intervals and to elevate the legs while sitting to prevent venous pooling in the extremities. The patient should avoid sitting in a chair for long periods (see Chapter 8 in *Foundations of Nursing*).

GASTROINTESTINAL STATUS

Abdominal distention frequently occurs after surgery. Because anesthesia, surgical manipulation, administration of narcotics, and introduction of carbon dioxide into the abdominal cavity during surgery slow peristalsis (i.e., the normal propulsion of food through the digestive tract), it may take 3 or 4 days for bowel activity to return. Auscultate for bowel sounds in the abdomen to assess the return of peristalsis. Normal peristalsis is indicated by hearing 5 to 30 gurgles per minute. Bowel sounds are auscultated in all four quadrants. If bowel sounds are absent (each quadrant must be assessed for 3 to 5 minutes to determine absence of bowel sounds), paralytic ileus (a significant decrease in or absence of intestinal peristalsis that may occur after abdominal surgery, peritoneal trauma, severe metabolic disease, and other conditions) may have developed. This finding can develop into a medical emergency within 24 to 48 hours. If inactivity continues, the physician usually orders placement of an NG or a nasointestinal tube to help remove any gas that has formed in the stomach and small intestine, as well as fluid that has accumulated. When listening for bowel sounds in patients who have an NG or a nasointestinal tube, turn off the suction machine during the assessment and then turn it back on.

If the patient has developed abdominal distention, it should be assessed by measuring the patient's abdominal girth. To ensure the measurement is accurate, mark the placement for the tape measure at the level of the umbilicus. Assess and chart the expelling of flatus, bowel sounds, and abdominal girth. On occasion, analgesics (meperidine) and other medications may slow peristalsis; charting the patient's GI habits helps identify causative factors.

Encouraging movement (turning every 2 hours, early ambulation) helps restore GI activity. The health care provider may order a rectal tube to be inserted to relieve pain from intestinal gas (see Chapter 15 in *Foundations of Nursing*). For the patient who has difficulty with flatus, limiting iced beverages and offering warm liquids may help resolve the discomfort. The patient may have fluids and food withheld until flatus is expelled. As the patient returns to previous eating habits, bowel function slowly resumes its preoperative state. Constipation is also a frequent problem after surgery. The same aids for abdominal distention assist in alleviating constipation. If the patient does not pass feces within 2 or 3 days after resuming solid foods, a suppository, stool softener, or a small-volume enema may be ordered.

Singultus (hiccup) is an involuntary contraction of the diaphragm followed by rapid closure of the glottis. Singultus results from irritation of the phrenic nerve. Sedatives may be necessary in extreme cases. Abdominal distention is sometimes the cause, so this is another important reason for thorough assessment of the patient's abdomen for proper GI function. Abdominal distention usually is caused by gas in the intestinal tract but may be related to internal bleeding. Proper assessment can help to determine the cause of abdominal distention.

FLUIDS AND ELECTROLYTES

Fluid is lost during surgery through blood loss and increased insensible fluid loss through the lungs and skin. For at least the first 24 to 48 hours after surgery, the body attempts to retain fluids as part of the stress response to trauma and the effect of anesthesia.

Sodium and potassium depletion can occur after surgery as a result of the loss of blood or body fluids during surgery or the loss of GI secretion because of vomiting and NG tubes. Potassium is also lost during catabolism (tissue breakdown), especially after severe trauma or crush injuries. Loss of gastric secretions can result in chloride loss, producing metabolic alkalosis. Electrolytes often are added to the IV solution in the form of potassium chloride (KCl).

The nurse is responsible for closely monitoring fluid tolerance and electrolyte values during the postoperative period. When the patient returns from the recovery room, IV therapy will be in progress. Until the patient is past the nausea and vomiting period and can tolerate oral fluids, parenteral therapy most likely will be maintained. The IV line must be assessed for patency and ordered fluid rate; the IV site also should be monitored for erythema, edema, heat, and pain. The IV solution may become infiltrated because of movement or inadvertent dislodgment of the needle when the patient ambulates; infiltration is indicated by the presence of swelling that is cool to the touch at the IV site, sluggish or absent flowing of the fluid, and/or absence of a blood return. The assessment for rate of infusion is extremely important for older patients or patients with cardiac and pulmonary disorders, who may quickly experience fluid overload and pulmonary edema.

Muscles and nerves require ongoing nourishment to function adequately, and parenteral fluids contain the necessary glucose and electrolytes. Depending on the type of surgery and the patient's nutritional needs, IV therapy lasts from a few hours to a few days. As long as the patient is receiving parenteral fluids, I&O status should be measured. If the patient's overall nutritional state is in question, daily weights should be obtained (see Chapter 19 in *Foundations of Nursing*).

As oral fluids are introduced, the patient should be encouraged to drink small amounts frequently (6 to 8 oz/h). A review of the diet history reveals fluids normally enjoyed by the patient. Unless otherwise ordered, patients usually begin by ingesting clear liquids (clear soda, water, tea, broth, gelatin) and progress as

the GI system returns to normal functioning. Unless the patient has other problems (e.g., decreased renal excretion because of renal failure or advanced age), encourage the patient to drink 2000 to 2400 mL in 24 hours. Because iced and carbonated beverages cause GI disturbances in some individuals, patients should avoid these fluids until active peristalsis is noted. If nausea and vomiting persist, an antiemetic such as promethazine (Phenergan), benzquinamide (Emete-Con), ondansetron (Zofran), or prochlorperazine (Compazine) may be ordered to be administered intravenously or rectally.

❖ NURSING PROCESS FOR THE SURGICAL PATIENT

The role of the LPN/LVN in the nursing process is that the LPN/LVN will:
- Participate in planning care for patients based on patient needs
- Review patients' care plans and recommend revisions as needed
- Review and follow defined prioritization for patient care
- Use clinical pathways, care maps, or care plans to guide and review patient care

◆ ASSESSMENT

General assessment of the preoperative patient includes obtaining a nursing history. This consists of any prior surgery, allergies, current medications, use of other drugs or alcohol, and smoking status. The patient's physical condition and at-risk data, emotional status of the patient and family members, and patient's preoperative diagnostic data also are assessed. It is important for the patient and family to understand the surgical procedure and the expected outcomes. In the intraoperative stage, any procedures such as skin preparation or catheterization are completed. During surgery and recovery, the patient's condition is assessed continually. Postoperative care should be tailored to prevent and detect postoperative complications and return the patient to wellness.

◆ PATIENT PROBLEMS

Determining patient problems establishes the direction for the care to be provided during one or all surgical phases (Boxes 2.11 and 2.12). Identification of the patient problems may focus on preoperative, intraoperative, and postoperative risks. Preventive care is essential for effective management of the surgical patient.

◆ EXPECTED OUTCOMES, GOALS, AND PLANNING

The care plan begins before surgery and follows through the postoperative period to provide the best nursing interventions possible. It is important to include the patient in health care planning. A patient informed about the surgical experience is less likely

---

| Box 2.11 | Preoperative Patient Problem Statements |

- Inability to Clear Airway
- Anxiousness
- Insufficient Knowledge
- Impaired Family Coping
- Impaired Role Functioning
- Fearfulness
- Insufficient Nutrition
- Potential for Compromised Skin Integrity

| Box 2.12 | Postoperative Patient Problem Statements |

- Compromised Oral Mucous Membrane, related to nothing by mouth (NPO) status, irritation of endotracheal tube or nasogastric (NG) tube
- Compromised Physical Mobility, related to pain, postoperative activity restrictions
- Compromised Verbal Communication, related to endotracheal tube placement
- Fluid Volume Overload, related to excess intravenous (IV) fluid replacement, decreased circulation
- Grief, related to patient's critical condition
- Impaired Coping, related to constraints imposed by surgery, postoperative condition
- Inability to Bathe Self, Dress Self, Feed Self, Toilet Self
- Inability to Clear Airway, related to diminished cough, prolonged sedation, retained secretions
- Inability to Maintain Adequate Breathing Pattern, related to incisional pain, effects of anesthetic, narcotic pain medications
- Potential for Compromised Skin Integrity, related to wound exudate, immobility, insufficient nutritional intake
- Potential for Inability to Regulate Body Temperature
- Potential for Inadequate Fluid Volume, related to wound drainage, decreased fluid intake
- Potential for Infection, related to surgical incision, indwelling catheter, wound drainage tubes
- Recent Onset of Pain

to be fearful and is better able to prepare for expected outcomes.

Goals and expected outcomes for the surgical patient may include the following:

Goal: Patient achieves physical comfort by demonstrating effective coughing and deep-breathing technique.

Outcome: Patient verbalizes relief of pain (optimally, 3 or less on a 10-point scale during the immediate postoperative phase), based on pain scale assessment.

◆ IMPLEMENTATION

Nursing interventions before surgery physically and psychologically prepare the patient for the surgical procedure. The nurse should act as an advocate for the patient during and after surgery to ensure that the patient's dignity and rights are protected at all times (Nursing Care Plan 2.1).

◆ EVALUATION

Evaluation of the effectiveness of the care plan is essential, and revision of the plan should be addressed as needed. An example of a goal and an evaluative measure is as follows:

Goal: Patient achieves physical comfort.

Evaluative measure: Observe patient for nonverbal signs of discomfort, such as guarding the painful area and grimacing. Also check that patient verbalizes decrease or elimination of pain based on pain scale assessment.

DISCHARGE: PROVIDING GENERAL INFORMATION

Preparation for the patient's discharge is an ongoing process throughout the surgical experience, beginning during the preoperative period. The informed patient therefore is prepared as events unfold and gradually assumes greater responsibility for self-care during the postoperative period. As discharge approaches, it is important that the patient be given certain vital information (Box 2.13). If the health care provider has not provided information about diet or activity restrictions, the nurse verifies this information with the health care provider before instructing the patient. Being careful to provide complete discharge instructions may prevent needless distress for the patient and prevent complications at home. Written instructions are important for reinforcing verbal information. The nurse must document specifically in the record the discharge instructions provided to the patient and family as well as any return demonstrations by the patient or caregivers that occur after discharge teaching. Documentation of information related to the patient's mental status (ability to understand importance of teaching for patient and family members) is necessary. For the patient, the postoperative phase of care continues into the recuperative period. Assessment and evaluation of the patient after discharge may involve a follow-up call or a visit from a home health nurse.

AMBULATORY SURGERY DISCHARGE

The patient leaving an ambulatory surgery setting must be able to provide a degree of self-care and must be mobile and alert. Postoperative pain and nausea and vomiting must be controlled. Overall, the patient must be stable and near the same level of functioning as before surgery. At discharge, the patient and family or responsible party are given specific and general instructions—verbally and reinforced with written directions. The patient may not drive and must be accompanied by a responsible adult at the time of discharge. Health care personnel often phone the patient to schedule a follow-up evaluation and to address any specific questions and concerns the day after discharge.

Nursing Care Plan 2.1   **The Postoperative Patient**

Mr. S. is a 40-year-old, obese patient weighing 280 lb who was admitted with bowel obstruction and a scheduled right hemicolectomy. Mr. S. has hypertension and a history of poor wound healing.

PATIENT PROBLEM

Inability to Clear Airway, related to incisional pain

Patient Goals and Expected Outcomes	Nursing Interventions	Evaluation and Rationale
Patient will cough deeply in 24 h. Patient's lung sounds will clear after coughing.	Medicate with analgesia to control pain. Raise head of bed to full Fowler position during exercises. Splint incision with rolled bath blanket. Have patient turn, cough, and deep-breathe q h while awake. Use incentive spirometer, 10 breaths hourly, if possible. Take vital signs q 4 h and note evidence of dyspnea or restlessness. Monitor intravenous fluids. Offer sips of fluid q h if permissible.	Providing pain relief enables patient to cough and breathe deeply without discomfort. In Fowler position the diaphragm falls, which permits lung expansion. Splinting incision provides abdominal support during coughing. Turning, coughing, and deep breathing aid in mobilizing secretions. Adequate lung expansion can prevent atelectasis. Increased fluid intake helps to prevent thickening of mucus.

PATIENT PROBLEM

Inability to Maintain Adequate Breathing Pattern, related to poor body mechanics

Patient Goals and Expected Outcomes	Nursing Interventions	Evaluation and Rationale
Patient will effectively use incentive spirometer.	Encourage deep breathing q 1–2 h while awake. Reposition q 2 h; support joints and incision. Continue oxygen at 2 L per cannula; cleanse nares q 4 h; post "No Smoking" sign. Encourage use of incentive spirometer, 10 breaths q h.	Adequate lung expansion helps prevent atelectasis. Turning promotes lung expansion. Additional oxygen ensures adequate tissue oxygenation. "No Smoking" sign promotes safety. Adequate lung expansion helps prevent atelectasis.
Patient's respirations will be even and unlabored.	Record respirations q 4 h, noting depth, rate, and quality. Assess skin and nail beds q 4 h; report slow blanching color and condition. Darken room; decrease stimuli, monitor pain, and offer analgesic prn (as needed).	Regular assessments help to detect early signs and symptoms of respiratory complications. A change in color of skin and nail beds signals poor oxygenation. Comfort measures promote rest and relaxation and decrease pain level.

PATIENT PROBLEM

Potential for Infection, related to open surgical incision and draining wound

Patient Goals and Expected Outcomes	Nursing Interventions	Evaluation and Rationale
Patient's wound will not be erythematous or produce purulent exudate. Patient's vital signs will remain within normal range.	Perform hand hygiene appropriately. Monitor wound q 4 h, noting amount and color of drainage; assess skin for warmth, color, and sensation. Mark drainage on dressing q 4 h; reinforce prn. Use surgical asepsis when changing dressing. Monitor vital signs q 4 h. Monitor white blood cell (WBC) level as ordered.	Hand washing helps to prevent transmission of microorganisms. Regular assessments reveal early signs and symptoms of wound infection. Containing wound drainage within dressing provides comfort to the patient and enables the nurse to correctly determine the type of drainage. Surgical asepsis prevents the transmission of microorganisms. Elevation of WBCs indicates an infectious process and its severity.

CRITICAL THINKING QUESTIONS

1. On the second postoperative day, Mr. S. is taking shallow breaths and having difficulty complying with coughing and deep breathing. His temperature is 101.8°F (38.8°C), and he has adventitious breath sounds bilaterally in the bases. List several nursing interventions to assist Mr. S.
2. In his third postoperative day, Mr. S. has an erythematous incision with moderate amounts of purulent exudate from the Penrose drain site. List the correct nursing interventions.
3. What signs and symptoms would the nurse note when assessing Mr. S. for dehydration secondary to elevated temperature and decreased fluid intake?

| Box **2.13** | **Vital Information for the Patient Being Discharged** |

- Action and possible side effects of any medications; when and how to take them
- Activities allowed and prohibited; when various physical activities can be resumed safely (e.g., driving a car, returning to work, sexual intercourse, leisure activities)
- Answers to any individual questions or concerns (allow time for questions)
- Care of wound site and any dressings
- Dietary restrictions or modifications
- Symptoms to be reported (e.g., development of incisional tenderness or increased drainage, discomfort in other parts of the body)
- Where and when to return for follow-up care

2019 NOVEL CORONAVIRUS (COVID-19)

At the time of updating the current edition of this text, it should be noted that normal surgery protocol is somewhat different due to the pandemic being experienced around the world. At this point, the 2019 novel coronavirus (COVID-19) continues to alter the way health care is delivered into the year 2021. For a period of time during the peaks of the virus, only emergency surgeries were performed, to keep down the footprint of people coming in and out of the hospital or surgery center. Visiting rules have differed depending on the number of cases in a given community. There have been times during the pandemic when patients' family members were not allowed to visit at any time during the hospitalization. Similarly, in surgery centers there have been periods when family could only drop off and pick up patients without entering the center. When cases have been lower in number, some facilities have allowed one visitor (the same visitor during the patient's entire stay in a facility) for a specified time period, or one person to accompany a patient in a surgery center. Patients undergoing any surgical procedure are tested for COVID-19 prior to their admission. Both patients and staff within a health care facility are required to wear masks at all times. The type of mask (cloth, surgical, or N95) is dependent on the facility. At the time of publication of this text, it is uncertain how the pandemic continues to change the face of health care. (See Chapter 7 in *Foundations of Nursing* for further infection control information.)

Get Ready for the NCLEX® Examination!

Key Points

- The time before, during, and after surgery is the perioperative period. It is divided into preoperative, intraoperative, and postoperative phases.
- Perioperative nursing interventions take place before, during, and after surgery.
- The ability to tolerate surgery is influenced by nursing interventions, previous illness, and past surgeries.
- Older adult patients are at surgical risk from their declining physiologic status.
- All medications taken before surgery are discontinued automatically after surgery unless a physician reorders the medications, except for medications for long-term conditions such as phenytoin for seizure control.
- Family members are important in assisting patients with physical limitations and in providing emotional support during the postoperative recovery.
- Preoperative assessment of vital signs and physical findings provides an important baseline for comparing perioperative and postoperative assessment data.
- A patient's feelings about surgery can have a significant effect on relationships with nursing staff and the patient's ability to participate in care.
- Clinical problems of the surgical patient may require interventions during one or all phases of surgery.
- Informed consent should not be obtained if a patient is confused, unconscious, mentally incompetent, or under the influence of sedatives. Know agency policy.
- Structured preoperative teaching positively influences postoperative recovery.
- A routine preoperative checklist is a guide for final preparation of the patient before surgery.
- Nurses in the OR focus on protecting the patient from potential harm.
- Assessment of the postoperative patient centers on the body systems most likely to be affected by anesthesia, immobilization, and surgical trauma.
- Because a surgical patient's condition may change rapidly during immediate postoperative recovery, monitor the patient's status at least every 15 minutes.
- The PACU nurse reports to the nurse on the postoperative unit information pertaining to the patient's current physical status and risk for postoperative complications.
- From the time of admission, plan for the surgical patient's discharge.
- Discharge planning identifies home care measures to promote recovery that involve patient and family.
- Evaluation of all perioperative care is sometimes difficult because the patient may be discharged from the nurse's care before the outcome is certain.
- The COVID-19 pandemic has changed the protocol normally used in hospitals and surgery centers.

Additional Learning Resources

SG Go to your Study Guide for additional learning activities to help you master this chapter content.

Be sure to visit the Evolve site at http://evolve.elsevier.com/Cooper/adult/ for additional online resources.

Review Questions for the NCLEX® Examination

1. A patient is being discharged, and the nurse is teaching the patient how to do daily dressing changes at home. What is the most important point to include in the teaching plan?

   1. Discussion of surgical asepsis
   2. Discussion of hand hygiene
   3. Instruction in sterilization
   4. Demonstration of gloving

2. The nurse is caring for a patient following a colon resection with a transverse colostomy. The patient is experiencing pain at the operative site and surrounding tissues. To assist this patient in the prevention of postoperative pulmonary complications, what interventions will be most helpful preoperatively? *(Select all that apply.)*

   1. Ask the surgeon to prescribe IPPB treatment.
   2. Teach and observe the patient perform leg exercises.
   3. Teach and observe the patient use an incentive spirometer correctly.
   4. Tell the patient that lack of an effective cough may result in pulmonary complications.
   5. Ask the patient to perform a return demonstration of controlled coughing.
   6. Assist the patient with splinting the incision during coughing and deep breathing.
   7. Medicate the patient with pain medication at least 30 minutes before ambulation or activity.
   8. Ambulate the patient as ordered by the surgeon.
   9. Ensure that the patient is consuming the suggested amount of fluids postoperatively.

3. A patient underwent surgery for lysis of adhesions. He is transferred from the PACU to his room on the surgical floor. During the immediate postoperative period on the surgical floor, how often should the nurse measure blood pressure, pulse, and respirations?

   1. Every 15 minutes
   2. Every 5 minutes
   3. Every 20 minutes
   4. Every 30 minutes

4. The nurse is assessing the bowel sounds of a patient who had a suprapubic prostatectomy 2 days ago. To confirm that no bowel sounds are present, the nurse would need to auscultate each quadrant for how long?

   1. 1 minute
   2. 3 minutes
   3. 10 minutes
   4. 15 minutes

5. A patient is recovering from a right lobectomy. The nurse is going to assist in splinting the patient's incision so that the patient can cough and breathe deeply. When should an intramuscular analgesic be administered to achieve the most therapeutic effect?

   1. After the procedure so the patient can rest
   2. 15 minutes before the procedure
   3. 1 hour before the procedure
   4. 30 minutes before the procedure

6. A patient reports being allergic to penicillin. Which question would elicit the most useful information?

   1. "When did the reaction occur?"
   2. "What infection did you have that required penicillin?"
   3. "What type of allergic reaction did you have?"
   4. "Did you notify your physician of the allergy?"

7. Which patient is at greatest risk for surgical and anesthetic complications?

   1. A 3-year-old patient scheduled for hernia repair
   2. An 80-year-old patient scheduled for exploratory laparotomy
   3. An 18-year-old patient scheduled for an appendectomy
   4. A 42-year-old patient scheduled for breast biopsy

8. An alert 75-year-old patient is to undergo elective surgery. Who must sign the operative permit?

   1. The patient
   2. The patient and the patient's spouse
   3. Either the patient or the patient's spouse
   4. The patient and the surgeon

9. What is the best nursing intervention to help a patient cope with fear of pain associated with surgery?

   1. Describe the degree of pain expected.
   2. Explain the availability of pain medication.
   3. Inform the patient of the frequency of pain medication.
   4. Divert the patient when talking about pain.

10. A patient tells the nurse that "using this tube thing [incentive spirometer] is a waste of time." Which statement by the nurse best explains the purpose of the incentive spirometer?

    1. "It helps by directly removing excess secretions from the lungs."
    2. "It increases pulmonary circulation."
    3. "It helps promote lung expansion and prevent pulmonary complications."
    4. "It helps stimulate the cough reflex and keeps your lungs working."

11. When a patient is prepared for surgery, which interventions are appropriate during the preoperative period? *(Select all that apply.)*

    1. Provide sips of water for a dry mouth.
    2. Remove the patient's makeup and nail polish.
    3. Remove the patient's gown before transport to the OR.
    4. Leave on all of the patient's jewelry.
    5. Teach the patient postoperative breathing and coughing exercises.

12. Which statement is accurate regarding a patient who receives general or regional anesthesia in an ambulatory surgery center?

    1. The patient will remain in the unit longer than a hospitalized patient.
    2. The patient is allowed to ambulate as soon as he or she is admitted to the recovery area.
    3. The patient's level of consciousness must be near the level of preoperative functioning before dismissal.
    4. The patient is immediately given liberal amounts of fluid to promote excretion of the anesthesia.

13. After abdominal surgery, a patient is suspected of having internal bleeding. Which finding is most indicative of this complication? *(Select all that apply.)*

    1. Increased blood pressure
    2. Incisional pain
    3. Increased abdominal distention
    4. Increased urinary output
    5. Increased respirations

14. An obese patient is at risk for poor wound healing postoperatively for what reasons? *(Select all that apply.)*

    1. Ventilation capacity is reduced.
    2. Fatty tissue has a poor blood supply.
    3. The risk for dehiscence is increased.
    4. Clotting factors are delayed.
    5. Thrombophlebitis risk is increased.

15. A patient asks the nurse why the nurse asked for the name and dosage of all prescription and over-the-counter medications (including herbal remedies) taken before surgery. Which response by the nurse is most accurate?

    1. "These medications may cause allergies to develop."
    2. "These medications are automatically ordered postoperatively."
    3. "These medications should be taken the morning of surgery with sips of water."
    4. "These medications may create a greater risk for complications or interact with anesthetic agents."

16. The nurse is correct when identifying a patient who smokes two packs of cigarettes per day as being at most risk for which postoperative complication?

    1. Infection
    2. Pneumonia
    3. Hypotension
    4. Cardiac dysrhythmias

17. A postoperative abdominal surgery patient complains that he "felt something give way" in his incision. On assessing the wound, the nurse notes a large amount of serosanguineous drainage and that wound edges are not approximated. Intestines are protruding from the wound. What nursing action is appropriate?

    1. Encourage the patient to turn, cough, and deep-breathe while splinting the opening.
    2. Cover the protruding internal organs with sterile gauze moistened with normal saline.
    3. Paint the open wound with an antimicrobial solution to prevent infection.
    4. Reinsert the organs and apply a pressure dressing to prevent further organ protrusion.

18. On admission of a patient to the PACU from surgery, on what should the nurse place the highest priority for assessment?

    1. Patient's level of consciousness
    2. Condition of the surgical site
    3. Adequacy of airway and breathing
    4. Fluid and electrolyte balance

19. The nurse is admitting a patient into the room on the surgical unit after abdominal surgery. There is a 1.5-cm–diameter spot of serosanguineous drainage on the dressing. What should the nurse do at this time?

    1. Notify the physician of bleeding from the wound.
    2. Note the amount of drainage and continue to monitor.
    3. Remove the dressing to check for bleeding from the suture line.
    4. Apply gentle pressure to the site for 5 minutes.

Care of the Patient With an Integumentary Disorder

Objectives

Anatomy and Physiology

1. Discuss the primary functions of the integumentary system.
2. Describe the differences between the epidermis and dermis.
3. Discuss the functions of the three major glands located in the skin.

Medical-Surgical

4. Discuss the general assessment of the skin.
5. Discuss the viral disorders of the skin.
6. Discuss the bacterial, fungal, and inflammatory disorders of the skin.
7. Identify common parasitic disorders of the skin.
8. Describe the common tumors of the skin.
9. Identify the disorders associated with the appendages of the skin.
10. State the pathophysiology involved in a burn injury.
11. Identify the methods used to classify the extent of a burn injury.
12. Discuss the stages of burn care with appropriate nursing interventions.
13. Discuss how to use the nursing process in caring for patients with skin disorders.
14. Identify general nursing interventions for the patient with a skin disorder.

Key Terms

alopecia (ăl-ō-PĒ-shē-ă, p. 92)
autograft (ĂW-tō-grăft, p. 99)
contractures (kŏn-TRĂK-chŭrz, p. 96)
Curling's ulcer (KŬR-lĭngz ŬL-sĕr, p. 96)
debridement (dă-BRĒD-mĕnt, p. 97)
eschar (ĔS-kăr, p. 97)
excoriation (ĕks-kŏr-ē-Ā-shŭn, p. 70)
exudate (ĔKS-ū-dāt, p. 67)
heterograft (xenograft) (HĔT-ĕr-ō-grăft; ZĒ-nō-grăft, p. 99)
homograft (allograft) (HŌ-mō-grăft; ĂL-ō-grăft, p. 99)
keloids (KĒ-loydz, p. 89)

macules (MĂK-ūlz, p. 74)
nevi (NĒ-vī, p. 89)
papules (PĂP-ūlz, p. 77)
pediculosis (pĕ-dĭk-ū-LŌ-sĭs, p. 87)
pruritus (prū-RĪ-tŭs, p. 58)
pustulant vesicles (PŬS-tū-lănt VĔS-ĭ-kŭlz, p. 74)
rule of nines (p. 93)
suppuration (sūp-ū-RĀ-shŭn, p. 75)
urticaria (ŭr-tĭ-KĂ-rē-ă, p. 79)
verruca (vĕ-RŪ-kă, p. 89)
vesicle (VĔS-ĭ-kl, p. 67)
wheals (wēlz, p. 79)

The skin, or *integument,* is a major organ and the outer covering of the body, making it essential to life. Together with its appendages—hair, nails, and special glands—it makes up the integumentary system. People spend a great deal of time and money on grooming hair, cleansing skin, applying cosmetics, and manicuring nails. However, beyond its value in appearance, the integument is the body's protector, its first line of defense against infection and injury.

ANATOMY AND PHYSIOLOGY OF THE SKIN

FUNCTIONS OF THE SKIN

By covering the body, the skin protects the internal organs. It works to maintain homeostasis by monitoring and adapting to changes in temperature and environmental conditions. The skin is subjected continuously to temperature variances, humidity, environmental changes, risk for exposure to pathogens, trauma, ecchymosis (bruising), and daily wear and tear. The skin carries out numerous functions to protect and maintain the body (Box 3.1).

Protection

Sensory receptors within the skin receive information about the environment. Messages about heat, cold, pressure, and touch are received and relayed to the central nervous system for interpretation. Healthy skin protects the body from absorbing many chemicals and foreign substances. In addition, as long as it remains intact, skin provides a barrier to many microorganisms in the environment. Internal organs are cushioned and protected by a subcutaneous layer of fat (adipose tissue). The skin aids in elimination of waste products, prevents dehydration, and serves as a reservoir for food and water. Keratin, a fibrous water-repellent protein found in skin, is tough and protects the skin from excessive fluid loss. It also helps the skin resist injury and prevents the entry of harmful substances. Melanin, another skin protein, forms a protective shield that guards the keratinocytes and nerve endings from ultraviolet light.

Temperature Regulation

Skin helps the body maintain a constant temperature under varying internal and external conditions. It allows blood vessels near the surface to constrict when the environment is cold to preserve heat and allows them to dilate when it is hot to release excess body heat. Sweat glands release moisture, which cools the body as it evaporates. A layer of adipose tissue insulates by retaining heat.

Vitamin D Synthesis

Cholesterol compounds in the skin are converted to vitamin D when bare skin is exposed to the sun's ultraviolet rays. Vitamin D is necessary for healthy bone development. Although exposure to the sun is important for vitamin D synthesis, prolonged exposure to the sun's rays, which include ultraviolet radiation, should be avoided due to the increased risk of developing skin cancer. Synthesis occurs with very limited periods of exposure. There is no universally established period of time recommended for exposure. Many factors, such as skin color, determine how much sunlight is needed. In addition to sunlight, our bodies rely on food sources for vitamin D.

STRUCTURE OF THE SKIN

Skin consists of two primary layers: the outermost layer, called the epidermis; and the innermost layer, called the dermis or corium. Beneath these layers of skin lies the subcutaneous layer, or superficial fascia (Fig. 3.1).

Epidermis

The *epidermis,* the outermost layer of the skin, is composed of stratified squamous (from the Latin *squama,*

Box 3.1   Functions of the Skin

- Aids in excretion of waste products
- Has nerve endings that provide the brain with sensory information related to pain, heat and cold, touch, pressure, and vibration
- Insulates body and protects from trauma through subcutaneous layer of fat
- Prevents excessive water loss (dehydration)
- Protects from pathogenic organisms and foreign substances; provides a natural barrier against infection
- Regulates temperature
- Synthesizes vitamin D

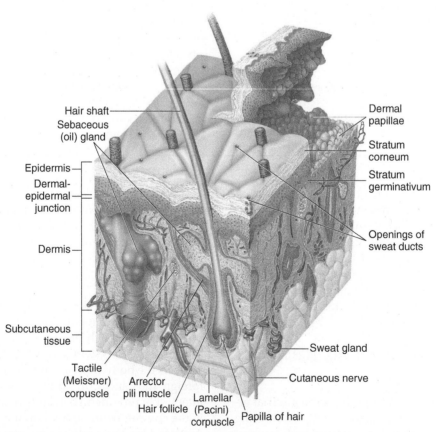

Fig. 3.1 **Structures of the skin.** (From Patton KT, Thibodeau GA: *The human body in health and disease,* ed 7, St. Louis, 2018, Elsevier.)

meaning "scale") epithelium. The cells of the epidermis are packed tightly and have no distinct blood supply (i.e., avascular). The epidermis is divided into layers, or strata: an outer, dead, cornified portion and a deep, living, cellular portion. The inner layer is called the *stratum germinativum*; it is the only layer of the epidermis able to undergo cell division and reproduce. It receives its blood supply and nutrition from the underlying dermis through a process called *diffusion*. The stratum germinativum provides a constant new supply of cells for the upper layer and enables the skin to repair itself after injury. As these cells push their way to the surface, their internal structures are destroyed, and the cells die. By the time they reach the outermost epidermal layer, called the *stratum corneum*, they are flat, and the cell structure is filled with a protein called *keratin*. The keratin makes the cells dry, tough, and somewhat waterproof.

Another layer in the epidermis contains highly specialized cells called *melanocytes*. These cells give rise to the pigment *melanin*, a black or dark brown pigment occurring naturally in the hair, the skin, and the iris and choroid of the eye. Melanin is responsible for the skin's color. Higher concentrations of melanin result in darker skin tones. Sometimes irregular patches with greater concentrations of melanin occur, producing freckles. Melanin levels are determined genetically. Although skin color is inherited, exposure to the sun and other factors can influence skin color.

Dermis

The *dermis*, or *corium*, often is called the true skin. It is well supplied with blood vessels and nerves and contains glands and hair follicles. It varies in thickness throughout the body but tends to be thickest on the palms and soles. The dermis is composed of connective tissue with cells scattered among collagen and elastic fibers. The dermis receives strength from the collagen and flexibility from the elastic connective fibers. The cells throughout this layer are bathed in tissue fluid, called interstitial fluid. The skin wrinkles with the normal aging process, as the dermis loses some of its elastic connective fibers, and the subcutaneous tissue directly beneath it loses some of its adipose tissue. Located in the upper portion of the dermis are small finger-like projections called *papillae* that project into the lower epidermal layer. Without the dermal papillae, the epidermal layer would be unable to survive.

Subcutaneous Layer

The subcutaneous layer, sometimes called the *superficial fascia*, is the layer of tissue directly beneath the dermis. The subcutaneous layer connects the skin to the muscle surface. This layer is composed of adipose tissue and loose connective tissue. It serves several important functions, including (1) storing water and fat, (2) insulating the body, (3) protecting the organs beneath it, and (4) providing a pathway for nerves and blood vessels. The distribution of subcutaneous tissue throughout the body provides shape and contour. A woman's body usually contains more subcutaneous tissue than a man's; thus, her body is softer and appears more rounded.

APPENDAGES OF THE SKIN

Sudoriferous Glands

The *sudoriferous* (sweat) *glands* are coiled, tubelike structures located in the dermal and subcutaneous layers. The tubes open into pores on the skin surface. Approximately 3 million sweat glands are located throughout the integumentary system. These glands excrete sweat, which cools the body's surface. Sweat is composed of water, salts, urea, uric acid, ammonia, sugar, lactic acid, and ascorbic acid.

Ceruminous Glands

Ceruminous glands are modified sudoriferous glands. They secrete a waxlike substance called *cerumen* and are located in the external ear canal. Cerumen is thought to protect the canal from foreign body invasion. However, too much cerumen, causing impaction in the ear canal, can cause difficulty with hearing and can make the ear canal a breeding ground for infection.

Sebaceous Glands

The *sebaceous* (oil) *glands* secrete *sebum* (an oily secretion) through the hair follicles distributed on the body. Their function is to lubricate the skin and hair that covers the body. Sebum also inhibits bacterial growth.

Hair and Nails

Hair is composed of modified dead epidermal tissue, mainly keratin. It is distributed all over the body in varying amounts. The root of the hair is enclosed in a follicle deep in the dermis. The shaft of the hair protrudes from the skin. Surrounding the hair follicle is a band of muscle tissue called *arrector pili* (see Fig. 3.1). A sensation of cold or fear causes these muscles to contract, making the hair stand upright and dimpling the skin surrounding it. The effect is called piloerection, "gooseflesh," or "goosebumps."

Nails also are composed mainly of keratin, but the keratin is more compressed. The base of the nail, the root, is made up of living cells and is covered mostly by the cuticle. Part of the root, the lunula, is exposed and looks like a white crescent. The remainder of the nail is called the *nail body*. It appears pink because of the blood vessels lying immediately beneath it.

ASSESSMENT OF THE SKIN

INSPECTION AND PALPATION

A thorough assessment of the skin helps identify many diseases. Skin assessment provides information about conditions taking place in other body systems.

Begin the assessment by obtaining a careful health history from the patient. Ask the patient about

(1) recent skin lesions or rashes, (2) where the lesions first appeared, and (3) how long the lesions have been present. Also ask questions about personal and family history. Inquire about conditions such as asthma, seasonal rhinitis, or allergies. Explore all complaints of pain, pruritus (the symptom of itching), tingling, or burning. Ask the patient about personal skin care and about (1) any recent skin color changes; (2) exposure to the sun, with or without sunscreen; and (3) family history of skin cancer.

Assess the skin under natural lighting, and use the senses of sight, touch, and smell while inspecting and palpating the skin. Expose the area to be assessed while maintaining privacy. Remember to wear gloves when inspecting the skin, mucous membranes, and any other involved area. Bathing the patient provides an excellent opportunity to assess the patient's skin without exposure or embarrassment.

Observe the color of the skin. The color depends on many physiologic factors, including the following:

- Amount of hemoglobin in the blood
- Amount of melanin in the epidermis
- Amount of substances such as bilirubin, urea, or other chemicals in the blood
- Oxygen saturation of the blood
- Quality and quantity of blood circulating in the superficial blood vessels

Skin lesion assessment includes a description of the appearance (size, shape, color), degree of moisture present, drainage, and location. Details assist the health care provider in determining the diagnosis and help the nurse to provide care. Disorders of the integument are characterized by the type of lesion involved. Most disorders have only one or two types of lesions. Some of the typical clinical manifestations of skin disorders are shown in Table 3.1.

Table 3.1   Primary Skin Lesions

DESCRIPTION	EXAMPLES
Macule	
Flat, circumscribed area that is changed in color; <1 cm in diameter	Freckles, flat moles (nevi), petechiae, measles, scarlet fever

Measles[a]

Papule	
Elevated, firm, circumscribed area; <1 cm in diameter	Warts (verrucae), elevated moles, lichen planus

Lichen planus[b]

Patch	
Flat, nonpalpable, irregularly shaped macule; >1 cm in diameter	Vitiligo, port-wine stains, mongolian spots, café-au-lait spots

Vitiligo[b]

Table 3.1   Primary Skin Lesions—cont'd

DESCRIPTION		EXAMPLES
Plaque		
Elevated, firm, rough lesion with flat-topped surface; >1 cm in diameter	Psoriasis, seborrheic keratosis, actinic keratosis	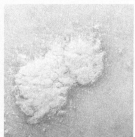 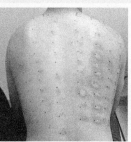 Plaque[a]
Wheal		
Elevated, irregularly shaped area of cutaneous edema; solid, transient; variable diameter	Insect bites, urticaria, allergic reaction	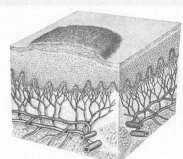 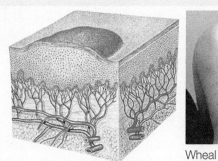 Wheal
Nodule		
Elevated, firm, circumscribed lesion; deeper in dermis than a papule; 1–2 cm in diameter	Erythema nodosum, lipomas	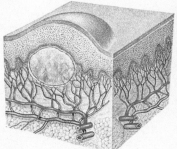 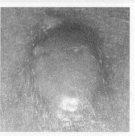 Hypertrophic nodule[a]
Tumor		
Elevated and solid lesion; may or may not be clearly demarcated; deeper in dermis; >2 cm in diameter	Neoplasms, benign tumor, lipoma, hemangioma	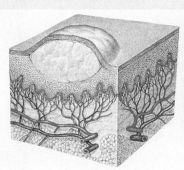 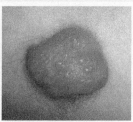 Hemangioma[b]

Continued

Table 3.1   Primary Skin Lesions—cont'd

DESCRIPTION	EXAMPLES	
Vesicle		
Elevated, circumscribed, superficial, not into dermis; filled with serous fluid; <1 cm in diameter	Varicella (chickenpox), herpes zoster (shingles)	Vesicles caused by varicella[b]
Bulla		
Vesicle >1 cm in diameter	Blister, pemphigus vulgaris	Blister[d]
Pustule		
Elevated, superficial lesion; similar to a vesicle but filled with purulent fluid	Impetigo, acne	Acne[b]
Cyst		
Elevated, circumscribed, encapsulated lesion; in dermis or subcutaneous layer; filled with liquid or semisolid material	Sebaceous cyst, cystic acne	Sebaceous cyst[b]
Telangiectasia		
Fine, irregular red lines produced by capillary dilation	Telangiectasia in rosacea	Rosacea

Table 3.1   Primary Skin Lesions—cont'd

DESCRIPTION		EXAMPLES
Scale		
Heaped-up keratinized cells; flaky skin; irregular; thick or thin; dry or oily; variation in size	Flaking of skin with seborrheic dermatitis after scarlet fever, or flaking of skin after a drug reaction; dry skin	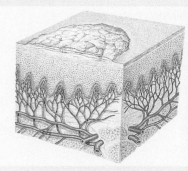 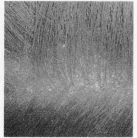 Fine scaling[c]
Lichenification		
Rough, thickened epidermis secondary to persistent rubbing, itching, or skin irritation; often involves flexor surface of extremity	Chronic dermatitis	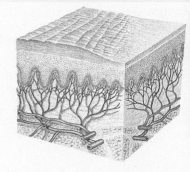 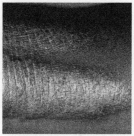 Stasis dermatitis in an early stage[b]
Keloid		
Irregularly shaped, elevated, progressively enlarging scar; grows beyond the boundaries of the wound; caused by excessive collagen formation during healing	Keloid formation after surgery	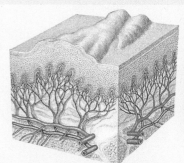 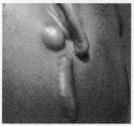 Keloid[b]
Scar		
Thin to thick fibrous tissue that replaces normal skin after injury or laceration to the dermis	Healed wound or surgical incision	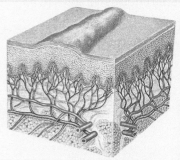 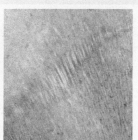 Incisional scar
Excoriation		
Loss of the epidermis; linear hollowed-out crusted area	Abrasion or scratch, scabies	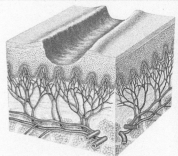 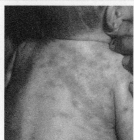 Scabies[b]

Continued

Table 3.1 **Primary Skin Lesions—cont'd**

DESCRIPTION	EXAMPLES	
Fissure		
Linear crack or break from the epidermis to the dermis; may be moist or dry	Athlete's foot, cracks at the corner of the mouth	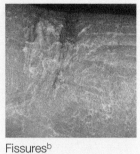 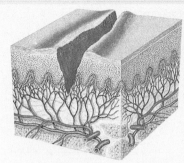 Fissures[b]
Erosion		
Loss of part of the epidermis; depressed, moist, glistening; follows rupture of a vesicle or bulla	Varicella, variola after rupture	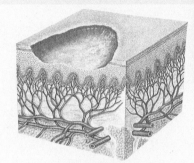 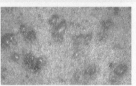 Erosion[d]
Ulcer		
Loss of epidermis and dermis; concave; varies in size	Pressure sores, stasis ulcers	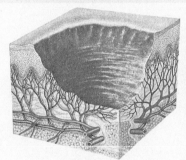 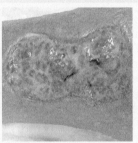 Stasis ulcer
Crust		
Dried serum, blood, or purulent exudate; slightly elevated; size varies: brown, red, black, or tan	Scab on abrasion, eczema	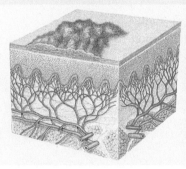 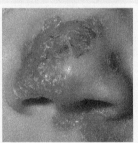 Scab[b]

Table 3.1	Primary Skin Lesions—cont'd	
DESCRIPTION	**EXAMPLES**	
Atrophy		
Thinning of skin surface and loss of skin markings; skin translucent and paper-like	Striae; aged skin	

Aged skin

[a]Zitelli BJ, McIntire SC, Nowalk AJ: *Zitelli and Davis' atlas of pediatric physical diagnosis*, ed 6, St. Louis, 2012, Saunders.
[b]Weston WL, Lane AT, Morelli JG: *Color textbook of pediatric dermatology*, ed 4, St. Louis, 2007, Mosby.
[c]Baran R, Dawber RPR, Levene GM: *Color atlas of the hair, scalp, and nails*, St. Louis, 1991, Mosby.
[d]Potter PA, Perry AG: *Fundamentals of nursing*, ed 7, St. Louis, 2009, Mosby.
[e]Cohen BA: *Pediatric dermatology*, London, 1993, Wolfe.
Modified from Thompson J, Wilson S: *Health assessment for nursing practice*, St. Louis, 1995, Mosby.

Assessment also includes noting the presence of rashes, scars, lesions, or ecchymoses and the distribution of hair. Assess temperature and texture by touch, using the palms of the hands to compare opposite body areas. For example, feel both legs before concluding that the left leg is cold. Use a cotton-tipped applicator to touch the sole of the foot and assess sensation. Inspect the nails for normal development, color, shape, and thickness. Clubbing (broadening) of the fingertips indicates decreased oxygenation (hypoxemia) and should be reported. Inspect the hair for thickness, dryness, or dullness. Assessment also includes inspecting the mucous membranes for pallor or cyanosis (blue discoloration). Document profuse sweating or any sign of impaired skin integrity. Examine the ceruminous and sebaceous glands for activity. Ask the patient to describe any occasions on which perspiration has been excessive or troubling as well as whether earwax has ever been removed by the health care provider.

A growing segment of the population has begun to embrace body art, such as piercing, tattoos, and carving/branding (used to facilitate the development of a keloid-type scar). Note the presence of any body art and its location. Allergic reactions to tattoo ink may occur years after application of the art.

The incidence of self-harm or non-suicidal self-injury (formerly known as self-mutilating) activities such as cutting, carving, or burning is increasing. The arms, legs, and anterior torso are the body areas most commonly affected. Persons who self-harm are most often female teens or young adults, but all patients need to be assessed for self-injury. Depression, personality disorders, or anxiety disorders may underlie such behavior. The presence of any injuries suspected as being self-inflicted must be documented (Mayo Clinic, 2018).

ASSESSMENT OF DARK SKIN

Skin color, which is determined genetically, depends on how much light is reflected when it strikes melanin, the underlying skin pigment. Melanin is produced by melanocytes deep in the epidermis. Melanocytes with increased activity, producing large amounts of melanin, account for darker skin colors. This increased melanin

Cultural Considerations

Skin Care

- The darker a person's skin, the more difficult it is to assess for changes in color. Establish a baseline in natural lighting if possible or with (at least) a 60-watt light bulb.
- Assess baseline skin color in areas with the least pigmentation, such as palms of the hands, soles of the feet, underside of forearms, abdomen, and buttocks.
- All skin colors have an underlying red tone. Pallor in black-skinned individuals is seen as ashen or gray. Pallor in brown-skinned individuals appears as yellowish. Assess pallor in mucous membranes, lips, nailbeds, and conjunctivae (i.e., the inner surface of the lower eyelids).
- To assess rashes and skin inflammation in dark-skinned individuals, rely on palpation for warmth and induration (i.e., an abnormally hard spot) rather than observation.
- Some folk remedies may be misdiagnosed as injuries. Three folk practices of Southeast Asia can leave marks on the body that can be mistaken for signs of abuse or violence. *Cao gio* is the rubbing of the skin with a coin to produce dark blood or ecchymotic strips; it is done to treat a thrombus or symptoms of the flu. *Bat gio* is skin pinching on the temples to treat headaches or on the neck for a sore throat. The treatment is considered a success if petechiae or ecchymoses appear. *Moxibustion* refers to the burning of the skin with a stick containing dried herbs. It is believed the burning will cause the noxious element that causes the pain to leave the body.[a]

[a]Marcia Carteret M, editor. © 2018. All rights reserved.

forms a natural sun shield, accounting for the lower incidence of skin cancer in people with dark skin.

The structures of dark skin are no different from those of lighter skin, but they are more difficult to assess due to their darker pigmentation. Practice is necessary. Assessment is easier in areas where the epidermis is thin, such as the lips and mucous membranes. Rashes are often difficult to observe and may have to be palpated.

Dark skin is predisposed to certain skin conditions, including pseudofolliculitis, keloids, and mongolian spots. Color cannot be used as an indicator of systemic conditions in darker-skinned individuals (e.g., flushed skin with fever) (see the Cultural Considerations box).

CHIEF COMPLAINT

When skin lesions accompanying a skin disorder are found, document the exact location, length, width, general appearance, and type. A helpful mnemonic for assessing the chief complaint is to remember *PQRST:*

P Provocative and **P**alliative factors (factors that cause the condition)

Q Quality and **Q**uantity (characteristics and size) of the skin problem

R Region of the body

S Severity of the signs and symptoms

T Time (length of time the patient has had the disorder)

An important objective in skin assessment is to identify possible malignancies. The three most common are melanoma, basal cell carcinoma, and squamous cell carcinoma. When assessing growths or changes in a mole, ask the following questions, using the mnemonic device *ABCDE:*

A Is the mole **A**symmetric?

B Are the **B**orders irregular?

C Is the **C**olor uneven or irregular?

D Has the **D**iameter of the growth changed recently?

E Has the surface area become **E**levated or is it **E**volving?

Promptly report a positive finding of any of these characteristics to a health care provider. After completing the assessment, document the findings. Proper assessment and identification serve as a baseline for evaluating nursing care and determining whether changes are needed.

PSYCHOSOCIAL ASSESSMENT

Integumentary disorders may be acute or chronic. Recovery may be lengthy with little visible outward improvement. A person's body image and self-esteem may be affected. Society's reaction to a skin condition has a significant effect on the patient. Personal appearance is a primary concern to many individuals. Others may think the condition is infectious and may isolate the patient socially. An integumentary disorder can have a negative effect on a patient's self-concept because of the value society places on a person's physical characteristics.

Assess the patient's coping abilities by using open-ended questions to encourage him or her to talk and ventilate feelings. Also assess the patient's interaction with family and others. Nonverbal behavior such as covering the involved area and avoiding eye contact may indicate a self-image problem. Validate or correct a patient's knowledge base. Be skilled and knowledgeable about skin care. Rarely are skin diseases fatal, and few are contagious. Work through your feelings about a patient's skin appearance before you can be a source of encouragement. Your attitude and interventions should be nonjudgmental, warm, and accepting.

A patient with a skin disorder may have a problem with anxiety. Decrease the patient's anxiety by implementing the following interventions:

- Provide the patient with consistent information related to his or her care plan.
- Include the family in the treatment plan. The family may be able to help the patient follow the instructions, which helps to decrease anxiety.
- Provide positive feedback concerning the patient's efforts and progress, no matter how large or small.
- Refer the patient to a support group as soon as possible (if appropriate).

PRESSURE INJURIES

The National Pressure Injury Advisory Panel (NPIAP) has announced that the term *pressure injury* will be used to replace the term *pressure ulcer* in the staging system. The NPIAP has determined that the term pressure injury more accurately describes injuries to intact and ulcerated skin, especially because previously stage 1 was referred to as a pressure injury and the remaining stages were referred to as ulcers. The numbering system also was changed at this time to Arabic numerals (NPIAP, 2018).

Skin breakdown can result from a variety of causes. Pressure injuries are responsible for many hospitalizations and health care–related expenses, in addition to the pain and suffering of patients. If a pressure injury is discovered, immediate action is required to ensure that the wound receives proper care and does not increase in size and develop additional complications.

The following sections summarize the revised stages of pressure injury development according to the NPIAP (2018). Additional information regarding pressure injuries can be found at www.npiap.org.

STAGE 1

A stage 1 pressure injury is a localized area of skin, typically over a bony prominence, that is intact with non-blanchable redness. Skin with darker tones may not have visible blanching, but its color is likely to differ from the surrounding area. The wound characteristics vary: areas may be painful, firm, soft, warm, or cool compared with adjacent tissue. This stage is typically difficult to detect in patients with dark skin tones.

STAGE 2

A stage 2 pressure injury involves partial-thickness loss of dermis. It appears as a shallow open injury, usually shiny or dry, with a red-pink wound bed without slough or bruising. (Bruising raises the suspicion of deep tissue injury.) Some stage 2 injuries manifest as intact or open (ruptured) serum-filled blisters. Do not use the term stage 2 to describe skin tears, tape burns, perineal dermatitis, maceration, or excoriation.

STAGE 3

A stage 3 pressure injury involves full-thickness tissue loss, in which subcutaneous fat is sometimes visible, but bone, tendon, and muscle are not exposed. If slough is present, it does not obscure the depth of tissue loss. Possible features are undermining and tunneling. The depth of a stage 3 pressure injury varies depending on its anatomic location. On the bridge of the nose, the ear, the occiput, and the malleolus—all of which lack subcutaneous tissue—these injuries are shallow. Extremely deep stage 3 pressure injuries develop in areas with significant layers of deep adipose tissue.

STAGE 4

A stage 4 pressure injury involves full-thickness tissue loss with exposed bone, tendon, cartilage, or muscle. Sometimes slough or eschar is present on some parts of the wound bed. The injury often includes undermining or tunneling. As with stage 3 pressure injuries, stage 4 pressure injuries vary in depth depending on their location. Because these injuries extend into muscle and supporting structures, the patient is at risk for osteomyelitis.

UNSTAGEABLE/UNCLASSIFIED

An unstageable pressure injury involves full-thickness tissue loss, a wound base covered by slough (yellow, tan, gray, green, or brown), and eschar in the wound bed that usually is tan, brown, or black. The true depth and stage of the injury cannot be determined until the base of the wound has been exposed. Stable eschar on the heels provides a natural biological cover. Do not remove it.

SUSPECTED DEEP TISSUE PRESSURE INJURY

During this stage, the wound appears as a localized purple or maroon area of discolored intact skin or a blood-filled blister. This is caused by underlying soft tissue damage from pressure or shear. Characteristics of the area range from painful, firm, mushy, boggy, or warm to cool compared with adjacent tissue. In patients with dark skin tones, deep tissue injury is sometimes difficult to detect but often starts with a thin blister over a dark wound bed. The wound sometimes becomes covered with thin eschar. Even with prompt treatment, some wounds evolve rapidly, exposing additional layers of tissue.

NURSING INTERVENTIONS

Nursing interventions for patients with pressure injuries include ongoing assessment and evaluation of improvement. Assessment data include the size and the depth of the injury, the amount and color of any exudate, the presence of pain or odor, and the color of the exposed tissue. Healing is a long-term process; therefore, make sure the plan of care is consistent over time and evaluate it for effectiveness.

WOUND CARE

The skin serves as the body's first defense. Impairments in the integument provide a portal for infection. Management of wounds and the prevention of their development are essential for health maintenance. During wound care, the type and size of the wound primarily will determine the dressing and treatment plans (Table 3.2).

VIRAL DISORDERS OF THE SKIN

HERPES SIMPLEX
Etiology and Pathophysiology

Herpes simplex virus (HSV) causes cold sores and genital herpes. It is one of the most common skin infections. Genital herpes affects an estimated one in six adults between the ages of 14 and 49 years (CDC, 2017). Two types of the virus are known:

- Type 1 (HSV-1) is the most common. It causes cold sores, often referred to as *fever blisters,* and usually is associated with febrile conditions. The infection is generally self-limiting, that is, it usually clears up by itself, requiring no treatment.
- Type 2 (HSV-2) causes lesions in the genital area known as genital herpes (Centers for Disease Control and Prevention [CDC], 2018a). HSV-2 is also a member of the herpesvirus family, as is HSV-1, and is discussed in Chapter 12.

Both types of viruses may be transmitted by direct contact with any open lesion. The primary mode of transmission for type 2 is through sexual contact. Lesions appear 2 days to 2 weeks after exposure. The lesions are usually present for 2 to 3 weeks and are most painful during the first week. Complications may be severe if the disease spreads to other body areas. HSV-1 herpes simplex is associated with oral lesions, but it may manifest anywhere on the body, including the perineal and genital regions. Most commonly found in the genital region, HSV-2 may present in facial or other areas of the body. Herpes simplex may have severe consequences in pregnancy. Miscarriage and premature delivery have been linked to herpes simplex. Herpesvirus may be fatal to the newborn when transmitted during childbirth. Studies indicate that the transmission rate of herpesvirus from an infected mother to a newborn is high, approximately 30% to 50% among women who acquire genital herpes near the time of delivery. The transmission rate is

Table 3.2   Characteristics and Uses of Wound-Dressing Materials

CATEGORY	EXAMPLES	DESCRIPTION	APPLICATIONS
Alginate	AlgiSite, Comfeel, Curasorb, Kaltogel, Kaltostat, Sorbsan, Tegagel	Alginate dressings are made of seaweed extract containing guluronic and mannuronic acids, which provide tensile strength; and calcium and sodium alginates, which confer an absorptive capacity. Some can leave fibers in the wound if they are not thoroughly irrigated. These dressings are secured with secondary coverage.	These dressings are highly absorbent and useful for wounds with copious exudate. Alginate rope is particularly useful to pack exudative wound cavities or sinus tracts.
Debriding agents	Hypergel (hypertonic saline gel), Santyl (collagenase), Accuzyme (papain urea)	These products provide some chemical or enzymatic debridement.	Debriding agents are useful for necrotic wounds as an adjunct to surgical debridement.
Foam	Lyofoam, Spyrosorb, Allevyn	Polyurethane foam has absorptive capacity.	These dressings are useful for cleaning granulating wounds with minimal exudate.
Hydrocolloid	CombiDERM, Comfeel, DuoDerm CGF Extra Thin, Granuflex, Tegasorb	Hydrocolloid dressings are made of a microgranular suspension of natural or synthetic polymers, such as gelatin or pectin, in an adhesive matrix. The granules change from a semi-hydrated state to a gel as the wound exudate is absorbed.	Hydrocolloid dressings are useful for dry necrotic wounds, wounds with minimal exudate, and for clean granulating wounds.
Hydrofiber	AQUACEL, AQUACEL-Ag, Versiva	An absorptive textile fiber pad, hydrofiber is also available as a ribbon for packing of deep wounds. This material is covered with a secondary dressing. The hydrofiber combines with wound exudate to produce a hydrophilic gel. Aquacel-Ag contains 1.2% ionic silver that has strong antimicrobial properties against many organisms, including methicillin-resistant *Staphylococcus aureus* and vancomycin-resistant enterococci.	Hydrofiber dressings are absorbent and used for exudative wounds.
Hydrogel	Aquasorb, DuoDerm, IntraSite gel, GranuGEL, Normlgel, Nu-Gel, Purilon gel, K-Y jelly	Hydrogel dressings are water-based or glycerin-based semipermeable hydrophilic polymers; cooling properties may decrease wound pain. These gels can lose or absorb water depending on the state of hydration of the wound. They are secured with secondary covering.	These dressings are useful for dry, sloughy, necrotic wounds (eschar).
Low-adherence dressing	Mepore, Skintact, Release	Low-adherence dressings are made of various materials designed for easy removal without damaging the underlying skin.	These dressings are useful for acute minor wounds, such as skin tears, or as a final dressing for chronic wounds that have nearly healed.
Transparent film	OpSite, Skintact, Release, Tegaderm, Bioclusive	Transparent films are highly conformable acrylic adhesive films with no absorptive capacity and little hydrating ability. They may be vapor permeable or perforated.	These dressings are useful for clean, dry wounds with minimal exudate. They also are used to secure an underlying absorptive material, to protect high-friction areas and areas that are difficult to bandage (e.g., heels), and to secure intravenous catheters.

From Daley BJ: Drugs, diseases, & procedures: Wound care treatment and management. Retrieved from https://emedicine.medscape.com/article/194018-treatment

much lower (<1%) in mothers who previously knew they were infected or those who were aware they contracted the infection during the first half of a pregnancy (CDC, 2017). Women who have active herpes lesions at the time of childbirth give birth by cesarean section.

Clinical Manifestations

HSV-1 is characterized by a vesicle (circumscribed elevation of skin filled with serous fluid; smaller than 0.5 cm) at the corner of the mouth, on the lips, or on the nose. It is commonly known as a *cold sore* (Fig. 3.2). At first, the involved area is usually erythematous and edematous (i.e., red and swollen). The vesicle then appears, ulcerates, and encrusts. When the vesicle ruptures, it produces a burning pain. The patient experiences general malaise and fatigue. Cold sores typically occur after an acute illness or infection.

Type 2, genital herpes, produces various types of vesicles that rupture and encrust, causing ulcerations. The cervix is the most common site in women, and the penis is the most common area in men. Flulike symptoms occur 3 or 4 days after the vesicles erupt. Headache, fatigue, myalgia, fever, and anorexia are common. Patients experiencing severe outbreaks in the genital region may experience difficulty voiding. In general, the initial outbreak is the most severe.

Assessment

Assessment involves primarily inspection of the skin. Obtain a complete health history to support assessment data. *Subjective data* (symptoms described by the patient, but that cannot be measured) include complaints of fatigue along with pruritus and burning pain in the mouth for HSV-1 and in the genital area for HSV-2. Patients experiencing a genital herpes outbreak may report pain with urination.

Objective data for HSV-1 include an edematous, erythematous area on the face. The most common location is the lips, but it may spread to the eyes. In HSV-2, the labia, vulva, or penis appears edematous and erythematous. The vesicular lesions may rupture, developing a dried exudate (fluid, cells, or other substances that have been slowly exuded, or discharged, from cells or blood vessels through small pores or breaks in cell membranes). Lymph nodes may be tender and enlarged.

Diagnostic Tests

Diagnosis of herpesvirus is made by laboratory assessment of cultures from the lesion. Inspection and health history support the diagnosis. Patients also should be assessed for human immunodeficiency virus (HIV).

Medical Management

Herpesvirus infection has no cure. Lesions spontaneously resolve if there are no complications. Treatment focuses on symptom relief. For HSV-1 outbreaks, over-the-counter topical treatments often are effective if used within the first 1 to 2 days of the outbreak. Antiviral drugs such as acyclovir—administered orally, topically, or intravenously—can shorten the outbreak and lessen its severity (Table 3.3). The initial outbreak often is treated for 7 to 10 days, and subsequent outbreaks are managed with a 5-day course of therapy. Oral acyclovir therapy can be continued safely and effectively for up to 5 years, but therapy should be interrupted after 1 year to assess the patient's rate of recurrent episodes. Adverse reactions to acyclovir are usually mild and include headache, occasional nausea and vomiting, and diarrhea. The safety of systemic acyclovir during pregnancy has not been established. Acyclovir ointment appears to be of no clinical benefit in treating recurrent lesions, either in speed of healing or in resolution of pain.

A patient with frequent outbreaks may be prescribed a daily suppressive therapy such as valacyclovir (Mayo Clinic, 2020b). Patients who are immunosuppressed are not candidates for suppressive therapies. Acetaminophen may be given for relief of discomfort. Pain may require a local anesthetic such as lidocaine or systemic analgesics such as codeine and aspirin. Nonsteroidal anti-inflammatory drugs such as ibuprofen may be used to manage inflammation.

Nursing Interventions and Patient Teaching

Nursing interventions focus primarily on treating symptoms and preventing spread of the disease. Lesions should be kept clean and dry. Loose, absorbent underclothing is usually more comfortable than tight-fitting clothing. The use of a sitz bath can decrease lesion discomfort and enhance urinary and bowel elimination. The patient can use warm compresses to relieve pain and severe pruritus. The specific patient problems related to herpes infection are based on the assessment data gathered. Type 2 herpesvirus (HSV-2; genital herpes) may be transmitted by viral shedding even during periods of remission. Open and direct discussions concerning safe sexual practices, including condoms, are indicated. Infection control and hand washing should be reviewed. How to manage recurrent outbreaks should also be reviewed.

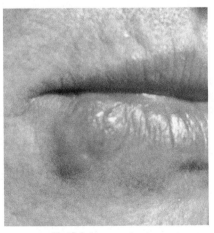

Fig. 3.2 Herpes simplex.

Table 3.3   Medications for the Integumentary System

GENERIC NAME (TRADE NAME)	ACTION	SIDE EFFECTS	NURSING IMPLICATIONS
acyclovir	Antiviral	*Topical:* Burning, rash, pruritus, stinging *Systemic:* Headache, seizures, renal toxicity, phlebitis at IV site	*Topical:* Use gloves to apply; cover lesion completely. *Systemic:* Ensure adequate hydration to prevent crystallization in kidneys; administer IV dose for at least 1 h.
Alpha Keri	Emollient	Local irritation, allergic reactions	For external use only; exercise caution when using in tub to avoid slipping.
Aluminum acetate solution (Burow's solution)	Astringent	Local irritation, allergic reactions	For external use only; do not use with occlusive dressings.
Antihistamines, including: diphenhydramine hydroxyzine	Blocks histamine at H$_1$ receptor site, inhibiting many allergic reactions	Drowsiness, dizziness, confusion, dry mouth, urinary retention	If drowsiness occurs, avoid activities that require concentration; avoid using with alcohol or other CNS depressants.
Benzoyl peroxide	Antiacne agent	Excessive drying of skin, allergic reactions	Discontinue use if excessive drying or peeling occurs; avoid contact with hair or fabric.
Calamine lotion	Astringent	Local irritation	For external use only.
chlorhexidine gluconate	Antimicrobial skin cleanser	Irritation, dermatitis, allergic reactions	For external use only; do not use on broken skin unless directed by a health care provider.
Coal tar	Treatment of pruritic dermatoses, including eczema and psoriasis	Photosensitivity, dermatitis, allergic reactions	Avoid exposure to sunlight for 72 h after use; may stain clothes and bathtub; for external use only.
Corticosteroids (topical), including: fluocinonide triamcinolone betamethasone	Anti-inflammatory agent	Local irritation, maceration, superinfection, atrophy, itching, and drying of skin (more severe local reactions and systemic effects possible with higher doses and potency or when used with occlusive dressings)	Do not use occlusive dressings unless directed by a health care provider; washing or soaking area before application increases drug penetration.
crotamiton	Scabicidal and antipruritic	Local irritation, allergic reactions	For external use only; do not apply to severely irritated skin.
Curel, Eucerin, Lubriderm	Emollient	Local irritation, allergic reactions	For external use only.
fluconazole	Antifungal	Headache, nausea, vomiting, diarrhea	May elevate liver function test results; monitor BUN, creatinine.
griseofulvin	Antifungal agent	Hypersensitivity reactions, photosensitivity, nausea, fatigue, mental confusion	Avoid exposure to sunlight; drug absorption increased when given with meals; clinical response may appear only after full course of therapy.
isotretinoin	Antiacne agent	Severe dryness of skin, mouth, eyes, mucous membranes, nose, and nails; skin fragility; epistaxis; joint and muscle pain; nausea; abdominal pain	Absolutely contraindicated in pregnant women or women contemplating pregnancy; women of childbearing age must practice contraception during therapy and 1 months before and after therapy; give drug with meals; do not give vitamin supplements containing vitamin A; avoid exposure to sunlight.
itraconazole	Antifungal agent	Hypertension, headache, nausea, anorexia	Give with food; check hepatic function; can increase PT.

Table 3.3   Medications for the Integumentary System—cont'd

GENERIC NAME (TRADE NAME)	ACTION	SIDE EFFECTS	NURSING IMPLICATIONS
lindane	Scabicide, ovicide	Local irritation, dizziness, seizures (rare)	For external use only; avoid applying to open skin lesions.
Lubriderm	Emollient	Local irritation, allergic reactions	For external use only; exercise caution when using in tub to avoid slipping.
methoxsalen	Skin-pigmenting agent	Severe photosensitivity, nausea, nervousness, insomnia, headache, hypopigmentation	Avoid all exposure to sunlight for 8h after oral ingestion and for several days after topical application; wear UVA-absorbing sunglasses for 24h after oral ingestion; use sunscreen to prevent exposure to sunlight; give agent with food or milk or in divided doses; clinical response may not appear for several months.
povidone-iodine	Topical antimicrobial agent	Local irritation	For external use only; may stain skin and clothing.
pyrethrin	Pediculicide	Local irritation	For external use only; do not use for infestations of eyebrows or eyelashes.
Salicylic acid	Keratolytic agent	Local irritation, erythema, scaling	For external use only; may damage clothing, plastic, wood, and other materials on contact.
terbinafine	Antifungal agent	Pruritus, local burning, erythema	For external use only; do not use occlusive dressings unless directed by a health care provider.
tetracycline	Antibacterial agent	*Topical:* Stinging, burning, slight yellowing of skin may occur *Systemic:* Nausea, diarrhea, photosensitivity	*Topical:* Avoid contact with sunlight *Systemic:* Give on empty stomach; avoid concomitant administration of dairy products, laxatives, antacids, and products containing iron; avoid contact with sunlight; may cause permanent tooth discoloration when used in children.
tolnaftate	Antifungal agent	Local irritation	For external use only.

BUN, Blood urea nitrogen; *CNS,* central nervous system; *IV,* intravenous; *PT,* prothrombin time; *UVA,* ultraviolet A.

Problem identification and interventions for the patient with herpes include, but are not limited to, the following:

PATIENT PROBLEM	NURSING INTERVENTIONS
Recent Onset of Pain, related to pruritus	Assess factors that precipitate pruritus Apply local anesthetic Apply drying agent to lesions Apply warm compresses Have patient wear loose-fitting, cotton clothing that does not constrict movement or occlude circulation
Compromised Skin Integrity, related to open lesions	Inspect lesions for drainage, color, and location Wash hands before and after contact Keep area dry Administer antiviral agents as ordered In genital herpes, a hair dryer can be used to dry the lesions and promote patient comfort

PATIENT PROBLEM	NURSING INTERVENTIONS
Potential for Infection, related to skin excoriation	Use standard precautions Teach patient proper skin care Wash hands before and after care Keep area dry Administer antiviral drugs as prescribed

Preventing infection is the priority when caring for a patient with an open skin lesion. Patient teaching focuses on the principles of medical asepsis and includes specific measures to prevent spread of the disease. Using good hygiene in all areas of care is critical to prevent secondary infections. Include the complications and precipitating factors in patient teaching and discharge planning.

Prognosis

Herpes simplex has no cure. The healing time for an HSV-1 infection is 10 to 14 days without treatment.

HSV-2 lesions are usually present for 7 to 14 days. After outbreaks, the virus goes dormant. Unfortunately, 75% of all patients have at least one recurrence, and two-thirds have one to five recurrences annually. However, the recurrences are often milder and of shorter duration than the primary infection. Triggers to an outbreak include fatigue, illness, emotional stress, and for HSV-2 lesions, genital irritation. Subsequent outbreaks are typically of shorter duration and less painful) (Mayo Clinic, 2020b).

HERPES ZOSTER (SHINGLES)

Etiology and Pathophysiology

Herpes zoster, commonly known as *shingles,* and chickenpox (varicella) are caused by the same virus: varicella-zoster virus (sometimes called human herpesvirus type 3). A person with shingles has a history of chickenpox infection. An estimated one in three people who have had chickenpox will also get shingles (CDC, 2019b). The varicella virus lies dormant until the person's resistance to infections becomes lowered. Risk factors for shingles include suppressed immunity, aging, infection, and stress. The virus causes an inflammation of the spinal ganglia and produces skin lesions of small vesicles along the peripheral nerve fibers of the spinal ganglia (Fig. 3.3). Sometimes the virus may affect a single nerve, such as the trigeminal nerve.

Clinical Manifestations

Eruption of the vesicles is preceded by pain. The rash generally occurs in the thoracic region but also may affect the lumbar, cervical, and cranial areas. Vesicles erupt in a line along the involved nerve. The vesicles rupture and form a crust, and the serous fluid in the vesicles may become purulent. This painful condition lasts 7 to 28 days.

The pain associated with herpes zoster is severe; most patients describe it as burning and knifelike. Extreme tenderness and pruritus occur in the affected area. The patient with herpes zoster needs frequent analgesic therapy during the acute episode.

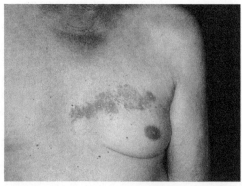

Fig. 3.3 Herpes zoster. (Courtesy Department of Dermatology, School of Medicine, University of Utah, Salt Lake City, UT.)

Herpes zoster is usually not permanently disabling to a healthy adult. The greatest risk is for a patient with a lowered resistance to infection, such as one receiving chemotherapy or large doses of prednisone. In a patient with a compromised immune system, the disease can be fatal.

Assessment

Assessment of the patient should include obtaining a thorough health history and performing a careful inspection to gather relevant data.

Subjective data include (1) sharp, burning pain, usually on one side; (2) severe pruritus of the lesions; (3) general malaise; and (4) a history of chickenpox (varicella).

Objective data include (1) evidence of skin **excoriation** (injury to the surface layer of skin caused by scratching or abrasion) related to scratching, (2) patches of vesicles on erythematous skin following a peripheral nerve pathway, and (3) demonstration of tenderness to touch in the involved area. Other objective signs may include frequent requests for analgesics.

Diagnostic Tests

The diagnostic test for herpes zoster is a culture that isolates the virus. Other diagnostic measures are physical examinations and a thorough health history obtained on admission to the health care facility.

Medical Management

Medical interventions are directed at controlling the pain and preventing secondary complications. Early diagnosis and initiation of treatment are key in the resolution of the outbreak. Oral and intravenous acyclovir, when administered early—ideally within 72 hours of onset of the development of symptoms—reduces the pain and duration of the virus. Analgesics, often opioids, are given for the pain. Steroids may be given to decrease inflammation and edema. Steroid lotions may be used to relieve pruritus, and corticosteroids may be used to relieve pruritus and inflammation. Recovery generally occurs in 2 to 3 weeks. Approximately 20% of patients experience some form of neuralgia after the episode. A vaccine to prevent herpes zoster is available. It is recommended for healthy adults over 50 years of age (CDC, 2018; CDC, 2019c).

Nursing Interventions and Patient Teaching

Nursing interventions are directed at education about the disease and plan of treatment, relieving pain and pruritus, and preventing secondary complications. Tranquilizers such as lorazepam are prescribed to decrease the anxiety associated with severe pain. Analgesics are given to control pain.

Nursing Care Plan 3.1   The Patient With Herpes Zoster

Ms. L., a 28-year-old teacher, is admitted with herpes zoster located around her left eye. She has several vesicles that have crusted and several vesicles that are still intact. She is complaining of pruritus and pain. She keeps asking the nurse if the lesions will leave a scar.

PATIENT PROBLEM

Compromised Skin Integrity, related to open lesions around the left eye

Patient Goals and Expected Outcomes	Nursing Interventions	Evaluation and Rationale
Patient's skin integrity will improve as shown by:		
• No signs of infection such as erythema, purulent drainage, and elevated white blood cell count during hospitalization	Assess skin, especially eye area, for changes in color, texture, turgor, and increase in lesion size. Assess lesions for signs of infection. Monitor albumin and white blood cell levels as ordered.	The patient showed no signs of erythema or purulent drainage. The patient showed improvement of vesicles.
• Remaining skin showing no signs of impairment during hospitalization	Use principles of aseptic technique.	No skin impairment noted in remaining skin.
• Decrease in the number of lesions within 72 h	Monitor status of lesions q 12 h.	The number of lesions increased during the first day of hospitalization but decreased during the next 48 h.
• Patient stating pain level has decreased from a "9" to a "4" within 24 h	Administer or apply medications as ordered to decrease pain or pruritus Teach patient importance of using medical asepsis in care of lesions.	Patient stated that pain was a "3" within 24 h of medication administration.

PATIENT PROBLEM

Distorted Body Image, related to location of lesions as manifested by continual remarks to the nurse, "Will these sores leave a scar?"

Patient Goals and Expected Outcomes	Nursing Interventions	Evaluation and Rationale
The patient will verbalize and demonstrate acceptance of appearance as manifested by:		
• Verbalizing positive feelings about body image	Assess patient's feelings about personal appearance by encouraging patient to express her feelings.	The goal was met: The patient stated she believed the lesions would not be permanent.
• Participating in normal activities	Encourage patient to ask questions about her health problem. Provide reliable information, and reinforce the information already given. Clarify any misconceptions about the care the patient is receiving. Provide privacy and avoid criticism. Teach patient about the disease and the course of the disease.	The goal was met: The patient returned to work after dismissal from the hospital before the lesions had completely healed.

CRITICAL THINKING QUESTIONS

1. Ms. L. turns on her call light. She is crying and states she is in severe pain. She describes the pain as a burning, stabbing pain over her left forehead and eye. She rates her pain as a 7 on a pain scale of 0–10. She also complains of pruritus. What would be the most appropriate nursing interventions to provide comfort and pain control for Ms. L.?
2. Ms. L. tells the nurse that a friend told her she could not visit because she has not had chickenpox. Her friend is afraid she might "catch chickenpox" from Ms. L.'s shingles. Describe the accurate patient teaching to give in response to Ms. L.'s statements.

The nurse must understand and be able to apply the principles of pain management to provide nursing interventions. Medicated baths and warm compresses may be ordered to soothe the skin. Use aseptic technique when caring for open lesions (Nursing Care Plan 3.1).

Problem identification and interventions for the patient with herpes zoster include, but are not limited to, the following:

PATIENT PROBLEM	NURSING INTERVENTIONS
Recent Onset of Pain, related to inflammation of the involved nerve pathways	Assess pain and pruritus for necessary relief measures Administer medications for pain and pruritus Teach stress relaxation techniques, and offer diversional activities
Potential for Infection, related to tissue destruction	Assess factors that contribute to infection, such as an immunocompromised patient (one who has decreased white blood cell count) Monitor for signs of infection, such as pyrexia and leukocytosis Stress aseptic hand hygiene technique Maintain aseptic technique when providing care Limit visitors

Begin patient teaching by assessing the patient's knowledge and readiness, including the following: (1) methods for controlling pain, (2) application of medication and wet dressings, (3) methods for inhibiting the spread of disease, (4) techniques to prevent secondary infections, and (5) proper diet with vitamin C to promote healing.

Health care staff who have received two doses of the varicella vaccine should be assessed for symptoms 8 to 21 days after exposure to a patient with shingles. Any staff member who develops symptoms consistent with herpes zoster should be removed from active duty. Health care staff who have not received the two doses of varicella vaccine may be contagious for 8 to 21 days and should be moved to another duty location, away from patient care (CDC, 2019c). Implementation of proper transmission-based precautions as directed by the infection control department prevent the transmission of the virus in the health care setting. The CDC suggests that immunocompromised patients should be placed in airborne and contact transmission-based precautions for disseminated herpes zoster until the infection is determined to be localized. If the infection is localized, standard precautions with the lesions covered are followed. For patients who are not immunocompromised, the CDC suggests using standard precautions with the lesions covered if the infection is localized; for disseminated herpes zoster, use airborne and contact precautions. Once the lesions are dry and crusted, the patient is no longer considered communicable (CDC, 2019c).

Prognosis

The prognosis is generally good; however, older adults are more susceptible to complications such as postherpetic neuralgia (PHN), which may persist for several months or even years after the skin lesions have cleared.

PHN is most common in adults older than age 60 years. Herpes zoster also can result in eye complications that can lead to blindness, deafness, brain inflammation, and death. Evidence indicates that the varicella-zoster virus remains latent in the body of a person once infected. A person lacking varicella (chickenpox) immunity or who is immunocompromised can acquire chickenpox from someone who has shingles (CDC, 2019c).

PITYRIASIS ROSEA

Pityriasis rosea is a skin rash that may affect people of any age but is noted most often in young adults. It is not known what causes the rash, but it is thought to be linked to a viral infection. It is not considered contagious.

Etiology and Pathophysiology

Pityriasis rosea is caused by a virus, but it is not clear which virus. Some studies indicate it may be linked to certain strains of the herpesvirus, but not the type 1 herpesvirus. The rash generally disappears without treatment within 4 to 8 weeks (Mayo Clinic, 2020c).

Clinical Manifestations

Pityriasis rosea begins as a single lesion referred to as a herald patch, a scaly area up to 4 inches in diameter (10 cm) with a raised border and a pink center that resembles ringworm (a fungal infection). Within 7 to 14 days after the initial eruption, smaller matching spots become widespread on both sides of the body. The rash consists of pink, oval-shaped spots that are ¼ to ½ inch across. The rash appears mainly on the chest, abdomen, back, groin, and armpits (axillae).

Assessment

Assessment involves inspecting the skin and gathering a detailed health history. Ask questions related to gathering subjective data.

Diagnostic Tests

Diagnosis of pityriasis rosea is based on inspection and subjective data provided by the patient. No specific laboratory tests support a definitive diagnosis.

Medical Management

Pityriasis rosea usually requires no treatment, but preventive interventions can control secondary infections related to pruritus. If the skin becomes dry, moisturizing cream may help. For pruritus, the patient should use 1% hydrocortisone cream two or three times a day. Ultraviolet light, such as sunbathing for 30 minutes, shortens the course of pityriasis rosea.

Nursing Interventions

The nursing interventions for pityriasis rosea include symptomatic relief of the symptoms such as pruritus. Analgesics and oatmeal baths may be ordered to help decrease the pain and pruritus. Antihistamines and topical steroids may be used to control the pruritus. Sun exposure aids in the resolution of the lesions.

Prognosis

The disease is self-limiting and resolves in a few weeks.

BACTERIAL DISORDERS OF THE SKIN

CELLULITIS

Etiology and Pathophysiology

Cellulitis, a potentially serious infection, involves the underlying tissues of the skin. Although it is not contagious, the bacteria that cause cellulitis can be spread by direct contact with an open area on a person who has an infection. The most common causes in adults are group A streptococci and *Staphylococcus aureus*; *Haemophilus influenzae* type B is more common in children. The risk is increased by venous insufficiency or stasis; diabetes mellitus; lymphedema; surgery; malnutrition; substance abuse; the presence of another infection; compromised immune function resulting from HIV; treatment with steroids or cancer chemotherapy; or autoimmune diseases, such as lupus erythematosus.

Cellulitis develops as an edematous, erythematous area of skin that feels hot and tender (Fig. 3.4). It occurs when bacteria enter the body through a break in the skin, such as a cut, scratch, or insect bite that is not cleansed with soap and water. The infection usually affects skin on the lower extremities or face, although cellulitis can occur on any part of the skin. The infection is usually superficial, but cellulitis may spread and become life threatening as the infection invades the deeper tissues, lymph nodes, and bloodstream.

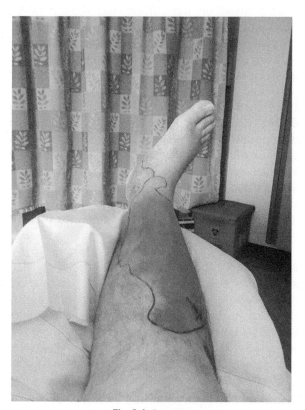

Fig. 3.4 Cellulitis.

Clinical Manifestations

Cellulitis is an infection of the skin and underlying subcutaneous tissues. The affected areas become erythematous, edematous, tender, and warm to the touch. Often a fever accompanies the other symptoms. The first signs and symptoms generally are erythema, pain, and tenderness over an area of skin. These signs and symptoms are caused by the bacteria and by the body's attempts to halt the infection. The infected skin may look slightly pitted, like an orange peel. Over time, the area of erythema spreads and small red spots may appear. Vesicles may form and burst, or large bullae may appear on the infected skin. As the infection spreads, nearby lymph nodes may become enlarged and tender (lymphadenitis). *Erysipelas* is one form of streptococcal cellulitis in which the skin is bright red and noticeably edematous, and the edges of the infected area are raised. Edema occurs because the infection occludes the lymphatic vessels in the skin. Most patients with cellulitis feel only mildly ill, but some have fever, chills, tachycardia, headache, hypotension, and confusion.

Assessment

Assessment involves primarily inspection of the skin. Collect a health history to support assessment data. Subjective data include complaints of fatigue, tenderness, pain, limited movement of the involved extremity, and general malaise. Objective data include edema, erythema, and areas that are warm to touch. Vesicles may be present. An elevated temperature accompanied by tachycardia and leukocytosis (elevated white blood cell count) often occurs.

Diagnostic Tests

Cellulitis is diagnosed by its appearance as well as the signs and symptoms. Cultures may be needed from blood, purulent exudate, or tissue specimens for laboratory identification of the bacteria. A complete blood count (CBC) reveals leukocytosis. A Gram stain can determine the appropriate antibiotic therapy. Sometimes tests are performed to differentiate cellulitis from deep vein thrombosis of the lower extremity because the signs and symptoms of these disorders are similar. X-ray examination, ultrasound, computed tomography, or magnetic resonance imaging may be used to determine the extent of inflammation and to identify abscess formation.

Medical Management

Prompt treatment with antibiotics can prevent cellulitis from spreading rapidly and reaching the blood and organs. Commonly used antibiotics include penicillin, cephalexin, and erythromycin. Most cases are treated with antibiotic therapy that is effective against streptococci and staphylococci (NLM, 2018). A patient with mild cellulitis may take oral antibiotics. If the patient has rapidly spreading cellulitis, high fever, or other evidence of a serious infection, the health care provider will order IV antibiotics.

Nursing Interventions and Patient Teaching

Nursing interventions involve treating the signs and symptoms and preventing the spread of the disease. Administer the antibiotic, monitor the patient's progress, assess pain, administer an analgesic, change dressings, and monitor the patient's nutrition and hydration status. The affected body part, when possible, should be immobilized and kept elevated to help reduce edema. Warm, moist dressings applied to the infected area may relieve discomfort.

Signs and symptoms of cellulitis usually disappear after a few days of antibiotic therapy. However, they may worsen before they improve because, as the bacteria die, they release substances that damage tissue. When this occurs, the body continues to react even though the bacteria are dead. Antibiotics are continued for a minimum of 10 days. Teach the patient that it is important to take the entire prescription of antibiotics and to monitor for signs and symptoms of secondary diseases such as yeast infections. The specific patient problems related to cellulitis depend on the assessment data gathered and the extent of the infection. Analgesics such as acetaminophen or oxycodone-acetaminophen help control the pain and fever associated with cellulitis. Patients who develop blistering, increasing temperatures, or red streaks in the affected extremity should be advised to contact their primary care provider.

Prognosis

Cure is possible with 7 to 10 days of treatment. Cellulitis may be more severe in people with chronic diseases and those who are susceptible to infection, such as those with immunosuppression. Complications from cellulitis include sepsis, meningitis, and lymphangitis.

IMPETIGO CONTAGIOSA

Etiology and Pathophysiology

Impetigo is caused by *S. aureus*, streptococci, or a mixed bacterial invasion of the skin. It is a highly contagious inflammatory disorder, seen at all ages but particularly common in children. The lesions start as macules (small, flat blemishes flush with the skin surface), develop into pustulant vesicles (small, circumscribed elevations of the skin that contain pus), and then rupture and form a dried exudate. The crust is honey-colored and easily removed. Under the dried exudate is smooth, red skin (Fig. 3.5).

Clinical Manifestations

The exposed areas of the body most often affected are the face, hands, arms, and legs. The pustulant lesions are distributed randomly over the involved area. The honey-colored dried exudate ranges from pinpoint to the size of a nickel or larger. Impetigo is highly contagious to a person who directly contacts the exudate of a lesion. The disease may be spread by touching personal articles, linens, and clothing of the infected person.

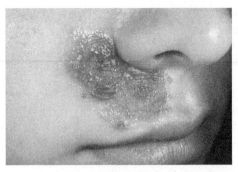

Fig. 3.5 Impetigo and herpes simplex. (Courtesy Department of Dermatology, School of Medicine, University of Utah, Salt Lake City, UT.)

Assessment

Subjective data include symptoms of (1) pruritus, (2) pain, (3) malaise, (4) spread of the disease to other parts of the body, and (5) the presence of other diseases.

Objective data include all or some of the following: (1) erythema; (2) pruritic areas; (3) honey-colored crust over dried lesions; (4) smooth, red skin under the crust; (5) low-grade fever; (6) leukocytosis; (7) positive culture for *Streptococcus* or *S. aureus*; and (8) purulent exudate.

Diagnostic Tests

The diagnosis is made by taking a culture of the exudate and identifying the specific bacterium. Inspection and symptoms are the standard means of identifying the condition.

Medical Management

The health care provider prescribes systemic antibiotics (such as erythromycin, dicloxacillin, or a cephalosporin) based on the culture and sensitivity test. Topical antibiotics, such as mupirocin, have proven effective when started early in the treatment, but most health care providers include a systemic antibiotic as well. Retapamulin may be used for topical treatment of impetigo for adults and children over 9 months old for methicillin-susceptible *Staphylococcus aureus* and *Streptococcus pyogenes* (CDC, 2020). Medical treatment emphasizes the use of antiseptic soaps to remove crusted exudate and cleansing agents to clean the involved area thoroughly before applying an antibiotic cream, ointment, or lotion. A primary goal is to prevent glomerulonephritis (inflammation of the glomerulus of the kidney), which may occur after streptococcal infections.

Nursing Interventions and Patient Teaching

Interventions are aimed at disrupting the course of the disease and preventing the spread of infection. Antibiotics are used to arrest the disease process. Systemic parenteral penicillin is one of the most commonly used antibiotics. Cephalosporins or beta-lactam/beta-lactamase inhibitor combination are also used in a first-line defense (Lewis and Steele, 2019). Wear gloves and wash the lesions with an antibacterial agent.

The lesions usually are soaked with an antiseptic solution, and the dried exudate is removed with special instruments. Topical antibiotics are applied several times a day using sterile technique.

Problem identification and interventions for the patient with impetigo include, but are not limited to, the following:

PATIENT PROBLEM	NURSING INTERVENTIONS
Compromised Skin Integrity, related to S. aureus, streptococci, or a mixed bacterial invasion as evidenced by crusted, open lesions	Inspect lesions every day for drainage, size, and extent of body area covered Keep area clean and dry
Insufficient Knowledge, concerning the cause and spread of the disease	Assess patient's knowledge level and readiness to learn Demonstrate appropriate care and application of topical medications Stress importance of individual personal items, such as linens and towels Involve family in patient teaching

Assess the patient's level of knowledge and instruct the patient and family members in the principles of hygiene. When demonstrating home care techniques, reinforce correct information and stress the importance of preventing the spread of the disease by contact.

Prognosis
With proper treatment, the prognosis is good. Emphasize that the patient should complete the prescribed medication therapies.

FOLLICULITIS, FURUNCLES, CARBUNCLES, AND FELONS
Etiology and Pathophysiology
Folliculitis is an infection of a hair follicle, generally by *S. aureus* bacteria. The infection may involve one or several follicles. It often occurs after men or women shave. A stye resulting from an infected eyelash is an example of folliculitis.

A *furuncle* (boil) is an inflammation that begins deep in the hair follicles and spreads to the surrounding skin. Irritation is a common predisposing factor. Common locations are the posterior area of the neck, the forearm, buttocks, and the axillae (Fig. 3.6).

A *carbuncle* is a cluster of furuncles. It is an infection of several hair follicles that spreads to surrounding tissue. Obesity, poor nutrition, untreated diabetes mellitus, and poor hygiene contribute to the formation of carbuncles.

A *felon* is an infection of the soft tissue under and around an area such as the fingernail. The involved finger becomes erythematous, edematous, and tender to touch.

Clinical Manifestations
The involved area is usually edematous, erythematous, painful, and pruritic. After several days, the infected area becomes localized. The exact area may become shiny. The lesion may begin to present with a pointed head and point up; in a furuncle or carbuncle, the center turns yellow. Carbuncles can have four or five cores with spontaneous rupture of the core. The pain stops immediately on rupture. A surgical incision and drainage can be performed if the core does not rupture.

Assessment
Subjective data include the patient's general symptoms, such as tenderness and pain with movement. Ask about a family history of diabetes mellitus or the wearing of improperly fitting clothing. Objective data include noting erythema and edema in the involved area. The patient is often overweight and may have poor body hygiene.

Diagnostic Tests
Diagnosis is based primarily on a thorough physical examination, health history, and inspection of the area. The drainage may be cultured.

Medical Management
Medical treatment is aimed at preventing the spread of infection. Patients in the hospital are isolated, using wound and secretion precautions. Surgical treatment may include draining the lesion and applying topical antibiotics.

Nursing Interventions and Patient Teaching
Warm soaks, 2 or 3 times a day, can speed the process of suppuration (production of purulent material). When the lesion ruptures, discontinue the soaks to prevent damage of the surrounding skin and spread of the infection. Use good medical asepsis while caring for these patients. In the hospital, follow isolation procedures for drainage and secretion. If the lesion is incised and drained, use sterile technique to apply topical antibiotics. The affected part must be immobilized to prevent pain and elevated to decrease the edema.

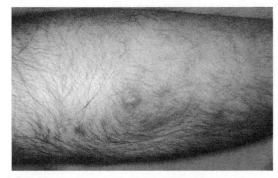
Fig. 3.6 Furuncle of the forearm. (Courtesy Department of Dermatology, School of Medicine, University of Utah, Salt Lake City, UT.)

Problem identification and interventions for the patient with bacterial disorders include, but are not limited to, the following:

PATIENT PROBLEM	NURSING INTERVENTIONS
Compromised Skin Integrity, related to infection of a hair follicle, as evidenced by exudates from wound	Assess wound daily for exudates and excoriation Apply skin protectant to opening
Recent Onset of Pain, related to infection of a hair follicle	Assess area for edema and tenderness Elevate involved body part above the level of the heart Apply hot soaks and immobilize affected part

Teach patients not to touch the exudate. Meticulous hand hygiene is a must before and after contact with the lesions. Demonstrate good hygiene practices and ask for return demonstrations by the patient and the family. Each family member needs his or her own toilet items and bath linens, which are not to be shared. They should be encouraged to use bacteriostatic soap and shampoo. Demonstrate proper disposal and cleaning of contaminated articles.

Prognosis
Patients make a full recovery when they follow the treatment plan. A follow-up examination with a health care provider may be needed to identify any underlying disease process, such as diabetes mellitus.

FUNGAL INFECTIONS OF THE SKIN

Fungal infections, which are known as *dermatophytoses,* are superficial infections of the skin. The most common types are tinea capitis, tinea corporis, tinea cruris, and tinea pedis.

Etiology and Pathophysiology
Tinea capitis is known commonly as ringworm of the scalp. *Microsporum audouinii* is the major fungal pathogen. The fungus is spread by contact with infected articles. Trauma or irritation breaks the skin and facilitates spread of the infection (Fig. 3.7).

Tinea corporis is known as ringworm of the body. It occurs on parts of the body with little or no hair.

Tinea cruris is known as jock itch. It is found in the groin area.

Tinea pedis is the most common of all fungal infections. Commonly known as athlete's foot, it occurs between the toes of people whose feet perspire heavily. The fungus also can be spread from contaminated public bathroom facilities and swimming pools.

Clinical Manifestations
Tinea capitis is usually an erythematous, round lesion with pustules around the edges (see Fig. 3.7). Temporary alopecia occurs at the site, and infected hairs turn blue-green under a Wood's lamp (an ultraviolet light).

Tinea corporis produces flat lesions that are clear in the center with erythematous borders. Scaliness also occurs, and pruritus is severe (Fig. 3.8).

Tinea cruris has brownish red lesions that migrate out from the groin area. Pruritus and skin excoriation from scratching are found.

Tinea pedis produces more skin maceration than the others. Commonly seen are fissures and vesicles around and below the toes, with occasional discoloration of the infected area.

Assessment
Subjective data include any symptoms of extreme pruritus and tenderness from excoriation of the area. Collection of objective data for tinea capitis includes an inspection and location of a round, scaled lesion that has pustules around the edges of the scalp. The involved area is erythematous and has no hair. In tinea corporis, the lesions are flat with clear centers and erythematous borders on nonhairy body parts. In tinea cruris, the groin area reveals brown to red lesions that radiate outward, with skin excoriation from intense scratching. In tinea pedis, fissures between the toes and soft skin are accompanied by vesicular lesions and thick toenails.

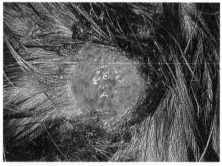

Fig. 3.7 Tinea capitis. (From Habif TP, Campbell JL Jr, Chapman MS, et al: *Skin disease: Diagnosis and treatment,* ed 3, St. Louis, 2011, Saunders.)

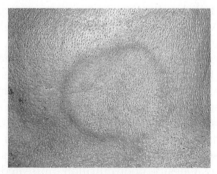

Fig. 3.8 Tinea corporis. (From Habif TP, Campbell JL Jr, Chapman MS, et al: *Skin disease: Diagnosis and treatment,* ed 3, St. Louis, 2011, Saunders.)

Diagnostic Tests

The diagnosis is primarily by visual inspection and, for tinea capitis, use of a Wood's lamp. The light causes hairs infected by the fungus to become brilliantly fluorescent. No other tests are performed, but a thorough health history supports the diagnosis of all fungal infections of the skin.

Medical Management

Medical treatment involves the use of topical or oral antifungal drugs. Griseofulvin is the most common oral drug given; topical drugs do not penetrate the hair bulb. Antifungal soaps and shampoos are recommended. Antifungal agents such as tolnaftate 1%, miconazole, and butenafine can be applied directly. Treatment may last from 2 to 6 weeks. See Table 3.3 for a list of drugs commonly used for fungal and other integumentary infections.

Nursing Interventions and Patient Teaching

Nursing interventions for fungal infections involve two primary principles: (1) protect the involved area from trauma and irritation by keeping it clean and dry and (2) alleviate the fungus through proper application of medications and warm compresses.

Tinea pedis should be treated with warm soaks, using Burow's solution (5% aluminum subacetate), and topical antifungal agents. Burow's solution has antiseptic properties, relieves itching, and aids in the reduction of bacterial and fungal growth. It is available without prescription. Excellent foot care is stressed. The feet should be cleaned and dried thoroughly, paying special attention to the toes. Wearing sandals or going barefoot helps decrease foot moisture. Footwear, such as stockings, must be made of an absorbent material. Wearing shower-shoes or sandals while in community locker rooms should also be emphasized.

Problem identification and interventions for the patient with fungal infections include, but are not limited to, the following:

PATIENT PROBLEM	NURSING INTERVENTIONS
Compromised Skin Integrity, related to fungal infection, as evidenced by: • Increased moisture • Pruritus	Keep involved area clean and dry Have patient wear loose-fitting clothing and shoes Apply medications as directed

Patient education involves teaching proper skin care and comfort measures to relieve pruritus. Review the medications to be taken and the procedures for the patient to do at home, emphasizing that fungal skin disorders may take months to cure. Stress general information about athlete's foot and clarify the many misconceptions.

Prognosis

Prognosis for recovery is good. Few complications result when treatment is followed.

INFLAMMATORY DISORDERS OF THE SKIN

Superficial infection of the skin is known as *dermatitis*. It can be caused by numerous agents, such as drugs, plants, chemicals, metals, and food. Regardless of the precipitating factor, the lesions associated with dermatitis develop along the same pattern. The nurse first observes erythema and edema, followed by the eruption of vesicles that rupture and encrust. Pruritus is always present, which promotes further skin excoriation.

CONTACT DERMATITIS
Etiology and Pathophysiology

Contact dermatitis is caused by direct contact with agents in the environment to which the individual is hypersensitive. The epidermis becomes inflamed and damaged by repeated contact with the physical and chemical irritants. Common causes of dermatitis are detergents, soaps, industrial chemicals, and plants such as poison ivy.

Clinical Manifestations

Lesions appear first at the point of contact with the irritant. Usually the patient feels burning, pain, pruritus, and edema. The involved area soon becomes erythematous, with papules (small, raised, solid skin lesions less than 1 cm in diameter) and vesicles appearing most often on the dorsal surfaces.

Assessment

Thoroughly research the patient's activities. If necessary, ask the patient to write a log of activities for the 48 hours before development of symptoms.

Subjective data usually reveal that the patient has (1) tried a new soap, (2) been traveling and using different personal items, or (3) been working with plants or flowers. The patient may have severe pruritus and difficulty moving the involved area.

Objective data should reveal (1) erythema, (2) papules and vesicles that generally ooze and weep a clear fluid, (3) scratch marks resulting from intense pruritus, and (4) edema of the area.

Diagnostic Tests

The primary diagnostic test is an accurate health history to identify the agent and inspection of the skin. Intradermal skin testing may identify plants and environmental agents, and elimination diets are used to identify food allergies. Elevated serum immunoglobulin E (IgE) levels and eosinophilia support the diagnosis. Both tests are thought to be related to abnormalities of T cell function.

Medical Management

Medical intervention involves identifying the cause of the hypersensitive reaction. Symptomatic treatment for the inflammation, edema, and pruritus may include topical application of corticosteroids and the oral administration of antihistamines such as diphenhydramine. If the patient has a history of asthma (reactive airway disease), he or she may experience an acute asthmatic episode. Hydroxyzine and inhalation treatments provide prophylactic treatment for asthma.

Nursing Interventions and Patient Teaching

The primary goal is to identify the offensive agent to protect the skin from further damage. Identify the cause by first describing the pattern of the reaction.

Wet dressings using Burow's solution help promote the healing process. To prevent infection, use aseptic technique when applying corticosteroids to the open lesions.

Pruritus is responsible for most of the discomfort. A cool environment with increased humidity decreases the pruritus. Cold compresses may be applied to reduce circulation to the area (vasoconstriction). The patient should take daily baths with an application of oil to cleanse the skin. Fingernails should be cut at the level of the fingertips to decrease excoriation from scratching. Clothing should be lightweight and loose to decrease trauma of the involved area.

Problem identification and interventions for the patient with inflammation of the skin include, but are not limited to, the following:

PATIENT PROBLEM	NURSING INTERVENTIONS
Compromised Skin Integrity, related to direct contact with agents in the environment as evidenced by scratching and the appearance of papules	Assess for signs of scratching Have patient keep fingernails short and wear mittens Apply medications as directed
Recent Onset of Pain, related to pruritus	Assess degree of pruritus and discomfort every shift Keep environment cool Apply cold compresses Apply antipruritic medications as prescribed

Teach the patient to keep an accurate history of possible predisposing offensive agents. As soon as the primary irritant has been identified, the patient should avoid it. Irritants may include certain soaps or excessive heat and friction at the site and should be avoided. Any time the skin is exposed to the primary irritant, the affected area should be washed thoroughly. Topical creams may be applied only as directed by a health care provider.

Prognosis

Removal of the offensive agent results in full recovery. Desensitizing the individual may be necessary if recurrences are frequent.

DERMATITIS VENENATA, EXFOLIATIVE DERMATITIS, AND DERMATITIS MEDICAMENTOSA

Etiology and Pathophysiology

Dermatitis venenata results from contact with certain plants, commonly *poison ivy* and *poison oak.* The signs and symptoms include mild to severe erythema with pruritus. Initial exposure causes the body to form sensitizing antigens, resulting in an immunologic change in certain lymphocytes. Subsequent exposure to the antigen causes the lymphocytes to release irritating chemicals, leading to inflammation, edema, and vesiculation. The lesions are found mainly on the body part exposed to the sensitizing agent.

Exfoliative dermatitis can be caused by the ingestion of certain heavy metals, such as arsenic or mercury, or by antibiotics, aspirin, codeine, gold, or iodine. The skin sloughs off, and the area becomes edematous and erythematous. If severe pruritus with fever occurs, the patient may require hospitalization. Treatment is individualized. If the cause can be determined, the source should be removed or treated appropriately. Careful monitoring is essential to prevent secondary infection, avoid further irritation, and maintain fluid balance.

Dermatitis medicamentosa occurs when people are given a medication to which they are hypersensitive. An individual may present with a skin reaction to a medication that was taken in the past without incident. Any drug can cause a reaction, but the common agents are penicillin, codeine, and cephalosporins (WebMD, 2019).

Clinical Manifestations

Clinical manifestations range from mild to severe erythema with vesicular eruptions. In severe reactions, respiratory distress may occur. Any type of lesion may be found.

Assessment

Subjective data for dermatitis include complaints of pruritus and a burning pain in the involved area.

Objective data include observation of lesions that are white in the center and red on the periphery. Vesicles are common in dermatitis venenata. Patients with dermatitis medicamentosa may have severe dyspnea caused by respiratory distress.

Diagnostic Tests

A careful patient history is paramount in the diagnosis of dermatitis venenata, exfoliative dermatitis, and dermatitis medicamentosa. A laboratory examination for serum IgE and eosinophilia is ordered.

Medical Management

The medical treatment for dermatitis ranges from therapeutic baths to administration of corticosteroids. The medical treatment is directed at the cause.

Nursing Interventions and Patient Teaching

Pruritus is the primary symptom in all types of dermatitis. Calamine lotion, a common over-the-counter medication, is used to reduce itching. Therapeutic baths using colloid solution, lotions, and ointments also help relieve the pruritus. Emotional support is necessary. The patient's physical appearance is difficult for the patient and family members to accept.

In dermatitis venenata, instruct the patient to wash the affected part immediately after contact with the offending allergen. After the lesions appear, only cool, open, wet dressings should be used.

In dermatitis medicamentosa, identifying the drug and discontinuing its use are paramount. If the offending allergen cannot be pinpointed, no drugs should be given. Notify the health care provider, who will determine which medication is responsible. The lesions will disappear after the medication is discontinued. More specific nursing intervention is directed by individual patient symptoms.

Problem identification and interventions for the patient with dermatitis include, but are not limited to, the following:

PATIENT PROBLEM	NURSING INTERVENTIONS
Compromised Skin Integrity, related to exposure to the antigen as evidenced by encrusted, open lesions	Inspect lesions every day for exudate, size, and specific body area involved Keep area clean and dry
Potential for infection, related to break in skin	Assess skin for signs of infection Identify interventions to prevent or reduce the risk of infection Monitor vital signs; assess for elevated temperature Stress medical aseptic hand hygiene technique Keep involved areas dry
Insufficient Knowledge, related to the cause and spread of the disease	Assess patient's knowledge level and readiness to learn Demonstrate appropriate care and application of topical medications Stress importance of individual personal items, such as linens and towels Involve family in patient teaching

Advise the patient to wear a medical alert bracelet or necklace showing the name of the allergen and to notify all health care personnel of the medication allergy.

Prognosis

Full recovery occurs when the offending agent is removed.

URTICARIA

Etiology and Pathophysiology

Urticaria is the presence of wheals or hives in an allergic reaction, commonly caused by drugs, food, insect bites, inhalants, emotional stress, or exposure to heat or cold. The wheals (round elevation of the skin; white in the center with a pale red periphery) (see Table 3.1) of urticaria appear suddenly. Urticaria, or hives, is caused by the release of histamine in an antigen-antibody reaction.

Clinical Manifestations

In addition to wheals, the increased histamine causes the capillaries to dilate, resulting in increased permeability. Respiratory involvement may occur.

Assessment

Subjective data include patient complaints of pruritus, edema, a burning pain, and sometimes dyspnea.

Collection of objective data identifies transient wheals of varying shapes and sizes with well-defined erythematous margins and pale centers. Intense scratching may be seen, and in some cases, respiration may be compromised. Assessment of respiratory status provides a baseline for future assessments.

Diagnostic Tests

A detailed health history is the primary tool to identify the cause of hives. An allergy skin test may be performed, using minute quantities of antigen, to identify the allergenic substances. A serum examination for IgE elevation may be ordered.

Medical Management

Administering an antihistamine—and sometimes epinephrine—provides relief from urticaria. Identification of the cause of the urticaria is important to prevent recurrence.

Nursing Interventions and Patient Teaching

Nursing interventions include helping the patient identify the cause of and decreasing the discomfort from the pruritus. Teach the patient about possible causes and prevention methods. Explain medications thoroughly and describe the procedure for therapeutic baths. Review the signs and symptoms of an anaphylactic reaction, including shortness of breath, wheezing, and cyanosis.

Prognosis

Patients recover fully when the offending agent is determined and avoided. Compliance with the therapeutic regimen influences the outcome.

ANGIOEDEMA

Etiology and Pathophysiology
Angioedema is a form of urticaria and is caused by the same offenders. It occurs in the subcutaneous tissue, whereas urticaria is a lesion of the skin and mucous membranes. Angioedema is characterized by local edema of an entire area, such as an eyelid, hands, feet, tongue, larynx, gastrointestinal (GI) tract, genitalia, or lips. Only a single edematous area usually appears at one time.

Assessment
Subjective data include symptoms of burning, pruritus, acute pain (if in the GI tract), or respiratory distress (if in the larynx).

The collection of objective data reveals edema (swelling); overlying skin appears normal.

Diagnostic Tests
A careful patient history is essential in the diagnosis of angioedema. Patients with a history of allergies are more likely to have angioedema.

Medical Management
Treatment to relieve angioedema may include antihistamine drugs such as diphenhydramine. Epinephrine injections and infusions of corticosteroids such as methylprednisolone also may be prescribed.

Nursing Interventions
A cold pack or cold compress may be used. Continual respiratory assessment is essential to detect respiratory distress. Instruct patients to wear a medical alert bracelet. Education is the key to prevent recurrent episodes.

Prognosis
With treatment, the prognosis is excellent.

ECZEMA (ATOPIC DERMATITIS)

Etiology and Pathophysiology
Eczema is a chronic inflammatory disorder of the integument. It usually is diagnosed in children, but exacerbations often continue into adulthood. There are associations with allergies to chocolate, wheat, eggs, and orange juice. The allergen causes histamine to be released, and an antigen-antibody reaction occurs.

Clinical Manifestations
Papular and vesicular lesions appear and are surrounded by erythema. The vesicles generally rupture, discharging a yellow, tenacious exudate that dries and encrusts. If the lesions become infected, the skin loses its pigment and becomes shiny with dry scales.

Assessment
Subjective data include complaints of pruritus and scratching. Children are generally fussy and irritable, and anorexia is common. The skin is sensitive to touch. A family history of allergies and asthma supports the findings in many cases.

Objective data include vesicles and papules found on the scalp, forehead, cheeks, neck, and surfaces of the extremities. The involved area is erythematous and dry. Tiny cracks in the epithelium allow fluid to escape and further promote dryness. The primary signs result from the scratching in response to pruritus. Scales accompanied by dryness in the involved area are a distinguishing characteristic of eczema.

Diagnostic Tests
The diagnosis generally is made during a thorough health history. Heredity is a prominent factor in the disease. An elimination diet and skin testing may be used to identify the specific substance to which the patient is hypersensitive. IgE serum tests provide data related to allergic response.

Medical Management
Medical treatment involves reducing the amount of allergen exposure. The eruptions and pruritus can be relieved if the aggravating factor is identified and controlled. The primary goal is to break the inflammation cycle.

Hydration of the skin is the key to treatment. The skin is dry because of tiny cracks that allow body fluids to escape. The skin may be hydrated by soaking the affected area in warm water for 15 to 20 minutes and then applying an occlusive ointment to retain the water. Examples of occlusive preparations are petrolatum and corticosteroid ointments. The skin should be patted dry after the bath and the occlusive preparation applied immediately to the damp skin.

Nursing Interventions and Patient Teaching
Nursing interventions are directed toward treatment of symptoms for the eczematous patient. Administer the therapeutic bath and occlusive preparations as directed. Use wet dressings to maximize hydration of the skin. Apply topical steroids to relieve discomfort.

When the lesions begin to heal, moisturizing lotions should be applied 3 or 4 times a day to add moisture to the skin. Wet wraps and occlusive preparations only hold water already present.

The emotional impact of having eczema ranges from anger to depression. The nurse provides an emotional outlet for these patients. Encourage the patient to share emotions by using effective listening skills and open-ended questions. This provides a means to establish a therapeutic rapport with the patient.

Before the development of steroids, coal tar products were used to reduce the skin inflammation. Coal tar products do not decrease inflammation as quickly as steroids, but they last longer and have fewer side effects, making them more suitable to treat chronic eczema. Preparations such as Estar gel and PsoriGel are applied once a day at bedtime with a moisturizer.

Problem identification and interventions for the patient with eczema include, but are not limited to, the following:

PATIENT PROBLEM	NURSING INTERVENTIONS
Compromised Skin Integrity, related to chronic inflammatory disorder as evidenced by open lesions	Assess skin for signs of secondary infection Monitor CBC for elevated white blood cell count Apply ordered medications, using medical aseptic technique
Potential for Impaired Self-Esteem due to Current Situation, related to change in body image	Assess patient's mental status Be an active listener Encourage verbalization of concerns the patient may be experiencing Observe interaction with family and staff members and assist in establishing a therapeutic rapport
Potential for Infection, related to open lesion	Report at once the signs of wound infection, such as erythema, especially beyond the wound margins Increasing edema, purulent exudates, change in the description of the pain or increased pain, and increased warmth in the involved area are signs and symptoms of infection

ACNE VULGARIS

Etiology and Pathophysiology
Acne is an inflammatory papulopustular skin eruption that involves the sebaceous glands; it occurs primarily in adolescents. The exact cause is unknown. Factors that may contribute to the condition include stress, hormone fluctuations, medications, diet, oil production, dead skin cells, clogged pores, and bacteria (Mayo Clinic, 2020a).

Acne develops when the oil glands become occluded. At puberty, androgens are secreted, increasing the size of the oil glands and causing the sebum to combine more readily with epithelial cells and bacteria. Sebum then may occlude a hair follicle, forming a comedo (plural, *comedones*). A comedo is a blackhead. It is dark because of the effect oxygen has on sebum, not because of the presence of dirt.

Clinical Manifestations
Acne is found most often on the face, neck, upper chest, shoulder, and back (Fig. 3.9). The first symptom is usually tenderness and edema in the area, followed by the comedo. The skin is oily and shiny, and the lesions last up to 10 days. Scarring results from large lesions that

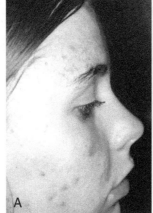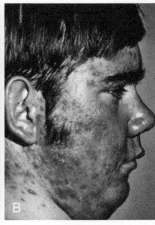

Fig. 3.9 Acne vulgaris. (A) Comedones with a few inflammatory pustules. (B) Papulopustular acne. (From Weston WL, Lane AT, Morelli JG: *Color textbook of pediatric dermatology,* ed 4, St. Louis, 2007, Mosby.)

are traumatized when the person tries to rupture the comedo.

Assessment
Acne can have psychological consequences that require treatment, so the collection of subjective data includes asking the adolescent how acne affects his or her lifestylewith questions such as, "Does it affect your participation in activities or group communication?" Most patients acknowledge that acne affects their self-image. Common locations for acne lesions are the face and chin, which are highly visible areas. The number of lesions increases with emotional upsets and stress.

Collection of objective data includes noting the presence of edema in the involved area. Comedones (blackheads) are found on the skin of the face, back, or chest.

Diagnostic Tests
The medical diagnosis is made primarily by inspection of the lesions and a health history that supports the diagnosis.

Medical Management
Medical management can involve topical, systemic, or intralesional medications. The medications prescribed will cleanse, dry, or reduce inflammation, bacterial count, or sebum production (Table 3.4). Women of childbearing age should receive counseling about the need for reliable methods of contraception with some medications. Some of the therapies may be teratogenic to fetal development.

Nursing Interventions and Patient Teaching
When planning nursing interventions, consider the compliance of adolescents. Assess and consider what acne means to them. The actual extent of the condition is not as important as the adolescent's feelings. Appearance and acceptance by peers are important to the adolescent. Self-esteem may be hindered with acne.

Table 3.4   **Treatments for Acne Vulgaris**

TREATMENT	APPLICATION	EFFECT	ADVERSE EFFECTS	COMMENTS
Retinoid therapies (tretinoin, adapalene, tazarotene)	Primarily topical for entire affected area	Reduces inflammation	Redness, burning, and sensitivity to sunlight Do not combine with OTC washes and medications	
isotretinoin	Oral	Reduces sebum production and abnormal keratinization of gland ducts	Destructive effect on fetal development Depression	Assess for: • Changes in behavior • Hepatotoxicity • Pregnancy prior to starting medication
benzoyl peroxide	Washes and soaps	Antimicrobial Reduces inflammation		
Antibiotic therapies (erythromycin, clindamycin, and tetracycline)	Oral	Reduce bacterial counts	Reduce effectiveness of oral contraceptives	Tetracycline may not be used for children under the age of 9 years or for those who are pregnant or breastfeeding
Salicylic acid	Ointment	Reduces inflammation		
Hormone therapy (combination contraceptives containing estrogen and progestin)ᵃ	Oral	Reduces sebum production		
benzoyl peroxide medications	Topical, spot treatment	Dry skin lesions		

ᵃUsed only in females.
OTC, Over the counter.
Based on data from WebMD: Skin condition and acne, 2020. Retrieved from https://www.webmd.com/skin-problems-and-treatments/acne/default.htm

In addition to psychological concerns, focus on preventive nursing interventions. The important areas are skin care, compliance, and emotional support. Prevention stresses identification of factors that directly exacerbate acne. Although poor hygiene may not be a cause, cleanliness decreases infection rate and promotes healing. The patient should keep the hands and hair away from the face, wear clothes that do not restrict affected areas, wash the hair daily, and wash the skin two or three times a day with medicated soap. Cosmetics must be water based. Improvement with the condition may take several weeks, making compliance difficult. Often 3 weeks of treatment are required before the patient, family, or friends notice improvement (see the Health Promotion box).

Problem identification and interventions for the patient with acne vulgaris include, but are not limited to, the following:

PATIENT PROBLEM	NURSING INTERVENTIONS
Compromised Skin Integrity, related to occluded oil glands	Assess extent of occluded oil glands by inspecting lesions for size, color, and location Monitor for signs of infection Wash involved areas 2 or 3 times a day Apply medications to decrease occlusion of oil glands

PATIENT PROBLEM	NURSING INTERVENTIONS
Impaired Self-Esteem due to Current Situation, related to change in body image	Assess primary cause of low self-esteem and depth of feelings Assess family support Encourage verbalization of feelings about cosmetic appearance and ways to deal with the situation Observe nonverbal communication to discover patient's perception of the illness Stress the importance of not comparing oneself with others Have patient list current successes and strengths Give positive reinforcement

Teaching should center on the patient's physical and emotional needs. Address diet, hygiene, stress reduction, makeup, and medications. Coping skills may have to be retaught and counseling referrals made. The extensive treatment time should be covered in minute detail because this disease is chronic, and exacerbations will occur. Helping the adolescent communicate about feelings will decrease any long-term effects that acne may have on his or her personality. The patient taking isotretinoin will develop dry skin; teach the patient measures to prevent it.

Health Promotion

Healthy Skin

- Adequate nutrition (fluids; protein; vitamins A, B complex, and C; iron; adequate calories; and unsaturated fatty acids) promotes healthy skin.
- Refrain from smoking to improve skin color and to prevent circulation difficulties.
- Drink eight glasses of water per day to help rid the skin of waste products.
- Exercise increases circulation and dilates blood vessels. Its psychological effects can improve one's appearance and mental outlook. Use caution to protect against overexposure to heat, cold, and sun during outdoor exercise.
- Wash the skin and hair often enough to remove excess oil and excretions and to prevent odor.
- The use of neutral soaps and avoidance of hot water and vigorous rubbing can noticeably decrease local irritation and inflammation.
- Older adults should avoid using harsh soaps and shampoos because of the increased dryness of their skin.
- Use moisturizers after bath or shower while the skin is still damp to seal in this moisture.
- Obesity has an adverse effect on the skin. Increased subcutaneous fat can lead to stretching and overheating. Overheating causes an increase in perspiring, which can impair normal or inflamed skin.

Prognosis

The prognosis for acne is good. However, lasting psychological effects can occur from the scarring that may result. In extreme cases, eczema may develop from taking medications such as isotretinoin for acne.

PSORIASIS

Etiology and Pathophysiology

Psoriasis is a noninfectious skin disorder. It is a hereditary, chronic, proliferative disease involving the epidermis and can occur at any age. No specific predisposing factors are known. In psoriasis, the skin cells divide much more rapidly than normal. The normal time for the entire skin to be replaced through sloughing and generation of new cells is 28 days; in psoriasis the time may decrease to 7 days. Severe scaling results from the rapid cell division.

Clinical Manifestations

The lesions appear as raised, erythematous, circumscribed, silvery scaling plaques. The primary lesion is papular. The papules become plaques, which are located on the scalp, elbows, chin, and trunk (see Plaques in Table 3.1). The condition may be classified as mild, moderate, or severe.

Assessment

Subjective data initially include symptoms of mild pruritus. Patients sometimes express feelings of depression, frustration, and loneliness. They report that others stare and avoid contact with them, thus increasing their self-consciousness about their appearance.

Objective data include the observation of dull, erythematous, sharply outlined plaques covered with silvery scales on the elbows, knees, and scalp. Fingernails can be affected and show pitting with yellowish discoloration.

Diagnostic Tests

No specific diagnostic tests exist for psoriasis. Primary diagnosis is made by observing the patient and the signs displayed.

Medical Management

Medical management is aimed at slowing the proliferation of epithelial layers of the skin. Topical steroids and keratolytic agents are used in occlusive wet dressings to decrease inflammation. Keratolytic agents such as tar preparations and salicylic acid decrease shedding of the outer layer of the skin. Topical steroids used are hydrocortisone and betamethasone valerate.

Another treatment, photochemotherapy, involves the use of a drug enhanced by exposure to light. This therapy combines methoxsalen, which is given orally, and the concurrent use of ultraviolet light A (UVA).

Methotrexate and vitamin D reduce epidermal proliferation in some cases. There are several systemic medications approved by the FDA to treat psoriasis, including methotrexate (an antimetabolite), cyclosporine (an immunosuppressant), and acitretin (a retinoid). Infliximab is an example of a biological classification drug used to control the severe plaque form of the disease (Mayo Clinic, 2020d).

Nursing Interventions and Patient Teaching

Nursing interventions include proper administration of the therapeutic modality. Additional rest and measures to promote psychological well-being, such as counseling, are necessary. The patient's emotional needs are as important as the physical needs. Because this disease is chronic, encourage the patient to focus on positive attributes.

Problem identification and interventions for the patient with psoriasis include, but are not limited to, the following:

PATIENT PROBLEM	NURSING INTERVENTIONS
Compromised Skin Integrity, related to proliferation of epithelial cells	Assess extent of the scale Administer treatment method correctly Use medical aseptic technique
Impaired Self-Esteem due to Current Situation, related to change in body image	Assess patient's concept of body Help patient focus on positive aspects Discuss with patient ways to conceal obvious lesions

PATIENT PROBLEM	NURSING INTERVENTIONS
Social Seclusion, related to decreased self-esteem	Assess activity pattern and social outlets Demonstrate ways to conceal lesions with clothes Involve patient in a support group

The primary points in patient teaching include the nature of the disease, correct application of the therapeutic modality, and compliance with medical care. The patient should be taught about factors associated with exacerbation of the condition.

Prognosis

Psoriasis is a chronic disease. The clinical course is variable, but fewer than half of the patients have a prolonged remission. Severity ranges from a minimal cosmetic problem to a life-threatening emergency.

SYSTEMIC LUPUS ERYTHEMATOSUS

The Latin word for wolf, *"lupus,"* is used to describe the skin changes that resemble the erythema of a red wolf (Fig. 3.10). Discoid lupus is an inflammatory condition with skin manifestations that can lead to the autoimmune disease, systemic lupus erythematosus (SLE) (Lupus Foundation of America, 2020).

Etiology and Pathophysiology

SLE is an autoimmune disorder characterized by inflammation of almost any body part. It is a chronic, multisystem inflammatory disorder that occurs when the body produces antibodies against its own cells. The resulting antigen-antibody complexes damage connective tissues. SLE is a disease of exacerbations and remissions. It is distinguished by an inflammatory lesion that affects several organ systems: the skin, joints, kidneys, and serous membranes.

SLE is chronic and incurable, and it has multiple causes. Although the disease's origin remains unknown, increasing evidence suggests that immunologic, hormonal, genetic, and possibly viral factors may contribute to its onset. Genetic predisposition seems to play a role in most cases, coupled with a precipitating agent or factor. The person with SLE has a decreased number of T-suppressor cells, and the remaining T-suppressor cells have a limited function in antibodies developed against antigens.

SLE usually is found in women of childbearing age; only about 10% of cases are men. African Americans are three times more likely than whites to be affected. Survival rates have increased to more than 15 years from diagnosis. Despite advances in treatment, SLE remains a serious illness.

Clinical Manifestations

Clinical manifestations include oral ulcers, arthralgias or arthritis, vasculitis, rash, nephritis, pericarditis, synovitis, organic brain syndromes, peripheral neuropathies, anemia, leukopenia, thrombocytopenia, coagulopathies, immunosuppression, and dermatitis. Anemia tends to be the most common complication (Box 3.2).

Diagnostic Tests

Diagnosis of SLE may require extensive evaluations over months or years. A detailed history, physical examination, and results of laboratory findings are required to confirm the diagnosis. Diagnostic tests for SLE (Box 3.3) often have positive results in the presence of inflammatory disease (Lupus Foundation of America, 2018). No single test is considered conclusive for diagnostic purposes. However, positive results for one or more diagnostic tests, along with at least three other criteria, lead to the diagnosis of SLE. Criteria for diagnosis include the following:

- Alopecia (hair loss), with frontal alopecia seen more frequently in women
- Erythematous butterfly rash (see Fig. 3.10) over the nose and cheeks and along the eyelids
- Hematologic disorders, such as hemolytic anemia, leukopenia, lymphopenia, or thrombocytopenia without other diagnostic reasons
- Immunologic disorder identified with positive lupus erythematosus prep, antinuclear antibody (ANA), or double-stranded DNA
- Neurologic signs, such as seizures of unknown cause
- Oral ulcers
- Other skin features, including bullae, patchy areas of purpura, or thickening of epidermis
- Photosensitivity
- Pleuritic pain, pleural effusion, pericarditis, and vasculitis
- Polyarthralgias and polyarthritis
- Positive ANA in the absence of patient use of drugs known to cause drug-induced lupus erythematosus
- Renal disorders as evidenced by protein or cellular casts in the urine

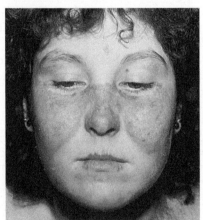

Fig. 3.10 Systemic lupus erythematosus flare. The classic butterfly rash occurs over the nose and cheek area in 10% to 50% of patients with acute cutaneous lupus erythematosus. (From Habif TP, Campbell JL Jr, Chapman MS, et al: *Skin disease: Diagnosis and treatment*, ed 3, St. Louis, 2011, Saunders.)

Box 3.2   Pathogenic Conditions and Clinical Manifestations in Body Systems of People With Systemic Lupus Erythematosus

MUSCULOSKELETAL

Inflammation of vessels, tendons, and muscle tissue occurs because of deposits of fibrin. Polyarthralgia and polyarteritis occur in approximately 90% to 95% of patients.

GASTROINTESTINAL

Ulceration occurs on mucosal membranes because of degeneration of collagen tissue, with gastrointestinal manifestations of hemorrhage, abdominal pain, pancreatitis, cholecystitis, and bowel infarction.

RENAL

Glomerular sclerosis and glomerulonephritis occur with persistent proteinuria or cellular casts in urine.

HEMATOLOGIC

Cells are destroyed, and interference with coagulation occurs because of circulating antibodies. Anemia, leukopenia, lymphopenia, thrombocytopenia, and elevated erythrocyte sedimentation rate result.

CARDIOVASCULAR

Pericarditis is the most common cardiac manifestation. It often is the first clinical problem the patient manifests. Pericardial rub, commonly associated with pericarditis, can lead to dysrhythmias. Vasculitis in the small vessels may occur.

PULMONARY

Pleurisy and pleural effusions resulting from inflammation of the pleura are relatively common.

INTEGUMENTARY

Classic characteristics include the erythematous butterfly rash over the bridge of the nose and on the cheeks and linear erythema along the eyelids (see Fig. 3.10). Other features may include bullae, patchy areas of purpura, urticaria, and subcutaneous nodules.

NEUROLOGIC

Mental and neurologic signs and symptoms occur in 35%–40% of patients with systemic lupus erythematosus. Signs and symptoms relate to the central nervous system, not to the peripheral nerves. Mental and behavioral changes may occur, as well as seizures, headaches, and strokes.

Box 3.3   Diagnostic Tests for Systemic Lupus Erythematosus

- Antinuclear antibody (ANA)
- Anti-Sm antibody
- Chest radiographic study
- Coagulation profile
- Complement
- Complete blood count (CBC)
- Coombs' test
- C-reactive protein (CRP)
- DNA antibody
- Erythrocyte sedimentation rate (ESR; not diagnostic, but used to monitor disease activity and effectiveness of therapy)
- Lupus erythematosus cell preparation (LE cell prep)
- Rapid plasma reagin (RPR)
- Rheumatoid factor (RF)
- Skin and renal biopsy
- Urinalysis

Medical Management

SLE treatment goals include relief of symptoms, remission of the disease, early alleviation of exacerbations, and prevention of untoward complications. Additional outcomes include therapeutic management of the signs and symptoms and suppression of inflammation.

Drug therapy includes nonsteroidal anti-inflammatory agents such as acetylsalicylic acid (ASA; aspirin) and ibuprofen, antimalarial drugs (hydroxychloroquine or chloroquine), and corticosteroids (such as prednisone) in low doses given several times a day. Methylprednisolone may be used intravenously in cases of exacerbation. Peak amounts of steroids help achieve remission. The steroid dosage is decreased slowly (tapered) until a maintenance dosage is reached. Topical corticosteroid creams are used to treat the distinctive SLE rash. Antineoplastic drugs, such as azathioprine or chlorambucil, may be used to achieve remission or to control signs and symptoms.

Antimalarial drugs (e.g., hydroxychloroquine) are used to control discoid and other skin lesions and rheumatic manifestations. Because retinal toxicity may occur at high doses, patients should receive pretreatment and annual ophthalmic examinations.

Anti-infective agents are used to treat and prevent infections in the patient with SLE. The specific antibiotic depends on the infection site. Urinary tract infections respond well to ciprofloxacin.

Peritoneal dialysis or hemodialysis may be indicated in patients who have moderate to severe renal involvement. Laboratory tests assessing blood urea nitrogen (BUN) and serum creatinine provide information regarding kidney function. Analgesics and diuretics may be used to treat symptoms often found in patients with SLE. Supportive therapy such as a balanced diet, a balance between rest and activity, and reduced exposure to the sun also may be indicated.

Nursing Interventions and Patient Teaching

Because SLE is a multisymptom disease, a thorough assessment is necessary. Tailor the care plan to include (1) skin care, including teaching avoidance of direct sunlight and use of protective clothing and sunscreen; (2) a balance between rest and activity; (3) recognition of signs of exacerbation (i.e., fever, rash, cough, or increasing muscle and joint pain); (4) early recognition of signs and symptoms of infection; (5) stress reduction and management; and (6) balanced nutrition and reduced sodium intake. Because the disease is one of exacerbation and remission, each exacerbation will intensify the patient's stress and decrease his or her ability to cope. Provide psychosocial, emotional, and spiritual support for the patient.

The patient with an impaired immune system function must endure the consequences of chronic or incurable disease. A caring, gentle, and understanding approach to patient care will help reduce the burden and stress of SLE (Nursing Care Plan 3.2). The nurse's responsibilities in patient education are related to the information needed to help the patient live a normal life. Focus on activity level, prevention of infection, and potential complications.

 Nursing Care Plan 3.2   **The Patient With Systemic Lupus Erythematosus**

Ms. T., age 34, is experiencing an acute exacerbation of systemic lupus erythematosus. She is admitted to the medical unit with severe joint pain, butterfly rash, generalized edema, and Sjögren's syndrome.

PATIENT PROBLEM
Compromised Skin Integrity, related to skin rash (butterfly across face), hair loss, skin atrophy, discoid lesions involving other parts of the body

Patient Goals and Expected Outcomes	Nursing Interventions	Evaluation and Rationale
Patient will verbalize understanding of skin care regimen and positioning schedule	Develop positioning schedule. Use appropriate devices such as air mattress, egg-crate mattress, sheepskin, or foam padding, where indicated.	Patient verbalizes understanding of the purpose of changing positions q 2 h to prevent skin impairment.
Patient will demonstrate behaviors to promote skin healing	Assess and monitor skin and mucous membranes and describe lesions' size, characteristics, and changes noted. Assess nutritional status and areas at risk for pressure. Measure intake and output. Provide optimum nutrition.	Patient states she understands skin care regimen to promote skin healing.
Patient will experience improved wound and lesion healing	Monitor for signs of infection. Encourage patient to minimize sun exposure by wearing long-sleeved blouses or shirts and wide-brimmed hats and by using sunscreens with a sun protection factor of at least 15. Teach skin care maintenance.	Patient's skin lesions are beginning to show signs of healing.

PATIENT PROBLEM
Distorted Body Image, related to baldness and pathologic skin pattern conditions

Patient Goals and Expected Outcomes	Nursing Interventions	Evaluation and Rationale
Patient will verbalize understanding of altered body image	Assess patient's perception of body image; investigate what aspects are not pleasing and how she perceives changes as deviating from social norms.	Patient states she understands that skin changes and hair loss are part of the disease process of systemic lupus erythematosus.
Patient will have a positive, accepting, and realistic body image	Teach patient ways to improve body image (e.g., improving personal hygiene, wearing makeup, changing type of clothes, protecting self from sun).	
Patient will perform self-care activities within level of own ability		
Patient will identify personal community resources that can provide assistance	Encourage family members and significant others to maintain open communication with patient. Assess and document emotional status. Set limits on maladaptive behavior.	Patient talks about importance of open communication with her family and significant other concerning her feelings of body image disturbance.

CRITICAL THINKING QUESTIONS
1. Ms. T. has painful, edematous joints that greatly decrease her mobility. She has 4+ pitting edema to the lower extremities secondary to the loss of protein through her kidneys. What are the most appropriate nursing interventions to decrease Ms. T.'s pain level and to increase her mobility?
2. On entering the room, the nurse notes Ms. T. crying. She says that her lifestyle is severely altered because she is unable to be in the sun to work in her beloved garden. What nursing interventions would be most beneficial?
3. Ms. T. confides that she fears that this severe increase in her symptoms will lead to an early death. What initial response to this statement would be of greatest assistance?

Prognosis

SLE has no known cure. Management of the disease depends on the nature and severity of the manifestations and the organs affected. Early treatment of SLE contributes to a better prognosis.

PARASITIC DISEASES OF THE SKIN

PEDICULOSIS

Etiology and Pathophysiology

Pediculosis (lice infestation) is a parasitic disorder of the skin. Although the condition is commonly associated with poor living conditions and poor personal hygiene, these are not prerequisites; it can occur anywhere. Lice are transmitted by close contact with either infected individuals or their personal items such as hats, clothing, and grooming items. Once lice find a host, they seek blood. Lice can live only 1 to 2 days without a blood source. They leave their eggs (nits) on the skin surface, attached to hair shafts (Figs. 3.11 and 3.12; CDC, 2019a).

Humans have three types of lice:

1. The head louse, causing pediculosis capitis
2. The body louse, causing pediculosis corporis
3. The pubic louse, causing pediculosis pubis

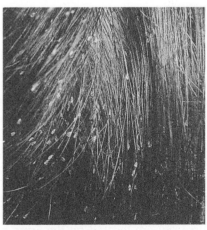

Fig. 3.11 Eggs of *Pediculus* (head lice) attached to shafts of hair. (From Baran R, Dawber RPR, Levene GM: *Color atlas of the hair, scalp, and nails,* St. Louis, 1991, Mosby.)

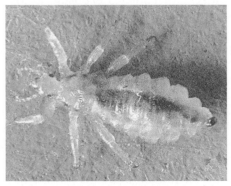

Fig. 3.12 Lice have six legs and are wingless. (From Habif TP: *Clinical dermatology,* ed 4, St. Louis, 2004, Mosby.)

In pediculosis capitis, the head louse attaches itself to the hair shafts. The adult has a relatively short lifespan of 30 days. The adult female may lay up to 10 eggs per day. The eggs are visible at the back of the neck as gray, shiny, oval bodies.

In pediculosis corporis, the body louse is found around the neck, waist, and thighs. The louse generally is found in the seams of clothing and causes severe pruritus and pinpoint hemorrhages.

The pubic louse, the parasite involved in pediculosis pubis, does not resemble the head or body louse. It looks like a crab with sharp pincers that attach to the pubic hair. Transmission can be through sexual contact or contact with infested bed linens or bath towels.

Clinical Manifestations

Nits or lice can be seen on the body. Pinpoints, raised red macules, pinpoint hemorrhages, and severe pruritus confirm the diagnosis. Excoriation is common because of the intense pruritus.

Assessment

Subjective data include complaints of pruritus in the area involved. Tenderness and difficulty wearing clothes also are noted.

Objective data include erythema, petechiae, and skin excoriation in the affected area.

Diagnostic Tests

The diagnostic test is a physical examination of the involved area. A health history supports the diagnosis. Removal of the parasite confirms the diagnosis.

Medical Management

Management may include over-the-counter (OTC) or prescription medications. Initial treatments traditionally begin with OTC preparations. Permethrin or pyrethrin with additives may be used. In the event the infestation is stubborn and repeated treatments are required, prescription strength medications will be employed. Prescription medications include benzyl alcohol, malathion, and lindane. A topical pediculicide such as lindane or pyrethrin is applied to any contaminated area. The specific technique for applying these products varies and should be followed closely to eliminate lice. Once the lice-killing shampoos and rinses are used, the lice and nits will not simply fall off. They must be picked off using a nit comb. The agents used to treat the conditions are pesticides. They cannot be used for children under the age of 2 years or for pregnant women. Occlusive (i.e., air- and water-tight) agents such as petroleum jelly are used to treat an infestation in these groups.

Nursing Interventions and Patient Teaching

The primary nursing intervention involves applying the medication to rid the patient of lice. Identify involved people and appropriate health teaching.

Stress the nature and transmission of the disease. Assess each family member for nits, and teach measures to reduce pruritus, such as cool compresses and corticosteroid ointments. Furniture, carpeting, and car interiors also must be cleaned to prevent reinfection. Bed linens should be washed in hot water and dried in a dryer. Children's stuffed animals may be placed in a hot dryer for a full cycle. Items that cannot be washed may be isolated and bagged in plastic trash bags for a period of time, allowing the lice to die. Assessment of the patient's emotional needs is also important.

Prognosis

The prognosis is good; proper treatment results in full recovery.

SCABIES

Etiology and Pathophysiology

Scabies is caused by the human itch mite *(Sarcoptes scabiei)*. The mite penetrates the skin and makes a burrow. Once under the skin, the mite lays eggs that mature and rise to the skin surface. Scabies is transmitted most often by prolonged contact with an infected individual or contact with infected items such as clothing and bedding. Overcrowded living conditions, poverty, changing sexual behaviors, and world travel have increased the incidence of scabies. Scabies occurs in all age groups and socioeconomic classes.

CLINICAL MANIFESTATIONS

Scabies causes wavy, brown, threadlike lines on the body, especially the hands, arms, body folds, and genitalia (see Table 3.1). Pruritus is severe, and secondary infections are common from the excoriation caused by scratching. The itching is more severe during the nighttime hours.

Assessment

Subjective data include the severe pruritus associated with scabies and the skin excoriation resulting from scratching.

Objective data include finding the wavy brown lines on the body and severe erythema from the scratching. The most common areas for the rash include the webbing between the fingers, wrists, elbows, arm pits, and waistline.

Diagnostic Tests

The condition is diagnosed most often by the presenting symptoms. Confirmation may involve a skin scraping, which may yield the mite.

Medical Management

Medical treatment attempts to eliminate the mite and prevent complications. Crotamiton and a 4% to 8% solution of sulfur in petrolatum may be prescribed to manage the condition. Treatment will also be extended to include sexual and other close contacts of the infected person. Treatment of pets is not necessary.

Nursing Interventions and Patient Teaching

Nursing interventions to restore skin integrity involve using medical aseptic techniques to improve hygiene and to apply medications. Proper application of medication is essential to destroy the parasite. The patient's emotional well-being is another focus of nursing care. Using open-ended questions and listening skills helps provide support.

A primary concern is to educate family members about the transmission of scabies. Each family member needs to treat the whole body with a scabicide. Clothing, bed linens, and bath articles should be washed in hot water and dried using the dryer's hot cycle. If clothes are line dried, they should be ironed. Stress the importance of compliance with the treatment. Parasitic infestations are often embarrassing and result in stress for the family. Conveying a nonjudgmental attitude is important.

Prognosis

The prognosis is good; with adequate treatment, full recovery results.

TUMORS OF THE SKIN

Overgrowth of the skin cells can develop from any layer or its appendages. Most skin tumors are benign. Outgrowths or tumors can be predisposing factors for skin cancer.

Etiology, Pathophysiology, and Clinical Manifestations

The specific signs and symptoms of skin tumors relate to the type of tumor. Keloids, which originate in scars, are hard and shiny. Angiomas resemble birthmarks. Warts (verrucae) are located on the arms and hands. Nevi are thought to predispose a person to cancer, and patients become anxious when they notice a color change. Skin cancers may be life threatening and occur wherever a patient's exposure to the sun was greatest.

Report any changes in a skin lesion to a health care provider, including changes in size, color, border, surface, or elevation. Also, report the development of pain, bleeding, or pruritus.

Assessment

Subjective data should include a good health history. First assess the patient's risk factors, such as lifestyle, occupation, family history, and geographic location.

Objective data include observation of the lesion in detail. The size, the location, and any pain are significant factors in determining the type of skin tumor. The lesion's appearance can take several forms.

Diagnostic Tests
The diagnostic test for skin tumors is biopsy of the lesion. A health history and visual inspection support the diagnosis.

Medical Management
The primary medical intervention for skin tumors is surgical removal. Other treatment modalities are radiation therapy to reduce the size of the tumor and application of topical medications such as corticosteroids to decrease tumor size and inflammation.

Nursing Interventions and Patient Teaching
Patients are understandably concerned about the potential threat of malignancy. Careful explanations of treatments, medications, and tests help decrease anxiety. Nursing interventions center on preparing the patient for the treatment needed. Skin tumors may be a threat to the patient's self-image. Emotional care is important; encourage the patient to verbalize feelings of fear or anxiety.

Problem identification and interventions for malignant melanoma, discussed in an earlier section (see "Assessment of the Skin: Chief Complaint"), are applicable to most skin cancers. Although the tumors previously mentioned are not all malignant, the problems posed are the same until a definitive diagnosis is made.

Discharge instructions include skin care, dressing changes, and follow-up care. Involve the family in teaching so that they can support the patient. Discuss the signs and symptoms of infection with the patient who had a tumor surgically removed.

KELOIDS
Keloids (an overgrowth of collagenous scar tissue at the site of a skin wound) are seen more often in individuals of African descent than in whites. Collagen tissue becomes raised, hard, and shiny. The keloid may be red, pink, or flesh-colored. Keloids usually originate from a scar and can be located anywhere on the body (see Table 3.1). Individuals who are susceptible may develop keloid scarring with ear piercing, surgical intervention, or other injuries to the integument. Management options for the scarring may include corticosteroid injections, cryotherapy, laser surgery, radiation, or surgical removal. The keloid may recur at the same site. Enlargement with return is also a possibility.

ANGIOMAS
An angioma develops when a group of blood vessels dilate and form a tumor-like mass. A common angioma is a birthmark, such as the port-wine birthmark. This discoloration is not elevated and may be found on one side of the face or any part of the body. Treatment involves electrolysis or radiation.

A spider angioma, or telangiectasia, is associated with liver disease. A group of venous capillaries dilate and branch out like a spider. Spider angiomas usually resolve as the disease improves.

VERRUCA (WART)
A verruca is a benign, viral, warty skin lesion with a rough, papillomatous (nipple-like) growth pattern. Warts occur in many forms: they may occur singly or in groups and are thought to be contagious. Common locations are the hands, arms, and fingers, but warts can occur anywhere on the body. The plantar wart develops on the sole of the foot and is extremely painful. Treatment of warts depends on the type, location, and number. Cauterization, solid carbon dioxide (i.e., dry ice), liquid nitrogen, and preparations of salicylic acid are used to remove warts.

NEVI (MOLES)
Nevi (singular, nevus), or moles, are pigmented, congenital skin blemishes that are usually benign but may become cancerous. They are nonvascular tumors, also called birthmarks. There are many types of nevi, and several may become malignant, especially if traumatized. The raised, black nevus is considered one of the most threatening, and removal is recommended to prevent it from becoming malignant. Any change in color, size, or texture or any bleeding or pruritus deserves investigation.

Basal Cell Carcinoma
Basal cell carcinoma is one type of skin cancer. Factors related to the development of skin cancer include frequent contact with certain chemicals, overexposure to the sun, and radiation treatment. Fair-skinned people are more likely to develop skin cancer, possibly because they have less melanin on the skin surface.

Basal cell carcinomas arise in the basal cell layer of the epidermis. They often are found on the face and upper trunk and may not be noticed by the patient. Metastasis is rare, but underlying tissue destruction can progress to include vital structures. Basal cell carcinoma is usually scaly in appearance. It may be a pearly papule with a central crater and waxy, pearly border.

With early detection and complete removal, the outcome is favorable; however, this type of cancer recurs in 40% to 50% of patients treated (Fig. 3.13).

SQUAMOUS CELL CARCINOMA
Squamous cell carcinoma arises in the epidermis. This cancerous neoplasm is a firm, nodular lesion topped with a crust or a central area of ulceration and indurated

margins (Fig. 3.14). Ten percent of patients have rapid invasion with metastasis by way of the lymphatic system, so early detection and treatment are important. Larger tumors are more prone to metastasis.

Sun-exposed areas, especially the head, neck, and lower lip, are common places of occurrence. The cancer also occurs on sites of chronic irritation or injury (scars, irradiated skin, burns, and leg ulcers).

MALIGNANT MELANOMA

Etiology and Pathophysiology

A malignant melanoma is a cancerous neoplasm in which pigment cells (melanocytes) invade the epidermis, dermis, and sometimes the subcutaneous tissue. Several types of melanomas occur, and they are categorized by location and description. Most melanomas arise from melanocytes in the epidermis, but some may appear in preexisting moles. A melanoma can metastasize to any organ, including the brain and heart.

Melanoma is the deadliest skin cancer, and its incidence has doubled in the past two decades, a faster rate of growth compared with any other cancer (Fig. 3.15).

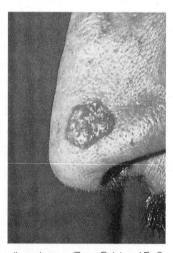

Fig. 3.13 Basal cell carcinoma. (From Belcher AE: *Cancer nursing*, St. Louis, 1992, Mosby.)

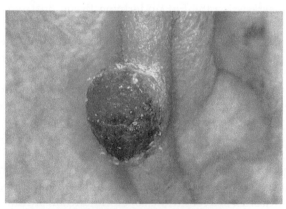

Fig. 3.14 Squamous cell carcinoma.

The increased occurrence is associated with recreational exposure to the sun (see the Evidence-Based Practice box). Heredity is also a factor, and any person who has a large number of moles with a variety of sizes and colors should be monitored. The person with a history of skin cancer is at greater risk.

Clinical Manifestations

Malignant melanomas are divided into four primary types: (1) superficial spreading melanomas, (2) lentigo malignant melanomas, (3) nodular melanomas, and (4) acral lentiginous melanomas.

Superficial spreading melanomas are the most common and may occur anywhere on the body. These melanomas are slightly elevated, irregularly shaped lesions in varying hues. Common colors are tan, brown, black, blue, gray, and pink. Lentigo malignant melanomas usually are found on the heads and necks of older adults. Characteristically these appear as tan, flat lesions that change in shape and size. Nodular melanomas appear as a blueberry-like growth, varying from blue-black to pink. The patient often describes the lesion as a blood blister that fails to resolve. Nodular melanomas grow and metastasize faster than the other types. Acral lentiginous melanomas occur in areas not exposed to sunlight and where no hair follicles are present. Common locations are the hands, soles, and mucous membranes of dark-skinned people.

Assessment

Subjective data should include a thorough health history related to skin cancer. Patients at greatest risk have fair complexions, blue eyes, red or blond hair, and freckles.

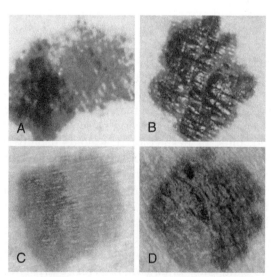

Fig. 3.15 The ABCDs of melanoma. (A) Asymmetry (one half unlike the other). (B) Border (irregularly scalloped or poorly circumscribed border). (C) Color varied from one area to another; shades of tan and brown, black, and sometimes white, red, or blue; change in shape, size, or color of mole. (D) Diameter larger than 6 mm as a rule (diameter of a pencil eraser). (From Habit TP: *Clinical dermatology*, ed 4, St. Louis, 2004, Mosby.)

Skin Cancer Prevention

RESEARCH SUMMARY

What is cancer? More specifically, what is skin cancer? Cancer is an uncontrolled growth and spread of abnormal cells. Therefore, skin cancer is characterized by abnormal skin cells, which can spread and invade other tissues. More importantly, what can we do about skin cancer? As nurses, it becomes our responsibility to assess for and educate our patients about all types of skin cancer, especially for the most serious form called melanoma. There are several risk factors for melanoma. The greatest risk is exposure to ultraviolet (UV) light. Additional factors include a family history of melanoma, a prior melanoma, and multiple or unusual moles. Other factors include a fair complexion/skin that is sensitive to the sun, and the use of tanning beds or booths.

Research has indicated that skin cancer, when detected early and treated properly, is highly curable. Overall survival rates for melanoma are 97% at 5 years and 95% at 10 years, so early intervention is of the utmost importance.

APPLICATION TO NURSING PRACTICE

The results of research studies have made it a nursing responsibility to screen patients and intervene when it is in their best interest. It is necessary that we promote self-screening for all patients and their family members. We also must educate the general public.

- Instruct patients to conduct a complete monthly self-examination of the skin and scalp, noting moles, blemishes, and birthmarks.
- Perform the examination after a bath or shower, including a head-to-toe check.
- Use a well-lit room and mirrors to examine all skin surfaces. If necessary, have the patient ask a family member/significant other to aid in the investigation.
- The American Cancer Society outlines the warning signs of skin cancer, using the ABCDE mnemonic: A is for Asymmetry—look for uneven shape; B is for Border irregularity—look for edges that are blurred, notched, or ragged; C is for Color—pigmentation is not uniform (blue, black, brown variegated and areas of pink, white, gray, blue, or red are abnormal); D is for Diameter—greater than the size of a typical pencil eraser; and E is for Evolving—in size, shape, or color.
- Teach your patients to contact their health care provider if a skin lesion or mole starts to bleed or ooze or feels different (swollen, hard, lumpy, itchy, or tender to the touch). Especially instruct older adults, who tend to have delayed wound healing.
- Inform your patients of ways to prevent skin cancer by avoiding overexposure to the sun:
  - Wear wide-brimmed hats and long sleeves.
  - Apply broad-spectrum sunscreens with a sun protection factor (SPF) of 15 or greater to protect against ultraviolet B (UVB) and ultraviolet A (UVA) rays approximately 15 minutes before going into the sun and after swimming or perspiring. Reapply every 2 hours.
  - Avoid tanning under the direct sun at midday (10 a.m. to 4 p.m.).
  - Do not use indoor sunlamps, tanning parlors, or tanning pills.
  - Inform patients who are on medications that make the skin more sensitive to the sun (e.g., oral contraceptives, antibiotics, anti-inflammatories, antihypertensives, immunosuppressives) to take extra precautions when spending time in the sun.
  - Advise patients to protect their children from the sun. Severe sunburns in childhood greatly increase melanoma risk later in life.

These interventions will provide the patient with self-screening measures to detect, prevent, and seek early treatment for skin cancer.

CDC, 2021; Cancer.net, 2021.

Objective data include the location, color, and appearance of the lesions.

Diagnostic Tests

Diagnosis depends primarily on the results of the tissue biopsy. The patient also is examined thoroughly for suspicious lesions. Monitor any lesion that is variegated in color or has an irregular border or surface. The tumor thickness at the time of diagnosis is a key factor in the prognosis of malignant melanoma.

Medical Management

Medical management depends on the site, level of invasion, thickness of the melanoma, and the patient's age and general health.

A wide surgical excision of the primary lesion with a margin of normal skin is the treatment of choice. Skin grafts sometimes are needed. Subsequent treatment modalities such as chemotherapy, nonspecific immunotherapy, chemoimmunotherapy, and radiation may be planned, depending on the stage of the disease.

Nursing Interventions and Patient Teaching

The major goals of nursing care include pain relief, reduction of anxiety, and palliative treatment of the disease. Fear of the unknown is a major concern for the patient with a melanoma. Explaining procedures and diagnostic tests in terms that the patient can understand may help decrease anxiety.

Problem identification and interventions for the patient with melanomas include, but are not limited to, the following:

PATIENT PROBLEM	NURSING INTERVENTIONS
Recent Onset of Pain, related to lesion	Use the mnemonic PQRST to assess the chief complaint[a]
	Provide nursing comfort measures, such as back rubs, to decrease pain
	Administer pain medication as needed
	Teach relaxation techniques

PATIENT PROBLEM	NURSING INTERVENTIONS
Anxiousness, related to cancer, its treatment, and prognosis	Listen to and accept expression of anger, sadness, and helplessness

aSee "Assessment of the Skin: Chief Complaint" earlier in this chapter.

Discharge instructions include wound care, medication, cleansing, and follow-up care. Assess the family's knowledge about the seriousness and treatment of the disease. Explain to the patient the need for regular physical examinations and regular skin self-assessment. Encourage the patient to protect skin from the sun by using sunscreens and protective clothing and by limiting exposure. Stress the use of medical aseptic techniques to prevent a secondary infection.

Prognosis

The key prognostic factor in malignant melanoma is the thickness of the lesion. Individuals with lesions less than 1 mm thick have a survival rate of almost 100%, whereas those with lesions 3 mm thick or thicker have survival rates of less than 50%. If the cancer spreads to regional lymph nodes, the patient has a 65% 5-year survival rate. The tumor may metastasize by vascular or lymphatic spread, with rapid movement of melanoma cells to other parts of the body. If metastasis occurs, treatment is largely palliative (American Cancer Society, 2020).

DISORDERS OF THE APPENDAGES

ALOPECIA

Alopecia is the loss of hair. The cause can be aging, drugs such as antineoplastics, anxiety, or disease processes. Unless it is related to aging, alopecia is usually not permanent; the hair usually grows back but can take several months. Any time a patient loses hair, body image and self-esteem are threatened.

HYPERTRICHOSIS (HIRSUTISM)

Hypertrichosis is an excessive growth of hair in a masculine distribution. It can be hereditary or acquired as a result of hormone dysfunction and medications. Treatment is removal by dermabrasion, electrolysis, chemical depilation, shaving, tweezing, or rubbing with pumice. Treatment of the cause usually stops growth of additional hair.

HYPOTRICHOSIS

Hypotrichosis is the absence of hair or a decrease in hair growth. Skin disease, endocrine problems, and malnutrition are associated factors. Treatment involves identifying and treating the cause.

PARONYCHIA

Paronychia is a disorder of the nails. The nails get soft or brittle, and the shape can change as they grow into the soft tissue (ingrown nails). In paronychia, an infection of the nail develops and spreads around the nail, thus giving it the nickname "runaround." The nails are painful as they loosen and separate from the tissue. Wet dressings or topical antibiotics may be used. Sometimes a surgical incision and drainage of the infected area are performed.

BURNS

Etiology and Pathophysiology

Between 2011 and 2015, approximately 486,000 people in the United States sought medical attention for burns. About 40,000 of them required hospitalization. The number of deaths from burn injuries or smoke inhalation was 3390 (American Burn Association, 2018). The survival rate for individuals admitted to burn facilities was 96.8% from 2011 to 2015 (American Burn Association, 2018). The high survival rate for burn patients stems from the creation of regional burn centers, as well as a national focus on fire safety, the use of smoke detectors, and occupational safety mandates.

Burns may result from thermal or nonthermal causes. Thermal burns are caused by flames, scalds, and thermal energy (heat) and are the most common type of burn injury. Nonthermal burns result from electricity, chemicals, and radiation. Skin destruction depends on the burning agent, temperature of the burning agent, condition of the skin before the injury, and duration of the person's contact with the agent.

 Safety Alert

Prevention of Burns

- The major cause of fires in the home is carelessness with cigarettes. Preventive education is imperative.
- Other causes of burns include hot water from water heaters set higher than 140°F (60°C), cooking accidents, space heaters, combustibles such as gasoline and charcoal lighter fluid, steam from radiators, and chemicals.
- Most burns can be prevented. The nurse is in a good position to conduct home safety assessments and to educate people about burn injuries before accidents occur. Home safety measures include using smoke alarms and fire extinguishers. Families should have fire drills, and each family member should know where to go and what to do in case of a fire.
- Local fire departments can inform the public of regional fire codes and perform home safety checks.
- Knowledge of potential sources of burn injury allows problem solving for burn prevention.

Teaching people the proper use of appliances (e.g., space heaters, electrical cords, wiring, outlets, outdoor grills, and water heaters) can prevent burn injury.

Burns cause dramatic changes in most physiologic functions of the body, beginning in the first few minutes to the first 12 to 24 hours after the burn injury. The burn's effect depends on two factors: the extent of the body surface burned and the depth of the burn injury.

The extent of burn is measured in terms of the total body surface area (TBSA) injured. Burns exceeding 20% TBSA result in massive evaporative water losses and fluid losses into the interstitial spaces. Depth depends on the layers of the skin involved.

With any burn injury, a pathophysiologic process ensues. In the damaged area, the capillaries dilate, resulting in capillary hyperpermeability that lasts for about 24 hours. The increased cell permeability causes the fluid to shift from the capillaries into the surrounding tissues (interstitial spaces), resulting in edema and vesiculation (blistering). A larger burned area results in a more rapid shift of fluid from the intravascular area into the interstitial area (sometimes known as third spacing). This shift poses the greatest threat to life because the cells become dehydrated. As a result, the body experiences hypovolemic shock and hyperviscosity. Blood pressure and blood flow to the kidneys decrease, symptoms of hypovolemic shock develop, and acute renal failure may result.

The pathophysiology and care of burns may be divided into three stages:

Stage 1, the emergent phase, is from the onset of the injury until the patient stabilizes. Hypovolemic shock is the major concern for up to 48 hours after a major burn.

Stage 2, the intermediate or acute (or diuretic) phase, begins 48 to 72 hours after the burn injury. In this stage, the greatest concern is circulatory overload. Circulatory overload may result from the fluid shift back from the interstitial spaces into the capillaries. The acute phase begins when the kidneys excrete large volumes of urine (hence the name diuretic stage).

Stage 3, the long-term rehabilitation phase, begins at the same time as burn wound treatment. In the third stage, the patient care outcome involves returning the patient to as normal a state as possible. A second outcome is freedom from wound infection.

In a burn injury, usually the greatest fluid loss occurs within the first 12 hours. The proteins, plasma, and electrolytes shift from the vascular compartment to the interstitial compartment. Red blood cells tend to remain in the vascular system, causing increased viscosity of the blood and a falsely elevated hematocrit level. Acute dehydration is present, and renal perfusion is seriously compromised. This fluid shift and the loss of intravascular fluids may lead to the development of burn shock. The rapid loss of fluid places a strain on the heart because the blood volume diminishes, and the heart can no longer supply enough blood to perfuse the vital organs. The body responds by increasing the peripheral resistance. Burn shock is characterized by hypotension, decreased urinary output, increased pulse (tachycardia), rapid and shallow respirations (tachypnea), and restlessness. Most deaths from burns result directly from burn shock.

Fluids begin to shift back to the vascular compartment in approximately 48 to 72 hours. Fluid return denotes the end of the hypovolemic stage and the beginning of the diuretic stage. Reabsorption of the interstitial fluid back into the intravascular area causes an increase in blood volume. As the blood volume increases, the cardiac output increases, resulting in increased renal perfusion. The result includes diuresis. Rapid movement of fluid back into the intravascular space puts the patient at risk for fluid overload. Monitor the patient's vital signs, urinary output, and level of consciousness. Patients with preexisting cardiac problems, as well as the very young and very old, run the greatest risk for circulatory overload.

A burn victim may experience smoke inhalation damage from breathing the chemicals produced by the burn. The fumes damage the cilia and the mucosa of the respiratory tract. Alveolar surfactant decreases, and atelectasis can occur. Breathing difficulties may take several hours to appear. While assessing a patient who has sustained any burn to the upper chest, neck, or face, consider the patient at high risk for respiratory distress. Signs of respiratory difficulty include a hoarse voice or a productive cough. Other physical findings suggesting an inhalation injury include the following:

- Singed nasal hairs
- Agitation, tachypnea, flaring nostrils, or intercostal retractions
- Brassy cough, grunting, or guttural respiratory sounds
- Erythema or edema of the oropharynx or nasopharynx
- Sooty sputum

Clinical Manifestations

Traditionally, burns were classified as first, second, or third degree (Table 3.5). However, using only the visual characteristics of the burn wound results in an inaccurate description. A more accurate classification is superficial thickness injuries, partial-thickness injuries, and full-thickness injuries. These terms graphically describe the burn and indicate the depth and severity of the tissue injury (Figs. 3.16 to 3.18).

Assessment

The nursing assessment includes (1) depth of the burn, (2) causative agent, (3) temperature and duration of contact, and (4) skin thickness. The patient's age and other disease processes affect the outcome of the burn. The rule of nines determines the TBSA burned (Fig. 3.19). The rule of nines divides the body into multiples of nine. The entire head is 9%; the anterior and posterior aspects of the arms are a total of 9% each; the legs are 9% anterior and 9% posterior; the chest and back are 18% each; and the perineum is 1%.

NOTE: The rule of nines does not take into account the different levels of growth and is not accurate for children.

Table 3.5   **Causes and Factors Determining Depth of Burn Injury**

DEPTH	CAUSE	APPEARANCE	COLOR	SENSATION
Superficial (first degree)	Flash flame, ultraviolet light (sunburn)	Dry, no vesicles Minimal or no edema Blanches with fingertip pressure, and refills when pressure is removed	Increased erythema	Painful
Partial thickness (second degree)	Contact with hot liquids or solids Flash flame to clothing Direct flame Chemicals Ultraviolet light	Large, moist vesicles that increase in size Blanches with fingertip pressure and refills when pressure is removed	Mottled with dull, white, tan, pink, or cherry red areas	Very painful
Full thickness (third degree)	Contact with hot liquids or solids Flame Chemicals Electrical contact	Dry with leathery eschar Charred vessels visible under eschar Vesicles rare, but thin-walled vesicles that do not increase in size may be present No blanching with pressure	White, charred, dark tan Black Red	Little or no pain Hair easily pulls out

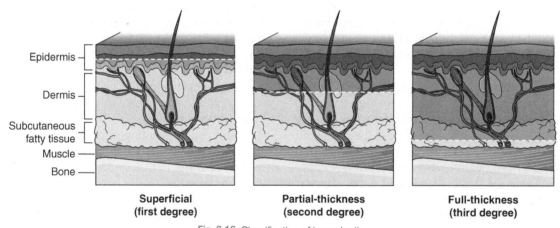

Epidermis

Dermis

Subcutaneous fatty tissue

Muscle

Bone

Superficial (first degree)   **Partial-thickness (second degree)**   **Full-thickness (third degree)**

Fig. 3.16 Classification of burn depth.

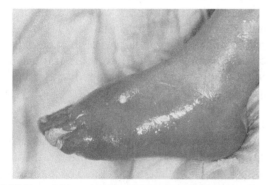

Fig. 3.17 Superficial partial-thickness injury. (Courtesy Intermountain Burn Center, University of Utah, Salt Lake City, UT.)

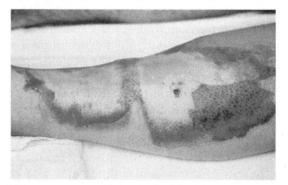

Fig. 3.18 Full-thickness thermal injury. (Courtesy Intermountain Burn Center, University of Utah, Salt Lake City, UT.)

Subjective data include the causative agent, other diseases present, the temperature and duration of contact, and the patient's age. If the patient is able to communicate, ask him or her to rate the pain on a scale from 0 to 10.

Objective data include the depth of the burn, the skin thickness involved, the percentage of TBSA burned, the specific location, and any other injuries

sustained. Any time a patient has a burn that involves the face, neck, or chest, observe for respiratory difficulty. Determine whether the victim has had a tetanus booster in the past 5 years.

The severity of the burn depends on several factors. Major burns require the most skilled nursing interventions. Moderate and minor burns require fewer

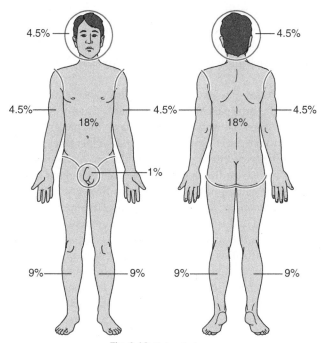

Fig. 3.19 Rule of nines.

nursing interventions. Factors determining a major, moderate, or minor burn are the (1) percentage of the TBSA burned, (2) victim's age, (3) specific location of the burn, (4) cause of the burn, (5) other diseases present, (6) depth of the burn, and (7) injuries sustained during the burn (Box 3.4).

Diagnostic Tests

The primary diagnostic test is a physical examination to determine the amount of burned area. Blood

---

Box **3.4**   **Classification of Severity of Burns**

MAJOR BURN INJURIES
- Burns complicated by inhalation injury or major trauma
- Burns in patients with preexisting disease (diabetes, heart failure, or chronic renal failure)
- Electrical burns
- Greater than 10% of total body surface area (TBSA), full thickness
- Greater than 25% of TBSA (greater than 20% in children younger than 10 years of age, and in adults older than 40 years of age)
- Involvement of face, eyes, ears, hands, feet, perineum

MODERATE BURN INJURIES
- 15%–25% TBSA in adults, partial thickness (10%–20% TBSA in children younger 10 years of age and adults older than 40 years of age)
- Burns in patients with no preexisting disease
- Burns with no concurrent injury
- Less than 10% TBSA, full thickness

MINOR BURN INJURIES
- Burns in patients with no preexisting disease
- Less than 15% TBSA in adults (less than 10% in children or older adults)
- Less than 2% TBSA, full thickness

---

assessments—such as those for electrolytes, CBC, serum chemistries, and arterial blood gases—may help establish the severity of dehydration. In inhalation burns, the carboxyhemoglobin level is evaluated. Most fatalities occur among survivors with severe asphyxiation or carbon monoxide intoxication. Carbon monoxide (CO) binds to hemoglobin with greater affinity than does oxygen, resulting in tissue hypoxia.

Medical Management

The medical treatment of burns is divided into three phases with differing priorities. Remember that these phases are not always clearly defined and may overlap.

Emergent Phase

The primary concern in the emergent phase is to stop the burning process, using the "stop, drop, and roll" technique. Also, removing clothing, shoes, and jewelry from the victim may eliminate the source of the burn to arrest skin damage. Do not apply ice to burns because it can cause rapid vasoconstriction, which may cause more trauma to the tissues by increasing the depth of the burn.

The second step is to provide an open airway; the third is to control bleeding. Fourth, remove all nonadherent clothing and jewelry (rings, watches). Fifth, cover the victim with a clean sheet or cloth. Sixth, transport the victim to the hospital. In the case of a chemical burn, it is important to rinse the skin generously with water to remove all chemicals. Electrical burns have an entry point and an exit point that must be identified. Most electrical burns result in cardiac arrest, and the patient requires cardiopulmonary resuscitation or astute cardiac monitoring.

During the primary survey assessment, quickly assess the ABCs (airway, breathing, and circulation) and look for life-threatening injuries, such as blunt chest trauma. Assessment of the patient's airway becomes and remains the priority of nursing care. Suspect an inhalation injury, especially if the burn occurred in a closed or confined area. Signs and symptoms of inhalation injury include singed facial hair, black-tinged sputum, soot in the throat, hoarseness, and neck or face burns. Stridor is a life-threatening sign.

Carbon monoxide (CO) poisoning is likely if the patient was in an enclosed area. CO displaces oxygen from hemoglobin. Do not rely on pulse oximetry to rule out CO poisoning. Oximeters cannot distinguish between oxyhemoglobin and carboxyhemoglobin. The carboxyhemoglobin level should be measured, when feasible, by means of a blood sample. Early signs of CO poisoning include headache, nausea, vomiting, and unsteady gait. Treatment includes administering 100% oxygen.

Once the patient is in the hospital, the severity of the burn dictates the care given. Perform a thorough assessment every 30 minutes to 1 hour in the emergent phase. Patients with major burns generally are transferred to burn care centers or units for treatment but must be stabilized first. Patients with moderate to severe burns are treated using the following steps:

1. Establish airway. Administer oxygen as ordered. Often the health care provider inserts an endotracheal tube to ensure a patent airway (Fig. 3.20).
2. Initiate fluid therapy. Begin intravenous fluid therapy with Ringer's lactate solution immediately. The amount of fluid given is related to the percentage of TBSA burned. Weigh the patient so that the health care provider can determine the amount of fluids needed.
3. Insert a Foley catheter to determine hourly urinary output. An hourly output of 30 to 50 mL is recommended. Intravenous fluids are given to maintain renal perfusion (Box 3.5).
4. Insert a nasogastric tube to prevent aspiration. Patients with severe burns often develop a paralytic ileus as a result of trauma.
5. Administer analgesics intravenously in small, frequent doses for pain control. Morphine may be used. Any degree of hypovolemia can increase the effects of medications. Carefully assess the patient's respiratory status when administering morphine.
6. Maintain airway and fluid status and monitor vital signs.
7. Give tetanus immunization prophylaxis as needed. (Patients who have been immunized against tetanus do not need a tetanus toxoid booster unless the last injection was more than 5 years ago. If the patient has never had a tetanus immunization, administer tetanus serum and active immunization in the emergency department.)

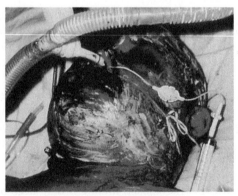

Fig. 3.20 Endotracheal intubation for patient with severe edema 5 hours after a burn injury. (Courtesy Burn Center, Cleveland Metropolitan General Hospital, Cleveland, OH.)

Box 3.5   Indications for Fluid Resuscitation

- Burns greater than 10% of total body surface area (TBSA) in children
- Burns greater than 20% of TBSA in adults
- Electrical burns
- Patient older than 55 or younger than 4 years of age
- Patient with preexisting disease that would reduce normal compensatory responses to minor hypovolemia (cardiac or pulmonary disease, diabetes)

The first 72 hours require diligent medical care. The primary goals in the emergent phase are to maintain respiratory integrity and to prevent hypovolemic shock, which may result in death (Box 3.6).

Acute phase. The acute phase begins when fluids shift back to the intravascular compartment, usually 72 hours after the burn. During the acute phase, the patient's metabolism increases. Urinary output also increases as the fluid shifts back into the blood circulation. As the urinary output increases, the edema in the tissues begins to decrease. The acute phase may last from 10 days to months. The two primary treatment goals are treatment of the burn wound and prevention and management of complications. Infection is the most common complication and cause of death after the first 72 hours. Other complications include heart failure, renal failure, **contractures** (shortening or tension of muscles that affects extension), paralytic ileus causing gastric dilation, and **Curling's ulcer** (a duodenal ulcer that develops 8 to 14 days after severe burns on the surface of the body; the first sign is usually vomiting of bright red blood).

Nursing Interventions. Prioritizing nursing care, using the ABCs, remains the most important nursing intervention. After completing the ABCs, gather data in a head-to-toe assessment concerning (1) respiratory pattern, (2) vital signs, (3) circulation, (4) intake and output, (5) ambulation, (6) bowel sounds, (7) inspection of the wound itself, and (8) mental status.

Fluid-reshifting complications may also develop during the acute phase if renal damage has occurred. Monitor the patient for signs of acute renal failure such as elevated serum creatinine and BUN. Electrolyte

---

Box 3.6   Patient Problems Seen in the Emergent Phase of Burns

- Compromised Skin Integrity, related to damage by the burns
- Compromised Swallowing Ability, related to mucosal edema
- Compromised Verbal Communication, related to breathing difficulties
- Inability to Clear Airway, related to edema of the respiratory passages
- Inadequate Fluid Volume (dehydration), related to shift of body fluids
- Inadequate Fluid Volume, related to capillary hyperpermeability with fluid moving out of the cells into the interstitial area
- Ineffective Sleep Pattern, related to hospital environment
- Insufficient Cardiac Output, related to hypovolemia
- Potential for Aspiration into Airway, related to decreased peristalsis
- Potential for Infection, related to impairment of skin integrity
- Recent Onset of Anxiousness, related to injury
- Recent Onset of Pain, related to loss of skin

levels also must be monitored closely. Serum potassium levels may rise sharply in the first 72 hours. Heart failure may develop as a result of the rapid increase in blood volume from the return of fluid from the interstitial spaces into the intravascular vessels. The primary goals in the acute phase include proper care of the burn wound to promote healing and prevent infection and the prevention and treatment of complications. Assessment for infection of the burn wound includes observing the wound for increasing erythema, odor, or a green or yellow exudate. Local and systemic infections complicate recovery and increase recovery time. Wound cultures and sensitivities help pinpoint the type of organism present and the most effective antibiotic for treatment. Report any signs of an infection.

Once the patient's vital signs and urinary output stabilize and the acute phase begins, complete a nutritional assessment. Provision for adequate nutrition remains a cornerstone of burn care during the acute phase. Increased amounts of protein, calories, and vitamins help repair the damaged tissue. Encourage oral intake of nutrients as soon as possible. The nutritional challenge includes providing enough nutrients to meet the body's increased metabolic requirement. Monitor nutritional status through daily measurement of weight, serum electrolytes, and serum albumin and through urinalysis. Adequate nutrition decreases healing time, whereas weight loss increases healing time. Skin grafts will not be successful unless nutrition is adequate.

Nursing interventions include measures to control pain and to support the patient's psychological well-being. Intravenous opioids in small, frequent doses provide relief from pain, but care must be taken to avoid jeopardizing respiratory integrity. Specific interventions include verbal support, unhurried care, truthful explanations, and effective listening. Excellent communication skills are essential.

Protective isolation is necessary when the skin is damaged. Wear a gown, mask, cap, and gloves during each contact with a patient with major burns. Follow strict surgical aseptic technique during dressing changes. Use of proper equipment and cleaning procedures is imperative. Hydrotherapy (e.g., whirlpool) can be a source of infection.

The standard treatment for partial-thickness burns includes debriding the wound, applying topical antibiotics, and changing dressings twice a day. A new treatment for burns includes temporary skin substitutes. Made from a variety of materials, skin substitutes promote faster healing for burn wounds and can eliminate painful dressing changes and minimize scarring. In 1997, TransCyte—a temporary bioengineered skin substitute—became the first such product to be approved by the FDA for burn treatment. TransCyte is designed as an alternative to silver sulfadiazine for patients with partial-thickness burns and to cadaver skin for full-thickness burns and deep partial-thickness

burns requiring surgical debridement. It is made from neonatal human fibroblast cells. The fibroblasts secrete human derma, collagen, matrix proteins, and growth factors. All these factors promote wound healing. TransCyte typically is applied only once, thus avoiding the frequent, painful dressing changes. TransCyte provides a temporary covering that helps protect against fluid loss and reduces the risk of infection.

A new and highly successful skin replacement therapy, based on the Integra Dermal Regeneration Template, is being used in the treatment of life-threatening, full-thickness, or deep partial-thickness burn wounds. Within the first few days of admission, the patient goes to surgery, the wound is debrided, and the Integra artificial skin is applied. The wound then is wrapped with dressings. The artificial skin stimulates regeneration of new dermis by the body. During a second surgical procedure, the artificial skin is removed and replaced by the patient's own autografts (US Food and Drug Administration, n.d.).

Traditional wound care involves the removal of the eschar that forms. Eschar is a black, leathery crust (i.e., a slough) that the body forms over burned tissue; eschar can harbor microorganisms and cause infection. It also may compromise circulatory status. An escharotomy often is done to relieve circulatory constriction (Fig. 3.21). Daily debridement (removal of damaged tissue and cellular debris from a wound or burn to prevent infection and to promote healing) and special cleansing support regeneration of the tissues. Hydrotherapy softens the eschar to make removal less painful. It also promotes range of motion to decrease contractures.

The specific wound care method depends on the severity of the burn. The open or exposure method may be used for burns of the face, neck, ears, and perineum. The area is cleaned and exposed to air. A hard crust forms, and regeneration of tissue follows.

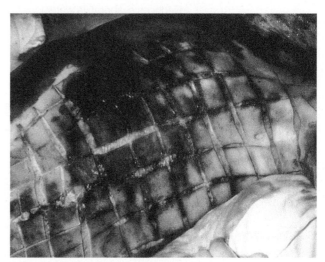

Fig. 3.21 Grid escharotomy used to alleviate circulatory and pulmonary constriction. (Courtesy Burn Center, Cleveland Metropolitan General Hospital, Cleveland, OH.)

Proper positioning and range-of-motion exercises (facilitated by the nurse and physical therapist) are vital for the burn patient's well-being. Special bed equipment is needed to prevent the burn from touching the linens. A bed cradle, a CircOlectric bed, or a Clinitron bed is recommended. Chilling may be controlled by keeping the room temperature at 85°F (29.4°C) and providing lights or heat lamps for additional warmth. Humidity should be between 40% and 50%.

Advantages to the open method are that (1) the wound can be observed more easily, (2) movement in bed is less restricted, (3) circulation of the body part is not restricted, and (4) exercises can be done more easily to prevent contractures. Disadvantages are (1) pain, (2) chilling, (3) contamination of wound by the health care provider, (4) unattractive appearance, which causes emotional distress, and (5) the need for protective isolation precautions for the immunocompromised patient.

Control the pain with intravenously administered opioids in the early days of the acute phase. Diazepam has been found to be effective, but morphine commonly is used.

The closed (or occlusive) method involves cleaning the burn, applying the prescribed medication, and dressing the wound as ordered. Advantages of the closed method are that (1) it protects the burn area from injury, and (2) it prevents contamination of the area by the health care provider. Circulation checks are important with pressure dressings to assess for adequate arterial perfusion to the involved areas.

The topical medications used to hasten healing and prevent infection vary. Topical administration is preferred because the capillaries are coagulated by the burn. Mafenide (Sulfamylon), silver sulfadiazine, and silver nitrate are drugs commonly used in burn care. Each drug has specific advantages and disadvantages (Table 3.6).

Burn care essentials include a lightweight dressing. A single layer of gauze covered with medication and a single wrap of Kerlix provide adequate coverage. When applying gauze to the burn area, place gauze between skin areas that touch to prevent skin-to-skin contact.

Changing burn dressings is painful. Therefore, 30 minutes before the procedure, administer an analgesic such as intravenous morphine sulfate or a sedative. Most dressings are changed after hydrotherapy. Remove all old medication and eschar before applying any new medication. Failure to debride promotes infection, delays healing, and increases scarring.

Table 3.6 Topical Medications for Burn Therapy Skin Grafts

GENERIC NAME (TRADE NAME)	ADVANTAGES	DISADVANTAGES
mafenide	Bacteriostatic against gram-negative and gram-positive organisms Penetrates thick eschar	Metabolic acidosis Pain on application Allergic rash
silver sulfadiazine	Broad antimicrobial activity against gram-negative, gram-positive, and *Candida* organisms No electrolyte imbalances Painless and somewhat soothing Not nephrotoxic	With repeated application, skin may develop slimy, grayish appearance, simulating an infection despite negative cultures Prolonged use may cause skin rash and depress granulocyte formation
silver nitrate	Bacteriostatic effect Lessens pain and eliminates odor Reduces evaporative water loss from burns	Electrolyte imbalances Stains everything it comes into contact with Does not penetrate eschar Pain on application
gentamicin sulfate	Broad antimicrobial activity Painless	Ototoxicity Nephrotoxicity Development of resistant bacterial strains
Neomycin	Broad antimicrobial activity Causes miscoding in the messenger RNA of bacterial cells	Serious toxic effects Ototoxicity Nephrotoxicity
Xeroform	Nonantiseptic Debrides and protects donor site Protects graft	Removal may be painful because it sometimes adheres to wound Neither antiseptic nor antimicrobial
sodium hypochlorite (Dakin's solution)	Chlorine-based solution that is bactericidal Aids in debriding wounds Aids cleaning of copious drainage	Dissolves blood clots May inhibit clotting May irritate the skin
Sutilains ointment	Topical enzymatic agent Dissolves necrotic tissue by proteolytic action Facilitates removal of eschar and purulent drainage	Mild, transient pain on application Paresthesia, bleeding, dermatitis Dressing must be kept moist at all times

RNA, Ribonucleic acid.
Based on data from Emedicine.com, 2019.

Skin grafts are used as soon as possible to cover full-thickness burns. Grafting promotes healing and prevents infection. Grafting generally occurs during the first 3 weeks of care. Four types of grafts may be used:

1. An autograft: Surgical transplantation of any tissue from one part of the body to another location in the same patient
2. A homograft (allograft): The transfer of tissue between two genetically dissimilar individuals of the same species, such as a skin transplant from another person who is not an identical twin (often a cadaver)
3. A heterograft (xenograft): Tissue from another species, such as a pig or a cow, used as a temporary graft
4. A synthetic graft substitute: The autograft is permanent, whereas the other types are temporary

Grafts are applied by either the pedicle method (the tissue is left partially attached to the donor site and the other portion of the tissue is attached to the burn site) or the freestanding method (the tissue is removed completely from the donor site and is attached to the burn site) (Chrysopoulo, 2017).

Graft sites are a nursing challenge. Any movement that results in pulling the graft area can dislodge the graft. Do not change dressings until ordered. The donor site resembles a partial-thickness burn after the graft. Donor site care is as important as care of the burn site. Inspect the donor site for signs of infection, such as erythema and malodor (see the Patient Teaching box). Pain is a primary complaint after the graft and should be treated.

Patient Teaching

Skin Grafts

- Do not remove dressing unless ordered.
- Keep surface of healed graft moistened daily with skin lotion for 6–12 months. (Grafted skin does not perspire; it dries and cracks easily.)
- Protect grafted skin from direct sunlight with a sunscreen lotion for at least 6 months.
- Report changes in the graft (hematoma, fluid collection) to health care provider.
- Wear a strong elastic stocking for 4–6 months for grafts on lower extremities.

The nutritional aspect of burn care is another nursing challenge. Destroyed body proteins and fluid loss present problems as the body increases metabolism to meet the extra demands for healing. Therefore, the body requires enough energy to maintain homeostasis while meeting the increased need for repairing the injury.

Burn patients should eat by mouth as soon as their condition permits. Protein requirements are increased. Normal protein intake is usually 0.8 g/kg of body weight, whereas the burned patient requires 1.5 to 2.0 g/kg[5] of body weight. Thus, a normal 150 lb. person needs 55 g of protein per day. If burned, the same person needs 102 to 158 g of protein, depending on the extent of the burn. Daily caloric requirements range from 2000 to more than 6000 calories,

depending on the burn. Meeting these enormous requirements requires diligent nursing interventions. Concentrated, high-calorie foods must be offered frequently. The body also requires additional amounts of vitamins A, B, and C to promote digestion, absorption, and repair of tissue. Increased amounts of calcium, zinc, magnesium, and iron are needed. Vitamin C and zinc aid in wound healing, and supplemental B complex vitamins help metabolize the extra protein and carbohydrate intake. Adding oral supplements such as Ensure and Sustacal can increase vitamin, mineral, and protein intake. Total parenteral nutrition provides an alternative to oral intake of proteins if the patient is unable to take in adequate nutrients by mouth (Americanburn.org, 2018).

Most burn victims have poor appetites and getting the patient to eat is difficult. Small, frequent feedings of high-calorie, high-protein, low-volume foods are the best way to meet the patient's nutritional needs. Some patients develop Curling's ulcer 8 to 14 days after the burn injury because of increased gastric acidity. The first sign is vomiting of bright red blood. The prophylactic treatment involves intravenous or oral administration of cimetidine, ranitidine, omeprazole, or famotidine. Box 3.7 lists patient problems commonly seen during the acute phase of burns.

Rehabilitation phase. Rehabilitation of the burn patient begins at admission. However, the third phase of burn care begins when 20% or less of the TBSA remains burned. The goal becomes to promote independence so

Box 3.7	Patient Problems Seen in the Acute Phase of Burns

- Compromised Physical Mobility, related to burns
- Distorted Body Image, related to disfigurement from burns
- Fearfulness, related to chronic illness
- Helplessness, related to prolonged recovery and loss of income
- Impaired Coping, related to seriousness of injury
- Impaired Family Processes, related to long-term hospitalization
- Impaired Role Functioning
- Impaired Self-Care (in ADLs), related to area of burn involved
- Insufficient Diversional Activity, related to confinement during care
- Insufficient Knowledge in all areas, related to expected care
- Insufficient Nutrition: less than body requirements, related to increased metabolic demands
- Potential for Infection, related to open skin wounds
- Prolonged Pain, related to procedures performed
- Recent Onset of Anxiousness, related to change in body image
- Social Seclusion, related to perceived change in body image

ADLs, Activities of daily living.

that the patient may have a productive life. The rehabilitation process addresses social and physical skills and may take years.

Mobility limitations constitute the major concerns. The patient requires a comprehensive physical therapy program for positioning, skin care, exercise, ambulation, and activities of daily living (ADLs). Contractures remain a concern in the care of a burn patient. Although physical therapists provide most of the rehabilitative care, the nurse helps to provide continuity of care. When planning the care, set realistic, short-term goals to motivate patients to try to achieve more.

Maintaining or restoring the patient's independence remains the primary rehabilitative goal. Given the possibility of a changed body image, encourage the patient to talk about fears and concerns. Working with others, such as social workers and counselors, develops a holistic care plan to provide the comprehensive care needed. During visiting hours, assess family interactions. Helping the family cope with the changes in their loved one is a major nursing intervention.

Patient problems commonly seen with burn victims, as listed in Box 3.8, encompass family, patient, and social roles.

Patient Teaching

Before discharge, the burn patient and family need education. Provide written instructions that are complete, comprehensive, easy to understand, and realistic. Return demonstrations are the best way to determine that learning has taken place. The major topics to cover are (1) wound care, (2) signs and symptoms of complications, (3) dressings, (4) exercises, (5) clothing, (6) ADLs, and (7) social skills (see the Home Care Considerations box).

🏠 Home Care Considerations

Burns

- Bathe twice a day with mild soap.
- Test the water temperature before getting into the shower because your skin is sensitive to extremes of hot and cold.
- Be certain to clean the tub well before each bath.
- If itching becomes severe, take a lukewarm bath with Alpha Keri lotion added to the bath water.
- Do not use lotions that contain lanolin or alcohol because they will cause blisters.
- Avoid direct sunlight. Wear light clothing to cover areas that have been burned because these areas burn easily.
- Discoloration and scarring are normal during healing. The color of the scar may remain red because of the healing process. Usually within 6 months to a year the scar loses its red color and becomes softer. Normal color to the area may take several months to return.
- Report to the health care provider:
- Any signs of infection
- Fever greater than 101°F (38.3°C)
- Feeling of inability to cope

Box 3.8 · Patient Problems Seen in the Rehabilitation Phase of Burns

- Anxiousness, related to role change
- Compromised Physical Mobility, related to splinting and dressings
- Distorted Body Image, related to scarring
- Excessive Demand on Primary Caregiver, related to prolonged recovery period
- Fearfulness, related to impending surgery
- Grief, related to loss of wellness
- Impaired Coping
- Impaired Coping, related to long-term rehabilitation
- Impaired Personal Identity, related to inability to return to previous lifestyle for prolonged period
- Impaired Self-Care (in ADLs)
  - Recent Onset of Pain
  - Lethargy or Malaise
- Inability to Clear Airway, related to edema of the respiratory passages
- Inability to Tolerate Activity, related to prolonged bed rest
- Insufficient Knowledge, related to impaired home maintenance management
- Post-Event Emotional Crisis, related to the cause of the burn
- Potential for Contractures or Muscle Atrophy, related to noncompliance
- Recent Onset of Pain

ADLs, Activities of daily living.

Evaluation

Evaluation depends on meeting the stated goals. In evaluating the burn patient, ask the following questions:
- Can the patient take care of self?
- Can the patient ambulate without difficulty?
- Can the patient and family cope?
- Does the patient have contractures?
- Does the patient understand the treatment process?

Burn care is extensive, and the exact nursing interventions for each patient are individualized. Many times, the patient must change vocation, and family relationships change. The degree of scarring—emotionally and physically—cannot be predicted; nor can the patient's acceptance by society.

Prognosis

The outcome for the patient with burns depends on the size of the burn, depth of the burn, the victim's age, the body part involved, the burning agent, and history of cardiac, pulmonary, endocrine, renal, or hepatic disease and other injuries sustained at the time of the burn.

❖ NURSING PROCESS FOR THE PATIENT WITH AN INTEGUMENTARY DISORDER

◆ ASSESSMENT

Assessment of the skin is an important aspect of patient care. Skin changes can reflect specific skin disorders, but they also may alert the nurse to a systemic disorder. Skin assessment allows the identification of obvious and subtle changes in the patient's state of health. Effective skin assessment takes a critical eye and knowledge of the expected normal findings.

Because the skin usually is assessed at the same time as other body systems, nurses tend to underestimate the valuable information that can be obtained. Assessing the skin provides a baseline knowledge of the patient's hygiene measures, nutritional status, circulatory status, and sensory perception. The skin is the first line of defense against infection. Ongoing assessment of the skin is important in the maintenance of health and the prevention of infection.

Assessment of the older adult can be challenging for the health care professional. Safe, effective patient care requires that the nurse understand the normal changes that occur with aging. The older patient population is growing, as are the opportunities for the student to assess the older patient (see the Lifespan Considerations box).

Lifespan Considerations

Older Adults

Effects of Aging on the Integumentary System

- Physiologic changes make the skin of the older adult more fragile and susceptible to impairment.
- Aging changes include decreases in tissue fluid, subcutaneous fat, and sebaceous secretions, resulting in dryness, flaking, pruritus, loss of elasticity, altered turgor, and a wrinkled appearance.
- Hyperkeratotic changes are typically seen in the nails, which make them thick and difficult to care for. Podiatric care is recommended for older adults, particularly those with circulatory impairments and diabetes mellitus.
- Circulatory changes and decreased mobility increase the risk of senile purpura and decubitus ulcers.
- Significant hair and scalp changes can occur with aging:
- Loss of pigmentation leading to graying
- Decreased hair thickness or balding
- Increased incidence of seborrheic dermatitis of the scalp requiring special care
- Growth of facial hair on women, which can damage self-image
- Localized clustering of melanocytes surrounded by areas of decreased pigmentation results in "age spots."
- The incidence of basal and squamous cell carcinoma increases with age, particularly in individuals who have had excessive sun exposure. Inspect aging skin closely for changes in the appearance of moles or warts.

◆ PATIENT PROBLEM

Assessment provides data to identify the patient's problems, strengths, potential complications, and learning needs. After defining the clinical problems, start formulating a care plan that meets the patient's needs, prioritizing problems from most to least important. Being able to prioritize nursing interventions

contributes to a more predictable recovery for the patient. Possible clinical problems that should be considered for the patient with a skin disorder are as follows:

PATIENT PROBLEM	NURSING INTERVENTIONS
Anxiousness, related to altered appearance	Assess anxiety level every shift Observe verbal and nonverbal behavior Encourage the patient to share feelings Teach relaxation techniques Assess patient for pain
Recent Onset of Pain, related to loss of superficial skin layers	Initiate nursing measures to minimize or relieve pain
Insufficient Knowledge, related to cause of skin disorder	Assess patient for learning needs daily Involve patient in setting goals Use audiovisuals as teaching aids Evaluate patient's success
Potential for Infection, related to impaired skin integrity	Assess patient daily for risk factors, such as abrasions, elevated white blood cell count, and temperature Implement nursing measures, such as using good hand hygiene and keeping patient's nails trimmed, to decrease risk factors
Insufficient Knowledge, related to treatment of pruritus	Assess factors contributing to pruritus Promote hydration of the skin by having patient avoid hot showers and apply emollients after bathing Encourage adequate fluid intake Implement nursing measures to decrease skin irritation, such as avoiding clothes made of rough weave Encourage patient to stop scratching by rubbing or applying pressure to the area Administer prescribed medications for pruritus such as corticosteroids and antihistamines
Potential for Trauma, related to excessive scratching	Assess onset and contributing factors of episodes of pruritus Encourage patient to stop scratching by rubbing or by applying pressure to the involved area
Social Seclusion, related to anticipated or actual response of others to disfiguring skin disorders	Encourage patient to discuss feelings of loneliness Identify available support systems to patient

PATIENT PROBLEM	NURSING INTERVENTIONS
Impaired Self-Esteem due to Current Situation, related to change in body image	Assess patient's feelings of self-worth by having patient describe feelings about self
	Implement nursing measures to assist patient in dealing with body image
	Accept feelings of anger or hostility from patient
	Suggest clothing to conceal changes in skin integrity

◆ EXPECTED OUTCOMES AND PLANNING

When planning patient care, look at the nursing diagnoses and establish the cause of the nursing problem. Determining the cause enables you to develop a care plan that includes nursing interventions to eliminate the cause if possible. Include the patient in this planning. Ascertain the patient's preferences and capabilities. Including the patient is one way to promote compliance. Most skin problems are chronic, and progress is often slow. Furthermore, many patients are older and require more time for healing.

Planning includes the development of realistic goals and outcomes that stem from the identified patient problems. Establish short- and long-term goals. Examples of measurable goals include the following:

Goal 1: Patient shows no signs of infection in abdominal wound as evidenced by the wound remaining free of erythema, purulent drainage, odor, and localized tenderness.

Goal 2: Patient is able to change dressing correctly as evidenced by the patient following the written guidelines during demonstration.

Goals should have a date when they will be evaluated. Failure to attain a goal means the nurse should reevaluate the chosen interventions and determine why the goals have not been met.

◆ IMPLEMENTATION

When providing nursing interventions related to the skin, (1) include ways to prevent skin problems, (2) provide education in home care management, and (3) provide safety tips for the patient. Patients with skin diseases usually are managed at home and need to be aware of the potential for infection because the skin is not intact (see Box 3.1 and the Home Care Considerations box).

Nursing measures for the skin include a variety of simple or complex interventions, including applying medications, dressings, and heat or cold application and teaching the patient how to perform these measures at home. The principles of surgical and medical asepsis are important when providing nursing interventions. Incorporate nutritional guidelines for the patient to follow. Patients need extra nutrients, such as protein, for the building and repair of tissues.

 Home Care Considerations

Home Care Guidelines for Baths and Soaks

- The water temperature should be comfortable, usually 90°F–100°F (32°C–38°C).
- Dissolve medication completely while tub is filling.
- The soak should last 20–30 min.
- When oils are added, assist the patient out of the water to prevent slipping.
- Pat the skin dry rather than rubbing to avoid skin irritation.
- Apply creams or ointments immediately after the bath to retain moisture.
- Drain water from the tub before the patient gets out.
- The door should not be locked, and a helper should be within hearing distance.
- Use a bathmat to prevent slipping.
- Handrails may be needed in the shower or tub.
- A seat may be needed in the shower or tub.
- After a medicated bath, pour one cup of bleach into used tub water, let stand 5 min, wipe sides and bottom of tub, drain tub, and clean as usual.

Consider the patient's cultural beliefs, personal values, and economic resources when selecting the appropriate care. More people are using forms of treatment for integumentary disorders other than traditional medical therapy (see the Complementary and Alternative Therapies box). To promote compliance with planned treatment, consider the patient's independence, dignity, privacy, and physical strengths and limitations.

 Complementary and Alternative Therapies

Integumentary Disorders

- The management of integumentary disorders is often difficult. Nutritional and herbal approaches to the treatment of skin problems have been shown to be effective for some disorders, often with fewer side effects than with conventional methods.
- Chinese herbs have long been used in Asian countries for the treatment of skin diseases. A landmark study in England showed the effectiveness of Chinese herbs in treating atopic dermatitis. This study was undertaken after dermatologists were impressed by the results in their patients who were also under the care of a Chinese herbalist. Participants in the study who received the active herbal formula reported decreases in the number of lesions and itching, as well as improved sleep.
- A traditional Australian plant remedy, tea tree oil (from *Melaleuca alternifolia*), has been effective in the treatment of acne.
- A topical mixture of the essential plant oils of thyme, rosemary, lavender, and cedarwood in a carrier of jojoba and grapeseed oils has been found to have significant effect in the treatment of alopecia areata.
- A published report from Taiwan states that acupuncture has been effective in the treatment of urticaria (hives).

From Sheehan MP, Rustin MH, Atherton DJ, et al: Efficacy of traditional Chinese herbal therapy in adult atopic dermatitis, *Lancet* 340:13–17, 1992.

◆ EVALUATION

During and after the planned nursing interventions, determine the outcomes. This is an ongoing process of continually trying to establish the most effective care plan.

Economic and home care implications are important. Patients are being discharged from the health care facility more quickly than in the past, and insurance companies are more selective in how they pay for the care and supplies the patient needs. Creativity and critical thinking are important skills to meet the needs of today's patient.

Evaluation involves determining whether the established goals have been met. The nurse and patient evaluate the goals to see whether the criteria for measurement have been met. For example, the goal is that the patient's wound would not become infected, as demonstrated by a lack of erythema, purulent drainage, and odor. If, at the end of the designated time frame, the wound shows no signs of infection, the goal has been met.

Get Ready for the NCLEX® Examination!

Key Points

- The skin, including nails, hair, and glands, makes up the integumentary system.
- The main functions of the integumentary system are protection, temperature regulation, and vitamin D synthesis.
- The two layers of true skin are the epidermis and dermis.
- The layer of tissue directly beneath the skin is the subcutaneous layer; it is composed of adipose tissue and loose connective tissue.
- The sudoriferous (sweat) glands release perspiration through the skin.
- The sebaceous (oil) glands secrete sebum, which lubricates the skin and prevents invasion of bacteria through the skin.
- Any injury to the skin poses a threat to a person's self-concept.
- It is important to establish a therapeutic relationship to meet the patient's psychological needs.
- Most skin disorders are not contagious and are rarely fatal. They are often chronic.
- Sterile technique and isolation techniques are required with any open, draining lesion.
- Wet dressings must be checked frequently. Constant moisture softens the skin and contributes to skin maceration.
- Medicines must be applied to clean skin.
- The nursing interventions for a skin disorder depend on the cause; however, common problems are decreased skin integrity, risk for infection, lack of knowledge concerning the disease, and ineffective coping.
- A primary nursing intervention is to teach the patient about the mode of transmission of the particular disease.
- The assessment of patients with skin disorders includes collection of subjective and objective data.
- Wet dressings and baths may be done to soothe, vasoconstrict, debride, or decrease pruritus.
- Before initiating heat and cold therapy, understand normal body responses to local temperature variations, assess the integrity of the body part, determine the patient's ability to sense temperature, and ensure proper operation of equipment.

- Prevent malignant skin diseases by educating the public about causes.
- Burns can be classified by depth and TBSA involved.
- The pathophysiology and care of burns involve three stages: the hypovolemic (emergent) phase, the acute (diuretic) phase, and the long-term (rehabilitation) phase.
- The three phases of burn care overlap, with different goals and nursing interventions in each.
- A primary nursing intervention for the burn patient in the emergent phase is to establish and maintain an open airway.
- The treatment method for a burn patient depends on age, body surface area involved, location, depth, and other diseases present.
- The primary causes of death in burn victims are hypovolemic shock in the first 72 hours and infection during the acute phase.
- Suspect inhalation injury if the burn injury occurred in a closed or confined area.
- A treatment for burns is use of temporary skin substitutes derived from human fibroblast cells.

Additional Learning Resources

SG Go to your Study Guide for additional learning activities to help you master this chapter content.

Be sure to visit the Evolve site at http://evolve.elsevier.com/Cooper/adult/ for additional online resources.

Review Questions for the NCLEX® Examination

1. The health care provider has ordered oral griseofulvin for tinea capitis. The patient's mother asks the nurse why an oral medication is used rather than a cream. What information should be provided by the nurse?

   1. Topical creams do not reach the root of the hair to kill the fungus.
   2. Oral medications are more economical.
   3. Topical medications cause more pain when applied.
   4. It is more convenient to take the medication once a day rather than applying the cream once a day.

2. The nurse is caring for a patient with an open skin lesion. Which patient goal is the highest priority?

   1. The patient understands the treatment regimen.
   2. The patient does not develop an infection of the lesion.
   3. The patient voices concern regarding the appearance of the lesion.
   4. The patient seeks assistance for care of the lesion upon discharge.

3. Which of the following assessments should the nurse report to the health care provider immediately for an adult patient with partial-thickness burns over 25% of his body?

   1. Complaints of pain every 4 to 6 hours
   2. Decreasing appetite over the past 2 days
   3. Hourly urinary output of 10 to 15 mL
   4. Edema at the intravenous (IV) site

4. A patient has a rash on her back that began about 10 days ago with a raised, scaly border and a pink center. Now she has similar eruptions on both sides of her back. With what condition are these manifestations most consistent?

   1. Impetigo contagiosa
   2. Pityriasis rosea
   3. Contact dermatitis
   4. Infantile eczema

5. A patient complains of a burning pain on his lower thoracic area. On inspection, the area is found to be erythematous and edematous with a cluster of vesicles. What condition is most likely to be diagnosed?

   1. Herpes zoster
   2. Herpes simplex
   3. Varicella
   4. Impetigo

6. A patient states that he has basal cell carcinoma and is going to die. When planning the best response to make, the nurse should include what knowledge?

   1. Basal cell carcinoma is rarely terminal.
   2. Without proper medication, it can result in melanoma.
   3. It is a hereditary disorder caused by decreased melanin.
   4. Treatment involves strong chemotherapeutic agents.

7. It is important to teach a patient the warning signs of skin cancer. Which characteristic(s) of a nevus is a warning sign of skin cancer? (Select all that apply.)

   1. Border irregularity
   2. Smooth surface
   3. Decreasing diameter
   4. Mole symmetry
   5. Delayed or prolonged lesional healing

8. A patient has an inhalation burn injury. Which is a medical emergency?

   1. Singed facial hair
   2. Neck or face burns
   3. Pallor
   4. Respiratory stridor

9. Which method of assessing burn size applies only to adults?

   1. Lund-Browder
   2. Rule of nines
   3. Parkland method
   4. Primary survey

10. The nurse just finished an assessment for a patient with systemic lupus erythematosus (SLE). Which clinical manifestation would the nurse expect to find? (Select all that apply.)

    1. Oral ulcers
    2. Urticaria
    3. Jaundice
    4. Diarrhea
    5. Erythematous rash over the nose and cheeks

11. The health care provider has scheduled a debridement for a patient who has partial-thickness burns on his chest and right upper leg. Which nursing intervention is most important?

    1. Ambulate the patient to increase the blood flow to the area.
    2. Administer an opioid analgesic intravenously before the debridement.
    3. Teach the patient to remove the old dressings, using clean technique.
    4. Explain to the patient that the procedure will be painful.

12. A patient is admitted with partial- and full-thickness burns on his right lower extremity. What is likely to be included in the plan of care initially?

    1. Closed dressing change every 3 hours
    2. Open dressing
    3. Temporary skin cover
    4. Incision and drainage of the wound

13. A patient is admitted with partial-thickness burns on his upper chest and face. What is the most important thing for the nurse to monitor in the patient on admission?

    1. Respiratory problems
    2. Burn shock
    3. Infection of the wound
    4. Cellulitis of the affected area

14. What should be included in the assessment of a patient with an electrical burn?

    1. Infection
    2. Cardiac irregularities
    3. Burn depth
    4. Hypovolemic shock

15. A patient is admitted with herpes zoster. The health care provider orders an antiviral medication to slow the progression of the virus. Which medication will the nurse administer?

    1. acyclovir
    2. cefaclor
    3. acetaminophen
    4. cimetidine

16. A patient has been diagnosed with scabies. What does the nurse anticipate to assess with this patient? *(Select all that apply.)*

    1. Wavy brown lines on the skin
    2. Nocturnal pruritus
    3. Localized pain
    4. Skin paresthesia
    5. Hives

17. An adolescent patient is seen in the clinic with a mild case of acne. What does the nurse expect to assess?

    1. The patient reports a plan for suicide.
    2. The patient reports a sense of low self-esteem.
    3. The patient reports an increased intake of fatty foods.
    4. The patient reports a drastic change in weight.

18. A patient with thermal burns over 30% of his body has maintained a urinary output of 250 mL for the past 8 hours. What can the nurse infer from this information?

    1. Patient is not improving as expected
    2. Stage of hypovolemic burn shock is resolving
    3. Pain is decreasing
    4. Nutritional status is improving

19. A patient tells the nurse she has not gone out of the house for weeks because she could not cover the lesions on her face with makeup. What would be an appropriate patient problem?

    1. Distorted Body Image, related to change in personal appearance
    2. Self-Protective Coping, related to lack of social contact
    3. Anxiousness, related to the fear of permanent disfigurement
    4. Inability to Tolerate Activity, related to lack of exercise

20. When teaching a patient to care for herpes zoster lesions at home, which is the most important instruction for the nurse to provide?

    1. Clean the lesions with sterile saline daily.
    2. Wash hands before and after applying medication.
    3. Report to the health care provider when the lesions are crusted.
    4. Launder all clothes in vinegar.

21. The nurse is reviewing the history for a patient who has been admitted with cellulitis. Which condition(s) would predispose the patient to cellulitis? *(Select all that apply.)*

    1. Malnutrition
    2. Treatment with chemotherapy
    3. Venous insufficiency of the lower legs
    4. Idiopathic hypertension
    5. Diabetes mellitus

22. A parent tells the dermatologist that her daughter seems to be losing interest in school. Which medication could have caused the patient's change in behavior?

    1. isotretinoin
    2. minocycline
    3. tazarotene
    4. penicillin

23. An African American patient is seen with impending shock after an accident. How would the nurse expect the skin to appear during the assessment of the patient?

    1. Ruddy blue
    2. Generalized pallor
    3. Ashen, gray, or dull
    4. Whitish, blue, or bright

24. The nurse planning the care for a patient who has impetigo expects to administer which topical drug to the patient?

    1. Acetaminophen
    2. Retapamulin
    3. Nystatin
    4. Corticosteroids

25. When teaching home care to a patient with recurrent genital herpes infection, it is important to include which information? *(Select all that apply.)*

    1. The infection is contagious only when lesions are visible.
    2. Antiviral agents are curative in the majority of cases.
    3. The patient will need to take antiviral agents daily for life.
    4. The patient will need to use protection even when no lesions are evident.
    5. Precautions for delivery must be made in the event of becoming pregnant.

26. The nurse is educating a patient about using the ABCD mnemonic for skin cancer. Which terms would the nurse use to describe what the ABCD's stand for? Select all that apply?

    1. Color
    2. Consistency
    3. Borders
    4. Asymmetry
    5. Diameter
    6. Dimensions
    7. Bulging
    8. Abrasion

27. The nurse is assessing a patient and notes a raised, fluid filled area that measures 1.3 cm in width. When documenting this finding, _____ is the term that would be used to describe this.

Care of the Patient With a Musculoskeletal Disorder

http://evolve.elsevier.com/Cooper/adult/

Objectives

Anatomy and Physiology

1. List the five basic functions of the skeletal system.
2. List the two divisions of the skeleton.
3. Describe the location of major bones and muscles of the body.
4. List the types of body movements.
5. Describe three vital functions muscles perform when they contract.

Medical-Surgical

6. List diagnostic examinations for musculoskeletal function.
7. Compare medical and nursing care for patients suffering from gouty arthritis, rheumatoid arthritis, and osteoarthritis.
8. List at least four healthy lifestyle measures people can practice to reduce the risk of developing osteoporosis.
9. Describe the medical and nursing care for the patient undergoing a total hip or knee replacement.
10. Discuss nursing interventions for a patient with a fractured hip after open reduction with internal fixation and bipolar hip prosthesis (hemiarthroplasty).
11. Discuss the physiology of fracture healing (hematoma, granulation tissue, and callus formation).
12. Describe the signs and symptoms of compartment syndrome.
13. List nursing interventions for a fat embolism.
14. List at least two types of skin and skeletal traction.
15. Compare methods for assessing circulation, nerve damage, and infection in a patient who has a traumatic insult to the musculoskeletal system.
16. List four nursing interventions for bone cancer.
17. Describe the phenomenon of phantom pain.
18. Define lordosis, scoliosis, and kyphosis.

Key Terms

ankylosis (ăng-kĭ-LŌ-sĭs, p. 121)
arthrocentesis (ăr-thrō-sĕn-TĒ-sĭs, p. 113)
arthrodesis (ăr-thrō-DĒ-sĭs, p. 131)
arthroplasty (ĂR-thrō-plăs-tē, p. 131)
bipolar hip replacement (hemiarthroplasty) (hĕ-mē-ĂR-thrō-plăs-tē, p. 137)
blanching test (p. 167)
callus (p. 139)
Colles' fracture (KŎL-ēz FRĂK-shŭr, p. 141)
compartment syndrome (p. 145)
crepitus (KRĔP-ĭ-tŭs, p. 139)

fibromyalgia (fī-brō-mĭ-ĂL-jă, p. 130)
kyphosis (kĭ-FŌ-sĭs, p. 166)
lordosis (lŏr-DŌ-sĭs, p. 166)
open reduction with internal fixation (ORIF) (p. 142)
paresthesia (păr-ĕs-THĒ-zē-ă, p. 157)
scoliosis (skō-lē-Ō-sĭs, p. 166)
sequestrum (sĕ-KWĔS-trŭm, p. 129)
subluxations (sŭb-lŭk-SĀ-shŭnz, p. 158)
tophi (TŌ-fī, p. 125)
Volkmann's contracture (VŎLK-mănz kŏn-TRĂK-shŭr, p. 146)

ANATOMY AND PHYSIOLOGY OF THE MUSCULOSKELETAL SYSTEM

Bones and joints form the framework of the body, and muscles contract and relax to allow movement. All movement of the body is orchestrated by the functioning of the bones, the joints, and the muscles attached to the bones. This chapter discusses the structure and the function of bones and muscles and how they serve the body.

FUNCTIONS OF THE SKELETAL SYSTEM

The human skeletal system is composed of 206 bones and has five basic functions.

1. *Support:* The skeleton is the body framework that supports internal tissues and organs.
2. *Protection:* The skeleton forms a firm, cage-like structure that protects many internal structures. The cranium (skull) protects the brain, the vertebrae protect the spinal cord, the ribs and the sternum

(breastbone) protect the lungs and the heart, and the pelvis protects the digestive and reproductive organs.

3. *Movement:* Skeletal muscles are attached to the bones, which enables the bones to provide leverage for movement. As a muscle contracts, it pulls on the bone and movement occurs.

4. *Mineral storage:* The bones serve as a storage area for various minerals, particularly calcium and phosphorus. When the body's intake of these minerals is inadequate, the bones release the minerals.

5. *Hematopoiesis:* Hematopoiesis (blood cell formation) takes place in the red bone marrow. The red bone marrow is spongy bone found in the ends of the long bones. A child's bones contain a proportionately larger amount of red bone marrow than an adult's. As a person ages, much of the red bone marrow converts to yellow bone marrow, which is composed of fat cells.

STRUCTURE OF BONES

Bones are classified into four groups, based on their form and shape: long, short, flat, and irregular. Long bones are found in the extremities, short bones are found in the hands and feet, flat bones are found in the skull and sternum, and irregular bones make up the vertebrae (backbone).

ARTICULATIONS (JOINTS)

Bones cannot bend without damage. To allow movement, individual bones articulate (join) at joint sites (Fig. 4.1). Bones are held together by flexible connective tissue. The joint is the point of contact between the individual bones. The structure of the individual bones depends on the function of the area. Every bone in the body (except the hyoid bone, which anchors the tongue) connects, or articulates, with at least one other bone.

Joints perform two important functions: they hold the bones together to form the skeleton, and they allow movement and flexibility of the skeleton.

The most common way to classify joints is according to the degree of movement they permit. There are three types of joints:

1. *Synarthrosis:* No movement
2. *Amphiarthrosis:* Slight movement
3. *Diarthrosis:* Free movement

A goniometer measures the angle of a joint. It is used to determine the degree of joint mobility.

DIVISIONS OF THE SKELETON

The skeleton is divided into the axial and the appendicular skeletons (Box 4.1). The axial skeleton is composed of the skull, hyoid bone in the neck, vertebral column, and thorax (chest). The appendicular skeleton is composed of the upper extremities, lower extremities, shoulder girdle, and pelvic girdle (excluding the sacrum) (Fig. 4.2).

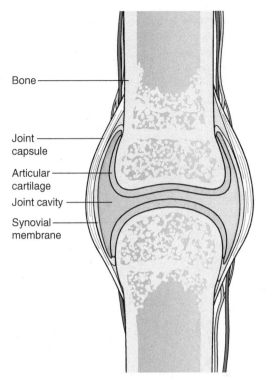

Bone
Joint capsule
Articular cartilage
Joint cavity
Synovial membrane

Fig. 4.1 Structure of a freely movable (diarthrotic) joint. Note these typical features: joint capsule, joint cavity lined with synovial membrane, and articular (hyaline) cartilage covering the end surfaces of the bones within the joint capsule.

Box 4.1 Main Parts of the Skeleton

AXIAL SKELETON	APPENDICULAR SKELETON
Skull	Upper extremities
• Cranium	• Shoulder (pectoral) girdle
• Ear bones	• Arms
• Face	• Wrists
Spine	• Hands
• Vertebrae	Lower extremities
Thorax	• Hip (pelvic girdle)
• Ribs	• Legs
• Sternum	• Ankles
	• Feet

FUNCTIONS OF THE MUSCULAR SYSTEM

The bones and joints provide the framework of the body, but the muscles are necessary for movement. This motion results from contraction and relaxation of the individual muscles. The body has more than 600 muscles, making up approximately 40% to 50% of the total body weight. They usually act in groups to execute a body movement (Table 4.1).

As muscles contract, they perform three vital functions: motion, maintenance of posture, and production of heat. Contraction also assists in return of venous blood and lymph to the right side of the heart.

All body movements rely on the integrated functioning of the bones, joints, and muscles. Muscle tissue is under voluntary or involuntary control. Voluntary muscle is under conscious control, whereas involuntary

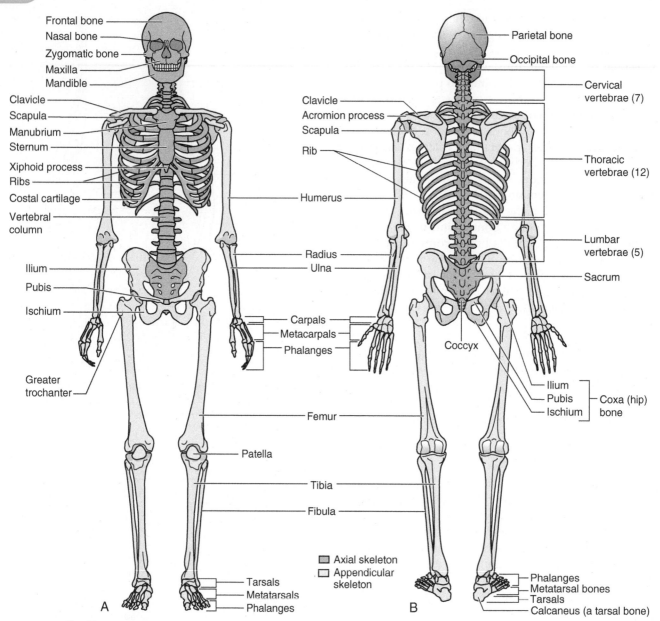

Fig. 4.2 Skeleton. Axial skeleton is shown in blue. Appendicular skeleton is bone colored. (A) Anterior view. (B) Posterior view.

muscle tissue responds to internal commands without any conscious control. Involuntary motions include activities conducted by the internal organs, such as the heart beating, the gallbladder releasing bile, and the stomach churning food.

The contraction of certain skeletal muscles gives the body proper posture. These muscles pull on various bones, allowing the body to sit or stand.

As skeletal muscles contract, they produce body heat. Approximately 85% of all body heat is generated by the contraction of the skeletal muscles.

Skeletal Muscle Structure

A skeletal muscle is composed of hundreds of muscle fibers (cells). Each skeletal muscle is surrounded by a covering of connective tissue called the *epimysium*. The

epimysium joins with two other inner coverings, the perimysium and the endomysium, and extends beyond the muscle to form a tough cord of connective tissue known as a *tendon*. Tendons anchor muscles to bones. As a muscle contracts, it pulls the corresponding tendon and bone toward it. This is how movement occurs. Tendons in the ankle and wrist are enclosed in *tendon sheaths*, which are sleeves or tube-like structures of connective tissue. Tendon sheaths contain synovial fluid and permit the tendons to slide easily; the sheaths also keep the tendons in place. All of the body's tendons, ligaments (which are like tendons, but anchoring bone to bone), and aponeuroses (very broad, flat, tendons) are composed of connective tissue in various sizes, shapes, and densities. These are known collectively as *fasciae*.

Table 4.1   Principal Muscles of the Body

MUSCLE	FUNCTION	INSERTION	ORIGIN
Muscles of the Head and Neck			
Frontal	Raises eyebrow	Skin of eyebrow	Occipital bone
Orbicularis oculi	Closes eye	Maxilla and frontal bone	Maxilla and frontal bone (encircles eye)
Orbicularis oris	Draws lips together	Encircles lips	Encircles lips
Zygomaticus	Elevates corners of mouth and lips	Angle of mouth and upper lip	Zygomatic bone
Masseter	Closes jaw	Mandible	Zygomatic arch
Temporal	Closes jaw	Mandible	Temporal region of the skull
Sternocleidomastoid	Rotates and extends head	Mastoid process	Sternum and clavicle
Trapezius	Extends head and neck	Scapula	Skull and upper vertebrae
Muscles That Move the Upper Extremities			
Pectoralis major	Flexes and helps adduct upper arm	Humerus	Sternum, clavicle, and upper rib cartilages
Latissimus dorsi	Extends and helps adduct upper arm	Humerus	Vertebrae and ilium
Deltoid	Abducts upper arm	Humerus	Clavicle and scapula
Biceps brachii	Flexes lower arm	Radius	Ulna
Triceps brachii	Extends lower arm (called "boxer's muscle"—straightens the elbow when a blow is delivered)	Ulna	Scapula and humerus
Muscles of the Trunk			
External oblique	Compresses abdomen	Midline of abdomen	Lower thoracic cage
Internal oblique	Compresses abdomen	Midline of abdomen	Pelvis
Transversus abdominis	Compresses abdomen	Midline of abdomen	Ribs, vertebrae, and pelvis
Rectus abdominis	Flexes trunk	Lower ribcage	Pubis
Muscles That Move the Lower Extremities			
Iliopsoas	Flexes thigh or trunk	Ilium and vertebrae	Femur
Sartorius	Flexes thigh and rotates lower leg	Tibia	Ilium
Gluteus maximus	Extends thigh	Femur	Ilium, sacrum, and coccyx
Gluteus medius	Abducts thigh	Femur	Ilium
Adductor group			
• Adductor longus	Adducts thigh	Femur	Pubis
• Gracilis	Adducts thigh	Tibia	Pubis
• Pectineus	Adducts thigh	Femur	Pubis
Hamstring group			
• Semimembranosus	Flexes lower leg	Tibia	Ischium
• Semitendinosus	Flexes lower leg	Tibia	Ischium
• Biceps femoris	Flexes lower leg	Fibula	Ischium and femur
Quadriceps group			
• Rectus femoris	Extends lower leg	Tibia	Ischium
• Vastus lateralis, intermedius, and medialis	Extends lower leg	Tibia	Femur
Tibialis anterior	Dorsiflexes foot	Metatarsals (foot)	Tibia
Gastrocnemius	Plantar flexes foot	Calcaneus (heel)	Femur
Soleus	Plantar flexes foot	Calcaneus (heel)	Tibia and fibula
Peroneus group			
• Peroneus longus and brevis	Plantar flexes foot	Tarsals and metatarsals (ankle and foot)	Tibia and fibula

Table 4.2 Muscles Grouped According to Function

PART MOVED	FLEXORS	EXTENSORS	ABDUCTORS	ADDUCTORS
Upper arm	Pectoralis major	Latissimus dorsi	Deltoid and latissimus dorsi contracting together	Pectoralis major
Lower arm	Biceps brachii	Triceps brachii	None	None
Thigh	Iliopsoas and sartorius	Gluteus maximus	Gluteus medius	Adductor group
Lower leg	Hamstrings	Quadriceps group	None	None
Foot	Tibialis anterior	Gastrocnemius and soleus	Peroneus longus	Tibialis anterior

Nerve and Blood Supply

Because of the physical demands placed on the skeletal muscles, they need a constant supply of oxygen and nutrition. They are well supplied with blood vessels that carry oxygen and nutrition to the area and remove the waste products of metabolism.

The skeletal muscles are voluntary, so they need a constant source of information. Nerve cells or fibers continuously send impulses that stimulate the muscle cells. These impulses enter at the neuromuscular junction, the point of contact between the nerve ending and the muscle fiber. As a nerve impulse passes through this junction, chemicals are released that cause the muscle to contract.

Usually one artery, two veins, and one nerve penetrate a particular muscle. Each muscle cell comes in contact with several capillaries and a portion of a nerve cell. The muscle cells, in union with the nerve cell that controls them, are called a *motor unit*.

The impulse from the nerve cell must travel across a small gap because the nerve cell and the muscle cell do not directly touch each other. This small gap is called a *synaptic cleft* and is filled with tissue fluid. A special chemical (*neurotransmitter*) travels through the fluid to stimulate the muscle fiber. Acetylcholine is the neurotransmitter for skeletal muscle tissue. An enzyme called *cholinesterase* breaks down the acetylcholine once it has transferred the message. This allows the muscle cell to relax between impulses.

Muscle Contraction

Muscle stimulus. Muscle cells are governed by the "all or none" law; that is, when a muscle cell is stimulated or shocked adequately, it will contract completely. Because each skeletal muscle is composed of thousands of muscle cells that react to many different nerve cells, the muscle as a whole contracts according to the principle of graded response. The strength of the muscle contraction therefore depends on the number of individual muscle cells responding. These muscle responses allow us to tenderly brush a baby's cheek or swat an irritating mosquito.

Muscle tone. The skeletal muscles are in a constant state of readiness for action. At any given time, several muscle cells within a certain muscle are contracted and the remainder are relaxed. Muscle tone is necessary for good posture but does not provide movement. To understand the importance of muscle tone, observe an extremity that has become paralyzed; the muscles are flaccid, limp, or atrophied (wasted) and incapable of producing movement because the cells no longer receive stimuli from the nerve fibers.

Types of body movements. Some muscles can move some body parts in only two directions, whereas others can move certain body parts in several directions. The body's more common movements include flexion, extension, abduction, adduction, rotation, supination, pronation, dorsiflexion, and plantar flexion (Table 4.2, Box 4.2, and Fig. 4.3).

Skeletal Muscle Groups

Skeletal muscles usually are classified into two broad categories: axial and appendicular. The axial muscle groups are located on the head, face, neck, and trunk. The appendicular muscle groups are in the extremities. Fig. 4.4 shows the location of the muscles of the body.

LABORATORY AND DIAGNOSTIC EXAMINATIONS

RADIOGRAPHIC STUDIES

The diagnostic study frequently used for determining musculoskeletal system integrity is the radiographic, roentgenographic, or (as it is more commonly known) x-ray examination or diagnostic imaging.

A radiographic examination of a joint reveals fluid, irregularity of the joint with spur formation, or changes in the size of the joint contour. Radiographic examination is used to determine the presence of a skeletal fracture. To avoid potential damage to a growing fetus it is vital to ask women of childbearing age if there is any possibility that they are pregnant before performing x-ray examinations.

Laminography or *planography* (also called *body section roentgenography*) is useful in locating small cavities, foreign bodies, and lesions that are overshadowed by opaque structures.

Scanography, a method of producing a radiograph of internal body organs by means of a series of parallel beams that eliminate size distortion, allows accurate measurement of bone length.

Myelogram

Myelographic examination involves injection of a radiopaque dye into the subarachnoid space at the lumbar spine to x-ray the spinal cord and the vertebral column. It is used to detect structural disorders such as a herniated disk, tumors, or the presence of infection. The test involves the same procedure as a lumbar puncture (spinal tap), which is discussed in Chapter 14. Contrast medium may be used. Assess for a history of allergies

to iodine or seafood. Allergies of this nature cause reactions to the contrast medium. Notify the health care provider if any allergies exist. The examination can be performed without the use of contrast medium.

This examination may involve the entire spine or just the cervical or lumbar area. After the myelogram has been obtained, the dye, if oil-based, is removed through the spinal needle to prevent meningeal irritation. Water-soluble dye is used most often and does not have to be removed; the body absorbs it and excretes it in the urine. Inform the patient that the test is performed with the patient on a tilting table that is moved during the test to allow contrast medium to flow up to the cervical area.

The most common discomfort after a myelogram is headache. If water-soluble dye is used, the patient should lie quietly in a semi-Fowler's position for approximately 8 hours. Patient positioning is important to keep the dye in the lower spine. During this time, encouraging fluid consumption helps the body absorb the dye from the spinal column. If oil-based dye is used, the patient rests in a flat position for up to 12 hours. Tell the patient to inform the nurse if he or she has a headache, stiff neck, leg weakness, or difficulty voiding. Rare complications include seizure, infection, drowsiness, severe headache, numbness, and paralysis.

Patients needing a myelogram may express concern that the needle insertion may damage the spinal cord. Provide instructions to the patient explaining that the needle is inserted below the level of the spinal cord at the fourth or fifth lumbar space (L4–L5).

Nuclear Scanning

Nuclear scanning tests are done in the nuclear medicine department, which has scanners or camera detectors that record images on radiographic film. Diagnostic

---

Box 4.2   Types of Body Movement

- *Abduction:* A movement of an extremity away from the midline of the body.
- *Adduction:* A movement of an extremity toward the axis of the body.
- *Extension* (see Fig. 4.3): A movement allowed by certain joints of the skeleton that increases the angle between two adjoining bones. For example, extending the leg increases the angle between the femur and the tibia. If the extension angle is more than 180 degrees, the extremity is *hyperextended.*
- *Flexion:* A movement allowed by certain joints of the skeleton that decreases the angle between two adjoining bones. For example, bending the arm at the elbow decreases the angle between the humerus and the ulna.
- *Rotation:* A movement of a bone around its longitudinal axis (e.g., a pivot motion, such as shaking the head "no").
- *Supination:* A movement of the hand and forearm that causes the palm to face upward or forward.
- *Pronation:* A movement of the hand and forearm that causes the palm to face downward or backward.
- *Dorsiflexion:* A movement that causes the top of the foot to elevate or tilt upward.
- *Plantar flexion:* A movement that causes the bottom of the foot to be directed downward.

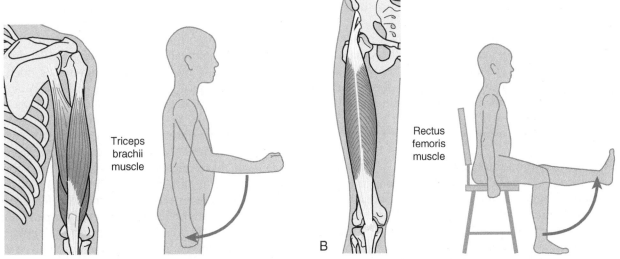

Fig. 4.3 Extension of the lower arm and lower leg. (A) When the triceps brachii muscle *(right)* contracts, it extends the lower arm at the elbow joint *(left)*. (B) When the rectus femoris muscle (part of the quadriceps femoris muscle group) *(right)* contracts, it extends the lower leg at the knee joint *(left)*.

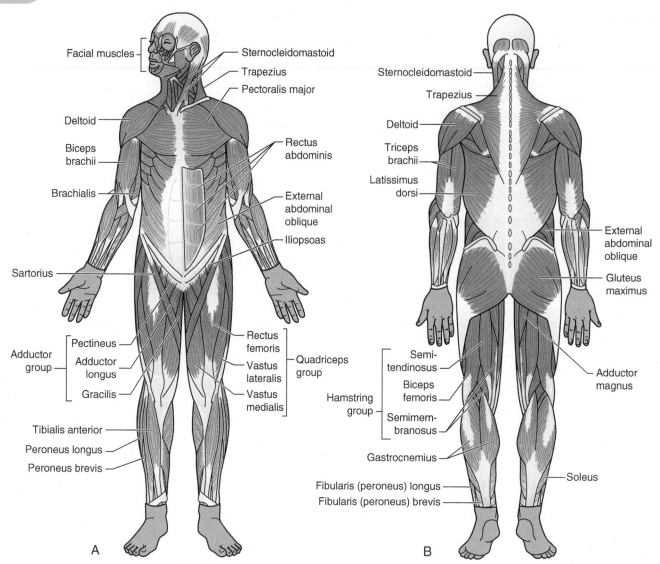

Fig. 4.4 (A) Anterior view of the body. (B) Posterior view of the body.

tests use low doses of radioactive isotopes; precautionary measures that are required for radium therapy are not necessary.

Nursing interventions required when patients are scheduled for nuclear scanning procedures include (1) obtaining written consent from the patient, (2) informing the patient that the radioactive isotopes will not affect family or visitors, and (3) following the nuclear medicine department's instructions for special preparations for specific scans.

Magnetic Resonance Imaging

Musculoskeletal magnetic resonance imaging (MRI) assists in diagnosing abnormalities of bones and joints and surrounding soft tissue structures, including cartilage, synovium, ligaments, and tendons. The test uses magnetism and radio waves to make images of cross sections of the body. MRI can give much more detailed pictures of fluid-filled soft tissue and blood vessels than any other test.

In preparation, ask the patient to remove any metal, such as jewelry, clothing with metal fasteners, glasses, and hair clips. Patients with metal prostheses such as heart valves, orthopedic screws, or cardiac pacemakers may not be allowed to undergo MRI, depending on the type of metal used. Certain metals, such as titanium, are typically safe during an MRI. Persons who have been involved in an explosion, such as military personnel, may be excluded from an MRI due to metal shrapnel embedded in the body.

The standard MRI machine looks like a narrow tunnel, which completely encloses the patient. Patients are required to lie still in this machine for 30 to 60 minutes. The patient enters the tunnel and may feel some anxiety or claustrophobia. The procedure is painless. Being enclosed in the machine may cause the patient to feel anxious. If the patient is extremely anxious, a sedative may be given if ordered by the provider. Encourage patients to use relaxation techniques, such as imagery, during the test. During the scanning procedure the patient will hear loud thumping and intermittent humming sounds. Headphones and ear plugs will be provided. Open MRIs are designed to be less confining and more comfortable than the traditional machine, but some providers feel that the closed MRI machine provides better images. Because the procedure requires the patient to be motionless, relaxation techniques that require flexing and relaxing the muscles are not appropriate during the test.

After the test, take routine vital sign measurements and allow the patient to resume pretest activities. There are no adverse effects.

Computed Tomography

Body sections can be examined from many different angles with a computed tomography (CT) scanner, which uses a narrow x-ray beam and produces a three-dimensional picture of the structure being studied. The CT scanner is approximately 100 times more sensitive than the radiograph machine and should not be used unnecessarily because of radiation exposure. Iodine contrast dye sometimes is used. The contrast dye allows for improved visualization of internal structures. A CT scan can be used for any part of the head and body. It is useful in locating injuries to the ligaments or tendons, tumors of the soft tissue, and fractures in areas difficult to define by other means.

Patient preparation includes (1) having the patient sign a consent form authorizing the examination if not included on the initial hospital consent form, (2) measuring vital signs to be sued as a baseline (3) asking the patient to void before the test, (4) removal of metal containing articles such as jewelry or hair pins. Patients who have the CT scan completed with contrast medium will also be questioned about allergies. They will be NPO for 3 to 4 hours before the test. An IV will be initiated. The contrast medium will be administered through the IV. The patient will report feelings of warmth or even burning in their upper torso as the infusion begins.

After the test, observe the patient for delayed allergic reactions (if contrast dye was used). Encourage fluids unless contraindicated. Pretest diet and activity usually can be resumed.

Bone Scan

The bone scan test is especially valuable in detecting metastatic and inflammatory bone disease (osteomyelitis). This test involves the intravenous (IV) administration of nuclides (atomic material) approximately 2 to 3 hours before the test is scheduled. There are no food or fluid restrictions, and patients are encouraged to drink water over the next 1 to 3 hours to aid renal clearance of any radioisotope not picked up by the bone. After the patient has voided, a scanning camera reveals the degree of radionuclide uptake; areas of concentrated nuclide uptake may represent a tumor or other abnormality. These areas of concentration can be detected days or weeks before an ordinary radiograph reveals a metastatic lesion. The test takes approximately 30 to 60 minutes and requires the patient to lie still.

Aspiration

An aspiration procedure is done to obtain a specimen of body fluid. The health care provider inserts a needle into a cavity with the patient under local anesthesia. This procedure is performed using sterile technique. Commonly, the health care provider takes a biopsy of tissue while doing the aspiration procedure. Nursing interventions are similar for all aspiration tests, with special emphasis on (1) having the consent form signed; (2) reinforcing the health care provider's explanation of the procedure; (3) encouraging the patient to remain immobile during the procedure; (4) having the patient void before the procedure; (5) maintaining sterile technique; (6) supporting the patient emotionally; (7) applying a sterile pressure dressing to the puncture site and maintaining the dressing until bleeding has stopped; (8) assisting with collecting, labeling, and transporting a specimen to the laboratory immediately; and (9) observing for emotional and physical distress after the procedure. Post procedure care involves resting and elevation of the affected area. Ice may be used to prevent inflammation. Observe for signs and symptoms of infection.

SYNOVIAL FLUID ASPIRATION

Arthrocentesis is the puncture of a patient's joint with a needle and the withdrawal of synovial fluid for diagnostic purposes. It is helpful in diagnosing trauma, systemic lupus erythematosus, gout, osteoarthritis (OA), and rheumatoid arthritis (RA). It also may be used to instill medications for the patient with septic arthritis or to remove fluid from joints to relieve pain. Normally a patient's synovial fluid is straw colored, clear, or slightly cloudy. If trauma or a disease is present, the synovial fluid appears cloudy, milky, sanguineous (i.e., containing blood), yellow, green, or gray.

After the procedure, provide proper support to the affected extremity. Placing it on a pillow and maintaining joint rest for approximately 12 hours may be indicated. Apply ice to the affected joint for 24 to 48 hours unless otherwise ordered. An anti-infective or corticosteroid may be prescribed. Assess the patient for signs of infection. After the pressure dressing is removed from the site, an adhesive bandage can be used.

ENDOSCOPIC EXAMINATION

For endoscopy, a lighted tube is used to visualize inside a body cavity. Although some procedures require general anesthesia, most require only local anesthesia. Emotional support and complete explanations help relieve the patient's anxiety. Preparation for an endoscopic examination is similar to that for surgical preparation: (1) have the patient sign a consent form;

(2) complete a preoperative checklist with special attention to removing jewelry, dentures, and contact lenses; (3) initiate NPO status 6 to 12 hours before the examination; (4) encourage the patient to void; (5) administer prescribed premedications, such as atropine and a sedative; (6) record vital signs; and (7) maintain bed rest with side rails up after giving the premedication.

Arthroscopy
Arthroscopy is an endoscopic examination that enables direct visualization of a joint. The procedure is used to (1) explore the joint to determine the presence of a disease process, (2) drain fluid from the joint cavity, and (3) remove damaged tissue or foreign bodies.

This examination is performed most commonly on the knee joint, with the synovium, articular surfaces, and meniscus (a curved, fibrous cartilage structure in the knee) visualized through the scope. The procedure involves insertion of a large-bore needle into the suprapatellar pouch and saline instillation into the joint. Arthroscopy also can be done on the hip or shoulder. The patient may be given a general or local anesthetic agent. After the arthroscopic examination, advise the patient to limit activities for several days.

Endoscopic Spinal Microsurgery
Surgeons can perform spinal surgery with less damage to surrounding tissues by passing endoscopic equipment through small incisions. Special scopes enable surgeons to successfully treat spinal column disorders (e.g., herniated disk, spinal stenosis) and spinal deformities (e.g., scoliosis, kyphosis). Spinal microsurgery can be performed with the patient under local anesthesia; discharge occurs after a brief stay. Candidates for microsurgery procedures are evaluated on the basis of information obtained from x-ray examinations, MRI scans, CT scans, and bone scans.

ELECTROGRAPHIC PROCEDURE
Electrographic procedures use electrodes to measure electrical activity in specific areas of the body.

Electromyogram
An electromyogram involves insertion of needle electrodes directly into the skeletal muscles so that electrical activity can be heard, seen on an oscilloscope (an instrument that displays a graphic representation of electron beams), and recorded on paper at the same time. Muscles do not produce an electrical charge at rest, but with neuromuscular disorders, unusual patterns can be observed. Nerves can be observed for neuropathy and muscles for myopathy. During the procedure the patient may experience varying degrees of discomfort as the needle electrodes are employed. The discomfort is quickly ended once the electrodes are removed. Conditions that may include electromyography in their diagnostic profile are chronic lower back pain and ulnar nerve dysfunction.

Laboratory Tests
Specific laboratory tests are ordered when musculoskeletal disorders are suspected (Table 4.3).

EFFECTS OF BED REST ON MINERAL CONTENT IN BONE
Bone requires exercise to remain healthy much like the rest of the human body. Weight-bearing exercises help maintain bone density. Immobility causes the body to lose calcium. Every day of bed rest leads to further loss of total bone density. Loss of activity will result in bone resorption, causing a loss of density. If immobilization is limited to 1 to 2 months, it is possible for the bone loss to be reversed totally once weight-bearing activities are resumed. Studies conducted on astronauts experiencing loss of gravity support these findings regarding bone loss. Patients who are immobile and thus experiencing lost bone density face an increased risk for pathologic fractures (NIH Osteoporosis and Related Bone Diseases National Resource Center, 2018).

DISORDERS OF THE MUSCULOSKELETAL SYSTEM

INFLAMMATORY DISORDERS
Arthritis is a disease involving inflammation of the joints. An estimated 54 million Americans are affected by arthritis. Nearly half report that their illness causes limitations in their daily lives. There are many types of arthritis, but the most common are RA, rheumatoid spondylitis, OA (degenerative joint disease [DJD]), and gout (gouty arthritis). Table 4.4 compares RA and OA.

RHEUMATOID ARTHRITIS
Etiology and Pathophysiology
RA, the most serious form of arthritis, can lead to severe joint deformity. It is a chronic, systemic inflammatory autoimmune disease that affects approximately 1.3 million people (Freeman, 2018). RA is more common in women, affecting nearly three times as many women as men. Although it can affect women of any age, women 30 to 60 years of age are affected most often. There is also a noted genetic link. Smoking significantly increases the risk of RA in men and women who are predisposed genetically to the disease. Additional risk factors include bacterial and viral diseases.

RA is a systemic disorder and can affect many organ systems (lungs, heart, blood vessels, muscles, eyes, skin). RA is characterized by a chronic inflammation of the synovial membrane (synovitis) of the diarthrodial joints (also called synovial joints: the freely movable joints in which continuous bony surfaces are covered by cartilage and connected by ligaments lined with synovial membrane).

Table 4.3 Laboratory Tests for Musculoskeletal Disorders

NORMAL VALUE	POSSIBLE CAUSE FOR INCREASE OR DECREASE
Calcium: 9.0–10.5 mg/dL	Increased in metastatic tumor in the bone, Addison's disease, Paget's disease of the bone, acromegaly, acute osteoporosis, hyperparathyroidism, vitamin D deficiency, renal failure, malabsorption, and rickets.
Phosphorus: 2.5–4.5 mg/dL	Increased in acromegaly, bone metastases, excessive levels of vitamin D, hypocalcemia, renal failure. Decreased in acute gout, hypercalcemia, vitamin D deficiency.
Vitamin D, 25–dihydroxy: 6–52 ng/mL	Increased in vitamin D intoxication. Decreased in bowel resection, malabsorption, rickets.
Vitamin D_1, 25–dihydroxy: 15–60 pg/mL	Increased in liver disease; bone disease; healing fractures; metastatic tumor in bone; osteogenic sarcoma; osteoporosis; cancer of breast, colon, lung, or pancreas. Decreased in severe anemia, folic acid deficiency, pernicious anemia.
Alkaline phosphatase: 30–120 units/L	Increased in skeletal muscle injury or myocardial infarction.
Myoglobin: 5–70 mcg/dL	Decreased in rheumatoid arthritis.
Erythrocyte sedimentation rate (ESR): • *Males:* Up to 15 mm/h • *Females:* Up to 20 mm/h	A nonspecific test used to detect inflammatory, neoplastic, infectious, and necrotic processes. Indicates the presence of inflammation as seen in rheumatoid arthritis and rheumatic fever. One of the most objective measurements of rheumatoid arthritis severity. Increased as the disease worsens. Increased in multiple myeloma, acute myocardial infarctions, toxemia, bacterial infections, and gout. Decreased in congestive heart failure, sickle cell anemia, polycythemia vera, infectious mononucleosis, degenerative arthritis, and angina pectoris.
Rheumatoid factor (RF): 40–60 units/mL	An immunoglobulin found in approximately 80% of adults with rheumatoid arthritis; other diseases such as systemic lupus erythematosus may cause a positive RF result.
Uric acid (blood): • *Males:* 2.1–8.5 mg/dL • *Females:* 2.0–6.6 mg/dL	Increased in patients with gout, kidney failure, alcoholism, leukemia, metastatic cancer, multiple myeloma, or dehydration.

Data from Pagana KD, Pagana TJ: *Mosby's manual of diagnostic and laboratory tests,* ed 5, St. Louis, 2014, Mosby.

Clinical Manifestations

RA is believed to involve an immune reaction caused when the body's immune system chooses to attack one of its own proteins. The immune response causes an inflammatory response. The repeated inflammation of the joints and surrounding tissue may lead to gross deformity and loss of function (Fig. 4.5).

RA is characterized by periods of remission and exacerbation. Arthritic flare-ups may be attributed to a precipitating stressful event such as infection, work stress, physical exertion, childbirth, surgery, or emotional upset. During remission the inflammation, pain, stiffness, and edema subside, and progression of tissue damage is halted or reduced.

Assessment

Collection of *subjective data* is important in helping diagnose RA. According to the Arthritis Foundation (2019) the symptoms of RA include the following:
• Joint pain, tenderness, swelling or stiffness for 6 weeks or longer
• More than one joint is affected
• Morning stiffness for 30 minutes or longer
• Small joints (wrists, certain joints of the hands and feet) are affected

• The same joints on both sides of the body are affected

Other symptoms include fatigue and low-grade fever. The patient with RA has periods of remission and exacerbation. The common terminology used for an exacerbation of RA is a "flare." RA flares can last for days up to months. If prolonged inflammation goes untreated or has frequent recurrences, RA can affect the patient systemically. Organs that are affected commonly include the eyes (dryness and light sensitivity), oral cavity (irritation and ulcerations), skin (RA nodules), lungs and blood vessels (inflammation), and bone marrow (anemia) (Arthritis Foundation, n.d.).

Collection of *objective data* includes observing the joints for edema, tenderness, subcutaneous nodules, limitation in range of motion (ROM), symmetric joint involvement, and fever.

Diagnostic Tests

No single test is definitive for RA. Diagnosis is based primarily on patient history and physical examination. The four classic symptoms most frequently reported are morning stiffness, joint pain, muscle weakness, and fatigue. Swelling of joints is not uncommon.

Table 4.4   Comparison of Rheumatoid Arthritis and Osteoarthritis

	RHEUMATOID ARTHRITIS	OSTEOARTHRITIS
Pathophysiology	Inflammation of synovial membrane; destruction of cartilage, joint capsule, bones, ligaments, and tendons	Degeneration of cartilage from wear and tear; bone spur formation
Joints most commonly affected	Symmetric joint involvement noted in wrists, knees, and knuckles	Often only one side of body affected with changes noted in hands, spine, knees, and hips
Clinical signs and symptoms	Edema, erythema, heat, pain, tenderness, nodule formation, fatigue, stiffness, muscle aches, and fever Systemic manifestations occur Vasculitis (inflammation of blood vessels) may be responsible for a variety of systemic complications, including peripheral neuropathy, myopathy, cardiopulmonary involvement, and ischemic ulcerations of the skin Potential complications include infection, osteoporosis, and Sjögren's syndrome. Dry mouth and decreased tearing occur in Sjögren's syndrome	Localized pain, stiffness, bony knobs of end joints of fingers (Heberden's nodes), edema (not as pronounced as in RA) No systemic involvement is present Constitutional symptoms such as fatigue or fever are not present Other organ involvement is absent as well, which is an important differentiation between OA and RA
Age at onset	Children nearing adolescence; adults between 20 and 50 years	Ages 45–90 years. Most people have some features with increasing age
Sex	Females affected more often than males, at a ratio of 3:1	Males and females affected equally
Heredity	Familial tendency	The form with knobby fingers can be hereditary
Diagnostic tests	Rheumatoid factor (RF) found in serum of about 85% of patients with RA. Erythrocyte sedimentation rate, C-reactive protein, complete blood count, x-rays, examination of joint fluid RF positive in 80% of patients	X-rays; no specific laboratory abnormalities are useful in diagnosing OA. RF negative
Treatment	Control inflammation and pain with medications Balance exercise with rest Provide joint protection; encourage weight control and stress reduction Surgically replace joints	Maintain activity level Control pain with medication Encourage exercise, joint protection, weight control, stress reduction Surgical joint replacement may be necessary

RA, Rheumatoid arthritis; *OA,* osteoarthritis.

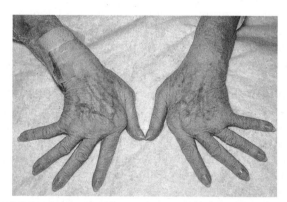

Fig. 4.5 Rheumatoid arthritis of the hands. (From Swartz MH: *Textbook of physical diagnosis,* ed 5, Philadelphia, 2006, Saunders.)

Radiographic studies reveal loss of articular cartilage and change in subchondral bone. The following laboratory tests are used often in supporting the diagnosis and in ruling out other diseases:

- *Anti-CCP (cyclic citrullinated peptide) antibody test:* Anti-CCP antibodies are found frequently in the blood of patients with RA. This test can identify RA before symptoms develop and identify the likelihood of patients developing severe RA.
- *Anti-nuclear antibody (ANA) titers and elevated C-reactive protein (CRP):* These are seen in some patients with RA.
- *C-reactive protein (CRP):* Indicates the presence of inflammation in the body.
- *Erythrocyte sedimentation rate (ESR):* An increase indicates the presence of an inflammatory reaction somewhere in the body.
- *Latex agglutination test:* This test detects the presence of the immunoglobulin M version of RF, which combines with antigen-coated latex particles to form a precipitate.
- *Red blood cell count:* This detects anemia, which is often present during chronic infection.
- *Rheumatoid factor (RF):* An elevation indicates an abnormal serum concentration of this protein. Positive RF occurs in approximately 80% of patients with RA.
- *Synovial fluid aspiration:* Normal fluid is usually clear and highly viscous; however, when inflammation is

present, the fluid is cloudy, yellow, less viscous, and contains increased protein.

- *Synovial fluid biopsy:* The biopsy shows changes in the synovial tissue.
- *X-rays:* To determine the presence of any joint damage.

Medical Management

The patient with RA benefits from aggressive treatment early in the course of the disease. The medical management of RA is directed toward (1) controlling the disease activity by administering disease-modifying and anti-inflammatory drugs (Table 4.5); (2) providing pain relief; (3) reducing clinical symptoms in days to weeks with the rapid anti-inflammatory effect of methotrexate; (4) prolonging joint function (often with physical therapy, traction, and splints); and (5) slowing the progression of joint damage by promoting activities of daily living (ADLs), an exercise program, and weight management.

Advances in cell and molecular biology have influenced the treatment of RA. Current medications actually target the pathophysiology of the disease. Disease-modifying antirheumatoid drugs (DMARDs) offer wider treatment options. These medications target a protein known as tumor necrosis factor (TNF). TNF is produced by the synovial cells and other cells of the body and is a proinflammatory substance—that is, it has the ability to produce signs and symptoms of inflammation (see Table 4.5). Complementary therapies to decrease inflammation include nonsteroidal anti-inflammatory drugs (NSAIDs); capsaicin, a non-opioid topical analgesic; fish oil; and antioxidants (vitamins C and E and beta-carotene). Musculoskeletal surgery in the form of joint replacement is another option.

Nursing Interventions and Patient Teaching

Patient education is essential to help the patient and family understand what is happening and what to expect as the disease progresses. Fatigue can be a major concern. Achieving restful sleep is important. Additional sleeping periods and naps are indicated only during disease exacerbation. Exercise helps prevent the joints from "freezing" and the muscles from weakening. An initial exercise program calls for two or three 10- to 15-minute daily sessions of "quiet" exercise that gently put joints through ROM. Heat is used often to relax and soothe muscles. Strength training, aerobic exercise, and yoga also may be included. Some patients achieve comfort from warm packs and heat lamps, and applications of hot paraffin wax may be helpful. Rehabilitation is aimed at helping the patient adapt to physical limitations and promoting normal daily activities.

Problem statements and interventions for the patient with RA include but are not limited to the following:

PATIENT PROBLEM	NURSING INTERVENTIONS
Prolonged Pain, related to joint inflammation	Administer prescribed salicylate or nonsteroidal anti-inflammatory drugs (NSAIDs)
	Assist patient with an exercise program prescribed by the health care provider
	Physical therapy referral as indicated to discuss proper body mechanics and use of a walker or cane
	During acute stages of disease, encourage patient to rest inflamed joints and maintain proper body alignment
	Application of heat (may include heating pads, warm compresses, heat patches, warm baths, or wax)
	Application of cold therapy (may include ice or cold packs)
	Assist and teach patient to extend joints as possible and to avoid external rotation of extremities; use sandbags or trochanter rolls
	Avoid use of pillow under knees and/or support joints
Prolonged Low Self-Esteem, related to negative self-evaluation about self or capabilities	Encourage patient to express feelings about health problems, progress, and prognosis concerning diagnosis
	Encourage patient to explore ways to remain active while experiencing limited mobility (e.g., doing tasks while sitting as opposed to standing or walking)

As with any chronic illness, patient teaching is perhaps the most important aspect of nursing interventions. Patient teaching includes providing information about joint protection and energy conservation techniques, proper balance of rest and activity, proper use of medications (i.e., names of drugs, dosages, precautions in administration, and side effects or toxic effects), plans for implementation of the exercise program prescribed by the health care provider or physical therapist, proper application of heat or cold packs, proper use of walking aids, safety measures to prevent injury, basics of good nutrition and the importance of avoiding weight gain, and the danger of following programs that promise a "cure."

Prognosis

The course of RA is variable but is marked by remissions and exacerbations. The prognosis is based on a variety of clinical and laboratory findings. Stage I represents early effects. Stage IV, the terminal category, includes marked joint deformity, extensive muscle atrophy, soft tissue lesions, bone and cartilage destruction, and fibrous or bony ankylosis.

Table 4.5   Medications for Rheumatoid Arthritis

GENERIC NAME	ACTION	SIDE EFFECTS/TOXIC EFFECTS	NURSING IMPLICATIONS
Salicylates			
aspirin, salsalate choline salicylate choline magnesium	Anti-inflammatory, analgesic, antipyretic; act by inhibiting synthesis of prostaglandins	GI irritation (dyspepsia, nausea, ulcer, hemorrhage) Prolonged bleeding time Exacerbation of asthma (aspirin-sensitive asthma) Tinnitus, dizziness with repeated large doses	Administer drug with food, milk, antacids as prescribed, or full glass of water; may use enteric-coated aspirin. Report signs of bleeding (e.g., tarry stools, bruising, petechiae, nosebleeds).
Nonsteroidal Anti-Inflammatory Drugs (NSAIDs)			
indomethacin	Analgesic, anti-inflammatory	Headache, vertigo, insomnia; confusion, GI irritation; can decrease effect of ACE inhibitors	Give with food, milk, or antacid. Discontinue if CNS symptoms develop and notify health care provider. Monitor BP. Report signs of bleeding.
ibuprofen	Analgesic, anti-inflammatory	Same as indomethacin but believed less irritating to GI tract Fluid retention Can cause hypertension	Know that delayed absorption occurs if taken with food. Monitor BP.
tolmetin sodium	Analgesic, anti-inflammatory	Same as ibuprofen	Give with food or milk.
naproxen	Analgesic, anti-inflammatory	Same as ibuprofen Causes drowsiness	Give with food, milk, or antacid. Tell patient to avoid driving until dosage effect is established.
meloxicam	Anti-inflammatory, analgesic, antipyretic	Dizziness, headache, insomnia, seizures, dysrhythmias, heart failure, hemorrhage, diarrhea, indigestion, nausea, pancreatitis, renal failure, leukopenia, thrombocytopenia, asthma, bronchospasm, angioedema Drug is contraindicated in women who are pregnant or plan to become pregnant	Monitor BP. Instruct patient to avoid using aspirin or products containing aspirin. Assess patient for history of allergic reactions to aspirin or other NSAIDs before starting drug. Tell patient the drug can be taken without regard to meals. Advise patient to report signs and symptoms of GI ulcers and bleeding. Advise patient to report any skin rash, weight gain, or edema. Alert patient with history of asthma that asthma may recur while taking the drug. Advise patient to avoid alcohol and tobacco products while taking the drug. NSAIDs can cause fluid retention; closely monitor patients with hypertension, edema, or heart failure. Inform patient that consistent pain relief may take several days of drug administration.
nabumetone	Analgesic, anti-inflammatory	Dizziness, anxiety, depression, gastric irritation, edema, prolonged bleeding, rash	Give with meals or antacids. Advise patient to avoid alcohol, aspirin, or aspirin products or acetaminophen without health care provider's consent. Arthritic relief noted in 1–2 weeks.
meclofenamate	Analgesic, anti-inflammatory	Gastric irritation, headache, dizziness, edema	Advise patients to avoid aspirin and aspirin products. Give 30 min before or 2 h after eating.
COX-2 Inhibitor			
celecoxib	Analgesic, anti-inflammatory	Mild to moderate indigestion, risk of GI bleeding, diarrhea, abdominal pain Has been linked to an increased risk of cardiovascular events, such as MI or stroke	Give medication orally. It can be taken with or without food. Celebrex is indicated for relief of the signs and symptoms of osteoarthritis and RA. Do not administer to patients who have asthma, urticaria, or allergic reactions to aspirin or other NSAIDs. Do not give to patients who are allergic to sulfonamide. Use cautiously with ACE inhibitors, warfarin, lithium, and furosemide. Monitor patients for signs of GI bleeding.

Table 4.5   Medications for Rheumatoid Arthritis—cont'd

GENERIC NAME	ACTION	SIDE EFFECTS/TOXIC EFFECTS	NURSING IMPLICATIONS
Potent Anti-Inflammatory Agents			
Adrenocorticosteroids (e.g., prednisone)	Interfere with body's normal inflammatory responses	Fluid retention, sodium retention, potassium depletion, hypertension, decreased healing potential, increased susceptibility to infection, GI irritation, hirsutism, osteoporosis, fat deposits, diabetes mellitus, myopathy. Adrenal insufficiency or adrenal crisis if abruptly withdrawn	Give with food, milk, or antacid. Do not increase or decrease dosage without health care provider supervision. Give in morning if given once a day.
Corticosteroids, intra-articular injections (e.g., methylprednisolone)	Suppression of inflammation and modification of the normal immune response	Decreased wound healing and increased susceptibility to infection	Check injection site for signs of infection. Inform patient joint improvement can last weeks to months. Advise patient to avoid overuse of joint.
Slow-Acting Anti-Inflammatory Agents			
Antimalarials			
hydroxychloroquine	Anti-inflammatory (mechanism unknown); effect not expected to be noted for 6–12 months after beginning therapy	GI disturbances. Retinal edema that may result in blindness	Instruct patient to obtain eye examination before beginning therapy and every 6 months thereafter. Monitor CBC.
Gold Salts (IM)			
Gold sodium thiomalate	Anti-inflammatory; effect not noted for 3–6 months after beginning therapy	Renal and hepatic damage, corneal deposits, dermatitis, ulcerations in mouth, hematologic changes	Monitor urinalysis and CBC before each injection. Report dermatitis, metallic taste in mouth, or lesions in mouth to health care provider.
Oral gold salts (auranofin)	Antirheumatic	Stomatitis (lesions in mouth); thrombocytopenia and leukopenia	Minimize exposure to sunlight and provide meticulous oral hygiene.
Antineoplastic			
methotrexate	Alters the way the body uses folic acid, which is necessary for cell growth; decreases inflammation	Upset stomach, nausea, vomiting, anorexia, diarrhea, or sore mouth; headache, blurred vision, dizziness	Drug is taken orally or by injection. Monitor vital signs, WBC, platelets, I&O, appetite. Advise patient to avoid pregnancy while taking this drug and not to get vaccinations without health care provider's consent. Keep patient well hydrated.
Disease-Modifying Antirheumatoid Drugs (DMARDs)			
etanercept	Blocks the normal and inflammatory immune responses seen in RA; binds tumor necrosis factor (TNF), which is involved in immune and inflammatory reactions	Pain at injection site, upper respiratory tract infections and sinusitis; in severe cases, tuberculosis possible	Give twice weekly subcutaneously in the thigh, abdomen, or upper arm. Refrigerate, but never freeze medication. Use with caution in patients with chronic infections. May cause or aggravate systemic lupus erythematosus.

Continued

Table 4.5   Medications for Rheumatoid Arthritis—cont'd

GENERIC NAME	ACTION	SIDE EFFECTS/TOXIC EFFECTS	NURSING IMPLICATIONS
leflunomide	Reduces signs and symptoms of RA and retards structural bone damage	Diarrhea, elevated liver enzymes, alopecia, rash	Medication is taken orally. Monitor urinary output. Do not use with patients with hepatic impairment or positive for hepatitis B or C.
infliximab	An antibody that binds specifically to proinflammatory enzymes produced by the synovial cells	Upper respiratory tract infections, headache, nausea, sinusitis, rash, cough	Administer intravenously at 2 and 6 weeks initially, then every 8 weeks thereafter. Do not give to patients with a clinically active infection.
adalimumab	Reduces infiltration of inflammatory cells	Increased risk of infection, headaches and rash; neutropenia; injection site reaction	Assess for signs of infection before injection. Do not give to patients with active infections. Monitor new infections closely.
sulfasalazine	Sulfonamide; anti-inflammatory; blocks prostaglandin synthesis	GI effects (anorexia, nausea, vomiting); bleeding, bruising, jaundice; headache; rash, urticaria, pruritus	Advise patient that drug may cause orange-yellow discoloration of urine or skin. Space doses evenly around the clock, taking drug after food with 8 oz of water. Treatment may be continued even after symptoms are relieved. Monitor CBC.
penicillamine	Anti-inflammatory; exact mechanism of action in RA unknown but may suppress cell-mediated immune response	GI irritation (nausea, vomiting, anorexia, diarrhea); reduced or altered taste; rash; proteinuria, hematuria; iron deficiency (especially in menstruating women)	Monitor WBC count, platelets, urinalysis. Advise patient to take medication 1 h before or 2 h after meals or at least 1 h away from any other drug, food, or milk.
anakinra	Blocks the action of interleukin-1, thus decreasing the inflammatory response	Injection site reaction, leukopenia, headache, abdominal pain, rash	Evaluate for relief of pain, swelling, stiffness; increase in joint mobility. Advise patient that injection site reaction generally occurs in first month of treatment and decreases with continued therapy. Evaluate renal function. Monitor for infection. Do not give drug with other TNF inhibitors.
abatacept	Modulates T cell activation; suppresses immune response	Headache, upper respiratory tract infection, nausea, sore throat, injection site reaction	Not recommended for concomitant use with TNF inhibitors. Evaluate for relief of pain, swelling, stiffness and increase in joint mobility.
rituximab	Monoclonal antibody that targets B cells	Dizziness, palpitations, fever, itching, difficulty breathing, sore throat	Give in combination with methotrexate. Monitor for infection and bleeding. Advise patient not to receive virus vaccines with treatment. Monitor for low BP if also taking BP medication.
Immunosuppressant			
azathioprine cyclophosphamide	Inhibits DNA, RNA, protein synthesis	GI irritation (nausea, vomiting, anorexia with large doses), rash	Evaluate for relief of pain, swelling, stiffness; increase in joint mobility. Advise patient to immediately report unusual bleeding or bruising. Advise patient that therapeutic response may take up to 12 weeks. Advise women of childbearing age to avoid pregnancy.

Table 4.5   Medications for Rheumatoid Arthritis—cont'd

GENERIC NAME	ACTION	SIDE EFFECTS/TOXIC EFFECTS	NURSING IMPLICATIONS
Topical Analgesics			
capsaicin cream 5% lidocaine	Depletes substance P from nerve endings, interrupting pain signals to the brain (substance P may participate directly or indirectly in the transmission process of certain neurons)	Rash, urticaria, localized burning sensation, erythema	Must be used regularly over time for maximal effect. Aloe vera cream may moderate burning sensation. Advise patient not to use cream with external heat source (heating pad) because of risk of burns. Available in OTC and prescription strengths. Advise patient to wear gloves when applying cream to other joints and to wash hands; avoid touching damaged or irritated skin, eyes, nose, and mouth.

ACE, Angiotensin-converting enzyme; *BP,* blood pressure; *CBC,* complete blood count; *CNS,* central nervous system; *DNA,* deoxyribonucleic acid; *GI,* gastrointestinal; *I&O,* intake and output; *IM,* intramuscular; *MI,* myocardial infarction; *OTC,* over the counter; *RA,* rheumatoid arthritis; *RNA,* ribonucleic acid; *WBC,* white blood cell count.
Data from Lewis SL, Heitkemper MM, Dirksen SR, et al: *Medical-surgical nursing: Assessment and management of clinical problems,* ed 10, St. Louis, 2016, Mosby, and Skidmore-Roth L: *Mosby's 2017 nursing drug reference,* ed 30, St. Louis, 2016, Elsevier.

ANKYLOSING SPONDYLITIS

Etiology and Pathophysiology
Ankylosing spondylitis (AS) is one of the types of arthritis that comprise the group of rheumatic disorders known as *spondyloarthritis,* or *SpA.* It is a chronic, progressive rheumatic disorder that affects primarily the spine. When other joints are involved, the disease commonly includes the sacroiliac and hip joints and the adjacent soft tissues. Another common type of arthritis that is part of the SpA group is psoriatic arthritis. This type of arthritis differs in that it largely effects the fingers and toes (causing swelling), back pain and stiffness, changes to the finger and toe nails (indentations or discoloration), and psoriatic lesions (Spondylitis Association of America, 2019). The exact cause of the disease is unknown. Genetic links are the strongest suspicion. A leading theory is that a trigger or stimulus from the environment or illness can trigger the disorder. Risk factors include testing positive for the HLA-B27 marker, a family history of the disease, and frequent gastrointestinal (GI) infections. It can affect both sexes but is seen more often in young men. The presence of human leukocyte antigen A and B27 (HLA-B27) in the serum of 90% of whites and 50% of African Americans with AS suggests a hereditary factor. The most common time for onset of AS is between 15 and 35 years of age. Women develop a milder form of AS than men, and fusion of the spine rarely is seen. It is sometimes referred to as *rheumatoid spondylitis* (Mayo Clinic, 2019a).

Clinical Manifestations
The characteristic spinal inflammation of AS results in the bones of the spine fusing (growing together). The accompanying fixation of the joint is referred to as ankylosis. This fixation is often in an abnormal position.

The inflammation typically is located where the ligaments and tendons attach to the bone. AS can affect joints such as the neck, jaw, shoulders, knees, and hips. Progression of the disease causes the ligaments to become ossified (hardened). The cardiovascular system can be involved, and heart enlargement and pericarditis can occur. If the costovertebral joints (i.e., where the ribs connect with the spine) are affected, kyphosis can occur, leading to a forward curvature of the upper back and altered respirations. The patient may have difficulty expanding the ribcage while breathing. Many patients with the disease also have inflammatory bowel disease. Vision loss occurs with chronic AS, and blindness may result from glaucoma and pupil damage. The condition is characterized by periods of remission and exacerbations or "flares."

Assessment
Subjective data include complaints of low backache, stiffness, and alternating or bilateral "sciatica pain" that lasts for a few days and then subsides. Pain is more pronounced when the patient is in an erect position. Inactivity exacerbates the pain, and exercise gives relief. Complaints of weight loss, abdominal distention, visual problems, and fatigue are common. AS is present in 3% to 10% of patients with inflammatory bowel disease.

Collection of objective data includes assessment for tenderness over the spine and sacroiliac region. Peripheral joint edema and decreased ROM may be seen. Assessment of vital signs may indicate elevated temperature, tachycardia, and hyperpnea. Respiratory difficulties arise if there is limited expansion of the chest, as often is seen in kyphosis.

Diagnostic Tests
Patients with AS often have the following laboratory test results: (1) low hemoglobin and hematocrit, indicative of

anemia; (2) elevated ESR and CRP, which are common in chronic inflammatory disease; (3) elevated serum alkaline phosphatase levels in patients who are immobilized or have bone resorption; and (4) presence of the HLA-B27 antigen. Radiographic examination often reveals sacroiliac joint and intervertebral disk inflammation with bony erosion and joint space fusion.

Medical Management

The health care provider usually prescribes oral analgesics and NSAIDs. Corticosteroid therapy with prednisone may be prescribed. TNF inhibitors are biological response modifiers. They target the immune cells. Examples include etanercept, infliximab, and adalimumab. Regular exercise is recommended. Exercise will help to prevent demineralization of bone and promote flexibility and improved posture. Swimming and walking are low-impact activities that may be considered for the regimen. Patients are encouraged to work toward exercising two or three times each week for 30 to 40 minutes. Patients who have been relatively sedentary will need to gradually build to this level of activity.

Surgery may be necessary to replace fused joints (commonly the hip or the knee). Cervical or lumbar osteotomy can be done for severe kyphosis.

Endoscopic microsurgery can be performed on select candidates. In microsurgery, the bone or tissue that is putting pressure on the spinal nerves is removed by using endoscopic equipment placed through small incisions. Most patients leave the hospital within 24 hours and start physical therapy within a few days.

Nursing Interventions and Patient Teaching

Nursing interventions are aimed at maintaining alignment of the spine. Providing a firm mattress, bed board, and back brace helps provide support. Encouraging the patient to lie on the abdomen for at least 15 to 30 minutes four times daily helps extend the spine. Turning and positioning every 2 hours helps prevent pressure sores. Postural and breathing exercises help compensate for the possibility of impaired gas exchange caused by the changes in posture and chest cavity size. Heat and cold also may be included in the plan of care. Heat will reduce pain and stiffness. Cold applications will aid in the reduction of inflammation and swelling.

Teach the patient the appropriate use of prescribed medications, postural exercises, and methods of applying heat to back and hips. Promote correct posture and prevent complications by encouraging the patient to use a firm mattress, sleep without a pillow, and do respiratory exercises.

Prognosis

AS is a chronic disease occurring in persons younger than age 30 years that will "burn itself out" after a course of 20 years in approximately 1% of affected people, entering long-term remission and leaving permanent, irreversible systemic involvement if not treated (National Institute of Arthritis and Musculoskeletal and Skin Diseases [NIAMS], 2020).

OSTEOARTHRITIS (DEGENERATIVE JOINT DISEASE)

Etiology and Pathophysiology

OA is the most common arthritis, and sometimes is referred to as DJD because it results from wear and tear on the joints. OA is a non-systemic, non-inflammatory disorder that begins with degeneration of the cartilage of joints, thus causing damage to bones. Obesity is a major contributing factor to OA. Degenerative joint changes traditionally are noticed beginning in middle age. By the age of 70 most adults have hypertrophic joint changes. Before age 55, OA occurs with similar frequency in men and women. Women begin to outpace men with incidence after that point (Box 4.3). The disease is a consequence of aging and is a major cause of severe chronic disability. OA takes two forms: primary (cause is unknown) and secondary (caused by trauma, infections, previous fractures, RA, stress on weight-bearing joints from obesity, occupations placing abnormal stressors on joints such as professional athletics, and occupations requiring excessive stooping and bending such as plumbers). A comparison of RA and OA is found in Table 4.4.

Clinical Manifestations

This disorder most commonly affects the joints of the hand, knee, hip, and cervical and lumbar vertebrae (Fig. 4.6) (NIAMS, 2019). Symptoms include pain and stiffness in the joints. The joints are stiffest in the morning hours upon awakening. With activity the stiffness reduces. Grating or cracking sounds may be noted with joint movement. The disease affects the hands in women more often, whereas in men the hips are affected.

Assessment

Collection of subjective data includes questioning the patient about pain and stiffness (rest usually relieves pain in the early stages). Past illnesses, surgical procedures, or trauma may be relevant, and information about excessive weight gain and occupation may be significant. Complaints regarding reduced grip strength are common.

Collection of objective data includes assessment for joint edema, tenderness, instability, and deformity. *Heberden's nodes* appear on the sides of the distal joints of fingers (Fig. 4.7), and *Bouchard's nodes* appear on the proximal joints of fingers; these nodes are hard, bony, and cartilaginous enlargements. The patient's gait reveals a limp, especially if the hips or legs are affected.

Diagnostic Tests

There is no specific test to diagnose OA. However, radiographic studies, MRI, arthroscopy, synovial fluid examination, and bone scans are used to provide supportive information.

Box 4.3   Osteoarthritis

- Osteoarthritis is the most common form of arthritis and the leading cause of disability in people older than age 65 years. Under age 55, men and women are affected equally. In older individuals, osteoarthritis of the hip is more common in men and osteoarthritis of the interphalangeal joints and the thumb is more common in women. Osteoarthritis occurs more frequently in people who are obese or who experience repetitive stress to the joints.
- More than 70% of total hip and knee replacements are for osteoarthritis.
- Overweight people have a higher risk of knee and hip osteoarthritis.
- Weight loss programs for overweight older adults lessen symptoms in those with the disease.
- Acetaminophen is recommended by the American College of Rheumatology for osteoarthritis pain because of fewer gastrointestinal and renal side effects compared with other drugs.
- Bicycling and swimming are considered good exercises for people with osteoarthritis of the knee; walking should be done on level ground.
- People with osteoarthritis of the knee or hip should avoid climbing stairs, bending, stooping, or squatting.

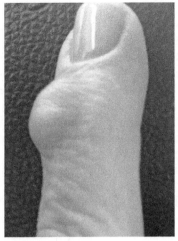

Fig. 4.7 Heberden's nodes.

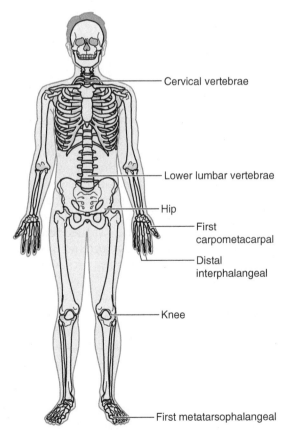

Fig. 4.6 Joints most frequently involved in osteoarthritis.

- Cervical vertebrae
- Lower lumbar vertebrae
- Hip
- First carpometacarpal
- Distal interphalangeal
- Knee
- First metatarsophalangeal

Medical Management

The primary care provider prescribes an exercise plan that is balanced with rest periods. Physical therapy using heat application helps reduce stiffness, pain, and muscle spasms. Gait enhancers—such as canes, walkers, and shoe inserts—help relieve discomfort while using weight-bearing joints. Pharmacologic therapies begin with lower doses of over-the-counter medications such as acetaminophen (Tylenol) and progress to NSAID therapies, including salicylates (aspirin) and ibuprofen (Motrin) (NIAMS, 2019). Dosages are increased as tolerance and/or the condition progresses. A corticosteroid (cortisone) sometimes is used in low doses or injected into joints to produce immediate pain relief and temporarily halt the destructive process. Patients with hypertension must be screened carefully while taking NSAIDs because certain NSAIDs elevate blood pressure. Patients need to inform their health care provider if they have been prescribed hypertensive medication by another health care provider so that a safe and effective combination of drugs can be chosen. Indomethacin (Indocin) can decrease the effect of enalapril (an angiotensin-converting enzyme inhibitor used for hypertension), and the combination of ibuprofen and lisinopril can trigger a hypertensive response. Acetaminophen is used commonly as an analgesic and does not affect the blood pressure. Tramadol hydrochloride is a synthetic analgesic used for moderate to severe pain and can be used for patients taking anti-hypertensives.

Alternatives to nonsteroidal anti-inflammatory drugs. The discomfort associated with acute or chronic RA, OA, gouty arthritis, and AS also may be decreased through the use of non-pharmacologic measures. Measures such as relaxation techniques, massage therapy, imagery, and therapeutic touch have been proven effective in reducing discomfort and decreasing the need for NSAIDs.

Glucosamine is found in the body and acts as a lubricant and shock absorber necessary for repairing and maintaining healthy joint function. The aging process has been linked to the loss of glucosamine and other substances in the cartilage. Taking supplements of natural glucosamine enables the body to manufacture collagen and proteoglycans and resupply lubricant found in the synovial fluid necessary for restoring healthy cartilage (see the Complementary and Alternative Therapies box). Glucosamine supplements have been linked with reductions in articular pain, joint tenderness, and restricted joint movement in people suffering from arthritis. People with chronic medical problems or women who are pregnant or lactating should not take supplemental glucosamine without conferring with a health care provider. Although glucosamine often is obtained from the shells of shrimp, crab, and lobster, there are no reports of allergic reactions by persons who are allergic to shellfish after using glucosamine (National Library of Medicine [NLM], 2021).

Complementary and Alternative Therapies

Musculoskeletal Disorders

- Alternative therapies being considered in the treatment of osteoarthritis include compounds such as glucosamine and chondroitin. These substances appear to provide pain relief, perhaps even slowing the disease process. Glucosamine apparently stimulates cartilage cells to manufacture proteoglycans, whereas chondroitin inhibits enzymes that break down cartilage. Few adverse effects have been seen with glucosamine used up to 3 years.
- Chiropractic adjustment has been effective in patients with some types of back pain. Many insurance companies allow for this form of therapy.
- Other manual healing methods—therapy that includes touch and manipulation of soft tissues or realignment of body parts to correct a dysfunction that affects other body parts—include the following:
  - Acupuncture
  - Massage and other physical healing methods
  - Reflexology (a system of treating certain disorders by massaging the soles of the feet or the palms of the hands)
  - Rolfing is a technique of deep massage intended to realign the body by altering the length and tone of myofascial tissues.

Cupping is treatment that involves the use of a flammable substance is put in a cup and ignited. The cup is then placed on the skin. The cup is held in place by suction. The resulting pressure brings increased circulation to the area, promoting healing and reduced pain and discomfort (Fig. 4.8).

Surgical intervention, such as osteotomy, may help correct malalignment. Joint replacement may be necessary to replace all or part of the joint's articulating surface. Arthroplasty of the hip and knee is the most common surgical intervention.

Nursing Interventions and Patient Teaching
Nursing interventions include encouraging the patient to maintain ADLs and adapt to limitations of

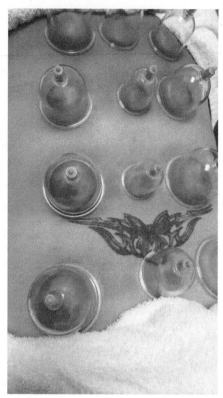

Fig 4.8 Cupping performed to manage back pain.

the disease. Alternating sitting, walking, and standing with periods of rest can help reduce joint discomfort and deterioration. Older patients may be physically capable of turning and moving in bed but may forget to do so because of alteration in their level of orientation. Assist the patient with a weight reduction plan if obesity is a problem. If splints are used to support a painful joint, assess for neurovascular impairment above and below the site of application. Also check gait enhancers for safety considerations, such as rubber tips on ends, proper size, and patient knowledge about use. If the patient has been taking aspirin over a period of time, GI bleeding may occur. It may be necessary to perform a guaiac test on stool and emesis to determine the presence of occult blood.

As with RA, teaching the person with OA about the disease process and the steps to control that process is the most important aspect of nursing interventions. Patient teaching should include the same information as for RA.

Prognosis
OA is a chronic disease that ultimately causes permanent destruction of affected cartilage and underlying bone with variable pain and disability. Bones rub against other bones because of the destruction of the cartilage between them; arthroscopic surgery to remove resultant bone spurs may help ease pain. Joint replacement is necessary for improved mobility and reduction in pain when severe OA is present.

GOUT (GOUTY ARTHRITIS)

Etiology and Pathophysiology

Gout is a metabolic disease resulting from an accumulation of uric acid in the blood. It is an acute inflammatory condition associated with ineffective metabolism of purines. Gout can be primary (linked with hereditary factors), secondary (resulting from use of certain medications or complication of another disease), or idiopathic (of unknown origin). It affects men approximately eight times more frequently than women and usually occurs in middle life. Women who experience gout traditionally are affected after menopause. Of all people with gout, 85% have a genetic tendency to develop the disease. Tophi (calculi containing sodium urate deposits that develop in periarticular fibrous tissue, typically in patients with gout) result in inflammation of the joint; it is unclear why this occurs. More than 75% of people with gout experience big toe involvement. Other joints such as the foot, fingers, and wrists are affected with lesser frequency.

Clinical Manifestations

Onset occurs at night, with excruciating pain, edema, and inflammation in the affected joint. The pain may last a short time but return at intervals, or it may be severe and continuous for 5 to 10 days. The patient may have repeated attacks or only one attack in a lifetime. Tophi are seen around the rim of the ear and can cause disfigurement. Surgical removal may be necessary.

Assessment

Collection of subjective data includes noting a complaint of pain occurring at night involving the great toe or other joints. Take a dietary history, with specific questions on consumption of alcohol and foods high in purines, such as organ meats (brain, kidney, liver, heart), anchovies, yeast, herring, mackerel, and scallops.

Collection of objective data includes assessment of joints (especially the great toe) for signs of edema, heat, discoloration (may appear erythematous or purple), and limited movement. Vital sign data may reveal an elevated temperature and hypertension, tachycardia, and tachypnea. Carefully assess urinary output because tophi can form in the kidneys and alter kidney function. Assess the patient for tophi (typically seen on the earlobes, fingers, hands, and toes).

Diagnostic Tests

Laboratory tests used to diagnose gout include serum (see Table 4.3) and urinary uric acid levels (elevation is significant), complete blood count (CBC) (leukocytosis and anemia may be present), and elevated ESR. Radiographic studies reveal cysts and toe bone pockets. Synovial fluid contains urate crystals.

Medical Management

Several drugs are used to treat gout. For acute attacks, colchicine is administered orally or intravenously. The drug is discontinued if GI symptoms develop or pain is not relieved. Indomethacin suspension and injectable is an effective anti-inflammatory drug in treating gout. Corticosteroids can be administered orally, intravenously, or intra-articularly and will relieve signs and symptoms within 12 hours. The health care provider may order allopurinol to decrease the production of uric acid. The medication probenecid is prescribed to inhibit renal tubular resorption of uric acid, which increases secretion of uric acid by the kidneys. The drug febuxostat has been prescribed to lower serum uric acid levels, but the US Food and Drug Administration (FDA) has warned that it has an increased risk for causing heart-related deaths and deaths from all causes (NLM, 2019). Aspirin inactivates the effect of uricosurics (e.g., probenecid), resulting in urate retention, and should be avoided while patients are taking uricosuric drugs.

Nursing Interventions and Patient Teaching

Nursing intervention is aimed at giving medications prescribed by the health care provider for relief of pain and inflammation. When giving colchicine, observe for side effects, such as diarrhea, nausea, and vomiting. Increasing the patient's fluid intake to at least 2000 mL daily helps eliminate the excess urinary urates. Approximately 10% to 20% of patients with gouty arthritis have uric acid kidney stones. Carefully document intake and output (I&O). Advise the patient to avoid excessive use of alcohol and consumption of foods high in purines, which include sardines, herring, anchovies, alcohol, and beer. Maintain bed rest and joint immobilization while the patient is symptomatic. Bed cradles prevent pressure from bed linens on the affected joints.

Problem statements and interventions for the patient with gout include but are not limited to the following:

PATIENT PROBLEM	NURSING INTERVENTIONS
Prolonged Pain, related to disease process	Maintain patient in a position of comfort with foot supported and in alignment; place bed cradle over foot; no weight-bearing Apply cold packs as ordered, keeping pressure off joint Administer analgesics and anti-gout and anti-inflammatory agents as ordered; observe for side effects
Insufficient Knowledge, related to lack of information concerning medications and home care management	Provide medication schedule, including name, dosage, purpose, and side effects Discuss importance of diet, exercise, and rest program Encourage follow-up visits with health care provider

Patient teaching is aimed at giving information about the disease and stressing the importance of keeping the serum uric acid levels within the normal range by taking the prescribed medications; following the prescribed diet; and avoiding infections, lack of sleep, and stress. The patient may need to take colchicine, probenecid, and allopurinol as a maintenance dose even when signs and symptoms are not present.

Prognosis

The signs and symptoms are recurrent; episodes become longer each year. The disorder is disabling and, if untreated, can progress to the development of tophi and destructive joint changes.

OTHER MUSCULOSKELETAL DISORDERS

OSTEOPOROSIS

Etiology and Pathophysiology

Osteoporosis is a disorder that results in a loss in bone density. This reduction is sufficient to interfere with the mechanical support function of the bone. Nearly 25% of women over the age of 65 and 5% of men in the United States have osteoporosis (CDC 2020). Women between the ages of 55 and 65 years are identified as a high-risk group for postmenopausal osteoporosis, and many researchers believe that this is related to the loss of the female hormone estrogen. Primary osteoporosis consists of the subcategories of juvenile and idiopathic. Juvenile osteoporosis traditionally impacts children and young adults. It is characterized by the sudden onset of bone pain and fracture or a fracture after a trauma. Idiopathic osteoporosis has two subcategories post-menopausal (type 1) and age-associated or senile (type 2). Post-menopausal osteoporosis results with the declining estrogen levels experienced by women as menopause results. Age-related osteoporosis is linked to the loss of bone mass as a result of aging. It is most common in people ages 70 to 85 years (Elam, 2021b). Both men and women are impacted. Each year, 700,000 people with osteoporosis experience compression fractures of the spine, and more than 2 million people overall experience some type of fracture related to the disease (Gagel, 2019). Genetic and environmental factors, such as small bone structure and lack of exercise, can contribute to the rate of bone loss. Osteoporosis affects the vertebrae, neck of the femur, pelvis, hands, and wrists. Risk factors can be categorized as modifiable or non-modifiable. Those factors an individual has not ability to control include age (over 50 years), menopause, gender, family history, broken bones or height loss. Ancestry also plays a role with an increased incidence in white (northern European descent) or Asian women. Body size is also implicated as small framed people face increased incidence. Risk factors that an individual can control include social behaviors such as smoking and alcohol use. Dietary habits are implicated with inadequate intake of calcium, Vitamin D, fruits and vegetables and excess intake of protein,

sodium, and caffeine are associated with the condition (National Osteoporosis Foundation, n.d.). Medical conditions associated with increased development of the disease include hyperthyroidism, chronic lung disease, cancer, inflammatory bowel disease, celiac disease, alcoholism, and vitamin D deficiency. Medications linked to the development of osteoporosis include steroids, anticonvulsants, immunosuppressant therapies, and heparin. Diets low in calcium or high in caffeine and protein also are implicated (see the Cultural Considerations box) (Mayo Clinic, 2019b).

Clinical Manifestations

Most patients with osteoporosis have no symptoms in the early stages of the disease. A fracture, usually of the vertebrae, is often the first symptom. Loss of height over time or a stooped posture may be an indication of the disease before a diagnosis is made.

Assessment

Collection of subjective data includes questioning the patient about lifestyle practices and complaints of pain (low thoracic and lumbar) that worsens with sitting, standing, coughing, sneezing, and straining.

Collection of objective data includes assessing the patient for dowager's hump (spinal deformity and height loss that result from repeated spinal vertebral fractures) and increased lordosis, scoliosis, and kyphosis (Fig. 4.9). Also assess gait impairment associated with inability to maintain erect posture.

Diagnostic Tests

The health care provider orders a CBC; serum calcium, phosphorus, and alkaline phosphatase; blood

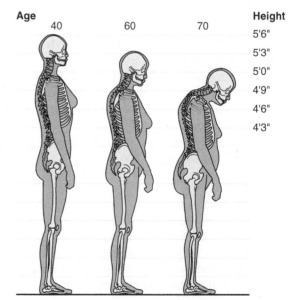

Fig. 4.9 A normal spine at age 40 years and osteoporotic changes at ages 60 and 70 years. These changes can cause a loss of as much as 6 inches in height and can result in the so-called dowager's hump *(far right)* in the upper thoracic vertebrae.

urea nitrogen (BUN); creatinine level; urinalysis; and liver and thyroid function tests. A bone mineral density (BMD) measurement is recommended for women around the time of menopause. BMD is determined by dual-energy x-ray absorptiometry (DEXA). The BMD test assesses the mass of bone per unit volume, or how tightly the bone is packed. Usually the hip and the spine are measured. The test takes about 10 minutes and involves low amounts of radiation. The World Health Organization has defined criteria for adult women as follows:

- Normal bones have a BMD within 1 standard deviation of the young female adult average.
- Low bone mass (osteopenia) is between 1 and 2.5 standard deviations below the young female adult average.
- Osteoporosis is 2.5 standard deviations or more below the young female adult average *of negative 1 or above* (International Osteoporosis Foundation, 2021).

Cultural Considerations

Osteoporosis

- White women have a higher incidence of osteoporosis than Asian women, followed by African American women (NIAMS, 2019).
- Like women, white and Asian men have a higher incidence of osteoporosis than other men; however, the rate of osteoporosis in men is significantly less than in women, 51% in men and 25% in women (CDC, 2020).
- Postmenopausal women are at the highest risk regardless of cultural background or ethnic group.
- Hispanic women are at a lower risk of osteoporosis than white and Asian women. The rate of osteoporosis for African American and Hispanic women is similar (NIAMS, 2019).

Medical Management

The health care provider orders a treatment regimen aimed at increasing bone density and retarding bone loss. Calcium supplements that bring the total calcium intake per day to 1200 mg for men and postmenopausal women are recommended, with 2000 mg being the maximum amount (as well as vitamin D, 800 international units daily). Alcohol intake should be limited because excessive intake interferes with absorption of calcium and vitamin D. Weight-bearing exercise programs to improve muscle tone, such as walking, help prevent further bone loss and stimulate new bone formation (Elam, 2021a).

Alendronate, zoledronic acid, and ibandronate are bone resorption inhibitors that assist in increasing bone density (Table 4.6). These drugs absorb calcium phosphate crystal in bone and are given orally to treat symptoms of osteoporosis. Administer these drugs first thing in the morning with 6 to 8 ounces of water at least 30 minutes before other medications, beverages, or food. Caution the patient to remain upright for 30 minutes after a dose to facilitate passage to the stomach and to minimize risk of esophageal irritation.

Risedronate is another bone resorption inhibitor. The drug adsorbs (i.e., binds) calcium phosphate crystal in bone and inhibits bone resorption without inhibiting bone formation or mineralization. It is given orally. The patient should sit upright for 30 minutes after a dose to prevent esophageal irritation. Another type of drug used in treating osteoporosis is selective estrogen receptor modulators, such as raloxifene. These drugs mimic the effect of estrogen on bone by reducing bone resorption.

Teriparatide is a form of parathyroid hormone approved for postmenopausal women who are at increased risk for osteoporosis fractures or who cannot use other treatments. The drug prevents sloughing of osteoblasts (bone cells that form new bone) in porous or spongy bones and increases bone mass in the spine and hip. Teriparatide treatment requires a daily subcutaneous injection of the drug and is limited to a 24-month period. The drug must be kept refrigerated. The most common side effects are nausea, dizziness, leg cramps, hypercalcemia, and orthostatic hypotension. The drug is not recommended for patients with an increased risk of osteosarcoma (Elam, 2021a).

Surgical interventions for osteoporosis. Women with severe osteoporosis who are unresponsive to an analgesic may be candidates for a surgical procedure to relieve the pain. Vertebroplasty and kyphoplasty may be successful in relieving pain from compression fractures of the spine. Vertebroplasty (plastic surgery on a vertebra) involves high-pressure injection of poly (methyl methacrylate) cement into the spine, which pushes the vertebrae apart. The procedure is performed with the patient under a general or local anesthetic. Major complications involve damage to the posterior vertebral walls from the high pressure used to inject the cement and movement of the cement out of vertebral spaces into the spinal canal.

Kyphoplasty (plastic surgery on dowager's hump) involves inserting a balloon into the center of the collapsed vertebrae, which restores the position of the vertebrae and creates a space for injection of poly (methyl methacrylate) cement. Porous bone is packed around the outside edge. This procedure is less risky than vertebroplasty because the balloon removes the need to use high pressure for the cement placement (Elam, 2021a).

Nursing considerations. Patients are admitted to the hospital and required to stay up to 24 hours after the procedure. Flat bed rest is ordered for the first 4 hours postoperatively, then patients are allowed to ambulate as able. A small dressing covers the operative site, and antibiotics and steroids typically are ordered for three doses after the procedure.

Table 4.6   Medications for Osteoporosis

GENERIC NAME (TRADE NAME)	ACTION	SIDE EFFECTS/TOXIC EFFECTS	NURSING IMPLICATIONS
Bisphosphonates: alendronate, risedronate, etidronate, pamidronate, ibandronate	Slow bone loss and increase bone density	Difficulty in swallowing, chest pain, severe or recurring heartburn	Administer first thing in the morning with 6–8 oz plain water, 30 min before other medications, beverages, or food.
calcitonin-salmon injection or calcitonin-salmon nasal spray	Increases bone mass, particularly in the spine	Injection site reaction, nasal irritation	Monitor for injection site reaction. Advise patient to take medication exactly as directed.
Estrogen receptor modulator: raloxifene	Prevents bone loss and spinal fractures	May increase tendency for deep vein thrombosis, myocardial infarcts, uterine bleeding, and breast abnormalities	Administer without regard to meals.
Parathyroid hormone: teriparatide	Prevents bone loss; promotes bone growth	Increased heart rate or dizziness	Administer subcutaneously into thigh or abdominal wall once daily.

Data from Skidmore-Roth L: *Mosby's 2017 nursing drug reference,* St. Louis, 2016, Mosby.

Nursing Interventions and Patient Teaching

Nursing interventions are aimed at preventing further bone loss and fractures. A diet rich in milk and dairy products provides most of the calcium in the diet (see the Patient Teaching box). Food and beverages that contain caffeine also contain phosphorus, which contributes to bone loss. Teach patients relaxation techniques and encourage them to stop smoking. Safety measures, such as side rails, hand rails, bedside commodes with seat elevators, and rubber mats in showers, can help prevent falls in older adults. Efforts are made to keep patients with osteoporosis ambulatory to prevent further loss of bone substance as a result of immobility. Encourage weight-bearing exercise to increase bone density.

Patient Teaching

Dietary Needs in Osteoporosis

- Calcium is a mineral that can slow bone loss and may decrease fractures.
- A total of 1200–2000 mg of calcium is needed daily in the diet or through supplements.
- Food sources of calcium include milk products, many green vegetables, calcium-fortified orange juice, and soy milk.
- Vitamin D helps calcium absorption and stimulates bone formation.
- A diet low in sodium, animal protein, and caffeine is recommended.
- Foods that are high in calcium include whole and skim milk, yogurt, turnip greens, cottage cheese, ice cream, sardines with bones, and spinach.

A patient problem statement and interventions for the patient with osteoporosis include but are not limited to the following:

PATIENT PROBLEM	NURSING INTERVENTIONS
Insufficient Knowledge, related to issues of home care	Stress importance of activity and rest; provide aerobic exercise schedule; caution patient to avoid jogging
	Advise patient to take recommended medications
	Instruct patient on how to maintain a healthy diet

To prevent osteoporosis, advise women to maintain an adequate daily intake of calcium and vitamin D; to avoid smoking; to decrease caffeine intake; to decrease excess protein in the diet; and to engage in moderate activity such as walking, bike riding, or swimming at least 3 days a week.

After menopause, the usual recommended daily allowance is 1000 mg of calcium in postmenopausal women taking estrogen and 1500 mg in postmenopausal women who are not taking estrogen. Vitamin D, which increases calcium absorption, may be added to the daily regimen of postmenopausal women according to the health care provider's orders. Encourage the patient to make follow-up visits to the health care provider for guidance on medication, diet, and exercise regimen.

Prognosis

Osteoporosis is a chronic disorder, but vitamin D and calcium, as well as pharmacologic therapy, may help stop the rate of bone loss. In postmenopausal women, therapy with estrogen decreases the rate of bone resorption but does not increase bone formation. Prevention of osteoporosis should begin before bone loss has occurred.

OSTEOMYELITIS

Etiology and Pathophysiology

Osteomyelitis (local or generalized infection of bone and bone marrow) can occur from bacteria introduced through trauma, such as a compound fracture or surgery. Bacteria also may travel by the bloodstream from another site in the body to a bone, causing an infection. Staphylococci are the most common causative agents. Other invading organisms include *Streptococcus viridans, Escherichia coli, Mycobacterium tuberculosis, Neisseria gonorrhoeae, Pseudomonas organisms,* salmonellae, and fungi.

Bacteria invade the bone, and bone tissue degenerates. Osteomyelitis can become chronic as a result of inadequate acute treatment. It is either a continuous persistent problem or a process of exacerbations and remissions. If osteomyelitis becomes chronic, the bone tissue often is weak and predisposed to spontaneous fractures. Over time, granulation tissue turns to scar tissue. This avascular scar tissue provides an ideal site for continued microorganism growth and is impenetrable to antibiotics.

Risk factors for osteomyelitis include severe injury involving a fracture or deep puncture, surgery involving orthopedic implants, poorly controlled diabetes, peripheral artery disease, medications that suppress the immune system, the presence of an indwelling device such as a central line or urinary catheter, smoking, and illicit IV drug use.

Clinical Manifestations

Clinical manifestations of osteomyelitis include fever, pain in the area of the infection, inflammation, and fatigue. The patient with osteomyelitis is subject to contractures in the affected extremity if positioned incorrectly. A new focus of infection can develop months and sometimes years after the initial infection is diagnosed.

Assessment

Take a complete history, along with a physical examination. Collection of subjective data includes a complete history of injuries, surgical procedures, and diseases. Assess the patient's complaints of persistent, severe, and increasing bone pain and tenderness, as well as regional muscle spasm. Also inquire about any allergies, especially to medications, because antibiotics are given long term.

Collection of objective data includes careful inspection of any wounds. Assess the drainage for color, amount, and odor. Monitor vital signs for signs of infection (temperature elevation, tachycardia, and tachypnea). Note any edema, especially in joints with limited mobility.

Diagnostic Tests

Radiologic tests may include radiographic studies, MRI, and CT scans. Laboratory studies may include a CBC (leukocytosis may be present), ESR, CRP, needle aspiration, and cultures of blood and drainage, if present (Cleveland Clinic, 2017).

Medical Management

Medical care for the patient with osteomyelitis includes wound management and antibiotic therapy. Necrotic tissue requires debridement. Drainage of pus from around the infected area may be indicated. Some patients, surgery may be performed to remove a fragment of necrotic bone that is partially or entirely detached from the surrounding or adjacent healthy bone (sequestrum). In the event the infection is at a site where orthopedic plates and screws have been placed, removal may be indicated. Hyperbaric oxygen therapy may be initiated. The administration of high levels of oxygen stimulates tissue growth and repair. Bed rest usually is prescribed.

Vigorous and prolonged IV antibiotic therapy will be used. These antibiotics may include penicillin, nafcillin, neomycin, cephalexin, cefoxitin, and gentamicin. Parenteral antibiotics are usually necessary for several weeks but may be prescribed for as long as 3 to 6 months. The involvement of multidrug-resistant bacteria requires a lengthier and more aggressive treatment regimen with a combination of antibiotics that may include vancomycin, linezolid, daptomycin and rifampin. As a last resort, infection that does not respond to treatment may require amputation of an affected limb.

Nursing Interventions and Patient Teaching

Nursing interventions include gentleness in moving and manipulating the diseased extremity, because pain is severe in the early phase of infection. The affected part may need absolute rest, with careful positioning using pillows and sandbags for good alignment. Wound irrigation with normal saline, an antiseptic, or antibiotic solution may be indicated. Sterile dressings are employed using strict surgical asepsis. Patients are placed on drainage and secretion precautions. Dietary planning includes a diet high in calories, protein, and vitamins. Monitor the patient for worsening infection. Assess vital signs. Review laboratory results.

Teaching includes information about the signs of infection, such as elevated temperature, and the importance of completing the antibiotic treatment as prescribed. Chronic osteomyelitis may last a lifetime. Warn the patient of the recurrence of signs and symptoms. Rarely pathologic fractures result to the affected bones.

Prognosis

Acute osteomyelitis may respond to treatment after several weeks. Abscess formation, deformity, sepsis, loss of mobility, and fractures are potential complications. Chronic osteomyelitis may persist for years with exacerbations and remissions. A recurrence of the infection is not uncommon.

FIBROMYALGIA SYNDROME

Etiology and Pathophysiology

Fibromyalgia is a chronic syndrome of unknown origin that causes pain in the muscles, bones, or joints. It is associated with soft tissue tenderness at multiple characteristic sites. It contributes to poor sleep, headaches, altered thought processes, and stiffness or muscle aches. Fibromyalgia affects approximately 4 million people; 80% to 90% of those diagnosed are women. The disorder is more common in people between ages 20 and 50 years. Fibromyalgia has been referred to as *fibrositis, fibromyositis, myofascial pain syndrome,* and *psychogenic rheumatism.* Clinical symptoms of fibromyalgia syndrome (FMS) can overlap those of chronic fatigue syndrome. It is not considered life threatening and does not cause permanent damage. It often is seen in patients who also have rheumatic conditions such as RA and lupus.

Clinical Manifestations

Patients with FMS frequently complain of a generalized achiness in axial locations, such as the neck and lower back, accompanied by stiffness that is worse in the morning. Factors that aggravate the condition include cold or humid weather, physical or mental fatigue, excessive physical activity, and anxiety or stress. Difficulty sleeping is common, as well as headaches, tingling or numbness in the hands and feet, and painful menstrual periods. Mental health concerns reported by fibromyalgia sufferers include cognitive difficulties, anxiety, and depression (Poindexter, 2017).

Assessment

Collection of subjective data includes questioning the patient about muscle pain, often described as muscle ache; tension or migraine headaches; premenstrual tension; jaw pain; excessive fatigue; anxiety; and depression. Include questions about sensations of numbness, tingling, and perception of insects crawling on or under the skin. Complaints of being forgetful and unable to recall recent information—such as appointments, location of parked car, or how to get to familiar places—are significant.

Collection of objective data includes noting periodic limb movement, especially at night, or a persistent need to move the lower extremities day and night. Ask about sleep deprivation and the patient's ability to complete self-care activities.

Diagnostic Tests

No specific laboratory and radiographic test diagnoses FMS. Diagnosis confirmation for patients with fibromyalgia may take months to years. The process is one that eliminates other potential conditions. Criteria used to affirm a diagnosis of fibromyalgia syndrome includes the widespread pain index (WPI). This tool is used to assess location of pain or tenderness and severity in 19 body locations. The duration of discomfort with no improvements for 3 months or longer is an additional criterion. Blood chemistry screening, a CBC, RF, and ESR are normal in patients with FMS. A sleep study may be ordered in patients with a history suggestive of particular types of sleep disturbances; however, sleep study findings are typically normal in patients with FMS. Research is focusing on the relationships between neurotransmitter levels and fibromyalgia syndrome.

Medical Management

There is no cure for fibromyalgia. The primary treatment approach includes patient education, emotional support and reassurance. Inform the patient with FMS that this is not a psychiatric disturbance and that symptoms are not uncommon in the general population. Pharmacological agents are combined with nonmedicinal therapies. Antidepressants, anticonvulsants, muscle relaxants and analgesics are utilized. Pain relief, improved sleep and lessened sleep may be seen with antidepressant use. Anticonvulsant medications can aid in the management of chronic pain. Analgesic use should not include opioids due to the risk of tolerance and addiction. Acetaminophen and NSAIDS are beneficial in the management of mild to moderate discomfort (Table 4.7).

Nursing Interventions and Patient Teaching

Nursing interventions are individualized, holistic, and goal oriented. Management of FMS focuses on functional goals that enable the patient to live as normal a life as possible. Treatment programs include education, exercise, and relaxation techniques. Patients are taught the basic principles of good sleep hygiene (see the Patient Teaching box). Exercise programs consist of gentle, progressive stretching, beginning with a muscle warm-up through either gentle exercise or warm baths. Stretching helps release tight muscles. Nonimpact exercise such as swimming, walking, or stationary cycling is helpful. Yoga benefits individuals in a variety of ways including promotion of relaxation, stress reduction, and increased flexibility.

 Patient Teaching

Sleep Hygiene

- Control environmental factors by avoiding large meals 2–3 h before bedtime and keeping the sleep environment dark, quiet, and comfortable.
- Exercise regularly each day.
- Keep a diary recording sleep patterns.
- Maintain regular sleep patterns by going to bed and awaking the same time each day; avoiding long naps, and taking a hot bath within 2 h of bedtime.
- Recognize how drugs such as nicotine, alcohol, and caffeine affect sleep.

Table 4.7 Medications for Fibromyalgia Syndrome

GENERIC NAME (TRADE NAME)	ACTION
Amitriptyline	Diminishes local pain and stiffness; improves sleep pattern
cyclobenzaprine	Diminishes local pain, improves sleep pattern, and decreases number of tender points
clonazepam	Decreases symptoms of constant leg movement, especially at night
acetaminophen and tramadol	Used together or given alone for management of moderate to severe pain. Bind opioid receptors, inhibit reuptake of norepinephrine and serotonin
pregabalin	An anticonvulsant that decreases pain severity and improves fatigue, sleep, and physical functioning
tizanidine	Eases pain by lowering substance P, which participates in the transmission process of certain neurons; improves sleep and physical functioning
sodium oxybate	Improves deep sleep and growth hormone levels and helps reduce pain and fatigue
duloxetine hydrochloride	Reduces pain in patients with fibromyalgia with or without having symptoms of major depression

Prognosis
Fibromyalgia is a challenging disorder to treat. Patients may have difficulty achieving remission of symptoms. Many patients report that the condition impacts their ability to successfully complete their ADLs. The emotional stressors of the condition affect their ability to maintain employment and remain active in family processes.

SURGICAL INTERVENTIONS FOR TOTAL KNEE OR TOTAL HIP REPLACEMENT

Surgical procedures can prevent progressive deformities; relieve pain; improve function; and correct deformities resulting from RA, OA, or other disorders. Tendon transplants can replace damaged muscles. Patients with RA may need a synovectomy (excision of synovial membrane) to maintain joint function. An osteotomy (cutting into bone to correct bone or joint deformities) can improve function and relieve pain. Arthrodesis (surgical fusion of a joint) can be performed when severe joint destruction has occurred. Total joint replacement arthroplasty (repair or refashioning of one or both sides, parts, or specific tissue within a joint) often is required on the elbow, hip, knee, or shoulder joint to restore or increase mobility.

KNEE ARTHROPLASTY (TOTAL KNEE REPLACEMENT)
The knee joint may be replaced to restore motion, relieve pain, or correct deformity. Figs. 4.10 and 4.11 show the tibial and femoral components of a knee prosthesis. Nursing interventions for the patient undergoing total knee replacement are shown in Box 4.4.

UNICOMPARTMENTAL KNEE ARTHROPLASTY
Unicompartmental knee replacement also is referred to as partial knee replacement. This modified surgical procedure is performed when only one of the compartments of the knee is affected by arthritic changes. If both sides of the bones in the knee, including the underside of the patella, are damaged, a total knee replacement is necessary (see Fig. 4.11).

The knee has three compartments: (1) the medial, or inside, compartment; (2) the lateral, or outside, compartment; and (3) the patellofemoral compartment, which is where the kneecap rests. Minimally invasive knee surgery removes only the most damaged areas of cartilage; a small plastic disk replaces the worn cartilage, providing a new cushion between the bones.

Partial knee surgery involves making a small incision over the knee and exposing the worn-out cartilage. The rough edges of the distal area of the femur and superior area of the tibia are cut flat and cleaned, and the unicompartmental device is put into place. Some of the devices are cemented in place.

Total knee arthroplasty (TKA) is performed on patients of all ages, from teenagers to patients in their nineties. The decision to perform TKA is based on the patient's overall health and expected outcome of the surgery. The patient must be able to withstand intensive physical therapy for several weeks to months after the replacement.

Assessment
Subjective data include a medical history of home medications, allergies, past surgeries, and significant medical problems. Assess the patient for complaints of pain on one or both sides of the knee with weight-bearing. Also gather information on the effectiveness of conservative treatments such as medications, cortisone injections, strengthening exercises, weight loss, and use of assistive devices such as gait enhancers.

Objective data include vital signs and weight. Patients who are obese or have significant inflammation are not candidates for the surgery. Blood tests, electrocardiogram (ECG), and chest x-ray examination are done to evaluate the patient's state of health. Also assess the patient's understanding of the surgical procedure.

Diagnostic Tests
An x-ray examination of the knee shows damage to the joint.

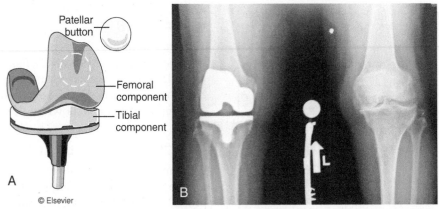

Fig. 4.10 (A) Tibial and femoral components of total knee prosthesis. Patellar button, made of polyethylene, protects the posterior surface of the patella from friction against the femoral component when the knee is moved through flexion and extension. (B) *(left)* Total knee prosthesis in place; *(right)* arthritic knee.

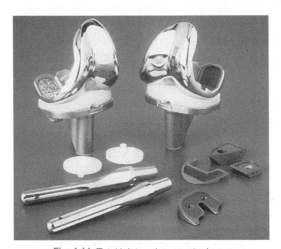

Fig. 4.11 Total joint replacements: knee.

Nursing Interventions and Patient Teaching

Nursing interventions are aimed at promoting healing and facilitating mobility. The typical postoperative stay for patients having TKA is one or two nights. Monitor pain and administer analgesics as needed. Help the patient deep breathe and cough every 2 hours. Encourage the encourage use of an incentive spirometer during waking hours. Begin clear liquids and advance to regular diet as tolerated. Monitor IV fluids and antibiotics. Change the dressing as needed.

Patients may resume weight-bearing postoperatively as soon as allowed by the surgeon, with some as soon as returning to their hospital room. Assess their ability to use an assistive device such as crutches or a walker. The day of surgery the physical therapist begins teaching basic postoperative exercises. Physical therapy continues either in a rehabilitation facility or at home upon discharge and then continues for several weeks or months. Also instruct the patient that prophylactic antibiotics are recommended before routine dental cleaning or any dental procedure up to 2 years after the surgery.

HIP ARTHROPLASTY (TOTAL HIP REPLACEMENT)

Hip arthroplasty, or total hip replacement, is performed commonly when arthritis involves the head of the femur and acetabulum. Additional indications for hip replacement include fractures, tumors, and injuries. The decision to have hip replacement surgery traditionally follows periods of lengthy pain and discomfort. The choice to have the surgery will in most cases result in reduced pain, improved mobility, and increased enjoyment of life.

Prosthetic devices may be cemented or uncemented. The cemented device is secured to the patient's healthy bone tissue with a gluelike adhesive (Fig. 4.12). Uncemented prosthetic devices are inserted and then the patient's body tissue grows into them for attachment. Several variations of hip replacement surgery are practiced, but each uses similar equipment. The Bechtol total hip system involves a white plastic cup cemented in place to replace the damaged acetabulum. A stainless steel or Vitallium ball on a stem replaces the head of the femur, which is removed surgically. The stem is cemented into the femoral canal, and the new head fits precisely into the plastic acetabulum, providing friction-free movement in the joint (FDA, 2019).

Assessment

Collection of subjective data includes assessing the patient's level of orientation, because older adults can become disoriented from a change in the environment (home to hospital setting) and the effects of anesthesia and other prescribed medications. Complaints of unrelieved pain and numbness, tingling, or paresthesia indicate neurovascular impairment.

Collection of objective data includes assessment of the patient's compliance with nursing interventions to promote circulation; prevent impairment of skin integrity; and prevent hypostatic pneumonia by such means as coughing, turning (to the unaffected side; additional pillows are used to keep the affected leg

Box 4.4   Nursing Interventions for the Patient Undergoing Total Knee Replacement

PREOPERATIVE INTERVENTIONS
Same as for any major surgery (see Chapter 2).

POSTOPERATIVE INTERVENTIONS
1. Positioning
   a. Elevate the operative leg on pillows to enhance venous return for the first 24 hours only. Place pillows with caution to avoid flexing the knee.
   b. The patient may be turned from side to back to side.
2. Wound care
   a. Care of drains (usually Hemovac) as for total hip replacement.
   b. Assess patient for systemic evidence of loss of blood (hypotension, tachycardia) if bulky compression dressing is used because it may hold large quantities of drainage before drainage is visible.
   c. Remove bulky dressings before the patient begins continuous passive motion (CPM) flexion greater than 20 degrees.
3. Activity
   a. Passive flexion in a CPM machine within prescribed flexion-extension limits may be started in the postanesthesia care unit (see Fig. 4.12). Patient's leg should remain in machine as much as tolerated (up to 22 hours per day) to facilitate even healing of tissue. The physical therapist increases extension on CPM as patient tolerates. (Once the large bulky dressing is replaced with a smaller dressing, flexion degree is increased.) Many surgeons are opting to not use CPM but rely on active patient flexion and extension exercises. When CPM is not occurring, patient's leg is extended with no pillow under leg.
   b. Encourage patient to perform active dorsiflexion of the ankles; quadriceps setting; and, after the drain is removed, straight leg–raising exercises.
   c. Patient begins active flexion exercises three or four times a day about the fifth postoperative day.
   d. Light weight-bearing with an assistive device may be started as early as upon arrival to the hospital room after surgery and increased as the patient tolerates.
   e. Sitting in a chair with the leg elevated may be started on the first postoperative day.
   f. Encourage patient to wear a resting knee extension splint (immobilizer) on the operated leg until able to demonstrate quadriceps control (independent straight leg–raising).
4. Pain control
   a. For initial control of pain, use opioids (usually with a patient-controlled epidural or patient-controlled analgesia) and positioning; gradually decrease medication to nonopioid analgesics as patient tolerates.
   b. Encourage patient to use cool applications at 40°F (4.4°C) continuously on knee.
5. Discharge instructions
   a. Patient must observe partial weight-bearing restriction and use ambulatory aid for approximately 2 months after discharge.
   b. Patient should continue active flexion and straight leg–raising exercises at home.

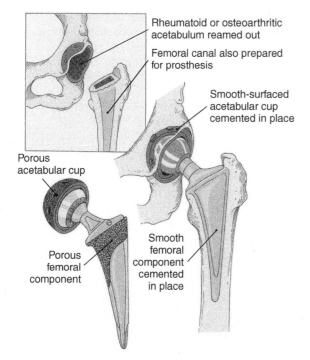

Rheumatoid or osteoarthritic acetabulum reamed out

Femoral canal also prepared for prosthesis

Smooth-surfaced acetabular cup cemented in place

Porous acetabular cup

Porous femoral component

Smooth femoral component cemented in place

Fig. 4.12 Hip arthroplasty (total hip replacement).

abducted), deep breathing every 2 hours, and using an incentive spirometer. Assess vital signs for evidence of excessive bleeding, including hypotension, tachycardia, and tachypnea. Decreased urinary output is indicative of hypovolemia. Carefully assess drainage of the surgical wound at least every 4 hours. Hemovacs or other suction devices are placed in the wound during surgery to provide closed-wound suction. Assess approximation of the incision line and signs of inflammation (erythema, edema, fever, and pain). Also assess traction (if used) for the correct amount of weight, the proper alignment, and maintenance of the affected leg in an abducted position. Look for any reaction to the cement, signs of phlebitis (edema, erythema, and pain), and urinary retention (indwelling catheters may be used for the first 24 to 48 hours).

Nursing Interventions and Patient Teaching
Nursing interventions are aimed at the assessment of potential complications, the promotion of healing, and facilitating mobility. Take vital signs at least every 4 hours. Document intake and output. Measure oral intake and urinary output as well as IV fluids and fluids from drainage devices such as the Hemovac. Thigh-high antiembolism stockings are used before and after surgery. Early in the postoperative period the surgeon orders a plan of weight-bearing and physical therapy. Nursing education should focus on reinforcing this plan to the patient and family.

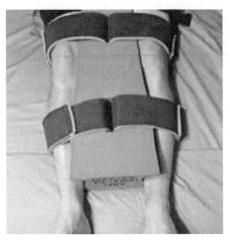

Fig. 4.13 Maintaining postoperative abduction after total hip replacement.

Encourage coughing and deep-breathing exercises at least every 2 hours. Give oxygen at 1 to 2 L per nasal cannula as needed. Instruct the patient in the use of the incentive spirometer every 2 to 4 hours.

Perform neurovascular checks every hour for 24 hours, then every 2 hours for the next 24 hours, and then every 4 hours. Check vital signs every 4 hours. Also carefully assess the patient for pain control. This includes monitoring patient-controlled epidural (PCE), patient-controlled analgesia (PCA), or oral medications, whichever is prescribed.

The surgical dressing will remain in place until removal is ordered by the surgeon; most surgeons prefer to remove the surgical dressing. Reinforce the dressing as needed. Report excessive drainage. Maintain the position of the operative area with a splint, an abduction pillow (Fig. 4.13), an immobilizer, or a brace; turn the patient to the non-operative side.

Begin clear liquids, and advance diet as tolerated. Encourage fluid intake and high-fiber foods (if tolerated) to prevent constipation.

Bed rest is maintained for approximately 24 hours postoperatively. Teach the patient to do isometric exercises on the quadriceps and gluteal muscles of the affected extremity by keeping the toes pointed up, flexing the ankles, and flexing and extending the knee of the unaffected extremity. Physical therapy exercises begin on the first or second postoperative day. The exercises are either active or passive to all joints, excluding the operated joint, and include quadriceps setting, straight leg–raising, flexion and extension, or other individually prescribed exercises. The patient should be up with walker or crutches four times daily; increase ambulation as the patient is able with up to 25 pounds of weight-bearing on the operative limb, gradually increasing to full weight-bearing with crutches or a walker. The patient should be up but not bearing weight on the operative limb after the bed rest order expires. Some health care providers may permit touch-down weight-bearing. Protection of the integrity of the new joint requires the avoidance of hyperflexion of the hip. Chair sitting initially is limited to 10 to 15 minutes two or three times daily for the first week, and then for 20 to 30 minutes four times daily. Use of a toilet-seat riser prevents hyperflexion of the hip after total replacement. Patient problem and interventions for the patient with a total hip replacement include but are not limited to the following:

PATIENT PROBLEM	NURSING INTERVENTIONS
Prolonged Pain, related to: • Preoperative arthritic pain necessitating surgery • Incisional pain • Soft tissue trauma of surgery	Explain analgesic therapy, including medication, dose, and schedule If patient is a candidate for patient-controlled analgesia or patient-controlled epidural, explain the concept and routine Respond quickly to pain complaints Obtain pain rating from patient Instruct patient to request analgesic before pain is severe Administer analgesics as ordered and per hospital policy or procedure Encourage use of analgesics 30–45 min before therapy; unrelieved pain hinders rehabilitation progress Change position (within hip precautions) q 2 h Document all responses to analgesics
Compromised Physical Mobility, related to surgical procedure and discomfort	Allow patient to dangle feet at bedside several minutes before getting out of bed Reinforce physical therapist's instructions for exercises and ambulation techniques and devices; consistent instructions from interdisciplinary team members promote safe, secure rehabilitation environment Maintain weight-bearing status on affected extremity as prescribed Keep abduction pillow between legs while turning in bed (see Fig. 4.14) Do not have the patient lie on the operative side Maintain the leg in abduction when the patient is lying supine or on the nonoperative side Encourage the patient to use trapeze in bed to assist in mobility

Discharge instructions include teaching the patient to use an ambulatory aid, avoid adduction, and limit hip flexion to 90 degrees for approximately 2 to 3 months. A raised toilet seat should be obtained and used at home until flexion restrictions are removed. The patient should avoid leaning forward and use assistive devices to avoid bending. The patient may need a long-handled shoehorn and reacher to facilitate ADLs within flexion restriction.

FRACTURES

FRACTURE OF THE HIP
Etiology and Pathophysiology
Hip fractures are the leading type of fracture requiring treatment in a hospital facility (see the Lifespan Considerations and Health Promotion boxes). Women are at greater risk for hip fracture because of their increased likelihood to develop osteoporosis and longer life expectancy compared with men.

Fractures of the hip include intracapsular fractures, in which the femur is broken inside the joint (subcapital) or in the femoral head or neck (transcervical and basal) (Fig. 4.14A–C). Intracapsular fractures may disrupt the blood supply to the head of the femur, which subsequently develops avascular necrosis (Figs. 4.15 and 4.16). Therefore, fractures of the head or proximal femoral neck may be treated with insertion of a femoral prosthesis (Fig. 4.17). The more common type of hip fracture is an extracapsular fracture, one that occurs outside the hip joint capsule. These are referred to as intertrochanteric or subtrochanteric fractures (see Fig. 4.14D). These fractures heal well, without vascular necrosis, with the use of compression screws or nails because the blood supply to the fracture site comes from the surrounding vessels outside the capsule (see Figs. 4.15 and 4.16). Side plates attached to the nails help maintain a stable reduction while healing progresses (Fig. 4.18A). An intertrochanteric fracture occurs below the lesser trochanter and frequently is seen in younger patients suffering from hip trauma (see Fig. 4.14D).

Clinical Manifestations
Signs and symptoms of hip fracture are severe pain and tenderness in the region of the fracture site or inability to move the leg voluntarily, and shortening or external rotation of the leg.

Assessment
Subjective data include an accurate history of the events before the injury. Assess the patient's level of orientation. Disorientation can occur, especially in older adults when they are in pain, are anxious, or are in an unfamiliar environment. The patient's medical and surgical history is significant, as is any family history of bone disease. Patients with gastroesophageal reflux disease who are taking antacids or using proton pump inhibitors are at increased risk of hip fractures, because these drugs cause malabsorption of calcium.

Signs and symptoms of a fracture vary with the type and location of the break. Usually the patient has some degree of discomfort that may be more pronounced with slight movement of the affected part. Most patients complain of pain in the affected leg after sustaining a fractured hip, although patients suffering from an impacted intracapsular fracture have little pain, if any, immediately after the fracture. Impaired sensation may indicate nerve damage from the bone fragments "pinching" or severing the nerve. Assess for edema, tenderness, muscle spasms, deformity, and loss of function. Patients may say they heard a "snap" or "pop" at the time the bone was injured. The patient may report simply sitting down and feeling or hearing the pop of the fracture.

Collection of objective data includes assessment for soft tissue injury, with erythema or ecchymoses noted. Look for differences between the injured limb and the uninjured limb. A change in the curvature or length of bone may indicate fracture. The affected leg is shorter, usually externally rotated approximately 90 degrees, and slightly flexed after an extracapsular hip fracture. With an intracapsular fracture, the upper thigh is more edematous than the area below it, and the affected leg is shortened with external rotation. Subtrochanteric fractures cause excessive bleeding into the soft tissue, and the affected leg is shortened and rotated anteriorly. Crepitus may be felt or heard as the broken bone ends rub together. Assess neurovascular status of the extremity (Box 4.5).

Keep the injured part still because movement of a fractured bone can cause additional damage and may turn a closed fracture into an open fracture. Assess the

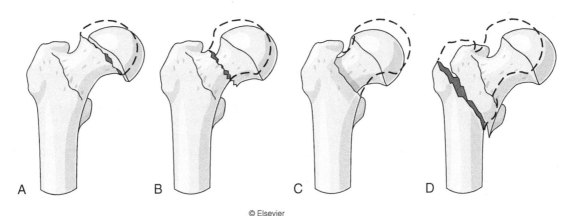

© Elsevier

Fig. 4.14 Fractures of the hip. (A) Subcapital fracture. (B) Transcervical fracture. (C) Impacted fracture of the base of the neck. (D) Intertrochanteric fracture.

patient's nutritional status. Thin and obese patients are at risk for impaired skin integrity if bed rest is ordered. After the fracture is reduced, regularly inspect skin areas in contact with cast edges or traction apparatus for signs of neurovascular compromise. Patients suffering from any trauma are at risk for shock. Treating the shock takes precedence over treating the fracture.

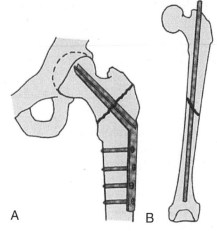

Fig. 4.18 (A) Neufeld nail and screws in repair of intertrochanteric fracture. (B) Küntscher nail (intramedullary rod) used in repair of midshaft femoral fracture. (From Monahan FD, Sands JK, Neighbors M, et al: *Phipps' medical-surgical nursing: Health and illness perspectives,* ed 8, St. Louis, 2007, Mosby.)

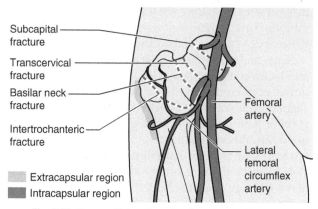

Fig. 4.15 Femur with location of various types of fractures.

- Subcapital fracture
- Transcervical fracture
- Basilar neck fracture
- Intertrochanteric fracture
- Femoral artery
- Lateral femoral circumflex artery
- Extracapsular region
- Intracapsular region

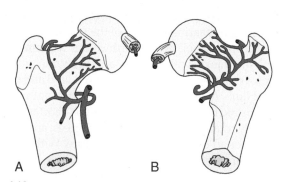

Fig. 4.16 (A) Anterior arterial blood supply to hip joint. (B) Posterior arterial blood supply to hip joint.

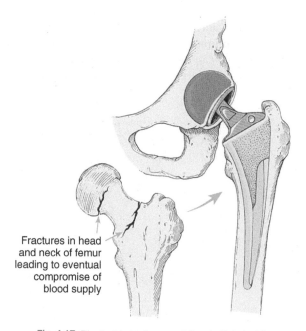

Fractures in head and neck of femur leading to eventual compromise of blood supply

Fig. 4.17 Bipolar hip replacement (hemiarthroplasty).

Box 4.5 Circulation Check (Neurovascular Assessment)

- A circulation check is also known as a neurovascular assessment. The mnemonic CMS indicates the need to check circulation, motion, and sensation. The assessment is made on patients after musculoskeletal trauma; postoperatively if damage to nerves and blood vessels is suspected; and after casting, splinting, or bandaging.
- Assess the patient every 15–30 min for several hours and every 3–4 h thereafter, with proper documentation of the findings.
- Subjective data include complaints of numbness or tingling not relieved by flexing the fingers and toes and repositioning the extremity. Objective data include cool, pale, or cyanotic skin above or below the altered site; edema; a capillary refill time greater than 2 s; and absent or diminished pulses.
- Remember the seven *P*s when completing the assessment:
  1. Pulselessness
  2. Paresthesia (numbness or tingling sensation)
  3. Paralysis or paresis
  4. Polar temperature
  5. Pallor
  6. Puffiness (edema)
  7. Pain
- Complaints of numbness or tingling may result from general decreased mobility and may be relieved by flexing the fingers and toes and repositioning the extremity. However, if the numbness and tingling are not relieved by these measures and the extremity feels cool to the touch, is slow in capillary refill, has diminished or absent pulses, and appears pale or cyanotic, these are significant symptoms of neurovascular impairment and the findings must be reported immediately.

Lifespan Considerations

Older Adults

Musculoskeletal Disorder

- Physiologic changes of aging result in decreased joint flexibility and muscular strength.
- Changes in bone mass with aging increase the risk of fractures. Hip fractures and compression fractures of the spine are noted most frequently.
- Degenerative joint disease related to "wear and tear" on joints is associated with aging. Joint replacement is no longer considered a last resort for older adults and provides an opportunity for improvement in the quality of life.
- Changes in the foot can occur with aging, poorly fitted shoes, or heredity. Bunions and hammertoe are seen with increasing frequency in older adults, causing pain and possibly decreased mobility. Encourage older adults to wear properly fitted shoes to reduce discomfort. If discomfort is severe, surgical correction may be necessary.
- Check the homes of older adults for safety hazards such as rugs that could cause falls.
- Older adults should avoid climbing unsteady or uneven surfaces because coordination and balance change with age and falls may result.
- Instruct older adults in the correct use of assistive devices such as canes or walkers. Encourage them to use these regularly to prevent injury.

Diagnostic Tests

Diagnosis is confirmed by radiographic examination of the injured part. Blood tests, such as hemoglobin values, often show decreased laboratory values because of bleeding at the fracture site; the blood glucose level may be elevated because of the stress of the trauma.

Medical Management

Surgical repair is the preferred method of managing intracapsular and extracapsular hip fractures. Surgical treatment enables the patient to get out of bed sooner and decreases the major complications associated with immobility.

The affected extremity may be immobilized temporarily by either Buck's or Russell's traction until the patient's physical condition is stabilized and surgery can be scheduled. The choice of fixation device depends on the fracture location and the potential for avascular necrosis of the femoral head and neck. Prosthetic implants, such as the bipolar hip replacement (hemiarthroplasty) (see Fig. 4.17), are used to replace the femoral head and neck in fractures when the vascular supply to the femoral head may be compromised. A Neufeld nail and screws are used in the repair of intertrochanteric fractures (see Fig. 4.18A). A Küntscher nail (intramedullary rod) is used to repair midshaft femoral fractures (see Fig. 4.18B). Sliding nails are used in repair of intertrochanteric fractures. Sliding nails usually permit the patient to bear weight to some degree because they "give" slightly without shifting their placement or penetrating the femur. The use of these

Health Promotion

Hip Fracture

- Factors that contribute to the incidence of hip fracture in older adults include an increased risk for falls, inability to correct a postural imbalance, inadequacy of local tissue to absorb shock (e.g., fat, muscle bulk), and underlying skeletal weakness.
- Factors that increase the risk of older adults falling include gait and balance problems, decreased vision and hearing, diminished reflexes, orthostatic hypotension, and medication use.
- Leading hazards that increase the risk of falls are loose rugs and slippery or uneven surfaces.
- Many falls are associated with getting in or out of a chair or bed.
- Falls to the side, the most common type in the frail elderly, are more likely to result in a hip fracture than forward falls.
- Two important factors influencing the amount of force imposed on the hip are the presence of energy-absorbing soft tissue over the greater trochanter and the state of leg muscle contraction at the time of the fall.
- Many older adults have poor muscle tone, an important factor in the severity of a fall.
- Older women often have osteoporosis and accompanying low bone density, which increases the risk of hip fracture.
- Targeted interventions to reduce hip fractures in older adults include a variety of strategies. Calcium and vitamin D supplementation, estrogen replacement, and drug therapy have been shown to decrease bone loss or increase bone density and decrease the likelihood of fracture. Be vigilant in planning interventions that are known to reduce the incidence of hip fracture in the older adult.

devices is called internal fixation. Bone grafts, either autograft (patient's bone) or allograft (cadaver bone), may be used with internal fixation devices when excessive bone is lost at the fracture site. If a stable reduction cannot be achieved, the health care provider may do an arthroplasty (surgical reconstruction of a joint). Immobilization devices, such as casts or splints, also may be used with open reduction.

Nursing Interventions and Patient Teaching

Nursing interventions for a fractured hip are concerned with preventing shock and further complications. A primary concern is to maintain proper alignment through traction and abduction of the hip when turning a patient with a fractured hip from side to side. Some health care providers do not want patients turned onto their sides for several days after surgery; others may order the patient to be turned only on the non-operative side. It is important to know the orders and to educate patients about activity restrictions. Patients who have had internal fixation for a fractured hip should avoid elevating the affected extremity when sitting. Elevate the head of the bed a maximum

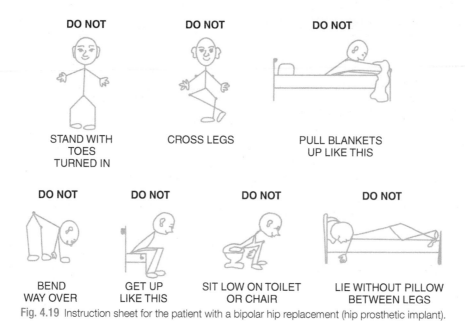

Fig. 4.19 Instruction sheet for the patient with a bipolar hip replacement (hip prosthetic implant).

of 45 degrees to avoid acute flexion of the hip and strain on the fixation device. Instruct the patient *not* to cross the legs because this can adduct the affected extremity and dislocate the hip. Limit weight-bearing on the hip by providing walking assists such as a walker or crutches.

Postoperative interventions for a patient with hip fracture repair include wound assessment with special attention to color, amount, and odor of exudate. Assess vital signs, as well as the suture line for approximation of skin edges and intact sutures or staples, at least every 8 hours. Jackson-Pratt or Hemovac drains often are used during the initial postoperative days and must be assessed for amount and color of wound drainage at least every 4 hours. Document intake and output. Encourage the use of incentive spirometers to aid in adequate respiratory ventilation and prevent pneumonia. Turn and move the patient on schedule to maintain skin integrity and promote circulation.

Leg manipulation during surgery and immobility afterward place the patient at risk for deep vein thrombosis and pulmonary embolism. Anti-embolism stockings, elastic wraps, or pneumatic compression stockings and foot and leg exercises increase venous flow to the heart. Remove the stockings once each shift to assess for compression points and skin integrity. Anticoagulation therapy with enoxaparin, aspirin, or warfarin often is prescribed.

Special postoperative instructions regarding proper positioning, sitting, and turning are required for patients who have had a prosthetic implant or bipolar hip replacement (Fig. 4.19; and the Patient Teaching box on postoperative care of the patient who had a fractured hip). Isometric exercises are done on the quadriceps and gluteal muscles to strengthen the muscles used for walking (see the Patient Teaching box on quadriceps setting exercises).

Patient Teaching

Quadriceps Setting Exercises

Quadriceps and gluteal muscles must be strong for ambulation. The quadriceps muscles stabilize the knee joint. Teach the patient to do the following exercises 10–15 times hourly:
- To strengthen quadriceps muscles, push the knee down against the mattress while raising the heel of the foot off the bed; maintain the contraction for a count of 5 and relax for a count of 5.
- For gluteal setting exercises, contract, or "pinch," the buttocks together for a count of 5, then relax for a count of 5.
- Strengthen the unaffected leg by pushing down against the footboard, holding for a count of 5, releasing for a count of 5, and repeating.

Nursing interventions also involve use of an abduction splint (a wedge-shaped foam bolster or pillow) for 7 to 10 days to ensure postoperative maintenance of leg abduction and to prevent dislocation of the prosthesis. Place the abduction splint between the patient's legs when in a supine position. Turn the patient with the extremities maintained in proper alignment by using the logrolling procedure with the assistance of at least two nurses. Most health care providers order the patient to be turned toward the unoperated side; check each order by the health care provider. Transfer the patient from bed to chair on the unoperated side by pivoting on the unaffected leg. The injured leg is kept extended forward to avoid extreme hip flexion and possible dislocation of the prosthesis. Provide a chair with a firm, nonreclining seat and arms; elevate the sitting surfaces as necessary with pillows or foam cushions to keep the angle of the hip within the prescribed limits when the patient is sitting. In general, patients who have had *any* kind of internal fixation for a fractured hip should avoid elevation of the operated leg when sitting in a chair because this puts excessive strain on the fixation device (Nursing Care Plan 4.1).

Prognosis

Complications of hip fractures are the most common cause of death after age 75. Hip fractures in older adults often are complicated by other medical conditions such as diabetes mellitus, cardiac problems (e.g., heart failure), and neurologic disorders (e.g., stroke). A large bone such as the hip heals slowly in older patients, and this predisposes them to various complications. They are at high risk for pneumonia, deep vein thrombosis, fat embolus, pulmonary embolus, impaired skin integrity, urinary retention, constipation, mental disorientation, and depression.

OTHER FRACTURES

Etiology and Pathophysiology

A fracture is a traumatic injury to a bone in which the continuity of the tissue of the bone is broken. Most fractures result from an insult to the bone, such as a forceful blow, twisting, or crushing, which places more stress on the bone than it can absorb. Fractures that occur without trauma are referred to as pathologic or spontaneous fractures and can be caused by a weakening of the bone by osteoporosis, metastatic cancer and tumors of the bone, Cushing's syndrome, malnutrition, and complications of long-term steroid therapy.

Fractures may result from (1) direct force, which causes a fracture at the site of the trauma; (2) torsion, as in a twisting injury in which the fracture occurs at a point remote from the trauma (e.g., forceful twisting of the wrist may fracture the arm); or (3) violent contractions involving highly developed muscles (e.g., severe muscle spasms may cause a fracture in a paraplegic patient).

The more than 150 types of fractures can be classified in various ways. First, they are described as either closed (simple) or open (compound) (Fig. 4.20). A closed fracture does not involve a break in the skin, and sometimes can be realigned by external manipulation rather than invasive surgery. Open fractures involve an open wound or break in the skin near the fracture in which the bone, or a part of the bone, may protrude. Open fractures are more serious because they involve more soft tissue damage, require surgical treatment to repair, and significantly increase the risk for infection.

Fractures sometimes are referred to as joint fractures if they involve or are close to a joint. An articulation fracture involves the surface of a joint. An extracapsular fracture involves a fracture near the joint but one that has not entered the joint capsule. An intracapsular fracture is a fracture within the joint capsule.

Fractures also can be described by their displacement. See Figs. 4.20 and 4.21 show that fragments may be displaced sideways, can override the opposite fractured surface, may angulate or create a bend in the bone, and may rotate away from the fracture site. When a bone is displaced, the bone fragments can cause soft tissue damage. The patient has severe pain, edema, and muscle spasms in the early stages of healing.

Bone is vascular; therefore, when a fracture occurs, bleeding occurs at the site of the fracture and in the surrounding tissue. A clot forms at the ends of the fractured bone. The next phase of healing occurs when the hematoma becomes organized as fibroblasts invade the area and a fibrin meshwork is formed. Inflammation is localized as the white blood cells wall off the area. Osteoblasts enter the fibrous area to help hold the union firm. Blood vessels develop, and collagen strands start to incorporate calcium deposits. Callus (bony deposits formed between and around the broken ends of a fractured bone during healing) forms when the osteoblasts continue to lay the network for bone buildup and osteoclasts destroy dead bone. The collagen strengthens and continues to incorporate calcium deposits. Remodeling is the final step and occurs when the excess callus is resorbed and trabecular bone is laid down along the lines of stress.

Clinical Manifestations

The signs and symptoms of fractures vary according to the location and function of the involved bone, the strength of its muscle attachment, the type of fracture sustained, and the amount of related damage. Pain, warmth over the injured area, and ecchymosis of the skin surrounding the injured area may not be present for several days. Some fractures may result in an obvious deformity and loss of normal function. The injured part may be incapable of voluntary movements; have a change in the curvature or length of bone (for a fractured hip, the affected leg will be shorter and externally rotated); and have a loss of sensation or paralysis distal to injury, which is indicative of nerve constricture. Crepitus, or a grating sound, may be heard if the limb is moved gently (do not attempt to verify this sign when fracture is suspected because it may cause further damage and increase pain). The patient also may demonstrate signs of shock related to tissue injury, blood loss, and severe pain.

Assessment

Rapid orthopedic and peripheral vascular assessment. Perform the *seven Ps of orthopedic assessment* to establish a baseline and monitor changes in the patient's muscular function, bone integrity, distal circulation, and sensation:

1. Pain: Does it seem out of proportion to the patient's injury? Does the pain increase on active or passive motion?
2. Pallor
3. Paresthesia, or numbness
4. Paralysis
5. Polar temperature: Is the extremity cold compared with the opposite extremity?

Nursing Care Plan 4.1   **The Patient With a Fractured Hip**

A female, age 72, fell in her kitchen while removing cookies from the oven. She sustained a subcapital fracture of the right hip. The patient is scheduled in the morning for a bipolar (hemiarthroplasty) prosthesis.

PATIENT PROBLEM

Compromised Tissue Perfusion, related to vascular injury or interruption of arterial and venous flow secondary to edema

Patient Goals and Expected Outcomes	Nursing Interventions	Evaluation and Rationale
Patient's circulation will be maintained to fulfill body requirements	Palpate site for warmth. Observe site for color. Apply moderate pressure to nailbed, and subsequently observe speed of capillary refill. Assess pedal pulse bilaterally q 4 h. Question patient regarding pain and paresthesia in injured part. Apply antiembolism stockings as ordered.	Distal pulses palpable; toes symmetric, warm, dry, and pink; sensation and mobility intact.
	Help and teach patient to cough q 2 h and deep breathe q h. Monitor vital signs q 2–4 h.	Able to cough and deep breathe with assistance; oxygen saturation 92%, lungs clear.

PATIENT PROBLEM

Insufficient Knowledge, related to home care management

Patient Goals and Expected Outcomes	Nursing Interventions	Evaluation and Rationale
Patient and/or significant other will demonstrate understanding of home care and follow-up instructions through interactive discussion and return demonstration	Stress importance of prescribed rehabilitation plan of activity, rest, and exercise.	Patient demonstrates ambulation with walker, exercises, transfers, and precautions, verbalizes understanding of discharge instructions and home care.
	Provide diet instructions on type and amount of food to eat, and advise patient to avoid weight gain if applicable.	Discusses correct foods to eat for therapeutic results.
	Discuss medications: name, purpose, schedule, dosage, and side effects.	Verbalizes knowledge of medications for purpose, dosage, side effects, and correct schedule to prevent any drug errors.
	Discuss signs and symptoms to report to health care provider: severe pain; changes in temperature, color, or sensation in extremity; malodorous drainage from wound.	Verbalizes knowledge of need to report abnormalities to the health care provider including severe pain, abnormal temperature, color, or tingling in affected extremity as well as abnormal wound drainage.
	Stress home safety factors such as elimination of throw rugs, use of safety bars on the bathtub, elevated toilet seats.	Discusses home preparations for safety to include removal of throw rugs, placement of safety bars on bathtub, and availability of toilet riser. Safety knowledge will prevent accidents.
	Encourage follow-up visits with health care provider.	Notes the importance of postoperative follow-up visits with health care provider. Promotes postoperative recovery.

CRITICAL THINKING QUESTIONS

1. The first postoperative evening, the patient is restless and disoriented. What nursing interventions are needed to prevent dislocation of her bipolar hip prosthesis?
2. On the third postoperative day the nurse notes an erythematous area on the patient's coccyx. What therapeutic measures can prevent skin impairment?
3. On the third postoperative day the patient complains of pain in the right calf when the nurse performs dorsiflexion. What is the most appropriate immediate action by the nurse?

Patient Teaching

Postoperative Care for the Patient Who Had a Fractured Hip

OPEN REDUCTION WITH INTERNAL FIXATION

Teaching for patients who had a fractured hip and received an internal fixation with nails or pins (see Fig. 4.19) would include the following:

- Assess patient's ability to understand instructions and limitations.
- Assist patient to dangle feet at bedside on first postoperative day and then to pivot to chair with no weight on operative leg, or touch-down weight if allowed.
- Stress that the operative foot should be placed on floor, but weight should be borne on the inoperative leg (refer to limb as either left or right leg so that the patient understands) to maintain safety in care.
- Turn patient every 2 h; prop with pillows between legs or under the back to maintain position.
- Assist with range-of-motion exercises to maintain muscle strength.
- Help physical therapist walk patient with walker and with limited weight placed on operative limb (if assistance is needed) for comfort and safety.
- Encourage patient and family members to walk together for patient's safety. Instruct family about weight-bearing techniques for clarity and safety.
- If a stable plate and screw fixation is used to repair the fractured hip, the patient should not bear weight for 6 weeks to 3 months to protect the fracture site.
- A telescoping nail fixation allows minimal to partial weight-bearing during the first 6 weeks to 3 months.

HIP PROSTHETIC IMPLANT

Teaching for patients who had a fractured hip and received a hip prosthetic implant (hemiarthroplasty) (see Fig. 4.18) includes the following:

- Avoid hip flexion beyond 60 degrees for approximately 10 days.
- Avoid hip flexion beyond 90 degrees for 2–3 months.
- Avoid adduction of the affected leg beyond midline for 2–3 months.
- Maintain partial weight-bearing status for approximately 2–3 months.
- Avoid positioning on the operative side in bed.

- Maintain abduction of the hip by using a wedge-shaped foam bolster or pillows arranged in a wedge; this will require nursing assistance.

Fractures can also be described in terms of appearance (Fig. 4.21).

- *Complete fracture:* Fracture line extends entirely through the bone, with the periosteum disrupted on both sides of the bone.
- *Comminuted fracture:* Bone is splintered into three or more fragments at the site of the break. There is more than one fracture line.
- *Transverse fracture:* Break runs directly across the bone at a right angle to the bone's axis.
- *Oblique fracture:* Break runs diagonally across the bone at approximately a 45-degree angle to the shaft of the bone.
- *Spiral fracture:* Break coils around the bone. This is sometimes called a torsion fracture and results from a twisting force.
- *Impacted fracture:* Sometimes called a *telescoped* fracture because one bone fragment is wedged forcibly into another bone fragment. In long bones, this can shorten the extremity.
- *Greenstick fracture:* Incomplete fracture in which the fracture line extends only partially through the bone. The bone is broken and bent but still secured at one side. This fracture is common in children because their bones are softer and more flexible than those of adults.

Fractures are described according to their location on the bone—for example, proximal, midshaft, or distal. Fractures also can be classified according to the force that caused the break. An example of this is the marching fracture, which can occur in the metatarsals as a result of a long march.

Fractures sometimes are named after the first health care provider to describe them. For example:

- **Colles' fracture:** Fracture of the distal portion of the radius within 1 inch of the wrist joint; commonly occurs when a person attempts to break a fall by putting the hands down.
- *Pott's fracture:* Occurs at the distal end of the fibula and is characterized by chipping off of a piece of the medial malleolus with a displacement of the foot outward.

---

6. Puffiness from edema or a hematoma
7. Pulselessness: A Doppler ultrasound device may be useful to determine the presence or absence of blood flow if unable to palpate distal pulses

Subjective data include pain at the site of the injury, loss of sensation or movement of the affected part, and cause of injury.

Objective data include warmth, edema, and ecchymosis; obvious deformity; loss of normal function in the injured part; signs of systemic shock; and signs of any circulatory, motor, or sensory impairment.

Diagnostic Tests

An accurate diagnosis of the fracture is made by radiographic examination.

Medical Management

Immediate management includes splinting and elevation to prevent edema of the affected part. Preservation of body alignment is also critical. Apply cold packs (during the first 24 hours) to reduce hemorrhage, edema, and pain. Administer analgesics as ordered. Observe the injured part for change in color, sensation, or temperature. Also observe the patient for signs of shock.

Secondary management for a closed fracture begins with optimal reduction: replacing bone fragments in their correct anatomic position. This can be accomplished through (1) closed reduction, which involves manual manipulations—moving bony fragments into position by applying traction and pressure to distal

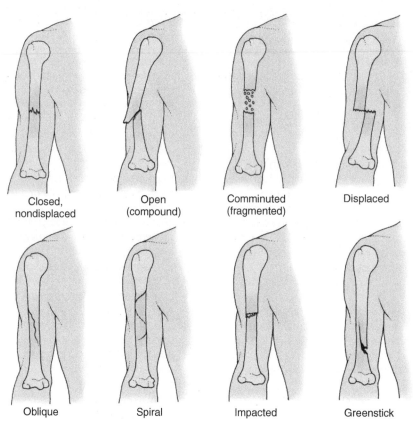

Fig. 4.20 Common types of fractures. (From Ignatavicius DD, Workman ML: *Medical-surgical nursing: Patient-centered collaborative care*, ed 8, St. Louis, 2016, Elsevier.)

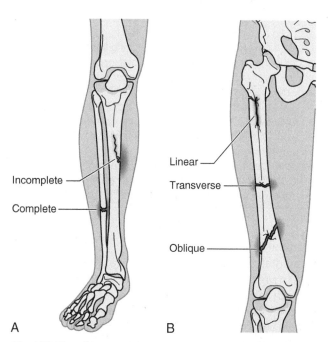

Fig. 4.21 Bone fractures. (A) Incomplete and complete. (B) Linear, transverse, and oblique.

fragments; (2) traction; (3) **open reduction with internal fixation (ORIF)**, a surgical procedure allowing fracture alignment under direct visualization while using various internal fixation devices applied to the bone; or (4) immobilization. Immobilization can be achieved through one or a combination of the following: (1) external fixation with a cast or splint; (2) traction; or (3) internal fixation devices such as pins, plates, screws, wires, and prostheses (see Fig. 4.19).

For an open fracture, additional measures are taken. The wound undergoes surgical debridement to remove dirt, foreign materials, devitalized tissue, and necrotic bone. The date of the last tetanus toxoid administration is needed. Patients having expired status must have the tetanus toxoid administered. A wound culture is indicated. Prophylactic antibiotic therapy is initiated. Observe the wound for signs of osteomyelitis, tetanus, or gangrene. Closure of the wound occurs when there is no sign of infection. Reduction and immobilization of the fracture then take place. Finally, observe for and treat any complications.

Nursing Interventions and Patient Teaching

The nursing interventions for patients with fractures are essentially the same as for any surgical patient. The care of the patient in traction and in a cast is discussed later in this chapter. Each healing phase after a fracture is enhanced by a balanced diet. Proteins, calcium, magnesium and other vitamins are essential. The patient should be instructed on good food sources for each. Protein-rich foods include lean meats, eggs, nuts, seeds, dairy products, tofu, and beans. Dark leafy green vegetables, low-fat dairy products, and soy are good sources for calcium. Vitamin D is found in many of the calcium-rich foods in addition to tofu, some seafood, and fortified cereals. Sources of magnesium are seeds, nuts, and greens. Fluids should be encouraged as with any well-balanced diet. Exercise of the unaffected joints, muscle-setting exercises, skin care, and elimination are important considerations in patient care. Internal fixation has simplified nursing intervention for many patients with fractures and shortened the period of hospitalization, but many patients require longer periods of hospitalization. If activity is restricted, anticipate and prevent the complications that result from immobility.

Patient teaching includes (1) how to move comfortably in bed; (2) how to transfer safely in and out of bed; (3) weight-bearing restrictions and activity limitations, including how long these must be observed; (4) proper use of ambulatory assistive devices; (5) how to avoid edema in the affected part by proper elevation; (6) how to control pain or discomfort in the affected part; (7) exercises to perform to maintain strength and enhance circulation; and (8) proper method of cleansing pins, using surgical asepsis per the health care provider's protocol.

Prognosis

Bone production and fracture healing depend on the patient's age and general health. The presence of other systemic diseases complicates the healing process. Nutrition is a major factor as well in the bone healing process.

FRACTURE OF THE VERTEBRAE

Etiology and Pathophysiology

Injuries such as diving accidents or blows to the head or body can result in fractures of the vertebrae. Motorcycle and car accidents (especially head-on collisions) occur more frequently with young men (ages 16 to 30 years). Patients with osteoporosis and metastatic cancer are at risk for vertebral fractures.

Fractures of the vertebrae may involve the vertebral body, lamina, and articulating processes and may occur with or without displacement. If the fracture has displaced the vertebral structures, pressure may be placed on spinal nerves. The sharp bone fragments also may sever the spinal cord nerves, causing permanent paralysis from the point of injury downward.

Clinical Manifestations

Signs and symptoms of vertebral fracture include pain at the site of the injury; partial or complete loss of mobility or sensation below the level of the injury; and evidence of fracture or fracture dislocation on routine radiographic examination, myelography, or CT scans.

Assessment

Collection of subjective data includes assessment for pain (if the fracture has injured the spinal cord, pain may not be present), numbness, tingling, and inability to move extremities from below the level of the trauma site.

Collection of objective data includes careful assessment of neurologic function, such as pupillary reaction to light, hand grip, ability to move extremities, level of orientation, vital signs, and reaction to painful stimuli (see Chapter 14). Observe for fecal and urinary retention and for signs of hemorrhage such as hypotension, tachycardia, tachypnea, and decreased renal functioning.

Diagnostic Tests

Radiographic studies are done to determine whether the vertebral bodies are compressed. A spinal cord injury may result from a fracture or dislocation of a vertebra; if this is suspected, the health care provider performs a spinal tap to evaluate the spinal fluid. Spinal fluid is normally clear, and the presence of blood indicates trauma (see Chapter 14).

Medical Management

Stable injuries to the vertebrae that are not a threat to spinal cord integrity are treated with pain medication and muscle relaxants. Anticoagulant therapy may be ordered as a prophylaxis for thromboembolic complications. Maintaining erect posture can be enhanced by the use of a back support, corset brace, or a cast. The patient may be allowed to ambulate with assistance (gait enhancers) once discomfort subsides.

Unstable fractures that involve displacement are more serious. Treatment is aimed at fracture reduction through postural positioning and traction. Cranial skeletal traction is used with cervical spine fractures (see Chapter 14). A halo brace (see Fig. 4.22), an external immobilization device in which a plaster or plastic brace that incorporates metal struts attached to pins is inserted into bone, is used to allow the patient to be mobile. Pelvic traction is used for lumbar spinal fractures. An open reduction may be necessary with internal fixation using a Harrington rod. After this surgical procedure, the patient is placed in a body cast.

Nursing Interventions and Patient Teaching

Nursing interventions are aimed at maintaining the stability of the fracture fixation by (1) logrolling the patient for position changes; (2) observing the correct procedure for turning a patient in a special bed, such as a Stryker frame or Foster bed; (3) elevating the head of the bed no more than 30 degrees; (4) using stabilization devices for the head and back. Assess the continuity of traction (e.g., weights hanging free and ropes not twisted) and surrounding traction equipment, as well as skin integrity (e.g., erythema, tenderness, and edema).

Patient problem statements and interventions for the patient with a vertebral fracture include but are not limited to the following:

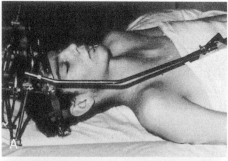

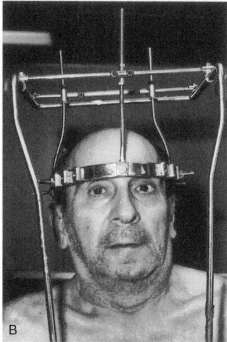

Fig. 4.22 Halo traction. (A) Halo attached to body cast. Metal strut will be anchored firmly into body cast with additional plaster. (B) Metal ring, or halo, that attaches to skull. (From Lewis SL, Heitkemper MM, Dirksen SR, et al: *Medical-surgical nursing: Assessment and management of clinical problems*, ed 7, St. Louis, 2007, Mosby.)

Patient teaching includes how to support the back by (1) using a firm mattress; (2) sitting in straight, firm chairs (for no longer than 20 to 30 minutes), when allowed; (3) using proper lifting techniques (using the leg muscles, not the back); and (4) doing back exercises to strengthen spinal extensor muscles.

Prognosis

Stable injuries to the vertebrae that are not a threat to spinal cord integrity have an excellent prognosis with full recovery. Unstable fractures are more serious, and the prognosis is guarded when spinal cord injury is involved.

FRACTURE OF THE PELVIS

Etiology and Pathophysiology

Most pelvic fractures result from trauma involving great force, such as falls from extreme heights, automobile accidents, or crushing accidents. When the trauma is severe enough to fracture the pelvis, vital abdominal organs, such as the bladder, vagina, uterus, liver,

PATIENT PROBLEM	NURSING INTERVENTIONS
Potential for Infection, related to immobility and/or surgical intervention	Monitor patient for signs and symptoms of infection (elevated temperature, increased pulse rate, malodorous exudates, erythema, cloudy urine, diminished breath sounds, and crackles and wheezes)
	Monitor laboratory values (such as complete blood count) and blood and wound cultures
	Protect patient from cross-contamination by practicing good hand-washing techniques, maintaining surgical asepsis when changing dressings, and using strict surgical asepsis with catheter care
	Encourage coughing, deep breathing, and leg exercises
	Encourage use of incentive spirometer
	Prevent people with infectious processes from coming in contact with patient
Compromised Physical Mobility, related to: • Discomfort • Neuromuscular skeletal impairment • Pain	Maintain bed rest in correct body alignment; avoid lifting or twisting body
	Place patient in immobilization device, such as cervical head halter, skeletal traction, Stryker frame, or CircOlectric bed, as ordered; maintain cervical spine in extension
	Assess neurovascular status q 2 h; monitor pulse, color, temperature, sensation, and mobility of all extremities
	Perform passive range of motion (ROM) or assist with and teach active ROM exercises for all extremities q 2 h
	As fracture heals, traction is replaced with cast
	Assist patient with ambulation when ordered; monitor for vertigo and weakness; progress slowly

spleen, intestines, or kidneys, also may be damaged. Extensive blood loss may result due to the rich blood supply of the pelvis. As much as 1 to 4 L may be lost in such an injury.

Clinical Manifestations

The patient with a fractured pelvis is unable to bear weight without discomfort. Local tenderness and edema are common at the trauma site. Hematuria (blood in the urine) may result from trauma to the bladder.

Hemorrhage is by far the most frequent life-threatening complication to a patient with a pelvic fracture.

Assessment

Subjective data include complaints of pelvic pain or tenderness and backache. Complaints of restlessness, anxiety, and progressive disorientation may be signs of shock.

Collection of objective data includes assessment of muscle spasms in the pelvic region; ecchymoses over the pelvis, perineum, groin, or suprapubic area; inability to raise the legs when supine; and external foot rotation on the affected side with noticeable shortening of one leg. Vital sign assessment may indicate shock (hypotension, tachycardia, tachypnea, oliguria, and diaphoresis). Careful observation for fat embolism syndrome is especially pertinent for patients with pelvic fractures. Assess bowel sounds in all four quadrants and document the findings; large bowel and rectal lacerations are possible in patients with pelvic fractures. Assess color and amount of urinary output because of the possibility of laceration of the bladder.

Diagnostic Tests

Abdominal radiographic studies are done with the patient in the supine and lateral positions. CT provides an evaluation of the bony pelvis and intra-abdominal contents. IV pyelogram is performed to determine kidney damage. Interpretation of laboratory values for hemoglobin and hematocrit, urinalysis, and stool for occult blood helps determine whether the patient is bleeding and anemic.

Medical Management

The patient often remains on bed rest for 3 weeks and then walks with crutches for approximately 6 weeks. If the patient has a symphysis pubis fracture and an iliac fracture on the same side, the health care provider performs surgery. After surgery, skeletal traction is applied for approximately 6 weeks to maintain the leg position. When traction is released, the patient may ambulate without bearing weight for approximately 3 months. For a bilateral fracture of the pelvis, the health care provider may order a pelvic sling to support the fracture. To treat severe fractures that totally disrupt the pelvic ring and dislocate the sacroiliac joints, the health care provider may apply an external skeletal fixation device. He or she also may apply a spica or body cast to support the fracture.

Nursing Interventions and Patient Teaching

Nursing interventions involve monitoring the patient for signs of progressive shock (hypotension, tachycardia, tachypnea, and decreased urinary output). Measure the abdominal girth at least every 8 hours for signs of increased abdominal pressure that could result from internal hemorrhaging. Monitor I&O for signs of hypovolemia, laceration of the bladder, and potential

kidney trauma. Insert a Foley catheter to monitor urinary output and color. Implement nursing interventions appropriate for impaired mobility, impaired skin integrity, fluid volume deficit, and pain management.

A patient problem statement and interventions for the patient with a pelvic fracture include but are not limited to the following:

PATIENT PROBLEM	NURSING INTERVENTIONS
Compromised Tissue Perfusion, related to: • Hemorrhage • Hypovolemia • Shock	Assess for ecchymosis over pelvis and perineum Monitor vital signs q 15 min for evidence of shock until stable Insert a Foley catheter per health care provider's order to monitor color and amount of urinary output Monitor parenteral fluids per health care provider's order Provide quiet, therapeutic environment Administer oxygen per health care provider's order Maintain bed rest per health care provider's order Monitor bowel sounds and measure abdominal girth to ascertain possible lacerated bowel

Reinforce the reasons for immobility and not bearing full weight; the patient may be too anxious to hear or understand initial explanations. Also explain measures for dealing with acute pain and changes in medications as pain decreases. In addition, explain turning and moving techniques to prevent skin impairment.

Prognosis

Chronic pain may linger long after the fracture has healed. Some patients may require referrals to a pain management specialist to develop a plan of care. Life-threatening complications may also be linked to pelvic fractures. Fatty embolus may result from pelvic and long bone fractures when traumatic injury is the root cause. Vascularity of the pelvic region elevates the risk for hemorrhage. The long-term prognosis depends on the immediacy of treatment, severity of the fracture, the patient's age, and the presence of other systemic disorders.

COMPLICATIONS OF FRACTURES

COMPARTMENT SYNDROME

Compartment syndrome is a pathologic condition caused by the progressive development of arterial vessel compression and reduced blood supply to one of the body's compartments, typically in an extremity. Muscle fascia lines the muscles, nerves, and blood vessels. It is a very fibrous, tough, and nonelastic structure. Fractures and traumatic crushing injuries may lead to inflammation and swelling. Expansion or inflammation of a compartment's contents can result in compression of the blood vessels, resulting in compartment syndrome. Compression of blood vessels may result from swelling or from a tight cast or dressing, resulting in deprivation of blood supply to the muscles and nerves because of the inability of the compartment to expand. Irreversible muscle ischemia can occur within 6 hours as a result of compression of the arteries, nerves, and tendons entering the compartment. Numbness, paralysis and sensory loss follow, with contracture and permanent disability of the extremity seen within 24 to 48 hours.

Assessment

Collection of subjective data includes pain assessment. Usually the patient complains of sharp pain that increases with passive movement of the hand or foot. The patient experiences deep, unrelenting, progressive, and poorly localized pain unrelieved by analgesics or elevation of the extremity. Numbness or tingling in the affected extremity is common.

Collection of objective data includes assessment of the patient's inability to flex the fingers or toes, coolness of the extremity, and absence of pulsation in the affected extremity. Assess skin color for signs of pallor or cyanosis. Gentle palpation of the extremity reveals slowing of the capillary refill time (blanching). Close monitoring and proper documentation of vital signs are essential (especially temperature to detect signs of tissue necrosis) (see Box 4.5).

Medical Management

Prompt management of compartment syndrome is indicated to avoid permanent neurovascular damage. Surgical intervention, a fasciotomy (incision into the fascia) to relieve pressure and allow return of normal blood flow to the area, is indicated. The incision is often left open to heal by granulation (healing by secondary intention) (Fig. 4.23).

Nursing Interventions

Nursing interventions include administration of analgesics with careful documentation of relief obtained. To slow further circulatory compromise, elevate the affected limb, no higher than heart level, to maintain arterial pressure. Apply cold packs and remove any constricting material, such as an elastic bandage. The most common complication when decompression is delayed is infection as a result of tissue necrosis. Purulent drainage from the dressing is a sign of infection and must be reported immediately. If drainage and secretion isolation are required, provide careful instructions to the patient, who may feel isolated. Encourage patients to express their fears and emotional needs. Volkmann's contracture is a permanent contracture (with claw hand, flexion of wrist and fingers, and atrophy of the forearm) that can occur as a result of compartment syndrome. Proper positioning and alignment can reduce the risk of this complication.

Box 4.6   Nursing Interventions for the Patient in Traction

- Maintain the patient's body in proper alignment. The force or pull on the extremities should be in alignment with the long axis of the bone.
- Ensure that weights hang freely from the bed and are never removed without a health care provider's order.
- Question patients as to their understanding of the purpose of the traction, and assess their ability to use a trapeze bar for self-movement. Elevate the foot of the bed to help prevent the patient from sliding down toward the foot of the bed (countertraction).
- Observe the condition of the traction cords, making sure they are not weakened or frayed. All knots used on the rope or cord are to be square knots.
- Center the ropes on the traction pulley.
- Assess, document, and report neurovascular impairment.
- Ensure that the weight used is the correct weight as ordered by the health care provider.
- Carefully observe the skin for signs of impairment. Use sheepskin heel protectors and bed pads to reduce impairment.
- If skeletal traction is used, assess the pin site for signs of infection. Cleanse the pin site every 8 hours with hydrogen peroxide or normal saline, as ordered.
- Assess the distal pulses bilaterally for circulatory integrity of the extremities.
- Inspect for loss of sensation in the dorsal area of the foot with weakness and inversion of the foot (inside surface turned outward).

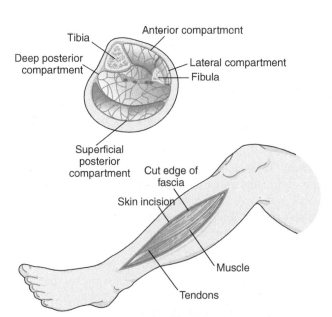

Fig. 4.23 Compartment syndrome. Often more than one compartment is involved, and the anterior compartment of the lower leg is especially vulnerable. Causes include trauma, severe burn, or excessive exercise. A single incision may open more than one compartment. (Courtesy Dr. Henry Bohlman, Cleveland, Ohio.)

Prognosis

Compartment syndrome can result in a variety of complications if not treated promptly. A permanent contracture deformity of the hand or foot, muscle necrosis, neurologic damage or infection may result.

SHOCK

Bone is vascular. Shock can occur as a result of blood loss from a fractured bone or from severed blood vessels, seen especially in open fractures. Pain and fear also can cause shock.

Assessment

Collection of subjective data includes monitoring the patient's level of consciousness. Restlessness or complaints of anxiety may suggest a decrease in cerebral perfusion, resulting in brain hypoxia. Complaints of weakness and lethargy are common.

Collection of objective data includes monitoring vital signs. Typical signs of shock include hypotension, tachycardia, diaphoresis, and tachypnea. As shock progresses, hypothermia occurs. The patient may have pale, cool, moist skin. Oliguria (diminished urinary output) is present with shock.

Medical Management

The health care provider's priority concern is to restore blood volume to ensure a rapid return of oxygen to the tissues. Blood volume can be expanded with rapid IV fluid administration. Lactated Ringer's solution and 5% dextrose in normal saline are common selections. Whole blood, plasma, or plasma substitutes also may be given. Respiratory assistance may be given by administering oxygen. A central venous catheter may be inserted for accurate monitoring of vital signs to prevent pulmonary edema.

Nursing Interventions

Nursing interventions for IV fluid administration include monitoring the IV insertion site for signs that infusion solution is seeping into the tissue surrounding the vein; this is called *infiltration*. Signs of infiltration include edema, pain, and induration (hardening of tissue) at the IV site. Monitor the patient's vital signs every 15 minutes until stable. Monitor urinary output every hour. Decreased renal perfusion is indicated by output less than 30 mL/h. The patient should remain flat in bed. If there are no head injuries, raise the lower extremities to improve venous return to the major body organs. Trendelenburg's position presses the abdominal organs against the diaphragm, reducing the effectiveness of heart and lung functions, and should be avoided. Keep the patient warm, but avoid external heat. Give nothing by mouth. Sedatives, tranquilizers, and narcotics may reduce the level of consciousness and mask neurologic changes and therefore should be avoided. Be aware that the patient's family will be anxious and provide them with brief explanations of the patient's condition.

Prognosis

Shock can lead to a loss of consciousness or coma. Shock can be fatal within a few hours of injury; therefore, immediate attention is required.

FAT EMBOLISM

Pulmonary fat embolism involves the embolization of tissue fat with platelets and circulating free fatty acids within the pulmonary capillaries. Fat embolism is rare but can be life threatening, because the fat droplets can occlude capillaries of the pulmonary circulation, causing brain hypoxia and tissue death. Risk factors include long bone and pelvic fractures, crush injuries, and hip replacement surgery. It can occur within 48 hours of the injuries. Pulmonary fat embolism syndrome is the most serious complication of long bone fractures.

Assessment

Collection of subjective data includes assessment of mental disturbances, such as irritability, restlessness, disorientation, stupor, and coma. These symptoms can result from effects of severe hypoxemia. The patient may complain of chest pain, especially on inspiration, and of localized muscle weakness, spasticity, and rigidity.

Collection of objective data includes assessing for tachypnea, dyspnea, hypoxemia, and auditory crackles and wheezes in the lung field. As the lung filters and traps embolic material, ventilation is disturbed. Assess the apical pulse to detect dysrhythmias. Patients are placed on cardiac monitoring for observation of dysrhythmias and cardiovascular collapse. Assess the patient for petechiae (a rash of red, pinpoint dots, especially in the buccal membranes, conjunctival sacs, hard palate, chest, and anterior axillary folds) caused by occlusion of capillaries. The appearance of petechiae on the conjunctiva of the eye, the neck, chest, or axillary region is a typical sign of a fat embolism (Kosova, 2015).

Diagnostic Tests

The diagnosis is based on clinical signs and symptoms, which appear within 24 to 48 hours of injury. Blood gases indicate hypoxemia. Hemoglobin and hematocrit laboratory values are decreased. Fat is present in the blood and urine. The sedimentation rate is increased, and the platelet count is decreased.

Medical Management

Treatment for fat embolism is directed at prevention. Careful immobilization of a long bone fracture is probably the most important factor in the prevention of fat embolism. The health care provider orders the administration of IV fluids to prevent shock and dilute free fatty acids. Use of corticosteroids to prevent or treat fat embolism is controversial. Digoxin often is ordered to increase the patient's cardiac output. Oxygen is administered if the arterial oxygen pressure (PaO_2) is less than 70 mm Hg. Intubation or intermittent positive-pressure ventilation may be considered if a satisfactory

PaO_2 cannot be obtained with supplemental oxygen alone. Incentive spirometry is ordered to improve lung expansion and oxygenation.

Nursing Interventions

Nursing interventions include close monitoring of the patient's arterial blood gases. Normal values include the following:

pH	7.35–7.45
$PaCO_2$	35–45 mm Hg
PaO_2	80–100 mm Hg
HCO_3	21–28 mEq/L
SaO_2	95%–100%

HCO_3, Bicarbonate; $PaCO_2$, arterial carbon dioxide pressure; PaO_2, arterial oxygen pressure; SaO_2, oxygen saturation of arterial hemoglobin.

Arterial hypoxia is present with fat emboli and may not be recognized clinically. If hypoxia is present, the health care provider orders the administration of oxygen. Check the liter flow of oxygen and educate patients and their families on safety precautions necessary when oxygen is administered (e.g., no smoking or use of electrical equipment). Respiratory failure is the most common cause of death. Careful stabilization and immobilization of long bone fractures are important steps in preventing fat embolism syndrome. Careful support when turning and positioning the patient can prevent the manipulation of the fracture and reduce the risk of fat embolism syndrome. Reposition the patient as little as possible before fracture immobilization because of the danger of dislodging more fat droplets into the general circulation. An accurate record of I&O and daily weights is essential to monitor fluid balance.

Prognosis

Fat embolism can be life threatening.

GAS GANGRENE

Gas gangrene is a severe infection of the skeletal muscle caused by gram-positive clostridial bacteria, particularly *Clostridium perfringens,* which may occur in the presence of open fractures and lacerated wounds. Clostridial bacteria in these injuries can produce exotoxins that destroy tissue. The onset is usually sudden, generally 1 to 14 days after injury. These organisms are anaerobic (i.e., they grow and function without oxygen) and are spore formers. They normally are found in soil and the intestinal tracts of humans. As the clostridial bacteria invade devitalized tissue (especially where blood supply is diminished), they multiply and produce toxins that cause (1) hemolysis (breakdown of red blood cells and release of hemoglobin); (2) vessel thrombosis; and (3) damage to the myocardium, liver, kidneys, and brain.

Assessment

Collection of subjective data includes observation of pain, which is usually sudden and severe at the site of the injury. A characteristic finding is toxic delirium.

Collection of objective data includes careful inspection of the skin for gas bubbles at the site of the wound. The various *Clostridium* species produce a characteristic cellulitis in which gas is present under the skin. This causes crepitation (a crackling sensation when the skin is touched). Observe for signs of infection, including elevated temperature, tachycardia, tachypnea, and edema around the wound. The skin around the wound becomes necrotic and ruptures, revealing necrotic muscle. The wound discharge is thin, watery, and foul smelling. Carefully document the patient's response to antibiotic therapy (e.g., decline in temperature and decrease in amount of wound drainage).

Medical Management

Treatment of gas gangrene involves establishing a larger wound opening to admit air and promote drainage. Antibiotics, such as penicillin G or cephalothin, are ordered intravenously and must be administered as scheduled. Observe the patient for adverse reactions.

Nursing Interventions

Nursing interventions include wound care, using strict medical asepsis. Spore-forming bacteria are not destroyed by ordinary disinfecting methods. Therefore, all contaminated equipment and linens must be autoclaved. Follow drainage and secretion isolation procedures to prevent the spread of the infection to other patients.

Prognosis

If left untreated, gas gangrene is rapidly fatal. Prompt treatment, including excision of gangrenous tissue and administration of penicillin G intravenously, saves 80% of patients. If massive gangrene develops, amputation is necessary.

THROMBOEMBOLISM

Etiology and Pathophysiology

Thromboembolism is a condition in which a blood vessel is occluded by an embolus carried in the bloodstream from the site of formation of the clot. It is associated with reduced skeletal muscle contractions and bed rest. The person with pelvic and hip fractures is at high risk for this complication.

Clinical Manifestations

The area supplied by an obstructed artery may tingle and become cold, numb, and cyanotic. An embolus in the lungs causes sudden, sharp thoracic or upper abdominal pain, dyspnea, cough, fever, and hemoptysis.

Assessment

Collection of subjective data includes careful investigation of complaints of pain in the lower extremities (especially the calf). A complaint of tenderness over the area is common. The patient may complain of a sharp pain in the thoracic area when an embolus is in the lung.

Collection of objective data includes assessing signs consistent with thromboembolism. The affected area may be erythematous, warm to the touch, and edematous. Assess for differences in leg size (circumference) bilaterally from thigh to ankle. (In the past, Homans' sign commonly was assessed and considered a positive finding for the condition. This involved the flexion of the foot. The presence of pain was consistent with a possible thromboembolus. This is not done in many facilities now because of fears of potentially dislodging the clot.) Also observe the patient for dyspnea and blood in the sputum if pulmonary embolus is present. When anticoagulant therapy is ordered, assess for signs of bleeding, such as petechiae, epistaxis, hematuria, hematemesis, and occult or gross blood in the stool.

Diagnostic Tests
A complete history is taken and a physical examination is performed. Laboratory studies, including a prothrombin time (PT), international normalized ratio (INR), D-dimer concentration, and CBC, may be performed. Diagnostic tests for deep vein thrombosis may include Doppler ultrasonography or duplex scanning. A spiral CT scan of the lung, a ventilation/perfusion scan, or a pulmonary arteriogram may be ordered to rule out pulmonary embolism.

Medical Management
Treatment includes administration of anticoagulants, such as heparin, enoxaparin, or warfarin. A surgical procedure known as a thrombectomy (removal of a thrombus from a blood vessel) may be done.

Nursing Interventions
Nursing interventions involve caring for the patient whose physical activity has been restricted. Often this involves bed rest with the foot of the bed elevated to aid venous return. Teach the patient to engage in active exercise, such as dorsiflexion (pointing backward) and plantar flexion (pointing forward) of the toes, several times each hour. This exercise stimulates circulation to the legs. Continuous hot, moist compresses usually are ordered. Antiembolism stockings and intermittent pneumatic compression devices are ordered while the patient is on bed rest and are maintained even after the patient is ambulatory. Assess lung sounds every 4 hours and adhere to the activity ordered. If the patient is receiving anticoagulants, closely monitor PT, INR, and partial thromboplastin times.

Prognosis
Obstruction of the pulmonary artery or one of its branches may be fatal (see the Safety Alert box). A thrombus in an extremity usually resolves with treatment, and a favorable prognosis is noted.

Safety Alert

Thromboembolism

Never massage a patient's lower extremities. A thromboembolus can be present without clinical signs and symptoms.

DELAYED FRACTURE HEALING
A *delayed union* is a fracture that fails to heal within the usual time. The healing is impaired but has not stopped completely and eventually will repair itself. *Nonunion* is when the ends of the fractured bone fail to unite and produce a stable union after 6 to 9 months. Potential causes of delayed union and nonunion include infection and poor perfusion. The calcification of cartilage and bone formation do not occur. Bone grafting, prosthetic implant, internal fixation, external fixation, or a combination of these methods can be used to correct the problem of delayed union or nonunion of bone fractures. Health care providers are using electrical stimulation as a new method of promoting healing of nonunion fractures. The use of electrical probes on bone stimulates bone production.

Prognosis
Bone production and fracture healing depend on the patient's age and general health. The presence of other systemic diseases complicates the healing process.

SKELETAL FIXATION DEVICES

EXTERNAL FIXATION DEVICES
External fixation devices are used to hold bone fragments in normal position. Casts, skeletal and skin traction, braces, and metal pins are examples of these devices.

Skeletal Pin External Fixation
One external fixation technique immobilizes fractures with pins inserted through the bone and attached to a rigid external metal frame (Fig. 4.24). This technique is becoming more popular because it provides rigid support of comminuted open fractures, infected nonunions, and infected unstable joints. The patient can use the muscles and joints above and below the fixation. Leaving the fracture open to air has the advantage of visibility of the area and accessibility for wound care.

This procedure is performed with the patient under general anesthesia. Reassure the patient that the pain after the insertion of the pins is minimal. Immediately after the procedure, the extremity is placed in balanced suspension traction to help relieve the edema. Assess the pins that are inserted through the bone at least every 4 hours. The position of each pin and surrounding skin should be documented in the assessment. Signs of infection, including drainage or odor, should be included. Remove dried exudate from around the pins as ordered, with the prescribed cleaning agent and surgical asepsis. Patients are permitted to ambulate on crutches when soft tissue edema is relieved. They are

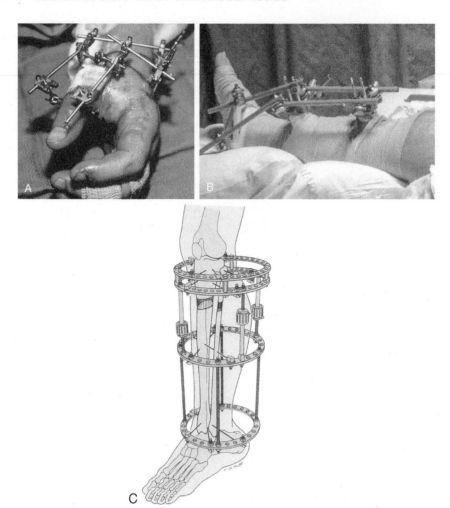

Fig. 4.24 External fixation apparatuses. (A) Hoffmann. (B) External fixation of tibia. (C) Ilizarov apparatus with corticotomies for lengthening lower leg. (A and C, From Beare PG, Myers JL: *Adult health nursing*, ed 3, St. Louis, 1998, Mosby.)

permitted to shower when the wounds have healed but must avoid salt or chlorinated water to prevent fixator corrosion.

NONSURGICAL INTERVENTIONS FOR MUSCULOSKELETAL DISORDERS

CASTS

Casts are immobilization devices. The materials most commonly used for casting are plaster and fiberglass. Material selection largely depends on the location of the fracture and the time needed for healing to take place. Body casts and long bones requiring more stabilization traditionally are casted with plaster, which is heavier and more durable. Fiberglass casts are relatively lightweight and are used commonly on arm fractures. Once the affected body part has been aligned, the casting material is applied. Alignment may be performed externally or internally through a surgical intervention. The process is relatively pain free. The patient experiences discomfort with the manipulation of the body part during the process. First a cotton or synthetic stockinette is applied to cover the length of

the extremity. Cotton sheeting or wadding is applied next, followed by the casting material. Most health care providers bring the stockinette up and over the distal and proximal edges of the cast. Inspect these edges for rough pieces of casting that may irritate the skin. Superficial burns can occur as the cast begins to set up, especially if the patient is not appropriately padded or too much fiberglass material is used.

The application is similar to that for an elastic bandage. The type of cast used is indicative of the part of the body immobilized. Examples include (1) short arm cast, which extends from below the elbow to the proximal palmar crease; (2) long leg cast, which extends from the upper thigh to the base of the toes; and (3) spica cast or body cast, which covers the trunk and one or both extremities (Fig. 4.25). A cast may be bivalved to relieve pressure. This involves splitting the cast down both sides and securing the pieces so that the extremity is supported (Skill 4.1, Step 8a).

Cast Brace

The cast brace is an alternative appliance to the traditional leg cast. It provides the support and stability of

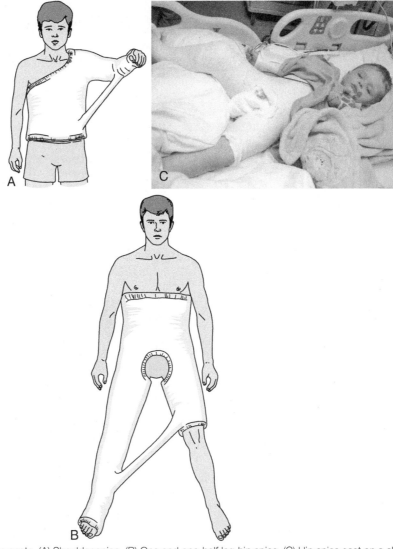

Fig. 4.25 Spica casts. (A) Shoulder spica. (B) One and one-half leg-hip spica. (C) Hip spica cast on a child (A and B, From Thompson JM, Hirsch JE, Tucker SM, et al: *Mosby's clinical nursing,* ed 5, St. Louis, 2002, Mosby.)

Skill 4.1   Care of the Patient in a Cast

NURSING ACTION *(RATIONALE)*

1. Patient teaching. *(Ensures patient cooperation; reduces patient anxiety.)*
   a. Explain why the cast is being applied and how it will be applied. *(Sudden movement during procedure could cause injury.)*
   b. Advise the patient that the plaster cast will feel warm as it dries.
   c. Explain the extent of immobilization.
   d. Explain care of the cast and expectations after discharge.
   e. Instruct patient not to insert sharp objects (coat hangers or pencils) under the cast. *(These may abrade the skin and lead to infection.)*

2. Handling the new cast. *(A fiberglass cast dries immediately after application; a plaster extremity cast dries in approximately 24 to 48 hours; a plaster spica or body cast dries in 48 to 72 hours [see Fig. 4.26].)*
   a. Support wet cast with the flat of the hands or on pillows. *(Avoids indentations that will cause pressure on underlying skin.)*
   b. Place cotton blankets or other absorbent material under the cast. *(Aids drying of cast.)*
   c. Expose the cast to air as much as possible. *(Aids drying of cast.)*
   d. Turn the patient frequently. *(Aids drying of cast.)*
   e. Use a cast dryer or hair dryer on a warm (not hot) setting. *(Circulates air over the cast.)*

Continued

Skill 4.1   Care of the Patient in a Cast—cont'd

f. Do not apply paint, varnish, or shellac to the cast. (*Plaster is a porous material that allows air to circulate to the skin.*)

3. Skin care. (*Decreases the chance of skin irritation or tissue injury.*)
    a. Inspect skin at edges of cast and underlying cast for erythema or skin impairment.
    b. Remove plaster crumbs from skin with a washcloth moistened with warm water.
    c. Use creams and lotions sparingly. (*They may soften the skin and cause the cast to stick to the skin.*)
    d. Apply waterproof material to cast around perineal area. (*Prevents soiling of and damage to cast and prevents skin impairment.*)
    e. Attend to patient's complaint of pain under the cast, particularly over bony prominences. (*This may indicate pressure on the skin.*) If discomfort is not relieved by repositioning, report to health care provider. (*Cast pressure may have to be relieved by windowing or bivalving [cutting into halves].*)

4. Turning: Turning to any position generally is permitted as long as the integrity of the cast is not compromised and the patient is comfortable; do not turn by grasping the abductor bar. (*It is not safe transport.*)

5. Toileting for a long leg or hip spica cast.
    a. Use a fracture pan with blanket roll or padding. (*Provides support under the small of the back.*)
    b. Elevate the head of the bed, if permitted, or place the bed in reverse Trendelenburg's position. (*Eases procedure.*)

6. Abdominal discomfort: Cast may be "windowed" (an opening cut into it). (*Provides relief of abdominal distention or a port for checking bladder distention.*)

7. Mobilization.
    a. The health care provider decides whether and how much weight-bearing is allowed.
    b. A cast shoe or a walking heel is incorporated into a lower extremity cast (see Fig. 4.25). (*Permits weight-bearing without damaging the cast.*)

8. Prevention of neurovascular problems: Establish baseline measurements and assess neurovascular status before cast application; palpate distal pulses; assess color, temperature, and capillary refill of the appropriate fingers or toes; assess neurologic function, including sensation and motion in the affected and unaffected extremity. (*Changes in neurovascular status may occur after casting, possibly further compromising already injured tissues. Note the baseline neurovascular status so that those changes, if they occur, can be assessed readily.*)
    a. Perform neurovascular checks every hour for at least 24 hours after cast application to detect difficulty from edema or pressure of cast on nerves or vessels; notify health care provider of color changes, alterations in sensation, or unrelieved discomfort; cast may need to be bivalved to relieve pressure.

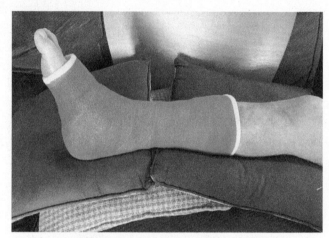

    b. Elevate affected extremity on pillows. (*Danger of edema is usually 24 to 48 hours.*)
    c. After mobilization of patient with lower extremity or upper extremity cast, avoid keeping extremity in dependent position for prolonged periods. (*Prevents edema.*)
    d. After lower extremity cast is removed, encourage patient to wear elastic stocking and elevate affected leg while at rest until full mobility is regained. (*After immobilization, the involved joints and muscles will be weak, and range of motion may be limited. Activity must be resumed slowly. Elastic stockings enhance deep vein circulation.*)

the plaster cast, with additional support and mobility provided by a hinged brace. The appliance is most effective for fractures of the shaft of the femur and permits early ambulation and weight-bearing. It is used approximately 2 to 6 weeks after fracture reduction.

Cast bracing is based on the concept that limited weight-bearing helps promote the formation of bone. A problem encountered frequently with cast bracing is edema around the knee. Instruct patients to elevate the leg when sitting to promote venous return. A cast shoe or walking heel incorporated into a lower extremity cast permits weight-bearing without damaging the cast (Fig. 4.26).

Assessment

Nursing assessment is similar regardless of what kind of casting material is used. Perform a neurovascular assessment, including capillary refill, every 15 to 30

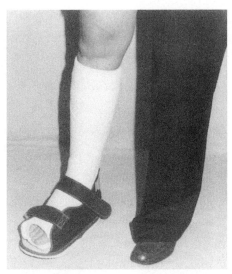

Fig. 4.26 Short leg walking cast with cast shoe. (Courtesy Dr. Henry Bohlman, Cleveland, Ohio.)

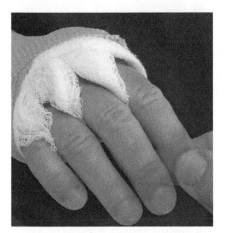

Fig. 4.27 Capillary refill assessment.

minutes for several hours after casting and every 4 hours the first few days (see Box 4.5). Capillary filling time is a way to assess arterial flow to the extremities; squeeze the patient's nailbeds to produce blanching and observe for the return of color. With normal arterial capillary perfusion, the color returns to normal within 2 seconds (Fig. 4.27). Observe the skin at the cast edges for erythema and irritation. Compare the temperature and skin appearance on the casted side and non-casted side for comparison purposes. Assess the ability of the patient to move the fingers or toes on the affected side. Complaints of pain or discomfort should be evaluated closely. Determine the specific location and assess the effectiveness of any analgesics administered.

Nursing Interventions and Patient Teaching

Nursing interventions for the patient in a cast (see Skill 4.1) include patient education on preventing infection, irritation, neurovascular pressure, and misalignment of bone ends. Handle a wet cast gently and support it with the flat of the hand or on pillows to avoid indentations that cause pressure on the skin and lead to skin impairment. Never use the bar in a spica cast as support when turning the patient. Turning the patient frequently aids the drying process. If a cast dryer is used, set it on warm, never hot (drying a plaster of Paris cast too quickly from the outside may weaken the cast). Elevating the casted extremity reduces edema (usually elevation is recommended for 24 to 48 hours). Instruct patients using crutches to support their weight on their hands; weight borne on the axillae can damage the brachial plexus nerves (crutch paralysis).

Cast syndrome (superior mesentery artery syndrome) can occur after the application of a spica (body) cast (see Fig. 4.25) and involves acute obstruction of the duodenum. If nausea occurs, place the patient prone to relieve pressure symptoms and alert the charge nurse. Gastric decompression may be necessary, and if conventional measures fail, surgical intervention (duodenojejunostomy—making an opening into the small intestine) may be necessary.

Patient teaching includes information about cleaning around the cast site with a mild soap and rinsing away excessive soap so that it does not accumulate around the cast and impair the skin. A synthetic (fiberglass) cast can be flushed with water if it becomes soiled. It must be dried afterward to prevent skin impairment and maceration (softening). A synthetic (fiberglass) cast can be dried by blotting it with a towel and then using a blow dryer on the cool or warm setting in a sweeping motion across the cast. Proper drying may take as long as 1 hour.

Patients often complain of pruritus (itching) of the skin that is covered by a cast (especially after having the cast for a few weeks). Recommend diversion activities when the pruritus begins. Also advise the patient to gently rub the area below and above the cast to decrease the desire to scratch. Warn patients not to stick sharp objects underneath the cast to relieve the pruritus. This may impair the skin and result in serious complications.

Cast Removal

Casts are removed with an electric vibrating saw rather than a cutting saw. Reassure patients that there is little risk of the saw injuring the skin beneath the cast, even though it is noisy and looks like a cutting saw. Prepare the patient for the sight of the skin beneath the cast. Patients may be distressed by the appearance of their extremity after the cast is removed. Health care providers removing the cast should opt to wear masks to avoid respiratory irritation from the powder released when the cast is cut. If this powder is inhaled over a period of time, the plaster deposits can build up in the lungs' small air sacs and cause respiratory distress.

After removal of a cast, eliminate the buildup of secretions and dead skin on the affected extremity by gently washing and applying lotion or cream to the area. This may take several days, but caution the patient against trying to remove the devitalized material rapidly to avoid causing skin impairment. Muscle atrophy is common. Reassure the patient that the muscle will increase in strength and size with proper exercise through either physical therapy or home exercise programs.

TRACTION

Traction is the process of putting an extremity, bone, or group of muscles under tension by means of weights and pulleys. Traction may be used to (1) align and stabilize a fracture site by reducing the fractured part, (2) relieve pressure on nerves as in the case of herniated disk syndrome, (3) maintain correct positioning, (4) prevent deformities, and (5) relieve muscle spasms. The two general types of traction are skeletal and skin. Traction may be continuous or intermittent. To stabilize a fracture, continuous traction is applied; it must not be disconnected unless ordered by the health care provider. Cervical and pelvic traction sometimes is ordered as intermittent traction.

Skeletal Traction

Skeletal traction (Fig. 4.28) is applied directly to a bone. It normally is used for longer periods and employs heavier weights than skin traction. A surgeon inserts wires and pins through the bone distal to the fracture site while the patient is under local or general anesthesia. The pin protrudes through the skin on both sides of the extremity, and traction is applied with weights attached to a rope that is tied to a spreader bar. Skeletal traction can be used for fractures of the femur (see Fig. 4.28A), tibia (see Fig. 4.28B), humerus, and cervical spine (see Chapter 14).

Skin Traction

Skin traction traditionally is intended for short-term use and uses lighter weights. The device is applied directly to the skin. Skin traction uses weight that pulls on sponge rubber, moleskin, and elastic bandage with adherent or plastic materials attached to the skin below the site of the fracture, with the pull exerted on the limb. Buck's, Russell's, and Bryant's are types of skin traction.

Buck's traction. Buck's traction (Fig. 4.29) is used as a temporary measure to provide support and comfort to a fractured extremity while waiting for more definitive treatment. Traction (pull) is in a horizontal plane with the affected extremity. This traction frequently is used to maintain the reduction of a hip fracture before surgery. It also can be used to treat muscle spasms and minor fractures of the lower spine.

Russell's traction. Russell's traction (see Fig. 4.29B) is set up similarly to Buck's traction. However, a knee sling supports the affected leg. It allows more movement in bed and permits flexion of the knee joint. Russell's traction is used commonly to treat hip and knee fractures.

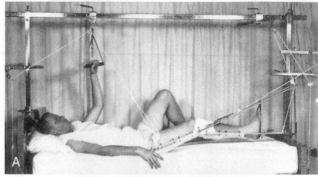

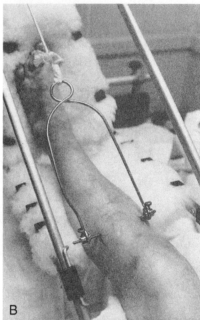

Fig. 4.28 (A) Balanced suspension skeletal traction to the femur. (B) Tibial pin traction with Steinmann pin used in treatment of distal femoral fracture. The bow attached to the pin provides a place of attachment for the rope that holds the traction weights. The pull exerted by the weight keeps the fracture fragments aligned. Pin sites must be inspected at least daily to detect signs of pin reaction or infection. (A, Modified from Mourad L: *Orthopedic disorders*, St. Louis, 1991, Mosby. B, From Monahan FD, Sands JK, Neighbors M, et al: *Phipps' medical-surgical nursing: Health and illness perspectives*, ed 8, St. Louis, 2007, Mosby.)

Nursing Interventions

Nursing interventions for patients in traction include measures to maintain the body in proper alignment and careful assessment of traction equipment. The pulleys must remain off the floor to ensure correct alignment. Care of a patient in skeletal traction involves assessment of the pin sites. Pin site care includes cleansing with a prescribed agent, using a sterile cotton-tipped applicator. Antibiotic ointment may be prescribed for the pin insertion sites. Traction care is summarized in Box 4.6.

Splints, *crutches*, and *braces* are used to immobilize and assist with ambulation. There are numerous types of splints and braces, and nurses must understand the procedure for the proper application for each kind.

Safety is the first concern when ambulatory devices such as crutches are used (see Safety Alert box on

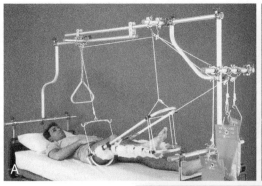
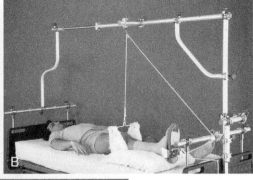
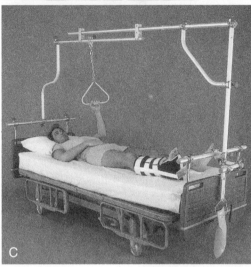

Fig. 4.29 (A) Balanced traction with a Thomas ring and a Pearson attachment. (B) Russell's traction. (C) Buck's traction. (Courtesy Zimmer, Inc., Warsaw, Indiana.)

> ### ⚠ Safety Alert
> #### Crutch Safety
>
> Crutch safety involves:
> - Proper measurement (with weight on hands, not axillae, to avoid nerve and blood vessel damage in the axillary region); leave a 2-inch width between the axillary fold and the arm piece on the crutches
> - Rubber tips on the ends of the crutches to prevent slippage
> - Adequate muscle strength in the upper extremities to support the patient's weight

crutch safety). Encourage the patient to do push-ups by pressing the hands against the mattress and lifting the upper body to gain muscle strength. Types of *crutch walking* depend on the number of points making contact with the floor (Fig. 4.30). For example, a three-point gait involves two crutch points plus one leg making contact with the floor (patient must have strong arms to support body weight). Instead of a three-point gait, patients may use the four-point gait (slower, but stable) or two-point gait (faster; requires balance). Another type of crutch walking is the swing-to or swing-through gait, in which the patient swings the body up to or beyond the two points of the crutch tips. Most crutch walking is taught by a physical therapist (Fig. 4.31). However, the nurse monitors the patient's progress.

Older patients are likely to use *cane walking* for balance and support. Instruct the patient to hold the cane in the opposite hand of the affected extremity and advance the cane at the same time the affected leg moves forward. An effective rubber tip on the point will help prevent slippage. Older adults also use walkers to maintain balance. Safety concerns are the same as those for the cane.

The Roll-A-Bout walker is a gait enhancer designed for patients who have an injury below the knee such as a fractured tibia, fibula, ankle, or foot. The Roll-A-Bout allows the patient to distribute weight evenly by placing the knee of the injured leg on the knee pad and propelling the Roll-A-Bout with the unaffected leg (Fig. 4.32).

TRAUMATIC INJURIES

Traumatic injuries to the musculoskeletal system can occur in all age groups. However, older adults may have disorders that predispose them to musculoskeletal injuries (see the Safety Alert box on preventing musculoskeletal trauma). The more serious injuries involving fractures are treated in a hospital, whereas the less serious—such as contusions, sprains, or strains—may be treated in an outpatient facility.

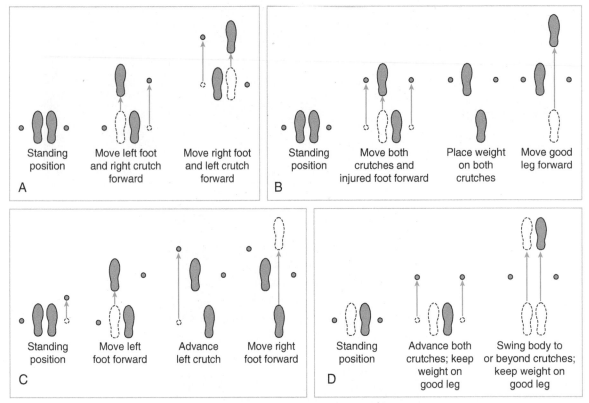

Fig. 4.30 Crutch walking. (A) Two-point gait. (B) Three-point gait. (C) Four-point gait. (D) Swing-through gait.

⚠ Safety Alert

Preventing Musculoskeletal Trauma

- Teach patients and community members to take appropriate safety precautions to prevent injuries while at home, at work, when driving, or when participating in sports.
- Be a vocal advocate for personal actions known to reduce injuries such as regularly using seatbelts, driving within posted speed limits, stretching before exercise, using protective athletic equipment (helmets and knee, wrist, and elbow pads), and not combining drinking and driving.
- Encourage older adults to participate in moderate exercise to aid in the maintenance of muscle strength and balance.
- To reduce falls, examine older adults' living environment to rule out the use of scatter rugs, to ensure adequate footwear and lighting, and to clear paths to bathrooms for nighttime use.
- Stress the importance of adequate calcium and vitamin D intake.

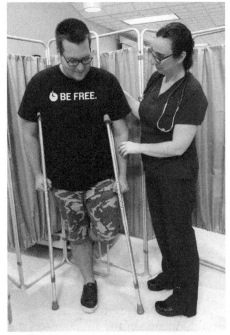

Fig. 4.31 Assisting the patient with crutch walking. Note how the therapist guards the patient and how the patient's elbows are at no more than 30 degrees of flexion.

CONTUSIONS

Etiology and Pathophysiology

Contusions are the most common soft tissue injury. An injury from a blow or blunt force causes local bleeding under the skin and possibly a hematoma (sac filled with blood). The severity of a contusion depends on the part of the body affected. A contusion of the brain is very serious, whereas a contusion of the arm is less serious. Large areas affected by soft tissue bleeding with slow absorption of the blood have a higher potential of developing into cellulitis (an infection of the subcutaneous tissue).

Medical Management

Most contusions are treated by applying ice bags or cold compresses for 15- to 20-minute periods over 12

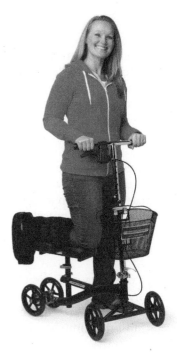

Fig. 4.32 The Roll-A-Bout walker. (Copyright 2013 Goodbye Crutches. Used with permission from Surgical Specialties Medical Devices, LLC.)

to 36 hours for the vasoconstrictive effects of cold. The involved extremity is elevated to reduce edema and suppress pain.

Prognosis
The prognosis is excellent.

SPRAINS

Etiology and Pathophysiology
Sprains can result from a wrenching or hyperextension of a joint, tearing the capsule and ligaments. A sprain can involve bleeding into a joint (hemarthrosis). Common sites include the knee, ankle, and cervical spine (whiplash). Sprains are often the result of a sudden, twisting injury. Medical management is similar to that for contusions. Treatment usually consists of rest, ice, compression, and elevation (RICE) of the affected area.

Prognosis
The prognosis is excellent.

WHIPLASH

Etiology, Pathophysiology, and Clinical Manifestations
Injury at the cervical spine, or whiplash, is classified as a type of cervical disk syndrome. This means that there is compression or irritation of one or more cervical nerves. Whiplash is caused by an injury that involves hyperextension and flexion, which results in compression of the anatomic structures. This type of injury usually occurs as a result of sudden acceleration

and deceleration, such as rear-end car collisions that cause violent back-and-forth movements of the head and neck. Symptoms of a whiplash (primarily pain) may not be obvious for a few days or even a week after the injury. Cervical fractures can accompany a whiplash injury.

Assessment
Collection of subjective data includes the patient's complaint of pain (the most common symptom), which usually begins in the cervical area but may radiate down the arm to the fingers and increase with cervical motion. The pain may increase sharply with coughing, sneezing, or any radical movement. Other signs and symptoms may be paresthesia (numbness or tingling), headache, blurred vision, decreased skeletal function, and weakened hand grip.

Objective data include edema in the cervical spine region with tightening of the muscles. Vital signs are usually within normal ranges. If the assessment findings indicate hypertension with widened pulse pressure and bradycardia, suspect increased intracranial pressure (ICP); report and document the findings immediately. Perform a neurologic assessment every 15 to 30 minutes to rule out increased ICP.

Diagnostic Tests
Physical examination and radiographic studies confirm the health care provider's diagnosis.

Medical Management
Symptoms commonly recur. A medical approach is used most often for the treatment of whiplash. Analgesics and muscle relaxants are prescribed, along with intermittent cervical traction. Surgery may be necessary if cervical fracture with displacement occurs (see "Herniation of Intervertebral Disk [Herniated Nucleus Pulposus]" later in this chapter).

Other treatments include special exercises, heat therapy, and administration of mild analgesics as ordered by the health care provider to control the pain. A soft foam rubber neck brace collar may be used for whiplash injuries to limit head movement.

Nursing Interventions
Nursing interventions include care of the patient with restricted activity to immobilize the cervical vertebrae, decrease irritation, and provide rest for the traumatized area. This is accomplished with cervical traction. If a neck brace is used, carefully inspect the skin around the neck and chin for signs of excoriation.

Prognosis
The prognosis depends on the extent of neurologic involvement. The prognosis is excellent with minor trauma, but because the spinal canal is full of neural tissue in the cervical area, more extensive injury can produce profound disability.

ANKLE SPRAINS

Etiology and Pathophysiology

An ankle sprain often is referred to as a twisted ankle and is caused by a wrenching or twisting of the foot and ankle (see Safety Alert box on strains and sprains). The ankles supporting ligaments are twisted or torn with the injury.

Clinical Manifestations

The ankle area becomes edematous quickly, with spasms of the muscles and pain on passive movement of the joint.

Assessment

Collection of subjective data includes assessment of pain and tenderness in the affected ankle that intensifies with movement of the foot or ankle.

Collection of objective data includes assessment of the traumatized ankle for signs of edema, limited movement and function of the joint, and ecchymosis of the soft tissue around the ankle.

Diagnostic Tests

A radiographic examination of the injured area is the only accurate way to ensure there is no bone injury.

Medical Management

Surgery may be indicated for severe sprains. The health care provider sutures torn ligament fibers together. If the ligaments have been torn from the bone, the surgeon reattaches them by drilling small holes in the medial malleolus (rounded bony protrusion on the medial area of the ankle).

Nursing Interventions

The injured area must be elevated and kept at rest. Application of ice for 15 to 20 minutes intermittently for 12 to 36 hours—followed after 24 hours by the application of mild heat for 15 to 30 minutes, four times daily—will promote absorption of blood and fluid from the area. Use compressive dressings and splinting to help support the injured area. A neurovascular assessment is necessary to detect impaired tissue perfusion.

 Safety Alert

Strains and Sprains

A strain and a sprain are not the same. Strains are produced by minute muscle tears and overstretching of tendons, whereas sprains are caused by a twisting of the joint.

Prognosis

With proper treatment, sprains and strains can be effectively treated. The prognosis is generally excellent.

STRAINS

Etiology and Pathophysiology

Strains are characterized by microscopic muscle tears as a result of overstretching muscles and tendons. An acute strain results when the muscles and tendons are overstretched in a forceful movement, such as unaccustomed vigorous exercise.

Assessment

Collection of subjective data includes noting the patient's complaint of sudden and severe pain away from the joint, which increases with activity. Chronic muscle strain can occur from repeated muscle overuse, and the pain may not appear for several hours. The patient typically complains of soreness, stiffness, and tenderness in the area.

Collection of objective data includes observation of stiffness, ecchymosis, and slight edema over the injury site. The most common sites are calf muscles, hamstrings, quadriceps, and the lumbosacral area. Edema can occur rapidly in the muscle and tendon area.

Diagnostic Tests

A radiographic study is necessary to rule out bone trauma.

Medical Management

Surgical repair is necessary if the muscle is ruptured completely. The health care provider orders analgesics and muscle relaxants. An exercise program almost always is prescribed if the strain is in the lumbosacral region. The exercises are aimed at strengthening the lower abdominal muscles.

Nursing Interventions

Nursing interventions for a strain are similar to those for a sprain. Ice application helps relieve pain, but some health care providers prefer heat application rather than ice. Back strains are among the most common strains. If the symptoms worsen, advise the patient to avoid strenuous activities, use a firm chair with rigid back support, avoid wearing high heels, use a firm mattress for sleep, and never sleep on the abdomen. Encourage the patient to do leg exercises to prevent development of thrombosis.

Prognosis

The prognosis is usually favorable.

DISLOCATIONS

Etiology and Pathophysiology

Dislocations usually involve tearing of the joint capsule; subluxations (partial or incomplete dislocations) involve stretching of the joint capsule. Both are temporary displacements of bones from their normal position within joints. A dislocation may be (1) congenital (e.g., congenital hip displacement), (2) caused by a disease process, or (3) caused by trauma. A dislocation or subluxation also may be accompanied by stretching and tearing of ligaments and tendons and by fractures. The displaced bone may rupture blood vessels. When subluxation occurs, the joint's articulating (movable) surfaces are partially separated.

Clinical Manifestations

Dislocation may or may not be visible. Sometimes a dislocation changes the length of an affected extremity. Pain and loss of function may be similar to those occurring with a fracture. However, dislocation partially immobilizes a joint, whereas a fracture site typically has abnormal free movement. Common dislocation sites include the shoulder, hip, and knee.

Assessment

Subjective data include the patient's description of the injury and pain. For shoulder dislocation, the patient complains of sensation loss and paresthesia.

Collection of objective data includes the assessment of any erythema, discoloration, edema, pain, tenderness, limitation of movement, and deformity or shortening of the extremity. Compare both sides for validation. Neurovascular assessment is important to determine whether vascular or nerve injury is present in the affected area. For shoulder dislocation, assess for an absent radial pulse, hypothermia of the hand, and wrist drop.

Diagnostic Tests

The diagnosis is based on complaints of discomfort, physical examination, and diagnostic radiographic examination of the injured site.

Medical Management

The health care provider may perform a closed reduction, which corrects the deformity through manipulation of the extremity. Surgical intervention to restore joint articulation sometimes is required.

Nursing Interventions and Patient Teaching

Nursing interventions include (1) reduction of edema and discomfort, (2) immobilization of the injured part to promote healing, and (3) patient education. Ice application is recommended for the first 24 hours after trauma. After 24 hours, heat may be used if there are no indications of bleeding. Elevation of the injured extremity on pillows and the application of elastic bandages help relieve edema. Immobilization of joints may involve application of a splint, sling, or elastic bandage. The air cast or air splint brace is an immobilization device. It is inflatable, lightweight, and conforms to the extremity's size and shape. When immobilization devices are used, perform a neurovascular assessment frequently (see Box 4.5 and the patient problem statements below). Administer analgesics as prescribed by the health care provider. Asking the patient to rate the pain on a scale from 0 to 10 is helpful in determining pain severity. For control of extreme pain, the health care provider may order an opioid, such as morphine. For mild to moderate pain, ibuprofen or acetaminophen (Tylenol) may be prescribed. Positioning and repositioning the injured part can help reduce discomfort.

Patient problem statements and interventions for the patient with impaired neurovascular integrity include but are not limited to the following:

PATIENT PROBLEM	NURSING INTERVENTIONS
Compromised Peripheral Tissue Perfusion, related to: • Injury • Treatment	Position extremities in alignment; elevate affected extremity Carefully monitor distal pulses, capillary refill, and temperature of involved area
Potential for Harm or Damage to the Body, related to neurovascular impairment	Compare affected extremity with unaffected extremity, using same hand for palpation Test capillary refill (blanching test) Check each digit for sensation and motion Document location and characteristics of pain Palpate pedal, tibial, or radial pulses, and compare with unaffected extremity Assess for edema with pallor, cyanosis, and coldness Ask patient to describe sensations Document all findings

Promoting an accident-free environment is essential. Areas of preventive medicine to explore with patients include the following:

- Grab bars mounted in the bathroom near the toilet or tub and rubber mats or slip guards in the tub and shower help prevent falls.
- Removing throw rugs and obstacles from the floor can prevent falls.
- A gait enhancer, such as a cane, crutches, or a walker, must be used correctly and with attention to safety precautions, such as using rubber tips on the points that make contact with the floor to prevent slippage.
- Patients in the hospital are at risk of falling out of bed if their disease, condition, or medication results in disorientation. Carefully assess their level of orientation, keep side rails up, and provide safety reminder devices to prevent self-injury.
- Using a safe ladder when climbing can help prevent a fall.
- Wearing protective clothing while engaging in dangerous work or contact sports is recommended.

Appropriate health teaching should be targeted for people at risk for musculoskeletal diseases, such as osteoporosis, which can predispose them to pathologic or nontraumatic fractures.

Prognosis

The prognosis is generally excellent.

AIRBAG INJURIES

Airbag deployment injuries include chemical burns, ocular trauma, cervical injury, soft tissue injury, and upper extremity and chest trauma. Orthopedic injuries tend to involve the upper extremities, especially the wrist, hand, and elbow. Injuries from airbag deployment can be life threatening in the very young. People at increased risk include older adults and small children. Airbag-induced injuries are associated with a rapid, forceful inflation, lasting less than 1 second from inflation to deflation. Management for these injuries will be based on the type and degree of injury. Treatments may include wound assessment and cleaning, application of ice to inflamed areas, and analgesic therapies.

MUSCULOSKELETAL DISORDER AND SURGICAL INTERVENTIONS

CARPAL TUNNEL SYNDROME
Etiology and Pathophysiology

Carpal tunnel syndrome is a painful disorder of the wrist and hand. It is caused by inflammation and edema of the synovial lining of the tendon sheaths in the carpal tunnel of the wrist. As a result, the tunnel space is narrowed, resulting in compression of the median nerve between the inelastic carpal ligament and other structures in the carpal tunnel (Fig. 4.33). The symptoms of *paresthesia* (any subjective sensation such as pricks of pins and needles) and *hypoesthesia* (a decrease in sensation in response to stimulation of the sensory nerves) of the thumb, index, and middle fingers may develop spontaneously or occur as a result of disease or injury.

This condition has a higher incidence in obese, middle-aged women and individuals employed in occupations involving repetitious motions of the fingers and hands (e.g., computing, hairdressing, manufacturing, basket weaving, meat carving, and typing). Carpal tunnel syndrome has become one of the three most common industrial or work-related conditions and is related to increased computer usage. Research also supports genetic links for the development of the condition. Edema of the tendon sheaths caused by RA can predispose a patient to carpal tunnel syndrome. Diabetes predisposes an individual to carpal tunnel syndrome due to the related risk of nerve damage. Pregnant women also develop the syndrome during their last trimester of pregnancy. Fluid retention and edema experienced during pregnancy are thought to be the likely cause by compressing the nerves. Medical conditions such as thyroid disorders, renal failure and lymphedema are linked to an increased occurrence of carpel tunnel syndrome.

Clinical Manifestations

The clinical manifestations include gradual to increased numbness and tingling in the thumb, index, and middle fingers. This sensation may travel from the wrist up the arm as the condition worsens. These symptoms initially may appear then disappear but then become increasingly persistent as the nerve becomes consistently compressed or becomes damaged. The affected hand has altered ability to grasp or hold small objects. Atrophy of the thenar eminence (the padded area of the palm below the base of the thumb) is noted as the disease progresses.

Assessment

Subjective data include the patient's description of discomfort, such as burning pain or tingling in the hands, relieved by vigorously shaking or exercising the hands. Pain may be intermittent or constant and is often more intense at night. The patient also may complain of numbness (hypoesthesia) of the thumb, index, and ring fingers, especially after prolonged flexion of the wrist; and inability to grasp or hold small objects.

Collection of objective data includes assessment of the hand, wrist, or fingers for edema; muscle atrophy; or a depressed appearance of the soft tissue at the base of the thumb on the palmar surface.

Diagnostic Tests

Physical examination reveals deficits in sensory mapping along median nerve innervation pathways; positive Tinel's sign; increased tingling with a gentle tap over the tendon sheath on the ventral surface of the central wrist; edema of the fingers; and thenar surfaces of the palm thinner than normal (wasting). Having the patient hold the wrists against each other in forced palmar flexion for 1 minute can elicit sensory changes of numbness and tingling, which is a positive Phalen's maneuver test (one indication of carpal tunnel syndrome).

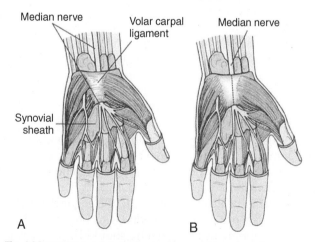

Median nerve   Volar carpal ligament   Median nerve

Synovial sheath

A   B

Fig. 4.33 (A) Wrist structures involved in carpal tunnel syndrome. (B) Decompression of median nerve. (From Thompson JM, Hirsch JE, Tucker SM, et al: *Mosby's clinical nursing*, ed 5, St. Louis, 2002, Mosby.)

An electromyogram shows a weakened muscle response to stimulation. MRI shows compression and flattening of the median nerve, increased signal intensity within the median nerve, and abrupt changes in diameter of the median nerve. A nerve conduction study will subject the median nerve to small shocks. Then the carpel tunnel is evaluated to assess the speed of nerve impulses.

Medical Management
If the symptoms are mild and surgery is not a desirable option, an immobilizer such as a splint can be used (Fig 4.34). Physical therapy and yoga have demonstrated improved strength and reduced discomfort. Hydrocortisone acetate suspension injected into the carpal tunnel can relieve mild symptoms. Surgery is indicated for severe symptoms with muscle atrophy. The standard surgical treatment is decompression of the median nerve by sectioning of the transverse carpal ligament. This can be accomplished by either an endoscopic technique or open surgery (Mayo Clinic, 2021).

Nursing Interventions and Patient Teaching
Education concerning the need for frequent position changes and stretching of the hands and fingers is helpful in preventing discomfort. There are specialized tools for the office and desk to prevent median nerve compression.

If surgery is not required, the nurse is involved in the application of an immobilizer to promote comfort. General nursing interventions are use of a wrist splint to relieve pressure and to lessen wrist flexion, elevation to relieve edema, ROM exercises to lessen sense of clumsiness, and restriction of twisting and turning activities of the wrist.

If surgery is required, postoperative interventions include (1) elevating the hand and arm for 24 hours; (2) implementing and evaluating active thumb and finger motion within limits imposed by the dressing; (3) administering prescribed analgesics as needed; (4) monitoring vital signs (temperature elevation could indicate infection); and (5) checking fingers for circulation, sensation, and movement every 1 to 2 hours for 24 hours.

Encourage patients to use the affected hand in normal activities as soon as 2 to 3 days after surgery.

Prognosis
Mild symptoms of carpal tunnel syndrome are relieved by nonsurgical treatment; severe symptoms require surgical intervention with excellent prognosis. If the patient is pregnant, symptoms usually are relieved after delivery.

HERNIATION OF INTERVERTEBRAL DISK (HERNIATED NUCLEUS PULPOSUS)
Etiology and Pathophysiology
Herniated nucleus pulposus is a rupture of the fibrocartilage surrounding an intervertebral disk, releasing the nucleus pulposus that cushions the vertebrae above and below. This displacement puts pressure on nerve roots. Lumbar and cervical herniations are most common (Fig. 4.35). Herniated nucleus pulposus can occur suddenly (from lifting, twisting, or trauma) or gradually (from degenerative changes, as seen with DJD, osteoporosis, aging, and chronic diseases affecting bones). Herniations of the lumbar spine usually affect people 20 to 45 years old; cervical herniations are seen most in people 45 years and older. Men are more prone to this disorder than are women.

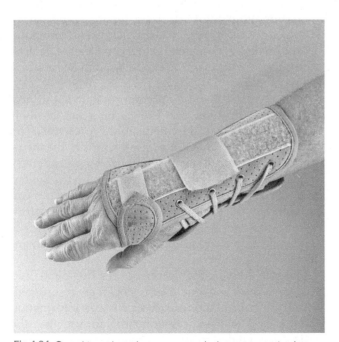

Fig 4.34 Carpal tunnel syndrome non-surgical management using a supportive splint.

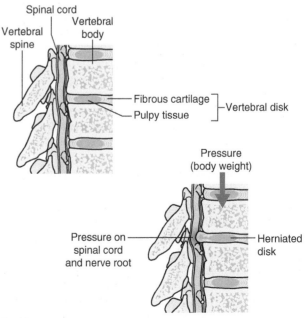

Fig. 4.35 Sagittal section of vertebrae showing normal (left) and herniated disks (right).

Clinical Manifestations

Low back pain that occurs with the slightest movement is the most common symptom of lumbar herniation. The pain radiates over the buttock and down the leg, following the sciatic nerve pathway *(radicular pain)*, causing numbness and tingling in the affected leg. Complaints of pain in the back radiating down the leg (sciatica) are common. Complaints about activity intolerance and alteration in bowel and bladder elimination (constipation and urinary retention) are significant.

A patient with cervical herniation may experience neck pain, headache, and neck rigidity. Pain, numbness, and tingling are not uncommon to radiate down one or both arms. Loss of strength in the arm or arms may occur as well.

Assessment

Collection of subjective data includes assessing pain and asking patient about measures used for relief and other possible symptoms, such as activity intolerance and altered bowel and bladder function. Pain often gets worse with activity.

Collection of objective data includes observing for signs of limited spinal flexibility (limited forward bending) and gait alteration (patient may support weight on one extremity). An ineffective breathing pattern may result from pain and decreased mobility. Assessment includes determination of bowel and bladder elimination and maintenance of traction equipment.

Diagnostic Tests

Obtain a complete history and physical examination. The health care provider orders radiographic studies, MRI, CT, myelography, and electromyelography to determine nerve involvement.

Medical Management

The patient may follow a conservative approach initially, which includes physical therapy; local heat or ice; ultrasound and massage; and transcutaneous electrical nerve stimulation (TENS). The patient typically is treated with NSAIDs and muscle relaxants. Epidural corticosteroid injections by a pain specialist are used commonly if other conservative approaches are not successful. If the patient demonstrates neurologic deterioration or continued pain, a surgical procedure may be required, such as one of the following:

- *Artificial disk replacement:* Replacement of a damaged intervertebral disk with an artificial disk. The artificial disk material is made of various materials, such as medical-grade metal or plastic. The goal of artificial disk replacement is the return of more natural movement of the spine.
- *Chemonucleolysis:* Can be done on patients who have no nerve involvement. The procedure involves administering a local anesthetic agent and then guiding a needle into the nucleus pulposus to inject chymopapain (a drug that dissolves the nucleus pulposus).

- *Diskectomy:* Removal of the extruded disk material, often with a microscope. Percutaneous lateral diskectomy—cutting a window around the anulus fibrosus—is performed with the patient under local anesthesia.
- *Endoscopic spinal microsurgery:* Can be performed with the patient under local anesthesia. Special scopes enable the surgeon to remove herniated disks successfully with minimal damage to surrounding tissues.
- *Laminectomy:* Surgical removal of the bony arches or one or more vertebrae performed to relieve compression of the spinal cord caused by bone displacement from an injury or degeneration of a disk, or to remove a displaced vertebral disk.
- *Spinal fusion* (arthrodesis; the surgical immobilization of a joint; artificial ankylosis): Removal of the lamina and several herniated nuclei pulposi. A portion of bone taken from the patient's iliac crest or from a bone bank is used as a bone graft in the vertebral spaces.

Postoperative laminectomy care includes assessing the incision site for signs of infection such as drainage, edema, odor, and temperature elevation. Use of surgical asepsis when changing dressings and handling drainage decreases the chance of infection. After chemonucleolysis, carefully assess for signs of allergic reactions to chymopapain, such as urticaria and respiratory difficulties.

Nursing Interventions and Patient Teaching

Nursing interventions are aimed at providing nursing care appropriate for the following patient problems:
- Anxiousness, related to discomfort, fear of the unknown, and lifestyle changes
- Recent Onset of Pain (back), related to muscle spasms and painful diagnostic tests
- Prolonged Infrequent or Difficult Bowel Elimination and Retaining Urine or Inability to Urinate, related to pain, analgesics, immobility, and neurologic involvement

Give the patient and family information about procedures and hospital protocol to help reduce their anxiety. Administer the medications prescribed on schedule, and document the effectiveness of the medication. Distraction, heat or ice application (if ordered), and moving (by logrolling) and positioning the patient every 2 hours (if not contraindicated because of need to maintain traction) can promote patient comfort. Dietary monitoring is important to ensure that the patient maintains a high-protein, iron- and vitamin-enriched diet.

Observe dressing for bleeding or cerebrospinal fluid leakage. Apply antiembolism stockings if ordered. Careful documentation of I&O provides information about bowel and bladder function. Ensure that the patient has voided in the first 8 hours, and use nursing measures to promote voiding before resorting to catheterization. Encourage the patient to sit in a straight, firm chair for no longer than 30 minutes at one time. Monitor the patient for evidence of respiratory distress and paralytic ileus, complications that may occur in laminectomy patients.

Patient problem statements and interventions for the patient with a herniated disk include but are not limited to the following:

PATIENT PROBLEM	NURSING INTERVENTIONS
Insufficient Knowledge, related to home care management	Stress importance of rehabilitation plan of activity, rest, and exercise Provide diet instructions related to type and amount of food and weight maintenance (no gain) if applicable Discuss medications: name, purpose, schedule, dosage, and side effects Discuss signs and symptoms to report to health care provider: severe pain; changes in temperature, color, or sensation in extremity; and malodorous drainage from wound Encourage follow-up visits with health care provider
Helplessness, related to: • Decreased mobility • Pain	Use active listening and permit verbalization of anger and weakness Assist patient in identifying coping mechanisms that will reduce feeling of powerlessness; use those that have been successful in the past Offer positive recognition for increased activity level Assist patient in identifying areas that can be controlled Involve patient in decision-making process for own care

The patient may begin activity out of bed as early as 1 day after a simple laminectomy or 2 to 4 days after a laminectomy and fusion. Transfer the patient out of bed with as little time spent in the sitting position as possible. The patient may be permitted to walk as much as tolerated, with assistance if necessary. Braces or corsets, if prescribed, are applied before the patient gets out of bed. Encourage the patient to participate in ADLs within prescribed limits of mobility.

Instruct the patient not to lift or carry anything heavier than 5 to 10 lb (about 2.25 kg) for at least 8 weeks, not to drive a car until permitted by the surgeon, and to avoid twisting motions of the trunk. Reinforce the importance of follow-up visits to the health care provider.

Prognosis
With conservative treatment, some patients receive relief of symptoms; if a neurologic pathologic condition develops, surgical intervention is needed. The prognosis is usually favorable.

TUMORS OF THE BONE
Etiology and Pathophysiology
Tumors of the bone may be primary or secondary and may be benign or malignant. As with other types of tumors, the cause of bone tumors is not always known. Carcinoma of the prostate, lung, breast, thyroid, and kidney may metastasize to the bones. Osteogenic tumors are primary malignant bone tumors that occur most often in young people.

Osteogenic sarcoma is a fast-growing and aggressive tumor that affects the long bones of the body, particularly the distal femur, the proximal tibia, and the proximal humerus. Osteogenic sarcoma can metastasize to the lungs and to the rest of the body via the bloodstream. It affects males between the ages of 10 and 25 more often than females.

Osteochondroma is the most common benign osteogenic tumor. The incidence is highest in males between 10 and 30 years of age. Osteochondromas can occur as a single tumor or as multiple tumors. They usually affect the humerus, tibia, and femur.

Clinical Manifestations
When healthy bone cells are replaced by cancer cells, the bone's strength is altered and spontaneous fractures can occur. Anemia occurs when cancer invades the long bones and interrupts the manufacture of red blood cells in the bone marrow. Cancerous bone tumors metastasize and invade other bones and lung tissue.

Benign bone tumors can grow large enough to put pressure on blood vessels and nerves. Benign tumors do not spread. However, they may undergo cancerous changes and become malignant.

Assessment
Malignant and benign bone tumors cause pain in the affected bone site. Subjective data include complaints of pain, especially with weight-bearing. Pain may result from a spontaneous fracture. The patient also may complain of tenderness at the affected site.

Collection of objective data includes assessment of the painful part, which may reveal edema and discoloration of the skin.

Diagnostic Tests
Diagnosis is confirmed with radiographic studies, bone scan, bone biopsy, and laboratory studies, such as a CBC (which reveals bone marrow involvement), serum protein levels (elevated in multiple myeloma), and serum alkaline phosphatase level (elevated in osteogenic sarcoma).

Medical Management

The health care provider evaluates the tumor type, size, and location and plans the treatment accordingly. Larger, symptomatic benign tumors and malignant tumors require surgical intervention. The surgical procedure depends on the tumor size, location, and extent of tissue involvement. The surgery may involve (1) wide excision or resection, (2) bone curettage, or (3) leg or arm amputation.

Treatment is aimed at destroying or removing the malignant lesion. Amputation of the affected extremity may be necessary. Radiation and chemotherapy may be used before surgery to decrease tumor size or tissue involvement. Limb-salvage surgical procedures in combination with radiation and chemotherapy are being used more frequently for treatment of malignant bone tumors.

Chemotherapy is aimed at destroying cancer cells at primary and metastatic sites. Patients usually receive chemotherapy in 3- or 4-week cycles. Radiation therapy may be given internally and externally. The nurse must know the safety precautions and side effects of chemotherapy and radiation therapy. (See Chapter 17 for a discussion of care of the patient with cancer.)

Nursing Interventions and Patient Teaching

Preoperatively the patient and family need complete and concise information about procedures and postoperative expectations. Postoperative nursing interventions include (1) performing a neurovascular assessment (see Box 4.5); (2) monitoring vital signs; (3) administering analgesics and evaluating the effectiveness; (4) providing cast care or dressing changes with careful documentation of drainage, odors, and signs of circulation impairment; (5) cooperating with physical and occupational therapists to promote mobility and ADLs; and (6) educating the patient and family about home health care and early detection of tumor recurrence.

A patient problem statement and interventions for the patient with a bone tumor include but are not limited to the following:

PATIENT PROBLEM	NURSING INTERVENTIONS
Anxiousness, related to: • Fear of cancer • Body image • Lifestyle change • Possibility of death	Establish therapeutic relationship: acknowledge fear, encourage patient to acknowledge and express feelings Give accurate information about condition and therapies Refer patient to other resources when necessary (e.g., social worker, religious counselor)

Prognosis

The prognosis for bone tumors has improved in recent years with the combination of local surgery, chemotherapy, and radiation. The combined survival rate for patients diagnosed with localized, regional, and distant osteosarcoma is 60% at 5 years with a 74% survival rate for localized and 27% for distant (American Cancer Society [ACS], 2021).

AMPUTATION

The amputation of a portion of or an entire extremity may be necessary because of malignant tumors, injuries, impaired circulation (caused by diabetes mellitus or arteriosclerosis), congenital deformities, and infections. Most amputations are elective surgery unless they are related to trauma. Advances in microsurgical techniques enable surgeons to reattach severed extremities. Therefore, traumatic amputations sometimes can be reversed by replantation if the severed limb is located, kept cooled, and presented to the emergency medical team.

Amputation of long bones can result in postoperative anemia. A traumatic or surgical amputation of an extremity can cause serious blood loss. Malignant bone tumors can metastasize via the bloodstream to other body systems.

Preoperative Assessment

Collection of subjective data includes questioning the patient about his or her understanding of the injury or disease process. Assess and document complaints of pain and symptoms of neurovascular impairment. Assess the patient's level of orientation, because many amputations occur in the older adult population as a result of impaired circulation.

Collection of objective data includes assessment of vital signs (temperature elevation, tachycardia, and tachypnea indicate infection). Assess arterial blood flow by palpation of bilateral pedal pulses and Doppler pressure measurements. Assess wound drainage for color, amount, and presence of odor. Evaluate upper body muscle strength and nutritional status.

Diagnostic Tests

A CBC is done to determine blood dyscrasias (i.e., an imbalance in the blood's cellular profile), such as anemia and bleeding tendencies, which could increase postoperative complications (such as hemorrhage, delayed wound healing, and disorientation). The health care provider orders laboratory studies such as BUN, potassium levels, and routine urinalysis. An ECG is performed to detect cardiac dysrhythmias, which are often present in older adult patients.

Medical Management

When the amputation results from traumatic injury to an extremity, the health care provider's interventions include measures to restore circulating blood volume, control pain, prevent infection in the wound, perform plastic surgical repair at the amputation site to facilitate the use of a prosthesis, and maintain adequate urinary output.

For elective amputations, the health care provider assesses the patient's physiologic, psychological, and emotional status. If infection is present in the body (gangrene may occur if circulation is impaired), treatment includes administration of antibiotics, and every attempt is made to control the infection before surgery. The health care provider discusses the possibility of the patient using a prosthesis. Much of the preoperative preparation focuses on the patient attaining a physical and emotional status conducive to wearing a prosthesis or achieving mobility through the use of a wheelchair or a gait enhancer such as crutches or a walker.

Postoperative Assessment, Nursing Interventions, and Patient Teaching

Collection of subjective data includes careful assessment of pain. *Phantom pain* (pain felt in the area of the missing extremity as if it were still present) may occur and be frightening to the patient. Phantom pain occurs because the nerve tracts that register pain in the amputated area continue to send a message to the brain; this is normal.

Collection of objective data includes observing for signs of hemorrhage, such as hypotension, tachycardia, tachypnea, pallor, decreased urinary output, restlessness, and progressive loss of consciousness. Monitor and document suction drainage, and assess and protect the remaining extremity. Observe for neurovascular impairment (done hourly in the immediate postoperative period) from tightly applied elastic wraps, dressings, or casts (see Box 4.5).

Nursing intervention is aimed at effective pain management and prevention of deformities (contractures, especially in the joint above the amputation, and abduction deformities are common). Flexion hip

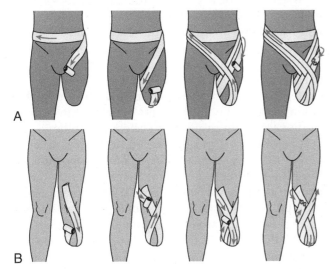

A

B

Fig. 4.36 Correct method of bandaging amputation stump. (A) Anchor bandage around patient's waist. (B) Method of bandaging midcalf stump, where bandage need not be anchored around waist.

contractures can be prevented postoperatively by raising the foot of the bed slightly to elevate the residual extremity (with care taken not to flex the patient's hips by elevating the stump on a pillow), encouraging movement from side to side, and placing the patient in a prone position at least twice a day. This will stretch the flexor muscles. Teach the patient how to strengthen the remaining muscles to facilitate mobility and prevent muscle atrophy (push-ups from a prone position and sit-ups from a seated position). Apply elastic wraps to shrink and reshape the residual extremity into a cone and facilitate the proper fit and use of a prosthesis (Fig. 4.36). A prosthesis may be fitted as early as 2 or 3 weeks postoperatively. Because many amputations are performed in people between 60 and 70 years of age, observe the patient carefully for pulmonary complications (such as pulmonary embolus) and cardiovascular collapse. Keep suction equipment and oxygen at the bedside.

Patient education concerning phantom limb sensation, and the fact that it is a normal physiologic response, can help relieve patient fears. The patient may feel pain or other sensations, such as burning, tingling, throbbing, or pruritus in the area of the amputated extremity. These sensations can last for months or decades on a consistent or intermittent basis. Recommend that patients gently rub the residual extremity or take analgesics for relief.

For persistent, severe phantom pain, the following measures may be employed:
- Stump revision with reamputation at a higher level
- Local infiltration of the stump with procaine
- Mechanical percussion by striking the sensitive digital stump against a solid object—believed to shrink neuromas (small tumors that form in the scar tissue of the stump)
- Sympathetic nerve block

Encourage the patient to share his or her feelings over the loss of the extremity. Discuss the importance of allowing the grieving process to occur.

Patient problem statements and interventions for the patient undergoing an amputation include but are not limited to the following:

PATIENT PROBLEM	NURSING INTERVENTIONS
Distorted Body Image, related to loss of limb	Assess effects of amputation on body image
	Encourage patient to express feelings of mutilation, grief, anger, and loss to aid adaptation processes
	Encourage patient to help with dressing changes and wrapping of stump as able
	Teach family member wrapping techniques if necessary to increase competence and independence

PATIENT PROBLEM	NURSING INTERVENTIONS
	Use prescribed pain management techniques
	Encourage family members to walk with patient to maintain strength and social contacts
	Encourage grooming and wearing of personal clothing to maintain individuality and personality
	Encourage activities for self-care and ambulation to maintain positive outlook and maximum strength
	Encourage or arrange for social services consultation for economic and employment aid
	Arrange for follow-up care referral to aid rehabilitation
Compromised Physical Mobility, related to loss of limb	Assess ability to use remaining limbs
	Turn and position on side, back, and abdomen (after 24 h) to maintain muscle and joint range of motion
	Teach adduction and extension exercises and help patient perform them q 4 h to prevent abduction and flexion contractures
	Assist with sitting in chair and ambulation with aid as able, to maintain muscle strength
	Prepare patient for physical therapy, transportation for exercises, and stump wrapping, if appropriate
	Encourage family members to walk with patient during initial ambulation periods, accompanied by health professionals, to increase independence
	Teach purposes of prone and extension positions to prevent contractures
	Assist prosthetist with prosthesis measurements and fitting as needed to aid rehabilitation

Before discharge, teach the patient and family proper positions, exercises, and ambulation techniques. Also demonstrate stump-wrapping techniques to the patient and family (see Fig. 4.36). Explain to them that prolonged phantom pain experiences are unusual and should receive medical attention. Discuss skin care with the patient and family so that they can take steps to prevent stump irritation or impairment. Also discuss the signs of a wound infection, and instruct them when it is necessary to call the health care provider.

Prognosis

The prognosis for successful adaptation to an amputation depends on the patient's age, the condition that resulted in amputation, other systemic disorders, emotional health, and support system.

❖ NURSING PROCESS FOR THE PATIENT WITH A MUSCULOSKELETAL DISORDER

The role of the licensed practical nurse/licensed vocational nurse (LPN/LVN) in the nursing process as stated is that the LPN/LVN will:

- Participate in planning care for patients based on patient needs
- Review patient's care plan and recommend revisions as needed
- Review and follow defined prioritization for patient care
- Use clinical pathways, care maps, or care plans to guide and review patient care

◆ ASSESSMENT

The musculoskeletal system provides protection, support, and movement for the body. Proper function of the musculoskeletal system is associated closely with proper function of the nervous and circulatory systems. Orthopedics is the branch of medicine that deals with the prevention or correction of disorders involving locomotor structures of the body. Permanent disability and crippling result if patients with musculoskeletal dysfunction do not receive prompt treatment.

Assess orthopedic function for all patients, especially those who are (1) having difficulty with gait; (2) experiencing muscle weakness; (3) suffering from trauma of soft tissue and bone; (4) unable to move and participate in activities for personal, economic, and social fulfillment; (5) experiencing diseases of the musculoskeletal system; or (6) chronically ill.

Assessment of a patient's mobility includes bone integrity, posture, joint function, muscle strength, gait, pain, and neurovascular disturbances related to pressure. Compare body symmetry. For example, assess both legs for same length and diameter and for comparable muscle strength. Observe the patient's gait for unsteadiness or irregular movements. Difficult ambulation associated with shortness of breath can indicate cardiovascular or respiratory system difficulties.

Assessment of posture and gait simply involves observing the patient walking. Common posture deformities include lateral (or S) curvature of the spine, known as scoliosis; a rounding of the thoracic spine (hump-backed appearance), known as kyphosis; and an increase in the curve at the lumbar space region that throws the shoulders back, resulting in a sway-backed gait, referred to as lordosis (Fig. 4.37). Rigidity of the spine can result from ankylosis, in which the vertebrae are fused with loss of mobility, producing a rigid gait or "poker spine" appearance.

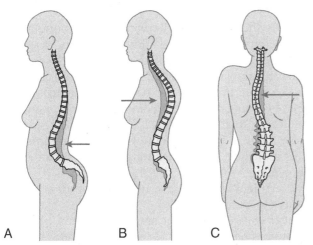

Fig. 4.37 Abnormal spinal curvatures. A, Lordosis. B, Kyphosis. C, Scoliosis.

Assessment of neurologic and circulatory function is important if the patient has experienced a traumatic injury; damaged blood vessels and nerves can cause permanent disabilities.

Assess the skin for signs of coolness, pallor, sensation, or cyanosis to help determine the patient's circulatory status. A faint or absent pulse in an extremity indicates impaired circulation. Palpating the femoral, popliteal, and dorsalis pedis pulses on both extremities provides pertinent data about the lower extremities. If the pulse is not palpated readily with a light touch of the finger, a Doppler instrument can be used to magnify the sound of the pulsation. The absence of a pulse is serious and must be reported to the charge nurse immediately. Assess the brachial and radial pulses to determine circulation in the upper extremities. Palpating a pulse may be difficult if the patient has a cast or bandage. Reach under the cast or bandage if possible. Assess the pulse in the unaffected extremity for comparison.

The blanching test (meaning to whiten or pale) is a test of the rate of capillary refill, which signals circulation status. This is also referred to as a *capillary nail refill test*. Compress each fingernail or toenail of the affected extremity (noting the white color as pressure is applied), release the pressure, and note how quickly the pink color returns to the nailbed. The nailbed color should return to normal within 2 or 3 seconds. If the color is slow to return, circulation is impaired and requires prompt attention (see Box 4.5).

Neurovascular assessments are made on patients with musculoskeletal trauma or damage to nerves and blood vessels resulting from surgery, tight bandages, splints, or casts. Impaired circulation resulting in alteration of nerve function can cause loss of the use of an extremity; this impairment generally is seen in the extremities. See Box 4.5 for information concerning neurovascular (circulation) assessment.

◆ **PATIENT PROBLEMS**

Nursing assessment establishes the patient's needs regarding mobility. Care of the patient is based on the following problem statements:
- Compromised Physical Mobility, related to musculoskeletal impairment
- Compromised Bed Mobility
- Inability to Tolerate Activity, related to musculoskeletal impairment
- Impaired Coping
- Anxiousness, related to changes in body integrity
- Prolonged Pain, related to musculoskeletal disorder
- Insufficient Knowledge, regarding therapeutic regimen
- Potential for Contractures or Muscle Atrophy

◆ **EXPECTED OUTCOMES AND PLANNING**

The plan for facilitating mobility must center on improving and restoring performance and preventing deterioration. Nursing interventions help the patient adapt, reduce, or eliminate activities that cause pain.

Consider the amount of assistance needed for ambulation. Assessment of ROM and muscle strength helps decide whether the patient can ambulate safely. Ambulation after surgery often requires physical assistance in addition to the use of mobility aids such as walkers, canes, and crutches.

The care plan focuses on accomplishing individual goals and outcomes that relate to the identified patient problems. Examples of these include the following:

Goal 1: Patient will demonstrate the correct use of adaptive devices to increase mobility.

Outcome: Patient demonstrates more independence in mobility with correct use of adaptive devices.

Goal 2: Patient will demonstrate ambulation for 20 feet with one assist before discharge from health care facility.

Outcome: Patient demonstrates ambulation skills for 23 feet with one assist before discharge.

◆ **IMPLEMENTATION**

Improving the patient's mobility requires awareness of the health care provider's orders specific to ambulation. Check mobility aids for the correct size. Educate patients on safety measures, such as rubber tips in good condition on canes. Shoes that are easy to put on, have nonslip soles, and provide foot and ankle support are safer than bedroom slippers or stockings.

Activities must be alternated with rest periods. Administer analgesics at least 30 minutes before ambulation for patients experiencing pain. Encourage patients to pace themselves. Patient assistance may be necessary to complete ADLs such as ambulating to the bathroom or to a bedside commode.

Specific principles are involved with mobility:
- Bone loss occurs when patients are confined to bed rest.

- The activities of the human body depend on effective interaction between normal joints and the neuromuscular parts that pilot them.
- Muscles, tendons, ligaments, cartilage, and bones do their share to ensure smooth function.

Nurses working with patient mobility needs must support physical therapy department activities and goals. Assess a patient's perceptions to help determine his or her motivation for mobility independence. For example, when older adults think they are too fragile to walk, they may be afraid of trying. Use a safety belt when a patient's stability is questionable. The belt encircles the patient's waist; grasp the belt in the middle of the back to help the patient stand, gain balance, and ambulate.

Patients may have difficulty coping with mobility aids and perceive them as a visible sign of weakness. Point out that devices to help mobility are not unlike glasses to help eyesight. Mobility aids increase proficiency of activities and promote joint rest and protection.

◆ EVALUATION

Evaluate the success of interventions by noting a patient's progress during and after ambulation, based on stated goals and outcomes. For example, if the patient is not able to walk to the bathroom, a shorter distance may be more practical. The patient may increase mobility by using a bedside commode. When patients are unable to meet expected outcomes, be ready to revise the care plan to promote success. Examples of goals and their corresponding outcomes include the following:

Goal 1: Patient will demonstrate the use of adaptive devices to increase mobility.
Evaluative measure: Patient ambulates within physical environment.
Goal 2: Patient will understand safety precautions concerning use of mobility aids.
Evaluative measures: Patient checks rubber tips on mobility aid and uses equipment correctly.

Get Ready for the NCLEX® Examination!

Key Points

- The skeletal system has five basic functions: support of the body, protection of internal organs, movement of the body, storage of minerals, and blood cell formation.
- The skeleton is divided into the axial and the appendicular skeletons. The axial skeleton is composed of the skull, vertebral column, and thorax. The appendicular skeleton is composed of the upper extremities, lower extremities, shoulder girdle, and pelvic girdle.
- The three types of joints and their movement are (1) synarthrosis: no movement; (2) amphiarthrosis: slight movement; and (3) diarthrosis: free movement.
- Joints hold the bones together and allow movement and flexibility. Differences in the structure determine the amount of flexibility.
- Some of the more common movements that the body produces are flexion, extension, abduction, adduction, rotation, supination, pronation, dorsiflexion, and plantar flexion.
- The bones and joints provide the framework of the body, but the muscles are necessary for movement. Movement results from contraction and relaxation of the individual muscles.
- An erythrocyte sedimentation rate is the most objective laboratory test for determining the severity of rheumatoid arthritis (RA).
- RA affects a young population (ages 30 to 55 years) with crippling changes in the synovial membrane of the joints.
- Salicylates and nonsteroidal anti-inflammatory drugs are used to treat RA and osteoarthritis.
- Osteoarthritis is a degenerative joint disease that affects the population older than 40 years of age and causes articular cartilage degeneration.
- Porous and brittle bones caused by a lack of calcium are one of the physiologic changes noted in osteoporosis.
- Osteoporosis-related fractures occur in one in two women, compared with one in eight men, over the course of a lifetime.
- Vertebroplasty and kyphoplasty are surgical procedures used to relieve pain in women with osteoporosis who do not respond to other pain management programs.
- Arthroplasty procedures (such as hip and knee arthroplasty) commonly are performed on patients suffering from severe arthritis.
- Unicompartmental knee arthroplasty, also referred to as partial knee replacement, is performed on patients who have only one of the compartments of the knee affected by arthritis.
- Nursing intervention specific to the care of a patient suffering from a fractured hip involves maintaining abduction of the affected leg.
- Fractured hip fixation devices—such as hip prosthetic implant, plate and screw fixation, and telescoping nail fixation—require some degree of non–weight-bearing for 6 weeks to 3 months.
- The use of antacids and proton pump inhibitors increases a patient's risk of hip fractures.
- A significant postoperative nursing intervention for a patient with an amputation is proper care of the stump to facilitate the use of a prosthetic device.
- Herniated nucleus pulposus is seen most often in the cervical and lumbar spinal regions and can be treated surgically (laminectomy and spinal fusion) or medically (medication, traction, and physical therapy).
- Osteogenic sarcoma is a common primary malignant tumor seen in young people; it can metastasize to the lungs.
- Compartment syndrome, shock, fat embolism, gas gangrene, thromboembolus, and osteomyelitis are complications resulting from a fractured bone.

- Petechiae on the conjunctiva of the eye, the neck, the chest, or the axillary region is a typical sign of a fat embolism.
- External fixation devices such as casts, braces, metal pins, and skeletal and skin traction are used to hold bone fragments in normal position.
- Whether the casting material is plaster of Paris or a synthetic material, proper drying, cleansing, handling, and assessing are required to prevent patient complications.
- The nurse caring for a patient in traction is responsible for knowing (1) the purpose of the traction (traction applied for fractures must be continuous), (2) the equipment needed and appropriate safety measures, (3) the amount of weight ordered, and (4) the patient's understanding of the traction.
- Crutches, canes, walkers, and the Roll-A-Bout are used as gait enhancers for patients with altered mobility.
- Crutch walking involving the three-point gait is used most commonly for patients wearing leg casts.

Additional Learning Resources

SG Go to the Study Guide for additional learning activities to help master this chapter content.

Be sure to visit the Evolve site at http://evolve.elsevier.com/Cooper/adult/ for additional online resources.

Review Questions for the NCLEX® Examination

1. Where does hematopoiesis take place?
   1. The lymph nodes
   2. The spleen
   3. The yellow bone marrow
   4. The red bone marrow

2. The nurse is repositioning a patient. During the movement the extremity is placed in a position away from the midline of the body. To document this position, what term is most appropriate?
   1. Adduction
   2. Pronation
   3. Flexion
   4. Abduction

3. A patient is suspected of having rheumatoid arthritis (RA). What diagnostic tests may be used to support the diagnosis? (Select all that apply.)
   1. Complete blood count
   2. Erythrocyte sedimentation rate
   3. Prothrombin time
   4. Urinary uric acid level
   5. C-reactive protein

4. The nurse is reviewing the assessment findings and medical history of a patient suspected of having gouty arthritis. What findings support the diagnosis?
   1. Heberden's nodes
   2. Pathologic fractures
   3. Tophi
   4. Homans' sign
   5. Metatarsophalangeal joint effusion

5. A 55-year-old patient mentions that she is postmenopausal and is not taking estrogen supplements. A review of her normal dietary intake indicates a high consumption of caffeine and limited dietary ingestion of calcium. Based on her history, she faces an increased risk for what condition?
   1. Osteomyelitis
   2. Osteoarthritis
   3. Osteogenic sarcoma
   4. Osteoporosis

6. What is an appropriate nursing intervention for a patient suffering from a fractured hip with bipolar hip repair? (Select all that apply.)
   1. Release traction weight every 4 to 6 hours.
   2. Maintain abduction of the affected extremity.
   3. Maintain adduction of the affected extremity.
   4. Encourage active range of motion in the affected extremity.
   5. Ensure the head of the bed is not elevated more than 45 degrees.

7. A patient is being discharged after a prosthetic hip implant. She asks when she can begin to bear weight on the affected leg. What is a correct response by the nurse?
   1. "You will not be able to bear weight on the affected leg for 6 to 12 months."
   2. "Most patients bear weight in 5 days. I will check your orders."
   3. "You will use a gait enhancer and keep the majority of weight off the unaffected leg."
   4. "You will most likely require some degree of non–weight-bearing for 6 weeks to 3 months."

8. A patient has been seeing the health care provider for complaints of osteoarthritis. Today the patient is discussing concerns about their condition and asks what has caused the osteoarthritis. Which response by the nurse is most correct?
   1. "We don't really know what causes osteoarthritis."
   2. "Everyone your age has arthritis; you are fortunate you are still able to walk."
   3. "Wear and tear over the years have most likely caused the joints to begin to degenerate."
   4. "You probably did not exercise as much as you should have, and you should start vigorous exercising now to prevent further complications."
   5. "Your diagnosis of osteoarthritis is a result of decreased estrogen and bone resorption."

9. When providing care to a patient in skeletal traction what priority action would be included in the nurse's plan of care?
   1. Provide cast care.
   2. Cleanse pin sites and observe for signs of infection.
   3. Place patient on drainage and secretion precautions.
   4. Encourage patient to sit in a straight, firm chair for no longer than 20 minutes each time.
   5. Logroll the patient for position changes.

10. After a fracture of the forearm or tibia, complaints of sharp, deep, unrelenting pain in the hand or foot unrelieved by analgesics or elevation of the extremity indicate which complication?

    1. Fat embolism
    2. Compartment syndrome
    3. Gas gangrene
    4. Cast syndrome

11. A patient suffered a knee injury while playing football. The patient is scheduled for an arthroscopic examination and asks the nurse to explain the procedure. What information should be included in the nurse's response?

    1. "Your health care provider will insert a small scope into your knee joint to visualize the joint for damaged tissue."
    2. "The test involves the use of magnetism and radio waves to make images of cross sections of the body."
    3. "The radiographic technician will inject your knee joint with an atomic material and take a radiograph of your affected knee."
    4. "The health care provider will insert needle electrodes into the knee muscle to document electrical activity of the knee."

12. A patient with RA asks if there is a cure. What response by the nurse is most appropriate?

    1. "Yes, new drugs offer a cure."
    2. "No, but new drugs can interfere with the body's reaction to inflammation and better control the disease process."
    3. "Yes, but the patient must take medication for at least 10 years."
    4. "No, most patients with RA also develop osteoarthritis."

13. A patient is scheduled for endoscopic spinal microsurgery to correct a herniated disk. Select the most accurate statement concerning this type of surgery.

    1. "Endoscopic spinal microsurgery requires a general anesthetic."
    2. "Special scopes are placed through small incisions, causing minimal damage to surrounding tissue."
    3. "Patients older than 80 years of age are always candidates for endoscopic spinal microsurgery."
    4. "Endoscopic spinal microsurgery is limited to the repair of herniated disks."

14. A patient has osteoarthritis of the knee and is seeking information about glucosamine supplements. What would be an appropriate response by the nurse?

    1. "Glucosamine is a natural substance in the body, and it is not necessary to take a supplement."
    2. "Glucosamine supplements are relatively safe in people younger than 40 years of age."
    3. "Studies suggest that glucosamine supplements may be helpful in maintaining healthy joint function."
    4. "A healthy lifestyle with high-impact exercise is more important than taking a supplement."

15. Select the priority nursing assessment for the patient problem of ineffective tissue perfusion, secondary to fractured hip.

    1. Assess for ecchymosis over pelvis and perineum.
    2. Protect patient from cross-contamination.
    3. Assess for adventitious lung sounds.
    4. Assess distal pulses.
    5. Assess for changes in LOC

16. A patient has just undergone total hip replacement. The patient asks why she cannot cross her legs when sitting but must do straight leg–raising exercises. What is the most correct response?

    1. "The exercises help strengthen the leg muscles; crossing your legs puts pressure on the joints and could damage the hip prosthesis."
    2. "The exercises keep you from getting too tired while you sit; when you want to cross your legs, it is time to rest."
    3. "The exercises strengthen the muscles in your upper legs to help you walk."
    4. "The health care provider ordered these exercises but did not order you to cross your legs."

17. Which objective signs will the nurse find during the assessment of a patient with compartment syndrome in the lower leg? *(Select all that apply.)*

    1. Hypotension
    2. Gas bubbles under the skin
    3. Positive Homans' sign
    4. Absence of pulsation in the affected extremity
    5. Pain that is unreleased by medication or elevation of the extremity

18. A patient had a compound fracture of his right femur 2 years before the present admission. His health care provider suspects osteomyelitis and has informed the patient that tests are needed to confirm the diagnosis. The patient wants to know what tests can be ordered to determine osteomyelitis. An appropriate response would include which test for osteomyelitis? *(Select all that apply.)*

    1. Goniometer
    2. BMX
    3. Bone scan
    4. Bone biopsy
    5. Erythrocyte sedimentation rate

19. A construction worker suffered a fracture of the femur 48 hours ago. The nurse notices that he has petechiae on the conjunctiva, chest, neck, and axillae. Petechiae in these locations are consistent with which condition?

    1. Compartment syndrome
    2. Deep vein thrombosis
    3. Gas gangrene
    4. Fat embolism

20. A woman, 33, visits her physician to request referral to a physical therapist. "I'm concerned about my posture," she says. "No matter how hard I work out with a personal trainer at the gym, my posture is still not great, especially my old-lady hump on the back of my neck. My mother had that, and I feel like I'm just way too young for it." Objective data shows no evidence of scoliosis. History reveals that she works as a fiction editor on average about nine hours a day at a desk and experiences lumbar pain that worsens with sitting and coughing. While she has no history of fractures, she does have a small frame. Her mother has not experienced any broken bones, but she has had some loss in height, and the patient's grandmother had several falls that resulted in a broken hip and a broken wrist. Patient history reveals inflammatory bowel disease. She doesn't mind fruit but eats very few vegetables. She used to smoke in high school but quit when she turned 20. CBC; serum calcium, phosphorus, and alkaline phosphatase; blood urea nitrogen (BUN); creatinine level; urinalysis; and liver and thyroid function tests. Because of her mildly hunched posture and concerns about maintaining good posture, a BMD (bone mineral density measurement) is ordered despite her youth.

Which possible explanations for this patient's ultimate diagnosis of osteopenia are most/least likely?

Check all that apply:

A. Presence of kyphosis
B. BMD 2 standard deviations below the young female adult average.
C. BMD 3 standard deviations below the young female adult average.
D. Risks due to weight-bearing exercise four mornings a week
E. Calcium intake of 1800 mg/day
F. Diet lacking in animal protein
G. Vitamin D deficiency

5

Care of the Patient With a Gastrointestinal Disorder

http://evolve.elsevier.com/Cooper/adult/

Objectives

Anatomy and Physiology

1. List in sequence each of the parts or segments of the alimentary canal and identify the accessory organs of digestion.
2. Discuss the function of each digestive and accessory organ.

Medical-Surgical

3. Discuss the laboratory and diagnostic examinations associated with the gastrointestinal system.
4. Identify nursing interventions associated with disorders of the gastrointestinal tract.
5. Explain the etiology and pathophysiology, clinical manifestations, assessments, diagnostic tests, medical-surgical management, and nursing interventions for the patient with disorders of the mouth, esophagus, stomach, and intestines.
6. Identify nursing interventions for preoperative and postoperative care of the patient who requires gastric surgery.

7. Compare and contrast the inflammatory bowel diseases of ulcerative colitis and Crohn disease.
8. Identify nursing interventions for the patient with a stoma for fecal diversion.
9. Discuss the etiology and pathophysiology, clinical manifestations, assessment, diagnostic tests, medical management, and nursing interventions for the patient with acute abdominal inflammations (appendicitis, diverticulitis, and peritonitis), for the patient with hernias, and for the patient with colorectal cancer.
10. Differentiate between mechanical and nonmechanical intestinal obstruction, including causes, medical management, and nursing interventions.
11. Explain the causes, medical management, and nursing interventions for the patient with fecal incontinence.

Key Terms

achalasia (ăk-ăh-LĀ-zhē-ă, p. 186)
achlorhydria (ă-khlŏr-HĪ-drē-ă, p. 172)
anastomosis (ă-năs-tŏ-MŌ-sĭs, p. 186)
cachexia (kă-KĔK-sē-ă, p. 216)
carcinoembryonic antigen (CEA) (kăr-sĭn-ō-ĕm-brē-ĂN-ĭk ĂN-tĭ-jĕn, p. 195)
dehiscence (dĕ-HĬS-ĕntz, p. 197)
dumping syndrome (DŬMP-ĭng SĬN-drōm, p. 196)
dyspepsia (dĭs-PĔP-sē-ă, p. 189)
dysphagia (dĭs-FĀ-jhē-ă, p. 182)
evisceration (ĕ-vĭs-ĕr-Ā-shŭn, p. 197)
exacerbations (ĕg-zăs-ĕr-BĀ-shŭnz, p. 202)
gluten (GLŪ-tĕn, p. 199)
hematemesis (hĕ-mă-TĔM-ĕ-sĭs, p. 188)

intussusception (ĭn-tŭs-sŭs-SĔP-shŭn, p. 179)
leukoplakia (lū-kō-PLĀ-kē-ă, p. 182)
lumen (LŪ-mĕn [adjectival, LŪ-mĕn-ăl], p. 179)
melena (MĔL-ĕh-nă, p. 178)
occult blood (ŏ-KŬLT, p. 179)
paralytic (adynamic) ileus (pă-ră-LĬ-tĭk ā-dī-NĂM-ĭk Ē-lē-ŭs, p. 214)
pathognomonic (păth-ŏg-nō-MŎN-ĭk, p. 180)
remissions (rĕ-MĬSH-ŭnz, p. 202)
steatorrhea (stĕ-ă-tō-RĒ-ă, p. 206)
stoma (STŌ-mă, p. 206)
tenesmus (tĕ-NĔZ-mŭs, p. 199)
volvulus (VŎL-vū-lŭs, p. 214)

ANATOMY AND PHYSIOLOGY OF THE GASTROINTESTINAL SYSTEM

DIGESTIVE SYSTEM

The digestive tract, or alimentary canal, is a muscular tube containing a mucous membrane lining that extends from the mouth to the anus (Fig. 5.1) and is approximately 9 m (30 ft) long. It consists of the mouth, pharynx, esophagus, stomach, small intestine, large intestine, and anus. *Peristalsis* is the coordinated, rhythmic, sequential contraction of smooth muscle that pushes food through the digestive tract, as well as bile through the bile duct.

Accessory organs aid in the digestive process but are not considered part of the digestive tract. They

172

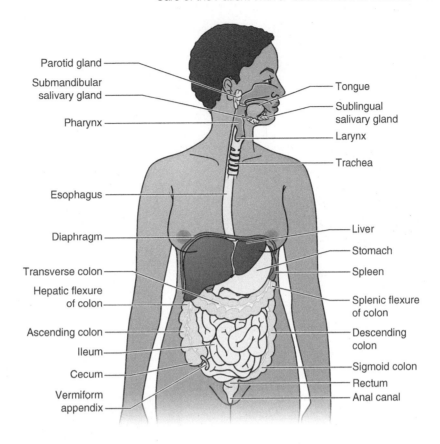

Fig. 5.1 Location of digestive organs.

release chemicals into the system through a series of ducts. The teeth, tongue, salivary glands, liver, gallbladder, pancreas, and appendix are considered accessory organs.

Organs of the Digestive System and Their Functions

Box 5.1 lists various organs of the digestive system and the accessory organs involved in digestion.

Mouth. The mouth marks the entrance to the digestive system. The floor of the mouth contains a muscular appendage, the tongue. The tongue is involved in chewing, swallowing, and the formation of speech. Tiny elevations, called *papillae,* contain the taste buds. They differentiate among bitter, sweet, sour, and salty sensations.

Digestion begins in the mouth. Here the teeth mechanically shred and grind food and enzymes begin the chemical breakdown of carbohydrates.

Teeth. Each tooth is designed to carry out a specific task. At the front of the mouth are the incisors, which are structured for biting and cutting. Posterior to the incisors are the canines, pointed teeth used for tearing and shredding food. The molars are to the rear of the jaw. These teeth have four cusps (points) and are used for mastication (the crushing and grinding of food).

Box 5.1	Organs of the Digestive System
ORGANS OF THE ALIMENTARY CANAL	• Sigmoid colon
• Mouth	• Rectum
• Pharynx (throat)	• Anal canal
• Esophagus (food pipe)	**ACCESSORY ORGANS**
• Stomach	• Teeth and gums
• Small intestine	• Salivary glands
• Duodenum	• Parotid
• Jejunum	• Submandibular
• Ileum	• Sublingual
• Large intestine (colon)	• Tongue
• Cecum	• Liver
• Ascending colon	• Gallbladder
• Transverse colon	• Pancreas
• Descending colon	• Vermiform appendix

Salivary glands. The three pairs of salivary glands are the parotid, submandibular, and sublingual glands (see Fig. 5.1). They secrete fluid called *saliva,* which is approximately 99% water with enzymes and mucus. Normally these glands secrete enough saliva to keep the mucous membranes of the mouth moist. Once food enters the mouth, the secretion increases to lubricate and dissolve the food and to begin the chemical process of digestion. The salivary glands secrete about 1000 to 1500 mL of

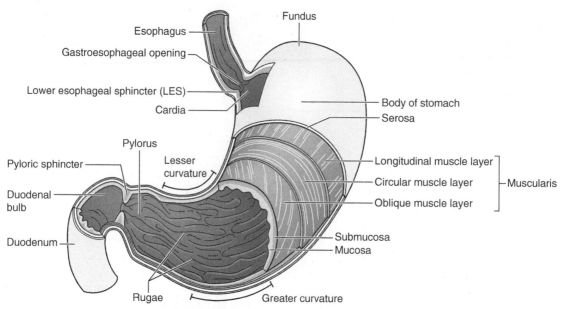

Fig. 5.2 Stomach. Cut-away sections show muscle layers and interior mucosa thrown into folds called *rugae*.

saliva daily. The major enzyme is salivary amylase (ptyalin), which initiates carbohydrate metabolism. Another enzyme, lysozyme, destroys bacteria and thus protects the mucous membrane from infections and the teeth from decay. After food has been ingested, the salivary glands continue to secrete saliva, which cleanses the mouth.

Esophagus. The esophagus is a muscular, collapsible tube that is approximately 25 cm (10 in) long, extending from the mouth through the thoracic cavity and the esophageal hiatus (a hole in the diaphragm) to the stomach. Digestion does not take place in the esophagus. Peristalsis moves the bolus (food broken down and mixed with saliva, ready to pass to the stomach) through the pharynx, to the esophagus, and then to the stomach in 5 or 6 seconds.

Stomach. The stomach is in the left upper quadrant of the abdomen, directly inferior to the diaphragm (Fig. 5.2). A filled stomach is the size of a football and can hold a volume of approximately 1 to 1.5 L. The stomach entrance is at the cardiac sphincter (so named because it is close to the heart); the exit is at the pyloric sphincter. As food leaves the esophagus, it enters the stomach through the relaxed cardiac sphincter. The sphincter then contracts, preventing reflux (splashing or return flow), which can be irritating to the esophagus.

Once the bolus has entered the stomach, the muscular layers of the stomach churn and contract to mix and compress the contents with the gastric juices and water. The gastric juices are secretions released by the gastric glands. Digestion of protein begins in the stomach. Hydrochloric acid softens the connective tissue of meats, kills bacteria, and activates pepsin (the chief enzyme of gastric juices that converts proteins into proteoses and peptones). Mucin is released to protect the

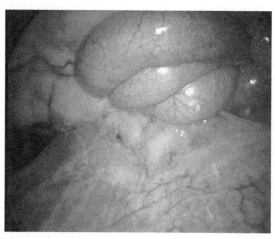

Fig. 5.3 Laparoscopic view of the small intestine. (From Abrahams P, Marks S, Hutchings R: *McMinn's color atlas of human anatomy,* ed 7, Philadelphia, 2013, Saunders.)

stomach lining. The intrinsic factor (a substance secreted by the gastric mucosa) is produced to allow absorption of vitamin B_{12}. The stomach breaks the food down into a viscous, semiliquid substance called *chyme.* The chyme passes through the pyloric sphincter into the duodenum for the next phase of digestion.

Small intestine. The small intestine (Fig. 5.3) is a tube that is 6 m (20 ft) long and 2.5 cm (1 in) in diameter. It begins at the pyloric sphincter, ends at the ileocecal valve, and is divided into three major sections: *duodenum, jejunum,* and *ileum.* Up to 90% of digestion takes place in the small intestine. The intestinal juices finish the metabolism of carbohydrates and proteins. Bile and pancreatic juices enter the duodenum. Bile from the liver breaks molecules into smaller droplets, which enables the digestive juices to complete their process. Pancreatic juices contain water, protein, inorganic salts, and enzymes. Pancreatic juices are essential in breaking down proteins into their amino acid components, in reducing dietary fats to glycerol and fatty acids, and in converting starch to simple sugars.

The inner surface of the small intestine contains millions of tiny finger-like projections called *villi,* which are clustered over the entire mucous membrane surface. The villi aid in the digestive process by absorbing the products of digestion into the bloodstream. They increase the absorption area of the small intestine by about 600 times. Inside each villus is a rich capillary bed, along with modified lymph capillaries called *lacteals.* The primary function of the lacteals is to absorb metabolized fats.

Large intestine. Once the small intestine has completed its tasks of digestion, the ileocecal valve opens and releases the contents of digestion into the large intestine. The large intestine is a tube that is larger in diameter (6 cm, or 2 in), but shorter at 1.5 to 1.8 m (5 to 6 ft), than the small intestine. The large intestine consists of the cecum; appendix; ascending colon, hepatic flexure, transverse colon, splenic flexure, descending colon, and sigmoid colon; rectum; and anus (Fig. 5.4). This is the terminal portion of the digestive tract, where the process of digestion is completed. The large intestine has four major functions: (1) completion of absorption of water, (2) manufacture of certain vitamins (such as vitamins K and B_7), (3) formation of feces, and (4) expulsion of feces.

Just inferior to the ileocecal valve is the cecum, a blind pouch approximately 2 to 3 in long. The vermiform appendix, a small, wormlike, tubular structure, dangles from the cecum. Research has revealed that the appendix functions as an area where nonpathologic bacteria live safely until they are needed for digestion, especially in the large intestine. In addition, the appendix houses immune system cells and tissue (Girard-Madoux, 2018). The open end of the cecum connects to the ascending colon, which continues upward on the right side of the abdomen to the inferior area of the liver. The ascending colon then becomes the transverse colon. It crosses to the left side of the abdomen, where it becomes the descending colon. When the descending colon reaches the level of the iliac crest, the sigmoid colon begins and continues toward the midline to the level of the third sacral vertebra.

Bacteria in the large intestine changes waste products from digestion (undigested food, fluid, and aged cells from the lining of the GI tract) into fecal material by releasing the remaining nutrients. The bacteria are also responsible for the synthesis of vitamin K, which is needed for normal blood clotting, and the production of some of the B-complex vitamins. As the fecal

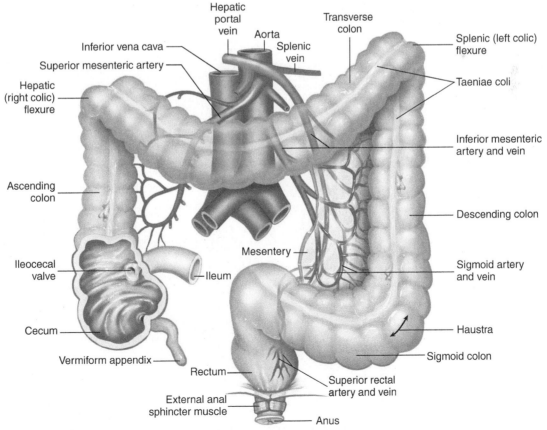

Fig. 5.4 Divisions of the large intestine. (From Patton KT, Thibodeau GA: *The human body in health and disease,* ed 7, St. Louis, 2018, Elsevier.)

material continues its journey, the remaining water and vitamins are absorbed into the bloodstream by osmosis.

Rectum. The rectum is the last 20 cm (8 in) of the intestine, where fecal material is expelled. The anus is the opening to the outside of the body, where feces are passed.

ACCESSORY ORGANS OF DIGESTION

Liver

The liver is the largest glandular organ in the body, weighing approximately 1.5 kg (3 to 4 lb) in the adult, and is one of the more complex organs in the body. It is located just inferior to the diaphragm, covering most of the upper right quadrant and extending into the left epigastrium, and it is divided into two lobes. The lobes are further divided into several lobules (smaller lobes) containing small blood vessels. Approximately 1500 mL of blood is delivered to the liver every minute by the portal vein and the hepatic portal artery. The cells of the liver produce a product called *bile,* a yellow-brown or green-brown liquid; bile is necessary for the emulsification of fats. The liver releases approximately 500 to 1000 mL of bile per day, which then travels to the gallbladder through hepatic ducts. The gallbladder is a sac about 8 to 9 cm (3 to 4 in) long, located on the right inferior surface of the liver. Bile is stored in the gallbladder until it is needed for fat digestion (Fig. 5.5).

In addition to producing bile, the liver's functions include managing blood coagulation; metabolizing proteins, fats, and carbohydrates; manufacturing cholesterol; manufacturing albumin to maintain normal blood volume; filtering out old red blood cells (RBCs) and bacteria; detoxifying poisons (alcohol, nicotine, drugs); converting ammonia to urea; providing the main source of body heat at rest; storing glycogen for later use; activating vitamin D; and breaking down nitrogenous waste (from protein metabolism) to urea, which the kidneys can excrete as waste from the body.

Gallbladder

The gallbladder is a pear-shaped organ measuring approximately 7 to 10 cm (3 to 4 in) long. Areolar connective tissue connects it to the underside of the liver. The gallbladder can store 30 to 50 mL of bile, and its primary function is to store and eject bile into the duodenum for digestion of fats.

Pancreas

The pancreas is an elongated gland, approximately 12 to 15 cm (6 to 9 in) long, which lies posterior to the stomach (see Fig. 5.4). It is involved in endocrine and exocrine duties. In this chapter, discussion of the pancreas is limited to its exocrine activities.

Each day the pancreas produces 1000 to 1500 mL of pancreatic juice to aid in digestion. This pancreatic juice contains the digestive enzymes protease (trypsin), lipase (steapsin), and amylase (amylopsin). These enzymes are important because they digest the three major components of chyme: proteins, fats, and carbohydrates. The enzymes are transported through an excretory duct to the duodenum. This pancreatic duct

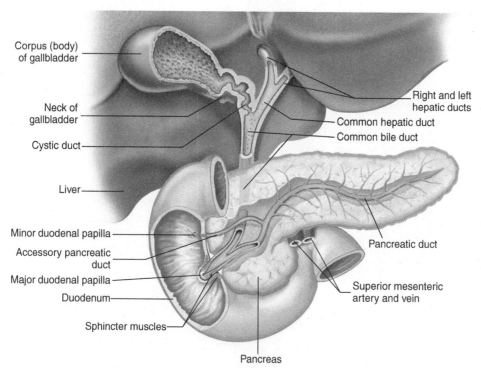

Fig. 5.5 Gallbladder and bile ducts. Obstruction of the hepatic or common bile duct by stone or spasm occludes the exit of the bile and prevents matter from being ejected into the duodenum. (From Patton KT, Thibodeau GA: *The human body in health and disease,* ed 7, St. Louis, 2018, Elsevier.)

connects to the common bile duct from the liver and gallbladder and empties through a small orifice in the duodenum called the *major duodenal papilla*. In addition, the pancreas contains an alkaline substance, sodium bicarbonate, which neutralizes hydrochloric acid in the gastric juices that enter the small intestine from the stomach.

REGULATION OF FOOD INTAKE

The hypothalamus, a portion of the brain, contains two appetite centers that affect eating. One center stimulates the individual to eat, and the other signals the individual to stop eating. These centers work in conjunction with the rest of the brain to balance eating habits. In addition to the hypothalamus, factors that also affect food intake include lifestyle, culture, eating habits, emotions, and genetics.

LABORATORY AND DIAGNOSTIC EXAMINATIONS

UPPER GASTROINTESTINAL STUDY (UPPER GI SERIES, UGI)
Rationale
The upper gastrointestinal (UGI) study consists of a series of radiographs of the lower esophagus, stomach, and duodenum, using barium sulfate as the contrast medium. A UGI series detects any abnormal conditions of the UGI tract, any tumors, or other ulcerative lesions.

Nursing Interventions
The patient should take nothing by mouth (NPO) and avoid smoking after midnight the night before the study. Explain the importance of rectally expelling all the barium after the examination. Feces (stools) are light in color until all the barium is expelled (up to 72 hours after the test). Eventual absorption of fecal water may cause a hardened barium impaction. Patients should be instructed to increase their fluid intake to help expel the barium, thus preventing constipation or blockage. The health care provider may order a laxative to be given in addition to increasing fluid intake.

TUBE GASTRIC ANALYSIS
Rationale
The stomach contents are aspirated to determine the amount of acid produced by the parietal cells in the stomach. The analysis helps determine the completeness of a vagotomy, confirm hypersecretion or achlorhydria (an abnormal condition characterized by the absence of hydrochloric acid in the gastric juice), estimate acid secretory capacity, or test for intrinsic factor.

Nursing Interventions
The patient should receive no anticholinergic medications for 24 hours before the test and should maintain NPO status after midnight to avoid altering the rate of gastric acid secretion. The patient also should be instructed that smoking is prohibited before the test because nicotine stimulates the flow of gastric secretions.

The nurse or radiology personnel inserts a nasogastric (NG) tube into the stomach to aspirate gastric contents. Specimens are labeled properly and sent to the laboratory immediately. The NG tube is removed, and the patient may eat and drink without restrictions unless otherwise ordered.

ESOPHAGOGASTRODUODENOSCOPY (EGD, UGI ENDOSCOPY, GASTROSCOPY)
Rationale
Endoscopy (from *endo*, within, inward; and *scope*, to look) enables direct visualization of a particular hollow organ or cavity by means of a long, flexible fiberoptic scope (Fig. 5.6). An EGD visualizes the esophagus, stomach, and duodenum for routine screening as well as for examination of tumors, varices (abnormally enlarged veins), mucosal inflammation, hiatal hernias, polyps (small tissue growths projecting from a mucous membrane), ulcers, *Helicobacter pylori*, strictures (narrowings), and obstructions. The endoscopist also can remove polyps, coagulate sources of active GI bleeding, and perform sclerotherapy (injection of a solution into the vein causing it to shrink and eventually disappear) of esophageal varices. Areas of narrowing can be dilated by the endoscope or by passing a dilator through the scope. Camera equipment can be attached to the viewing lens to photograph a pathologic condition. The endoscope also can obtain tissue specimens for biopsy or culture to determine the presence of *H. pylori*.

Endoscopy enables evaluation of the esophagus, stomach, and duodenum. A longer fiberoptic scope allows evaluation of the upper small intestine. This is referred to as *enteroscopy*.

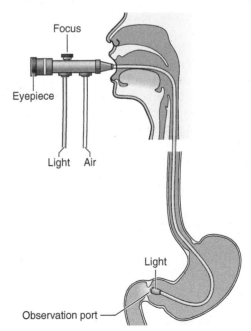

Fig. 5.6 Fiberoptic endoscopy of the stomach.

Nursing Interventions

The patient should maintain NPO status after midnight before the test, and an informed consent form must be signed. The patient usually is given a preprocedure intravenous (IV) sedative such as midazolam or diprivan, and the patient's pharynx is anesthetized by spraying it with lidocaine hydrochloride. After the procedure the patient will not be allowed to eat or drink until the gag reflex returns, which is usually soon after the procedure and can be assessed by placing a tongue blade to the back of the pharynx. Monitor the patient's vital signs and oxygen saturation after the procedure and assess for any signs and symptoms of perforation, including abdominal pain and tenderness, guarding, oral bleeding, melena (tarlike, fetid-smelling stool containing undigested blood), and hypovolemic shock.

CAPSULE ENDOSCOPY

Rationale

For capsule endoscopy, the patient swallows a capsule (approximately the size of a large vitamin) containing a camera that provides endoscopic evaluation of the GI tract. It commonly is used to visualize the small intestine and diagnose diseases such as Crohn disease, celiac disease, and malabsorption syndrome. It also helps identify sources of possible GI bleeding in areas not accessible by upper endoscopy or colonoscopy. The camera takes tens of thousands of images during an 8-hour examination. The capsule relays images to a data recorder that the patient wears on a belt. After the examination, images are viewed on a monitor (Mayo Clinic, 2019).

Nursing Interventions

The patient is NPO for approximately 12 hours before the test and should not smoke for 24 hours before the test. The patient may need to stop taking some medications before the procedure. The health care provider determines which, if any, medications must be halted before the patient ingests the capsule. The patient swallows the video capsule and usually is kept NPO for 2 hours and usually can eat a light meal 4 hours after swallowing the capsule. The procedure is comfortable for most patients. Peristalsis causes passage of the disposable capsule with a bowel movement, usually within 2 to 3 days or sooner, depending on the patient's rate of peristalsis. The pill camera does not have to be retrieved (Mayo Clinic, 2019).

BARIUM SWALLOW AND GASTROGRAFIN STUDIES

Rationale

A barium swallow study allows a clearer view of the esophagus than that provided by most UGI examinations; this is because the esophageal movements do not show up well on x-rays. When the patient swallows barium, however, the outline of the esophagus is clear. As in most barium contrast studies, defects in luminal filling and narrowing of the barium column indicate tumor, scarred stricture, or esophageal varices. A barium swallow allows easy recognition of swallowing difficulties resulting from conditions such as cerebrovascular accidents (stroke or brain attack), and of anatomic abnormalities, such as hiatal hernia. Cancers of the esophagus, gastroesophageal reflux disease (GERD) and ulcers, and muscle disorders are other reasons for performing a barium swallow study (Johns Hopkins University, n.d.).

Gastrografin (diatrizoate meglumine and diatrizoate sodium) is a product used in place of barium for patients who are susceptible to bleeding from the GI tract and who are being considered for surgery. Gastrografin is water soluble and rapidly absorbed, so it is preferable when a perforation is suspected. Gastrografin facilitates imaging through radiographs, but if the product escapes from the GI tract, it is absorbed by the surrounding tissue. In contrast, if barium leaks from the GI tract, it is not absorbed and can lead to complications (Drugs.com, 2020).

Nursing Interventions

The patient is NPO after midnight. Food and fluid in the stomach prevent barium from accurately outlining the GI tract, and the radiographic results may be misleading. Explain the importance of rectally expelling all barium. Stools will be light in color until this occurs. Eventual absorption of fecal water may cause a hardened barium impaction. The patient should be instructed to increase his or her fluid intake to help in expelling the barium, thus preventing constipation or blockage. The health care provider may order a laxative to be given in addition to increasing fluid intake.

ESOPHAGEAL FUNCTION STUDIES (BERNSTEIN TEST)

Rationale

The Bernstein test, an acid perfusion test, is an attempt to reproduce the symptoms of gastroesophageal reflux. It helps differentiate esophageal pain caused by esophageal reflux from that caused by angina pectoris. If the patient suffers pain with the instillation of hydrochloric acid into the esophagus, the test is positive and indicates reflux esophagitis (National Library of Medicine [NLM], 2020a).

Nursing Interventions

The patient is NPO for 8 hours before the examination, and any medications that may interfere with the production of acid, such as antacids and analgesics, are withheld. An NG tube is inserted, and mild hydrochloric acid is instilled followed by saline. The patient should be asked if any pain or discomfort is felt during instillation of the hydrochloric acid.

EXAMINATION OF STOOL FOR OCCULT BLOOD

Rationale

Tumors of the large intestine grow into the lumen (the cavity or channel within a tube or tubular organ) and are subject to repeated trauma by the fecal stream. Eventually the tumor ulcerates and bleeding occurs. Sometimes the bleeding is so slight that gross blood is not seen in the stool. If this occult blood (blood that is obscure or hidden from view) is detected in the stool, a benign or malignant GI tumor is suspected. Tests for occult blood include the stool guaiac test, Hemoccult test, and Hematest.

Occult blood in the stool also may occur in ulceration and inflammation of the upper or lower GI system, as well as with internal hemorrhoids that are bleeding. Other causes include swallowing blood of oral or nasopharyngeal origin. For specimen collection the patient usually is asked to collect stool in an appropriate container.

Nursing Interventions

The patient is instructed to keep the stool specimen free of urine or toilet paper, because either can alter the test results. The nurse or patient should don gloves and use tongue blades or an appropriate specimen collection device for stool to transfer the stool to the proper receptacle. The patient should not eat any organ meat for 24 to 48 hours before a guaiac test. Use a specimen slide and developer to test the stool for occult blood. The health care provider sometimes orders that three consecutive stools be tested for occult blood.

SIGMOIDOSCOPY (LOWER GI ENDOSCOPY)

Rationale

Endoscopy of the lower GI tract allows visualization of the inner lining of the sigmoid colon and, if indicated, access to obtain biopsy specimens of tumors, polyps, or ulcerations of the anus, rectum, and sigmoid colon. The lower GI tract is difficult to visualize radiographically, but sigmoidoscopy allows direct visualization. Microscopic review of tissue specimens obtained using this procedure leads to diagnoses of many lower bowel disorders.

Nursing Interventions

The patient should maintain NPO status after midnight before the test, and an informed consent form must be signed. The specific bowel preparation is determined by the health care provider performing the procedure, usually a gastroenterologist, and usually consists of laxatives, enemas, or a combination of both. After the examination, observe the patient for evidence of bowel perforation (abdominal pain, tenderness, distention, and bleeding) and instruct the patient to watch for these symptoms at home.

BARIUM ENEMA STUDY (LOWER GI SERIES)

Rationale

The barium enema (BE) study consists of a series of x-rays of the colon used to detect the presence and location of abnormalities such as polyps, tumors, and diverticula. Barium sulfate also assists in visualization of mucosal detail. Therapeutically, a BE may be used to reduce (treat) a nonstrangulated ileocolic intussusception (infolding of one segment of the intestine into the lumen of another segment) in children (Chahine, 2018). The contrast agent causes the infolded portion to move back into its normal position.

Nursing Interventions

The evening before the BE, cathartics such as magnesium citrate, or other cathartics designated by facility policy, are administered. A cleansing enema the evening before or the morning of the BE is administered if directed by the health care provider's order or facility policy. Fluids should be encouraged, and a laxative may be ordered after the BE to stimulate evacuation of the barium.

After the BE study, assess the patient for complete evacuation of the barium, or instruct the patient to monitor stools at home. Patients typically expel most of the barium before leaving the radiology department. Retained barium may cause constipation or a hardened impaction. Stool will be light in color until all the barium has been expelled.

COLONOSCOPY

Rationale

The development of the fiberoptic colonoscope has enabled examination of the entire colon, from the anus to the cecum, in most patients. Colonoscopy visualizes the mucosa of the colon and can detect lesions in the proximal colon, which would not be found by sigmoidoscopy. Benign and malignant neoplasms, mucosal inflammation or ulceration, and sites of active hemorrhage also can be visualized. Biopsy specimens can be obtained and small tumors removed through the scope. Actively bleeding vessels can be coagulated.

A less invasive test than a standard colonoscopy is called virtual colonoscopy. This test uses computed tomography (CT) scanning or magnetic resonance imaging (MRI) with computer software to produce images of the colon and rectum. For both procedures a small tube is inserted through the anus and into the rectum. With the CT procedure, the colon is expanded by instillation of carbon dioxide gas to aid in visualization. For the MRI method, a contrast medium is given to expand the colon. The colon preparation is similar to that for a regular colonoscopic examination. Sedatives are not required and no scope is needed. One disadvantage of this procedure is that it does not allow for biopsies, removal of polyps, or coagulation of vessels

(National Institute of Diabetes and Digestive and Kidney Diseases [NIDDK], 2016). Patients who have had cancer of the colon are at high risk for developing a subsequent colon cancer; patients who have a family history of colon cancer are also at high risk. For these patients, colonoscopy allows early detection of any primary or secondary tumors.

Nursing Interventions

Informed consent is necessary for a colonoscopy to be performed. Dietary restrictions include a clear liquid diet for 1 to 3 days before the procedure to decrease the residue in the bowel, and then NPO status is maintained for 8 hours before the procedure. Laxatives and/or enemas, and premedication, such as a stool softener, are ordered to cleanse the bowel. The bowel preparation will depend on the health care provider's preference and the patient's condition.

After the colonoscopy, monitor the patient for evidence of bowel perforation (abdominal pain, guarding, distention, tenderness, excessive rectal bleeding, or blood clots). The stools should be examined for gross blood. Monitor the patient for hypovolemic shock.

STOOL CULTURE

Rationale

The feces (stool) can be examined for the presence of bacteria, ova, and parasites (a plant or animal that lives on or within another living organism and obtains some advantage at its host's expense). The health care provider may order a stool for culture of bacteria or of ova and parasites (O&P). Many bacteria (such as *Escherichia coli*) are indigenous in the bowel. Bacterial cultures usually are done to detect enteropathogens (such as *Staphylococcus aureus*, *Salmonella* or *Shigella* organisms, *E. coli* O157:II7, or *Clostridium difficile*) (Centers for Disease Control and Prevention [CDC], 2019; CDC, 2021).

When a patient is suspected of having a parasitic infection, the stool is examined for O&P. Usually at least three stool specimens are collected on consecutive days. Because culture results are not available for several days, they do not influence initial treatment, but they do guide subsequent treatment if bacterial infection is present.

Nursing Interventions

If an enema must be administered to collect specimens, only normal saline or tap water is used. Soapsuds or any other substance could affect the viability of the organisms collected.

Stool samples for O&P are obtained before barium examinations. Be sure that urine is not mixed with feces in the sample. Wear gloves for sample collection. The specimen is taken to the laboratory within 30 minutes of collection in a specified container.

OBSTRUCTION SERIES (FLAT PLATE OF THE ABDOMEN)

Rationale

The obstruction series is a group of radiographic studies performed on the abdomen of patients who have suspected bowel obstruction, paralytic ileus, perforated viscus (a *viscus* is any large interior organ in any of the great body cavities), or abdominal abscess. The series usually consists of at least two radiographic studies. The first is an erect abdominal radiographic study that allows visualization of the diaphragm. Radiographs are examined for evidence of free air under the diaphragm, which is pathognomonic (signs or symptoms specific to a disease condition) of a perforated viscus (hollow organ). This radiographic study also is used to detect air-fluid levels within the intestine (NLM, 2019a).

Nursing Interventions

For adequate visualization, ensure that this study is scheduled before any barium studies.

DISORDERS OF THE MOUTH

Common disorders of the mouth and esophagus that interfere with adequate nutrition include poor dental hygiene, infections, inflammation, and cancer.

DENTAL PLAQUE AND CARIES

Etiology and Pathophysiology

Dental decay is an erosive process that results from the action of bacteria on carbohydrates in the mouth, which in turn produce acids that dissolve tooth enamel. Many Americans experience tooth decay at some time in their life. Dental decay can be caused by several factors:

- Dental plaque, a thin film on the teeth made of mucin and colloidal material found in saliva and often secondarily invaded by bacteria
- The strength of acids and the inability of the saliva to neutralize them
- The length of time the acids are in contact with the teeth
- Susceptibility of the teeth to decay

Medical Management

Dental caries are treated by removal of affected areas of the tooth and replacement with some form of dental material. Treatment of periodontal disease focuses on removal of plaque from the teeth. If the disease is advanced, surgical interventions on the gingivae and alveolar bone may be necessary.

Nursing Interventions and Patient Teaching

Proper technique for brushing and flossing the teeth at least twice a day is the primary focus for teaching patients. Plaque forms continuously and must be removed periodically through regular visits to the dentist. Stress the importance of prevention through continual care. Because carbohydrates create an environment in which caries develop and plaque accumulates more easily, include proper nutrition in patient teaching. When the patient is ill, the mouth's normal cleansing action is impaired. Illnesses, drugs, and irradiation interfere with the normal action of saliva. If the patient is unable to manage oral hygiene, assume this responsibility.

Patient problems and interventions for the patient with dental plaque and caries include but are not limited to the following:

Patient Problem	Nursing Interventions
Insufficient Knowledge, related to: • Inability to prevent dental caries • Periodontal disease	Assess and observe the oral cavity for moisture, color, and cleanliness Stress importance of meticulous oral hygiene Explain the need to see a dentist at least yearly for an examination

Modified from Ackley BJ, Ladwig GB: *Nursing diagnosis handbook: An evidence-based guide to planning care*, ed 12, St. Louis, 2020, Mosby.

The prevention and elimination of dental plaque and caries are related directly to oral hygiene, dental care, nutrition, and heredity. All but heredity are controllable factors. The prognosis is more favorable for people who brush, floss, regularly visit the dentist for removal of affected areas, eat low-carbohydrate foods, and drink fluoridated water.

CANDIDIASIS

Etiology and Pathophysiology

Candidiasis is any infection caused by a species of *Candida*, usually *C. albicans*. *Candida* is a fungal organism normally present in the mucous membranes of the mouth, intestinal tract, and vagina; it also is found on the skin of healthy people. This infection also is referred to as *thrush* or *moniliasis.*

This disease appears more commonly in the newborn infant, who becomes infected while passing through the birth canal. In the older individual, candidiasis may be found in patients with leukemia, diabetes mellitus, or alcoholism, and in patients who are taking antibiotics (chlortetracycline or tetracycline), are undergoing corticosteroid inhalant treatment, or are immunosuppressed (e.g., patients with acquired immunodeficiency syndrome [AIDS] or those receiving chemotherapy or radiation therapy).

Clinical Manifestations

Candidiasis appears as pearly, bluish white "milk-curd" membranous lesions on the mucous membranes of the mouth, tongue, and larynx. One or more lesions may be on the mucosa, depending on the duration of the infection (see Chapter 16, Fig. 16.5 for illustration). If the patch or plaque is removed, painful bleeding can occur.

Assessment

Assessment of the patient with oral candidiasis may reveal subjective complaints of soreness and difficulty swallowing. Angular cheilitis (cracks at the corners of the mouth) is an objective sign of oral candidiasis. Failure to eat is an objective common sign of candidiasis of the GI tract that is seen in infants and adults.

Medical Management

Nystatin or amphotericin B (an oral suspension) or buccal tablets of anidulafungin or fluconazole, one-third–strength hydrogen peroxide, and saline mouth rinses may provide some relief. In addition, eating unsweetened yogurt or taking acidophilus capsules or liquid can restore normal bacterial flora (Hidalgo, 2020).

Nursing Interventions

Meticulous hand hygiene should be used to prevent spread of the infection. For infants, hand hygiene, care of feeding equipment, and cleanliness of the mother's nipples are important to prevent spread. The infant's mouth should be assessed regularly.

For adults, encourage the patient to use a soft-bristled toothbrush and to avoid hot, cold, spicy, fried, or citrus foods. Many patients find that a topical anesthetic such as a lidocaine or benzocaine oral solution eases the discomfort of eating and drinking if taken approximately an hour prior.

Prognosis

If the host has a strong defense system and medical treatment is initiated early in the course of the disease, the prognosis is good.

CARCINOMA OF THE ORAL CAVITY

Etiology and Pathophysiology

Oral (or oropharyngeal) cancer may occur on the lips, the oral cavity, the tongue, and the pharynx. The tonsils occasionally are involved. Most of these tumors are squamous cell epitheliomas that grow rapidly and metastasize to adjacent structures more quickly than do most malignant tumors of the skin. An estimated 532,600 new cases and 10,750 deaths from oral cavity and pharynx cancer are expected to occur in 2020. The number of new cases has been consistent in the male population but has risen with women. The rise in the incidents of oral cancer in women is linked to infection with the human papilloma virus (HPV). Death rates have been decreasing over the past 30 years (American Cancer Society [ACS], 2021c).

Tumors of the salivary glands occur primarily in the parotid gland and are usually benign. Tumors of the submaxillary gland have a high incidence of malignancy. These malignant tumors grow rapidly and may be accompanied by pain and impaired facial function.

Kaposi sarcoma is a malignant skin tumor that occurs primarily on the skin or on mucosal surfaces such as in the mouth. It is seen at a rate of 6 cases per million people infected with AIDS, and at a rate of 1 in 200 for patients receiving immunosuppressive therapy after organ transplantation. The lesions are purple and nonulcerated. Irradiation is the treatment of choice (ACS, 2018).

The types of cancers of the lip that usually are seen are basal cell carcinoma and squamous cell carcinoma. Cancer of the lip occurs most frequently as a chronic ulcer of the lower lip in men over the age of 50. The cure rate for cancer of the lip is high because the lesion is apparent to the patient and to others, so patients often seek early treatment. If early detection and treatment do not occur, metastasis to regional lymph nodes may occur. In some instances a lesion may spread rapidly and involve the mandible and the floor of the mouth by direct extension. On occasion, the tumor may be a basal cell lesion that starts in the skin and spreads to the lip (Skin Cancer Foundation, 2020).

Cancer of the anterior tongue and floor of the mouth may seem to occur together because their spread to adjacent tissues is so rapid. Because of the tongue's abundant vascular and lymphatic drainage, metastasis to the neck may occur. There is a higher incidence of cancers of the mouth and throat among people who are heavy drinkers and who have a history of tobacco use (e.g., cigar, cigarette, pipe, chewing tobacco) and exposure to human papillomavirus (HPV) (National Cancer Institute, n.d.). Also, data show that men are twice as likely to be diagnosed with cancer of the tongue (ACS, 2021d).

Clinical Manifestations

Leukoplakia (a white, firmly attached patch on the mouth or tongue mucosa) may appear on the lips and buccal mucosa. These nonsloughing lesions cannot be rubbed off by simple mechanical force. They can be benign or malignant. A small percentage develop into squamous cell carcinomas, and biopsy is recommended if the lesions persist for longer than 2 weeks.

Assessment

Collection of subjective data includes understanding that malignant lesions of the mouth may be asymptomatic. The patient may feel only a roughened area with the tongue. As the disease progresses, the first complaints may be (1) difficulty in chewing, swallowing, or speaking; (2) edema, numbness, or loss of feeling in any part of the mouth; and (3) earache, facial pain, and toothache, which may become constant. Cancer of the lip is associated with discomfort and irritation caused by a nonhealing lesion, which may be raised or ulcerated. Malignancy at the base of the tongue produces

less obvious symptoms: slight dysphagia (difficulty in swallowing), sore throat, and salivation. Most oral cancers occur in males over the age of 60, but do not overlook symptoms based on age and gender.

Diagnostic Tests

Direct and indirect laryngoscopy are important diagnostic tests for examination of the soft tissue. This procedure allows direct visualization of the oral cavity, and both can be performed in the health care provider's office. If necessary, panendoscopy—a more invasive form of laryngoscopy—may be performed with an endoscope. Radiographic evaluation of the mandibular structures is another essential part of the head and neck examination to rule out cancer. Excisional biopsy is the most accurate method for making a definitive diagnosis. Oral exfoliative cytology, in which a scraping of a lesion provides cells for cytologic examination, is used to screen intraoral lesions (ACS, 2021c).

Medical Management

Treatment depends on the location and staging of the malignant tumor. Stage I oral cancers are treated by surgery or radiation. Stage II and III cancers require surgery and radiation. Chemotherapy also may be used when surgery and radiation therapy fail or as the initial therapy for smaller tumors. Treatment for stage IV cancer may include all three treatment modalities, or treatment may be palliative if metastasis is extensive. The 5-year survival rate for patients with oral cancers that have metastasized depends on the degree of metastasis. For lip cancer the 5-year survival rate is 60% for regional metastasis and 28% for distal metastasis. The 5-year survival rate for cancer of the tongue is 68% for regional metastasis and 39% for distal metastasis. If the cancer is in the floor of the mouth, the 5-year survival rate is 38% for regional metastasis and 20% for distal metastasis (ACS, 2021h).

Small, accessible tumors can be excised surgically. Surgical options include a glossectomy, removal of the tongue; hemiglossectomy, removal of part of the tongue; mandibulectomy, removal of the mandible; and total or supraglottic laryngectomy, removal of the entire larynx or the portion above the true vocal cords.

Large tumors usually require more extensive and traumatic surgery. In a functional neck dissection of neck cancer with no growth in the lymph nodes, the surgeon removes the lymph nodes but preserves the jugular vein, the sternocleidomastoid muscle, and the spinal accessory nerve. In radical neck dissection, all these structures are removed, and reconstructive surgery is necessary after tissue resection. Patients may have drains in the incision sites that are connected to suction to aid healing and reduce hematomas. A tracheostomy also may be performed, depending on the degree of tumor invasion.

Because of the location of the surgery, complications can occur. These include airway obstruction, hemorrhage, tracheal aspiration, facial edema, formation of fistulas (abnormal passages connecting internal organs, or to the surface of the body), and necrosis of the skin flaps. If the patient has difficulty swallowing, a percutaneous endoscopic gastrostomy (PEG) tube may be inserted to allow for adequate nutritional intake. Neurologic complications can occur because of nerves being severed and manipulated during surgery.

Radiation therapy may involve (1) external radiation beam radiation therapy or (2) internal radiation by means of needles or seeds. The purpose of radiation therapy is to shrink the tumor. It can be given preoperatively or postoperatively, depending on the health care provider's preference and the patient's disease process. In more advanced cases, chemotherapy may be combined with radiation postoperatively to make the patient more comfortable. Other treatment options include laser excision.

Nursing Interventions and Patient Teaching

A holistic approach to patient care includes awareness of the patient's level of knowledge regarding the disease, emotional response and coping abilities, and spiritual needs. Nursing interventions must be individualized to the patient—beginning with the preoperative stage, continuing through the postoperative stage, and ending after the patient's rehabilitation in the home environment. Family members, hospice workers, close friends, social workers, and pastoral care staff may provide information and support during this potentially fatal disease.

Patient problems and interventions for the patient with oral cancer include but are not limited to the following:

Patient Problem	Nursing Interventions
Distorted Body Image and Impaired Personal Sense of Identity, related to: • Disfiguring appearance of an oral lesion • Reconstructive surgery	Provide alternative methods for communication if radiation therapy results in dysarthria (difficult, poorly articulated speech, resulting from interference in the control over muscles of speech) Provide information to the patient and family to help with difficult decisions related to surgery, radiation, or chemotherapy Provide support to the patient and family

Modified From Ackley BJ, Ladwig GB: *Nursing diagnosis handbook: An evidence-based guide to planning care*, ed 12, St. Louis, 2020, Mosby.

Prevention is the key to successful treatment or cure for cancer of the oral cavity and should include education on avoiding excess exposure to sun and wind on the lips, eliminating smoking or chewing tobacco, eliminating plaque and caries through good oral and dental care, and decreasing the intake of excessive amounts of alcohol. Individuals infected with HPV also should be

monitored for the development of oral cavity cancer. Early detection of oral cancer can increase the patient's chance of survival. Any person with a mouth lesion that does not heal within 2 to 3 weeks is urged to seek medical care.

Provide instruction regarding preoperative and postoperative care, with full explanations regarding potential speech loss and alternative methods of nutritional intake if warranted by the extent of cancer or anticipated surgical procedure. Explanation of tracheostomy care and other tubes the patient may have on discharge helps reduce anxiety and increases the patient's sense of control over the situation.

Prognosis

Staging and biological characterization of the neoplasm provide prognostic information. The prognosis of carcinoma in the oral cavity is related directly to the size of the primary tumor, the involvement of regional lymph nodes, and the presence or absence of metastasis. The patient's immunologic response and general condition also influence the prognosis and the choice of therapy.

Carcinomas of the lip generally can be detected early by the patient, the health care provider, or the dentist during examination, and the prognosis for cure is good. If the carcinoma is difficult to detect, as on the anterior tongue and the floor of the mouth, it is often in a more advanced stage when detected, making the prognosis poor.

DISORDERS OF THE ESOPHAGUS

GASTROESOPHAGEAL REFLUX DISEASE

Etiology and Pathophysiology

GERD is a backward flow of stomach acid up into the esophagus. Symptoms typically include burning and pressure behind the sternum, often described by patients as heartburn. Most cases are thought to be caused by the inappropriate relaxation of the lower esophageal sphincter (LES) in response to an unknown stimulus. Symptoms of GERD develop when the LES is weak or experiences prolonged or frequent transient relaxation, conditions that allow gastric acids and enzymes to flow into the esophagus. Reflux is much more common in the postprandial state (after meals) because this position allows more reflux of gastric juices when the LES is relaxed. GERD occurs in all age groups and is one of the most common upper GI problems seen in adults.

Clinical Manifestations

The clinical manifestations of GERD are consistent but vary substantially in severity. The irritation of chronic reflux produces the primary symptom, which is heartburn (*pyrosis*). Heartburn often is described as a substernal or retrosternal burning sensation that tends to radiate upward and may involve the neck, the jaw, or the back. Heartburn usually is experienced after eating.

An atypical pain pattern that closely mimics angina also may occur and must be differentiated carefully from true cardiac disease. The second major symptom of GERD is regurgitation. The individual experiences a feeling of warm fluid moving up the throat and may experience a sour taste in the mouth. Symptoms also may include a dry cough, a feeling of a lump in the throat, dysphagia, and hoarseness or a sore throat (Mayo Clinic, 2020a).

GERD can produce symptoms such as dysphagia or odynophagia (painful swallowing), dry cough, hoarseness, and a sore throat. Eructation (belching) and a feeling of flatulence are other common complaints. The frequency and severity of reflux episodes usually determine the severity of the symptoms.

Assessment

Subjective data include heartburn, a substernal or retrosternal burning sensation that may radiate to the back or jaw (in some cases the pain may mimic angina), and regurgitation, which causes a sour or bitter taste in the pharynx. Frequent eructation, flatulence, and dysphagia or odynophagia usually occurs only in severe cases.

Objective data include nocturnal cough, wheezing, and hoarseness.

Diagnostic Tests

When a mild case of GERD is suspected, treatment is initiated on the basis of the presumptive diagnosis. More involved cases may require other screening tools, such as an esophageal pH test. In this test the patient is fitted with a small NG tube that remains in place and is connected to a small computer that may be worn on the belt or on a shoulder strap. The probe, in the esophagus, monitors acid levels for 24 to 48 hours. An esophageal motility test and Bernstein test can be performed in conjunction with pH monitoring to evaluate LES competence and the response of the esophagus to acid infusion. The barium swallow with fluoroscopy is used widely to document the presence of hiatal hernia. Endoscopy is performed routinely to evaluate for LES competence, potential scarring and strictures, the presence and severity of esophagitis, and to rule out malignancy (Cleveland Clinic, 2019).

Medical Management

In its simplest form, GERD produces mild symptoms that occur infrequently (twice a week or less). In these cases, encouraging the patient to avoid problem foods or beverages, stopping smoking, elevating the head of the bed, or losing weight may solve the problem. Medication therapy for GERD focuses on improving LES function, increasing esophageal clearance, decreasing volume and acidity of reflux, and protecting the esophageal mucosa. Treatment with antacids or acid-blocking medications called H_2 receptor antagonists—such as cimetidine, ranitidine, famotidine, or nizatidine—also may be used. More severe and

frequent episodes of GERD can trigger asthma attacks, cause severe chest pain, result in bleeding, or promote a narrowing (stricture) or chronic irritation of the esophagus. In these cases, more powerful inhibitors of stomach acid production called proton pump inhibitors (PPIs), such as omeprazole, esomeprazole, pantoprazole, rabeprazole, and lansoprazole, may be added to the treatment prescribed. Sucralfate is an antiulcer drug that may be used in patients with GERD for its protective properties by forming a complex that adheres to an ulcer. Metoclopramide is used in moderate to severe cases of GERD. It is in a class of drugs called *promotility agents,* which increase peristalsis and therefore promote gastric emptying and reduce the risk of gastric acid reflux.

If conventional treatments fail, the health care provider may suggest a surgical procedure to treat the condition. *Nissen fundoplication* is a surgical procedure that can be performed to strengthen the sphincter. The procedure involves wrapping a layer of the upper stomach wall (fundus) around the sphincter and terminal esophagus to lessen the possibility of acid reflux (see Fig. 5.14). Surgery also may be performed to create a barrier that will prevent the backup of gastric acid. A device called an *EsophyX* folds the tissue at the base of the stomach, acting as a sphincter valve. Another surgical approach is the *Stretta procedure.* This procedure uses electrodes to heat the tissue in the esophagus to create scar tissue that strengthens the esophagus. The *LINX* is another surgical device that is used to treat GERD; it consists of a band of titanium beads with magnetic cores that, when implanted around the LES, strengthens it by closing the sphincter when necessary. If GERD is left untreated, serious pathologic (precancerous) changes in the esophageal lining may develop—a condition called *Barrett esophagus* (esophageal metaplasia). In Barrett esophagus the normal squamous epithelium of the esophagus is replaced by columnar epithelium. Because patients with Barrett esophagus are at higher risk for esophageal cancer, they may need to be monitored regularly (every 6 to 12 months) by endoscopy and biopsy (Mayo Clinic, 2020d).

Nursing Interventions and Patient Teaching

Nursing interventions involve educating the patient about diet and lifestyle modifications that may alleviate symptoms of GERD.

Dietary instructions include the following: (1) eat four to six small meals daily; (2) follow a low-fat, adequate-protein diet; (3) reduce intake of chocolate, tea, and other foods and beverages that contain caffeine; (4) limit or eliminate alcohol intake; (5) eat slowly, and chew food thoroughly; (6) avoid evening snacking, and do not eat for 2 to 3 hours before bedtime; (7) remain upright for 1 to 2 hours after meals when possible, and never eat in bed; (8) avoid any food that directly produces heartburn; and (9) reduce overall body weight if needed.

Numerous lifestyle changes also are indicated in the treatment of GERD. Patients who smoke should be encouraged to stop. Cigarette smoking has been associated with decreased acid clearance from the lower esophagus. Advise patients to avoid constrictive clothing over the abdomen and avoid activities that involve straining, heavy lifting, or working in a bent-over position. Also, patients should be instructed never to sleep flat in bed. They should elevate the head of the bed at least 6 to 8 inches for sleep, using wooden blocks or a thick foam wedge.

Prognosis

If GERD is not controlled successfully, it can progress to serious and even life-threatening problems. Esophageal ulceration and hemorrhage may result from severe erosion, and chronic nighttime reflux is accompanied by a significant risk of aspiration. Adenocarcinoma can develop from the premalignant tissue (termed *Barrett esophagus*). Gradual or repeated scarring can permanently damage esophageal tissue and produce strictures (NLM, 2020b).

CARCINOMA OF THE ESOPHAGUS

Etiology and Pathophysiology

Carcinoma of the esophagus is a malignant epithelial neoplasm that has invaded the esophagus and has been diagnosed as a squamous cell carcinoma or an adenocarcinoma. In 2017, 16,940 new esophageal cancer cases were diagnosed, 13,360 in men and 3580 in women. Recent statistics reveal that about 15,690 deaths from esophageal cancer occur with 12,720 in men and 2970 in women. Risk factors for esophageal cancer include alcohol and tobacco use, acid reflux, and obesity. Environmental carcinogens, nutritional deficiencies, chronic irritation, and mucosal damage also have been considered as causes of esophageal cancer. Another risk factor is Barrett esophagus. The longer a person has Barrett esophagus, the greater the chance that it will progress to esophageal adenocarcinoma (ACS, 2021g) (see Health Promotion box on prevention or early detection of esophageal cancer).

🏃 Health Promotion

Prevention or Early Detection of Esophageal Cancer

- Patients with diagnosed gastroesophageal reflux disease and hiatal hernia need counseling regarding regular follow-up evaluation.
- Health teaching should focus on elimination of smoking and excessive alcohol intake.
- Maintenance of good oral hygiene and dietary habits (intake of fresh fruits and vegetables) may be helpful.
- Patients diagnosed with Barrett esophagus must be monitored because this is considered a premalignant condition. Regular endoscopic screening with biopsy is required.
- Encourage patients to seek medical attention for any esophageal problems, especially dysphagia.

Unfortunately, early esophageal cancer typically has no symptoms, making early diagnosis difficult. The stage of esophageal cancer greatly affects the 5-year survival rate. The overall 5-year survival rate for a person with a localized cancer of the esophagus is approximately 40%; regional metastasis is approximately 20%; and distant metastasis is 4%. Less than 15% of all cases of esophageal cancer occur before the age of 55, and it is more prevalent in men (ACS, 2021g).

Clinical Manifestations

The most common clinical symptom is progressive dysphagia over a 6-month period. The patient may have a substernal feeling, as though food is not passing through the esophagus.

Assessment

Collection of subjective data includes noting that initially the patient may have difficulty swallowing when eating bulky foods such as meat; later the difficulty occurs with soft foods and finally with liquids and even saliva. Another symptom is odynophagia (painful swallowing). Pain is a late symptom and indicates local extension of the malignancy. Additional subjective symptoms include chest pain, pressure, or burning; indigestion; heartburn; and fatigue.

Collection of objective data includes observing the patient for regurgitation (backward flowing or casting up of undigested food), vomiting, hoarseness, chronic cough, choking, and iron deficiency anemia. Weight loss may be related directly to the cancer or to the difficulty in swallowing. Hemorrhage may occur if the cancer erodes through the esophagus. Esophageal perforation may result in the formation of a tracheoesophageal fistula (an abnormal passage between two internal organs), causing the patient to cough when swallowing anything, including saliva. Esophageal tumors may enlarge enough to cause esophageal obstruction, causing increased dysphagia. The cancer spreads via the lymph system; the liver and lung are common sites of metastasis.

Diagnostic Tests

A barium swallow examination with fluoroscopy and endoscopy is used to detect esophageal cancer. An endoscopy with biopsy and cytologic examination provides a highly accurate diagnosis. Endoscopic ultrasonography is an important tool used to stage esophageal cancer. CT, positron emission tomography (PET), and MRI also are used to assess the extent of the disease.

Medical Management

The treatment of esophageal cancer depends on the tumor's location and whether invasion or metastasis has occurred. Tumor staging must be determined to guide patient management. For esophageal cancer that has not metastasized, a wide excision removing the tumor and enough surrounding tissue to leave cancer-free margins may be effective. For more advanced cases an esophagectomy may be necessary. If the cancer has spread from the esophagus to the stomach, an esophagogastrectomy is performed. A description of these surgeries is described below (Mayo Clinic, 2020c).

Radiation therapy may be curative or palliative. Problems associated with radiation therapy include the development of a tracheoesophageal fistula and burning. The burning that occurs may result in sunburned-like skin when external radiation is used, or damage to nearby organs such as the lungs and heart if internal radiation therapy is used. Aspiration from the fistula and edema from the radiation are common as well. Chemotherapeutic agents such as cisplatin, paclitaxel (Taxol), and fluorouracil (5-FU) are used currently, as well as other chemotherapy agents, in combination with radiation before and/or after surgery (ACS, n.d.). Because of the extreme toxicity of these drugs, expect the patient to experience side effects of respiratory and liver dysfunction, nausea and vomiting, leukopenia, and sepsis. If the tumor is in the upper third of the esophagus, radiation is indicated. A tumor in the lower third usually is resected surgically.

The following four types of surgical procedures can be performed:

1. *Esophagogastrectomy:* Resection of a lower esophageal section with a proximal portion of the stomach, followed by anastomosis (surgical joining of two ducts, blood vessels, or bowel segments to allow flow from one to the other) of the remaining portions of the esophagus and stomach. Surrounding lymph nodes also are removed.
2. *Esophagogastrostomy* or *esophagectomy:* Resection of a portion of the esophagus with anastomosis to the stomach. Surrounding lymph nodes also are removed.
3. *Esophagoenterostomy:* Resection of the esophagus and anastomosis to a portion of the small intestine. Surrounding lymph nodes also are removed.
4. *Gastrostomy:* Insertion of a catheter into the stomach and suture to the abdominal wall; performed when the patient cannot take food orally because inoperable cancer of the esophagus interferes with swallowing

Nursing Interventions and Patient Teaching

Patient problems and nursing interventions for the patient with esophageal carcinoma include but are not limited to the following:

Patient Problem	Nursing Interventions
Inability to Maintain Adequate Breathing Pattern, related to: • Incisional pain • Proximity of incision to diaphragm	Monitor respirations carefully because of proximity of incision to diaphragm and patient's difficulty in carrying out breathing exercises
Insufficient Nutrition, related to: • Dysphagia • Decreased stomach capacity • Anorexia	Monitor intake and output and daily weights to determine adequate nutritional intake Assess which foods patient can and cannot swallow to select and prepare edible foods Administer tube feedings through gastrostomy, if present

Discuss with the patient and family all aspects of care, including surgery, radiation, and chemotherapy. Psychological adjustment of the patient who cannot ingest food orally, whether temporary or permanent, is difficult. Thorough explanations of all diagnostic tests, medications, procedures, and the treatment plan help relieve the patient's anxiety. Give support to the patient with this serious diagnosis by allowing time for questions.

Prognosis

In carcinoma of the esophagus, the disease is often well advanced by the time symptoms appear. The delay between the onset of early symptoms and when the patient seeks medical advice may be extensive. High mortality rates among these patients are affected by the following issues: (1) the patient is generally older; (2) the tumor usually has invaded surrounding structures by the time diagnosis is made; (3) the malignancy tends to spread to nearby lymph nodes; and (4) the esophagus is close to the heart and lungs, making these organs accessible to tumor extension.

The esophagus has an extensive lymphatic network, which facilitates the rapid spread of malignant cells to various local and distant sites. As discussed earlier in this section, the stage of the disease when diagnosed directly affects the survival rate.

Collection of objective data includes observing for premalignant lesions, including leukoplakia. Unusual bleeding in the mouth, some blood-tinged sputum, lumps or edema in the neck, and hoarseness may be observed.

ACHALASIA

Etiology and Pathophysiology

Achalasia, also called *cardiospasm*, is an abnormal condition characterized by the inability of a muscle to relax, particularly the cardiac sphincter of the stomach. Although the cause is unknown, nerve degeneration, esophageal dilation, and hypertrophy are thought to contribute to the disruption of the esophagus's normal neuromuscular activity. This results in decreased motility and dilation of the lower portion of the esophagus, along with an absence of peristalsis. Thus little or no food can enter the stomach, and in extreme cases the dilated portion of the esophagus holds as much as a liter or more of fluid. This disease may occur in people of any age but is more prevalent in middle-aged to older adults (NLM, 2019b).

Clinical Manifestations

The primary symptom of achalasia is dysphagia. The patient has a sensation of food sticking in the lower portion of the esophagus. As the condition progresses, the patient complains of regurgitation of food, which relieves prolonged distention of the esophagus. The patient also may have substernal chest pain.

Assessment

Observe for loss of weight, poor skin turgor, and weakness.

Diagnostic Tests

Radiologic studies show esophageal dilation above the narrowing at the cardioesophageal junction. The diagnosis is confirmed by manometry, which shows the absence of primary peristalsis. Esophagoscopy also is used to confirm the diagnosis.

Medical Management

Conservative treatment of achalasia includes drug therapy and forceful dilation of the narrowed area of the esophagus. Anticholinergics, nitrates, and calcium channel blockers reduce pressure in the LES.

Dilation is done by first emptying the esophagus. Then a dilator with a deflated balloon is passed down to the sphincter. The balloon is inflated and remains so for 1 minute; it may have to be reinflated once or twice.

The preferred surgical approach is a cardiomyotomy. The muscular layer is incised longitudinally down to but not through the mucosa. Two-thirds of the incision is in the esophagus, and the remaining one-third is in the stomach; this permits the mucosa to expand so that food can pass easily into the stomach.

Nursing Interventions and Patient Teaching

Nursing interventions for esophageal surgery are presented in Box 5.2.

A patient problem and interventions for the patient with achalasia include but are not limited to the following:

Discuss home care and follow-up care in preparation for dismissal. Include a family member or support

Patient Problem	Nursing Interventions
Insufficient Nutrition, related to difficulty swallowing both liquids and solids	Encourage fluids with meals to increase lower esophageal sphincter pressure and to push food into stomach. Monitor liquid diet for 24 h after dilation procedure

person if possible and involve the patient as an active participant in the planning. Explain the need to eat high-calorie, high-protein foods, and provide printed

---

Box 5.2   Nursing Interventions for the Patient Experiencing Esophageal Surgery

PREOPERATIVE NURSING INTERVENTIONS
1. Encourage improved nutritional status.
   a. Offer a high-protein, high-calorie diet if oral diet is possible.
   b. Total parenteral nutrition may be necessary for severe dysphagia or obstruction.
   c. Gastroscopy tube feedings may be indicated.
2. Give meticulous oral hygiene; breath may be malodorous.
3. Give preoperative preparation appropriate for thoracic surgery.
4. Give prescribed antibiotics before esophageal resection or bypass, as ordered.

POSTOPERATIVE NURSING INTERVENTIONS
1. Promote good pulmonary ventilation.
2. Maintain chest drainage system as prescribed.
3. Maintain gastric drainage system.
   a. Small amounts of blood may drain from nasogastric tube for 6–12 h after surgery.
   b. Do not disturb nasogastric tube (to prevent traction on suture line).
4. Maintain nutrition.
   a. Start clear fluids at frequent intervals when oral intake is permitted.
   b. Introduce soft foods gradually, increasing to several small meals of bland foods.
   c. Have patient maintain semi-Fowler's position for 2 h after eating and while sleeping if heartburn (pyrosis) occurs.

---

material in support of such a diet. Explain the need to sleep with the head elevated and to avoid bending over and stooping. Discuss medications if prescribed (including name, dose, time of administration, purpose, and side effects). Discuss ways to avoid constipation by eating high-fiber foods (if tolerated) and natural laxatives. Explain the importance of follow-up care with the health care provider. Finally, discuss symptoms of recurrence or progression of disease and the need to report these to the health care provider.

PROGNOSIS

Surgical separation, in addition to bag dilation, permits the return of normal peristalsis in approximately 10% of patients with achalasia.

DISORDERS OF THE STOMACH

GASTRITIS (ACUTE)

Etiology and Pathophysiology

Gastritis is an inflammation of the lining of the stomach. Acute gastritis is a temporary inflammation associated with alcoholism, smoking, and stressful physical problems, such as burns; major surgery; food allergens; viral, bacterial, or chemical toxins; chemotherapy; or radiation therapy. Changes in the mucosal lining from gastritis damages the cells that secrete acid and pepsin. Acute gastritis is often a single incident that resolves when the offending agent is removed.

Clinical Manifestations

If the condition is acute, the patient may experience fever, epigastric pain, nausea, vomiting, headache, coating of the tongue, and loss of appetite. If the condition results from ingestion of contaminated food, the intestines are usually affected, and diarrhea may occur. Some patients with gastritis have no symptoms.

Assessment

Collection of subjective data includes observing for anorexia, nausea, discomfort after eating, and pain.

Collection of objective data includes observing for vomiting, hematemesis (vomiting blood), and melena caused by gastric bleeding.

Diagnostic Tests

Diagnosis is based on testing the stools for occult blood, noting white blood cell (WBC) differential increases related to certain bacteria, evaluating serum electrolytes, and observing for elevated hematocrit related to dehydration.

Medical Management

If medical treatment is required, an antiemetic—such as prochlorperazine, promethazine, or trimethobenzamide—may be prescribed. Antacids and cimetidine or ranitidine may be given in combination. Antibiotics are given if the cause is a bacterial agent. IV fluids are used to correct fluid and electrolyte imbalances. Patients who experience GI bleeding from hemorrhagic gastritis require fluid and blood replacement and NG lavage.

Nursing Interventions and Patient Teaching

Monitor and record the patient's I&O. Withhold oral foods and fluids as prescribed until signs and symptoms of gastritis subside. Monitor tolerance to oral feedings and administer IV feedings as prescribed. Clear liquids are increased to a diet as tolerated when the patient's symptoms improve.

A patient problem and interventions for the patient with gastritis include but are not limited to the following:

Patient Problem	Nursing Interventions
Inadequate Fluid Volume, related to vomiting, diarrhea, and blood loss	Keep patient nothing by mouth or on restricted food and fluids as ordered, and advance as tolerated
	Monitor laboratory data for fluid and electrolyte imbalance (potassium, magnesium, sodium, and chloride)
	Maintain intravenous feedings
	Record intake and output

Patient education includes explanations of (1) the effects of stress on the mucosal lining of the stomach; (2) how salicylates, nonsteroidal anti-inflammatory drugs (NSAIDs), and particular foods may be irritating; and (3) how lifestyles that include alcohol and tobacco may be harmful. Assist the patient in locating self-help groups in the community to deal with these behaviors.

Prognosis

Because of the many classifications and causes of gastritis, prognosis is variable. In general, the prognosis is good for individuals who are willing to change their lifestyles and follow a medical regimen.

PEPTIC ULCER DISEASE

Etiology and Pathophysiology

Peptic ulcers are ulcerations of the mucous membrane or deeper structures of the GI tract. They most commonly occur in the stomach (*gastric ulcer*) and duodenum (*duodenal ulcer*). The term *peptic ulcer* refers to acid in the digestive tract eroding the mucosal lining of the stomach, esophagus, or duodenum.

The stomach normally is protected from autodigestion by the gastric mucosal barrier. The GI tract has a high cell turnover rate, and the stomach's surface mucosa is renewed about every 3 days. As a result, the mucosa continuously repairs itself except in extreme instances when cell breakdown surpasses the cell renewal rate. In such cases, peptic ulcers can occur. The most common causes of peptic ulcer disease include the presence of *H. pylori* bacteria in the stomach, regularly taking NSAIDs, smoking or chewing tobacco, and excessive alcohol intake.

Understanding of the factors that contribute to ulcer formation is developing rapidly. The 30% to 50% of the people in the United States have the bacteria in their stomachs. The incidence of *H. pylori* has dramatically decreased in the United States. *H. pylori* has been identified in 14% to 17% of patients with gastric ulcers and 21% to 25% of those with duodenal ulcers. In the United States, only about 10% of the population have *H. pylori* (Saltzman, 2020).

Stress ulcers develop as the result of physiologic trauma to the body. Examples of patients who develop stress ulcers include patients with burns, sepsis, or those who have prolonged stays in the hospital or intensive care units. A stress ulcer is a form of erosive gastritis. It is believed that the gastric mucosa of the stomach undergoes a period of transient ischemia in association with hypotension, severe injury, extensive burns, and complicated surgery. The ischemia is due to decreased capillary blood flow as blood is shunted away from the GI tract, so blood flow bypasses the gastric mucosa. This occurs as a compensatory mechanism in hypotension or shock. The decrease in blood flow produces an imbalance between the destructive properties of hydrochloric acid and pepsin and protective factors of the stomach's mucosal barrier, especially in the fundus portion. Multiple superficial erosions result, and these may bleed. Because of the possibility of development of physiologic stress ulcers and high morbidity, patients at risk receive prophylaxis with anti-secretory agents, including H_2 receptor blockers and PPIs.

Clinical Manifestations
Gastric and duodenal ulcers may have similar symptoms but may differ in timing, degree, or factors that worsen or alleviate the symptoms. Pain is the characteristic symptom and is described as dull, burning, or gnawing; it is located in the epigastric region.

Assessment
Collection of subjective data requires awareness that in patients with gastric ulcers, the pain is associated closely with food intake and usually does not awaken the patient at night. With duodenal ulcers the patient often complains of pain 1 to 2 hours after eating. Nausea, weight loss, eructation (belching), and distention are also common complaints made by patients with PUD. Upset stomach and other vague GI complaints are referred to as dyspepsia.

Collection of objective data includes observing for signs of complications of PUD. Hemorrhage is a potential complication.

- *Hematemesis and melena:* When GI bleeding occurs, one sign is the vomiting of blood (hematemesis) that is either bright red or has a "coffee grounds" appearance resulting from the action of the gastric acid on hemoglobin. The patient may produce melena (stool that is black and tarry with undigested blood), which occurs when the blood passes through the digestive tract. Salicylates and alcohol aggravate bleeding in patients with a history of peptic ulcers.
- *Hemorrhage:* Bleeding from a gastric ulcer can worsen quickly into an emergency situation if erosion is extensive. Hemorrhage, with accompanying symptoms of shock, occurs when the ulcer erodes into a blood vessel. Surgical intervention is indicated if the patient remains unstable after receiving blood over several hours.
- *Perforation:* Perforation occurs when the ulcer crater penetrates the entire thickness of the wall of the stomach or duodenum. The release of air, gastric acid, pancreatic enzymes, or bile into the peritoneal cavity causes pain, emesis, fever, hypotension, and hematemesis. Perforation is considered the most lethal complication of peptic ulcer. Bacterial peritonitis may occur within hours. The severity of the peritonitis is proportional to the amount and duration of the spillage through the perforation.
- *Gastric outlet obstruction:* Gastric outlet obstruction is a complication of benign peptic ulcer disease. It is a blockage, located close to the pylorus (the part of the stomach that connects to the duodenum) and is caused by acute inflammation or edema. The most common symptom is vomiting undigested food. Symptoms may be relieved by constant NG aspiration of stomach contents due to the inability for digestion to occur. This also helps relieve edema and inflammation of the pylorus. Medications to treat inflammation of the pylorus may be administered intravenously. If conservative treatment is not successful, surgery may be warranted to address the stenosis.

Diagnostic Tests
Fiberoptic endoscopy can detect gastric and duodenal ulcers. This is called *esophagogastroduodenoscopy (EGD)*. Fiberoptic endoscopy is more reliable than barium contrast studies because of the maneuverability of fiberoptic scopes and direct visualization of the entire esophagus and gastric and duodenal mucosa. This procedure also can be used to determine the degree of ulcer healing after treatment. During endoscopy, specimens can be obtained for identification of *H. pylori* or tissue specimens for biopsy. The patient is sedated but remains conscious throughout the endoscopy procedure. Local anesthetics in the throat are used to decrease the gag reflex and minimize pain during the procedure. No liquids or food are allowed after the procedure until the patient's gag reflex returns.

A noninvasive test used for diagnostic purposes is a breath test to detect *H. pylori*. The test calls for the patient to drink a solution containing carbon-13–enriched urea, a natural, nonradioactive substance. If *H. pylori* infection is present, it breaks down the compound and releases carbon-13 dioxide ($^{13}CO_2$). Thirty minutes after drinking the solution, the patient exhales into a collection bag, which is sent to the manufacturer for analysis. A finding of $^{13}CO_2$ confirms *H. pylori* infection. The test may prove especially useful in determining whether antibiotic therapy eradicated an *H. pylori* infection. A fecal assay antigen test for *H. pylori* is another test that is especially useful to determine eradication of the bacteria after antibiotic treatment. An additional noninvasive way to confirm *H. pylori* infection is a serum or whole blood antibody test, in particular, immunoglobulin G. This test is approximately 90% to 95% sensitive for *H. pylori* infection but cannot distinguish active from recently treated disease (Johns Hopkins Medicine, n.d.b).

Barium contrast studies (UGI) are not as accurate as endoscopy, especially for small lesions, but still are used occasionally. Testing of feces for occult blood in the intestinal tract also is used for diagnosis.

Medical Management
The health care provider may order insertion of an NG tube to remove gastric contents and blood. Surgery usually is indicated for complications of perforation, penetration, or obstruction, or for PUD that is no longer responding to medical management.

Scar tissue builds up with repeat episodes of ulceration and healing, causing obstruction, particularly at the pylorus. The patient may experience gastric dilation, vomiting, and distention. When fluid and electrolyte balance is achieved, surgical intervention is possible.

The primary treatment for peptic ulcers is to reduce signs and symptoms by decreasing or neutralizing normal gastric acidity with drug therapy. The types of drugs most commonly used include the following (Table 5.1):

• *Antacids:* Neutralize or reduce the acidity of stomach contents (e.g., magnesium hydroxide, aluminum hydroxide, calcium carbonate, and magaldrate).

• *Antisecretory and cytoprotective agent:* Inhibits gastric acid secretion and protects gastric mucosa (misoprostol). Misoprostol is approved in the United States for the prevention of gastric ulcers induced by NSAIDs and aspirin (NLM, 2017).

• *Histamine receptor blockers:* Decrease acid secretions by blocking histamine (H_2) receptors (e.g., cimetidine, ranitidine, famotidine, and nizatidine). Do not give within 2 hours of antacids.

• *Mucosal healing agent:* Heals ulcers without antisecretory properties. Sucralfate is a cytoprotective drug. It accelerates ulcer healing, presumably

Table 5.1   Medications for Gastrointestinal Disorders

GENERIC NAME (TRADE NAME)	ACTION	SIDE EFFECTS	NURSING IMPLICATIONS
Antacids, e.g., aluminum, calcium, magnesium salts, and sodium bicarbonate	Neutralizes gastric acid; aluminum and calcium antacids also bind phosphates in patients with renal failure	Aluminum: Constipation, hypophosphatemia Calcium: Constipation, rebound hyperacidity, hypercalcemia Magnesium: Diarrhea, hypermagnesemia Sodium bicarbonate: Sodium and water retention, alkalosis, rebound hyperacidity	Monitor serum electrolytes with long-term use; do not give antacid simultaneously with other medications because absorption of the other medication may be affected; best to separate administration by 2 h; magnesium salts are contraindicated in patients with renal disease
Antispasmodics, including atropine, scopolamine, hyoscyamine, dicyclomine, clidinium	Anticholinergic agents that decrease GI motility by relaxing GI smooth muscle	Dry mouth and skin, constipation, paralytic ileus, urinary retention, tachycardia, drowsiness, dizziness, confusion, altered vision	Avoid using other CNS depressants or alcohol at the same time; avoid driving or other potentially hazardous tasks until accustomed to sedating effects
bismuth subsalicylate	Antidiarrheal agent; also used in peptic ulcer disease caused by *Helicobacter pylori*	Fecal impaction, tinnitus	May turn stools dark gray to black; avoid use with aspirin; consult health care provider if diarrhea is accompanied by high fever or lasts more than 2 days
cimetidine	H_2 receptor antagonist; inhibits gastric acid secretion	Confusion, headache, gynecomastia, bone marrow suppression (rare)	Increases serum levels and clinical effects of oral anticoagulants, theophylline, phenytoin, some benzodiazepines, and propranolol (these medications may require dosage reduction)
dimenhydrinate	Antiemetic agent; blocks central vomiting center	Drowsiness, dry mouth, constipation	Avoid use with other CNS depressants and alcohol; avoid driving or other hazardous activities until accustomed to sedating effects
diphenoxylate with atropine	Antidiarrheal agent (diphenoxylate: narcotic; atropine: anticholinergic)	Drowsiness, sedation, constipation, dry mouth, urinary retention	Avoid use with other CNS depressants and alcohol; avoid driving or other hazardous activities until accustomed to sedating effects; do not use in infectious diarrhea
famotidine	H_2 receptor antagonist; inhibits gastric acid secretion	Headache, dizziness, constipation, thrombocytopenia (rare)	Unlike cimetidine, does not affect serum levels of hepatically metabolized drugs (warfarin, phenytoin, theophylline)

Table 5.1 **Medications for Gastrointestinal Disorders—cont'd**

GENERIC NAME (TRADE NAME)	ACTION	SIDE EFFECTS	NURSING IMPLICATIONS
kaolin-pectin	Antidiarrheal agent	Constipation	Shake well before using
ketoconazole	Antifungal agent	Gynecomastia, impotence, hepatotoxicity, abdominal pain	Requires acid environment for absorption; do not use with antacids, H_2 receptor blockers, or omeprazole; do not use with loratadine (has caused dysrhythmias and death); monitor liver function tests often; monitor serum levels and clinical effects of warfarin, cyclosporine, and theophylline
lansoprazole	Binds to an enzyme in the presence of acid gastric pH, preventing the final transport of hydrogen ions into the gastric lumen	Drowsiness, abdominal pain, diarrhea, nausea	Sucralfate decreases absorption of lansoprazole (take 30 min before sucralfate); administer before meals. Assess patient routinely for epigastric or abdominal pain. May cause abnormal liver function test results
loperamide	Antidiarrheal agent	Drowsiness, dry mouth, constipation	Monitor for dehydration; do not use in infectious diarrhea
mesalamine	GI anti-inflammatory agent	Abdominal cramps and gas, rash, headache, dizziness	Swallow tablets whole; give enema at bedtime, retain 10–15 min
misoprostol	Prostaglandin analog that acts as gastric mucosal protectant against NSAID-induced ulcers	Diarrhea, nausea, vomiting, flatulence, uterine cramping	Absolutely contraindicated in pregnant women; women of childbearing age must use reliable contraception
nizatidine	H_2 receptor antagonist, inhibits gastric acid secretion	Drowsiness, headache, dizziness, sweating, thrombocytopenia (rare)	Does not affect serum levels of hepatically metabolized drugs (warfarin, phenytoin, theophylline)
nystatin	Antifungal agent, available as oral suspension and topical product	*Oral:* Nausea, vomiting, diarrhea *Topical:* Local irritation	Long-term therapy may be needed to clear infection; use for entire course
olsalazine	GI anti-inflammatory agent	Diarrhea, abdominal pain and cramps, nausea, allergic reactions, arthralgia, rash, anaphylaxis	Take with food; notify health care provider if severe diarrhea occurs
	Proton pump inhibitor; totally eradicates gastric acid production	Headache, dizziness, abdominal pain, nausea, vomiting, rare bone marrow suppression	Inhibits hepatic metabolism of warfarin, phenytoin, benzodiazepines, and other drugs metabolized by liver; do not crush or chew capsule contents
	H_2 receptor antagonist; inhibits gastric acid secretion	Headache, abdominal discomfort; granulocytopenia and thrombocytopenia (both rare)	Minimal effect on serum levels of hepatically metabolized drugs (phenytoin, warfarin, theophylline)
sucralfate	Gastric mucosal protectant agent; adheres to site of ulcer	Constipation, hypophosphatemia	Do not give with other drugs; coating action may interfere with the absorption of other drugs—separate by 2 h
sulfasalazine	GI anti-inflammatory agent	Nausea, vomiting, abdominal pain, photosensitivity, rash, Stevens-Johnson syndrome (rare), renal failure, bone marrow suppression (rare), allergic reactions, anaphylaxis	Ensure adequate hydration to prevent crystallization in kidneys; avoid exposure to sunlight; women taking oral contraceptives need to use alternative methods because of decreased effectiveness of oral contraceptives; monitor CBC and renal function; take with meals

CBC, Complete blood count; *CNS,* central nervous system; *GI,* gastrointestinal; *NSAID,* nonsteroidal anti-inflammatory drug.
Data from Skidmore-Roth L: *Mosby's 2021 nursing drug reference,* ed 34, St. Louis, 2020, Elsevier.

because of the formation of an ulcer-adherent complex that covers the ulcer and protects it from erosion by pepsin, acid, and bile salts.

- *Proton pump inhibitors:* Anti-secretory agents that inhibit secretion of gastrin by the parietal cells of the stomach (e.g., omeprazole, lansoprazole, pantoprazole, rabeprazole, and esomeprazole).

Antibiotic therapy eradicates *H. pylori*. The drugs used include metronidazole , tetracycline, amoxicillin, and clarithromycin. The combination of nitroimidazole and tetracycline has also proved to be successful in the treatment of H. pylori. These medications are packaged as a kit containing a 14-day supply of nitroimidazole and tetracycline, with each daily dose packaged on a blister card to improve patient compliance. Antibiotic treatment typically is combined in a therapeutic regimen with other medications, such as bismuth or omeprazole.

Among patients whose *H. pylori* is treated with antibiotics, the peptic ulcer recurrence may be as low as 10%. Patients who do not receive antibiotics have a relapse rate of 75% to 90%.

Dietary modification may be necessary to avoid foods and beverages that irritate the ulcer. There is considerable controversy over the therapeutic benefits of a bland diet because the rationale is not supported by scientific evidence. It is recommended that the patient eat smaller meals more frequently throughout the day to decrease the degree of gastric motor activity.

Smoking has an irritating effect on the mucosa, increases gastric motility, and delays mucosal healing. Smoking should be eliminated completely or severely reduced. The combination of adequate rest and cessation of smoking accelerates ulcer healing. Because caffeinated and decaffeinated coffee, tobacco, alcohol, and aspirin aggravate the mucosal lining of the stomach and duodenum, educate patients with ulcers about the need for lifestyle change.

Surgical intervention has decreased drastically with more effective diagnosis and medical treatment with medications. Approximately 20% of patients with ulcers require surgical intervention. These are patients who are unresponsive to medical management, raising concerns about gastric cancer; patients whose ulcers are drug induced but who cannot be withdrawn from the drugs (e.g., patients with rheumatoid arthritis); or patients who develop complications. Surgical procedures that may be performed are the same as those listed for cancer of the stomach.

Nursing Interventions and Patient Teaching

NG or intestinal tube insertion, irrigation, and intermittent suctioning often are performed while the patient is feeling ill and uncomfortable from PUD. In addition to being skilled and knowledgeable in performing these procedures, the nurse is responsible for easing the patient's fears and anxieties. Patient cooperation not only

makes the procedures easier but also reduces patient discomfort.

Helping patients through the experience of GI intubation requires understanding of the following points:

- For most patients, NG or intestinal tube placement is a new and frightening experience. Explain the rationale for this therapy to the anxious patient and family. Help the patient and family understand that the advantages far outweigh the discomfort.
- Inability to chew, taste, and swallow food and liquids may contribute to patient anxiety during GI intubation.
- A patient with an NG or intestinal tube is usually on NPO status. On occasion, ice chips are allowed.
- An NG or intestinal tube is connected to either continuous or intermittent suctioning, usually at 100 to 125 mm Hg for decompression.
- An NG or intestinal tube is a constant irritant to the nasopharynx and nares, requiring frequent care to the mouth and nose.
- A patient with a GI tube may be afraid that moving will dislodge the tube. Implement frequent position changes to enhance tube functioning and prevent complications of immobility.

An NG tube is inserted through the nose, pharynx, and esophagus into the stomach. Various tubes are available, depending on the purpose (Table 5.2).

Nursing interventions depend on the stage of the ulcer disease. The emphasis in patient care always should be on prevention and early detection of

Table 5.2	Purposes of Nasogastric Intubation	
PURPOSE	**DESCRIPTION**	**TYPE OF TUBE**
Decompression	Removal of secretions and gaseous substances from GI tract; prevention or relief of abdominal distention	Salem sump, Miller-Abbott
Feeding (gavage)	Instillation of liquid nutritional supplements or feedings into stomach for patients unable to swallow fluid	Duo, Dobhoff
Compression	Internal application of pressure by means of inflated balloon to prevent internal GI hemorrhage	Sengstaken-Blakemore
Lavage	Irrigation of stomach in cases of active bleeding, poisoning, gastric dilation, or intestinal obstruction	Ewald, Salem sump

GI, Gastrointestinal.

pain in the epigastric region, hematemesis, melena, or tenderness and rigidity of the abdomen (see the Communication box on gastrointestinal bleeding and Nursing Care Plan 5.1).

Patient problems and interventions for the specific stages of ulcer care include but are not limited to the following:

Patient Problem	Nursing Interventions
Insufficient Knowledge, related to: • Medications • Diet • Signs and symptoms of bleeding, perforation, or gastric outlet obstruction	Provide verbal and written instructions on exact dosage and time intervals for medications and whether medication is taken with or without food Have dietitian provide instructions on therapeutic diet Explain that repeat episodes are not uncommon; listen carefully for aggravating factors
Nonconformity, related to: • Risk behaviors (use of tobacco or alcohol) • Dietary patterns	Assess patient's level of knowledge regarding food and other irritants to mucosal lining Teach preventive measures, such as quitting smoking Explain need for small and frequent meals Caution patient to avoid high-fiber foods, sugar, salt, caffeine, alcohol, and milk Remind patient to take fluids between meals, not with meals Explain the need to eat slowly and chew food well Discuss importance of adequate rest and exercise
Insufficient Nutrition, related to preoperative food and fluid restrictions	Maintain nothing by mouth status Connect nasogastric tube to intermittent suction apparatus Note color and amount of gastric output q 4 h Do not reposition tube Maintain patency of tube by irrigation with measured amounts of saline only if ordered NOTE: After gastrectomy, output is minimal Monitor parenteral fluids with electrolyte additives as ordered Measure intake and output When bowel sounds return and flatus is expelled, administer clear liquids as ordered Progress to small, frequent meals of soft food as ordered. Avoid milk because it may cause dumping syndrome

Communication

Patient With Gastrointestinal Bleeding

Nurse: You look like you are resting better, Mrs. S. How have you been feeling? *(Reaffirming a relationship that was begun yesterday.)*

Patient: My stomach pain is much better. The medicine helped.

Nurse: If you are comfortable, perhaps you and your husband have some questions about why you are here. *(Trying to determine whether the patient is receptive to patient teaching. A knowledge deficit was suspected on admission.)*

Patient: I was scared when I started to vomit blood. It has happened before but not this much. Where does the blood come from?

Nurse: You have a diagnosis of GI bleeding with questionable duodenal ulcer. This means that the bleeding is coming from somewhere in your digestive tract or from an ulcer that has formed in the first part of your small intestine. The ulcer is an erosion of the lining of your stomach or small intestine. Do you understand what I have said so far? *(The nurse begins with the admitting diagnosis and explains one thing at a time, making sure the patient verbalizes understanding before continuing. It is beneficial for the nurse to show the patient a diagram of the GI system.)*

Patient: Well, I understand where the bleeding is coming from, but why am I bleeding there?

Nurse: We are not sure yet, Mrs. S., but you are scheduled for a procedure that will allow the health care provider actually to look at the surface of the stomach and a portion of the intestine. It is called an endoscopy, and it will be done tomorrow morning. Did someone explain this to you? *(The nurse answers the patient's question openly and honestly and uses her answer to lead into further patient education.)*

It is necessary to form a trusting relationship with the patient with an ulcer because of the severity of the condition and the need for long-term treatment. Include the family in patient education sessions to increase understanding and support, and involve the patient in goal setting to increase compliance (see the Home Care Considerations box).

Instruct the patient to seek medical attention immediately if severe and sudden pain occurs. Assist the patient in describing signs and symptoms of weakness, anorexia, nausea, diarrhea, constipation, anxiety, or restlessness. When medications are prescribed, the patient must understand fully (1) the purpose of taking antibiotic therapy to eradicate *H. pylori*; (2) the importance of taking all medications such as H_2 receptor antagonists, antiulcer drugs, prostaglandin E analog, and PPIs as prescribed; (3) why the antacids are taken in specific dosages and at the specific times ordered; and (4) the known side effects (diarrhea and constipation). Preventive teaching includes identifying high-risk behaviors, such as the use of tobacco, caffeine, and alcohol. Emphasize that the patient should eat six smaller meals daily and avoid any foods that cause noticeable stomach discomfort.

Home Care Considerations

Peptic Ulcer Disease

- The patient who has recurrent ulcer disease after initial healing must learn to live with a chronic disease.
- The patient may be angry and frustrated, especially if he or she has faithfully followed the prescribed therapy but failed to prevent the recurrence or extension of the disease process.
- Unfortunately, many patients do not comply with the care plan and experience repeated exacerbations.
- Changes in lifestyle are difficult for most people and may be resisted.
- The patient who is instructed to stop smoking or avoid alcohol may resist.

- The goal should be to adhere to the prescribed therapeutic regimen, including nutritional management, cessation of smoking, and decreased use of alcohol and caffeine.
- A patient with chronic ulcers needs to be aware of the complications that may result from the disease, the clinical manifestations indicating their presence, and what to do until the health care provider can be seen.
- Teach the patient to take all medications as prescribed. This includes antisecretory and antibiotic drugs. Failure to take prescribed medications can result in relapse.

 Nursing Care Plan 5.1   **The Patient With Gastrointestinal Bleeding**

Mr. D., 33 years of age, is admitted with pain in the epigastric region and copious hematemesis. He appears anxious; his skin is pale, cool, and clammy; and he is breathing rapidly. This patient has a history of recurrent episodes of vomiting blood that has a coffee grounds appearance. He denies passing blood rectally but admits his stools have changed in consistency.

PATIENT PROBLEM

Potential for Inadequate Fluid Volume, related to hemorrhage, vomiting, and diarrhea

Patient Goals and Expected Outcomes	Nursing Interventions	Evaluation
Patient will have normal fluid balance as evidenced by balanced intake and output (I&O) within 24 h, including stable weight Blood pressure, pulse, and respiratory rate will be within normal limits Patient will have normal tissue turgor within 24 h	Monitor IV and blood transfusion therapy as ordered. Accurately record I&O q h until stable: emesis, urine, and stool. Document fluid losses for possible imbalance; urinary output less than 30 mL/h may indicate hypovolemia. Monitor for signs and symptoms of dehydration and fluid and electrolyte imbalance (dry mucous membranes, poor skin turgor, thirst, decreased urinary output, and changes in behavior) q 15 min until stable, then q 2 h. Document characteristics of output. Test all emesis and fecal output for presence of blood as ordered. Prepare to assist with inserting a nasogastric (NG) tube and connecting it to wall suction. Irrigate NG tube with saline as ordered to promote clotting; irrigation removes old blood from the stomach.	Patient has urinary output of 1500 mL for prior 24-h period. Patient's blood pressure, pulse, and respiratory rate are within patient's pre-gastrointestinal bleeding baseline levels. Patient's tissue turgor is normal.

PATIENT PROBLEM

Anxiousness, related to hospitalization and illness

Patient Goals and Expected Outcomes	Nursing Interventions	Evaluation
Patient will demonstrate decrease in anxiety as evidenced by ability to sleep or rest at frequent intervals, verbalization of feelings, and blood pressure and pulse within normal limits	Assess physiologic components of anxiety (restlessness, increased pulse and respirations, diaphoresis, and elevated blood pressure) at least q 8 h. Provide concise explanations for all procedures; prepare patient for surgery if indicated. Develop rapport with patient and family members with each contact.	Patient is sleeping 5–6 h during the night and resting at intervals during the day. Patient verbalizes a feeling of less stress and anxiety. Therapeutic rapport with nurse, patient, and family members is noted.

CRITICAL THINKING QUESTIONS

1. Mr. D. has an NG tube connected to wall suction that is draining sanguineous fluid. He complains of severe fatigue and epigastric pain. He is pale and drawn, with a hemoglobin level of 5.1 g/dL. Mr. D. puts his call light on and requests the nurse to assist him to the bathroom for a bowel movement. What appropriate interventions will ensure Mr. D.'s safety?
2. During assessment of Mr. D., what signs and symptoms would indicate inadequate fluid volume?
3. Mr. D. says to the nurse that he fears he may die. He appears anxious and tremulous. What is the most therapeutic approach to help decrease his fears?

If surgery is required, explain the procedures thoroughly, including the reasons for them. Explain immediate postoperative care, including deep breathing; coughing; position changes; frequent monitoring of vital signs; IV tubing, NG tubing, catheters, and other drainage tubes; and the use of patient-controlled analgesia (PCA) or other medications for pain relief. The patient's ability to eat normally after healing depends on the type of surgery and when peristalsis returns. Help the patient realize that symptoms often recur and that he or she should seek medical care if they do.

Prognosis for Peptic Ulcers

Recurrence of an ulcer may happen within 2 years in about one-third of all patients. Among patients whose *H. pylori* is treated with antibiotics, the peptic ulcer recurrence drops to 20%. Patients who do not receive antibiotics have a relapse rate of 85% to 90%. The likelihood of recurrence is lessened by eliminating foods that aggravate the condition and following prescribed therapies such as taking PPIs and avoiding NSAIDs. If symptoms recur, the prognosis is better in patients who seek immediate medical treatment and comply with the prescribed regimen (Anand, 2017).

CANCER OF THE STOMACH

Etiology and Pathophysiology

Stomach, or gastric, cancer saw its peak in the 1930s, when it was the leading cause of death. Although those numbers have decreased significantly over the years, the American Cancer Society estimates that 2020 will see 27,600 new cases of stomach cancer in the United States and nearly 11,010 people will die from the disease. Of the new cases diagnosed, 16,980 will be in men and 10,620 in women. The incidence and mortality rate are much higher outside of the United States, especially in less developed areas. Rates are highest in Japan, China, Southern and Eastern Europe, and South and Central America. Gastric cancer affects mostly the elderly population: nearly two-thirds of those diagnosed are over the age of 65, and the average age is 69 (ACS, 2021a). The most common neoplasm or malignant growth in the stomach is adenocarcinoma. The primary location is the pyloric area, but the incidence of proximal tumors seems to be rising. Because of its location, the tumor may metastasize to lymph nodes, liver, spleen, pancreas, or esophagus.

Many factors have been implicated in the development of stomach cancer, yet no single causative agent has been identified. Stomach carcinogenesis probably begins with a nonspecific mucosal injury as a result of aging; autoimmune disease; or repeated exposure to irritants such as bile, anti-inflammatory agents, or smoking. Other factors include history of polyps, pernicious anemia, hypochlorhydria (deficiency of hydrochloride in the stomach's gastric juice), chronic atrophic gastritis, and gastric ulcer. Because the stomach has prolonged contact with food, cancer in this part of the body is associated with diets that are high in salt, smoked and preserved foods (which contain nitrites and nitrates), and carbohydrates, and low in fresh fruits and vegetables. Whole grains and fresh fruits and vegetables are associated with reduced rates of stomach cancer. Infection with *H. pylori*, especially at an early age, is considered a definite risk factor for gastric cancer.

Clinical Manifestations

The patient may be asymptomatic in early stages of the disease. Stomach cancer often spreads to adjacent organs before any distressing symptoms occur. With more advanced disease, the patient may appear pale and lethargic if anemia is present. With a poor appetite and significant weight loss, the patient may appear cachectic (weak and emaciated).

Assessment

Subjective data include complaints of vague epigastric discomfort or indigestion, early satiety, and postprandial (after meal) fullness. Some patients complain of an ulcer-like pain that does not respond to therapy. Anorexia and weakness are also common.

Objective data include weight loss, blood in the stools, hematemesis, and vomiting after drinking or eating. Anemia is common. It is caused by chronic blood loss as the lesion erodes through the mucosa or as a direct result of pernicious anemia, which develops when intrinsic factor is lost. The presence of ascites is a poor prognostic sign.

Diagnostic Tests

Endoscopic or gastroscopic examinations are the best tools for diagnosing stomach cancers because direct visualization aids in removing tissue samples for biopsy. The stomach can also be distended with air during the procedure to stretch mucosal folds for better visualization of the mucosa. Endoscopic ultrasound and CT and PET scans can be used to stage the disease. Stool examination provides evidence of occult or gross bleeding. Carcinoembryonic antigen (CEA) and carbohydrate antigen 19-9 tumor markers usually are elevated in advanced gastric cancer. Serum tumor markers correlate with the degree of invasion, liver metastasis, and cure rate. Laboratory studies of RBCs, hemoglobin, hematocrit, and serum B_{12} assist in the detection of anemia and determination of severity.

Medical Management

Treatment depends on the staging of the disease. Often a combination of treatments, including surgery, chemotherapy, radiation therapy, and targeted drug therapy, is beneficial. Surgery may be done as an exploratory celiotomy to determine involvement. The surgical interventions used in treating gastric cancer are typically the same procedures used for peptic ulcer disease.

A partial or total gastric resection is the treatment of choice for an extensive lesion. Surgery for advanced gastric cancer carries high morbidity and mortality rates (Mayo Clinic, 2021). Types of surgical procedures include the following:

- *Antrectomy:* Removal of the entire antrum, the gastric-producing portion of the lower stomach, to eliminate the main stimulus to acid production.
- *Gastroduodenostomy (Billroth I)* (Fig. 5.7A): Direct anastomosis of the fundus of the stomach to the duodenum; used to remove ulcers or cancer located in the antrum of the stomach.
- *Gastrojejunostomy (Billroth II)* (Fig. 5.7B): Closure of the duodenum, and anastomosis of the fundus of the stomach into the jejunum; used to remove ulcers or cancer located in the body of the fundus.
- *Pyloroplasty:* Surgical enlargement of the pyloric sphincter to facilitate passage of contents from the stomach; commonly done after vagotomy or to enlarge an opening that has been constricted from scar tissue. A vagotomy decreases gastric motility and subsequently gastric emptying. A pyloroplasty accompanying vagotomy increases gastric emptying (Johns Hopkins Medicine, 2013).

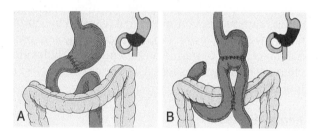

Fig. 5.7 Types of gastric resections with anastomoses. A, Billroth I. B, Billroth II.

- *Total gastrectomy:* Removal of the entire stomach; rarely used for patients with gastric cancer.
- *Vagotomy:* Removal of the vagal innervation to the fundus, decreasing acid produced by the parietal cells of the stomach (Fig. 5.8); usually done with a Billroth I or II procedure or with a pyloroplasty.

The choice of which procedure to use is difficult and depends on the surgeon's preference and results of diagnostic testing. Regardless of the procedure selected, postoperative complications are possible. Bleeding may occur up to 7 days after gastric surgery. Abdominal rigidity, abdominal pain, restlessness, elevated temperature, increased pulse, decreased blood pressure, and leukocytosis are possible indications of postoperative bleeding. Note the amount and type of drainage from the incision. Surgical intervention may be necessary to correct the bleeding.

Dumping syndrome is a rapid gastric emptying of undigested food from the stomach to the small intestine, causing distention of the duodenum or jejunum. Increased intestinal motility, peristalsis, and changes in blood glucose levels occur. Patients may report diaphoresis, nausea, vomiting, epigastric pain, explosive diarrhea, borborygmi (rumbling noises made by gas passing through the liquid of the small intestine), and dyspepsia. Dumping syndrome is the direct result of surgical removal of a large portion of the stomach and the pyloric sphincter. Approximately one-third to one-half of patients experience dumping syndrome after peptic ulcer surgery. Treatment includes eating six small meals daily that are high in protein and fat and low in carbohydrates, eating slowly, and avoiding fluids during meals. Treatment also includes (1) anticholinergic agents to decrease stomach motility, and (2) reclining for approximately 1 hour after meals. To increase long-term

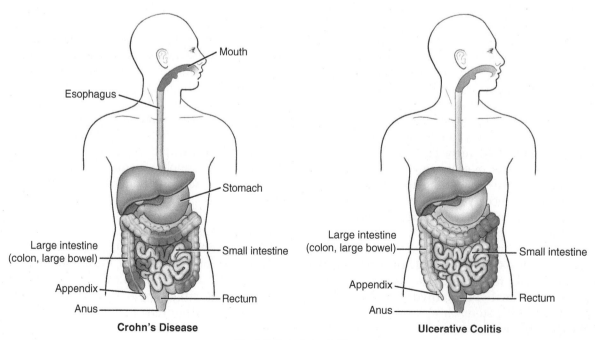

Crohn's Disease   **Ulcerative Colitis**

Fig. 5.8 Crohn's vs. Colitis.

compliance, reassure patients that following the recommended treatment will decrease symptoms within a few months. The symptoms are self-limiting and often disappear within several months to a year after surgery.

Several other complications after gastric surgery present serious health threats. Diarrhea is common and usually responds to conservative treatment of controlled diet and antidiarrheal agents. Diphenoxylate with atropine, loperamide, paregoric, or codeine is often used. Reflux esophagitis and nutritional deficits—leading to weight loss, malabsorption, anemia, and vitamin deficiency—can also be life threatening.

Pernicious anemia is a serious potential complication for any patient who has had a total gastrectomy or extensive resections. This is caused by a deficiency of intrinsic factor, produced exclusively by the stomach, which aids intestinal absorption of vitamin B_{12}. Recommend that all patients with a partial gastrectomy have a blood serum vitamin B_{12} level measured every 1 to 2 years so that replacement therapy of vitamin B_{12} via a monthly injection, weekly via the nasal route, or sublingually can be instituted before anemia appears.

Wound healing may be disrupted by dehiscence (a partial or complete separation of the wound edges) or by evisceration (protrusion of viscera through the disrupted wound). Dehiscence and evisceration may be caused by problems in suturing the wound or by poor tissue integrity. Excessive coughing, straining, malnutrition, obesity, and infection also may increase the chances of dehiscence. Nursing interventions for dehiscence include instructing the patient to remain quiet, to cover the wound with a dry sterile dressing, and to avoid coughing or straining. Keep the patient in a dorsal recumbent position (on the back with the knees flexed) to remove stress on the wound and notify the surgeon. If evisceration occurs, keep the patient on bed rest and loosely cover the protruding viscera with a warm sterile saline dressing. Notify the surgeon immediately because treatment consists of reapproximating (i.e., drawing together) the wound edges.

Chemotherapy yields greater response and longer survival rates than radiation. Because the radiosensitivity of stomach cancer is low, radiation therapy is of little value. Radiation therapy may be used as a palliative measure to decrease tumor mass and temporarily relieve obstruction. The combination of chemotherapy and radiation therapy sometimes is used for patients who are at high risk for disease recurrence after surgery. These treatment modalities often are used in conjunction with surgery (Mayo Clinic, 2021).

Nursing Interventions and Patient Teaching
Provide the patient and family with further clarification about the disease and the surgical intervention. Preoperative preparation includes improving the patient's nutritional status by monitoring total parenteral nutrition (TPN; complete nutrition provided intravenously) and providing supplemental feedings.

Postoperative teaching is necessary to relieve anxiety and promote understanding of drainage tubes, feeding tubes, dressing changes, weakness, medications, and other routine care. Close monitoring of intake and output, maintenance of TPN, and being alert to weight loss are important in the postoperative period for surgeries involving the stomach.

Patient problems and interventions for the patient with cancer of the stomach include but are not limited to the following:
Because care encompasses so many areas, instruction

Patient Problem	Nursing Interventions
Potential for Harm or Damage to the Body, related to: • Aspiration • Infection • Hemorrhage • Anemia or vitamin deficiency	Monitor closely for elevated temperature, bleeding from incision, pallor, dyspnea, cyanosis, tachycardia, increased respirations, and chest pain Monitor laboratory results and activity tolerance because of possible anemia Change dressings, using sterile technique

should be (1) planned according to the patient's needs and level of understanding, (2) given when the patient is free of pain, and (3) communicated verbally and in print. Address areas such as surgery, chemotherapy, radiation therapy, continued nutritional needs, pain relief, and support groups for psychosocial needs.

Weight loss indicates the need for additional caloric intake and can be measured by monitoring weight and comparing it with the patient's normal weight before illness. If a gastrostomy tube (G-tube) is necessary, prevention of skin excoriation around the G-tube site should be ensured. Hypermotility or diarrhea that follows radiation therapy can be treated with dietary therapy and/or medication. The debilitated patient and family may require referral for hospice care.

Prognosis
The prognosis for patients with gastric cancer depends on the stage at which the cancer was detected. If found and treated in the early stages, the 5-year survival rate is approximately 65%. For gastric cancer that has metastasized to nearby tissue or lymph nodes, the 5-year survival rate is approximately 30%. Distant metastasis has a 5% survival rate in 5 years. The overall average 5-year survival rate is about 30% (ACS, 2021e).

DISORDERS OF THE INTESTINES

INFECTIONS
Etiology and Pathophysiology
Intestinal infections are the invasion of the alimentary canal (both the small and large intestine) by pathogenic

microorganisms that reproduce and multiply. The infectious agent can enter the body by several routes. The most common way is through the mouth in contaminated food or water. Some intestinal infections occur as a result of person-to-person contact. Fecal–oral transmission occurs through poor hand hygiene after elimination.

Bacterial flora grow naturally in the intestinal tract and help the immune system combat infection. Long-term antibiotic therapy can destroy the normal flora, resulting in pathogenic microorganisms entering the intestines. The impaired immune response in some individuals delays the body's attempt to destroy invading pathogens.

Infectious diarrhea causes secretion of fluid into the intestinal lumen. *Clostridium, Salmonella, Shigella,* and *Campylobacter* bacteria are associated with intestinal infections (American Academy of Family Physicians, 2018). These bacteria produce toxic substances, and the mucosal cells respond by secreting water and electrolytes, causing an imbalance. The colon normally absorbs water to be recirculated in the body but since these pathogens induce extra fluid to be secreted, diarrhea results.

One strain of *E. coli*—serotype O157:H7—often has a virulent course. Unlike other strains, *E. coli* O157:H7 is not part of the normal flora of the human intestine. Found in the intestines of approximately 1% of food cattle, in turkeys, and rarely in pigs, this strain can, even in small amounts, contaminate a large amount of meat, especially ground beef (Mayo Clinic, 2020b). It is transmitted in contaminated, undercooked meats such as hamburger, roast beef, ham, and turkey; in produce that has been rinsed with water contaminated by animal or human feces; or by a person who has been handling contaminated food. The bacterium also has been cultured in an unpasteurized milk, cheese, and apple juice and can be found in lakes and pools that have been contaminated by fecal matter. Hemorrhagic colitis (which results in bloody diarrhea and severe cramping accompanied by diffuse abdominal tenderness) develops between the second and fourth days. Antidiarrheals should not be given because these medications prevent the intestines from getting rid of the *E. coli* pathogen. Antimotility drugs such as diphenoxylate with atropine or antibiotic therapy are not recommended because they increase the likelihood of developing hemolytic-uremic syndrome, a pathologic condition of the kidney. Poisoning with *E. coli* O157:H7 can be life threatening, particularly in the very young and in older adults. Usually little or no fever is present, and the illness resolves in 5 to 10 days. In approximately 2% to 7% of infections, particularly in young children, hemolytic-uremic syndrome occurs and the kidneys fail.

Sigmoidoscopic or colonoscopic examination and stool specimens are used to diagnose a type of inflammation or colitis called *antibiotic-associated pseudomembranous colitis* (AAPMC). Immunosuppressed patients and older adults are particularly susceptible. *C. difficile* is a facility-acquired infection, because hospitalized patients are often immunosuppressed, antibiotic therapy is common, and the spores can survive for up to 70 days on inanimate objects. *C. difficile* spores have been found on commodes, telephones, thermometers, bedside tables, floors, and other objects in rooms, as well as on the hands of health care workers. Health care workers who do not adhere to infection control precautions can transmit *C. difficile* from patient to patient. Washing hands with soap and water is necessary because antiseptic hand rub does not destroy *C. difficile*. This type of colitis is a complication of treatment with a wide variety of antibiotics, including lincomycin, clindamycin, ampicillin, erythromycin, tetracycline, cephalosporins, and aminoglycosides. A *C. difficile* test is ordered on stool specimens to aid in the diagnosis of AAPMC in inpatients and outpatients. Characteristic lesions of AAPMC are identified on tissues obtained through endoscopic examination.

Treatment with antibiotics (especially clindamycin, ampicillin, amoxicillin, and the cephalosporins) inhibits normal bacterial growth in the intestine. This inhibition of normal flora can lead to the overgrowth of other bacteria such as *C. difficile*. Under the right conditions, *C. difficile* produces two toxins, A and B. Toxins A and B are produced by *C. difficile* at the same time, and these toxins cause the tissue damage seen in AAPMC. The incidence of *C. difficile* toxin found in the stool ranges from 1% to 2% in a normal population to 10% in hospital inpatients and up to 85% to 90% in patients with proven AAPMC. The *C. difficile* test alone is not conclusive but does aid in the diagnosis of AAPMC.

Because the level of *C. difficile* antigens associated with the disease state may vary, a negative *C. difficile* test result alone may not rule out the possibility of *C. difficile*–associated colitis. Signs and symptoms of the disease such as the duration and severity of diarrhea should be monitored. These observations, along with the duration of antibiotic treatment and the presence of colitis or pseudomembranes, are factors the health care provider must consider when diagnosing AAPMC disease.

The health care provider treats a mild case of antibiotic-related *C. difficile*–associated diarrhea by simply discontinuing the antibiotic and providing fluid and electrolyte replacement. For mild to moderate cases of the infection, the antibiotic is discontinued and oral metronidazole is recommended as initial treatment. In more severe cases, the health care provider discontinues the antibiotic and starts antimicrobial therapy with fidaxomicin or vancomycin (CDC, 2020).

A treatment that is being used in some cases is fecal microbial transplantation. In this procedure a patient is prepped for a colonoscopy, a sample of feces is obtained from a donor (who has been screened for any infection) and is sent to the laboratory for processing, and the sample then is placed into the sigmoid colon of the recipient. The goal of this therapy is to promote growth of normal flora in the intestine that has been lost.

Clinical Manifestations
Diarrhea is the most common manifestation of an intestinal infection. The fecal output has increased water content, and if the intestinal mucosa is directly invaded, the feces may contain blood and mucus.

Assessment
Collection of subjective data includes noting complaints of diarrhea, rectal urgency, tenesmus (ineffective and painful straining with defecation), nausea, and abdominal cramping.

Objective data include fever and vomiting. History taking provides useful information regarding number and consistency of bowel movements, recent use of antibiotics, recent travel, food intake, and exposure to noninfectious causes of diarrhea. Noninfectious diarrhea may be caused by heavy metal poisoning, shellfish allergy, and ingestion of toxins from mushrooms or fish. Diarrhea from noninfectious causes usually is characterized by a short incubation period (minutes to hours after exposure).

Diagnostic Tests
The key laboratory test for patients with intestinal infections is a stool culture. Stools are examined for blood, mucus, and WBCs. A blood chemistry study to monitor changes in the patient's fluid and electrolyte status may be included.

Medical Management
Usually the treatment of intestinal infections is conservative, letting the body limit the infection. Antibiotics rarely are used to treat acute diarrhea but may be given in cases of prolonged or severe diarrhea with a stool positive for leukocytes. If fluid and electrolyte replacement is necessary to offset the losses from diarrhea, the oral route is usually sufficient. The IV route is indicated if the patient cannot take sufficient fluids orally.

The use of antidiarrheals and antispasmodic agents actually may increase the severity of the infection by prolonging the contact time of the infectious organism with the intestinal wall. The health care provider determines when and if such medications should be prescribed.

Nursing Interventions and Patient Teaching
Perform a thorough assessment to aid the health care provider in determining the seriousness of the intestinal infection. Determining the onset of the disease and the number of people exposed is important, because the majority of GI infections are communicable and represent a community health problem. Also, assessment for fluid imbalance is important, including measurement of postural changes in blood pressure, skin turgor, mucous membrane hydration, and urinary output.

Patient problems and interventions for the patient with intestinal infections include but are not limited to the following:

Patient Problem	Nursing Interventions
Inadequate Fluid Volume, related to excessive losses from diarrhea and vomiting	If oral intake is tolerated, offer apple juice, clear carbonated beverages, clear broth, plain gelatin, and water
	If intravenous feedings are required to maintain intravascular volume, these fluids should have electrolytes added
	Maintain accurate intake and output

Instruct the patient to report the number, color, consistency of bowel movements, abdominal cramping, and pain. Ensure that the patient and family understand the importance of hand hygiene after bowel movements to interrupt the fecal–oral route of transmission. Information should be given to family members responsible for food preparation about the importance of proper methods of food preparation and storage to reduce the growth of infecting organisms. The patient at home may benefit from drinking water and rehydration solutions such as Gatorade (adults) or Pedialyte (infants and children).

Prognosis
Intestinal infections. The body may be able to defend itself successfully against the infection without medical intervention. In severe cases, medications and fluid replacement may be necessary. Prognosis is favorable unless the patient is severely debilitated by other conditions.

Antibiotic-associated pseudomembranous colitis. The prognosis for AAPMC is better when the disease is diagnosed early and the antibiotics are changed. This allows the normal growth of bacteria in the intestine to resume. The prognosis depends on the patient's overall condition.

CELIAC DISEASE (CELIAC SPRUE)
Etiology and Pathophysiology
Celiac disease is a genetic disorder that most commonly affects the small intestine but can affect any part of the GI system. It is considered an autoimmune disease that disrupts the absorption of nutrients from foods in response to the ingestion of gluten (a protein primarily found in wheat, rye, and barley). When these proteins are ingested, the immune system begins damaging the inner lining of the small intestine and destroying the villi (finger-like protrusions lining the intestine). Celiac disease affects approximately 1 in 100 people in the world. Among first-degree relatives of patients with

celiac disease, the incidence increases to 1 in 10 people (Celiac Disease Foundation, n.d.).

Clinical Manifestations

The patient with celiac disease experiences very individualized clinical manifestations. Commonly, abdominal pain and diarrhea after ingesting foods containing gluten is experienced. Malabsorption occurs because the damage to the lining of the small intestine prevents digestion from occurring. This manifestation may result in weight loss and vitamin deficiencies. Vitamin deficiencies may be so severe that the brain, peripheral nervous system, bones, liver, and other vital organs are affected.

Assessment

Subjective data include complaints of abdominal pain and bloating, irritability and depression, joint pain, muscle cramps, neuropathic complaints such as tingling in the legs and feet, and general weakness and fatigue.

Objective data include chronic intermittent diarrhea, weight loss, osteoporosis, mouth sores, dental problems, unexplained iron deficiency anemia, and pale, foul-smelling stools that contain a large amount of fat.

Diagnostic Tests

Blood tests for the presence of specific autoantibodies (anti–tissue transglutaminase antibodies [TGAs] or anti-endomysial antibodies [EMAs]) are performed while the patient still is ingesting gluten. False negatives may occur if gluten already has been eliminated from the diet. Intestinal biopsy via an endoscopy is performed if blood tests are positive for the disease (Celiac Disease Foundation, no date).

Medical Management

There is no medical treatment for celiac disease other than following a gluten-free diet. Referral to a dietitian is most beneficial for a patient newly diagnosed with the disease. Vitamins and supplements may be ordered by the health care provider for severe deficiencies. Steroids also may be prescribed to treat extensive inflammation of the intestinal lining.

Nursing Interventions and Patient Teaching

The patient diagnosed with celiac disease must understand how to incorporate a gluten-free diet into his or her life. Foods containing wheat, rye, and barley are prohibited. Foods that commonly contain these ingredients are made with wheat flour, which includes most grains, cereal, pasta, and many processed foods. Replacing these foods with potato, rice, soy, amaranth, quinoa, buckwheat, and bean flour prevent the autoimmune response of celiac disease. In 2006, the Food Allergen Labeling and Consumer Protection Act (FALCPA) required that food labels identify wheat and other common food allergens in the list of ingredients. Many food labels clearly identify gluten-free products. Plain meat and fish, fruits, vegetables, and rice can be included into the diet because they do not contain gluten.

Prognosis

Patients who follow a strict gluten-free diet typically notice improvement in symptoms within a few days of changing their diet, and the damage to the intestine often is resolved within 3 to 6 months. Small amounts of gluten can damage the intestine even if symptoms are not apparent.

IRRITABLE BOWEL SYNDROME

Etiology and Pathophysiology

Irritable bowel syndrome (IBS) is considered a functional disorder characterized by episodes of altered bowel function and intermittent and recurrent abdominal discomfort and pain. Patients with IBS experience diarrhea, constipation, or a combination of both that occurs for months or years, and the cause of the disorder is not known.

IBS affects about 10% to 15% of the American population. More women than men are affected by IBS (two of three individuals with the disorder), and most people with IBS are under the age of 50.

The actual cause of IBS is unknown, but there are several commonalities among those diagnosed with the disorder and theories regarding the cause. One theory is that the brain, intestine, and nervous system interact in a way that causes greater than normal discomfort when stool passes through the colon. Another theory is that peristalsis contractions last longer and are stronger than normal, causing more discomfort, bloating, and frequency of stools. The opposite problem of slowed peristalsis, leading to hardened feces and causing discomfort, may be attributed to episodes of constipation. . Risk factors for developing IBS include having a family member with IBS, stress, and a history of severe intestinal infection (NIDDK, 2017).

Clinical Manifestations

Alterations of bowel function include abdominal pain relieved after a bowel movement; more frequent bowel movements with pain onset; a sense of incomplete evacuation; flatulence; and constipation, diarrhea, or both. Stress is not considered a cause of IBS but can exacerbate symptoms of diarrhea (usually weight loss does not occur). The physical examination is generally normal, and nocturnal symptoms are rarely present. The symptoms of IBS are deceptive and are frustrating for the patient to manage.

Assessment

Subjective data include complaints of abdominal distress, pain at onset of bowel movements, abdominal pain relieved by defecation, and feelings of incomplete emptying after defecation.

Objective data include the presence of mucus in stools, visible abdominal distention, and frequent or unformed stools.

Diagnostic Tests
The key to accurate diagnosis of IBS is a thorough history and physical examination. Emphasize symptoms, health history (including psychosocial aspects such as physical or sexual abuse), family history, and drug and dietary history.

Diagnosis of IBS occurs by exclusion. Patients who see the health care provider with symptoms of intermittent or chronic abdominal pain and altered bowel motility are screened for pathologic conditions such as Crohn disease, ulcerative colitis, colorectal cancer, diverticulitis, and infections such as *Salmonella*. When no pathologic or structural abnormality is detected, IBS is a probable diagnosis. Symptom-based criteria for IBS have been standardized and are referred to as the *Rome criteria*. Rome III criteria include abdominal discomfort that occurs at least 3 days per month within the past 3 months and that has at least two of the following characteristics: (1) relieved with defecation, (2) onset associated with a change in stool frequency, and (3) onset associated with a change in stool appearance.

Medical Management
Stress management and behavioral therapy. Although stress does not cause IBS, it can make the symptoms worse. Stress management techniques, biofeedback, relaxation therapy, and hypnosis are some of the cognitive therapies used to manage IBS. Keeping a diary also may help with identifying lifestyle and diet issues that may worsen symptoms, thus allowing modifications of these issues.

Diet and bulking agents. Increasing dietary fiber may help to increase stool bulk and frequency of passage and to reduce bloating. Adequate fiber may be provided more reliably with over-the-counter bulking agents than with diet alone. The bulking agents seem to be most effective in treating constipation-predominant IBS, although they may alleviate mild diarrhea. If the patient's symptoms are exacerbated consistently after eating certain foods, those foods should be avoided. Advise the patient whose primary symptoms are abdominal distention and increased flatulence to eliminate common gas-producing foods (e.g., broccoli, cabbage) from the diet and to substitute yogurt for milk products to help determine whether he or she is lactose intolerant.

Medication. Anticholinergic drugs may help relieve abdominal cramps caused by spasm of the colon, and antidiarrheal medications may be necessary for bouts of diarrhea. Antianxiety drugs may help patients suffering from panic attacks associated with IBS. Antidepressants may be used sparingly for diarrhea-predominant IBS in

patients with severe discomfort who have not responded to other measures, or for those experiencing depression from living with IBS. New drug therapies are in development. Drugs that affect serotonin receptors hold promise in the treatment of IBS. Newer medications that have been approved for the treatment of select patients with IBS include alosetron and lubiprostone. Alosetron is a nerve receptor antagonist that helps in relaxing the colon and slowing the movement of stool through the colon, and lubiprostone is a chloride channel activator that works for those suffering from constipation by increasing fluid secretion in the small intestine to help with the passage of stool.

Some patients have reported benefits from the use of complementary therapies such as acupuncture, herbal therapy, chiropractic techniques, and yoga (see the Complementary and Alternative Therapies box). Although some studies have examined the use of such therapies in the treatment of IBS, clinical trial data are inadequate to determine their efficacy or to recommend any one as the sole therapy in the treatment of the syndrome.

Complementary and Alternative Therapies
Irritable Bowel Syndrome
- Peppermint oil, an herbal extract, has been studied for its use in irritable bowel syndrome. It acts by relaxing smooth muscle in the colon. Peppermint may cause heartburn, so the patient should be advised to take enteric-coated tablets.
- Biofeedback is a relaxation training method that gives individuals a greater degree of awareness and control of physiologic function. Computer-based biofeedback equipment gives immediate feedback to the patient on changes in certain parameters, such as muscle electrical activity and skin temperature.
- Similar interventions have used various psychotherapy, stress management, and relaxation exercises, often in combination.
- Herbs that patients should avoid because they can cause GI upset include milk thistle (*Silybum marianum*), goldenseal (*Hydrastis canadensis*), ginger (*Zingiber officinale*), kelp (*Fucus vesiculosus*), comfrey (*Symphytum officinale*), chaparral (*Larrea divaricata*), cayenne (*Capsicum*), and alfalfa (*Medicago sativa*).
- Some people find that acupuncture or acupressure provides relief from nausea and vomiting and relaxation of muscle spasms in the colon.
- Some people experience improved blood flow to digestive organs and improved digestion after chiropractic adjustment.
- Probiotics are "good" bacteria that are found in the intestinal tract. One theory is that people with IBS have an insufficient amount of good intestinal bacteria. Therefore foods that are high in probiotics, such as yogurt, or dietary supplements sometimes are added to the diet as a complementary treatment method.
- Regular exercise, massage, yoga, and meditation may help in managing stress.

Nursing Interventions and Patient Teaching

Many patients with IBS learn to cope with their symptoms enough to live in reasonable comfort. It is the nurse's role to assist in identifying those patients with IBS who need management. The nurse's skill in history taking, listening, nutrition planning, and understanding psychological effects on the body can assist the patient in setting goals to manage the disease. Emphasize the importance of keeping a daily log showing diet; number and type of stools; presence, severity, and duration of pain; side effects of medication; and life stressors that aggravate the disorder. This information assists in the diagnosis and treatment of IBS.

Patient problems and interventions for the patient with an irritable bowel include but are not limited to the following:

Patient Problem	Nursing Interventions
Discomfort, related to diet consumed and bowel evacuation	Have patient log the type of food consumed in terms of fiber content, consistency of stool, and degree of pain
Insufficient Knowledge, related to the effect of fiber content on spastic bowel	Educate patient regarding the relationship of fiber to constipation and diarrhea. Teach patient about the use of bulking agents

IBS involves many personal feelings that the patient must recognize and be comfortable with before a care plan can be established. It is important to establish a strong relationship with the patient before patient teaching begins. Patient teaching includes diet management and ways to control anxiety in daily living. The goal of patient teaching is to empower the patient to control the disorder. Provide community resources for counseling if psychological problems seem related to increased or decreased elimination accompanied by pain and discomfort.

Prognosis

IBS does not damage the bowel. It is a functional problem that if managed well, can interfere minimally with a person's daily life.

INFLAMMATORY BOWEL DISEASE

Ulcerative colitis and Crohn disease are chronic, episodic, inflammatory bowel diseases. These are immunologically related disorders that commonly affect adults usually between the ages of 15 and 35, and 55 to 70 years. These diseases are distributed evenly between males and females; ulcerative colitis is slightly more prevalent in females, whereas Crohn's is slightly more prevalent in males. There also seems to be a familial tendency for both disorders .

The causes of ulcerative colitis and Crohn disease are unknown. Theories involve genetic and environmental factors, including bacterial infection, immunologic factors, and psychosomatic disorders. The fact that people with ulcerative colitis commonly have a relative with Crohn disease and vice versa supports the existence of a common gene. Inflammatory bowel diseases are characterized by exacerbations (increases in severity of the disease or any of its symptoms) and remissions (decreases in severity of the disease or any of its symptoms).

The two diseases require similar nursing interventions but different surgical interventions and medical treatment. Certain criteria are used to differentiate ulcerative colitis from Crohn disease (Table 5.3), but the diseases have much in common and cannot be differentiated in some cases. Patients have been known to have features of both diseases, making a definite diagnosis difficult.

ULCERATIVE COLITIS

Etiology and Pathophysiology

Because of difficulty in diagnosing and misclassification of the diseases, the data may not be completely accurate, but the incidence of ulcerative colitis appears to be higher than that of Crohn disease. The causes of IBD may be attributed to the immune system and/or genetics. Regarding the immune system, it is believed that either a virus or bacterium invades the immune system, resulting in inflammation from the immune response; or an autoimmune reaction occurs, causing inflammation, with no pathogen provoking this response. Genetics are suspected because the disease is seen frequently among first-degree relatives.

Ulcerative colitis is confined to the mucosa and submucosa of the colon. The disease can affect segments of the entire colon, depending on the staging (phases or periods in the course of the disease). This disease usually starts in the rectum and moves in a continuous pattern toward the cecum. Although sometimes mild inflammation of the terminal ileum occurs, ulcerative colitis is a disease of the colon and rectum. The inflammation and ulcerations occur in the mucosal layer of the bowel wall. Because it does not extend through all bowel wall layers, fistulas and abscesses are rare. Capillaries become friable and bleed, causing the characteristic diarrhea containing pus and blood. Pseudopolyps (tissue that resembles polyps because of the cratering effect of surrounding ulcerations) are common in chronic ulcerative disease and may become cancerous. With healing and the natural formation of scar tissue, the colon may lose elasticity and absorptive capability.

Clinical Manifestations

The person diagnosed with ulcerative colitis often has periods of exacerbation and remission, and the degree of the illness can vary from mild to severe. Patients with severe ulcerative colitis may have as many as 15 to 20 liquid stools per day, containing blood, mucus,

Table 5.3   **Comparison of Ulcerative Colitis and Crohn Disease**

FACTOR	ULCERATIVE COLITIS	CROHN DISEASE
Cause of disorder	Unknown; autoimmune; genetic factors and environment play a role; various bacteria have been proposed	Unknown; possible cause is an altered immune state; autoimmune; various bacteria have been proposed Genetic and environmental factors play a role
Usual age at onset	Teenage years and early adulthood; second peak in sixth decade	Early adolescence; second peak in sixth decade
Area of involvement	Confined to mucosa or submucosa of the colon	Can occur anywhere along the gastrointestinal tract from the mouth to the anus Most common site is terminal ileum and proximal cecum
Area of inflammation	Mucosa and submucosa	Transmural (pertaining to the entire thickness of the wall of an organ)
Characteristics of inflammation	Tends to be continuous, starting at the rectum and extending proximally; limited to the mucosal lining	May be continuous or interspersed between areas of normal tissue; may extend through all layers of the bowel
Character of stools	Blood present No fat 15–20 liquid stools daily	No blood present Steatorrhea (fat in stool) 3 or 4 semisoft stools daily
Major complication	Toxic megacolon, fistulas, and abscesses (rare)	Malabsorption, bowel obstruction, fistulas, tissue abscesses
Major complaints	Rectal bleeding, abdominal cramping	Right lower abdominal pain with mass present
Reason for surgery	Poor response to medical therapy	Indicated to remove diseased areas that do not respond to aggressive medical therapy. Surgery does not cure the disease
Response to surgery	Removal of the colon cures the intestinal disease, but not extraintestinal symptoms, such as inflammation of joints and liver disease	Alleviation of symptoms caused from diseased portion of intestine
Cancer potential	Increased risk after 10 years of disease	Small intestine incidence increased; colon incidence increased, but not as much as in ulcerative colitis
Biopsy findings	Architectural changes consistent with chronic inflammation	Architectural changes consistent with chronic inflammation; may show granulomas
Weight loss	May develop weight loss depending on severity	Cobblestoning of mucosa is common; may be severe
Malabsorption and nutritional deficiencies	Minimal incidence	Common; may be severe; frequent

and pus. With severe diarrhea, losses of sodium, potassium, bicarbonate, and calcium ions may occur. Abdominal cramps may occur before the bowel movement. The urge to defecate lessens as scarring within the bowel progresses. This results in involuntary leakage of stool. In mild to moderate ulcerative colitis, diarrhea may consist of two to five stools per day with some blood present.

Complications are seen less in ulcerative colitis than with Crohn disease. Complications of ulcerative colitis include bleeding from ulcerations of the colon, rupture of the bowel, and severe abdominal bloating. A less common complication is toxic megacolon (toxic dilation of the large bowel). The bowel becomes distended and so thin that it could be perforated at any time.

Clinical manifestations of toxic megacolon include fever, abdominal pain and tenderness, severe abdominal distention, and shock. The patient with ulcerative colitis is at increased risk for colon cancer. Surgical interventions for treatment of this complication are usually necessary.

Assessment
Subjective data include complaints of rectal bleeding and abdominal cramping. Lethargy, a sense of frustration, and loss of control result from painful abdominal cramping and unpredictable bowel movements.

Objective data include weight loss, abdominal distention, fever, tachycardia, leukocytosis, and observation of frequency and characteristics of stools.

Diagnostic Tests

Double-contrast BE studies of the intestine, sigmoidoscopy and colonoscopy with biopsy, and stool testing for melena aid the health care provider in diagnosis. Additional studies include radiologic examination of the abdomen, serum electrolytes and albumin levels, liver function studies, and other hematologic studies.

Medical Management

The medical interventions chosen depend on the phase of the disease and the individual response to therapy. Common treatment modalities include medication, diet intervention, and stress reduction.

Drug therapy. The four major categories of drugs used are (1) those that affect the inflammatory response, (2) antibacterial drugs, (3) drugs that affect the immune system, and (4) antidiarrheal preparations.

Sulfasalazine is a common medication used for mild chronic ulcerative colitis. Sulfasalazine is broken down by bacteria in the colon into sulfapyridine and 5-aminosalicylic acid (5-ASA). It affects the inflammatory response and provides some antibacterial activity. It is effective in maintaining clinical remission and in treating mild to moderately severe attacks. Newer preparations have been developed to deliver 5-ASA to the terminal ileum and colon (e.g., olsalazine, mesalamine, and balsalazide). These drugs are as effective as sulfasalazine and are better tolerated when administered orally. Immune system suppressants such as cyclosporine, infliximab, methotrexate, and ustekinumab commonly are prescribed.

Non-sulfa drugs such as mesalamine can be given by retention enema.

Corticosteroids are anti-inflammatory drugs effective in relieving symptoms of moderate and severe colitis; they can be given orally or intravenously if inflammation is severe.

Antidiarrheal agents are recommended over anticholinergic agents because anticholinergic drugs can mask obstruction or contribute to toxic colonic dilation. Loperamide may be used to treat cramping and diarrhea of chronic ulcerative colitis. Azathioprine is also beneficial (Crohn's & Colitis Foundation, n.d.b.).

Nutrition therapy. Diet is an important component in the treatment of inflammatory bowel disease, and a dietitian should be consulted. The goals of diet management are to provide adequate nutrition without making symptoms worse, to correct and prevent malnutrition, to replace fluid and electrolyte losses, and to prevent weight loss. Patients with inflammatory bowel disease must eat a balanced, healthy diet with sufficient calories, protein, and nutrients. Patients can use MyPlate guidelines to ensure that they get adequate portions from all the food groups. The diet for each patient is individualized.

Patients with diarrhea often decrease their oral intake to reduce the diarrhea. The anorexia that accompanies inflammation also results in decreases in food intake. Blood loss leads to iron deficiency anemia.

Inflammatory bowel disease has no universal food triggers, but patients may find that certain foods initiate diarrhea. A food diary helps them identify problem foods to avoid. Many patients are lactose intolerant and improve when they avoid milk products. High-fat foods also tend to trigger diarrhea. Cold foods and high-fiber foods (cereal with bran, nuts, and raw fruit) may increase GI transit. Smoking stimulates the GI tract (increases motility and secretion) and should be avoided. Patients with significant fluid and electrolyte losses or malabsorption may need parenteral nutrition or enteral feedings, such as elemental diets. Elemental diets are high in calories and nutrients, lactose free, and absorbed in the proximal small intestine, which allows the more distal bowel to rest.

Stress control. Ulcerative colitis is aggravated by stress. Identifying the factors that cause stress is the first step in controlling the disease. Working with the patient to find healthful coping mechanisms is part of the holistic approach in nursing interventions.

Surgical intervention. If an acute episode does not respond to treatment, if complications occur, or if the risk of cancer becomes greater because of chronic ulcerative colitis, surgical intervention is indicated (Box 5.3). Most surgeons prefer a conservative approach, removing only the diseased portion of the colon. The operations of choice may be a single-stage total proctocolectomy with construction of an internal reservoir and valve (Kock pouch, or Kock continent ileostomy) (Fig. 5.9); total proctocolectomy with ileoanal anastomosis with or without construction of an internal reservoir; and temporary ileostomy. In the case of a high-risk patient, a subtotal colectomy may be performed with ileostomy. After the patient's recovery (approximately 2 to 4 months), removal of the rectum or construction of an internal reservoir is possible.

Nursing Interventions

Nursing interventions include a thorough assessment of the patient's bowel elimination, support systems, coping abilities, nutritional status, pain, and understanding of the disease process and treatment required. Patients need a complete understanding of the care plan so that they can make informed choices. Prevention of future episodes is a goal for the patient with ulcerative colitis.

Preoperative care for these patients includes (1) selecting a stoma site, (2) performing additional diagnostic tests if cancer is suspected, (3) helping the patient accept that previous treatments were unsuccessful in curing the disease, and (4) preparing the bowel for surgery. The bowel is prepared 2 or 3 days preoperatively. A bland to clear liquid diet is ordered, along with a bowel prep of laxatives. Antibiotics, such as

Box 5.3 Surgical Interventions for Ulcerative Colitis

- *Colon resection:* Removal of a portion of the large intestine and anastomosis of the remaining segment
- *Ileoanal anastomosis:* Removal of the colon and rectum but leaving the anus intact, along with the anal sphincter; anastomosis formed between the lower end of the small intestine and the anus
- *Ileostomy:* Surgical formation of an opening of the ileum onto the surface of the abdomen, through which fecal matter is emptied
- *Kock pouch (Kock continent ileostomy):* Surgical removal of the rectum and colon (proctocolectomy) with formation of a reservoir by suturing loops of adjacent ileum together to form a pouchlike structure, nipple valve, and stoma
- *Proctocolectomy:* Removal of anus, rectum, and colon; ileostomy established for the removal of digestive tract wastes

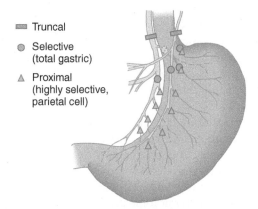

■ Truncal

● Selective (total gastric)

△ Proximal (highly selective, parietal cell)

Fig 5.9 Types of vagotomies: truncal, selective, and proximal or parietal cell. (From Black JM, Hawks JH: *Medical-surgical nursing: Clinical management for positive outcomes*, ed 8, St. Louis, 2009, Saunders.)

erythromycin and neomycin, frequently are given to decrease the number of bacteria in the bowel.

Postoperative nursing interventions depend on the type of procedure performed and the individual's response. Areas of concern are bowel and urinary elimination; fluid and electrolyte balance; tissue perfusion; comfort and pain; nutrition; gas exchange; infection; and, in the case of ostomy construction, assessment of the ileostomy and peristomal skin integrity.

A patient problem and interventions for the patient with chronic inflammatory bowel disease include but are not limited to the following:

Patient Problem	Nursing Interventions
Helplessness, related to loss of control of body function	Assist weakened patient with activities of daily living (bathing, oral hygiene, shaving, and other grooming needs) Offer choices to patient, when possible, to provide a sense of control

Patient problems for the surgical patient include *Potential for Impaired Coping, Impaired Self-Esteem due to Current Situation,* and *Distorted Body Image.* Nursing interventions include reinforcing the health care provider's explanation of the surgical procedure and expected outcomes. Providing reading material and demonstrating the care of an ostomy pouch when the patient seems ready reduces anxiety. A visitor from the United Ostomy Associations of America can provide hope as a recovered and productive role model. Surgical intervention and the subsequent stoma are often difficult for the patient to cope with initially. Be supportive and encourage the patient to share fears. Box 5.4 lists postoperative nursing interventions.

Peristomal area integrity. Assess the peristomal skin for impaired integrity. Four primary factors contributing to loss of peristomal skin integrity are allergies, mechanical trauma, chemical reactions, and infection:

- Allergies to pouches, adhesives, skin barriers, powders, and paste are rare but are evident at areas of contact. The skin may appear erythematous, eroded, weeping, and bleeding. Changing the type of pouch, tape, or adhesive may resolve the problem.
- Mechanical trauma caused by pressure, friction, or stripping of adhesives and skin barriers can be avoided by changing the pouch less frequently, using adhesive tape sparingly, and using skin preparation solutions. The skin must be protected when the pouch is removed.
- The most common chemical irritant is the stool from the stoma. Protect the skin from these digestive enzymes by using skin barriers before applying the pouch. Skin barriers include adhesives (Stomahesive), powders (Stomahesive powder), liquid skin barriers (Skin Prep), and caulking paste (Stomahesive paste).
- A common cause of infection of the peristomal skin is *Candida albicans.* People who have been taking antibiotics for 5 or more days may be prone to this problem. Treatment is the application of nystatin powder or cream, by health care provider order. A skin barrier should be applied over the medicated area to ensure that the adhesive sticks.

Patient Teaching

The patient and/or the caregiver must be taught the appropriate care of the ileostomy or colostomy to foster independence. This includes pouch change, cleansing, irrigation, and skin care. Providing a list of foods known to cause constipation, diarrhea, blockage, odors, and flatus is helpful. Before discharge, the patient should be given a list of resource people; phone numbers; and supplies, including where to obtain them.

Prognosis

The prognosis for patients with chronic ulcerative colitis is related directly to the number of years they have

Box 5.4 **Postoperative Nursing Interventions for Ulcerative Colitis**

1. Monitor nasogastric (NG) suction for patency until bowel function is resumed. Maintain correct wall suctioning. Accurately record color and amount of output. Irrigate NG tube as needed. Apply water-soluble lubricant to nares. Assess bowel sounds, being certain to turn off NG suction during auscultation.
2. Initiate ostomy care and teaching when bowel activity begins. Be sensitive to patient's pain level and readiness for teaching of ostomy care.
3. Observe **stoma** (an artificial opening of an internal organ on the body's surface) for color and size (should be pink/red and slightly edematous). Document assessment (e.g., "stoma pink and viable").
4. Select appropriate pouching system that has skin-protective barrier, accordion flange to ease pressure applied to new incisional site, adhesive backing, and pouch opening no more than ¹⁄₁₆ inch larger than the stoma. Stomas change in size over time and should be measured before new supplies are ordered.
5. Empty pouch when it is approximately one-third to one-half full to prevent breaking the seal, resulting in pouch leakage.
6. Explain that initial dark green liquid will change to yellow-brown as patient is allowed to eat.
7. Teach patient to care for the stoma; this includes having patient look at stoma and gradually assist with emptying, cleaning, and changing pouch. Teach patient that normal grieving occurs after loss of rectal function. Be supportive of patient's concerns.
8. Promote independence and self-care to decrease state of denial.
9. Instruct on follow-up home care, including changing skin barrier (a piece of pectin-based or Karaya wafer with measurable thickness and hydrocolloid adhesive properties) every 5–7 days. Using antacids, skin protective paste, and liquid skin barrier may be appropriate if skin excoriation is observed.
10. Patient may shower or bathe with or without pouch on.
11. Patient should avoid lifting objects heavier than 10 lb until health care provider says it is allowed.
12. A special diet is not necessary, but patients should drink 8–10 glasses of water a day, chew food well, and limit or avoid certain gas-forming foods.
13. Sexual relationships can be resumed when health care provider feels it is not harmful to the surgical area. Counseling may be appropriate if patient has fear of resuming this activity.

had the disease and the severity. The incidence of carcinoma increases when the colon is extensively involved over time. The disease carries a higher mortality rate among patients who have had the disease for an extended period of time.

CROHN DISEASE

Etiology and Pathophysiology

Crohn disease, although not as prevalent as ulcerative colitis, is increasing in incidence. Crohn disease is characterized by inflammation of segments of the GI tract. The cause of the disease is not known, but there seems to be a strong association between Crohn disease and altered immune mechanisms. Genetic and environmental factors seem to play a role. It most commonly occurs during adolescence and early adulthood but is also seen developing in patients between 50 and 60 years of age. Crohn disease can occur anywhere in the GI tract from the mouth to the anus but occurs most commonly in the terminal ileum and proximal colon. The inflammation involves all layers of the bowel wall. It may involve only one segment of the bowel, or segments of diseased tissue may alternate with healthy tissue. In the early stages of the disease, tiny ulcers form on various parts of the intestinal wall. Over time, horizontal rows of these ulcers fuse with vertical rows, giving the mucosa a cobblestone appearance. Inflammation, fibrosis, and scarring often involving the entire thickness of the intestine are characteristics of Crohn disease. Patients with Crohn disease are likely to have a bowel obstruction, fistulas, fissures, and abscesses. In some patients, the disease may involve the colon without any changes in the small intestine.

Malabsorption is the major problem when the small intestine is involved, and this contributes to nutritional problems. Pernicious anemia may result from decreased absorption of vitamin B_{12} in the small intestine. Fluid and electrolyte disturbances with acid-base imbalances can occur, particularly with depletion of sodium or potassium associated with diarrhea or with excessive small intestine drainage through fistulas associated with the pathologic process.

Clinical Manifestations

The manifestations depend largely on the anatomic site of involvement, extent of the disease process, and presence of complications. The onset of Crohn disease is usually insidious, with nonspecific complaints such as diarrhea, fatigue, abdominal pain, weight loss, and fever. As the disease progresses, the patient experiences weight loss, malnutrition, dehydration, electrolyte imbalance, anemia, and increased peristalsis.

Assessment

Collection of subjective data for the patient with Crohn disease includes noting the patient's list of complaints, including weakness, loss of appetite, abdominal pain and cramps, intermittent low-grade fever, sleeplessness caused by diarrhea, and stress. Right-lower-quadrant abdominal pain is characteristic of the disease and may be accompanied by a tender mass of thickened intestines in the same area.

Objective data include complaints of diarrhea—three or four semisolid stools daily, containing mucus and pus, but usually no blood. **Steatorrhea** (excess fat in the feces) also may be present if the ulceration extends high in the small intestine. With small intestine involvement, weight loss occurs from malabsorption.

Scar tissue from the inflammation narrows the lumen of the intestine and may cause strictures and obstruction, a frequent complication. Intestinal fistulas are a cardinal feature and may develop between segments of bowel. Cutaneous fistulas, common in the perianal area, and rectovaginal fistulas may occur. Fistulas communicating with the urinary tract may cause urinary tract infections. Poor absorption of bile salts by the ileum may lead to watery stools. Fever and unexplained anemia also may occur.

Diagnostic Tests

The most definitive test to differentiate Crohn disease from ulcerative colitis is colonoscopy with multiple biopsies of the colon and terminal ileum. The appearance of the mucosa in Crohn disease can range from normal to severely inflamed, and areas of inflammation may be continuous or interspersed with areas that appear normal. The small bowel mucosa may show abnormalities such as a cobblestone appearance, as well as fistulas and strictures of the ileum. Blood tests for anemia also may be ordered. Because viewing the entire small intestine may be limited with traditional endoscopy, capsule endoscopy may be beneficial in the diagnostic process (Crohn's and Colitis Foundation, n.d.a.).

Medical Management

Medications. Treatment is individualized depending on the patient's age, the location and severity of the disease, and any complications present. Once Crohn disease has been diagnosed, the patient is started on drug therapy to try to get the disease in remission. Those with mild to moderate disease usually take anti-inflammatory agents such as sulfasalazine, mesalamine, olsalazine, or balsalazide. When inflammation is severe, corticosteroids such as prednisone may be prescribed. Patients are weaned off steroids as soon as possible to prevent dependency and long-term complications. Multivitamins and B_{12} injections often are recommended to correct deficiencies. If first line fails, treatment with second-line drugs becomes necessary. These include immunosuppressive agents such as azathioprine; cyclosporine (Neoral; methotrexate; and IV immunoglobulin. Biological response modifiers such as infliximab, adalimumab, and certolizumab pegol may be used to treat Crohn disease.

Diet intervention, stress reduction, and surgery also are used to manage Crohn disease.

Diet. Bowel symptoms and diarrhea may be minimized by excluding from the diet (1) lactose-containing foods in patients suspected of having lactose intolerance; (2) certain gas-causing vegetables (e.g., cauliflower, broccoli, asparagus, cabbage, Brussels sprouts); (3) caffeine, beer, monosodium glutamate, and sugarless (sorbitol-containing) gum and mints; and (4) highly seasoned foods, concentrated fruit juices, carbonated beverages, and fatty foods.

Diets high in protein (100 g/day) are recommended for patients with hypoproteinemia caused by mucosal loss, malabsorption, maldigestion, or malnutrition. Some patients find small frequent meals to be beneficial to limiting symptoms. Liquids, especially water, should be increased to replace fluid lost. Placing the patient on NPO status and starting TPN may be necessary when the patient with Crohn disease is having severe symptoms so that the colon can be allowed to rest.

Complications of inflammation with fibrous scarring, obstruction, fistula formation in the small intestine, abscesses, and perforation are indications for surgical excision and anastomosis. Resection is the preferred surgery because the bypass procedure has a greater failure rate.

Surgical treatment. Surgical intervention for patients' with Crohn disease is not uncommon. Although surgery produces remission, recurrence rates are high. Surgical removal of large segments of the small intestine can lead to short-bowel syndrome, a condition in which the absorption surface is inadequate to maintain life and parenteral nutrition is used. Surgery is reserved for emergency situations (excessive bleeding, obstruction, peritonitis) or when medical treatment has failed. One surgical technique for Crohn disease is strictureplasty to widen areas of narrowed bowel. It is sometimes necessary to resect the diseased bowel and anastomose the ends. Unfortunately, the disease commonly recurs at the area of anastomosis. Emergency surgery is necessary when perforation allows bowel contents to drain into the abdominal cavity. Surgery to cleanse the peritoneal cavity and create a temporary ostomy frequently is performed.

Nursing Interventions

In caring for the patient with Crohn disease, consider nutrition, fluid balance, elimination, medications, psychological aspects, and sexuality. Total parenteral nutrition may be ordered in cases of severe disease and marked weight loss. Tube feedings that allow rapid absorption in the upper GI tract are begun, and then oral intake of a low-residue, high-protein, and high-calorie diet is introduced gradually. Vitamin supplements are frequently necessary, and vitamin B_{12} is given when there is a marked loss of ileum. When anemia is present, iron dextran is given by Z-track injection (because of irritation to the tissues) because oral intake of iron is ineffective because of intestinal ulceration.

Oral diets of 2500 mL/day to replace fluids and electrolytes lost from diarrhea are not uncommon. Monitor the patient for weight loss or gain. Monitor daily skin condition and I&O. A urinary output of at least 1500 mL/day is desired.

When a patient is hospitalized, a bedside commode or a bedpan must be accessible at all times because of the urgency and frequency of stools. Emptying the bedpan immediately and deodorizing the room maintain an aesthetic environment. The anal region may become excoriated from frequent stools. Assess the anal area regularly and keep it clean, using medicated wipes and sitz baths. These nursing interventions promote comfort and hygiene for the patient.

Most patients with Crohn disease require emotional support from all health care personnel. The onset of the disease often occurs at a young age, before the person has the emotional development and maturity to cope. The support groups sponsored by the CCFA can play a major role in helping patients. Antidepressants and psychology or psychiatry services may be required when managing the disease. Current evidence suggests that Crohn disease is not caused by psychological stress but that psychiatric disturbances are the result of the disease's symptoms and chronicity.

Patient problems and interventions for patients with Crohn disease include but are not limited to the following:

Patient Problem	Nursing Interventions
Helplessness, related to exacerbations and remissions	Explore with patient factors that aggravate the disease Assist patient in listing factors that can be controlled: diet, stressors, medication compliance, self-monitoring of symptoms
Insufficient Nutrition, related to: • Bowel hypermotility • Decreased absorption	Emphasize the importance of weighing daily, following special diets, and assessing energy levels

Nursing Interventions and Patient Teaching

The patient must understand how diarrhea and rapid emptying of the small intestine affect the body's nutritional needs. This leads to acceptance of special diets and the ability to retain some personal control of the disease. The patient must also understand the relationship of emotional feelings to Crohn disease. Identifying resources for emotional support in the family and community and among health professionals promotes coping skills and mental hygiene.

Prognosis

Crohn disease is a chronic disorder; it has a high rate of recurrence, especially in patients younger than 25 years of age. Prognosis depends on the extent of involvement, duration of illness, and success of medical interventions. No known therapy keeps a patient with Crohn disease in remission.

ACUTE ABDOMINAL INFLAMMATION

APPENDICITIS
Etiology and Pathophysiology

Appendicitis is the inflammation of the vermiform appendix, usually acute. If undiagnosed, it leads rapidly to perforation and peritonitis. Appendicitis is most likely to occur in persons between the ages of 10 and 30 years.

The vermiform appendix is a small tube in the right lower quadrant of the abdomen. The lumen of the proximal end is shared with that of the cecum, whereas the distal end is closed. The appendix fills and empties regularly in the same way as the cecum. However, the lumen is tiny and easily obstructed. The most common causes of appendicitis are obstruction of the lumen by a fecalith (accumulated feces), foreign bodies, and tumor of the cecum or appendix. If it becomes obstructed and inflamed, pathogenic bacteria (*E. coli*) begin to multiply in the appendix and cause an infection with the formation of pus. If distention and infection are severe enough, the appendix may rupture, releasing its contents into the abdomen. The infection may be contained within an appendiceal abscess or may spread to the abdominal cavity, causing generalized peritonitis.

Clinical Manifestations

Light palpation of the abdomen elicits rebound tenderness in the right lower quadrant (increased pain felt when using the fingertips to press on the abdomen on the opposite side of the suspected problem, then quickly releasing pressure). The abdominal musculature overlying the right lower quadrant may feel tense because of voluntary rigidity. The patient often lies on the back or side with knees flexed in an attempt to decrease muscular strain on the abdominal wall.

Assessment

Subjective data include the most common complaint of constant pain in the right lower quadrant of the abdomen, around McBurney's point (halfway between the umbilicus and the crest of the right ileum). The pain may be accompanied by nausea and anorexia.

Objective data include vomiting, fever, an elevated WBC count, rebound tenderness, a rigid abdomen, and decreased or absent bowel sounds.

Diagnostic Tests

The health care provider orders a WBC count with differential. Most patients have a WBC level above $10,000/mm^3$ (the normal range is 4500 to $11,000/mm^3$). An abdominal CT scan and abdominal ultrasound are excellent diagnostic tools. Urinalysis also may be performed to rule out a urinary tract infection as the source of pain.

Medical Management

Emergency surgical intervention is the preferred treatment for acute appendicitis, or surgery may be performed when a patient is having another abdominal surgical procedure. Because mortality correlates with perforation and peritonitis, and perforation correlates with duration of symptoms, early diagnosis and appendectomy are essential. Antibiotic therapy is given when perforation is likely. Complications include infection, intra-abdominal abscess, and mechanical small bowel obstruction (see the Safety Alert box).

> ⚠ **Safety Alert**

Appendicitis

- Encourage the patient with abdominal pain to see a health care provider and to avoid self-treatment, particularly the use of laxatives and enemas.
- The increased peristalsis of laxatives and enemas may cause perforation of the appendix.
- Until the patient is seen by a health care provider, he or she should remain nothing by mouth to ensure the stomach is empty in case surgery is needed.
- An ice bag may be applied to the right lower quadrant to decrease the flow of blood to the area and impede the inflammatory process.
- *Heat is never used* because it could cause the appendix to rupture.
- Surgery usually is performed as soon as a diagnosis is made.

Nursing Interventions and Patient Teaching

Nursing interventions include following general preoperative procedure. Explain diagnostic tests and possible surgical procedures to relieve anxiety. Maintain bed rest and NPO status, provide comfort measures for pain relief so that symptoms are not masked by medication, and replace fluids and electrolytes. The patient's vital signs are monitored and documented every hour because of the threat of perforation resulting to peritonitis.

Administer prescribed opioids after the health care provider has assessed the patient. Opioids can mask symptoms of acute appendicitis. In some cases, an ice bag to relieve pain is given; no heat is applied because this increases circulation to the appendix and could lead to rupture. A cleansing enema is not ordered because of the danger of rupture. General postoperative care is performed.

Patient problems and interventions for the patient with appendicitis include but are not limited to the following:

Patient teaching may include the reason for IV fluids with gradual advancement of the diet from clear

Patient Problem	Nursing Interventions
Recent Onset of Pain, related to inflammation	Support the patient and the family by listening and by explaining tests and procedures
	Administer opioids as soon as indicated after the health care provider assesses the patient
	Monitor for increases in pain, rebound tenderness (Rovsing sign), and abdominal rigidity
	Take vital signs frequently (q h)

liquids to regular diet as peristalsis returns. If antibiotics or oral medications are continued postoperatively, ensure the patient understands the name, purpose, and side effects of each medication. If complications occur, necessitating an NG tube or drainage tubes, explain the reason for these interventions to the patient.

Prognosis

The rate of cure through surgical intervention is high in patients with appendicitis. The patient's prognosis is altered if peritonitis complicates this diagnosis.

DIVERTICULOSIS AND DIVERTICULITIS

Etiology and Pathophysiology

Diverticular disease has two clinical forms: *diverticulosis* and *diverticulitis*. Diverticulosis is the presence of pouch-like herniations through the circular smooth muscle of the colon, particularly the sigmoid colon (Fig. 5.10). Diverticulitis is the inflammation of one or more of the diverticular sacs.

The incidence of diverticulosis is increased after the age of 40. Several factors are linked to the incidence of the diseases. Aging may lead to decreased strength and elasticity of the colon, resulting in the outward pouching. Lack of fiber in the diet and an increase in refined carbohydrates is also thought to be a contributing factor, causing high pressure in the lumen of the colon. Other contributing factors include lack of exercise, obesity, and smoking. Penetration of fecal matter through the thin-walled diverticula causes inflammation and abscess formation in the tissues surrounding the colon. With repeated inflammation, the lumen of the colon narrows and may become obstructed. When one or more diverticula become inflamed, diverticulitis results, which is a complication of diverticulosis. This inflammation can lead to perforation, abscess,

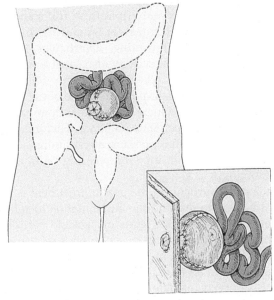

Fig. 5.10 Kock pouch (Kock continent ileostomy).

peritonitis, obstruction, and hemorrhage. Diverticulitis is the most common cause of lower GI hemorrhage.

Clinical Manifestations

When diverticula perforate and diverticulitis develops, the patient complains of mild to severe pain in the left lower quadrant of the abdomen, has a fever, and has an elevated WBC count and erythrocyte sedimentation rate. If the condition goes untreated, septicemia and septic shock can develop. This patient is generally hypotensive and is tachycardic. Intestinal obstruction can occur, causing abdominal distention, nausea, and vomiting.

Assessment

Collection of subjective data includes an awareness that the patient with diverticulosis may not display any problematic symptoms. Complaints of constipation and diarrhea accompanied by pain in the left lower quadrant are common. Other common symptoms include increased flatus and chronic constipation alternating with diarrhea, anorexia, and nausea.

Objective data include abdominal distention, low-grade fever, leukocytosis, vomiting, blood in the stool, abdominal tenderness on palpation, and sometimes a palpable abdominal mass.

Diagnostic Tests

Ultrasound and CT scan with oral contrast are used to confirm the diagnosis and evaluate the severity of the disease. A complete blood count (CBC), urinalysis, and fecal occult blood test should be performed. A BE occasionally is used to determine narrowing or obstruction of the colonic lumen. Colonoscopy may help rule out polyps or a malignancy. A patient with acute diverticulitis should not have a BE or colonoscopy because of the possibility of perforation and peritonitis.

Medical Management

A diet high in fiber, mainly from fresh fruits and vegetables, and decreased intake of fat and red meat are recommended for preventing diverticular disease. High levels of physical activity also seem to decrease the risk.

Weight reduction is important for the obese person. Patients should avoid increased intra-abdominal pressure, which may precipitate an attack. Factors that increase intra-abdominal pressure are straining at stool; vomiting; bending; lifting; and wearing tight, restrictive clothing.

In acute diverticulitis, the goal of treatment is to allow the colon to rest and the inflammation to subside. Observe the patient for signs of possible peritonitis. Administer broad-spectrum antibiotics as ordered. Monitor the WBC count. Frequently, diverticulitis can be managed in an outpatient setting, and hospitalization is reserved for older adults or those with severe symptoms.

When the acute attack subsides, oral fluids are given initially, progressing to semisolids. The patient should be observed for a recurrent exacerbation. If the patient has a bowel resection or colostomy, the nursing care is the same as previously discussed.

Although diverticular disease is common, complications are rare. Bowel rest and antibiotic therapy are usually adequate. Surgical treatment is advised if long-term problems do not respond to medical management and is likely if complications (e.g., hemorrhage, obstruction, abscesses, or perforation) occur. In elective surgery, a thorough bowel preparation is most important. Laxatives, enemas, or intestinal lavage are given to cleanse the bowel, depending on the surgeon's preference. Antibiotics are given orally and parenterally.

In cases of perforation, abscess, peritonitis, or fistula, resection of the bowel with a temporary colostomy is needed. Either the one-stage procedure (resection of the affected bowel with anastomosis and no diverting colostomy) or the two-stage procedure (resection of the diseased bowel with diverting colostomy) is performed.

The bowel diversion can be accomplished by Hartmann's procedure (Fig. 5.11A), in which the descending colon is resected, the proximal end is brought to the abdominal wall surface, and the distal bowel is sealed off for later anastomosis. Other procedures are the double-barrel colostomy, in which the bowel is brought up through the abdominal surface (Fig. 5.11B), and transverse loop colostomy, in which a loop is formed and the bowel is held in place with a plastic butterfly bridge between the bowel and the abdomen (Fig. 5.11C). The bowel can be opened at the time of surgery or postoperatively. Removal of the affected bowel segment and reanastomosis of the bowel are included in the initial procedure.

Closure of the temporary colostomy is the desired goal in the case of diverticular disease. Usually this takes place 6 weeks to 3 months after the initial surgical procedure. Again, the bowel must be prepared for

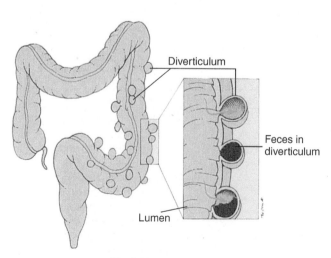

Fig. 5.11 Diverticulosis.

closure by a liquid diet; laxatives; antibiotics; intestinal lavage as mentioned; and a cleansing colostomy irrigation of the proximal and, in the case of the loop or double-barrel colostomy, distal end of the stoma.

Nursing Interventions and Patient Teaching

The return of bowel activity after closure may take several days. The patient will have IV fluids and an NG tube for the first few days postoperatively.

Nursing interventions include teaching the patient about the disease process and surgery, if planned. Assess the patient's nutritional status and reinforce the prescribed diet. Assess the patient's pain so that comfort measures or medication can be administered. Include the patient and family in setting goals for the teaching plan.

Patient problems and interventions for the patient with diverticular disease include but are not limited to the following:

Patient Problem	Nursing Interventions
Insufficient Knowledge, related to disease process and treatment	Instruct patient and family in disease process and signs and symptoms of acute diverticulitis attack
Insufficient Nutrition, related to decreased oral intake	Instruct patient about dietary fiber (for prevention) or bland, low-residue diet (for inflammatory phase) Assess daily weights, calorie counts, and intake and output Monitor serum protein and albumin

When a colostomy is performed, ask the patient or family member to verbalize and demonstrate understanding of ostomy care. The teaching of colostomy care must not be rushed; the patient should be free of pain and receptive to learning. A family member may be taught to help until the patient is able to assume self-care, keeping in mind that the goal is patient independence. A home care referral may be needed so that the teaching process may continue after discharge.

Prognosis

With diverticulosis, the prognosis is good. Most patients have few symptoms except for occasional bleeding from the rectum. Diverticulitis has a good prognosis; some patients need bowel resection of the affected part in acute cases to reduce mortality and morbidity.

PERITONITIS

Etiology and Pathophysiology

Peritonitis is an inflammation of the abdominal peritoneum. This condition occurs after fecal matter seeps from a rupture site, causing bacterial contamination of the peritoneal cavity. Some examples are diverticular abscess and rupture, acute appendicitis with rupture, and strangulated hernia. Peritonitis also can be caused by chemical irritants, such as blood, bile, necrotic tissue, pancreatic enzymes (pancreatitis), and foreign bodies. Ascites that occurs with cirrhosis of the liver provides an excellent liquid environment for bacteria to flourish. Patients who use continuous ambulatory peritoneal dialysis are also at high risk. No matter what the cause, the resulting inflammatory response leads to massive fluid shifts (peritoneal edema and adhesions as the body attempts to wall off the infection). Sepsis can occur if peritonitis is not treated early enough or if it is not treated successfully.

Clinical Manifestations

Generalized peritonitis is an extremely serious condition characterized by severe abdominal pain. The patient usually lies on the back with the knees flexed to relax the abdominal muscles; any movement is painful. Rebound tenderness, muscular rigidity, and spasm are major symptoms of irritation of the peritoneum. The abdomen is usually tympanic and extremely tender to the touch.

Assessment

Collection of subjective data includes observing for severe abdominal pain. Nausea and vomiting occur, and as peristalsis ceases, constipation occurs with no passage of flatus. Chills, weakness, and abdominal tenderness (local and diffuse, often rebound) are other symptoms.

Collection of objective data includes noting a weak and rapid pulse, fever, and lowered blood pressure. Leukocytosis and marked dehydration occur, and the patient can collapse and die.

Diagnostic Tests

An abdominal x-ray is ordered to find out whether free air is present under the diaphragm as a result of visceral perforation. A CBC with differential is ordered to determine the degree of leukocytosis. A blood chemistry profile helps determine renal perfusion and electrolyte balance. Peritoneal aspiration may be performed and the fluid analyzed for blood, bile, pus, bacteria, or fungus. Ultrasound and CT scans may help identify ascites and abscesses.

Medical Management

Aggressive therapy includes correction of the contamination or removal of the chemical irritant by surgery and parenteral antibiotics. NG intubation is ordered to prevent GI distention. IV fluids and electrolytes are administered to prevent or correct imbalances. Analgesics are provided intravenously via PCA pump. The patient may be placed on TPN because of increased nutritional requirements. Early treatment to prevent severe shock from the loss of fluid into the peritoneal space is essential.

Nursing Interventions and Patient Teaching

Nursing interventions for the patient with peritonitis include the following:

- Place patient on bed rest in semi-Fowler's position to help localize purulent exudate in lower abdomen or pelvis.
- Give oral hygiene to prevent drying of mucous membranes and cracking of lips from dehydration.
- Monitor fluid and electrolyte replacement.
- Encourage deep-breathing exercises; patient tends to have shallow respirations as a result of abdominal pain or distention.
- Use measures to reduce anxiety.
- Use meticulous surgical asepsis for wound care.

Instruct the patient about the importance of ambulation, coughing, deep breathing, use of an incentive spirometer, and leg exercises. If the patient has a draining wound at discharge, teach surgical asepsis for dressing changes. Encourage a nutritious diet. Instruct the patient not to lift more than 10 lb. until the health care provider approves it. Stress the importance of keeping health care provider follow-up appointments.

Prognosis

The mortality rate among patients with generalized peritonitis depends on how quickly the infection is diagnosed, as well as age, cause of the peritonitis, and overall condition of the patient. Early recognition and treatment yield a 5% mortality rate, whereas later treatment yields a mortality rate of greater than 30%. Up to 70% of patients who have bacterial peritonitis experience a recurrent episode within 1 year. Delayed treatment often leads to gastrointestinal bleeding, renal dysfunction, and liver failure (Daley, 2019).

HERNIAS

EXTERNAL HERNIAS
Etiology and Pathophysiology

A hernia is the protrusion of a viscus through an abnormal opening or a weakened area in the wall of the cavity in which it normally is contained. Most hernias result from congenital or acquired weakness of the abdominal wall or a postoperative defect, coupled with increased intra-abdominal pressure from coughing, straining, or an enlarging lesion within the abdomen.

The various types of hernias include ventral hernia, femoral hernia, inguinal hernia, and umbilical hernia. A ventral, or incisional, hernia is due to weakness of the abdominal wall at the site of a previous incision. It is found most commonly in patients who are obese, who have had multiple surgical procedures in the same area, and who have inadequate wound healing because of poor nutrition or infection. An inguinal hernia is caused by a weakness in the lower abdominal wall opening, through which the spermatic cord emerges in men and the round ligament of the uterus emerges in women. A femoral hernia also is caused by a weakness in the lower abdominal wall, resulting in a bulging of tissue in the patient's groin.

A hernia may be reducible (able to be returned to its original position by manipulation) or irreducible (or incarcerated; unable to be returned to its body cavity). When the hernia is irreducible, it may obstruct intestinal flow. The hernia is strangulated when it occludes blood supply and intestinal flow. To prevent anaerobic infection in the area, immediate surgical intervention is performed when a hernia strangulates.

Factors such as age, wound infection, malnutrition, obesity, increased intra-abdominal pressure, or abdominal distention can affect whether a hernia forms after surgical incisions. Fewer hernias occur with transverse incisions than with longitudinal incisions. Also, upper abdominal incisions are associated with fewer hernias than lower abdominal incisions.

Assessment

Collection of objective data includes palpation of the hernia area, revealing the contents of the sac as soft and nodular (omentum; the layer of tissue that surrounds the abdominal organs) or smooth and fluctuant (bowel). Never attempt to push a hernia back into place, because this can lead to complications such as rupture of the strangulated contents.

Subjective and objective signs and symptoms depend on where the hernia occurs. With an inguinal hernia, the patient may complain of pain, urgency, and a mass in the groin region.

Objective data include a visible protruding mass or bulge around the umbilicus, in the inguinal area, or near an incision; this is the most common objective sign. If complications such as incarceration or strangulation follow, the patient may have bowel obstruction, vomiting, and abdominal distention.

Diagnostic Tests

The diagnosis is aided by palpation of the weakened wall. Radiographs of the suspected area may be ordered.

Medical Management

Hernias that cause no discomfort can be left unrepaired unless strangulation or obstruction follows. Teach the patient to seek medical advice promptly if abdominal pain, distention, changing bowel habits, temperature elevation, nausea, or vomiting occurs. If the hernia can be reduced manually, an abdominal binder keeps the hernia from protruding and holds the abdominal contents in place.

Elective surgery for hernia repair may be done because of inconvenience to the patient or constant risk of strangulation. A procedure to close the hernial defect by approximating and suturing the edges of adjacent muscles or using a synthetic mesh is done on either an inpatient or outpatient basis.

Nursing Interventions and Patient Teaching

Nursing interventions for external hernia require observation of the hernia's location and size and tissue perfusion to the area. The patient may be limited in activity and the type of clothing worn.

Herniorrhaphy (surgical hernia repair) usually is performed by a laparoscopic procedure on an outpatient basis. Open abdominal surgery may be necessary for the patient with a strangulated hernia. The patient should be prepared for a longer hospitalization, which may include NG suctioning, IV antibiotics, fluid and electrolyte replacement, and parenteral analgesics until peristalsis returns.

Postoperatively, the patient is monitored for urinary retention; wound infection at the incision site; and, with inguinal hernia repair, scrotal edema. If scrotal edema is present, the scrotum is elevated on a rolled pad with an ice pack applied, and a supportive garment (scrotal support, jockstrap, or briefs) provided. The patient should deep breathe every 2 hours, but many surgeons discourage coughing. Teach the patient how to support the incision by splinting the area with a pillow or pad. This support, along with analgesics, helps relieve pain.

Patient problems and interventions for the patient with a hernia include but are not limited to the following:

Patient Problem	Nursing Interventions
Insufficient Knowledge, related to disease process	Instruct patient to observe and report hernias that become irreducible or edematous Instruct patient to report increased pain, abdominal distention, or change in bowel habits Explain reason to avoid prolonged standing, lifting, or straining Instruct patient to support weakened area by use of truss or manually as needed (as when coughing)
Compromised Blood Flow to Tissue, related to strangulation or incarceration of hernia	Monitor patient for increased pain, distention, changing bowel habits, abnormal bowel sounds, temperature elevation, nausea, and vomiting Report changes in appearance and signs and symptoms to health care provider

Follow-up care includes teaching the patient to limit activities and avoid lifting heavy objects or straining with bowel movements for 5 to 6 weeks. In addition, the patient should report to the health care provider immediately any erythema or edema of the surgical area or increased pain or drainage.

HIATAL HERNIA

A hiatal hernia (esophageal hernia or diaphragmatic hernia) results from a weakness of the diaphragm. Hiatal hernia is a protrusion of the stomach and other abdominal viscera through an opening, or hiatus, in the diaphragm (Fig. 5.12). A hiatal hernia is a problem of the diaphragm that affects the alimentary tract. It is an anatomic condition, not a disease. This condition occurs predominantly in individuals over the age of 50 (NLM, 2021). The major difficulty in symptomatic patients is gastroesophageal reflux, manifested as pyrosis (heartburn) after overeating. Complications of strangulation, infarction, or ulceration of the herniated stomach are serious and require surgical intervention. Factors contributing to the development of these hernias include obesity, trauma, and a general weakening of the supporting structures as a result of aging (see the Lifespan Considerations box).

Lifespan Considerations
Older Adults

Gastrointestinal Disorders

- Loss of teeth and resultant use of dentures can interfere with chewing and lead to digestive complaints.
- Dysphagia commonly is seen in the older adult population and may be caused by changes in the esophageal musculature or by neurologic conditions.
- Hiatal hernias and esophageal diverticula are increased significantly with aging because of changes in musculature of the diaphragm and esophagus.
- Older adults have decreased secretion of hydrochloric acid (hypochlorhydria and achlorhydria) from the parietal cells of the stomach. This results in an increased incidence of pernicious anemia and gastritis in the older adult population.
- Peptic ulcers are common, but often the symptoms are vague and go unrecognized until there is a bleeding episode. Medications such as aspirin, nonsteroidal anti-inflammatory drugs, and steroids that are taken for the chronic degenerative joint conditions common with aging should be used with caution because they can contribute to ulcer formation.
- Frequency of diverticulosis and diverticulitis increases dramatically with aging and can contribute to malabsorption of nutrients.
- Constipation is a problem for many older adults. Inactivity, changes in diet and fluid intake, and medications can contribute to this problem. Monitor bowel elimination and establish a bowel regimen to prevent impaction.

Medical Management

The health care provider may perform (1) a posterior gastropexy, in which the stomach is returned to the abdomen and sutured in place; or (2) a laparoscopically performed Nissen fundoplication, in which the fundus of the stomach is wrapped around the lower part of the esophagus and sutured in place (Fig. 5.13). The use of laparoscopic techniques has reduced the

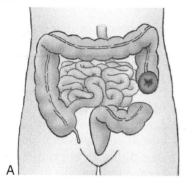
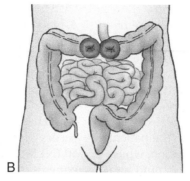
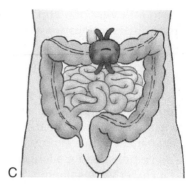

Fig. 5.12 (A) Hartmann pouch. (B) Double-barrel transverse colostomy. (C) Transverse loop colostomy with rod or butterfly. (Modified from Black JM, Hawks JH: *Medical-surgical nursing clinical management for positive outcomes*, ed 8, St. Louis, 2009, Saunders.)

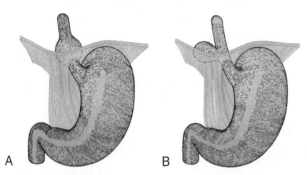

Fig. 5.13 Hiatal hernia. (A) Sliding hernia. (B) Rolling hernia.

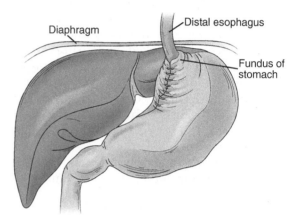

Fig. 5.14 Nissen fundoplication for hiatal hernia, showing fundus of stomach wrapped around distal esophagus and sutured to itself.

overall morbidity, complications, and cost of hospitalization associated with a thoracic or open abdominal approach. However, a thoracic or open abdominal approach may be used in selected cases.

Nursing Interventions
Nursing care of the patient after surgery is similar to that after gastric surgery or thoracic surgery, depending on the procedure performed.

Prognosis
The prognosis for hernias is good because surgical intervention is usually successful. The result can be altered if the patient is a poor surgical risk or has other complications.

DISORDERS OF THE SMALL AND LARGE INTESTINES

INTESTINAL OBSTRUCTION
Etiology and Pathophysiology
Intestinal obstruction occurs when intestinal contents cannot pass through the GI tract. Intestinal obstructions are considered mechanical (e.g., a tumor blocking the intestinal lumen) or nonmechanical (e.g., paralytic ileus after surgery). No matter the cause, an intestinal obstruction can become a life-threatening condition. Prompt assessment of symptoms by the nurse is vital. An obstruction may be partial or complete.

Mechanical obstruction. Mechanical obstruction may be caused by an occlusion of the lumen of the intestinal

tract. Most obstructions occur in the ileum, which is the narrowest segment of the small intestine. Adhesions (Fig. 5.14A) from previous abdominal surgeries account for approximately 60% of all intestinal obstructions. Other mechanical obstructions include incarcerated hernias. Additional causes include impacted feces, diverticular disease, tumor of the bowel, intussusceptions, volvulus (Fig. 5.14B) (a twisting of bowel onto itself), or the strictures of inflammatory bowel disease. Residues from foods high in fiber, such as raw coconut or fruit pulp, also can obstruct the small bowel.

Nonmechanical obstruction. Nonmechanical obstruction may result from a neuromuscular or vascular disorder, or it may be the result of a general anesthetic during surgery. The cause is something that decreases the muscle action of the bowel and affects the ability of fecal matter and fluid to move through the intestines. Paralytic (adynamic) ileus (lack of intestinal peristalsis and bowel sounds) is the most common form of nonmechanical obstruction. It occurs to some degree after any abdominal surgery. Other causes include inflammatory responses (e.g., acute pancreatitis, acute appendicitis), electrolyte abnormalities (especially hypokalemia), and thoracic or lumbar spinal trauma from either fractures or surgical intervention. Vascular obstructions are rare and are due to an interference with the blood supply to a portion of the intestines. The most common causes are emboli and atherosclerosis of the mesenteric arteries. The celiac, inferior, and superior mesenteric arteries supply blood to the bowel. Emboli may originate from thrombi in patients with chronic atrial fibrillation, diseased heart valves, and prosthetic valves.

When the small intestine is obstructed, it interrupts the normal process of secretion and reabsorption of 6 to 8 L of electrolyte-rich fluid. Large amounts of fluid, bacteria, and swallowed air build up in the bowel proximal to the obstruction. Water and salts shift from the circulatory system to the intestinal lumen, causing distention and further interfering with absorption. As the fluid increases, so does the pressure in the lumen of the bowel. The increased pressure leads to an increase in capillary permeability and extravasation of fluids and electrolytes into the peritoneal cavity. Edema, congestion, and necrosis from impaired blood supply and possible rupture of the bowel may occur. The retention of fluid in the intestine and peritoneal cavity can lead to a severe reduction in circulating blood volume and result in hypotension and hypovolemic shock.

Clinical Manifestations

The signs and symptoms of intestinal obstruction vary with the site and degree of obstruction. During partial or early phases of mechanical obstruction, auscultation of the abdomen reveals loud, frequent, high-pitched sounds. However, when smooth muscle atony (weak, or lack of normal tone) occurs, bowel sounds are absent.

Assessment

Subjective data include the pattern of the patient's pain, including onset, frequency, and characteristics. Nausea and the inability to pass flatus are common symptoms. Early complaints of obstruction of the small intestine include spasms of cramping abdominal pain as peristaltic activity increases proximal to the obstruction. As the obstruction progresses, the intestine becomes fatigued, with periods of decreased or absent bowel sounds and increased abdominal pain. Note any history of previous bowel disorders or abdominal surgeries and changes in bowel elimination.

Collection of objective data begins with assessing the abdominal surface for evidence of distention, hernias, scars indicating previous surgeries, or visible peristaltic waves. Bowel sounds may be high pitched when assessed in early obstruction, progressing to hypoactive or absent bowel sounds later. Other objective data include vomiting; signs of dehydration caused by the fluid shift; abdominal distention, tenderness, and muscle guarding; and decreased blood pressure.

Obstruction of the colon causes less severe pain than obstruction of the small intestine, marked abdominal distention, and constipation. The patient may continue to have bowel movements, because the colon distal to the obstruction continues to empty.

Diagnostic Tests

Abdominal x-rays are the most useful diagnostic aids. Flat, upright, and lateral x-rays show gas and fluid in the intestines. Intraperitoneal air (sometimes referred to as *free air under the diaphragm*) indicates perforation. Radiographic examination reveals the level of obstruction and its cause. Sigmoidoscopy or colonoscopy may provide direct visualization of an obstruction in the colon. CT scans also may be used in diagnosis. The fluid and electrolyte balance are evaluated through laboratory test results. Elevated blood urea nitrogen and decreased serum sodium, chloride, potassium, and magnesium are common. The patient's hemoglobin and hematocrit levels may increase because of hemoconcentration associated with the fluid volume deficit.

Medical Management

Treatment is directed toward decompression of the intestine by removal of gas and fluid, correction and maintenance of fluid and electrolyte balance, and relief or removal of the obstruction. Treatment may include the evacuation of intestinal contents by means of an intestinal tube. An NG or nasojejunal tube is inserted and connected to wall suction rto decompress the intestine. A long intestinal tube (10 ft. [300 cm]; e.g., Miller-Abbott) may be used instead of an NG tube to decompress the bowel; however, its use is controversial and limited because it is more difficult and time consuming to insert and may not be more effective than an NG tube. Surgical repair is necessary to relieve mechanical obstructions caused by adhesions, volvulus, and strangulated hernias or if obstruction does not resolve within 48 hours after less invasive therapies have been initiated. Restore fluid and electrolyte balance by carefully monitoring IV infusion. Nonopioid analgesics usually are prescribed to avoid the decrease in intestinal motility that often accompanies the administration of opioid analgesics.

Nursing Interventions and Patient Teaching

Unless surgery is indicated, nursing interventions include carefully monitoring fluids and electrolytes, measuring the patient's urinary output, observing the function of tubes used to decompress and relieve distention, and administering analgesics.

For the patient with intestinal obstruction undergoing surgery, preoperative preparation includes explaining the procedure at a level the patient can understand. Provide emotional support for the patient because he or she is experiencing the stressors of pain and vomiting plus the added stressor of emergency surgery.

Postoperative nursing interventions are similar to those for any patient who has had abdominal surgery. Place the patient in a Fowler's position for greater diaphragm expansion. Encourage the patient to breathe through the nose and not swallow air, which would increase distention and discomfort. Encourage deep breathing and coughing. Continue nasointestinal suctioning until bowel activity returns. Assess for bowel sounds and abdominal girth and expulsion of flatus and stool to help determine the return of peristalsis. When the patient is ready to eat, usually within 24 to 48 hours after surgery or at the first sounds of peristalsis, provide a progressive diet as tolerated. Some patients require temporary bowel diversion via a double-barrel or loop colostomy to manage the obstruction.

To manage pain, administer all medications as prescribed. Medications may include opioids or opioid derivatives.

Patient problems and interventions for the patient with an intestinal obstruction include but are not limited to the following:

Patient Problem	Nursing Interventions
Recent Onset of Pain, related to increased peristalsis	Reposition patient frequently to help intestinal tube advance Irrigate suction tubing with 30 mL of sterile saline to keep tube patent Explain purpose of all procedures Provide comfort measures Administer analgesics as ordered

Follow-up teaching focuses on prevention, including diet and prevention of constipation, as well as early symptoms of recurrence and the need to seek prompt medical care. For the patient with a temporary ostomy, follow-up care is necessary as plans are made for closure of the stoma.

Prognosis

The prognosis depends on early detection of the obstruction and the type and cause of the obstruction, as well as the success of medical interventions. The prognosis is poorer for patients who develop complications such as hypovolemic shock.

CANCER OF THE COLON AND RECTUM (COLORECTAL CANCER)

Etiology and Pathophysiology

Malignant neoplasms that invade the epithelium and surrounding tissue of the colon and rectum are the third most prevalent internal cancers in the United States and the second leading cause of cancer deaths. The American Cancer Society estimates 104,270 new cases of colon cancer and 45,230 new cases of rectal cancer will be diagnosed in 2021. An estimated 53,200 deaths will result from these cancers (ACS, 2021b).

Most growths are seen in the sigmoid and rectal areas of the colon. Cancer occurs with the same frequency in men and women; 9 of 10 colorectal cancer cases occur in people 50 years of age and older.

The cause of colorectal cancer remains unknown, but certain conditions appear to make patients more susceptible to malignant changes. These conditions are termed *predisposing* or *risk factors.* Fortunately, a vast majority of colorectal cancers arise from adenomatous polyps, which can be detected and removed from the rectum and sigmoid colon by sigmoidoscopy or colonoscopy. Some diseases, including ulcerative colitis and diverticulosis, increase the risk of colorectal cancer over time. Recent research has isolated a gene that causes colon cancer in certain families. Hereditary diseases (e.g., familial adenomatous polyposis) account for about 5% to 10% of colorectal cancer cases. Lynch syndrome and familial adenomatous polyposis (FAP) are the most common inherited forms of hereditary colorectal cancer (The University of Texas Southwestern Medical Center, n.d.). History-taking and regular checkups are important preventive measures.

Other factors implicated in colorectal cancer include lack of bulk in the diet, high fat intake, and high bacterial counts in the colon. It is theorized that carcinogens are formed from degraded bile salts, and the stool that remains in the large bowel for a longer period as a result of too little fiber to stimulate its passage may overexpose the bowel to these carcinogens. Another theory is that the increased transit time for low-fiber foods to pass through the intestine is related to malignancy. These factors support certain dietary changes: decreased animal fat, reduced red meat, and increased high dietary fiber found in fruits, vegetables, and bran may have a protective effect and act as a primary preventive measure. Smoking, excessive intake of alcohol, obesity, and diabetes, have also been identified as risk factors.

Clinical Manifestations

Signs and symptoms of cancer of the colon vary with the location of the growth. During the early stages, most patients are asymptomatic. Clinical manifestations are usually nonspecific or do not appear until the disease is advanced.

Assessment

Subjective data include changes in bowel habits alternating between constipation and diarrhea, excessive flatus, and cramps. Constipation is more likely with descending colon cancer, whereas ascending colon cancer may produce no change in bowel habits. Another complaint may be rectal bleeding (the most common sign of colorectal cancer), with the color varying from dark to bright red, depending on the location of the neoplasm. Later stages of colon cancer may involve subjective symptoms of abdominal pain, nausea, and cachexia (weakness and emaciation associated with general ill health and malnutrition).

Collection of objective data includes observing for vomiting, weight loss, abdominal distention or ascites, and test results that are compatible with the diagnosis. The most common clinical manifestations are chronic blood loss and anemia.

Diagnostic Tests

Early diagnosis of the tumor, including identification of the cell type involved, is the most important factor in treating the disease. Fecal occult blood tests are an early screening test used to assist in colon cancer detection. Because half of all cases are found in areas of the colon that are inaccessible by sigmoidoscopy, colonoscopy is considered the gold standard for colorectal cancer screening and the detection and removal of precancerous polyps. Other procedures include endorectal ultrasonography and CT scan of the abdomen and pelvis to localize the lesion or determine its size.

A baseline colonoscopy before age 50 should be performed on those who have a family history of colon cancer. Individuals with known gene mutations need to be monitored by colonoscopy every year.

The American Cancer Society has established guidelines for colorectal cancer screening (see the Health Promotion box). In addition to these recommendations, other laboratory and diagnostic studies include an UGI series, radiologic abdominal series, and BE. Hemoglobin, hematocrit, and electrolyte levels are examined and, if cancer and metastasis are suspected, a blood test is done to detect antibodies to CEA (an oncofetal glycoprotein, found in colonic adenocarcinoma and other cancers and in nonmalignant conditions; *oncofetal* means occurring in both cancerous tissue and fetal tissue). Because the CEA level can be elevated in benign and malignant diseases, it is not considered a specific test for colorectal cancer. Its use is limited to determining the prognosis and monitoring the patient's response to antineoplastic therapy. Newer diagnostic studies used in colorectal cancer screenings and diagnostics include stool DNA testing. Cologuard DNA testing method was approved by the US Food and Drug Administration (FDA) in 2014 (Nelson, 2014). It detects minute amounts of blood in the stool. It also detects nine DNA biomarkers and three genes that have been found in colorectal cancers. The disadvantage of Cologaurd testing is that the interior of the colon is not being visualized as with a colonoscopy and polyps and tissue cannot be biopsied.

Health Promotion

Screening for Colorectal Cancer

Current recommendations from the American Cancer Society for colorectal cancer screening are as follows:
- Starting at the age of 45 years, individuals at an average risk of developing colon cancer should begin screening by either fecal testing or colonoscopy
- Flexible sigmoidoscopy every 5 years (colonoscopy if test results are positive)
- Colonoscopy every 10 years
- CT colonography (virtual colonoscopy) every 5 years
- Tests that are done mainly to find cancer:
- Fecal occult blood test (FOBT) every year
- Fecal immunochemical test (FIT) every year
- Stool DNA (sDNA) test every 3 years
- Screening for high-risk patients beginning before age 45, usually by colonoscopy

Data from American Cancer Society (ACS): American Cancer Society guideline for colorectal cancer screening, 2020. Retrieved from https://www.cancer.org/cancer/colon-rectal-cancer/detection-diagnosis-staging/acs-recommendations.html

Medical Management

Medical treatment includes radiation, chemotherapy, and surgery. Radiation therapy often is used before surgery to decrease the chance of cancer cell implantation at the time of resection. Radiation can reduce the size of the tumor and decrease the rate of lymphatic involvement. Radiation before surgery has few side effects but some potential complications.

Postoperatively, those patients at high risk for recurrence or people whose disease has progressed may receive radiation administered over 4 to 6 weeks.

Chemotherapy is given (1) to patients with systemic disease that is incurable by surgery or radiation alone; (2) to patients in whom metastasis is suspected (e.g., when a patient has positive lymph node involvement at the time of surgery); or (3) for palliative therapy to reduce tumor size or relieve symptoms of the disease, such as obstruction or pain. Health care provider opinion and individual patient response vary regarding use of chemotherapy for colorectal cancer.

Surgical interventions depend on the tumor's location, presence of obstruction or perforation of the bowel, possible metastasis, the patient's health status, and the surgeon's preferences. When obstruction has not occurred, a portion of the bowel on either side of the tumor is removed and an end-to-end anastomosis (EEA) is done between the divided ends. When obstruction of the bowel occurs, the commonly used procedures are as follows:
- One-stage resection with anastomosis
- Two-stage resection with (1) the ends of the bowel brought to the surface and creation of a temporary colostomy and mucus fistula or Hartmann pouch (see Fig. 5.11A); (2) a double-barrel colostomy (see Fig. 5.11B); or (3) a temporary loop colostomy (see Fig. 5.11C), for closure later
- Surgical procedures for colorectal cancer include the following:
  - *Right hemicolectomy:* Resection of ascending colon and hepatic flexure (Fig. 5.15A); ileum anastomosed to transverse colon
  - *Left hemicolectomy:* Resection of splenic flexure, descending colon, and sigmoid colon (Fig. 5.15B); transverse colon anastomosed to rectum
  - *Anterior rectosigmoid resection:* Resection of part of descending colon, the sigmoid colon, and upper rectum (Fig. 5.15C); descending colon anastomosed to remaining rectum

In carcinoma of the rectum, the surgeon makes every effort to preserve the sphincter, often with an EEA. The use of EEA staplers allows lower and more secure anastomosis. The stapler is passed through the anus, where the colon is stapled to the rectum. This technique makes it possible to resect lesions as low as 5 cm from the anus. If the surgeon is unable to perform an anastomosis, an abdominoperineal resection may be done.

In the abdominoperineal resection, an abdominal incision is made and the proximal sigmoid is brought

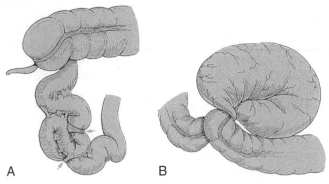

Fig. 5.15 Intestinal obstructions. (A) Adhesions. (B) Volvulus.

through the abdominal wall in a permanent colostomy. The distal sigmoid, rectum, and anus are removed through a perineal incision (Fig. 5.16). The perineal wound may be closed around a drain or left open with packing to allow healing by granulation. Possible complications are delayed wound healing, hemorrhage, persistent perineal sinus tracts, infections, and urinary tract and sexual dysfunction.

Nutritional status is important because of the threat of infection and a compromised postoperative healing process as a result of constipation, diarrhea, nausea, vomiting, and possible obstruction.

Nursing Interventions and Patient Teaching

Nursing interventions include assessment of bowel and urinary elimination, fluid and electrolyte balance, tissue perfusion, nutrition, pain, gas exchange, infection, and peristomal skin integrity, as discussed previously.

Preoperative care. The patient has some type of bowel preparation, which usually includes 2 or 3 days of liquid diets; a combination of laxatives, or enemas; and oral antibiotics to sterilize the bowel. The antibiotic of choice may be neomycin, kanamycin, or erythromycin; each suppresses anaerobic and aerobic organisms in the colon.

Before surgery, provide instruction in turning, coughing, and deep breathing; use of an incentive spirometer; wound splinting; and leg exercises. Inform the patient that he or she will have IV lines, a Foley catheter, possibly an NG tube, a Hemovac or Jackson-Pratt drain, and abdominal dressings after surgery.

If a stoma is planned, the enterostomal therapist should be notified so that the stoma site can be marked before surgery. The stoma should be placed at the best site for the patient.

Postoperative care. Assess the patient for stable vital signs and return of bowel sounds. Check the dressings for drainage or bleeding and change them as needed as per the health care provider's order. Monitor the NG tube, any wound drains, and the Foley catheter for rate of flow and color of output. Keep accurate I&O records to maintain the fluid and electrolyte balance. Other postoperative

care includes coughing, deep breathing, early ambulation, adequate nutrition, pain control, and meticulous wound and stoma care.

Paralytic ileus, a common complication of abdominal surgery, produces the classic signs of increased abdominal girth, distention, nausea, and vomiting. Interventions include decompression of the bowel with an NG tube connected to wall suction, NPO status, and increased patient activity (refer to *Foundations of Nursing,* Chapter 15, Skill 15.5).

Long-term complications of abdominal resection with permanent colostomy are urinary retention or incontinence, pelvic abscess, failure of perineal wound healing, wound infection, and sexual dysfunction.

In addition to monitoring the stoma for color, size, location, and the condition of the peristomal skin, watch for possible complications, including necrosis and abscess. Necrosis results from compromised blood flow to the stoma; the stoma appears pale and dusky to black. Abscess caused by stoma placement too close to the wound, retention sutures, and drains must be assessed promptly. Report all complications promptly to the surgeon and document them in the medical record.

Patient problems and interventions for the patient with cancer of the colon include but are not limited to the following:

Patient Problem	Nursing Interventions
Distorted Body Image, related to loss of normal body function (colostomy)	Allow time for grieving. Assist patient and family in accepting ostomy. Encourage verbalization. Observe for signs of denial, grief, or anger. Answer all questions, and explain treatment and procedure. Provide care in positive manner; always avoid facial expressions connoting distaste. Provide privacy and a safe environment. Encourage self-care and independence when patient demonstrates readiness. Facilitate contact with individuals with similar changes in body image to provide realistic experiences of having ostomy

The patient with a permanent end colostomy (Fig 5.17) can be taught two forms of colostomy management: (1) emptying and cleansing the pouch as needed and (2) managing colostomy irrigation. In planning patient teaching, consider past bowel habits; location of the colostomy; and the patient's age, general health, and personal preference (refer to *Foundations of Nursing,* Chapter 15, Skills 15.11 and 15.12).

Nerves that control the bladder may be damaged when a large amount of tissue is removed in an

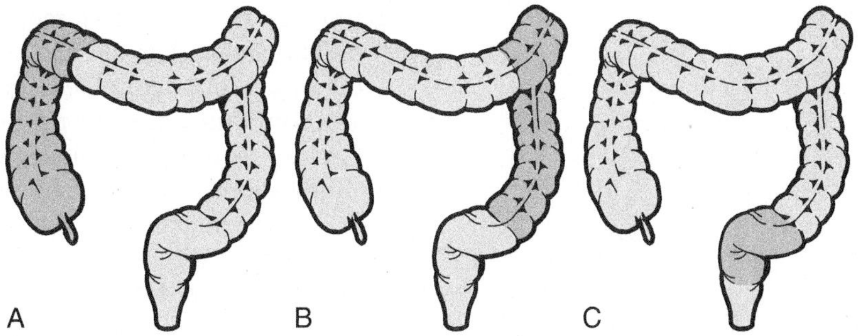

Fig. 5.16 Bowel resection. (A) Right hemicolectomy. (B) Left hemicolectomy. (C) Anterior rectosigmoid resection.

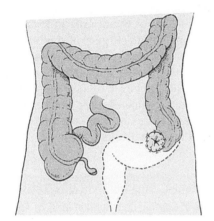

Fig. 5.17 Descending or sigmoid colostomy.

abdominoperineal resection or if radiation therapy has occurred. When the Foley catheter is removed after surgery, the patient may be unable to void or empty the bladder completely. If the problem does not resolve, the patient may need a Foley catheter and a urology consultation.

When a large amount of tissue is removed, as in an abdominoperineal resection, the cavity left is a reservoir for bacteria, increasing the risk of infection. Monitor the drain site for increased pain, erythema, and purulent drainage, and monitor for elevated body temperature. The perineal wound may be closed using various techniques. The wound may be closed with a drain to suction. The semi-closed wound usually has either a Jackson-Pratt or Hemovac drain. The open wound (in which packing is used and later removed) may need irrigation and sitz baths to facilitate healing. Any changes in exudate color and odor and temperature elevation are reported to the surgeon.

Sexual dysfunction for men and women is related to removal of the rectum. Contributing factors may be partial to complete disruption of the nerve supply to the genital organs, psychological factors, or decreased activity associated with age. When the nurse and the patient have a comfortable relationship, it is easier to introduce the topic of sex. Exploring the patient's and the partner's fears and providing information on penile prosthesis surgery and simple suggestions to both partners help decrease anxiety concerning intercourse. Counseling may be necessary if the patient's and the partner's perceptions of body image have been altered. Support groups are available to the cancer patient in most communities. Above all, the nurse's silent communication of touch and eye contact can give the patient a message that he or she is accepted and valued.

Prognosis
The 5-year survival rate for localized colon cancer is approximately 90%. For regional metastasis, the 5-year relative survival rate is about 71%; the distant metastasis survival rate is about 14%. Survival rates at the 5-year mark for rectal cancer are nearly the same as colon cancer (ACS, 2021f).

HEMORRHOIDS
Etiology and Pathophysiology
Hemorrhoids are varicosities (dilated veins) that may occur outside the anal sphincter as external hemorrhoids or inside the sphincter as internal hemorrhoids. This is one of the most common health problems, with the greatest incidence from ages 20 to 50 years. Etiologic factors include straining at stool with increased intra-abdominal and hemorrhoidal venous pressures. With repeated increased pressure and obstructed blood flow, permanent dilation occurs. Hemorrhoids may be caused by constipation, diarrhea, pregnancy, congestive heart failure, portal hypertension, and prolonged sitting and standing.

Clinical Manifestations
The most common symptoms associated with enlarged, abnormal hemorrhoids are prolapse (protrusion outside the anal sphincter) and bleeding. The bright red bleeding and prolapse usually occur at time of defecation.

Assessment
Subjective data include complaints of constipation, pruritus, severe pain when dilated veins become thrombosed, and bleeding from the rectum that is not mixed with feces.

Collection of objective data includes observing external hemorrhoids and palpating internal hemorrhoids. Because bleeding and constipation are signs of cancer of the rectum, all patients with these symptoms should have a thorough examination to rule out cancer.

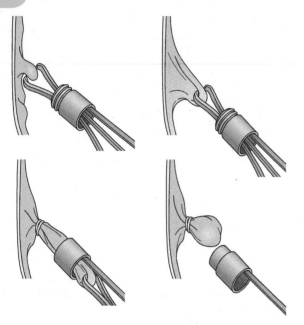

Fig. 5.18 Rubber band ligation of an internal hemorrhoid.

Diagnostic Tests

Internal hemorrhoids are diagnosed by digital examination, anoscopy, and sigmoidoscopy. External hemorrhoids can be diagnosed by visual inspection and digital examination.

Medical Management

Therapy is directed toward the causes and the patient's symptoms. A high-fiber diet and increased fluid intake prevent constipation and reduce straining, which allows engorgement of the veins to subside. Conservative interventions include the use of bulk stool softeners, as well as bran, and natural food fibers to relieve straining. Topical creams with hydrocortisone relieve pruritus and inflammation, and analgesic ointments relieve pain. Sitz baths usually are given to relieve pain and edema and promote healing.

Rubber band ligation is a popular and easy method of treatment (Fig. 5.18). Tight bands are applied with a special instrument in the health care provider's office, causing constriction and necrosis. The destroyed tissue sloughs off in about 1 week, and discomfort is minimal. Sclerotherapy (with a sclerosing agent injected at the apex of the hemorrhoid column), cryotherapy (tissue destruction by freezing), infrared photocoagulation (destruction of tissue by creation of a small burn), laser excision, and operative hemorrhoidectomy are additional interventions.

Hemorrhoidectomy, the surgical removal of hemorrhoids, can be performed if other interventions fail to relieve the distressing signs and symptoms. Surgery is indicated for patients with prolapse, excessive pain or bleeding, or large hemorrhoids. In general, hemorrhoidectomy is reserved for patients with severe symptoms related to multiple thrombosed hemorrhoids or marked protrusion. Surgical removal may be done by cautery,

clamp, or excision. After removal of the hemorrhoid, wounds can be left open or closed, although closed wounds are reported to heal faster. Hemorrhoidectomy is not considered a major procedure, but the pain may be acute, requiring opioids and analgesic ointments. Complications include hemorrhage, local infection, pain, urinary retention, and abscess.

Nursing Interventions and Patient Teaching

Rectal conditions can be embarrassing to the patient, and the nurse's direct but concerned attitude can decrease this embarrassment. Assess the knowledge level by asking patients about their condition, what they have been told about treatment, and what treatments have been done before surgery and why.

Observe the patient with a prolapsed hemorrhoid for edema, thrombosis, and ischemia. Ischemic tissue is dark red to necrotic (black). Explain that a low-bulk diet can produce chronic constipation (see the Evidence-Based Practice box on managing chronic constipation in older adults).

🔍 Evidence-Based Practice

Management of Chronic Constipation in Older Adults

EVIDENCE SUMMARY

For adults over the age of 60, chronic constipation is a common occurrence. Primary, or functional, constipation refers to the passage of hard stools with normal frequency, infrequent defecation, or infrequent defecation along with bloating and discomfort. Secondary constipation refers to constipation that is related to disease conditions, medications, or psychosocial concerns. Approximately 50% of nursing home residents experience constipation. The study indicates that if a patient has constipation, there are two pathways to address the problem. If the assessment of the patient indicates a disorder may be present, the patient must be referred to a gastroenterologist. If there is no indication of a disorder, then the suggested line of treatment is (1) behavioral changes (increase fiber and fluids, schedule toileting after meals), if no improvement; (2) administer polyethylene glycol (Miralax), if no improvement; and (3) stool softeners and stimulant laxatives.

Application to Nursing Practice

- Note the subjective and objective assessment findings and communicate these findings to the health care provider.
- If the health care provider determines that there is no disorder present, first implement nursing measures to address the constipation.
- Ensure the patient receives a fiber intake of 20–35 g/day along with an adequate fluid intake, depending on the patient's condition.
- Ensure a toileting schedule is followed, including toileting after meals when the defecation impulse is generally high.
- Initiate health care provider orders if constipation continues, including polyethylene glycol (osmotic agent that causes water to be retained with the stool), and stool softeners and stimulant laxatives as needed.

Information from Management of Constipation in Older Adults, Sept 15, 2015, Vol 92(6), American Family Physician Copyright© 2003 American Academy of Family Physicians. All Rights Reserved.

For the surgical patient, take vital signs frequently for the first 24 hours to rule out internal bleeding. Sitz baths are given several times daily. Early ambulation and a soft diet facilitate bowel elimination. The patient may have a great deal of anxiety concerning the first defecation; discuss this and provide an analgesic before the bowel movement to reduce discomfort. A stool softener such as docusate (Colace) usually is ordered for the first few postoperative days.

Patient problems and interventions for the patient with hemorrhoids include but are not limited to the following:

Patient Problem	Nursing Interventions
Recent Onset of Pain, related to edema, prolapse, and surgical interventions	Instruct patient to wash anal area after defecation and pat dry Sitz baths or local heat applied to site may be soothing Use of local anesthetics (dibucaine ointment or Tucks pads) may give relief Apply ice packs to hemorrhoids if thrombosed to prevent edema and pain Use cushion for sitting postoperatively
Anxiousness, related to: • Previous experiences • Fear of first bowel movement postoperatively • Lack of knowledge regarding diet	Establish a supportive relationship with patient Explain need for high-residue diet Administer laxatives and oil-retention enema as ordered Give analgesics before first bowel movement and a sitz bath for pain relief

Advise the patient to include bulk-forming foods in the diet, such as fresh fruits, vegetables, and bran cereals, as well as 8 to 10 glasses of fluid a day unless contraindicated. If the patient is anemic, discuss foods high in iron, such as red meats, liver, and dark green leafy vegetables. Sitz baths are recommended for 1 to 2 weeks postoperatively. Emphasize the need for moderate exercise and a routine time for a daily bowel movement. In addition, instruct the patient to report any signs of infection or delayed healing.

Prognosis
There are several preferred methods of treatment for hemorrhoids. Conservative modes of treatment and surgical intervention for hemorrhoids have good prognostic rates.

ANAL FISSURE AND FISTULA
An anal fissure is a linear ulceration or laceration of the skin of the anus. Usually it is the result of trauma caused by hard stool that overstretches the anal lining. The fissure is aggravated by defecation, which initiates spasm of the anal sphincter; pain; and, at times, slight bleeding. If the lesion does not heal spontaneously, the tract is excised surgically.

An anal fistula is an abnormal opening on the cutaneous surface near the anus. Usually this is from a local crypt abscess; it is also common in Crohn disease. A perianal fistula may or may not communicate with the rectum. It results from rupture or drainage of an anal abscess. This chronic condition is treated by a fistulectomy (removal) or fistulotomy (opening of the fistula tract).

The postoperative care required for repair of an anal fissure or fistula is similar to that for the patient who has had a hemorrhoidectomy.

Prognosis
The prognosis for anal fissures and fistulas is good, whether the patient is treated with conservative measures or with surgical intervention.

FECAL INCONTINENCE
Etiology and Pathophysiology
Fecal incontinence is a complex problem that has a variety of causes. The external anal sphincter may be relaxed, the voluntary control of defecation may be interrupted in the central nervous system, or messages may not be transmitted to the brain because of a lesion within or external pressure on the spinal cord. The disorders that cause breakdown of conscious control of defecation include lesions of the cerebral cortex, spinal cord lesions or trauma, and trauma to the anal sphincter (e.g., from fistula, abscess, or surgery). Perineal relaxation and actual damage to the anal sphincter often are caused by injury from perineal surgery, childbirth, or anal intercourse. Relaxation of the sphincter usually occurs with the general loss of muscle tone in aging. The normal changes that occur with aging are usually not significant enough to cause incontinence, however, unless concurrent health problems predispose the patient to the disorder.

Normally the contents of the bowel are moved by mass peristaltic movements toward the rectum. The rectum then stores the stool until defecation occurs. Distention of the rectum initiates nerve signals that are transmitted to the spinal cord and then back to the descending colon, initiating peristaltic waves that force more feces into the rectum. The internal anal sphincter relaxes, and if the external sphincter is relaxed, defecation results. Defecation is a reflex response to the distention of the rectal musculature, but this reflex can be inhibited voluntarily. Voluntary inhibition of defecation is learned in early childhood, and control typically lasts throughout life. The rectum is emptied when the external anal sphincter (under cortical control) relaxes, while the abdominal and pelvic muscles contract.

Reflex defecation continues to occur even in the presence of most upper or lower motor neuron lesions, because the musculature of the bowel contains its own nerve centers that respond to distention through peristalsis. Therefore, even when the patient has motor paralysis, reflex defecation often persists or can be stimulated. Defecation occurs primarily in response to mass peristaltic movements that follow meals or distention of the rectum. Any physical, mental, or social problem that disrupts any aspect of this complex learned behavior could result in incontinence.

Medical Management and Nursing Interventions

Biofeedback training is the cornerstone of therapy for patients who have motility disorders or sphincter damage that causes fecal incontinence. The patient learns to tighten the external sphincter in response to rectal distention. This technique has been proven effective with alert, motivated patients.

Bowel training is the major approach used with patients who have cognitive and neurologic problems resulting from stroke or other chronic diseases. If a person can sit on a toilet, he or she may be able to defecate automatically given a pattern of consistent timing, familiar surroundings, and controlled diet and fluid intake. This approach allows many patients to defecate predictably and remain continent throughout the day. Surgical correction is possible for a small group of patients whose incontinence is related to structural problems of the rectum and anus.

Patient Teaching

Bowel training requires significant amounts of time and effort on the part of the nursing staff, family, and patient. Incontinence is a major issue in home care and frequently is cited as the most common reason for older adults to be admitted to nursing homes.

To plan the most effective approach, gather specific information concerning the person's general physical and cognitive condition, ability to contract the abdominal and perineal muscles on command, and awareness of the need or urge to defecate. Also, collect data about the nature and frequency of the incontinence problem, particularly its relationship to meals or other regular activities.

Teach the family about the training program and how they can assist and support the patient. This includes the importance of providing a high-fiber diet and ensuring that the patient has a sufficient fluid intake. Evaluate the need for a regular stool softener or bulk former. When an optimal time for defecation has been established, usually after breakfast, a glycerin suppository may be inserted to stimulate defecation.

Despite efforts by family members, staff, and patient, fecal incontinence may remain uncontrolled. Efforts then shift to odor control, prevention of skin impairment, and support for the patient's psychological integrity. Commercially available protective briefs are expensive, but they can reduce the burden of care for the family substantially and provide the patient with a sense of security and dignity.

❖ NURSING PROCESS FOR THE PATIENT WITH A GASTROINTESTINAL DISORDER

◆ ASSESSMENT

To care for the patient admitted with a GI disorder, a thorough, immediate, and accurate nursing assessment is an essential first step. The assessment includes the patient's level of consciousness; vital signs; skin color; edema; appetite; weight loss; nausea; vomiting; and bowel habits, including color and consistency of stools. Assess the abdomen for distention, guarding, and peristalsis. Also, obtain a past history of smoking or alcohol use, medications, epigastric or abdominal pain, and acute or chronic stressors and coping/stress tolerance.

◆ PATIENT PROBLEMS

Assessment provides the data for identifying the patient's problems, strengths, potential complications, and learning needs. Once the patient problem statements are defined, assist in formulating a care plan that meets the patient's needs and prioritizing nursing interventions. Possible patient problem statements that should be considered for the patient with a GI disorder include but are not limited to the following:

- Anxiousness
- Compromised Maintenance of Health
- Compromised Tissue Perfusion
- Discomfort
- Distorted Body Image
- Fearfulness
- Frequent, Loose Stools
- Impaired Coping
- Inability to Tolerate Activity
- Inefficient Sleep Pattern
- Infrequent or Difficult Bowel Elimination
- Insufficient Nutrition: Less Than Body Requirements
- Potential for Compromised Skin Integrity
- Potential for Inadequate Fluid Volume
- Social Seclusion

◆ EXPECTED OUTCOMES (GOALS) AND PLANNING

Care planning for the patient with a GI disorder involves looking at the patient problems and establishing nursing interventions to assist in eliminating the problems. Include the patient in planning to promote compliance with the nursing interventions.

The care plan may be based on one or both of the following goals:

Goal 1: Patient will have no evidence of excoriation around stomal area.

Goal 2: Patient will begin to adjust to disturbed body image.

◆ IMPLEMENTATION

Nursing interventions for the patient with a GI disorder may be simple or complex. Interventions include assessment, monitoring nutritional status, administering medications, promoting health, relieving pain, maintaining skin integrity, managing fluid and electrolyte imbalance, promoting normal bowel elimination patterns, preventing wound infection, health counseling to focus on elimination of smoking and excessive alcohol intake, and patient teaching for enterostomal therapy.

◆ EVALUATION

Determining the outcomes of the nursing interventions is an ongoing process that helps the nurse to establish the most effective care plan. The nurse and the patient evaluate the goals to see whether the criteria for assessment have been met. Examples of goals and the corresponding evaluative measures are as follows:

Goal 1: Patient will have no evidence of excoriation around stomal area.

Evaluative measure: There is no impairment of skin integrity around stoma.

Goal 2: Patient will begin to adjust to disturbed body image.

Evaluative measures: Patient demonstrates adjustment to disturbed body image by expressing feelings about stoma and is beginning to assume some stoma and pouch care. Goal met.

Get Ready for the NCLEX® Examination!

Key Points

- The digestive tract begins with the mouth, extends through the thoracic and abdominal cavities, and ends with the anus.
- The major processes of digestion and absorption take place in the small intestine.
- The large intestine is responsible for the preparation and evacuation of feces.
- Diet therapy has an important role in the treatment of GI disorders.
- Treatment of esophageal disorders often involves providing the patient with a means of eating in addition to treating the disorder.
- Common causes of gastric disorders are alcohol, tobacco, aspirin, and anti-inflammatory agents.
- Duodenal ulcers are the most common type of peptic ulcer disease.
- A relatively new diagnostic examination is capsule endoscopy, in which the patient swallows a capsule equipped with a camera to visualize the small intestine and diagnose diseases such as Crohn disease.
- Surgical procedures are available as alternatives to the traditional ileostomy and colostomy.
- A nursing goal for the patient with an ileostomy or a colostomy is to foster patient independence in daily care when the patient demonstrates readiness.
- Keeping the surgical area free of contamination is paramount after rectal surgery.
- The approximate location of GI bleeding may be determined by the characteristics of the emesis or the fecal material.
- Explain the purpose of any diagnostic procedure, how the procedure is performed, and the preparation necessary for the procedure, and help the patient understand the results.
- *Helicobacter pylori* has been identified in patients with gastric ulcers and duodenal ulcers.
- Individuals with inflammatory bowel disease have a greater risk of developing cancer of the bowel.
- Early detection of cancer in the GI system facilitates early treatment and a better prognosis.

- An NG tube is inserted to keep the stomach empty until peristalsis resumes after a general anesthetic or any condition that interferes with peristalsis.
- Effective postoperative care begins with patient teaching during the preoperative period.

Additional Learning Resources

SG Go to your Study Guide for additional learning activities to help you master this chapter content.

Be sure to visit the Evolve site at http://evolve.elsevier.com/Cooper/adult/ for additional online resources.

Review Questions for the NCLEX® Examination

1. The nurse is caring for a patient who has had a partial gastrectomy. Which vitamin will the nurse anticipate educating the patient about?
   1. A
   2. B_{12}
   3. C
   4. K

2. The nurse is caring for several patients on a medical-surgical unit. Which patient is the nurse most concerned may develop a paralytic (adynamic) ileus?
   1. The patient with impacted feces, tumor of the colon, or pancreatitis
   2. The patient with an electrolyte imbalance, or acute inflammatory reactions
   3. The patient with adhesions or a strangulated hernia
   4. The patient with volvulus, intussusceptions, or electrolyte imbalances

3. The nurse is caring for a patient scheduled for an esophagogastroduodenoscopy. Which intervention should the nurse include in the patient's plan of care? *(Select all that apply.)*

   1. Allow the patient to drink fluids up to 4 hours before the examination.
   2. Withhold any anticholinergic medications before the procedure.
   3. Encourage the patient to not smoke before the examination.
   4. Maintain NPO status until the gag reflex returns postprocedure.
   5. Instruct the patient to contact the health care provider if intense abdominal pain occurs postprocedure.

4. A patient has been admitted with a diagnosis of peptic ulcers. Which drugs would the nurse expect this patient to be prescribed to decrease gastric acid secretion? *(Select all that apply.)*

   1. sodium polystyrene sulfonate
   2. ranitidine
   3. erythromycin
   4. sucralfate
   5. famotidine

5. A patient is scheduled for a hemicolectomy for removal of a cancerous tumor of the ascending colon. The patient asks the nurse why he is taking intestinal antibiotics preoperatively. Which response by the nurse is correct?

   1. To decrease the bulk of colon contents
   2. To reduce the bacteria content of the colon
   3. To prevent pneumonia
   4. To eliminate the risk of postoperative wound infection

6. A patient was admitted during the evening shift with a tentative diagnosis of cancer of the esophagus. What complaint does the nurse anticipate finding in the initial assessment of the patient?

   1. Dysphagia
   2. Malnutrition
   3. Pain
   4. Regurgitation of food

7. When caring for a patient admitted with a bleeding peptic ulcer, the nurse will include what intervention in the patient's acute plan of care?

   1. Measuring the blood pressure and pulse rates each shift
   2. Frequently monitoring arterial blood levels
   3. Observing vomitus for color, consistency, and volume
   4. Checking the patient's stools for occult blood

8. A patient has undergone numerous diagnostic tests to determine whether a gastric malignancy is present. The patient asks the nurse what test will be most definitive for diagnosis. **Choose the *most likely* options for the information missing from the statements below by selecting from the list of options provided.**

Your health care provider has ordered a/an _____ in order to perform a _____ to determine if you have cancer in your stomach.

OPTIONS
Radiographic GI study
Biopsy
Breath test for *Helicobacter pylori*
Esophagogastroduodenoscopy
Barium swallow
Colonoscopy
CT scan
Complete blood count
Cholangiogram

9. A patient has been prescribed infliximab for the treatment of Crohn disease. What information should the nurse include in patient teaching regarding this medication?

   1. "This medication is given to suppress your immune system's overactive response."
   2. "This medication has been prescribed to treat the infection in your colon."
   3. "This medication is given to cure your Crohn disease."
   4. "This medication will decrease the inflammation in your intestine."

10. During assessment of a patient with esophageal achalasia, what does the nurse expect the patient to report when the health history is obtained?

    1. A history of alcohol use
    2. A sore throat and hoarseness
    3. Dysphagia, especially with liquids
    4. Relief of pyrosis with the use of antacids

11. What nursing intervention is most appropriate to decrease postoperative edema and pain in a male patient after an inguinal herniorrhaphy?

    1. Applying a truss to the hernial site
    2. Allowing the patient to stand to void
    3. Supporting the incision during routine coughing and deep breathing
    4. Elevating the scrotum with a support or small pillow

12. The nurse is preparing a presentation on the differences between ulcerative colitis and Crohn disease. What should the nurse include in the presentation? *(Select all that apply.)*

    1. Ulcerative colitis causes more nutritional deficiencies than Crohn disease.
    2. Ulcerative colitis is confined to the mucosa and the submucosa of the colon.
    3. The intestinal disease of ulcerative colitis is curable with a colectomy, whereas Crohn disease often recurs after surgery.
    4. Blood is often present in the stools with ulcerative colitis; fat is usually present in the stools with Crohn disease.
    5. Patients with ulcerative colitis may have 3 or 4 semisoft stools per day; 15 to 20 liquid stools per day are common with Crohn disease.

13. Which type of medication order should the nurse question when caring for a patient with *E. coli* 0157:H7?

1. Antiemetics
2. Antimotility drugs
3. Antilipidemic agents
4. Beta blockers

14. The nurse is discharging a patient after a hemorrhoidectomy. Which teaching point should the nurse include in the discharge instructions?

1. Do not use the Valsalva maneuver.
2. Eat a low-fiber diet to rest the colon.
3. Administer an oil-retention enema to empty the colon.
4. Use a prescribed analgesic before a bowel movement.

15. The student nurse is teaching a patient about his Crohn disease. The student is correct in identifying what complication as being the result of granulomatous cobblestone lesions of the small intestine?

16. After a transverse loop colostomy, the nurse inspects the patient's stoma. The stoma appears pale pink with some dusky discoloration at the lower border. What is the most appropriate action by the nurse?

1. Clean the area around the stoma and record the observation in the nurses' notes.
2. Carefully place a clean pouch over the stoma to prevent any tissue damage.
3. Cover the stoma with petroleum gauze to prevent any further irritation to the stoma.
4. Clean the area around the stoma, apply a clean pouch, and notify the health care provider about the discoloration.

17. The nurse is teaching a postgastrectomy patient about dumping syndrome. Which statement indicates that the patient needs further instruction?

1. "I will lie down after eating a meal."
2. "I will eat smaller portions of food, more frequently."
3. "I will not drink liquids when I eat."
4. "I will avoid fats and increase carbohydrates."

18. A patient has recently been diagnosed with celiac disease. What patient statement indicates the need for further teaching regarding the disease? *(Select all that apply.)*

1. "I should add pasta and bread back into my diet gradually."
2. "There is no cure for my disease, but I can manage it well with my diet."
3. "I will likely need to have surgery to repair the damage to my intestine."
4. "My children are at a higher risk for developing celiac disease because I have it."
5. "I will need to eliminate foods containing wheat flour from my diet."

19. While obtaining the patient's health history and reviewing the medical records, which information will alert the nurse that the patient has an increased risk of developing peptic ulcer disease? *(Select all that apply.)*

1. Excess of gastric acid or a decrease in the natural ability of the GI mucosa to protect itself from acid and pepsin
2. Invasion of the stomach and/or duodenum by *Helicobacter pylori*
3. Viral infection, allergies to certain foods, immunologic factors, and psychosomatic factors
4. Taking certain drugs, including corticosteroids and anti-inflammatory medications
5. Having allergies to foods containing gluten in their ingredients

Objectives

1. Discuss nursing interventions for the diagnostic examinations of patients with disorders of the gallbladder, liver, biliary tract, and exocrine pancreas.
2. Explain the etiology, pathophysiology, clinical manifestations, assessment, diagnostic tests, medical management, and nursing interventions for the patient with cirrhosis of the liver, carcinoma of the liver, hepatitis, liver abscesses, cholecystitis, cholelithiasis, pancreatitis, and cancer of the pancreas.
3. Discuss specific complications and teaching content for the patient with cirrhosis of the liver.
4. Define jaundice and describe signs and symptoms that may occur with jaundice.
5. State the six types of viral hepatitis, including their modes of transmission.
6. List the subjective and objective data for the patient with viral hepatitis.
7. Discuss the indicators for liver transplantation and the immunosuppressant drugs to reduce rejection.
8. Discuss the two methods of surgical treatment for cholecystitis and cholelithiasis.

Key Terms

ascites (ă-SĪ-tēz, p. 233)
asterixis (ăs-tĕr-ĬK-sĭs, p. 236)
biliary atresia (BĬL-ē-ăr-ē ă-TRĒZ-yă, p. 231)
esophageal varices (ē-sŏf-ă-JEL VAR-ĭ-sēz, p. 234)
flatulence (FLĂT-ū-lĕns, p. 244)
hepatic encephalopathy (hĕ-PĂT-ĭk ĕn-sĕf-ă-LŎP-ă-thē, p. 236)
hepatitis (hĕp-ă-TĪ-tĭs, p. 229)

jaundice (JĂWN-dĭs, p. 233)
occlusion (ŏ-KLŪ-zhĕn, p. 249)
paracentesis (pă-ră-sĕn-TĒ-sĭs, p. 233)
parenchyma (pă-RĔN-kĭ-mă, p. 231)
sclerotherapy (SKLĔR-ō-THĔR-ă-pē, p. 235)
spider telangiectases (SPĪ-dĕr tĕl-ĂN-jē-ĕk-TĂ-sēz, p. 233)
steatorrhea (stē-ăt-ŏ-RĒ-ă, p. 245)

Chapter 5 discussed the anatomy and function of the organs of the gastrointestinal system, as well as care of the patient with disorders involving the gastrointestinal system. This chapter discusses the care of the patient with disorders involving the accessory organs of the digestive system; specifically, the liver, the gallbladder, and the exocrine pancreas. These organs assist in digestion in various ways.

LABORATORY AND DIAGNOSTIC EXAMINATIONS IN THE ASSESSMENT OF THE HEPATOBILIARY AND PANCREATIC SYSTEMS

SERUM BILIRUBIN TEST

Bilirubin is the pigment that gives bile its yellow-orange color. It is formed when old or damaged red blood cells disintegrate and release their hemoglobin, which is broken down into its component parts, including heme. The heme in turn is converted into bilirubin. Unconjugated (water-insoluble; also called *indirect*) bilirubin passes through the bloodstream to the liver, where it is converted into conjugated (water-soluble;

also called *direct*) bilirubin. From here the bilirubin is expelled into the bile. Normal values are as follows:
Direct bilirubin: 0.1 to 0.4 mg/dL
Indirect bilirubin: 0.2 to 0.8 mg/dL
Total bilirubin: 0.3 to 1.2 mg/dL

Rationale

Total serum bilirubin determination measures direct and indirect bilirubin. The total serum bilirubin level is the sum of the direct and indirect bilirubin levels. Testing for bilirubin in the blood provides valuable information for the diagnosis and evaluation of liver disease, biliary obstruction, and hemolytic anemia. Jaundice, the discoloration of body tissues caused by abnormally high blood levels of bilirubin, is visible when the total serum bilirubin exceeds 2.5 mg/dL.

Nursing Interventions

Keep the patient on NPO (nothing by mouth) status until after the blood specimen is drawn. Inform the patient about blood draws and what test is being performed. Monitor the venipuncture site for bleeding.

LIVER ENZYME TESTS

The normal values for liver enzyme test results are as follows:

- *Alkaline phosphatase:* Adult: 30 to 120 units/L. The alkaline phosphatase level is elevated in obstructive disorders of the biliary tract, hepatic tumors, cirrhosis, hepatitis, primary and metastatic tumors, hyperparathyroidism, metastatic tumor in bones, and healing fractures.
- *ALT* (alanine aminotransferase; formerly serum glutamic-pyruvic transaminase [SGPT]): Adult or child: 4 to 36 units/L. The ALT level is elevated in hepatitis, cirrhosis, hepatic necrosis, and hepatic tumors and by hepatotoxic drugs.
- *AST* (aspartate aminotransferase; formerly serum glutamic oxaloacetic transaminase [SGOT]): Adult: 0 to 35 units/L. The AST level is elevated in myocardial infarction, hepatitis, cirrhosis, hepatic necrosis, hepatic tumor, acute pancreatitis, and acute hemolytic anemia.
- *GGT* (gamma-glutamyl transpeptidase): Males and females older than age 45 years: 8 to 38 units/L; females younger than age 45 years: 5 to 27 units/L. Levels are elevated in liver cell dysfunction such as hepatitis and cirrhosis; in hepatic tumors; with the use of hepatotoxic drugs; in jaundice; and in myocardial infarction (4 to 10 days after), heart failure, alcohol ingestion, pancreatitis, and cancer of the pancreas.
- *LDH* (lactic acid dehydrogenase): Adult: 100 to 190 units/L. Values are increased in myocardial infarction, pulmonary infarction, hepatic disease (e.g., hepatitis, active cirrhosis, neoplasm), pancreatitis, and skeletal muscle disease.

Rationale

The liver is a storehouse of many enzymes. Injury or diseases affecting the liver cause release of these intracellular enzymes into the bloodstream, and their levels become elevated. Some of these enzymes also are produced in other organs, and injury or disease affecting these organs raises the serum level. Therefore, although elevation of these serum enzymes is found in pathologic liver conditions, the test is not specific for liver diseases alone.

Nursing Interventions

Provide information to the patient regarding blood draws and what test is being performed. Monitor the venipuncture site for bleeding.

SERUM PROTEIN TEST

The normal values for serum protein test results are as follows:

Total protein: 6.4 to 8.3 g/dL
Albumin: 3.5 to 5 g/dL
Globulin: 2.3 to 3.4 g/dL
Albumin/globulin (A/G ratio): 1.2 to 2.2 g/dL

Rationale

One way to assess the liver's functional status is to measure the products it synthesizes. One of these products is protein, especially albumin. When a disorder or disease affects liver cells (i.e., hepatocytes), they lose their ability to synthesize albumin and the serum albumin level falls markedly. A low serum albumin level also may result from excessive loss of albumin into urine (as in nephrotic syndrome) or into third-space volumes (as in ascites), as well as in liver disease, increased capillary permeability, or protein-calorie malnutrition.

Nursing Interventions

Provide information to the patient regarding blood draws and what tests are being performed. Monitor the venipuncture site for bleeding.

CHOLECYSTOGRAPHY

Rationale

The oral cholecystogram (OCG) provides roentgenographic visualization of the gallbladder after the oral ingestion of a radiopaque, iodinated dye. Adequate visualization requires concentration of the dye within the gallbladder. This test is used much less frequently than in the past. More often, the test is performed via a T-tube with contrast agents such as Hypaque or Renografin. Other options include using a CT scan using the iodine based dye Biliscopin intravenously to evaluate the biliary tree.

Nursing Interventions

To prevent an allergic reaction, determine whether the patient is allergic to iodine, because the dyes typically used for these tests are iodine based. The patient is put on NPO status from midnight. The patient may be given a high-fat meal or beverage to stimulate emptying of the gallbladder after the test has begun. No other food or fluids are allowed until after the examination.

INTRAVENOUS CHOLANGIOGRAPHY

Rationale

In intravenous cholangiography, intravenously administered radiographic dye is concentrated by the liver and secreted into the bile duct. The intravenous cholangiogram (IVC) allows visualization of the hepatic and common bile ducts and the gallbladder if the cystic duct is patent. An IVC is used to demonstrate stones, strictures, or tumors of the hepatic duct, common bile duct, and gallbladder. Intravenous cholangiography is a less commonly used method of visualizing the biliary tree. It should not be used in the jaundiced patient unless it is determined that there are no blocked ducts.

OPERATIVE CHOLANGIOGRAPHY

In operative cholangiography the common bile duct is injected directly with radiopaque dye. Stones appear as radiolucent shadows, and the presence of tumors causes partial or total obstruction of the flow of dye into the duodenum. Visualization of the biliary duct structures provides the surgeon with a "road map" of a difficult anatomic area. This reduces the possibility of inadvertently injuring the common duct.

If common duct stones are suspected, a cholecystectomy and a common duct exploration (CDE) are necessary. When intraoperative cholangiography is used routinely, CDE is performed only on those with positive cholangiograms.

T-TUBE CHOLANGIOGRAPHY
Rationale
T-tube cholangiography (postoperative cholangiography) is performed to diagnose retained ductal stones postoperatively in the patient who has undergone a cholecystectomy and a common bile duct (CBD) exploration to demonstrate good flow of contrast into the duodenum. The test is performed through a T-shaped rubber tube that the surgeon places in the bile duct during the operation. The end of the T tube exits through the abdominal wall, where dye is injected and radiographic films are taken.

Nursing Interventions
During the preoperative phase ensure the patient is not allergic to iodine. Preparation of the patient also includes maintaining NPO status after midnight and until the examination is completed. Administer a cleansing enema on the morning of the examination, if ordered.

Postoperatively, the patient is protected from sepsis by connecting the T tube (if left in place) to a sterile closed-drainage system. If the T tube is removed, cover the T tube tract site with a sterile dressing to prevent bacteria from entering the ductal system.

ULTRASONOGRAPHY OF THE LIVER, THE GALLBLADDER, AND THE BILIARY SYSTEM
Rationale
Ultrasonography (ultrasound, echogram) is an imaging technique that visualizes deep structures of the body by recording the reflections (echoes) of ultrasonic waves directed into the tissues. This diagnostic test is not effective in examining all tissue, because ultrasound waves do not pass through structures that contain air, such as the lungs, the colon, or the stomach. Although fasting is preferred, it is not necessary for ultrasonography. Because ultrasound requires no contrast material and has no associated radiation, it is especially useful for patients who are allergic to contrast media or are pregnant. Ultrasound is used to corroborate data already obtained by "questionable positive" cholangiograms, liver scans, and OCGs. Gallstones are detected easily with ultrasound.

Nursing Interventions
The patient is on NPO status from midnight before the test. If the patient has had recent barium contrast

studies, request an order for laxatives because ultrasound cannot penetrate barium, and the study will not be adequate.

GALLBLADDER SCANNING
Rationale
The biliary tract can be evaluated safely, accurately, and noninvasively by intravenous (IV) injection of technetium (^{99}Tc; technetium-99m), and positioning the patient under a camera to record distribution of the tracer in the liver, biliary tree, gallbladder, and proximal small bowel. The primary use of this study is in the diagnosis of acute cholecystitis. This procedure is superior to oral cholecystography, ultrasonography, and computed tomography (CT) scanning of the abdomen for the detection of acute cholecystitis. Hepatobiliary iminodiacetic acid (HIDA) scanning is also useful for identifying diffuse hepatic disease (such as cirrhosis or neoplasm) and a nonfunctioning gallbladder.

Nursing Interventions
Reassure the patient that exposure to radioactivity is minimal, because only a trace dose of the radioisotope is used. The patient is on NPO status from midnight until the examination is complete.

NEEDLE LIVER BIOPSY
Rationale
Needle liver biopsy is a safe, simple, and valuable method of diagnosing pathologic liver conditions. A specially designed needle is inserted through the skin (making it a *percutaneous* procedure), between the sixth and seventh or eighth and ninth intercostal space, and into the liver. The patient lies supine with the right arm over the head. The patient is instructed to exhale fully and not breathe while the needle is inserted. This procedure often is done using ultrasound or CT guidance. A piece of hepatic tissue is removed for microscopic examination. The tissue sample is placed into a labeled specimen bottle containing formalin and sent to the pathology department. Percutaneous liver biopsy is used in the diagnosis of various liver disorders, such as cirrhosis, hepatitis, drug-related reactions, granuloma, and tumor.

Nursing Interventions
After the health care provider has explained the procedure to the patient, verify the patient has signed the consent form. Ensure that measurements of platelets, clotting or bleeding time, prothrombin time, and international normalized ratio (INR) have been ordered; report any abnormal values to the health care provider. After the procedure observe the patient for symptoms of bleeding. Monitor the patient's vital signs every 15 minutes (two times), then every 30 minutes (four times), and then every hour (four times). Keep the patient lying on the right side with a rolled towel against the puncture site for at least 2 hours to splint the puncture site. In this position, the liver capsule (a connective

tissue layer covering the liver) is compressed against the chest wall, decreasing the risk of hemorrhage or bile leak.

Some pain is common. When leakage involves a large quantity of blood or bile, the peritoneal reaction is great and the resulting pain severe. Assess the patient for pneumothorax (collapsed lung) caused by improper placement of the biopsy needle into the adjacent chest cavity or for bile peritonitis. Immediately report to the health care provider signs and symptoms of pneumothorax such as shortness of breath, change in respiratory and cardiac rate, or decreased breath sounds on the affected side.

RADIOISOTOPE LIVER SCANNING

Rationale

A radioisotope liver scan is a procedure used to outline and detect structural changes of the liver. A radioisotope (also called a *radionuclide*) is given intravenously. Later, a gamma ray–detecting device (Geiger counter) is passed over the patient's abdomen. This records the distribution of the radioactive particles in the liver. The spleen also can be visualized by the detector when technetium-99m sulfur is used.

Nursing Interventions

The patient is on NPO status from midnight before the test. Assure patients that they will not be exposed to a large amount of radioactivity, because only trace doses of isotopes are used.

SERUM AMMONIA TEST

The normal serum ammonia test value is 10 to 80 mcg/dL.

Rationale

Ammonia is a by-product of protein metabolism. Most of the ammonia is made by bacteria acting on proteins in the intestine. By way of the portal vein, ammonia goes to the liver, where it normally is converted into urea and then excreted by the kidneys. When the patient has severe liver dysfunction or altered blood flow to the liver, ammonia cannot be catabolized, the serum ammonia level rises, and the blood urea nitrogen level decreases. The serum ammonia level is used primarily as an aid in diagnosing hepatic encephalopathy and hepatic coma. Elevated serum ammonia levels suggest liver dysfunction as the cause of these signs and symptoms.

Nursing Interventions

Notify the laboratory of any antibiotics the patient is currently taking. Certain broad-spectrum antibiotics such as neomycin can cause a decreased ammonia level, thus giving inaccurate test results.

HEPATITIS VIRUS STUDIES

A normal laboratory test result is negative for hepatitis-associated antigen.

Rationale

Hepatitis is an inflammation of the liver caused by viruses, bacteria, and noninfectious causes such as alcohol ingestion and drugs. Five viruses, designated A through E, can cause this disease. Hepatitis A, B, and C viruses are the most common hepatitis viruses. Hepatitis D virus is carried by the hepatitis B virus (HBV). Hepatitis D and E viruses are seen less frequently in the United States than are the hepatitis A, B, or C viruses. The various types of hepatitis virus can be detected by their antigen and antibody levels, and their different incubation periods must be considered.

Nursing Interventions

Use standard precautions and handle the serum specimen as if it were capable of transmitting viral hepatitis. Don gloves when handling any blood or body fluids, and wash hands carefully after handling equipment.

SERUM AMYLASE TEST

The normal serum amylase test value is 60 to 120 Somogyi units/dL, or 30 to 220 units/L (SI units).

Rationale

The serum amylase test can aid in quickly diagnosing pancreatitis in its early stages. Damage to pancreatic cells (as in pancreatitis) or obstruction to the pancreatic ductal flow (as in pancreatic carcinoma) causes an outpouring of this enzyme into the intrapancreatic lymph system and the free peritoneum. Blood vessels draining the free peritoneum and absorbing the lymph pick up this excess amylase. An abnormal rise in the serum level of amylase occurs within 2 hours of the onset of pancreatic disease. Because amylase is cleared rapidly by the kidney, serum levels may return to normal within 36 hours. Persistent pancreatitis, duct obstruction, or pancreatic duct leak (e.g., pseudocysts) cause persistent elevated serum amylase levels.

Nursing Interventions

Note on the laboratory order whether the patient is receiving intravenous dextrose or any medications, because these can cause a false-negative result.

URINE AMYLASE TEST

The normal urine amylase test value is up to 5000 Somogyi units/24 h, or 6.5 to 48.1 units/h.

Rationale

Levels of amylase in the urine remain elevated for 7 to 10 days after the onset of pancreatitis. Urine amylase is particularly useful in detecting pancreatitis late in the disease course. This fact is important for diagnosing pancreatitis in patients who have had symptoms for 3 days or longer.

Nursing Interventions

Record the exact time at the beginning and end of the collection period. A 2-hour spot urine or 6-hour, 12-hour, or 24-hour collection can be performed, depending on the health care provider's order. The collection begins after the patient empties the bladder and discards that specimen. All subsequent urine is collected, including the voiding at the end of the collection period. Keep the specimen on ice or refrigerated until it is sent to the laboratory.

SERUM LIPASE TEST

The normal value for serum lipase test results is 10 to 140 units/L.

Rationale

Like serum amylase, serum lipase is elevated in acute pancreatitis and is a helpful complementary test because other disorders (e.g., mumps, cerebral trauma, and renal transplantation) also may cause an increase in serum amylase. Lipase appears in the bloodstream after damage to the pancreas. The lipase levels rise a little later than amylase levels (4 to 48 hours after the onset of pancreatitis), peak around 24 hours, and remain elevated for at least 14 days. Because lipase peaks later and remains elevated longer than amylase, it is more useful in the diagnosis of acute pancreatitis later in the course of the disease.

Nursing Interventions

Instruct the patient to remain on NPO status from midnight, except for water.

ULTRASONOGRAPHY OF THE PANCREAS

Rationale

With the use of reflected sound waves, ultrasonography of the pancreas provides diagnostic information about this inaccessible abdominal organ. Ultrasound examination of the pancreas is used mainly to diagnose carcinoma, pseudocyst, pancreatitis, and pancreatic abscess. Because abnormalities seen on ultrasound persist from several days to weeks, it can support the diagnosis of pancreatitis even after the serum amylase and lipase levels have returned to normal. Furthermore, a follow-up ultrasound study is used to monitor the resolution of pancreatic inflammation and a tumor's response to therapy. A newer procedure using ultrasound is endoscopic ultrasound of the pancreas. In this procedure an ultrasound probe is passed through the patient's mouth and into the small intestine. The sound waves emitted by the probe allow examination of the structures surrounding the pancreas and for fine needle biopsy of the pancreas (the needle is passed through the stomach wall to the pancreas) or lesions of the pancreas to differentiate benign lesions from malignancies. The procedure is an esophagogastroduodenoscopy (EGD) (see Chapter 5) with a camera. In the event that a lesion is cancerous, this procedure also provides staging of the cancer by visualization via ultrasound of the surrounding structures.

Nursing Interventions

Fluids and food are withheld for 8 hours before the examination. If an endoscopic ultrasound is being performed, implement the same interventions as for an EGD (see Chapter 5). If the patient's abdomen is distended with gas or if the patient has had a recent barium examination, the study should be postponed, because gas and barium interfere with sound wave transmission.

COMPUTED TOMOGRAPHY OF THE ABDOMEN

Rationale

A CT scan of the abdomen is a noninvasive, accurate radiographic procedure used to diagnose pathologic pancreatic conditions such as inflammation, tumors, pseudocyst formation, ascites, aneurysms, cirrhosis, abscesses, trauma, cysts, and anatomical abnormalities. The recognizable cross-sectional image produced by a CT scan is especially important for studying the pancreas, because this organ is well hidden by the overlying peritoneal organs.

Nursing Interventions

Fluids and food are withheld from midnight until the examination is complete; however, this test can be performed on an emergency basis on patients who have eaten recently. If possible, show the patient a picture of the machine and encourage the patient to verbalize fears, because some patients suffer claustrophobia when enclosed in the machine.

ENDOSCOPIC RETROGRADE CHOLANGIOPANCREATOGRAPHY OF THE PANCREATIC DUCT

Rationale

Endoscopic retrograde cholangiopancreatography (ERCP) enables visualization not only of the biliary system but also of the pancreatic duct. The test involves inserting a fiberoptic duodenoscope through the oral pharynx, through the esophagus and the stomach, and into the duodenum (Fig. 6.1). Dye is injected for radiographic visualization of the common bile duct and pancreatic duct. ERCP of the pancreas is a sensitive and reliable procedure for detecting clinically significant degrees of pancreatic dysfunction. It also can be used to evaluate obstructive jaundice, remove common bile duct stones, and place biliary and pancreatic duct stents to bypass obstruction. Localized pancreatic duct narrowing indicates the presence of a tumor. Chronic pancreatitis is demonstrated by multiple areas of ductal narrowing, which can be visualized by ERCP.

Nursing Interventions

Withhold food and fluids for 8 hours before the examination and obtain the patient's signature on a consent

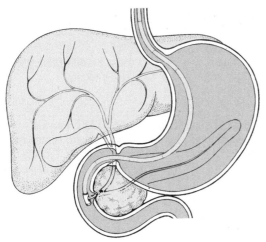

Fig. 6.1 Endoscopic retrograde cholangiopancreatography (ERCP). (From Pagana KD, Pagana TJ: *Mosby's diagnostic and laboratory test reference*, ed 12, St. Louis, 2015, Elsevier.)

form. Assess prothrombin time and INR before the procedure. Tell patients that the test takes approximately 1 to 2 hours, during which time they must lie completely motionless on a hard x-ray table, which may be uncomfortable. After the procedure, keep the patient on NPO status until the gag reflex returns; assess for abdominal pain, tenderness, and guarding, which could be signs of perforation. Assess for signs and symptoms of pancreatitis (the most common ERCP complication), including increasingly intense abdominal pain, nausea, fever, chills, vomiting, and diminished or absent bowel sounds. Assess for signs of hypovolemic shock, including decreased blood pressure, increased pulse and respirations, shortness of breath, cool and clammy skin, and decreased urine output.

DISORDERS OF THE LIVER, BILIARY TRACT, GALLBLADDER, AND EXOCRINE PANCREAS

The liver, gallbladder, and exocrine pancreas are organs that assist with digestion. Review the anatomy and physiology of the accessory organs of digestion (see Chapter 5) and the hepatic portal circulation. Refer to Table 6.1 for medications used for disorders of the accessory organs of digestion.

CIRRHOSIS

Etiology and Pathophysiology

Cirrhosis is a chronic, degenerative disease of the liver in which the lobes become covered with fibrous (scar) tissue, the parenchyma (i.e., the functional tissue of an organ, as opposed to supporting or connective tissue) degenerates, and the lobules are infiltrated with scar tissue or fat. The liver normally can regenerate itself, but not when cirrhosis is present. In the early stages of the disease the liver can function, but as the disease progresses, the liver fails to perform its normal functions. The overgrowth of new and fibrous tissue restricts the flow of blood to the organ, which contributes

to its destruction. Hepatomegaly (enlargement of the liver) and liver contraction (occurs later in the disease) cause loss of the organ's function (National Institutes of Diabetes and Digestive and Kidney Diseases [NIDDK], n.d.).

Cirrhosis and chronic liver disease is ranked as the ninth leading cause of death in the United States. Approximately 42,838 people die each year from the disease. Slightly more men are diagnosed with cirrhosis than women; more than 4.5 million people have cirrhosis or chronic liver disease (Centers for Disease Control and Prevention [CDC], 2021).

There are several forms of cirrhosis, caused by different factors. *Alcohol-related liver disease* may occur with heavy alcohol consumption. The amount of alcohol that causes damage to the liver differs among individuals. The chances for developing alcohol-related cirrhosis increase for women when they ingest more than two or three alcoholic drinks per day, and for men when they drink three or four drinks per day. *Postnecrotic cirrhosis,* which occurs worldwide, is caused by viral hepatitis (especially hepatitis C, but also hepatitis B and D), exposure to hepatotoxins (e.g., industrial chemicals, drugs, medications), or infection. *Biliary cirrhosis* results from destruction of the bile ducts as a result of inflammation. The resulting damage to the ducts leads to bile backing up into the liver. Conditions such as chronic biliary tree obstruction from gallstones, chronic pancreatitis, a tumor, cystic fibrosis, or biliary atresia (the absence of or underdevelopment of biliary structures that is congenital in nature) in children lead to biliary cirrhosis. *Cardiac cirrhosis* results from longstanding, severe right-sided heart failure in patients with cor pulmonale, constrictive pericarditis, and tricuspid insufficiency. *Nonalcoholic fatty liver disease (NAFLD)* results from fat building up in the liver. The incidence of NAFLD is increasing as a result of the growing obesity population. NAFLD also is associated with diabetes, coronary artery disease, and use of corticosteroids.

The cause of cirrhosis is not always known. Alcoholism is by far the greatest factor leading to cirrhosis. It is believed to result from the combination of alcohol's hepatotoxic effect on the liver coupled with the common problem of protein malnutrition seen in alcoholics. Cirrhosis of the liver from severe malnutrition without alcoholism also has occurred.

With repeated insults, the liver progresses through the following stages: destruction, inflammation, fibrotic regeneration, and hepatic insufficiency. Although liver cells have great potential for regeneration, repeated scarring decreases their ability to replace themselves. As the blood supply continues to diminish and scar tissue increases, the organ atrophies.

Functions of the liver are altered in several ways. The liver's ability to synthesize albumin is reduced as a result of liver cell damage. Obstruction of the portal vein as it enters the liver results in portal

Table 6.1   Medications for Disorders of the Gallbladder, Liver, Biliary Tract, and Exocrine Pancreas

GENERIC NAME	ACTION	SIDE EFFECTS	NURSING IMPLICATIONS
cholestyramine	Binds bile acids in the GI tract, forming an insoluble complex; relief of pruritus associated with elevated levels of bile acids	Nausea, constipation, abdominal discomfort	Assess severity of pruritus and skin integrity
gemcitabine hydrochloride	Exhibits antitumor activity; indicated as first-line treatment of locally advanced or metastatic adenocarcinoma of the pancreas	Myelosuppression; nausea and vomiting; macular papular pruritic rash	Monitor CBC. Provide antiemetic to control nausea and vomiting. Provide relief measures to control pruritus
lactulose	Acidifies colonic contents, thus decreasing absorption of ammonia from gut; also has cathartic laxative properties; primarily used in hepatic encephalopathy	Nausea, vomiting, diarrhea	Titrate dose to three or four loose stools per day; monitor for dehydration; monitor for serum ammonia levels and improved mental status
meperidine	Binds to opiate receptors in CNS; alters perception of and response to painful stimuli, while producing generalized CNS depression; used for biliary pain because morphine may cause spasms of the sphincter of Oddi	Sedation, confusion, respiratory depression, hypotension, bradycardia, nausea, vomiting, urinary retention	Assess type, location, intensity of pain before and 1 h after administration. If respiratory rate is <10 breaths/min, assess level of sedation
neomycin	Inhibits protein synthesis in bacteria at the level of the 30S ribosome subunit; decreases the number of ammonia-producing bacteria in the gut as part of management of hepatic encephalopathy	Ototoxicity; local stinging, burning; nephrotoxicity	Monitor neurologic status and renal function
pancrelipase	Increased digestion of fats, carbohydrate, and proteins in the GI tract; treatment of pancreatic insufficiency associated with chronic pancreatitis, pancreatectomy	Diarrhea, nausea, stomach cramps, abdominal pain	Assess patient's nutritional status; monitor stools for high fat content; assess patient for allergy to pork; administer immediately before meals or with meals
propantheline	Antisecretory and antispasmodic agent; slows GI motility through anticholinergic activity; decreases pancreatic activity	Drowsiness, confusion, dry mouth, constipation, urinary retention, tachycardia, blurred vision	Avoid use with other CNS depressants or alcohol; avoid driving or other activities until accustomed to effects; may cause hypotension when given intravenously; do not use in patients with Parkinson's disease
spironolactone	Competes with aldosterone at receptor sites in distal tubule, resulting in excretion of sodium chloride and water and retention of potassium and phosphate; used in cirrhosis of the liver with ascites	Headache, confusion, diarrhea, bleeding, dysrhythmias, impotence, hypokalemia	Assess electrolytes, sodium, chloride, potassium, BUN, serum creatinine. Weigh daily; monitor I&O. Administer in the morning to avoid interference with sleep
vasopressin	Synthetic pituitary agent; antidiuretic effects on kidney; a potent vasoconstrictor; used to treat bleeding esophageal varices	Hypertension; ischemia to heart, mesenteric organs, and kidneys; angina; myocardial infarction; water retention; hyponatremia	Use with caution in older adults and in patients with known coronary artery disease or known CHF; discontinue if chest pain develops; monitor urinary output and serum sodium

BUN, Blood urea nitrogen; *CBC*, complete blood count; *CHF*, congestive heart failure; *CNS*, central nervous system; *GI*, gastrointestinal; *I&O*, intake and output.
From Skidmore-Roth L: *Mosby's 2021 nursing drug reference*, ed 34, St. Louis, 2020, Mosby.

hypertension—increased venous pressure in the portal circulation caused by compression or occlusion of the portal or hepatic vascular system. In most instances, portal hypertension that is caused by cirrhosis is irreversible.

This increased pressure causes ascites (an accumulation of fluid and albumin in the peritoneal cavity). The damaged liver cannot metabolize protein in the usual manner; therefore protein intake may result in an elevation of blood ammonia levels. Reduced synthesis of protein and the leaking of existing protein result in hypoalbuminemia (reduced protein or albumin level in the blood), which reduces the blood's ability to regain fluids through osmosis. Protein must be present in adequate amounts to create colloidal osmotic pressure and "attract" the fluid to pass back into the blood vessels after it escapes in the capillaries. As fluid leaves the blood and the circulating volume decreases, the receptors in the brain signal the adrenal cortex to increase secretion of aldosterone to stimulate the kidneys to retain sodium and water. The normal liver inactivates the hormone aldosterone, but the damaged liver allows its effect to continue (hyperaldosteronism). Retention of fluid and sodium results in increased pressure in blood vessels and lymphatic channels, resulting in portal hypertension. Ascites is thus a result of portal hypertension, hypoalbuminemia, and hyperaldosteronism.

Hepatic insufficiency gradually causes distention of veins in the upper part of the body, including the esophageal vein. Esophageal varices develop and may rupture, causing severe hemorrhage.

Clinical Manifestations

Clinical manifestations of cirrhosis of the liver differ, depending on the stage of the disease. In the early stages the liver is firm and therefore easier to palpate, and abdominal pain may be present because rapid enlargement produces tension on the organ's fibrous covering. Later stages of the disease are characterized by dyspepsia, changes in bowel habits, gradual weight loss, ascites, enlarged spleen, malaise, nausea, jaundice, ecchymoses, and spider telangiectases (small, dilated blood vessels with a bright red center point and spiderlike branches). Spider telangiectases occur on the nose, cheeks, upper trunk, neck, and shoulders. These later manifestations are the result of scarring of liver tissue that produces chronic failure of liver function and fibrotic changes that cause obstruction of the portal circulation.

When enough cells of the liver become involved to interfere with its function and obstruct its circulation, the GI organs and the spleen become congested and cannot function properly. Anemia occurs because of the body's decreased ability to produce red blood cells (RBCs). The cirrhotic liver cannot absorb vitamin K or produce the clotting factors VII, IX, and X. These factors cause the patient with cirrhosis to develop bleeding tendencies.

Assessment

Subjective data in the early stages include the patient's description of flulike symptoms (loss of appetite, nausea and vomiting, general weakness, and fatigue), indigestion, abnormal bowel function (either constipation or diarrhea), flatulence, and abdominal discomfort. The anatomic area most commonly affected is in the epigastric region or the right upper quadrant of the abdomen.

Subjective data in the later stages typically include the same early stage symptoms, but now more intense in the later stages. The patient may complain of dyspnea, pruritus, and severe fatigue that interfere with the ability to carry out routine activities. Pruritus results from an accumulation of bile salts under the skin, the result of jaundice.

Collection of objective data in the early stages includes observing low hemoglobin, fever, weight loss, and jaundice (yellow discoloration of the skin, mucous membranes, and sclera of the eyes [scleral icterus], caused by greater than normal amounts of bilirubin in the serum). Collection of objective data in the later stages includes noting epistaxis, purpura, hematuria, spider angiomas (telangiectases), and bleeding gums. Late symptoms include ascites, hematologic disorders, splenic enlargement, and hemorrhage from esophageal varices or other distended GI veins. The patient also may appear mentally disoriented and display abnormal behaviors and speech patterns because of increased ammonia levels in the brain. Any prolonged interference with gas exchange leads to hypoxia, coma, and ultimately death.

Diagnostic Tests

Many diagnostic tests aid in the diagnosis of cirrhosis. Poor liver function may be manifest as abnormal electrolyte values; elevated serum bilirubin, AST, ALT, LDH, and GTT; decreased total protein and serum albumin; elevated ammonia; low blood glucose (hypoglycemia) from impaired gluconeogenesis; prolonged prothrombin time; increased INR; and decreased cholesterol levels. Visualization through ERCP (to detect common bile duct obstruction), esophagoscopy with barium esophagography to visualize esophageal varices, scans and biopsy of the liver, and ultrasonography are used to diagnose cirrhosis. Paracentesis (a procedure in which fluid is withdrawn from the abdominal cavity) relieves ascites and also provides fluid for laboratory examination.

Medical Management

When possible causes have been identified, the initial treatment is to eliminate those causes, decrease the buildup of fluids in the body, prevent further damage to the liver, and provide individual supportive care. Eliminating alcohol, hepatotoxins (e.g., acetaminophen [Tylenol]), or environmental exposure to harmful chemicals is essential to prevent further damage to the liver. Diet therapy is aimed at correcting malnutrition, promoting the regeneration of functional liver tissue, and compensating for the liver's inability to store vitamins, while avoiding fluid retention and hepatic encephalopathy. A diet that is well balanced, high in calories (2500 to 3000 calories/day), moderately high in protein (75 g of high-quality protein per day), low in fat, low in sodium (1000 to 2000 mg/day), and with additional vitamins and folic acid usually meets the needs of the patient with cirrhosis and improves deficiencies. A protein-restricted diet may be prescribed for a patient recovering from an acute episode of hepatic encephalopathy.

Antiemetics may be prescribed to control nausea or vomiting. Monitor the patient closely for toxicity, which develops quickly when the poorly functioning liver cannot clear these drugs from the system. Diphenhydramine or dimenhydrinate may be given, whereas prochlorperazine maleate, hydroxyzine pamoate, ondansetron hydrochloride, and hydroxyzine hydrochloride are contraindicated in severe liver dysfunction.

Later manifestations may be severe and result from liver failure and portal hypertension. Jaundice, peripheral edema, esophageal varices, hepatic encephalopathy, and ascites develop gradually (Fig. 6.2).

Complications and treatment. The severity of fluid retention from ascites and edema determines the treatment. Initially the patient is placed on bed rest with accurate monitoring of intake and output (I&O). Restrictions are placed on the amount of fluid (500 to 1000 mL/day) and sodium (1000 to 2000 mg/day) consumed. Diuretic therapy may be added if the diet does not control the ascites and edema. Spironolactone at 100 to 400 mg/day may be used to obtain the desired diuresis. Other diuretics may be added, including furosemide or hydrochlorothiazide. Vitamin supplements include vitamin K, vitamin C, and folic acid. Salt-poor albumin may be administered in an attempt to restore plasma volume if the intravascular volume is decreased significantly. Complications of diuretic therapy include plasma volume deficit, decreased renal function, and electrolyte imbalance.

Another method of treatment for ascites and edema is the LeVeen continuous peritoneal jugular shunt (Fig. 6.3). This procedure allows the continuous shunting of ascitic fluid from the abdominal cavity through a one-way, pressure-sensitive valve into a silicone tube that empties into the superior vena cava. Patients with this shunt are monitored for complications, which include congestive heart failure, leakage of ascitic fluid, infection at the insertion sites, peritonitis, septicemia, and shunt thrombosis.

Paracentesis (see *Foundations of Nursing,* Chapter 23), in which fluid is removed from the abdominal cavity by either gravity or vacuum, provides temporary relief from ascites. It is imperative that patients urinate immediately before the procedure to prevent puncture of

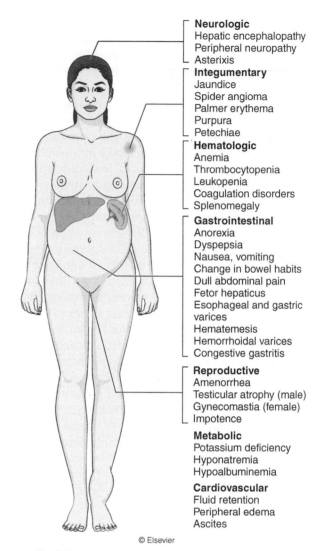

Neurologic
Hepatic encephalopathy
Peripheral neuropathy
Asterixis

Integumentary
Jaundice
Spider angioma
Palmer erythema
Purpura
Petechiae

Hematologic
Anemia
Thrombocytopenia
Leukopenia
Coagulation disorders
Splenomegaly

Gastrointestinal
Anorexia
Dyspepsia
Nausea, vomiting
Change in bowel habits
Dull abdominal pain
Fetor hepaticus
Esophageal and gastric varices
Hematemesis
Hemorrhoidal varices
Congestive gastritis

Reproductive
Amenorrhea
Testicular atrophy (male)
Gynecomastia (female)
Impotence

Metabolic
Potassium deficiency
Hyponatremia
Hypoalbuminemia

Cardiovascular
Fluid retention
Peripheral edema
Ascites

© Elsevier

Fig. 6.2 Systemic clinical manifestations of liver cirrhosis.

the bladder. The patient should sit on the side of the bed or be placed in a high Fowler's position. An incision is made in the skin, and a hollow trocar, cannula, or catheter is passed through the incision and into the cavity. The fluid is removed over a period of 30 to 90 minutes to prevent sudden changes in blood pressure, which could lead to syncope. Monitor the patient closely for signs of hypovolemia and electrolyte imbalances. Apply a dressing over the insertion site, and observe for bleeding and drainage.

Esophageal varices (a complex of longitudinal, tortuous veins at the lower end of the esophagus) enlarge and become edematous as the result of portal hypertension. They are susceptible to ulceration and hemorrhage; avoiding this is a main goal of treatment. For patients who have not bled from esophageal varices, prophylactic treatment with nonselective beta blockers (e.g., propranolol) has been shown to reduce the risk of bleeding and bleeding-related deaths. Varices can rupture as a result of anything that increases abdominal venous pressure, such as coughing, sneezing, vomiting, or the Valsalva maneuver. Rupture may

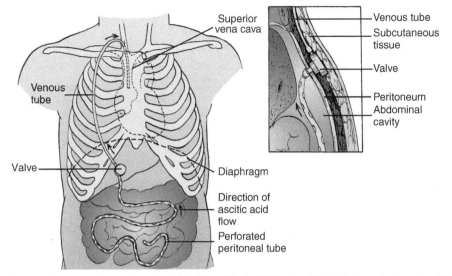

Fig. 6.3 LeVeen continuous peritoneal jugular shunt. (From Black JM, Hawks JH: *Medical-surgical nursing: Clinical management for positive outcomes*, ed 8, St. Louis, 2009, Mosby.)

occur slowly over several days or suddenly and without pain. An endoscopy may be performed to identify varices or to rule out bleeding from other sources. Endoscopic therapies include sclerotherapy (the injection of chemicals used to cause inflammation, followed by fibrosis and destruction of the vessels causing the bleeding) and ligation of varices.

Therapeutic management of a ruptured esophageal varix is a medical emergency. The patient's airway must be maintained, the bleeding varix controlled, and IV lines established for fluids and blood replacement as needed. The hormone vasopressin (VP), administered intravenously or directly into the superior vena cava, is used to decrease or stop the hemorrhaging. VP produces vasoconstriction of the vessels, decreases portal blood flow, and decreases portal hypertension. Current drug therapy in some institutions is a combination of VP and nitroglycerin (NTG). NTG reduces the detrimental effects of VP, which include decreased coronary blood flow and increased blood pressure. VP should be avoided or used cautiously in the older adult because of the risk of cardiac ischemia (i.e., a restriction in blood supply to the heart). If the VP drip does not stop or control bleeding, a Sengstaken-Blakemore tube with openings at the tip may be inserted. This triple-lumen tube has a lumen for inflating the esophageal balloon, one for inflating the gastric balloon, and one for gastric lavage (Fig. 6.4). The tube is passed through the nose, and the balloon in the stomach, the one in the esophagus, or both are inflated to press against the bleeding vessels and control the hemorrhage. The gastric aspiration is attached to low, intermittent suction. When either balloon is inflated, a Levin tube is passed into the esophagus through the mouth and attached to low suction to drain the saliva that cannot drain into the stomach. The balloon must be deflated periodically to

prevent necrosis. Give the patient nothing by mouth and elevate the head of the bed 30 to 45 degrees to help prevent aspiration of stomach contents and help the patient breathe.

Gastric lavage is performed to remove any swallowed blood from the stomach. Some facilities use iced isotonic saline solutions for the lavage to facilitate vasoconstriction. Endoscopic sclerotherapy also may be used to control the bleeding.

Other methods used to treat bleeding esophageal varices include band ligation. In this procedure an endoscope is passed into the esophagus and elastic bands are placed to tie off bleeding vessels. This procedure also is performed to prevent esophageal varices from bleeding. Band ligation has a small risk of causing scarring of the esophagus. The medication octreotide sometimes is used in combination with band ligation when treating bleeding varices. Octreotide slows the flow of blood from internal organs to the portal vein. This helps to reduce pressure in the portal vein and is administered for 5 days after an esophageal hemorrhage (Mayo Clinic, 2019).

Patients suffering from portal hypertension and esophageal varices may benefit from surgical shunting procedures that divert blood from the portal system to the venous system. The portacaval shunt diverts blood from the portal vein to the inferior vena cava. The splenorenal shunt requires the removal of the spleen, and the splenic vein is anastomosed to the left renal vein. The mesocaval shunt involves anastomosis of the superior mesenteric vein to the inferior vena cava. These procedures are associated with a high mortality rate. They may be performed in an emergency to control acute esophageal varix bleeding or in a therapeutic situation when a patient already has bled. Complications of surgical shunting procedures are hepatic encephalopathy, GI bleeding, ascites, and liver failure.

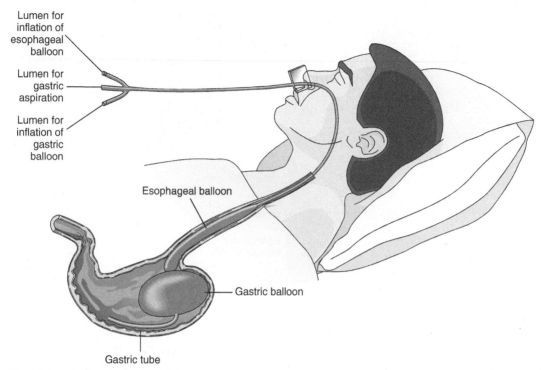

Lumen for
inflation of
esophageal
balloon

Lumen for
gastric
aspiration

Lumen for
inflation of
gastric
balloon

Esophageal balloon

Gastric balloon

Gastric tube

Fig. 6.4 Esophageal tamponade accomplished with a Sengstaken-Blakemore tube. (From Copstead-Kirkhorn LE, Banasik J: *Pathophysiology*, ed 5, St. Louis, 2013, Mosby.)

Care of the patient who has hemorrhaged from an esophageal varix includes maintenance of oxygen content levels within the blood and administration of fresh frozen plasma and packed RBCs, vitamin K, histamine (H_2) receptor blockers such as cimetidine, and electrolyte replacements as needed without fluid overload. Ammonia buildup is avoided with the use of cathartics (e.g., lactulose) and neomycin. Preventing ammonia buildup prevents hepatic encephalopathy.

Hepatic encephalopathy is a type of brain damage caused by liver disease and consequent ammonia intoxication. It is thought to result from a damaged liver being unable to metabolize substances that can be toxic to the brain, such as ammonia. The patient's signs and symptoms progress from inappropriate behavior, disorientation, asterixis, and twitching of the extremities to stupor and coma. **Asterixis** is a hand-flapping tremor in which the patient stretches out an arm and hyperextends the wrist with the fingers separated, relaxed, and extended. A rapid, irregular flexion and extension (flapping) of the wrist occurs in the patient who is acutely ill. Treatment of the patient with hepatic encephalopathy consists of supportive care to prevent further damage to the liver.

In the past, a low-protein diet often was prescribed for patients with cirrhosis of the liver. Restricting protein intake was thought to decrease the amount of ammonia produced in the intestine, thus preventing hepatic encephalopathy. The current belief is that protein and calories should not be restricted, because these patients often have existing malnutrition. On occasion, protein is decreased in the diet of a patient with

an exacerbation of hepatic encephalopathy, but this is rarely seen with current treatment because this can put the patient at risk for muscle wasting. If the patient is unable to consume enough nutrients with food, liquid dietary supplements may be added to the diet. The content of supplements varies, so the health care provider should be consulted when choosing the proper supplement.

Teach the patient to avoid potentially hepatotoxic over-the-counter drugs such as acetaminophen and to abstain from alcohol. Medications may be given to cleanse the bowel and help decrease the serum ammonia level. Lactulose decreases the bowel's pH from 7 to 5, thus decreasing the production of ammonia by bacteria within the bowel. Lactulose may be administered orally, as a retention enema, or via nasogastric (NG) tube. It also functions as a cathartic. The lactulose traps ammonia in the gut, and the drug's laxative effect expels the ammonia from the colon. Antibiotics such as neomycin, which are poorly absorbed from the GI tract, are given orally or rectally. They reduce the bacterial flora of the colon. Bacterial action on protein in feces results in ammonia production. Because neomycin may cause renal toxicity and hearing impairment, lactulose frequently is preferred.

Nursing Interventions and Patient Teaching
Check vital signs every 4 hours or more often if evidence of hemorrhage is present. Observe the patient for GI hemorrhage as evidenced by hematemesis, melena, anxiety, and restlessness.

Most patients require a well-balanced, moderate, high-protein, high-carbohydrate diet with adequate vitamins. With impending liver failure, fluids and sodium may be restricted. Sodium restriction can make providing a palatable diet more difficult. Provide frequent oral hygiene and a pleasant environment to help the patient increase food intake.

A major nursing focus for many patients is to help them deal with alcoholism. This requires establishing trust that the health team is interested in the patient's well-being. Patients must admit that they have a drinking problem before they can be helped. Provide information regarding community support programs, such as Alcoholics Anonymous, for help with alcohol abuse.

Because of pruritus, malnutrition, and edema, the patient with cirrhosis is prone to skin lesions and pressure sores. Initiate preventive nursing interventions to avoid impairment of skin integrity, such as an alternating pressure air mattress, frequent turning, and back rubs. Apply soothing lotion to relieve pruritus.

Observe the patient's mental status and report changes such as disorientation, headache, or lethargy. Assist in activities of daily living (ADLs) as needed to promote good hygiene while allowing the patient to conserve energy. Observe for edema by measuring ankles daily, and observe for ascites by measuring abdominal girth. Record accurate I&O and daily weight. Nursing intervention with concern and warmth regardless of physical changes is essential in helping the patient maintain self-esteem.

Refer to Nursing Care Plan 6.1 for a sample nursing care plan for the patient with cirrhosis of the liver. The patient with cirrhosis must understand the need for getting adequate rest and avoiding infections. Plan activity around complete bed rest until strength is regained. Turning the patient at least every 2 hours and providing range-of-motion exercises help avoid infection and prevent thrombophlebitis. Instruct the patient to use a soft-bristled toothbrush, use an electric razor, blow the nose cautiously, and avoid straining at stools to prevent bleeding as a result of a lack of vitamin K and certain clotting factors. Avoid soap, perfumed lotion, and rubbing alcohol, because they dry the skin. For pruritus caused by dry skin, administer diphenhydramine (Benadryl). Explain the relationship of the therapeutic diet to the diagnosis and the liver's ability to function.

Help the patient and family identify community resources for home health care and alcohol rehabilitation to assist them in dealing with problems that arise after discharge. Because of the seriousness of the disease, the patient and the family need understanding and support throughout the treatment (see the Home Care Considerations box).

Home Care Considerations

CIRRHOSIS OF THE LIVER

- The patient and the family need to understand the importance of continual health care and medical supervision.
- Encourage measures to achieve and maintain remission. These include proper diet, rest, avoidance of potentially hepatotoxic over-the-counter drugs (e.g., acetaminophen), and abstinence from alcohol.
- Provide information regarding community support programs, such as Alcoholics Anonymous, for help with alcohol abuse.
- Help the patient maintain the highest level of wellness possible and initiate and maintain necessary lifestyle changes.
- Ensure the patient and caregivers understand the importance of a well-balanced diet. Provide sample diets for reference.

Prognosis. Cirrhosis of the liver cannot be cured; the patient's prognosis depends on many factors. If the cause of the liver damage can be treated or eliminated, the prognosis improves. Discontinuing drinking alcohol and treating the hepatitis help to slow and even stop the progression of cirrhosis. The patient's adherence to prescribed treatment also is a determining factor in the prognosis. Liver transplantation is an option for some patients, but this depends on many factors, including the cause of the cirrhosis and the patient's overall health status.

LIVER CANCER

Etiology and Pathophysiology

The American Cancer Society (ACS) estimates that *primary liver cancer* will be diagnosed in nearly 43,000 people in the year 2020 (30,170 in men and 12,640 in women). Of these newly diagnosed cases it is estimated that almost 30,160 will die of the disease. The type of primary liver cancer seen most frequently is hepatocellular carcinoma; the other primary tumors are intrahepatic cholangiomas or biliary duct carcinomas (ACS, 2021a). Cirrhosis of the liver and infection with hepatitis C or hepatitis B are high-risk factors for primary liver cancer. Being infected with both hepatitis B and C increases the chances of liver cancer even more. Further increasing the risk are those individuals who drink alcohol excessively (at least 6 drinks per day). It is estimated that 2.4 million people in the United States have hepatitis C and 862,000 have hepatitis B, with many not even realizing that they are infected. Increasing age, obesity, type 2 diabetes, male gender, cirrhosis, and hepatotoxins are some of the risk factors tied to liver cancer (CDC, 2021c).

Metastatic carcinoma of the liver, or *secondary liver cancer,* occurs more often than primary liver cancer. The amount of blood flow through the portal vein and the extensive capillary structure make the metastasis of cancer cells to the liver more likely than to other organs. The pancreas, colon, stomach, breast, and lung

Nursing Care Plan 6.1   The Patient With Cirrhosis of the Liver

Mr. K., 49 years of age, is admitted with loss of appetite, generalized edema, pruritus, flappy tremors of the hands, ascites, and lethargy. He appears disoriented. His skin has areas of excoriation caused by scratching and a sallow appearance. His wife states that he has been unable to concentrate, appears confused and listless, and has been eating poorly. Mr. K. has been an alcoholic for the past 18 years. His total bilirubin is 4.5 mg/dL, GGT is 65 units/L, total protein is 4.8 g/dL, albumin is 2.8 g/dL, and blood ammonia is 160 mcg/dL. He is demonstrating signs and symptoms of hepatic encephalopathy.

PATIENT PROBLEM

Insufficient Nutrition, related to anorexia, nausea, and impaired utilization and storage of nutrients, as demonstrated by lack of interest in food, aversion to eating, inadequate food intake

Patient Goals and Expected Outcomes	Nursing Interventions	Evaluation/Rationale
Patient will eat 50% of meal Patient will maintain baseline body weight	Monitor weight to determine whether weight loss occurs Provide oral care before meals to remove foul taste and improve taste of food Administer antiemetics as ordered to relieve nausea and vomiting Provide small, frequent meals at times the patient can best tolerate them to prevent feeling of fullness and to maintain nutritional status Determine food preferences and allow these whenever possible to increase appeal of food for patient	Patient is eating 50% - 75% of his meals Patient has no weight loss, indicating maintaining satisfactory nutritional balance

PATIENT PROBLEM

Recent Onset of Confusion, related to increased formation of ammonia as demonstrated by inability to concentrate, lethargy, disorientation, and asterixis (hand flapping tremors)

Patient Goals and Expected Outcomes	Nursing Interventions	Evaluation
Patient will be oriented to person, place, time, and purpose	Monitor for hepatic encephalopathy by assessing patient's general behavior, orientation to time and place, speech, and ammonia levels, because liver is unable to convert accumulating ammonia to urea for renal excretion Encourage fluids (if not restricted), and give laxatives and enemas as ordered to decrease ammonia production Provide prescribed protein-restricted diet until acute clinical signs and symptoms of hepatic encephalopathy are decreased Administer lactulose or neomycin as prescribed Limit physical activity because exercise produces ammonia as a by-product of metabolism. Control factors known to precipitate hepatic coma	Patient responds appropriately to assessment of person, place, time, and purpose

CRITICAL THINKING QUESTIONS

1. Mr. K. is thrashing about in his bed and has attempted to climb over the side rails. He is disoriented to time and place. What appropriate nursing interventions will ensure Mr. K.'s safety?
2. Mrs. K. notes that her husband has a low-protein diet. She confides to the nurse that she thinks he needs more meat, eggs, and cottage cheese to improve his nutrition. What is the most appropriate response?

are common primary sites of cancer that metastasizes to the liver.

Clinical Manifestations and Diagnostic Tests

Diagnosing carcinoma of the liver is difficult. In its early stages many of the clinical manifestations (e.g., hepatomegaly, weight loss, peripheral edema, ascites, portal hypertension) are similar to those of cirrhosis of the liver. Other common manifestations include dull abdominal pain in the epigastric or right upper quadrant region, jaundice, anorexia, nausea and vomiting, and extreme weakness. Palpation may reveal an enlarged, nodular liver. Patients frequently have pulmonary emboli. Tests to assist in the diagnosis are a liver scan, ultrasound, CT scan, magnetic resonance imaging, hepatic arteriography, ERCP, and needle liver biopsy. Serum liver function tests can be an early indication that the liver is not functioning properly, but this is not always a routine lab test. Alpha-fetoprotein (AFP) is a protein made in the liver. In adults, this level should be very low. Increased levels may be an indication of liver cancer or other diseases of the liver.

Medical Management and Nursing Interventions

Treatment of cancer of the liver is largely palliative. Surgical excision (lobectomy) sometimes is performed if the tumor is localized to one portion of the liver. Only a small percentage of patients have surgically resectable disease; usually the cancer is too advanced for surgery when it is detected. Surgical excision or transplantation offers the only chance for cure. Medical management is similar to that for cirrhosis of the liver. Chemotherapy may be used, but the response is usually poor. Portal vein or hepatic artery perfusion with chemotherapy agents such as 5-fluorouracil (5-FU) may be attempted.

Nursing interventions for the patient with liver carcinoma focus on keeping the patient as comfortable as possible. Because the problems are the same as with advanced liver disease, the nursing interventions discussed for cirrhosis of the liver apply.

Prognosis

The 5-year survival rate for liver cancer depends on the extent of the cancer when it is diagnosed. Localized liver cancer (cancer has not spread past the liver) 5-year survival rate is approximately 33%. Regional stage liver cancer (involves the liver and nearby lymph nodes and organs) 5-year survival rate is 11%. Unfortunately, the 5-year survival rate for distant liver cancer (metastases to distant organs or tissues) is 2%. If liver cancer is detected early and the patient has a liver transplant, the 5-year survival rate is 60% to 70% (ACS, 2021a).

HEPATITIS

Etiology and Pathophysiology

Hepatitis is an inflammation of the liver resulting from several types of viral agents or exposure to toxic substances. Rarely, hepatitis is caused by bacteria, such as streptococci, salmonellae, or *Escherichia coli*.

The five major types of viral hepatitis are caused by distinct but similar viruses that produce almost identical signs and symptoms in some of the strains but vary in their incubation period, mode of transmission, and prognosis. Hepatitis A (formerly called infectious hepatitis) is the most common form today and is a short-incubation virus (10 to 40 days). Hepatitis B (formerly called serum hepatitis) is a long-incubation virus (28 to 160 days). Hepatitis C has an incubation period of 2 weeks to 6 months (commonly 6 to 9 weeks). Hepatitis D (also called delta virus) only occurs in people infected with hepatitis B and may progress to cirrhosis and chronic hepatitis. The incubation period is 2 to 10 weeks. Hepatitis E (also called enteric non-A–non-B hepatitis) is transmitted through fecal contamination of water, primarily in developing countries. It is rare in the United States. The incubation period is 15 to 64 days. Hepatitis G virus is a little known strain that infects only 2% to 5% of the population. It frequently coexists with other hepatitis viruses, such as hepatitis C.

Health officials are required by law to report all cases of viral hepatitis to the Centers for Disease Control and Prevention (CDC) in Atlanta, Georgia. Modes of transmission for the various types of hepatitis are listed in Box 6.1.

The basic pathologic findings in the six forms of viral hepatitis are similar. A diffuse inflammatory reaction occurs, liver cells begin to degenerate and die, and the liver's normal functions slow down. The outcome may be affected by the virulence of the virus, the liver's preexisting condition, the health care given when the disease is diagnosed, and patient compliance with treatment.

BOX 6.1   Modes of Transmission of the Six Types of Viral Hepatitis

- Hepatitis A spreads by direct contact through the oral-fecal route, usually by food or water contaminated with feces. The incidence of the infection in the United States has decreased significantly because of the availability of the hepatitis A vaccine. People traveling outside the United States should avoid untreated water sources and uncooked food.
- Hepatitis B is transmitted by contaminated serum via blood transfusion, contaminated needles and instruments, needlesticks, illicit intravenous (IV) drug use, and by direct contact with body fluids from infected people, such as breast milk and sexual contact. An ever-increasing risk comes from improper disposal of used needles and syringes. Sharing toothbrushes, razor blades, or personal items with an infected person also may lead to exposure.
- Hepatitis C (HCV) is transmitted through needlesticks, blood transfusions, illicit IV drug use, and unidentified means. HCV also can be transmitted by sharing contaminated straws used for snorting cocaine. In the past, hepatitis C could not be detected in banked blood, so it was transmitted more easily through transfusion. The advent of routine blood screening in 1992 greatly reduced the number of cases of transfusion-related hepatitis C.
- Hepatitis D is transmitted in the same way as hepatitis B; it appears as a coinfection with hepatitis B.
- Hepatitis E is transmitted by the oral-fecal route; it spreads through the fecal contamination of water.
- Hepatitis G is seen frequently as a coinfection with hepatitis C; it spreads through bloodborne exposure. Hepatitis G has been found in some blood donors and can be transmitted by transfusion. Transmission occurs through contaminated injectable drugs; contaminated blood, organs, or tissues; or unsafe methods of tattooing or body piercing.

From World Health Organization: https://www.who.int/health-topics/hepatitis#tab=tab_1.

Safety Alert

PREVENTION OF ACUTE VIRAL HEPATITIS

Hepatitis A
- Hand washing is imperative. Hepatitis A virus (HAV) is transmitted when people eat food that is contaminated with fecal material (called "fecal–oral transmission"). Teach patients the importance of good hand hygiene after using the bathroom or changing a diaper, as well as proper food preparation, to prevent the spread of HAV. There are several documented cases of HAV being linked to food preparation and handling in restaurants.
- The best protection against HAV transmission is the two-dose HAV vaccine.

Hepatitis B
- Wash hands.
- One of the best preventive measures against hepatitis B virus (HBV) is the HBV vaccine.
- Hepatitis B is transmitted via blood and body fluids containing blood.
- Children younger than 19 years of age are vaccinated routinely.
- People who are at risk for the virus, such as health care workers, should be vaccinated.
- Others that should be vaccinated include: Individuals who have sex with partners susceptible to hepatitis B or are having sex in a relationship that is not a long-term monogamous relationship; men who have sex with men; IV drug users; public safety workers; people who travel outside the US; patients on hemodialysis.
- Risk factors do not have to be identified for an individual to get vaccinated for hepatitis B
- People who are positive for HBV should not donate blood, organs, or tissue, and should not breastfeed.
- Ensure proper disposal of needles.
- Use standard precautions when handling blood products.

- Use needleless IV access devices if available.

Hepatitis C
- Wash hands.
- Hepatitis C virus is transmitted by needle sharing among illicit IV drug users.
- Other significant risk factors include receipt of clotting factor made before 1987, hemodialysis, receipt of blood or solid organs donated before 1992, maternal-fetal transmission, and multiple or infected sex partners.
- Ensure proper disposal of needles.
- Use standard precautions when handling blood products.
- Use needleless IV access devices if available.

Hepatitis D
- Hepatitis D is a viral liver infection that only occurs in people with hepatitis B.
- Modes of hepatitis D virus (HDV) transmission are similar to those of HBV. Sexual transmission of HDV is less efficient than for HBV. Educate patients regarding risky behavior.

Hepatitis E
- Educate patients to avoid drinking water or beverages with ice in areas with uncertain water quality. They should refrain from eating raw shellfish and avoid raw produce unless it is prepared with purified water.
- Hepatitis E is seen most often in Southeast and Central Asia, the Middle East, Africa, and Mexico.

Hepatitis G
- Hepatitis G has been detected in blood samples in Europe, Asia, and Australia.
- Transmission of hepatitis G virus occurs when tainted injectable drugs are used; tainted blood, organs, or tissues are received; or unsafe methods are used for tattooing or body piercing.

Centers for Disease Control and Prevention (CDC), 2021b. Retrieved from: https://www.cdc.gov/hepatitis/index.htm.

Clinical Manifestations

The clinical manifestations for viral hepatitis vary greatly; some patients are asymptomatic, whereas others develop hepatic failure or hepatic encephalopathy.

Assessment

Subjective data include patients' reports of general malaise, aching muscles, photophobia, lassitude, headaches, and chills. Abdominal pain, dyspepsia, nausea, diarrhea, and constipation are reported also. The patient may complain of pruritus from the buildup of bile salts in the skin. The patient complains of tenderness in the liver and remains fatigued for several weeks.

Collection of objective data includes observing hepatomegaly, enlarged lymph nodes, and weight loss. Jaundice appears because of the damaged liver's inability to metabolize bilirubin; the resultant signs are yellowish skin; discoloration of the sclera (scleral icterus) and mucous membranes; dark, tea-colored urine; and clay-colored stools. Relapses are common in the convalescent stage.

Diagnostic Tests

Changes in the liver caused by viral hepatitis result in elevated direct bilirubin, GGT, AST, ALT, LDH, and alkaline phosphatase levels; a prolonged prothrombin time and increased INR; and, in severe hepatitis, decreased serum albumin. Leukopenia (low white blood cell count) is common in these patients, followed by lymphocytosis (high white blood cell count). Hypoglycemia is present in approximately 50% of patients with hepatitis. Serum is examined for the presence of antigens associated with hepatitis A, B, C, D, or G. A CT scan of the abdomen reveals hepatomegaly.

Medical Management

Providing supportive therapy for existing signs and symptoms and preventing transmission of the disease are important aspects of treatment of the patient with viral hepatitis. Hospitalization is an option for patients whose bilirubin concentrations in the blood are more than 10 mg/dL and for those with a prolonged prothrombin time and increased INR, but usually patients are cared for at home. Bed rest for several weeks commonly is prescribed.

Gamma globulin or immune serum globulin is given as soon as possible to people who have been in direct contact with a person with hepatitis A during the infectious period (2 weeks before and 1 week after onset of symptoms). A dose of 0.1 to 0.2 mL/kg of body weight, given intramuscularly, is effective in preventing hepatitis A in 80% to 90% of cases. Vaccines used to prevent hepatitis A include Havrix and Vaqta. Primary immunization consists of a single dose administered intramuscularly in the deltoid muscle. A booster is recommended between 6 and 12 months after the primary dose to ensure adequate antibody titers and long-term protection. However, primary immunization provides immunity within 30 days after a single dose (CDC, 2020a).

Until routine vaccination of children is feasible, people who are at risk for infection should be vaccinated for hepatitis A. This includes people traveling to countries where hepatitis A is endemic; sexually active homosexual and bisexual men; patients with chronic liver disease; injecting drug users; and people at risk for occupational infection, such as those who work with hepatitis A in research laboratory settings.

Drug therapy for chronic hepatitis B focuses on decreasing the viral load, decreasing the rate of disease progression, and monitoring for detection of drug-resistant HBV. Drugs that are considered first line treatment for chronic HBV include pegylated interferon alfa, entecavir, and tenofovir disoproxil fumarate. These are antiviral medications used to stop or reverse the progression of HBV. A serious side effect that is associated with these medications is lactic acidosis that is caused by the buildup of lactic acid in the bloodstream. Common symptoms of lactic acidosis include nausea, abdominal pain, elevated heart rate, muscle ache and weakness, and unintentional weight loss. Liver failure can result from this condition.

In chronic hepatitis C, drug therapy also is directed at reducing the viral load, decreasing progression of the disease, and promoting seroconversion. Treatment options for HCV are interferon alfa-2b, ribavirin, and pegylated interferon alfa-2a. This combination therapy eradicates the virus more effectively than monotherapy. Another treatment option is liver transplantation. In fact, half of all liver recipients are HCV positive. Most transplanted livers eventually become infected with HCV, but recipients can increase quantity and quality of life by avoiding risky behaviors (CDC, 2020b).

The patient is not allowed alcohol for at least 1 year and may need supportive care from the community to comply. Most patients tolerate small, frequent meals of a low-fat, high-carbohydrate diet. If the patient is dehydrated, IV fluids are given with addition of vitamin C for healing, vitamin B complex to assist the damaged liver's inability to absorb fat-soluble vitamins,

and vitamin K to combat prolonged coagulation time. Avoid all unnecessary medications, particularly sedatives.

Individuals who have been exposed to HBV via a needle puncture or sexual contact should be protected with hepatitis B immune globulin. A dose is administered intramuscularly as quickly after exposure as possible. This dose is repeated 1 month later.

The hepatitis B vaccination series can be given at any age, but the CDC (2019) recommends making hepatitis B vaccine a part of routine vaccination schedules for all newborns and adolescents. The protection program consists of three vaccinations: an initial vaccination, a vaccination 1 month later, and a third vaccination 6 months after the first injection. The first injection of the series is given within 12 hours of birth. It is hoped that universal vaccination will lead to eventual prevention and control of hepatitis B. A titer can be drawn to determine immunity in anyone who has received the series. A titer greater than 10 mIU/mL indicates adequate immunity. It is hopeful that the vaccination series will yield lifetime immunity, but studies thus far show immunity for as much as 30 years. Studies will continue to determine if lifetime immunity is achieved.

Hepatitis B, C, D, and G are spread through blood transfusions. The blood used should be screened for elevated ALT and anti–hepatitis B core, and for anti–hepatitis C, anti–hepatitis D, and anti–hepatitis G antigens.

Liver transplantation. Liver transplantation has become a practical therapeutic option for many people with end-stage liver disease, generally improving their quality of life. Indications for liver transplantation include congenital biliary abnormalities, inborn errors of metabolism, hepatic malignancy (confined to the liver), sclerosing cholangitis, and chronic end-stage liver disease. Liver disease related to chronic viral hepatitis is the leading indication for liver transplantation. Liver transplants are not recommended for patients with widespread malignant disease. In 2017 there were approximately 11,500 people waiting for liver transplants. Approximately 8000 transplants are performed annually (Mayo Clinic, 2021).

The major postoperative complications are rejection and infection. Liver transplant candidates must go through a rigorous presurgery screening. However, the liver seems to be less susceptible to rejection than the kidney.

The source of a liver used for transplantation may be a deceased donor or a live donor. The live donor donates only a portion of his or her liver to the recipient. Within weeks the recipient and the donor's liver will grow to the size the body needs. The donor faces potential risks, such as liver and biliary problems, postoperative infection, and other common postoperative complications (see Chapter 2).

The most common complications for the recipient of a liver transplant include rejection of the new liver tissue and infection. The use of cyclosporine, an effective immunosuppressant drug, has been a major factor in improving the success rate of liver transplantation. It does not cause bone marrow suppression and does not impede wound healing. Other immunosuppressants used include azathioprine, corticosteroids, tacrolimus, and mycophenolate mofetil. The interleukin-2 receptor antagonists basiliximab and daclizumab, are being used in combination with other immunosuppressive agents to reduce rejection. Other factors in the improved success rate are advances in surgical techniques, better selection of potential recipients, and improved management of the underlying liver disease before surgery.

Patients who receive liver tissue transplantation from a living donor have better short-term survival rates than those who receive a liver transplant from a deceased donor. It is thought that this could be due to the shorter time period for awaiting a transplant if a living donor is used. Approximately 75% of patients survive more than 5 years after transplantation. (Mayo Clinic, 2021).

NURSING INTERVENTIONS AND PATIENT TEACHING

The patient who has a liver transplant requires competent and highly skilled nursing interventions, in either an ICU or another specialized unit. Postoperative nursing care includes assessing neurologic status; monitoring for signs of hemorrhage; preventing pulmonary complications; monitoring drainage, electrolyte levels, and urinary output; and monitoring for signs and symptoms of infection and rejection. Common respiratory problems include pneumonia, atelectasis (collapsed lung), and pleural effusions. Have the patient use measures such as coughing, deep breathing, incentive spirometry, and repositioning to prevent these complications. Measure and record drainage from the Jackson-Pratt or Hemovac drain, NG tube suctioning, and T tube, and note the color and consistency of drainage. A critical aspect of nursing interventions after liver transplantation is monitoring for infection. The first 2 months after the surgery are critical. Infection can be viral, fungal, or bacterial. Fever may be the only sign of infection. Emotional support and teaching the patient and family are essential.

The care of the patient with viral hepatitis includes ensuring rest, maintaining adequate nutrition, providing adequate fluids, and caring for the skin. The care of the patient with hepatitis continues over time, and support and patient education are necessary throughout the entire illness.

Preventing transmission of the disease is paramount in caring for the patient with viral hepatitis. The patient, family, and health care providers must be knowledgeable about routes of transmission of the virus and take steps to avoid such transmission. Proper personal hygiene and good sanitation, as well

as hepatitis A vaccination, help prevent the spread of hepatitis A. Thoroughly explain to patients the reasons for the precautions, and instruct them in the proper handling of their own secretions and body wastes and in thorough methods of hand hygiene. Wear gown and gloves when handling excreta, giving enemas, taking rectal temperatures, handling food waste, handling needles, disposing of urine, or carrying out any other procedure or hygiene measure that involves direct contact with the patient's body fluids.

Not all patients know they are infected with hepatitis, so following standard precautions with all patients prevents the spread of all bloodborne pathogenic diseases. Health care personnel always should take the utmost care in handling syringes, needles, and other instruments that are contaminated with the patient's serum. Maintaining standard precautions while exposed to blood and body fluids such as saliva, semen, and vaginal secretions is essential to prevent the transmission of hepatitis B. Follow appropriate transmission-based precautions as designated by facility policy. Use enteric precautions for 7 days after the onset of hepatitis A. Use standard precautions for all patients.

Patient problems and interventions for the patient with hepatitis include but are not limited to the following:

PATIENT PROBLEM	NURSING INTERVENTIONS
Potential for Harm or Damage to the Body, related to: • Poor nutrition • Prolonged clotting times	Pad side rails if necessary Assist weakened patient with activities Encourage use of electric razor and soft toothbrush
Insufficient Nutrition, related to: • Anorexia • Nausea • Vomiting • Altered metabolism of nutrients by the liver	Provide diet high in carbohydrates and low in fats, and encourage total fluid intake of 2500–3000 mL daily Monitor I&O Monitor daily weight Note color and consistency of stool and color and amount of urine Administer antiemetics as ordered Offer support and understanding Promote adequate rest

For the patient with viral hepatitis being cared for at home, teach the family necessary precautions. Patients should avoid sexual activity during the acute stage of hepatitis B, C, and D. Sexual precautions should be taken, and needles and razors should not be shared. Patients with hepatitis A must wash their hands thoroughly after toileting, must disinfect feces-soiled articles (boil for 1 minute), and must not prepare foods for others while symptomatic. If possible, the patient should use separate bathroom facilities. Personal care items and drinking glasses should not be shared. The patient's clothes should be laundered separately in hot water. Contaminated items should be disposed of properly. Sexual intercourse should be avoided while in the acute stage of hepatitis A.

Inform the patient and family about signs and symptoms associated with hepatitis, including light-colored stools, dark-colored urine, jaundice, fever, GI disturbances, unusual bleeding that may be indicative of a prolonged prothrombin time and increased INR, and tenderness or pain in the abdomen. The danger of alcohol use and its effect on the liver should be clearly understood.

Prognosis
The prognosis for the patient with hepatitis differs, depending on the causative agent. Recovery from hepatitis A is high, because the virus does not remain in the body after the infection has resolved. Within 3 months after diagnosis most people recover and nearly all recover within 6 months. For this reason, the mortality rate for hepatitis A is very low. The acute stage of the illness typically lasts up to 3 weeks, and it is usually 4 to 6 months before the liver returns to normal function. A small percentage of patients develop chronic hepatitis and cirrhosis as a result of hepatitis B infection. Patients who do develop chronic hepatitis are at a higher risk for liver cancer. Hepatitis B has a higher mortality rate than hepatitis A, but not as high as hepatitis C. Hepatitis C often progresses to chronic hepatitis, and the majority develop chronic infection. Cirrhosis and liver cancer are not uncommon with hepatitis C. The prognosis for patients with chronic hepatitis C infection has increased the demand greatly for liver transplants. The acute phase of hepatitis D typically improves within 2 to 3 weeks, and liver enzymes return to normal within 16 weeks. Almost all patients with hepatitis E recover completely. Hepatitis G infections frequently coexist with other hepatitis infections, such as hepatitis C. However, most hepatitis G infections are not associated with chronic hepatitis; thus the association of hepatitis G virus with liver disease is, at this time, uncertain.

Recovery from acute toxic hepatitis is rapid if the hepatotoxin is identified early and removed or if exposure to the agent has been limited. However, the prognosis is poor if the period between exposure and the onset of signs and symptoms is prolonged, because there are no effective antidotes.

LIVER ABSCESSES
If an infection develops anywhere along the GI tract, there is a chance of the infecting organisms reaching the liver through the biliary system, portal venous system, or hepatic arterial or lymphatic systems, and creating an abscess (a collection of pus). If an abscess is allowed to progress, it can become life threatening, with the mortality rate for undiagnosed liver abscesses being 100% because of the vague clinical symptoms, inadequate diagnostic tools, and inadequate surgical drainage. The current mortality rate for patients diagnosed with a liver abscess who are treated promptly is 5% to 30%.

Etiology and Pathophysiology
If the body does not successfully destroy the bacteria, the bacterial toxins attack neighboring liver cells, and the necrotic tissue produced is a protective wall for the organism. Meanwhile, leukocytes migrate into the infected area. The result is an abscess: a cavity full of a liquid containing living and dead leukocytes and bacteria. Pyogenic (pus-producing) abscesses of this type may be single or multiple. Common sources of liver abscess include abdominal infections such as appendicitis, diverticulitis, and perforated colon. Other causes include any infection in the blood or bile ducts, and trauma to the liver.

Clinical Manifestations
Patients with liver abscess often have vague signs and symptoms. Fever accompanied by chills, abdominal pain, and tenderness in the right upper quadrant of the abdomen are common complaints. Unintentional weight loss, jaundice, anorexia, and malaise are additional symptoms. Some patients experience cough and/or hiccups due to irritation of the diaphragm from the infected liver.

Assessment
Subjective data are related to the infection and to the inability of the liver to function normally. Symptoms include chills, complaints of dull abdominal pain, abdominal tenderness, and discomfort.

Objective data also are related to the infection and impaired function of the liver. Signs of liver abscess include fever, hepatomegaly, jaundice, and anemia. Clay-colored stools and dark urine also are commonly present because of the decreased amount of bile being excreted.

Diagnostic Tests
The diagnosis is established by demonstrating a space-occupying lesion in the liver radiographically (radiograph, ultrasound, CT, and liver scan). CT scans are 95% to 100% accurate in identification of the abscess. Liver biopsy may be performed to determine the presence of an abscess, and a culture may be initiated to determine the infective agent. Common laboratory testing that helps establish the diagnosis includes bilirubin levels, liver enzymes, blood cultures for bacteria, and a complete blood count (CBC).

Medical Management
Usually liver abscesses are managed by medical therapy. Treatment includes IV antibiotic therapy specific to the organism identified. Antibiotic therapy often is continued for 4 to 6 weeks.

Percutaneous (performed through the skin) drainage of a liver abscess is reserved for patients who do not respond to medical therapy or are at high risk for rupture. Open surgical drainage has been the standard in patients whose liver abscesses have ruptured into the peritoneal space, but some of these patients now are managed with percutaneous drainage. All patients require a full course of antibiotic therapy.

Nursing Interventions and Patient Teaching
Continuous monitoring and supportive care are indicated because of the seriousness of the patient's condition. Monitoring objective and subjective symptoms is important. Notify the health care provider if signs and symptoms increase in severity.

The patient's response to drug therapy is determined by a decrease in fever, tenderness and rigidity of the abdomen, chills, and discomfort. If percutaneous or open surgical drainage is instituted, observe the drainage for amount, color, and consistency.

A patient problem and interventions for the patient with a liver abscess include but are not limited to the following:

PATIENT PROBLEM	NURSING INTERVENTIONS
Potential for Inability to Regulate Body Temperature, related to infectious state	Check temperature as ordered by health care provider or as indicated by the patient's worsening condition, and report findings to health care provider Encourage fluids to prevent dehydration. Monitor IV fluids Explain how fever and drainage can deplete fluids in the body Record I&O Monitor oral mucous membranes and skin turgor

In addition to the relationship of infection and nutrition, teach preoperative and postoperative procedures if the patient requires percutaneous or open surgical drainage. A thorough explanation and assessment for the patient's understanding are necessary. The seriously ill patient becomes less anxious as the knowledge base increases and the patient feels more in control of the situation.

Prognosis
The prognosis for patients with liver abscesses was very poor in the past, with an extremely high mortality rate. Sepsis was commonly the cause of death. The prognosis today is much improved because of enhanced diagnostic tests, including CT and liver scans, and aggressive medical and nursing interventions.

CHOLECYSTITIS AND CHOLELITHIASIS
Etiology and Pathophysiology
Disorders of the biliary system are common in the United States and are responsible for the hospitalization of hundreds of thousands of people each year. The two most common conditions are cholecystitis (inflammation of the gallbladder) and cholelithiasis (presence of gallstones in the gallbladder). These two diseases are seen more commonly in women than men; in Native Americans, white Americans, and African Americans; and in obese people, pregnant women, multiparous women (i.e., women who have given birth to two or more babies), women who use birth control pills, and people with diabetes.

Cholecystitis can be caused by an obstruction, a gallstone, a nonfunctioning gallbladder, or a tumor. The exact cause of stone formation in the gallbladder and the common bile duct is not known. However, altered lipid metabolism and female sex hormones play a role in the disease. The stones usually occur in multiples but can occur singly (Fig. 6.5).

When an obstruction is caused by gallstones or a tumor prevents bile from leaving the gallbladder, the trapped bile acts as an irritant, causing inflammatory cells to infiltrate the gallbladder wall after 3 to 4 days. A typical inflammatory response occurs, and the gallbladder becomes enlarged and edematous. The vascular occlusion along with bile stasis causes the mucosal lining of the gallbladder to become necrotic. At first, the bile in the gallbladder is sterile. Within a few days bacteria infiltrate and begin to grow. When the disease is severe enough, the gallbladder may become gangrenous, rupture, and spread infection to the hepatic duct and liver.

Clinical Manifestations
The condition may be acute, with a sudden onset of indigestion; nausea and vomiting; and severe, colicky pain in the right upper quadrant of the abdomen. The pain may be referred to the right shoulder and scapula. Pain resulting from cholecystitis or cholelithiasis sometimes is mistaken for a cardiac problem because of the pain that is felt in the epigastric region and radiating to the back. If the condition is chronic, the patient usually has had several milder attacks of pain and a history of fat intolerance. When gallstones move through the biliary ducts, the patient often complains of pain being intensified.

Assessment
Subjective data include complaints of indigestion after eating foods high in fat. The pain of acute cholecystitis is abrupt in onset, reaches peak intensity quickly, and remains at that level for 2 to 4 hours. It localizes in the right upper quadrant epigastric region. The pain radiates around the mid-torso to the right scapular area. Anorexia, nausea, vomiting, and flatulence (excess formation of gases in the stomach or intestine) also are noted. This pain is caused by the gallbladder contracting in an attempt to secrete bile for fat digestion. Patients may experience increased heart and respiratory rates and become diaphoretic (sweaty), leading them to think they are having a heart attack. These symptoms are decreased or absent in patients with chronic cholecystitis.

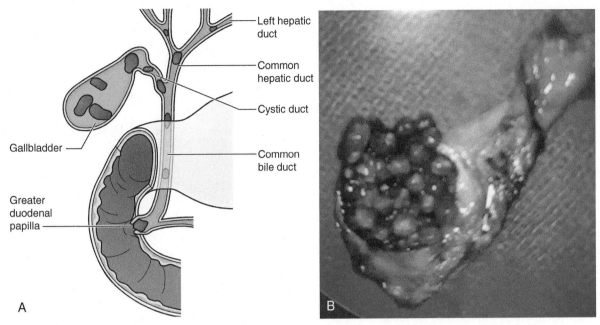

Fig. 6.5 (A) Common sites of gallstones. (B) Gallbladder with stones removed via laparoscopic cholecystectomy

Objective data include a low-grade fever, increased pulse and respirations, nausea, vomiting, an elevated leukocyte count, mild jaundice, stools that contain fat (steatorrhea), and clay-colored stools caused by a lack of bile in the intestinal tract. The urine may be dark amber to tea colored and contain urobilinogen as the kidneys try to remove excess bilirubin from the bloodstream.

Diagnostic Tests

A number of diagnostic studies are performed to confirm a diagnosis of cholecystitis and cholelithiasis. Fecal studies, serum bilirubin tests, ultrasound of the gallbladder and biliary system, a HIDA scan, and an OCG may be done. Ultrasound of the gallbladder is extremely accurate in diagnosing cholelithiasis. HIDA scanning is helpful in assessing the patency of the cystic and common bile ducts as well as the ability of the gallbladder to function efficiently. Operative cholangiography is a procedure in which the common bile duct is injected directly with radiopaque dye. This frequently is done at the time of gallbladder surgery.

Medical Management

If the attack of cholelithiasis is mild, the patient is treated conservatively. Bed rest is prescribed, an NG tube is inserted and connected to low suction, and the patient is placed on NPO status. This allows the GI tract, including the gallbladder, to rest. IV fluids are given to rehydrate the patient and to replace drainage from the NG tube.

Antispasmodic and analgesic drugs may be given to decrease pain. Meperidine and ketorolac are used commonly for pain management. An antispasmodic such as dicyclomine may be used to decrease the incidence of spasms of the sphincter of Oddi (which controls the flow of pancreatic juices and bile into the duodenum). Morphine generally is not used for pain management because it often increases the tone of the sphincter of Oddi. Antibiotics may be given (1) prophylactically to prevent infection; (2) to treat an existing infection; and (3) after perforation, should it occur. A diet that is low in fat and cholesterol may be prescribed (see the Complementary and Alternative Therapies box).

Complementary and Alternative Therapies

GALLBLADDER, BILIARY, AND PANCREATIC DISORDERS
- Fresh black root is used as an emetic. The dried root has a gentler action and is used to treat constipation and liver and gallbladder disease and to increase bile flow. Caution patients with gallstones or bile duct obstruction to avoid using it because it may worsen these diseases.
- Blessed thistle is used orally to treat digestive problems such as liver and gallbladder diseases.
- Dandelion traditionally is used as a bile stimulator to treat gallbladder ailments.
- Onion is used as a gallbladder stimulant. It increases the risk of hypoglycemia, so monitor patients with diabetes closely.
- Autumn crocus (active ingredient: colchicine) has been used to treat hepatic cirrhosis and primary biliary cirrhosis. Because of the plant's toxicity, internal use is not recommended.
- Papaya (pawpaw) is used to treat gastrointestinal tract disorders such as pancreatic insufficiency.
- Royal jelly (bee pollen complex) is used in treating liver disease and pancreatitis. Do not confuse royal jelly with bee pollen and honeybee venom. (Royal jelly should be used with extreme caution by patients with asthma, because allergic reactions to royal jelly have led to asthma attacks, anaphylaxis, and death.)

Lithotripsy. Extracorporeal shock wave lithotripsy is used to treat a patient who has mild or moderate symptoms caused by a few stones. The machine discharges a series of shock waves through water or a cushion that breaks the stones into fragments. The natural flow of bile carries the stone fragments out of the gallbladder and into the intestine for eventual excretion. Nursing intervention after the procedure is similar to that for patients undergoing liver biopsy.

Surgical intervention. The treatment of choice is cholecystectomy (removal of the gallbladder) with ligation of the cystic duct, vein, and artery. A laparoscopic cholecystectomy and open abdominal cholecystectomy are the two surgical procedures (Fig. 6.6 for stone retrieval). A Jackson-Pratt or Hemovac drain (which promotes drainage and prevents pressure and fluid accumulation under the diaphragm) may be inserted if an open cholecystectomy is performed. If the stones are in the common bile duct and edema is present, a biliary drainage tube, or T tube, is inserted to keep the duct open and allow drainage of the bile until the edema resolves. The short end of the tube is placed in the common bile duct, and the longer end is brought to the surface through a stab wound (Fig. 6.7). The long end is attached to a closed drainage system (bile bag) that is placed below the level of the common bile duct.

The T tube also provides a route for postoperative cholangiography if desired (T-tube cholangiogram) to assess the patency of the common bile duct. The T tube is removed 24 hours after the cholangiogram if the edema is resolved and the common bile duct appears normal. The T tube is removed by cutting the anchoring stitches and pulling the tube out. The small opening is covered with an adhesive bandage or gauze dressing and heals on its own within a few days. The 24-hour period allows the dye to drain out of the common bile duct. If the edema does not resolve in this time, the patient may be discharged with the T tube in place.

The most common treatment for cholecystitis and cholelithiasis is with an endoscopic technique called *laparoscopic cholecystectomy,* in which a laser or cautery is used to remove the gallbladder. This procedure replaces the open surgical procedure 90% of the time. It involves removing the gallbladder through one of four small punctures in the abdomen (a comparatively minor procedure). During surgery, the abdominal cavity is inflated with 3 to 4 L of carbon dioxide to improve visibility. A laparoscope, which has a camera attached, is inserted into the abdomen. The surgeon removes the deflated gallbladder through the laparoscope. If the organ contains so much bile or gallstones that it cannot be collapsed, its contents will be aspirated first. Laparoscopic cholecystectomy offers several advantages over the common open abdominal cholecystectomy, including the following:

- It is less invasive (and thus there is less chance of wound infection or respiratory impairment) and

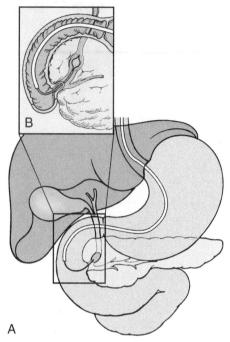

A

Fig. 6.6 (A) During endoscopic sphincterotomy, a flexible endoscope is advanced through the mouth and the stomach until its tip sits in the duodenum opposite the common bile duct. (B) After widening the duct mouth by incising the sphincter muscle, the health care provider advances a basket attachment into the duct and retrieves the stone. (From Lewis SL, Dirksen SR, Heitkemper MM, et al: *Medical-surgical nursing: Assessment and management of clinical problems,* ed 10, St. Louis, 2017, Elsevier.)

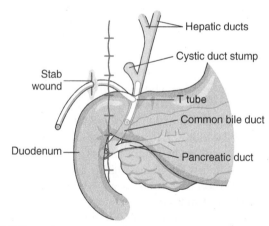

Fig. 6.7 T tube in common bile duct. (From Beare PG, Myers JL: *Adult health nursing,* ed 3, St. Louis, 1998, Mosby.)

has a shorter healing time and a shorter recuperative time.
- There is no unsightly scar.
- There is less pain and thus more rapid return to normal activities.

When a medical history, physical examination, and blood studies are complete, an ultrasound is done to locate gallstones and detect any dilation of the hepatic bile ducts. If *choledocholithiasis* (stones in the common bile duct) is confirmed, a sphincterotomy and stone extraction (see Fig. 6.6) are performed before laparoscopic surgery.

It is important to obtain informed consent for endoscopic and open cholecystectomy in case converting from one procedure to the other is necessary. The conversion may be necessary if an extensive adhesion, gallstones within the common bile duct, unusual vascular or ductal anatomy, unsuspected pathologic condition of the abdomen, or excessive bleeding complicates the endoscopic procedure.

Postoperative care for laparoscopic cholecystectomy. A small number of patients report minor discomfort at the laparoscopic insertion site or mild shoulder or neck pain resulting from diaphragmatic irritation secondary to abdominal stretching or residual carbon dioxide. Oral analgesics or anti-inflammatory agents relieve these symptoms.

Oral liquids and a light meal are given the first night after surgery. The patient has bandages at the puncture sites on the abdomen. Assess vital signs routinely. The patient is usually ambulatory immediately after surgery.

Most patients are discharged the same day as surgery. Patients are usually able to resume moderate activity within 48 to 72 hours. Depending on their occupation, most patients are released to return to work and normal activity 2 weeks postoperatively.

Patient teaching. Before discharge, patients should be able to eat without difficulty and walk and should have no abdominal distention, evidence of bleeding, or bile leakage. Instruct them to immediately report to the health care provider any severe pain, tenderness in the right upper quadrant, increase in abdominal girth, leakage of bile-colored drainage from the puncture site, increase in pulse, or symptoms of low blood pressure.

Nursing Interventions and Patient Teaching

Nursing interventions begin with careful assessment of the characteristics of pain (if it is present) and any signs of jaundice of the skin, sclera, and mucous membranes. Observe the patient's urine and stool for alterations in the presence of bilirubin.

When the patient is treated conservatively, nursing interventions center on keeping the patient comfortable by carefully administering the medications prescribed and monitoring the patient's response to the medications. The patient is kept on NPO status or on clear liquids. Administer antiemetics if nausea is present. Observe IV infusions for patency, correct rates, and entry sites that are free from erythema and edema. Measure I&O and describe carefully.

Preoperative care includes teaching the patient to turn, cough, and deep breathe and to use an incentive spirometer to facilitate air movement in and out of the lungs to prevent pneumonia and atelectasis. To enable the patient to follow postoperative instructions more easily, teach him or her how to splint the abdomen with the hands, small pillow, or rolled bath blanket before attempting a cough; practice repositioning in the hospital bed; and assume a sitting position from a standing or lying position. If an open cholecystectomy is anticipated, explaining the IV tubing and urinary catheter and their functions helps relieve patient anxiety. The patient should be familiar with any medications that may be used to relieve pain and nausea and should understand that vitamin K and antibiotics may be given preoperatively to prevent hemorrhage and infection.

Postoperative care for open cholecystectomy includes monitoring vital signs and observing dressings frequently and carefully for exudate or hemorrhage. The dressings usually require reinforcement at the drain site. Place the patient in a semi-Fowler's position to facilitate drainage. Monitor the Jackson-Pratt or Hemovac drain for patency. Notify the surgeon if the drainage is excessive, contains bile, or is bright red.

The patient needs encouragement to perform deep breathing and coughing and to use an incentive spirometer, because of the location of the incision. Provide analgesics frequently in the early postoperative period to facilitate movement and deep breathing. Help the patient to dangle (i.e., sit up with the legs hanging over the side of the bed) the night of surgery and ambulate the first postoperative day. Monitor the patient's neurologic status by checking ability to be aroused easily, orientation to the environment and family, and ability to move extremities equally on command.

Maintain fluid balance with IV therapy; potassium usually is added to compensate for loss from surgery. Check the health care provider's order before giving ice or clear liquids to the patient, and allow the patient to rinse the mouth frequently.

The nurse is responsible for the care of the T tube if one is placed. The drainage bag for the T tube is placed below the level of the common bile duct to prevent the reflux of bile. Position the bag so that the tube is not kinked and bile can drain from the liver. Frequently check the position of the bag and tube and the color and amount of exudate during the first 24 hours and record the results. Place a gauze roll under the tube, anchoring it to the patient's abdomen and preventing tension and pull on the tube from the weight of the bag. The T tube drains as much as 500 mL during the first 24 hours. The amount should decrease as the edema resolves and bile begins flowing through the common bile duct. Be careful not to dislodge the T tube when changing the patient's dressings, as prescribed by the health care provider.

After oral intake is resumed, the health care provider may order the T tube clamped for 1 to 2 hours before meals and unclamped 1 to 2 hours after the patient eats, to aid in the digestion of fat. While the T tube is clamped, the patient may show signs of distress, including abdominal pain, nausea, vomiting, light brown urine, and clay-colored stools. If distress occurs, unclamp the tube immediately. Increase the time that the T tube remains clamped as the patient tolerates the procedure. The tube may be left in place for as long as 10 days. The health care provider removes the tube when the common bile duct is patent for drainage of bile.

Check bowel sounds every 8 hours for the return of peristalsis by auscultating the abdomen. Ask the patient if he or she is passing flatus. A clear liquid diet usually is ordered immediately or within the first 24 hours postoperatively and increased as tolerated. When the patient begins eating solid food, usually low-fat foods are best. Flatulence or nausea after eating certain foods may persist after surgery; instruct the patient to experiment with different foods.

The patient who undergoes a cholecystectomy must be observed for complications. These include jaundice (from an occluded common duct) and hemorrhage (indicated by decreased blood pressure, increased pulse, and increased exudate at the dressing site). An elevated temperature could indicate peritonitis or wound infection. Pancreatitis may occur after cholecystectomy.

Patients at high risk of not surviving a cholecystectomy may need a cholecystostomy (forming an opening into the gallbladder through the abdominal wall). This can be done using a local anesthetic. The opening provides a means of removing purulent exudate and possibly the stone. It also allows drainage of bile.

Patient problems and interventions for the patient with open cholecystectomy or cholecystostomy include but are not limited to the following:

PATIENT PROBLEM	NURSING INTERVENTIONS
Potential for Compromised Skin Integrity, related to: • Wound drainage • Accidental obstruction of bile drainage	Maintain patency and prevent tension on T tube; promote drainage of T tube by placing patient in low Fowler's to semi-Fowler's position Observe, describe, and record amount and character of drainage from T tube at least q 8 hr Empty bile bag when half full Clamp T tube as ordered by health care provider 3 to 4 days postoperatively Reinforce primary dressing and observe exudates; change and apply sterile, dry dressing as ordered; use Montgomery straps to secure if drainage is profuse Cleanse skin thoroughly at insertion site before applying sterile dressing Apply skin barriers as needed for added protection

Dietary teaching is necessary for the patient who is treated conservatively for cholecystitis, as well as for the patient who undergoes surgery. The patient who is treated conservatively must continue to avoid fatty foods, including fried foods, cream, whole milk, butter, margarine, peanut butter, nuts, chocolate, pastries, and gravies. For the postsurgical patient, provide instructions to try small amounts of foods that previously caused discomfort and gradually eliminate those that continue to do so. The patient usually can resume a normal diet without difficulty.

The patient should understand that stones may recur elsewhere in the biliary system. Teach the patient to identify the signs of complications that should be reported. These include jaundice caused by occlusion or stricture of a duct, hemorrhage or leakage of bile, elevated temperature, pain, and dietary intolerance associated with another attack. The patient also should be able to demonstrate care of the T tube, if present on discharge; identify activity restrictions; and identify a date for a return visit to the health care provider.

Prognosis

To prevent complications from cholecystitis or cholelithiasis, assess the patient for signs and symptoms of infection within the gallbladder, which can lead to death of the gallbladder from gangrene infection if the initial infection is not treated or does not respond to therapy. Other complications include abscess formation, and rupture of the gallbladder (which can lead to peritonitis). Stones may also lodge in various biliary ducts, including the common bile duct, leading to pancreatitis or obstructive jaundice.

With prompt treatment of cholecystitis and cholelithiasis, the prognosis is excellent. Laparoscopic surgery also has decreased the number of complications. The prognosis is not as favorable in patients who develop pancreatitis (see the Lifespan Considerations box).

 Lifespan Considerations

Older Adults

Gallbladder, Liver, Biliary Tract, or Exocrine Pancreatic Disorder

- The incidence of cholelithiasis increases with aging. Closely observe older adults with histories of this disease for changes in the color of urine and stool or other signs and symptoms of gallbladder problems.
- As the body ages, the number and size of hepatic cells decrease, which results in an overall reduced size and weight of the liver. The liver also has decreased ability to regenerate after injury or from hepatotoxic injury. Detoxification of substances is delayed.
- Older adults have a decrease in protein synthesis in the liver and possible changes in the production of enzymes that assist in the metabolism of drugs, particularly anticonvulsants, psychotropics, and oral anticoagulants.
- Be alert to the signs and symptoms of drug toxicity, even when the drugs are administered in normal doses, because the decreased metabolism in the liver can cause an accumulation of the drugs.
- The pancreas exhibits ductal hyperplasia and fibrosis with aging, but these changes are not necessarily associated with altered functioning. The output of pancreatic secretions steadily declines after age 40, but related problems with absorption cannot be documented.

PANCREATITIS

Etiology and Pathophysiology

Pancreatitis is an inflammatory condition of the pancreas that may be acute or chronic. The degree of inflammation varies from mild edema to severe hemorrhagic necrosis. Although the exact cause of pancreatitis remains unknown, many predisposing factors have been identified. Acute or chronic pancreatitis is generally the result of damage to the biliary tract (most common in women), alcohol consumption (most common in men), trauma, infectious disease, or certain drugs. Alcoholism and biliary tract disease are the two factors most commonly associated with pancreatitis. Pancreatitis can develop as a postoperative complication in patients who have had surgery of the pancreas, stomach, duodenum, or biliary tract. Pancreatitis also can occur after undergoing ERCP (see Fig. 6.1).

In the pathophysiologic process of pancreatitis, the enzymes cannot flow out of the pancreas because of occlusion (an obstruction or closing off) of the pancreatic duct (duct of Wirsung) by edema, stones, or scar tissue. The pancreatic enzymes build up and increase pressure within the duct. The duct ruptures, releasing enzymes that begin digesting the pancreas (autodigestion). In chronic pancreatitis, the enzyme-producing acinar tissue atrophies and is replaced with fibrotic tissue, resulting in the pancreas becoming necrotic.

The development of pseudocysts or abscesses in pancreatic tissue is a serious complication. After autodigestion occurs, the pancreas and occasionally the surrounding organs form walls around cystic fluid, including pancreatic enzymes, and necrotic debris. These pseudocysts can develop into an abscess.

Clinical Manifestations

Manifestations include severe abdominal pain radiating to the back. The pain usually is located in the left upper quadrant. The pain is sometimes relieved by leaning forward, taking the stomach weight off the pancreas. Jaundice may be noted if the common bile duct is obstructed.

Assessment

Pain is the most common subjective data associated with pancreatitis. Pain may be gradual or have a sudden onset and is often severe. The pain is caused by the enlargement of the pancreatic capsule, an obstruction, or chemical irritation from enzymes. The pain usually is decreased by flexing the trunk, leaning forward from a sitting position, or by assuming the fetal position. It is increased by eating or lying down. Other complaints include nausea and vomiting, anorexia, malaise, and restlessness. The patient often displays a fever, increased white blood cell count, fat in the stools (steatorrhea), and weight loss.

Diagnostic Tests

Acute and chronic pancreatitis are diagnosed by radiologic studies (abdominal CT scan and ultrasound of the pancreas), endoscopy, and laboratory analysis of the pancreatic enzymes in the serum and urine. Laboratory tests reveal an increased level of serum amylase and lipase during the first few days and increased urine amylase thereafter. Amylase and lipase levels that are three times above normal are considered most definitive for pancreatitis. The amylase level is not a specific indicator for pancreatitis; abnormal levels also can be seen in cases of perforated peptic ulcer, perforated bowel, and diabetic ketoacidosis. Elevation of the pancreatic amylase level is a better indicator of pancreatitis. The level of lipase is more specific for diagnosing acute pancreatitis. The lipase level typically remains elevated for 12 days with pancreatitis. In chronic pancreatitis the serum lipase levels often remain elevated, and the serum amylase remains normal. Leukocytosis, an elevated hematocrit level, hypocalcemia, hypoalbuminemia, and hyperglycemia also may be present. Pancreatic insulin production may be diminished if the islets of Langerhans become infected, and some patients develop diabetes mellitus.

Medical Management

Treatment is medical unless the precipitating cause is biliary tract disease; then surgery may be indicated. Food and fluids are withheld to avoid stimulating pancreatic activity, and IV fluids are administered. The patient is on NPO status, and an NG tube is inserted to decrease pancreatic stimulation, to treat or prevent nausea and vomiting, and to decrease abdominal distention. Analgesics prescribed by the health care provider should be administered as needed to control the pain associated with pancreatitis. Analgesics may be combined with an antispasmodic to achieve optimum pain control.

Parenteral anticholinergic medication, such as atropine or propantheline, helps decrease pancreatic activity. This medication is contraindicated in paralytic ileus. Antacids or antihistamine H_2 receptor antagonists, such as cimetidine, may be given to prevent stress ulcers caused by decreased gastric pH. Some health care providers prescribe antibiotics to treat secondary infections.

Enteral feeding (i.e., tube feeding) is begun 24 to 48 hours after the onset of acute pancreatitis and is administered via the jejunum to prevent the release of pancreatic enzymes. Enteral feeding is preferred to the IV route because it is more nutritionally sound, is less costly, and has fewer complications. However, if enteral feeding is not tolerated in 5 to 7 days, the patient may need to be switched to total parenteral nutrition (TPN, intravenous feeding).

A clear liquid diet with gradual progression may be started once the patient's pain is under control for at least 24 hours. The diet should be low in fat and protein. The diet also should be free of caffeinated beverages because caffeine acts as a gastric stimulant. If the patient experiences increased pain from oral nutrition, hold all food and fluids and contact the health care provider. Oral hypoglycemic agents or insulin may be needed if there is destruction of the islets of Langerhans.

Nursing Interventions and Patient Teaching

Determine the presence and location of pain, as well as what aggravates or relieves the pain. Keep the patient as comfortable as possible through proper administration of analgesic and antispasmodic medications. The patient is usually on bed rest with bathroom privileges to decrease the flow of pancreatic enzymes. Nutritional needs are met by enteral feeding via the jejunum as long as necessary. If enteral feedings fail, the patient may need parenteral feedings. The patient who is addicted to alcohol may go through withdrawal while in the hospital. Be prepared to protect the patient from injury and provide supportive care to the patient and the family. Carefully monitor all replacement fluids and medications for proper administration.

Patient problems and interventions for the patient with pancreatitis include but are not limited to the following:

PATIENT PROBLEM	NURSING INTERVENTIONS
Recent Onset of Pain, related to stimulation of nerve endings caused by enlargement of pancreatic capsule, obstruction, or chemical irritation from enzymes	Administer medications as prescribed and monitor the response Restrict diet as necessary to prevent aggravation of pain (eliminate fats, alcohol, caffeine) Use alternative comfort measures: Repositioning, positive imagery, and time for listening Monitor NG tube hookup to wall suction for functioning to prevent abdominal distention
Insufficient Nutrition, related to: • Anorexia • Nausea • Vomiting • Loss of enzymes necessary for the digestive process	Administer enteral feeding via jejunum as ordered Weigh patient daily at same time and using same scale Record I&O, including NG tube suctioning output Administer antacids and antiemetics as prescribed Instruct patient to follow a diet that is low in fat and high in protein and carbohydrates when tolerated

The patient remains on a low-fat, high-calorie, high-carbohydrate diet after discharge. Alcohol and beverages or foods containing caffeine are not allowed if full recovery is desired. Ensure that the patient understands the disease process and the severity of the disease and related complications.

Prognosis

The prognosis of pancreatitis depends on the course of the disease and complications, including pseudocysts and abscesses. In most patients, acute pancreatitis is mild, requiring less than 1 week of hospitalization. However, 5% to 25% of patients have a more complicated course with recovery time taking weeks to months. The severity of the disease varies according to the extent of pancreatic destruction. Some patients recover completely; others have recurring attacks. The overall mortality rate for acute pancreatitis is 10% to 15%. The mortality rate for patients with severe disease resulting in organ failure is approximately 30%. Complications can occur with mild, acute, chronic, or severe pancreatitis. Mortality rates for acute necrotizing pancreatitis are 20% and higher, depending on other organs that become involved (Mathew, 2021).

CANCER OF THE PANCREAS

Although once considered relatively rare, pancreatic cancer is now the fourth leading cause of cancer death in the United States and Canada. According to the American Cancer Society, it is estimated that more than 57,600 Americans will be diagnosed with pancreatic cancer during 2020 and that more than 47,050Americans will die of the disease (ACS, n.d.). A major factor in the high death rate from pancreatic cancer is the difficulty in diagnosing it at an early, curable stage. The disease usually occurs after middle age. The risk increases with age, with peak incidence occurring between 65 and 80 years of age.

Etiology and Pathophysiology

The most common environmental risk factor for pancreatic cancer is cigarette smoking. Smoking is seen in 25% of patients diagnosed with the disease. Other risk factors include exposure to chemical carcinogens, diabetes mellitus, cirrhosis, and chronic pancreatitis. Diets high in red meat and pork (especially processed meat such as bacon), fat, and coffee also are linked to pancreatic cancer. Obesity, genetics, and being an African American male increase the risk of developing pancreatic cancer.

The cancer may originate in the pancreas or be the result of metastasis from cancer of the lung, the stomach, the duodenum, or the common bile duct. Most often the head of the pancreas is involved and causes jaundice by compressing and obstructing the common bile duct. As the cancer spreads, it may invade the posterior wall of the stomach, the duodenal wall, the colon, and the common bile duct. Biliary obstruction and gallbladder dilation are subsequent complications. It is not uncommon for the tumor to grow rapidly and invade the vascular and lymphatic systems. Many patients live only 4 to 6 months after diagnosis because of the common late diagnosis.

Clinical Manifestations

The insidious onset of the disease with initially vague symptoms generally accounts for delays in diagnosis. Complaints of anorexia, malaise, nausea, and fatigue are common. Abdominal pain in the mid-epigastric region or back occurs in many of the patients. About half the patients develop diabetes mellitus if islet cells are involved.

Assessment

A psychosocial history taken during patient assessment may reveal that the patient belongs to one of the at-risk populations such cigarette smokers, coal- and gas-plant employees, chemists, and workers exposed to beta-naphthol and benzidine. Subjective data include anorexia; fatigue; nausea; flatulence; a change in stools; and steady, dull, and aching pain in the epigastrium or referred to the back. The pain is usually worse at night.

Objective data include weight loss, often gradual and progressive, which is one of the earliest signs. Jaundice usually is progressive and may occur late. Pruritus accompanies the jaundice. Many patients have recent onset of diabetes mellitus.

Diagnostic Tests

Diagnosis of pancreatic cancer is based on the patient's history, signs and symptoms, and diagnostic studies. Diagnostic studies include transabdominal ultrasound and CT, endoscopic ultrasound (EUS) with fine needle biopsy to obtain specimens for cytologic examination, ERCP, and pancreatic scans. ERCP allows for visualization of the pancreatic duct and biliary system. With ERCP, pancreatic secretions and tissues can be collected for analysis of various tumor markers (see Fig. 6.1).

The level of one tumor marker, cancer-associated antigen CA 19-9, is elevated in patients with pancreatic cancer. It is the most commonly used tumor marker to diagnose pancreatic adenocarcinoma and to monitor the patient's response to treatment. However, CA 19-9 can be elevated in other diseases such as cancer of the gallbladder and acute pancreatitis. Also, it is less sensitive in the early stages of the disease. CA 19-9 has proven to be more helpful for staging purposes and monitoring the patient posttreatment.

Medical Management

Often malignant tumors of the pancreas are inoperable by the time they are diagnosed. Treatment of pancreatic cancer is primarily surgical and has been associated with a high mortality rate. Cancer of the head of the pancreas usually is treated by pancreatoduodenectomy; the Whipple procedure involves resection of the

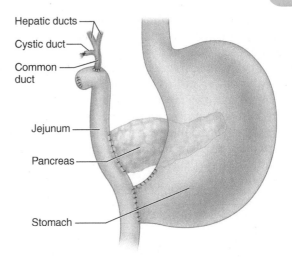

Fig. 6.8 The Whipple procedure, or radical pancreaticoduodenectomy. This surgical procedure involves resection of the proximal pancreas, adjoining duodenum, distal portion of the stomach, and distal portion of the common bile duct. The pancreatic duct, common bile ducts, and stomach are anastomosed to the jejunum.

antrum of the stomach, the gallbladder, the duodenum, and varying amounts of the pancreas. Anastomoses are constructed between the stomach, the common bile duct and the pancreatic ducts, and the jejunum (Fig. 6.8). In most cases, this procedure is performed by surgeons who are specially trained and experienced.

Another procedure is total pancreatectomy with resection of parts of the GI tract. Subtotal pancreatic resection has complications of postoperative pancreatic fistulas and is not recommended.

Combinations of drugs such as fluorouracil and gemcitabine (Gemzar) may produce a better response than a single chemotherapeutic agent. Gemcitabine is a main treatment for pancreatic cancer that has metastasized. The current role of chemotherapy in pancreatic cancer is limited. Adjuvant therapy—using surgical resection, radiation, and chemotherapy—is believed by some to be the most effective way to manage the almost always fatal cancer of the pancreas.

Nursing Interventions and Patient Teaching

Pancreatic surgery is radical and requires critical care nursing. Postoperative care focuses on maintaining fluid and electrolyte balance, preventing hemorrhage, preventing respiratory complications, and monitoring endocrine and exocrine functions of the pancreas.

Palliative care is crucial for the patient who is not a candidate or elects not to have treatment or surgery for pancreatic cancer. The patient may receive long-acting narcotic analgesics for chronic pain, supplemented by quick-acting opioids for breakthrough pain. Tricyclic antidepressants as well as antiemetics often are administered with the narcotic analgesic to potentiate (enhance) their effects. Nerve blocks or lysis of nerves of the celiac ganglia can be performed if pain control cannot be achieved with medications. Radiation therapy also is used to treat the pain associated with pancreatic cancer.

The health care provider caring for the patient with pancreatic cancer must offer compassionate physical and emotional assistance. Refer the patient and the family to social services and support groups. Hospice care is very beneficial to the family and patient.

A patient problem and interventions for patients with cancer of the pancreas include but are not limited to the following:

PATIENT PROBLEM	NURSING INTERVENTIONS
Potential for Compromised Skin Integrity, related to drainage from wound	Monitor for excoriation and infection; use skin barriers and disposable postoperative pouches and appliances to prevent enzymatic contact with the skin and to aid in the accurate collection and measurement of pancreatic drainage

The patient is facing a life-threatening illness, and family members and close friends are important for the patient's well-being. If the patient has an inadequate support system, it is important to use the resources that are available. Health care personnel, support groups, and hospice care are essential resources for supportive care.

Prognosis

The prognosis for patients with cancer of the pancreas is very poor because of the often late diagnosis. Median survival after diagnosis is only 5 to 12 months. The 5-year survival rate for localized pancreatic cancer is 37%. Regional metastasis results in a 12% 5-year survival rate, and distant metastasis results in a 5-year survival rate of 3%. Prognosis is related to the tumor's location and the stage at which the disease is diagnosed (ACS, 2021b).

❖ NURSING PROCESS FOR THE PATIENT WITH A GALLBLADDER, LIVER, BILIARY TRACT, OR EXOCRINE PANCREATIC DISORDER

◆ ASSESSMENT

Nursing assessment of the patient with a gallbladder, liver, biliary tract, or exocrine pancreatic disorder must be performed accurately. Perform a head-to-toe assessment. Also assess the patient's knowledge of the disease process, nutritional status, pain, discomfort, current health problems, and signs and symptoms. Note changes in appetite and weight. Measure vital signs, noting any alterations from normal, such as hyperthermia, hypotension, hypertension, tachycardia, or tachypnea. Observe the skin, the sclerae, the mucous membranes, the urine, and the stool for alterations in the presence of bilirubin. Inspect, auscultate, and palpate the abdomen. Document any abdominal tenderness, pain, or abnormal bowel sounds.

◆ PATIENT PROBLEMS

Assessment provides data for identifying the patient's problems, strengths, potential complications, and learning needs. Patient problems for patients with disorders of the liver, biliary tract, or exocrine pancreas include but are not limited to the following:
- Compromised Maintenance of Health
- Compromised Skin Integrity
- Helplessness
- Inability to Maintain Adequate Breathing Pattern
- Inability to Tolerate Activity
- Inadequate Fluid Volume
- Insufficient Knowledge
- Insufficient Nutrition
- Noncooperation or Nonconformity
- Potential for Harm or Damage to the Body
- Prolonged Pain
- Recent Onset of Confusion
- Recent Onset of Pain

◆ EXPECTED OUTCOMES AND PLANNING

When planning care, look at the identified patient problem(s) and establish interventions. The overall goals for patients with disorders of the gallbladder, liver, biliary tract, and exocrine pancreas include (1) relief of pain and discomfort; (2) stabilization of fluid and electrolyte balance; (3) minimal to no complications; (4) ability to resume normal activities; (5) a return, if possible, to normal pancreatic and liver function without complications; and (6) a return to as normal a lifestyle as possible.

Planning includes the development of realistic goals and outcomes from the identified patient problems. Establish short- and long-term measurable goals. Examples of measurable goals are the following:
- Patient will feel rested enough to assist in ADLs.
- Patient will have increased activity tolerance by walking 100 ft.
- Patient will report that pain is less than a 4 on a scale of 0 to 10.

◆ IMPLEMENTATION

Maintaining the patient's optimal level of health is important in reducing biliary and pancreatic symptoms. Nursing interventions may include nutritional management, pharmacologic management, and health promotion and maintenance to prevent complications. Encourage the early diagnosis and treatment of liver, biliary tract, and pancreatic disease. Nursing interventions involve supportive care with special attention to nutrition, hydration, skin care, and pain relief.

◆ **EVALUATION**

During and after the planned nursing interventions, determine the outcomes of the interventions. This is an ongoing process of continually trying to establish the most effective care plan.

Evaluation involves determining whether the established goals have been met. Involve the patient in evaluating the goals to see whether the criteria for measurement have been met. Goals and evaluative measures for disorders of the liver, biliary tract, and exocrine pancreas may include the following:

Goal 1: Patient voices and demonstrates improved activity tolerance.

Evaluative measure: Observe patient exercise.

Goal 2: Patient remains free of bodily injury.

Evaluative measure: Ask patient to list factors that increase the risk of injury.

GET Ready for the NCLEX® Examination!

Key Points

- Planned nursing interventions must be individualized according to each patient's and family's unique needs.
- The most common cause of cirrhosis of the liver is alcohol ingestion.
- Clinical manifestations of cirrhosis of the liver differ, depending on whether the patient is in the early or later stages of the disease.
- An important aspect of nursing interventions in patients with hepatitis and cirrhosis of the liver is the relief of pruritus.
- Prevention of the spread of viral hepatitis is a primary concern of health care professionals.
- Vaccines are available to prevent the development of hepatitis A and hepatitis B.
- If an infection develops anywhere along the GI tract, there is danger that the infecting organism may reach the liver through the biliary system, portal venous system, or hepatic arterial or lymphatic system and result in a liver abscess.
- Cholecystectomy (removal of the gallbladder by means of a laparoscopic or open abdominal procedure) is one of the most commonly performed surgical procedures.
- Pancreatic disorders may cause diabetes mellitus because of interference with insulin production.
- Clinical manifestations of acute pancreatitis include severe abdominal pain radiating to the back; the pain is sometimes relieved when the patient leans forward, taking the weight of the stomach off the pancreas.
- Tumor markers are used to establish the diagnosis of pancreatic adenocarcinoma and to monitor the response to treatment of cancer; CA 19-9 is elevated in pancreatic cancer and is the most commonly used tumor marker.

Additional Learning Resources

SG Go to your Study Guide for additional learning activities to help you master this chapter content.

Be sure to visit the Evolve site at http://evolve.elsevier.com/Cooper/adult/ for additional online resources.

Review Questions for the NCLEX® Examination

1. A patient is admitted with common bile duct obstruction related to cancer of the pancreas. Which clinical manifestations would the nurse expect to find? *(Select all that apply.)*

   1. Brown feces
   2. Scleral icterus
   3. Dark, tea-colored urine
   4. Jaundice
   5. Mid-epigastric pain
   6. Left upper quadrant abdominal pain
   7. Anorexia
   8. Weight loss
   9. Headache
   10. Loss of taste

2. The nurse is caring for a postoperative open cholecystectomy patient. The nurse includes coughing and deep breathing in the patient's care plan based on what criteria?

   1. The patient is obese.
   2. The patient smokes.
   3. The patient is on bed rest for a prolonged period.
   4. The patient tends to take shallow breaths due to the location of the incision.

3. The nurse is caring for a patient with hepatic encephalopathy. While assessing the patient, the nurse notes rapid, irregular flexion and extension (flapping) of the wrist when the nurse requests that the patient stretch out the arm and hyperextend the wrist with fingers separated. How should the nurse document this finding?

   1. "Patient demonstrates the presence of varices."
   2. "Patient demonstrates the presence of asterixis."
   3. "Patient demonstrates the presence of pruritus."
   4. "Patient demonstrates the presence of bacterial toxins."

4. A patient has advanced cirrhosis of the liver with an acute exacerbation of hepatic encephalopathy. What type of food may be limited for a short time in his diet?

   1. Fruits
   2. Vegetables
   3. Meats
   4. Carbohydrates

5. The nurse is assessing a newly admitted patient. Which findings are most indicative of a liver abscess?

   1. Asterixis, ascites, and esophageal varices
   2. Fever accompanied by chills, abdominal pain, and tenderness in the right upper quadrant
   3. Enlarged spleen and spider telangiectases
   4. Constipation; left quadrant abdominal cramping; and loud, high-pitched abdominal sounds on auscultation

6. While discharging a patient after a laparoscopic cholecystectomy, the nurse hears the patient report mild shoulder pain. The nurse is aware that the pain is likely caused by which factor?

1. Paralytic ileus with mesenteric irritation
2. Incision along the rectus abdominis muscle
3. Diaphragmatic irritation secondary to residual carbon dioxide
4. Spasm of the duct of Wirsung

7. A patient has been admitted with right upper quadrant pain and has been placed on a low-fat diet. Which tray would be acceptable for the patient?

1. Whole milk, veal, rice, and pastry
2. Liver, fried potatoes, gelatin, and avocado
3. Skim milk, lean fish, steamed carrots, and fruit
4. Ham, mashed potatoes, creamed peas, and gelatin

8. The nurse is preparing a presentation on hepatitis types B and C. What should the nurse include in the presentation regarding the most common methods of becoming infected with the disease? *(Select all that apply.)*

1. Recent blood transfusions
2. Contaminated needles and instruments
3. Direct contact with body fluids from infected people, such as through sexual contact
4. Eating food prepared by someone with unclean hands
5. Drinking contaminated water

9. A patient is scheduled for surgery for a common bile duct exploration. The nurse would expect the patient to return from surgery with which device in place?

1. An underwater-seal drainage
2. A T tube connected to gravity drainage
3. A Penrose drain
4. A nephrostomy tube

10. The nurse is caring for a patient with cholecystitis associated with cholelithiasis. Which statement by the nurse is most accurate when answering patient questions?

1. "The disorder can be successfully treated with oral bile salts that dissolve gallstones."
2. "Analgesics are usually not necessary to relieve the pain of bile duct spasms during an acute attack."
3. "A heavy meal with a high fat content may precipitate the signs and symptoms of the disease."
4. "A low-cholesterol diet is indicated to reduce the availability of cholesterol for gallstone formation."

11. Discharge teaching in relation to home management after a laparoscopic cholecystectomy should include which instructions?

1. Keeping the bandages on the puncture sites for 48 hours
2. Reporting any bile-colored drainage or pus from any incision
3. Using over-the-counter antiemetics if nausea and vomiting occur
4. Emptying and measuring the contents of the bile bag from the T tube every day

12. The student nurse asks the nurse why a patient with advanced cirrhosis has an abdomen that is so swollen. Which response by the nurse is correct?

1. "A lack of clotting factors promotes the collection of blood in the abdominal cavity."
2. "Portal hypertension and hypoalbuminemia cause a fluid shift into the peritoneal space."
3. "Decreased peristalsis in the GI tract contributes to gas formation and bowel distention."
4. "Bile salts in the blood irritate the peritoneal membranes, causing edema and pocketing of fluid."

13. When caring for a patient with acute exacerbation of hepatic encephalopathy, the nurse may give a lactulose enema, provide a low-protein diet, and limit physical activity. The nurse explains to the patient that these measures are taken for what reason?

1. To promote fluid loss
2. To eliminate potassium ions
3. To decrease portal pressure
4. To decrease ammonia production

14. If a patient is scheduled for an ultrasound of the pancreas, which situation would cause the examination to be postponed? *(Select all that apply.)*

1. Low serum albumin
2. MRI of abdomen
3. ERCP examination
4. Recent barium enema examination

15. The surgical procedure for cancer of the pancreas involves resection of the antrum of the stomach, the gallbladder, the duodenum, and varying amounts of the pancreas. Anastomoses are constructed between the stomach, the common bile and pancreatic ducts, and the jejunum. The nurse correctly identifies this procedure with which name?

1. Whipple procedure
2. Pancreatectomy
3. Billroth I
4. Billroth II

16. A patient's brother asks the nurse why the patient's pancreatic cancer is at stage IV so early after hearing the diagnosis. The nurse correctly identifies the late diagnosis and high mortality rates as being attributed to what factors? *(Select all that apply.)*

1. It is difficult to diagnose pancreatic cancer at an early, curable stage.
2. Patients with pancreatic cancer are often in denial.
3. The majority of cancers have metastasized at the time of diagnosis.
4. Early tumors often remain asymptomatic, or "silent," until their growth is advanced.
5. Patients often attribute the vague early symptoms of pancreatic cancer to problems that do not warrant seeking medical attention.

17. While caring for a patient with hepatitis A, the nurse expects the stools of the patient to appear what color?

1. Dark brown
2. Black
3. Clay-colored
4. Green

Care of the Patient With a Blood or Lymphatic Disorder

7

Objectives

Anatomy and Physiology

1. Describe the components of blood.
2. Discuss factors necessary for the formation of erythrocytes.
3. Differentiate between the functions of erythrocytes, leukocytes, and thrombocytes.
4. Define the white blood cell differential.
5. Describe the blood-clotting process.
6. List the basic blood groups.
7. Describe the generalized functions of the lymphatic system and list the primary lymphatic structures.

Medical-Surgical

8. List common diagnostic tests for evaluation of blood and lymph disorders, and discuss the significance of the results.
9. Compare and contrast the various types of anemia in terms of etiology and pathophysiology, clinical manifestations, assessment, diagnostic tests, medical management, nursing interventions, patient teaching, and prognosis.
10. List six signs and symptoms associated with hypovolemic shock.
11. Discuss important issues to cover in patient teaching and home care planning for the patient with pernicious anemia.
12. Discuss the etiology and pathophysiology, clinical manifestations, assessment, diagnostic tests, medical management, nursing interventions, patient teaching, and prognosis for patients with acute and chronic leukemia.
13. Compare and contrast the disorders of coagulation (thrombocytopenia, hemophilia, disseminated intravascular coagulation) in terms of etiology and pathophysiology, clinical manifestations, assessment, diagnostic tests, medical management, nursing interventions, and prognosis.
14. Discuss the primary goal of nursing interventions for the patient with lymphedema.
15. Discuss the etiology and pathophysiology, clinical manifestations, assessment, diagnostic tests, medical management, nursing interventions, patient teaching, and prognosis for the patient with multiple myeloma, malignant lymphoma, and Hodgkin lymphoma.
16. Apply the nursing process to the care of the patient with disorders of the hematologic and lymphatic systems.

Key Terms

anemia (ă-NĒ-mē-ă, p. 266)

disseminated intravascular coagulation (DIC) (dĭ-SĔM-ĭ-năt-ĕd, p. 286)

erythrocytosis (ĕ-rĭth-rō-sī-TŌ-sĭs, p. 276)

erythropoiesis (ĕ-rĭth-rō-pō-Ē-sĭs, p. 257)

hemarthrosis (hē-mär-THRŌ-sĭs, p. 283)

hemophilia (hē-mō-FĒL-ē-ă, p. 283)

heterozygous (hĕt-ĕr-ō-ZĪ-gŭs, p. 273)

idiopathic (ĭd-ē-ō-PĂTH-ĭk, p. 268)

leukemia (lū-KĒ-mē-ă, p. 278)

leukopenia (lū-kō-PĒ-nē-ă, p. 279)

lymphangitis (lĭm-făn-GĪ-tĭs, p. 289)

lymphedema (lĭm-fĕ-DĒ-mă, p. 289)

multiple myeloma (MŬL-tĭ-pŭl mī-ĕ-LŌ-mă, p. 287)

pancytopenia (păn-sī-tō-PĒN-ĭk, p. 268)

pernicious anemia (pĕr-NĬSH-ŭs, p. 271)

recombinant (p. 286)

Reed-Sternberg cells (rēd–STĔRN-bĕrg, p. 291)

thrombocytopenia (thrŏm-bō-sīt-ō-PĒ-nē-ă, p. 263)

ANATOMY AND PHYSIOLOGY OF THE HEMATOLOGIC SYSTEM

The hematologic system consists of bone marrow and a fluidic substance known as blood. Bone marrow and blood serve vital functions that drive metabolic processes and protect the body from pathogens. Even minor changes in the way in which bone marrow or blood functions can create disease within the hematological system. Since the workings of the hematological system results in the transport of oxygen and nutrients to cells and the removal of waste products, disease can potentially impact other organ systems within the body. Patients suffering from hematological disease may then manifest widespread symptoms in other body systems and disturbances in homeostasis.

BONE MARROW

Bone marrow is made up of soft, spongy tissue that is found within the bones of the sternum, vertebrae, ribs, and pelvis in adults. It consists of two components known as yellow marrow and red marrow. The yellow marrow is largely made up of fat that does not produce any cell line. However, under times of stress, this yellow marrow can again be replaced by active red marrow. Red marrow is highly vascular and actively produces cells that exist within blood. The production of cell types arises from the differentiation of stem cells that exist within the bone marrow. Stem cells have two remarkable qualities. One, they can self-replicate, thus ensuring the presence of stem cells throughout life. Two, stem cells are totipotent, meaning they can differentiate into any of the cell types that exist in blood. Differentiation of stem cells occurs on a continuous basis to replenish damaged and dying cells, and in response to chemical messengers. Stem cells differentiate into either myeloid cells or lymphoid cells and then further differentiate to eventually produce red blood cells (RBCs), white blood cells (WBCs), and platelets.

Myeloid cells give rise to RBCs, platelets, and all WBCs except lymphocytes. Lymphoid cells give rise to lymphocytes that then become B cells and T cells. Damage to stem cells, bone tumors, or administration of chemotherapy are just a few examples that can alter production of cell lines within the bone marrow. Any alteration in the functioning of bone marrow will then result in hematological disease as it will affect the quality and quantity of cells produced.

Characteristics of Blood

Blood is a substance that is contained within the intravascular space and perfused by the heart. The fluid contained in the intravascular space is commonly known as blood, though it is actually an accumulation of multiple substances held in suspension within fluid, including all cell types produced from the bone marrow, electrolytes, proteins, fats, sugars, microminerals, and hormones. The fluid contained in blood consists of approximately 20% of the body's total water content. This water content is called plasma and is yellowish in appearance. Plasma contains electrolytes, dissolved gasses, hormones, coagulation factors, proteins including albumin that maintains osmotic pressure, and antibody proteins, etc. Plasma accounts for 55% of the total volume circulating within blood vessels. The remaining 45% volume circulating in blood vessels is made up of RBCs, WBCs (Fig 7.1), and platelets, and these cell lines are held in suspension within plasma. Together, the plasma and its contents including cell lines is what constitutes blood.

The average adult has a circulating blood volume of 5 to 6 L. It is this circulation that allows blood to perform some of its critical functions. Blood transports oxygen and nutrients to cells; vital components of the

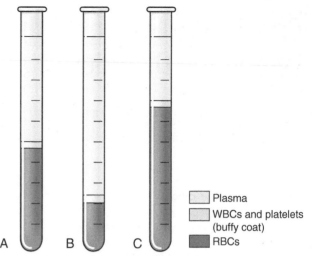

Fig. 7.1 Hematocrit (Hct) tubes showing normal blood, anemia, and polycythemia. Note the buffy coat located between the packed red blood cells (RBCs) and the plasma. (A) A normal percentage of RBCs. (B) Anemia (a low percentage of RBCs). (C) Polycythemia (a high percentage of RBCs). *WBCs,* White blood cells.

immune system to injured areas of the body or sites of infection; coagulation factors to prevent blood loss and initiation of clotting; hormones released by endocrine glands to their target tissues; and waste products released by cells to other organs for further processing and/or excretion. Blood maintains a slightly alkaline pH of 7.35 to 7.45. This pH is maintained via the regulation of substances dissolved in blood known as buffers.

Components of Blood Relevant to the Hematological System

Erythrocytes or Red Blood Cells. A RBC is known as an *erythrocyte* in its mature form. Immature RBCs are known as *reticulocytes* and may be released from the bone marrow in times of stress. Erythrocytes make up the major cellular component circulating in blood. These cells differentiate from stem cells, and as they differentiate, they eventually lose their nucleus and obtain a biconcave disk shape. The biconcave disk shape is vital to their function, as it allows for better maneuverability through capillary beds. Erythrocytes consist of cytoplasm and mainly the protein hemoglobin that contains iron. The presence of hemoglobin allows erythrocytes to perform their essential function of gas exchange. When the hemoglobin in erythrocytes is saturated with oxygen molecules, blood appears a brighter red than when it is carrying carbon dioxide. Therefore, arterial blood is a brighter red in color than venous blood.

The lifespan of an erythrocyte is 120 days. Aged and damaged erythrocytes are removed from circulation by the spleen and liver. The hemoglobin and iron contained within the erythrocyte are mostly recycled to make new erythrocyte cells. The rest of the hemoglobin is broken down into bilirubin and secreted in bile which is then excreted in fecal matter and urine. Iron is lost in fecal matter, urine, and monthly menstrual flow.

Aged and damaged erythrocytes are replaced by the production of new ones from the bone marrow. This means that the bone marrow is actively producing new erythrocytes. The production of erythrocytes is known as *erythropoiesis*. The bone marrow requires certain essential vitamins, proteins, and minerals to produce healthy mature erythrocytes. When the nutrient needs are not met, the production of erythrocytes is altered, which results in hematological disease, mainly anemias.

Erythrocytes may also be produced from the bone marrow in response to alterations in oxygen saturation levels. As blood filters through the kidney, specialized cells in the kidney sense oxygen levels. When oxygen levels are low, the kidney produces a hormone known as *erythropoietin*. Erythropoietin is then transported via blood to the bone marrow where it stimulates the bone marrow to increase production of erythrocytes. Healthy mature erythrocytes are produced in response to this stimulation as long as the bone marrow has an available and healthy supply of folic acid, iron, vitamin B_{12}, pyridoxine (vitamin B6), amino acids, etc. In addition, disease within the kidney can result in alterations in sensing oxygen saturation levels or its ability to produce and release erythropoietin. Thus, patients with kidney disease may suffer from anemia known as anemia of chronic kidney disease.

Leukocytes or White Blood Cells. WBCs are known as leukocytes and are the body's primary defense mechanism against foreign invaders. There are five types of leukocytes, which are divided into two broad categories—granulocytes and agranulocytes. Granulocytes are so named because these cells contain granules inside of them that become apparent when stained in a laboratory with Wright's stain. Agranulocytes, on the other hand, contain no granules and do not absorb Wright's stain.

Granulocytes. There are three types of leukocytes that are granulocytes. These are neutrophils, basophils, and eosinophils. Basophils and eosinophils are further discussed in the immune chapter (Chapter 15), as their primary role involves allergic and hypersensitivity reactions. Neutrophils are also called polymorphonuclear neutrophils (PMNs or polys) or segmented neutrophils (segs). Mature neutrophils differentiate from the myeloid stem cell and contain a multi-lobed nucleus that is connected by thin filaments. On microscopic examination, this nucleus appears segmented, thus leading to a name of segmented neutrophils. Immature neutrophils are referred to as band cells, as their nucleus on microscopic examination consists of one elongated nucleus that is not "cut" into multiple lobes. As in the case of reticulocytes, band cell numbers may increase in blood supply during times of stress. An increase in band cells within the blood may be referred to as a shift to the left,

as typically band cell numbers are recorded on the left side of the paper.

Segmented neutrophils produced and released from the bone marrow circulate within blood for a few short hours before migrating into body tissues. Here, they surveil for inflammation and possible invasion by bacteria and fungi. Neutrophils are primary defenders and arrive at the site of inflammation within an hour of onset. They ingest pathogens and dispose of dead tissue using phagocytosis. Neutrophils also release lysozyme from their granules, which is an enzyme that destroys the cell wall of bacteria, thereby causing bacterial contents to leak out, resulting in cessation of the bacterial cell cycle and death. Once recruited in the immune response, a neutrophil dies within 1 to 2 days. The bone marrow is constantly producing neutrophils, and their numbers remain stable in a healthy person; however, when challenged by serious infections, the bone marrow can quickly produce and release large numbers of neutrophils into circulation.

Agranulocytes. Leukocytes are comprised of two cell lines that are agranulocytes or without granules—monocytes and lymphocytes. Monocytes originate from the myeloid stem cell line. They remain in blood circulation for a few hours after being released from the bone marrow and then travel to various tissues in the body such as liver, spleen, and lungs. Once monocytes reach these tissues, they differentiate into macrophages. Macrophages are scavenger cells that fight infection, help other WBCs remove dead or damaged tissues, destroy cancer cells, and regulate immunity against foreign substances. Lymphocytes are cells that are derived from differentiation of stem cells to lymphoid cells. There are two types of lymphocytes—B-cells and T-cells. B-cells leave the bone marrow as mature cells while T-cells leave the bone marrow in an immature form and migrate to the thymus where thymic hormones help bring them to maturity (Kumar, Connors, & Farber, 2018). T-cells or T-lymphocytes are responsible for killing foreign cells directly by releasing substances that enhance their phagocytic activity. They also serve as primary cells that destroy tumors within the body. The process by which they defend the body is known as cellular immunity. B-cells or B-lymphocytes differentiate into plasma cells. Plasma cells, when exposed to foreign particles on the cells of pathogens, produce antibodies that bind with those foreign particles. This in essence "tags" the pathogen as a foreign entity within the body. Once tagged, the foreign substance can be attacked by other immune defender cells in the body or destroyed by the B-cell itself. The process of producing antibodies to defend the body from foreign invaders is termed *humoral immunity*.

Thrombocytes (Platelets). Thrombocytes or platelets arise from the myeloid line of stem cells and differentiate into giant cells known as megakaryocytes.

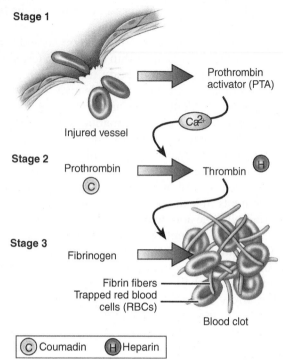

Stage 1

Injured vessel

Prothrombin activator (PTA)

Ca²⁺

Stage 2

Prothrombin

C

Thrombin H

Stage 3

Fibrinogen

Fibrin fibers
Trapped red blood
cells (RBCs)

Blood clot

C Coumadin   H Heparin

Fig. 7.2 Blood clotting. The extremely complex clotting mechanism can be distilled into three basic stages: *stage 1*, release of clotting factors from injured tissue cells and sticky platelets at the injury site; *stage 2*, formation of thrombin; and *stage 3*, formation of fibrin and trapping of red blood cells to form a clot. (From Herlihy B: *The human body in health and illness*, ed 6, St. Louis, 2018, Elsevier.)

Megakaryocytes then fragment into granular cells that are released into circulation. These cells are anucleated and the smallest of all cells in the blood. The production of megakaryocytes within the bone marrow is partly regulated by the release of a hormone known as thrombopoietin. Thrombopoietin is released by cells in the kidney and liver. Thrombocytes have a lifespan of 5 to 9 days after being released into blood circulation. These cells are vital to the maintenance of homeostasis within the body, which is accomplished by preventing blood loss. In times of injury, thrombocytes collect at the injured site and adhere to each other to create a plug that stops further bleeding. Thrombocytes also release granules that activate coagulation factors in blood that help form a stable clot at the site of injury (Fig. 7.2).

Hemostasis. Hemostasis is a body process that arrests the flow of blood and prevents hemorrhage. Three actions take place: (1) vessel spasm, (2) platelet plug formation, and (3) clot formation. When a vessel has a tear or rupture, the smooth muscle in the walls of the vessel causes it to contract. Platelets rush in and attempt to seal the area, which is effective in small vessel tears. The third process, clot formation, is more detailed and occurs in larger injuries. This process can be summarized as follows (see Fig. 7.2):
1. Injury occurs, and a blood vessel is damaged.
2. Hemorrhage begins.

3. Platelets are activated and clump at the site of damage.
4. Thromboplastin, released from platelets, reacts with calcium ions.
5. In the presence of thromboplastin and calcium, prothrombin is converted to thrombin.
6. Thrombin links with fibrinogen.
7. Fibrinogen forms fibrin.
8. Fibrin traps RBCs and platelets, forming a blood clot.
9. The blood clot seals the damaged blood vessel.

ANATOMY AND PHYSIOLOGY OF THE LYMPHATIC SYSTEM

The lymphatic system is a subdivision of the cardiovascular system and a transverse network used by immune cells that defend the body against foreign invaders. It consists of lymphatic capillaries, lymph fluid, lymphatic vessels, lymph nodes, tonsils, spleen, and the thymus gland. The lymphatic system is responsible for maintaining fluid levels within the body, absorbing fats from the digestive tract, protecting the body against foreign invaders, transporting and removing waste products, and transporting abnormal cells to various sites for destruction.

Lymph Capillaries, Vessels, and Lymph Fluid
At its smallest level, the lymphatic system consists of lymph capillaries. Lymph capillaries exist between cells and within the interstitial tissues of the body. Their structure is special in that it allows fluid and proteins to move from interstitial spaces into the lymphatic capillaries but not out of them. Via arteries and arterioles, the heart pumps and perfuses approximately 20 L of blood throughout our body bringing cells nutrients needed to drive metabolic processes. At the capillary bed level, RBCs deliver oxygen in single file while the plasma contained in blood delivers nutrients such as proteins, fats, carbohydrates, minerals, etc. Blood and plasma bathe cells and their surrounding tissue spaces with nutrients and oxygen and then recede back into venules to reenter the cardiovascular system. Approximately 17 L of the 20 L of blood and plasma recede back into the venous system. The remaining 3 L contained within the interstitial tissue spaces is re-collected to rejoin the cardiovascular system via lymph capillaries. The fluid remaining in the interstitial spaces along with proteins, waste products of cells, carbon dioxide, and abnormal cells move into lymph capillaries and stay there based on pressure inside the lymph capillary. The fluid contained in lymph capillaries is now called lymph and is delivered into larger lymphatic vessels. Lymphatic vessels, like veins, have one-way valves that do not allow lymph to back flow. Lymphatic vessels carry lymph to lymph nodes that exist throughout the body.

Lymph Nodes

The body contains approximately 500 to 600 lymph nodes connected by lymph vessels. Lymph carried by lymphatic vessels flows through these lymph nodes on its way to the right and left subclavian veins. Lymph nodes are small, soft, bean-shaped cells occurring in clusters. They are found all over the body but are particularly concentrated in areas such as the cervical, inguinal, axillary, thorax, and abdominal areas of the body. The inner structure of lymph nodes is complex and consist of two functional divisions. Within these divisions, lymph nodes house B-cells, T-cells, dendritic cells, and macrophages. As lymph flows through lymph nodes, cells of the immune system work to destroy foreign pathogens, damaged cells, and cancer cells. After lymph fluid is processed through a lymph node, it continues on its journey via lymphatic vessels to lymph ducts that eventually empty into the subclavian veins.

Tonsils

The tonsils are a set of lymphoid organs or soft tissue masses that are located at either side of the pharynx. Their tissue resembles that of lymph nodes, and like lymph nodes, tonsils work to defend the body against pathogens entering the body through the oropharynx or nasopharynx. Like lymph nodes, they house cells of the immune system, in particular T-cells, B-cells, and macrophages. Most of the time, tonsils protect the body without any issues. However, like lymph nodes, when overwhelmed with infection, tonsils enlarge and cause pain and severe discomfort.

Spleen. The spleen is a soft, roughly ovoid, highly vascularized organ located in the left upper quadrant of the abdominal cavity, just below the diaphragm (Fig. 7.3). The spleen is 5 to 6 in (12.7 to 15.2 cm) long and 2 to 3 in (5 to 7.6 cm) wide. It is the largest of the organs in the lymphatic system. The spleen contains two main regions referred to as red pulp and white pulp. The red pulp contains venous sinuses filled with blood and connective tissue that contains red cells and white cells. The white pulp consists of B-cells and T-cells. As blood flows into the spleen, it enters a maze of passages. Within these passages, blood is surveilled for healthy and damaged/dying RBCs. Healthy RBCs continue to flow through the passages while damaged/dying RBCs are taken out of circulation and broken down by macrophages. When breaking down RBCs, hemoglobin and iron are stored by the spleen to be reused by the bone marrow when making more RBCs. In addition to processing and removing damaged RBCs from circulation, the spleen also stores roughly 500 mL of blood, which it will release into circulation in the event of an emergency. The storing of blood is what gives the spleen its deep purple color. The white pulp of the spleen is instrumental in destroying pathogens that enter the spleen via blood, thereby cleaning the blood supply as it flows through the spleen.

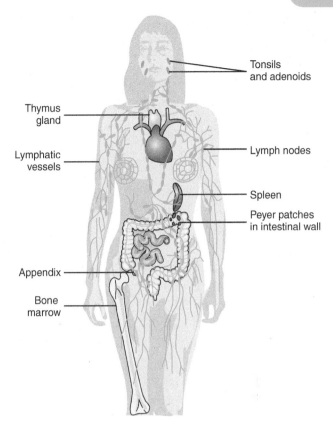

Fig. 7.3 Principal organs of the lymphatic system. (From Copstead-Kirkhorn LE, Banasik J: *Pathophysiology*, ed 5, St. Louis, 2013, Mosby.)

Thymus. The thymus gland (see Fig. 7.3) is a specialized lymphoid organ that is soft and roughly triangular in shape. It is located in the mediastinum, anterior and superior to the heart, posterior to the sternum. It houses immature T-cells known as thymocytes and contains specialized epithelial cells that help thymocytes mature into T-cells. These T-cells then migrate to the spleen and lymph nodes where they play a critical role in immune defense. The thymus gland plays the largest role in immunity during neonatal and pre-adolescent years. In pre-teen years, it starts to atrophy in size and activity. In adults, the thymus gland is mostly replaced by fatty tissue, though the maturation of T-cells continues throughout life.

Laboratory and Diagnostic Tests

Complete blood count. The complete blood count (CBC) is an important screening tool. It is used to confirm and investigate for many disease processes. The CBC detects many disorders of the hematologic system and provides data for diagnosing and evaluating disorders in other body systems. A CBC can be ordered as a CBC or a CBC with differential. Most of the times it is ordered as a CBC with differential, which gives the values of the five types of WBCs separately. Further details of this important screening tool are displayed in Table 7.1. A CBC includes red cells, white cells, and platelets; hematocrit (Hct) and hemoglobin (Hgb) levels; erythrocyte indexes; differential WBC count; and

Table 7.1   Diagnostic Blood Studies

BLOOD TEST	NORMAL VALUES	DESCRIPTION
White Blood Cells		
White Blood Cells (WBCs) or Leukocytes	5000–10,000 cells/mm^3	Actual cell count
Leukocytopenia—total WBC cells count is lower than 5000 cells/mm^3 Present in chemotherapy, radiation, aplastic anemia	Low High	Leukocytosis—total WBC count is higher than 10,000 cells/mm^3 Present in infections caused by a variety of pathogens, inflammatory disorders, trauma, and leukemia
Neutrophils	60%–70% 3000–7000 cells/mm^{3a} (60% × 5000) to (70% × 10,000)	Cell count based on normal percentage values for neutrophils; calculated by taking 60%–70% of WBC high and low range
Neutropenia—percentage of neutrophils present among total WBC count is less than 60% Present in patients exposed to chemotherapy and radiation, agranulocytosis, and autoimmune diseases	Low High	Neutrophilia—percentage of neutrophils present among total WBC count is higher than 70% Present in burns, crushing injuries, diabetic ketoacidosis, infections
Eosinophils	1%–4% 50–400 cells/mm^{3a} (1% × 5000) to (4% × 10,000)	Cell count based on normal percentage values for eosinophils; calculated by taking 1%-4% of WBC high and low range
A concern if low along with other white blood cells, with alcohol intoxication, or excessive cortisol production	Low High	Increased in allergic reactions and with parasitic disorders
Basophils	0.5%–1% 25–100 cells/mm^{3a} (0.5% × 5000) to (1% × 10,000)	Cell count based on normal percentage values for basophils; calculated by taking 0.5%-1% of WBC high and low range
May indicate a severe allergic reaction	Low High	Can occur due to chronic inflammation
Lymphocytes	20%–40% 1000–4000 cells/mm^{3a} (20% × 5000) to (40% × 10,000)	Cell count based on normal percentage values for lymphocytes; calculated by taking 20%-40% of WBC high and low range
Lymphocytopenia—percentage of lymphocytes present among total WBC count is lower than 20% Present in AIDS, SLE, and Hodgkin lymphoma.	Low High	Lymphocytosis—percentage of lymphocytes present among total WBC count is higher than 40% Present in infectious mononucleosis, measles, infectious hepatitis, and lymphocytic leukemia.
Monocytes	2%–6% 100–600 cells/mm^{3a} (2% × 5000) to (6% × 10,000)	Cell count based on normal percentage values for monocytes; calculated by taking 2%-6% of WBC high and low range
Monocytopenia—percentage of monocytes present among total WBC count is lower than 2% Present with aplastic anemia, hairy leukoplakia, thermal injuries, and treatment with corticosteroids	Low High	Monocytosis—percentage of monocytes present among total WBC count is higher than 6% Present with recovery phase from bacterial infections and chronic inflammatory conditions
Platelets		
Platelets or thrombocytes	150,000–400,000 cells/mm^3	Actual cell count
Thrombocytopenia—number of circulating platelets is less than 150,000 cells/mm^3. Present in thrombocytopenia and aplastic anemia.	Low High	Thrombocytosis—number of circulating platelets is more than 400,000 cells/mm^3. Present in granulocytic leukemia; bone marrow suppression, such as with chemotherapy or radiation therapy

Table 7.1   Diagnostic Blood Studies—cont'd

BLOOD TEST	NORMAL VALUES	DESCRIPTION
Red Blood Cells		
Red Blood Cells or erythrocytes	Males 4.7–6.1 million cells/µL Females 4.2–5.4 million cells/µL	Actual cell count
Erythrocytopenia or erythropenia—number of circulating red blood cells is less than 4.7 (Males) or 4.2 (Females) million cells/uL Present in anemia due to bleeding, iron deficiency anemia, megaloblastic anemia, sick cell, and hemophilia; kidney disease or damage Decreased number of red blood cells directly impacts the amount of cells present that can carry oxygen and therefore results in reduced oxygen carrying capacity. Since there are fewer red blood cells, the hemoglobin count will also be decreased.	Low High	Erythrocytosis—number of circulating red blood cells is more than 6.1 (Males) or 5.4 (Females) million cells/uL Present in polycythemia vera Causes blood to be more viscous which can lead to clotting
Hemoglobin	Males: 13.5–17.5 g/dL Females: 12–15.5 g/dL	Actual count of the amount of hemoglobin in grams per deciliter of blood
Oxygen-carrying capacity in the blood is directly impacted, as oxygen is carried in blood by binding to hemoglobin Present in iron deficiency anemia, folate deficiency anemia, vitamin B 12 deficiency anemia, blood loss such as hemophilia, sickle cell anemia	Low High	Usually high because the red blood cell count is also higher. This indicates a compensatory mechanism. Present in thalassemia, renal disease, dehydration, pulmonary problems, and polycythemia vera
Hematocrit	Males: 42%–52% Females: 35%–47%	Volume of red blood cells divided by the total volume of the sample multiplied by 100%
Low hematocrit indicative of fluid overload, blood loss, leukemia, iron deficiency anemia, vitamin B_{12} deficiency anemia, sickle cells anemia, hemophilia	Low High	High hematocrit indicative of dehydration, polycythemia vera, pulmonary disease, renal disease
Mean Corpuscular Volume[b]	80–100 fL (femtoliters)	Measure of the average size and volume of a red blood cell
Average size and volume of a red blood cell are smaller than normal, indicating microcytic anemia; conditions classified as microcytic anemia include iron deficiency anemia, sideroblastic anemia, and thalassemia's (Maner & Mosavi, 2020).	Low High	Average size and volume of a red blood cell are larger than normal, indicating macrocytic anemia; conditions classified as macrocytic anemia include megaloblastic anemia (folate deficiency, vitamin B_{12} deficiency, orotic aciduria) and non-megaloblastic anemia due to hepatic insufficiency, chronic alcoholism, and Diamond Blackfan anemia (Maner & Mosavi, 2020)
Red Cell Distribution Width	Males: 12.2%–16.1% Females: 11.8% -14.5%	Measures the variance of the volume and size of red blood cells; the difference in volume and size from the biggest to the smallest red blood cell
Indicates all red blood cells are about the same volume and size Not associated with any hematological disorder (May, Marques, Reddy, et al., 2019).	Low High	Indicates red blood cells vary in size from small to big at a higher percentage than normal Usually caused by nutritional deficiencies such as Vitamin B_{12}, folate, and iron; hallmark of iron deficiency anemia in the early stages of the disease; can also indicate acute hemorrhage or hemolysis

Continued

Table 7.1	Diagnostic Blood Studies—cont'd	
BLOOD TEST	NORMAL VALUES	DESCRIPTION
Mean Corpuscular Hemoglobin (MCH)[b]	27.5–33.2 pg (picograms)	Average mass of hemoglobin that is in each red blood cell, which is determined by iron
As the mass of hemoglobin depends on iron content, low MCH is indicative of iron deficiency anemia	Low High	Occurs with macrocytic anemias, as the cells are too big, and so the average mass of hemoglobin increases Occurs with folic acid deficiency or vitamin in B_{12} deficiency
Mean Corpuscular Hemoglobin Concentration (MCHC)[b]	33.4–35.5 g/dL	Average weight of the hemoglobin in a volume of red blood cells
Indicative of iron deficiency anemia	Low High	Indicative of sickle cell anemia

[a]Calculating the number of cells present based on percentages of total white blood cell values is known as the absolute count.
[b]The mean corpuscular volume, mean corpuscular hemoglobin, and mean corpuscular hemoglobin concentration together are known as the erythrocyte indices and these values together help give clues as to the etiology of anemias.

examination of the peripheral blood cells. Prepare the patient by explaining that a blood sample will be taken from a vein. The hand and arm (usually the antecubital fossa) are used commonly as sites for blood collection.

Peripheral blood smear. A peripheral blood smear, along with the differential CBC, allows examination of the size, shape, and structure of individual blood cells and platelets. This information is useful in differentiating various forms of anemias and dyscrasias (any abnormal physiologic condition, especially of the blood). All three hematologic cell lines (RBCs, WBCs, and platelets) can be examined. When adequately prepared and examined microscopically by an experienced technologist, a peripheral blood smear is the most informative of all hematologic tests.

Schilling test and megaloblastic anemia profile. The Schilling test was developed by Dr. Robert F. Schilling to aid in diagnosing a vitamin B_{12} deficiency. Vitamin B_{12} deficiency can occur due to deficiencies in diet, lack of intrinsic factor, or due to lack of absorption. The Schilling test aids in pinpointing the cause of the deficiency. In stage 1 of the test, patients suspected to have vitamin B_{12} deficiency are given radio-cobalt-labeled vitamin B_{12} orally and are put on a 24-hour urine collection. Patients with diet deficiencies in vitamin B_{12} will have a normal result of 8% to 40% of radioactive cobalt vitamin B_{12} excretion in urine within 24 hours. Patients with either a lack of intrinsic factor or absorption issues will have low levels of radioactive-labeled vitamin B_{12} in the excreted 24-hour urine collection. In stage 2 of the test, patients are again given radiolabeled vitamin B_{12} orally along with an oral dose of intrinsic factor and are again put on a 24-hour urine collection. If the 24-hour urine collection shows a normal result of 8% to 40% of radioactive vitamin B_{12} excretion, then the patient is lacking intrinsic factor and has pernicious anemia. If, however, the 24-hour urine collection shows an abnormal level of excreted radiolabeled

vitamin B_{12}, the patient has absorption issues in the terminal ileum, and other disease processes need to be investigated to determine the cause of vitamin B_{12} deficiency (Ramphul & Mejias, 2019). Despite the diagnostic value of this, it is no longer used to diagnose the etiology of vitamin B_{12} deficiency due to the decreased availability of radiolabeled cobalt and as advances in science have allowed for other laboratory studies to be performed. Today, vitamin B_{12} deficiency is diagnosed using a CBC, serum vitamin B_{12} levels, and methylmalonic acid and homocysteine levels (both of which are converted to other substances only in the presence of vitamin B_{12}). Together, these four tests are known as the *megaloblastic anemia profile.*

Radiologic studies. Radiologic studies of the hematologic system involve primarily the use of computed tomography (CT) or magnetic resonance imaging (MRI) for evaluating the spleen, liver, and lymph nodes. In the past, lymphangiography (i.e., x-ray analysis of lymphatic vessels and nodes) with contrast dye was a common procedure for evaluating lymph nodes deep inside the body.

Bone marrow aspiration or biopsy. Bone marrow aspiration and biopsy can help establish a diagnosis when there is a suspected hematologic issue. These are invasive procedures, therefore they are used judiciously. Bone marrow aspiration and biopsy are used to investigate anemias, penia or cytosis in WBCs or platelets, cancers within the bone marrow, and fevers of unknown origin. The most common site for this procedure is the posterior iliac crest due to a lack of vital organs, major blood vessels, and nerves in this area. In some cases the sternum can be used as well, though when used, it is mostly to perform an aspiration as opposed to a biopsy.

Normal bone marrow is soft and semifluid and can be removed by aspiration through a specialized needle device. Bone marrow aspiration is most commonly performed in people with marked anemia, neutropenia (decreased number of certain WBCs), acute leukemia, and thrombocytopenia (decreased number of platelets). The aspirate is examined for cell types, numbers, and degree of maturation. Because the aspirate is a sample of cells, it may not provide the degree of detail that can be gained from a biopsy, therefore it is possible that a biopsy may be necessary after an aspiration procedure. In a bone marrow aspiration, 5 mL of blood and marrow is aspirated. If a biopsy is needed, it is best performed after an aspiration in a slightly different location. A bone marrow biopsy garners a core sample that better represents the cells in the marrow than an aspiration procedure and has a greater diagnostic value. Patients undergoing either of these procedures need an explanation of the procedure and a signed informed consent. Patients undergoing an aspiration or biopsy procedure experience a pressure sensation as the needle is advanced. Aspiration causes brief but sharp pain, while biopsy causes a pressure sensation but no pain. Post procedure, complications include a risk of bleeding and an ache at the site of the biopsy for 1 to 2 days. The needle insertion site is usually covered with a small sterile dressing.

Hematological Therapies

Splenectomy. A splenectomy is the surgical removal of the spleen and a treatment option for patients with various hematological disorders. Hypersplenism, overactive spleen, is a condition where the spleen destroys excessive numbers of RBCs and platelets instead of just destroying damaged or dead cells, thus resulting in anemia and clotting disorders. The removal of the spleen ceases this excessive destruction, thus causing a rebound in the numbers of circulating RBCs and platelets. A splenectomy is a treatment of choice for patients with immune thrombocytopenia purpura (ITP), cancers such as Hodgkin and non-Hodgkin lymphoma, genetic conditions such as sickle cell disease and thalassemia, splenomegaly, presence of tumors, abdominal injury that results in trauma and subsequent bleeding to the spleen, and in incidences of splenic infarction or aneurysm.

A splenectomy can be performed either open or laparoscopically. Open splenectomy is preferred in gross enlargement of the spleen and if the patient has experienced abdominal trauma. In most cases, a splenectomy is performed laparoscopically. Preoperative assessment includes the status of major organ systems such as cardiovascular, respiratory, and gastrointestinal (GI). Drugs such as aspirin, blood thinners, and anti-inflammatory medications must be stopped at least 1 week prior to surgery. Time permitting, patients are also advised to receive the pneumococcal pneumonia vaccine, as post splenectomy this infection poses the greatest risk, especially in children. The Centers for Disease Control and Prevention (CDC) also recommends scheduled vaccinations for influenza, Haemophilus influenza type B (Hib), meningococcal, HPV, MMR, varicella, and Tdap (tetanus, diphtheria, and pertussis) (CDC, 2016). Postoperative assessment includes comparison of major organ system functions with baseline data recorded during the preoperative assessment. The patient is also monitored for signs and symptoms of complications such as infection, hemorrhage, blood clots, paralytic ileus, and injury to adjacent organ structures. Post splenectomy, patients are at a greater risk of getting serious infections, and it takes them longer to recover from injuries or illness. Patients are taught to notify the provider at the first sign of an infection.

Hematopoietic stem cell transplant. A hematopoietic stem cell transplant (HSCT), more commonly known as a bone marrow transplant, may potentially be a life-saving procedure for patients with diseases such as leukemia, aplastic anemia, myelodysplastic syndrome, thalassemia, and many more. The process starts by first identifying the source of the stem cells to be transplanted. Autologous HSCT occurs when the bone marrow to be transplanted is taken from the patient afflicted with the disease. Allogenic HSCT occurs when a patient is given stem cells from a donor. Patients suffering from diseases that afflict the bones and bone marrow are generally given allogenic HSCT donations rather than undergoing an autologous transplant.

Allogenic hematopoietic stem cell transplant. Prior to stem cell transplant, a human lymphocyte antigen (HLA) donor match is identified. Stem cells are harvested from the allogenic donor by either conducting a bone marrow harvest or using peripheral blood stem cell (PBSC) harvesting technique. In a bone marrow harvest, stem cells are removed from the pelvic bones of the donor under general anesthesia. A surgeon harvests stem cells by inserting a large needle in multiple places in the pelvic bone and aspirating stem cells. Roughly 1 L of stem cells are harvested using this technique, which takes about 2 hours. Complications experienced by the donor may include bleeding, infection, and nerve damage. PBSC harvesting is a procedure that has been in use for about 10 years and is an effective means of collecting stem cells as a small quantity of stems cells circulate in blood. Donors may or may not be administered cytokines prior to PBSC harvest. Two cytokines (filgrastim and sargramostim) are FDA approved for PBSC harvest and cause an increase in the number of circulating stem cells in the blood by 100-fold. Once peripheral venous access is secured, the donor blood flows from the venous catheter into an apheresis machine where stem cells are separated from the rest of the donor's blood and the donor's blood minus stem cells is returned to the donor's circulatory system. Stem cells are recognized and differentiated from other cells in blood, as they contain a special antigen on their cell surface known as CD34+ antigen. A donor may undergo multiple harvest sessions with the goal of collecting 2 million stem cells/kg of patient weight (Sheth, Jain, Gore, et al., 2020).

Autologous hematopoietic stem cell transplant. Autologous donation is a choice for patients who do not have a suitable allogenic HSCT donor and/or for those with healthy bone marrow but requiring bone marrow ablative chemotherapy prior to transplantation. Autologous HSCT is the preferred donor type for patients with myeloma, non-Hodgkin lymphoma (Sheth, Jain, Gore, et al., 2020), Hodgkin lymphoma, and plasma cell disorders (Mayo Clinic, 2019). Patients receiving an autologous HSCT undergo a PBSC procedure to harvest stem cells. PBSC procedure is preferred over standard bone marrow harvest technique, as it is easier to access and as blood cell counts recover quicker. Patients are given a stem cell mobilizer (cytokines—filgrastim and sargramostim) that increases the amount of circulating stem cells in the blood supply 100-fold. After harvesting the stem cells from the blood via apheresis, stems cells are frozen and the patient is readied for the next step in a HSCT.

Allogenic versus autologous. Donor type used has advantages and disadvantages. Allogenic stem cell transplant is advantageous to the patient, as the stem cells are foreign to the patient's body, and this allows for cancer cells to be tagged as foreign and destroyed more easily. The ability of stem cells from the donor to more effectively kill a patient's cancer cells is called the graft-versus-tumor effect. The disadvantage of using an allogenic donor is that the donor's stem cells may recognize normal cells in the patient as foreign and destroy them as well. In this case, the patient would have graft-versus-host disease (GVHD). GVHD is a complication of allogenic stem cell transplant that can be mild, moderate, or severe. The occurrence and severity of GVHD can be controlled by prescribing immunosuppressive medications. Another disadvantage of using an allogenic donor is the possibility of graft failure. When allogenic donor stem cells are infused into a patient, the stem cells need to migrate to the bone marrow and start producing RBCs, WBCs, and platelets. Successful production of cell lines means that engraftment has occurred, while failure to produce cell lines means the stem cell transplant resulted in graft failure. Allogenic stem cell transplants have the disadvantage of possibly resulting in graft failure, whereas graft failure is extremely rare in an autologous donation. Autologous stem cell transplant also carries the advantage of no GVHD but has the disadvantage of being less effective at killing cancer cells, as the transplanted cells are from the patient. Therefore, the graft-versus-tumor effect may be reduced.

Transplanting stem cells. Patients, whether they are receiving an allogenic or autologous HSCT, undergo either myeloablative or nonmyeloablative chemotherapy and/or radiation. In myeloablative chemotherapy, the patient receives high doses of chemotherapy with the aim of eradicating the existing bone marrow and any malignant cells. In nonmyeloablative chemotherapy, the aim is to destroy malignant cells without completely eradicating all the stem cells in the bone marrow. After administration of chemotherapy, patients are placed in neutropenic precautions and watched closely for signs and symptoms of infection as the cells capable of fighting off infections have been reduced greatly or destroyed. The time frame between chemotherapy/radiation and stem cell transplant depends on the patient's ability to rest and recover from the ablative therapy. Once recover occurs, stem cells are transplanted via a central venous catheter. Patients may experience side effects from chemicals used to preserve the stem cells and from the effects of an allogenic transplant.

Blood Transfusions. According to the American National Red Cross (2020), less than 38% of the United States population is eligible to donate blood and platelets, and one donation can save potentially three lives. Blood transfusions are conducted every 2 seconds in the United States for a multitude of reasons including surgeries, trauma, GI bleeding, sickle cell disease, hemophilia, and anemias.

ABO blood group. The process of blood transfusions starts with blood typing (see Fig. 7.4). Blood types or groups are inherited from parents. There are four major blood types: type A, type B, type AB, and type O, known collectively as the ABO blood group system. Type A blood contains A antigen on their cell surface, type B blood contains B antigen on their cell surface, type AB blood contains both A and B antigens on their cell surface, and type O blood contains no antigens on their cell surface. When conducting blood typing, a sample of the patient's blood is mixed with antibody A and antibody B. Type A blood will clump together when exposed to antibody A and have no reaction when exposed to antibody B. Type B blood will clump together when exposed to antibody B and have no reaction to antibody A. Type AB blood will clump together when exposed to both antibody A and B. Type O blood will not clump together when exposed to either antibody A or antibody B.

Patients with type O blood do not have A or B antigens on their cell surface and therefore contain anti-A and anti-B antibodies. They can only be given type O blood in a transfusion, but because they do not have antigens A or B, type O blood can be transfused to patients with type A, type B, and type AB blood. For this reason, type O blood is known as the universal donor. Patient's with type A blood have A antigens on their cell surface but also contain anti-B antibodies. Therefore, a patient with type A blood can be given type A or O blood, and giving type B blood would cause a blood transfusion reaction. Patients with type B blood have B antigens on their cell surface but also contain anti-A antibodies. Transfusion of type A blood to a person with type B blood would cause the anti-A antibodies to start killing the transfused blood cells, resulting in a

Recipient's blood		Reactions with donor's blood			
RBC antigens	Plasma antibodies	Donor type O	Donor type A	Donor type B	Donor type AB
None (Type O)	Anti-A Anti-B				
A (Type A)	Anti-B				
B (Type B)	Anti-A				
AB (Type AB)	(None)				

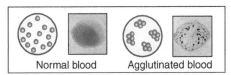

Normal blood   Agglutinated blood

Fig. 7.4 Results of various combinations of donor and recipient blood. The *left columns* show the recipient's blood characteristics, and the *top row* shows the donor's blood type. (From Patton KT, Thibodeau GA: *The human body in health and disease*, ed 7, St. Louis, 2018, Elsevier.)

transfusion reaction. Patients with type B blood can be transfused with type B or O blood. Patients with type AB blood contains both A and B antigens and have no antibodies for either type of blood. These patients can be transfused type A blood, type B blood, and type O blood. For this reason, type AB blood is known as the universal recipient.

Blood typing is extremely important, as transfusion of incorrect blood types can cause hemolysis (rupturing of RBCs). Hemolysis occurs when the antibodies in the patient receiving the blood attach to the antigens on the donor's cell surface, causing RBCs to rupture, release cell contents into the blood supply, and die. Symptoms include fever, chills, hypotension, bronchospasm, and low back pain. The blood transfusion must be stopped immediately. There is no rescue medication for this reaction, only prevention through meticulous attention to detail on the part of all health care personnel. Blood transfusions can also cause allergic reactions that are triggered due to plasma proteins within the blood that is being transfused. In an allergic reaction, patients may experience hives (urticaria), flushing, and itching. If this occurs, stop the blood transfusion and resume it again if treatment with antihistamines is successful. Patients who have had multiple transfusions in the past and have a history of known allergic reactions can be given antihistamines prior to the transfusion.

Rh factor. Besides ABO blood grouping, blood typing also determines the Rh factor. The Rh- antigen, sometimes known as Rh (D), is also found in the cell membranes of RBCs. Patients that have the Rh factor are said to be Rh positive while patients who do not have the Rh factor are said to be Rh negative. Similar to ABO typing, Rh factor is determined by exposing a sample of the patient's blood to Rh antibodies. If the Rh antigen is present, the blood cells will clump and the patient will be recorded as being Rh positive. Patients who are Rh+ may receive blood from a patient that is Rh+ or Rh-, but Rh- patients can only receive Rh- blood. Unlike in ABO blood type, Rh+ antibodies develop in people who are Rh- only on exposure. Subsequent exposures of Rh+ blood in people who are Rh- will cause an antibody reaction and thus a transfusion reaction. The transfusion reaction that occurs when Rh- recipient is exposed to Rh+ blood is less severe than ABO transfusion reactions but not without consequence. Rh incompatibility is seen most commonly in pregnancy. Fortunately, this incompatibility can be prevented. The first step in preventing hemolytic disease of the newborn (HDN) is to find out the Rh types of the expectant parents. If the mother is Rh negative and the father is Rh positive, the baby is at risk for developing HDN. The next step is to test the mother's serum to make sure she does not already have anti-Rh (also called anti-D) antibodies from a previous pregnancy or transfusion. Finally, the Rh-negative mother is given an injection of Rh immune globulin (RhIg) at 27 to 28 weeks of gestation, and again after delivery, if the baby is Rh positive. The RhIg attaches to any Rh-positive cells from the baby in the mother's bloodstream, preventing them from triggering anti-D antibody production in the mother. An Rh-negative woman also should receive RhIg after a miscarriage, abortion, or ectopic pregnancy.

DISORDERS OF THE HEMATOLOGIC SYSTEM

The hematologic and lymphatic systems include the blood and the organs of blood production, the bone marrow, and lymphatic tissue. Disorders of blood production, bone marrow, or lymphatic tissues affect all body systems. Disturbances in this delicate balance can produce life-threatening signs and symptoms, severe pain, and incapacitation.

DISORDERS ASSOCIATED WITH ERYTHROCYTES

ANEMIA

Anemia is a condition in which there is a below-normal amount of RBCs, causing a decrease in Hgb and Hct. These decreases directly impact all body systems as oxygen carrying capacity is reduced. Anemias can occur due to a deficiency in the production of erythrocytes, destruction of the erythrocytes, or due to bleeding. Impaired production of RBCs can occur due to bone marrow depression, bone marrow disease, or nutritional deficiencies, acting alone or in combination. Bone marrow depression and disease may be of shorter relative duration when occurring with cancer treatments or may be longer depending on disease process. Likewise, nutritional-related anemias can give rise to the onset of long-term anemias. Destruction of erythrocytes may occur due to mismatched blood transfusions and diseases such as sickle cell anemia and thalassemia. It is also possible for destruction of erythrocytes to occur due to autoimmune processes as is the case with autoimmune hemolytic anemia. Another cause of anemias is bleeding, which can occur from the GI tract (peptic ulcers, diverticulosis, ulcerative colitis, colon cancer), due to prolonged menstrual periods, during surgeries, and traumatic events.

Anemias can be classified as chronic or acute. Chronic anemias occur when there is a gradual decline in RBCs, Hct, and Hgb. The gradual decrease allows for the body's compensatory mechanisms to take effect. Thus, patients with chronic anemias may be asymptomatic or show few symptoms on exertion such as tachycardia and fatigue. Acute anemias cause a rapid decline in RBCs, Hct, and Hgb. This rapid decline does not allow for the body's compensatory mechanisms to take effect, causing symptoms in patients. Normally, healthy patients experiencing acute anemias can lose up to 20% blood volume without experiencing symptoms, as their body will compensate via reflex vasospasm and redistribution of blood flow to vital organs (Adler & Tambe, 2020).

Clinical Manifestations

Clinical manifestations for anemias are dependent on patient health status, patient activity level, and whether the anemia experienced is acute or chronic. Patients with chronic anemias may show no symptoms and the anemia may be discovered incidentally on routine labs. Some common symptoms experienced in anemias include general malaise, heart palpitations, shortness of breath on exertion, dizziness, and lightheadedness. Patients may also notice that their extremities are colder than before the onset of anemia.

Symptoms of acute anemias will also depend on patient condition prior to the onset of the anemia. Patients who are active and have no comorbid conditions may not manifest symptoms until after 20% blood loss. Symptoms experienced include hypotension, respiratory distress, changes in mental status, chest pain, and cold and clammy extremities. Without correction, patients experience hypovolemic shock, myocardial infarction (MI), stroke, and death.

Assessment

Subjective data commonly include complaints of weakness, dyspnea, fatigue, and vertigo. Anorexia and dyspepsia may accompany headache and insomnia, but the patient generally does not link these complaints to the condition unless questioned. In older adult patients with impaired cardiopulmonary reserves, be alert to complaints of chest pain, dyspnea on exertion, palpitations, and dizziness.

Collection of objective data includes observing signs of bleeding or shock (hypovolemic anemia). Laboratory values show a low RBC count along with low Hct and Hgb levels. Skin and mucous membranes are pale, and cardiac symptoms are related to anemia.

Diagnostic Tests

The CBC of a patient with anemia typically shows a low RBC count and below-normal Hgb and Hct levels. Serum iron, total iron-binding capacity, and serum ferritin levels also may be below normal. Serum folate (also called *folic acid*) may be measured if certain types of anemia are suspected. The reticulocyte (i.e., immature RBC) count may be increased because of the presence of high numbers of immature RBCs. A bone marrow study shows a deviation from normal findings. Peripheral blood smears enable identification of abnormalities in the shape and color of blood cells. A megaloblastic anemia profile reveals decreased levels of vitamin B_{12}.

Medical Management

Intervention depends on the cause. Correction of the disease process may correct or lessen the anemic condition. Transfusion is appropriate for blood loss; iron, folate, or vitamin B_{12} are replaced if these are deficient. Treatment is often specific to the particular anemia (see the Cultural Considerations box).

Cultural Considerations

Jehovah's Witness Opposition to Blood Transfusion

The nurse providing culturally appropriate nursing interventions to a Jehovah's Witness has many factors to consider. It should be noted that individuals of this religion may vary in their choice. It is important for the nurse to determine the preference for every patient. Jehovah's Witnesses, typically, are opposed to homologous blood transfusion (blood obtained from a blood bank or through donations). This is based on religious beliefs and not fear of potential risks of receiving a transfusion. Some Jehovah's Witnesses may agree to certain types of autologous blood transfusions (sometimes called *autotransfusions*). One type of autologous transfusion that may be acceptable is blood retrieved through induced hemodilution at the start of surgery. This blood conservation technique involves removing blood from a patient—either immediately before or shortly after induction of anesthesia—while simultaneously replacing the blood with an equivalent volume of a blood volume expander (e.g., crystalloid [sodium chloride] and/or colloid). The withdrawn blood is anticoagulated and maintained at room temperature in the operating room for up to 8 hours. It is reinfused into the patient as needed during or after the surgical procedure (JPAC, 2020).

The consensus of the US Supreme Court has been that an adult—that is, a person who has reached the age of majority—has the right to refuse treatment but does not have the right to withhold a potentially life-saving treatment from a minor child.

Some Jehovah's Witnesses allow the use of certain blood volume expanders (colloids). Many Jehovah's Witnesses carry a document called an Advance Decision Document with the types of blood volume expanders permitted. Ask the patient for this card or, if the patient is unconscious, examine the patient's personal belongings to find this extremely important card (JPAC, 2020).

Nursing Interventions and Patient Teaching

Patient problems and interventions for the patient with anemia include but are not limited to the following:

PATIENT PROBLEM	NURSING INTERVENTIONS
Compromised Blood Flow to Tissue (cardiovascular), related to reduction of cellular components necessary for delivery of oxygen to the cells	Monitor changes in vital signs and change in LOC; Monitor for cardiac rhythms; Monitor Hgb, Hct, and RBCs; Assess baseline arterial blood gases and electrolytes; Note presence and degree of dyspnea, cyanosis; Administer blood products as ordered; Monitor for blood transfusion reactions

PATIENT PROBLEM	NURSING INTERVENTIONS
Insufficient Oxygenation, related to deficient: RBCs, Hgb, Hct	Evaluate ability to manage activities of daily living (ADLs), related to oxygen decrease; Assess activity tolerance, dyspnea, heart rate, oxygen saturation, nail beds for cyanosis; Observe for cyanosis, hypoxia, and hypercapnia; Maintain bed rest as necessary and provide range-of-motion (ROM) exercise; Monitor oxygen saturations frequently by pulse oximetry; Administer oxygen as ordered; Explain activity–oxygen deficit relationship
Inability to Tolerate Activity, related to: Tissue hypoxia, Dyspnea	Plan care to conserve energy after periods of activity; Encourage the patient to limit visitors, phone calls, and unnecessary interruptions to conserve energy; Assist the patient with self-care activities as needed; Place articles within easy reach of the patient to reduce physiologic demands on the body; Administer oxygen as ordered to relieve dyspnea; Monitor Hgb and Hct levels

Hct, Hematocrit; *Hgb,* hemoglobin; *LOC,* level of consciousness; *RBCs,* red blood cells.

Tailor patient education to the individual's condition and needs.

Hypoproliferative anemias. A hypoproliferative anemia occurs when the bone marrow fails to produce an adequate number of RBCs. RBC production requires healthy and functioning bone marrow and a supply of nutrients. Anemias that fall into this category include aplastic anemia, iron deficiency anemia, and megaloblastic anemia.

Aplastic Anemia

Etiology and pathophysiology. Aplastic anemia is a rare disorder that is more common in teens, young adults, and older adults, though it can occur at any age. The incidence of aplastic anemia is low, affecting approximately 0.7 to 4.1 per million population each year, and is two to three times more prevalent in Asia than North America and Europe (Zhu, Gao, Hu, et al., 2020). It can occur as an inherited disorder, but it is mostly acquired. The acquired forms of aplastic anemia can occur due to any number of reasons including exposure to toxins, medications, radiation, hepatitis, HIV, Epstein-Barr virus, and pregnancy (Medline Plus, 2018). However, the majority of cases are idiopathic (unknown cause) and thought to occur as an autoimmune condition where the body's T-cells attack stem cells in the bone marrow, causing damage (Zhu, Gao, Hu, et al., 2020). In aplastic anemia, stem cells in the bone marrow are damaged or destroyed. This causes either a reduction or cessation in the production of erythrocytes, thrombocytes, and leukocytes, a condition known as pancytopenia.

Clinical manifestations. The signs and symptoms of aplastic anemia may have an acute onset or may develop slowly over several weeks to months. These signs and symptoms are directly related to the decreased levels of erythrocytes, thrombocytes, and leukocytes in circulation. Decreased erythrocyte levels cause a concomitant decrease in hemoglobin levels, thus decreasing oxygen carrying capacity. Patients experience the symptoms of anemia such as fatigue, shortness of breath, dizziness, headaches, cold hands and feet, and pallor. A reduction in leukocytes within the circulation results in more frequent and recurrent infections causing symptoms such as fevers, rashes, and flu-like symptoms. Thrombocytopenia results in petechiae, easy bruising or bleeding including from the nose and gums, and blood in the stool. The smallest injury may cause prolonged bleeding to occur.

Assessment. Subjective data include a detailed interview and history relating to chemical exposures, medications the patient may be taking, incidences of infections, and potential exposure to radiation.

Collection of objective data includes monitoring the patient for pallor, shortness of breath, fatigue, tachycardia, chest pain, cold extremities, signs of infection, and bleeding tendencies.

Diagnostic tests. The diagnosis of aplastic anemia begins with a CBC that reveals pancytopenia. A definitive diagnosis can be made with a bone marrow aspiration and biopsy that will show either a hypoplastic or aplastic bone marrow replaced with fat. Post bone marrow studies, aplastic anemia is staged based on the number of cells present into either moderate, severe, or very severe (Johns Hopkins Medicine, n.d.). Other tests conducted include viral studies, liver and kidney studies, levels of vitamin B_{12} and folic acid, CT, and ultrasound scans. These tests help clinicians navigate through potential causes of aplastic anemia, including perhaps an idiopathic cause.

Medical management. When medications such as cimetidine, anticonvulsants, sulfonamides, or chloramphenicol are identified as the cause of aplastic anemia,

the patient is treated by immediately stopping these medications. Bone marrow suppression is expected with certain antineoplastic medications or radiation therapy. In these cases, patients are treated with drugs known as colony-stimulating factors. Filgrastim, pegfilgrastim, and sargramostim stimulate the bone marrow to produce more WBCs; epoetin alfa stimulates stem cells in the bone marrow to produce RBCs; and eltrombopag stimulates production of platelets.

Patients diagnosed with moderate aplastic anemia are generally not treated and monitored via symptoms and lab values. Patients with severe or very severe aplastic anemia, without a HLA-matched sibling donor, and over the age of 35 are treated with immunosuppressive medications (Zhu, Gao, Hu, et al., 2020). Common immunosuppressive therapies used include anti-thymocyte globulin (which kills T-cells) and cyclosporine (which inhibits T-cell proliferation) (Shetty, Narendra, Adiraju, et al., 2016). Patients experiencing complications such as petechiae and bleeding are treated with platelet transfusions, and those experiencing symptoms of anemia due to low RBC levels are transfused packed red blood cells (PRBCs). Multiple blood transfusions carry the complication of iron overload that requires chelation therapy or the possibility of the patient developing antibodies to the transfused blood. Infections are treated and prevented with the use of antibiotics and antivirals.

Patients with severe or very severe aplastic anemia, with a HLA-matched sibling donor, and under the age of 35 are treated with a HSCT (discussed earlier) (Zhu, Gao, Hu, et al., 2020).

Nursing interventions and patient teaching. Proper observation and care after bone marrow study are essential. Patients with aplastic anemia are highly susceptible to infection; thus nursing interventions should be directed toward prevention. Adhere to strict aseptic techniques for dressing changes and intravenous (IV) site care. To prevent impaired skin and mucous membranes, avoid intramuscular injections, administration of rectal medications, and measurement of rectal temperatures. An air mattress can help protect the patient's skin. In the presence of thrombocytopenia, observe carefully for any signs of bleeding and prevent any risk for injury. Monitor the patient's urine and stool for occult or gross blood.

Patient problems and interventions for the patient with aplastic anemia include, but are not limited to, Inability to Tolerate Activity, related to inadequate tissue oxygenation; and Potential for Infection, related to increased susceptibility.

Patients with aplastic anemia need to know how to protect themselves from excessive bleeding. Help the patient maintain a balance between rest and activity. Discuss with the patient how to avoid infection, especially of the respiratory or urinary tract (see the Safety Alert box).

Safety Alert

Aplastic Anemia

- Avoid contact with those who have infection.
- Avoid enemas or other rectal insertions.
- Avoid excessive workload or heavy lifting, and ask for assistance with strenuous activity.
- Avoid intramuscular injections.
- Avoid picking or blowing the nose forcefully.
- Avoid sharing eating utensils and bath linens.
- Avoid trauma, falls, bumps, and cuts; avoid contact sports.
- Avoid use of aspirin or over-the-counter (OTC) aspirin preparations (anticoagulant effect).
- Bathe or shower every day (or every other day if skin is dry); keep perineal area clean.
- Decrease activity if shortness of breath, dizziness, or sensation of heaviness in extremities occurs.
- Eliminate intake of raw meats, fruits, or vegetables.
- Immediately report signs of infection to health care provider.
- Increase time necessary for routine care.
- Keep mouth clean and free of debris.
- Observe for signs such as blood in urine or stool and petechiae, and report these to health care provider.
- Prevent fatigue.
- Prevent hemorrhage.
- Prevent infection.
- Report signs of increased fatigue.
- Take frequent rest periods between activities of daily living (ADLs).
- Use a soft toothbrush or swab for mouth care.
- Use adequate lubrication and gentleness during sexual intercourse.
- Use an electric razor.
- Use good hand hygiene technique.
- Use good oral hygiene.

Box 7.1 Signs of Hypovolemia

- Anxiety or agitation
- Confusion
- Cool, clammy skin
- Decreased or no urine output
- Diaphoresis
- General weakness
- Hypotension
- Low body temperature
- Pale skin color (pallor)
- Pulse weak and thready
- Rapid breathing
- Tachycardia
- Unconsciousness

Box 7.2 Causes of Iron Deficiency Anemia

- Blood loss is a major cause of iron deficiency in adults. The major sources of chronic blood loss are from the gastrointestinal (GI) and genitourinary systems. Common causes of GI blood loss are peptic ulcers, gastritis, esophagitis, diverticulitis, hemorrhoids, and neoplasms. The average monthly menstrual blood loss is about 45 mL and causes the loss of 22 mg of iron.
- Daily iron intake from food and dietary supplements is adequate to meet the needs of men and older women, but it may be inadequate for those with higher iron needs (e.g., menstruating or pregnant women).
- Iron deficiency may develop from inadequate dietary intake, malabsorption, blood loss, or hemolysis (breakdown of red blood cells).
- Malabsorption of iron may occur after certain types of GI surgery and in malabsorption syndromes. Iron absorption occurs in the duodenum. Malabsorption of iron may involve disease of the duodenum, in which the absorption surface is altered or destroyed.

Prognosis. The prognosis for the patient with aplastic anemia depends on the cause. Aplastic anemia caused due to medications, toxins, and viruses is short term, and any complications can be treated. Aplastic anemia may or may not resolve in pregnant patients after delivery, and women may be susceptible to the disease during future pregnancies. Patients receiving bone marrow transplants fair better, but immunosuppressive therapies work well for patients unable to get a bone marrow transplant. Patients with severe chronic aplastic anemia that doesn't respond to treatment has the poorest prognosis.

Iron Deficiency Anemia

Etiology and pathophysiology. Iron deficiency anemia is a condition that occurs when the mineral iron is not available to make healthy RBCs. Iron is a key ingredient in the construction of hemoglobin, which is a protein on the RBC and the carrier of oxygen. A decrease in the amount of hemoglobin in RBCs creates a concomitant decrease in oxygen saturation in blood, which then decreases the amount of oxygen available to all cells within the body. Common causes of iron deficiency anemia are excessive iron loss, a diet low in iron sources, bleeding from gastric or duodenal ulcers, esophageal varices, hiatal hernias, colonic diverticula, and tumors. The major sources of chronic blood loss are from the GI and genitourinary systems (Box 7.2).

GI bleeding is often not apparent and may exist for a considerable time before being identified. Loss of 50 to 75 mL of blood from the upper GI tract is required for stools to appear black, or *melenic*. The color results from the iron in the RBCs. Blood losses related to menstruation or pregnancy are common causes of iron deficiency anemia in young women. Rarely, excessive losses occur through microhemorrhages into lung tissue or from intestinal parasites. Even without excessive blood loss, iron deficiency anemia can result when the body's demand for iron exceeds its absorption, which commonly occurs in infants, young adolescents, and pregnant women. Iron deficiency anemia also may result from malabsorption of iron caused by diseases such as celiac disease and sprue. Subtotal gastrectomy may lead to iron deficiency caused by *achlorhydria* (loss of hydrochloric acid), occult bleeding, and decreased iron in post gastrectomy diets. Deficiency caused by poor dietary intake is rare in middle-aged adults.

Approximately 1 mg of every 10 to 20 mg (5% to 10%) of iron ingested is absorbed in the duodenum. For example, the average daily iron requirement for infants (older than 6 months), children, adolescents, and adults is between 7 mg and 11 mg. This amount of dietary iron meets the needs of men and older women, but it may be inadequate for people who have higher iron needs (e.g., ill children, pregnant and lactating women).

Clinical manifestations. Symptoms specific to iron deficiency anemia are pallor, glossitis (red, smooth tongue), and brittle nails. Patients may also crave non-nutritive substances such as ice, dirt, and starch, known as Pica. Other signs and symptoms for iron deficiency anemia are those common to all other types of anemias as discussed previously.

Assessment. Collection of subjective data includes complaints of fatigue, cold hands and feet, headache, dizziness or lightheadedness, and reports of craving non-nutritive substances. Patients may also report chest pain and palpitations.

Collection of objective data includes noting the signs, including pallor and tachycardia. Fingernails may be fragile and shaped like the head of a spoon with a central depression and raised borders. Mucous membranes of the mouth may be inflamed (stomatitis), and sore lesions at the corners of the mouth known as angular cheilosis may be present.

Diagnostic tests. The peripheral blood counts show that RBCs, Hgb levels, and Hct are decreased, which points to the presence of anemia. The mean corpuscular volume (MCV) that measures the size and volume of the RBC is low. A low ferritin level is diagnostic for iron deficiency anemia as ferritin stores iron.

Medical management. Administration of iron salts such as ferrous sulfate often is required. In 3 weeks the Hct level should rise 5% to 15%, and the Hgb level should rise by 2 to 5 g/dL. For the body to incorporate 100 mg of iron per day, 900 mg/day is administered. Iron is administered orally or by injection. For patients unable to swallow pills, liquid ferrous sulfate can be administered. Ascorbic acid (vitamin C) has been shown to enhance iron absorption. Food sources of iron include meat, fish, poultry, eggs, green leafy vegetables, whole grains, and dried beans (Box 7.3).

When the patient cannot tolerate oral preparations of iron, parenteral iron therapy is used. The Z-track method of giving iron dextran intramuscularly is preferable to prevent skin staining. Iron sucrose is an IV drug frequently used to treat iron deficiency anemia.

Nursing interventions and patient teaching. Because treatment is directed toward diagnosis and alleviation of the cause, the patient interview is important. Medication therapy for iron replacement is initiated as ordered. Plan for rest periods when fatigue is present. Education about nutritional needs relative to the condition may prevent this anemia (see Box 7.3).

Box 7.3   Food Sources of Nutrients Needed for Erythropoiesis

IRON
- Dark green vegetables: spinach, Swiss chard, kale, greens (dandelion, beet, and turnip)
- Dried fruits: apricots, dates, figs, prunes, and raisins
- Eggs
- Iron-enriched or iron-fortified breads and cereals
- Legumes and nuts
- Muscle meats, especially dark meat from poultry
- Organ meats: liver, kidney, heart, and tongue
- Shellfish
- Whole-grain breads and cereals

FOLIC ACID
- Asparagus, broccoli
- Enriched and fortified breads and cereals
- Fish
- Green, leafy vegetables
- Legumes
- Meat
- Organ meats: Liver
- Whole-grain breads and cereals

VITAMIN B$_{12}$
- Eggs
- Milk and cheese
- Muscle meats
- Organ meats: liver and kidney

AMINO ACIDS
- Eggs
- Fish
- Legumes
- Meat
- Milk and milk products (cheese, ice cream)
- Nuts
- Poultry

VITAMIN C
- Cantaloupe
- Citrus fruits
- Leafy, green vegetables
- Strawberries

Explanation of the side effects of iron therapy is essential to alleviate distress and to extend the therapy for the necessary time (see the Health Promotion box). The patient must know which signs and symptoms are significant and must be reported to the health care provider. Diarrhea or nausea is significant, but black, tarry stools are not (these are expected with iron therapy).

Prognosis. The prognosis is usually good with correction of the underlying cause and compliance with the medical treatment.

Megaloblastic Anemia

Etiology and pathophysiology. Megaloblastic anemia, a type of macrocytic anemia, occurs due to the deficiency of two important vitamins, folic acid (also known as folate, folacin, and vitamin B9) and vitamin B$_{12}$ (cyanocobalamin). In the absence of either folic acid, vitamin B$_{12}$, or both, cells within the bone marrow undergo impaired DNA synthesis, which results in the production of cells that are too big (megaloblasts), not fully developed, and cells that do not live as long as normal RBCs. These megaloblasts crowd the bone marrow, resulting in self-death, as well as the crowding out of and destruction of WBCs and platelets. The cells that do manage to make it out of the bone marrow are fewer in numbers, thus resulting in the finding of pancytopenia (decreased levels of leukocytes,

🏃 Health Promotion

Iron Administration

- Check for constipation or diarrhea. Record color (iron turns stools green to black) and amount of stool.
- Dilute liquid iron preparations in juice or water, and administer with a straw to avoid staining teeth. Provide oral hygiene after taking.
- Do not administer with antacids, because they reduce the absorption of iron.
- Dosages are determined by the elemental iron content of the preparation.
- If a dose is missed, continue with the schedule; do not double a dose.
- If side effects develop, the dose and type of iron supplement may be adjusted. Some people cannot tolerate ferrous sulfate because of the effects of the sulfate base. Ferrous gluconate may be an acceptable substitute.
- Iron is absorbed best from the duodenum and proximal jejunum. Therefore enteric-coated or sustained-release capsules, which release iron farther down in the GI tract, are counterproductive; they are also more expensive.
- Iron is best absorbed in an acidic environment. To avoid binding the iron with food, iron should be taken about an hour before meals, when the duodenal mucosa is most acidic. Taking iron with vitamin C (ascorbic acid) or orange juice, which contains ascorbic acid, also enhances iron absorption. Gastric side effects, however, may necessitate ingesting iron with meals.
- Iron is toxic, and caution must be taken to store iron preparations out of a child's reach.
- Iron may interfere with absorption of oral tetracycline antibiotics (quinolones). Do not take within 2 hours of each other.
- Iron preparations supplement the body's natural iron stores.
- Iron supplements may be contraindicated in peptic ulcer disease.
- Side effects include gastrointestinal (GI) upset (nausea, vomiting), constipation or diarrhea, and green to black stools. Elixir may stain teeth.

thrombocytes, and erythrocytes) on CBC examination. The large RBCs that are released into circulation carry less hemoglobin, which means there is a concomitant decrease in the amount of oxygen carried.

Folic acid is present in foods such as green vegetables (broccoli, Brussel sprouts, kale, cabbage, and spinach), fruits (mango, kiwi, and pomegranate), and liver. Patients who rarely consume uncooked vegetables are at higher risk for folic acid deficiency. The recommended average intake for adults is 400 µg and pregnant women 600 µg. Approximately 5 mg of folic acid is stored in the liver. This store is depleted in 3 to 4 months' time if diet is deficient of all folic acid. Besides an inadequate diet, folic acid deficiency can occur in the presence of alcoholism, malabsorption disorders (celiac disease, jejunal resection), malnutrition, due to medications such as anticonvulsants or

anticancer agents, hemodialysis, and hemolysis (Hariz & Bhattacharya, 2020).

Vitamin B_{12} is obtained through dietary sources such as meat, fish, eggs, and dairy products. Two to 3 mg of vitamin B_{12} is stored in the liver and in the absence of dietary vitamin B_{12}, the amount of vitamin B_{12} stored in the liver would deplete over the span of 2 to 4 years. Vitamin B_{12} deficiency can develop in patients who are strict vegans who do not consume any dairy or meat products. Another cause of vitamin B_{12} deficiency is malabsorption. Oral absorption of vitamin B_{12} occurs with the help of intrinsic factor that is produced by the parietal cells in the gastric mucosa. Vitamin B_{12} and intrinsic factor travel to the duodenum and jejunum where they are bound together. The bound intrinsic factor-vitamin B_{12} complex is then absorbed by the terminal portion of the ileum. Diseases such as Crohn affect the ileum and would lead to a decrease in the absorption of vitamin B_{12}. Other disorders that affect vitamin B_{12} absorption include bariatric surgery, gastrectomy, chronic use of histamine blockers, overuse of antacids or proton pump inhibitors, Zollinger-Ellison syndrome, and pancreatic insufficiency. Patients may also be deficient in vitamin B_{12} due to a deficiency in the production of intrinsic factor. Without intrinsic factor, orally consumed vitamin B_{12} is unable to be absorbed. Anemia that occurs due to a lack of intrinsic factor is known as **pernicious anemia**.

Clinical manifestations. The symptoms from megaloblastic anemia are insidious and may not manifest until the stores of folic acid, vitamin B_{12}, or both are depleted. Symptoms common to all types of anemia are also present in megaloblastic anemia, such as weakness, fatigue, lightheadedness, and palpitations. These symptoms may not manifest until later. Most of the symptoms of folic acid and vitamin B_{12} deficiency are similar except that vitamin B_{12} deficiency includes neurological symptoms.

Symptoms common to folic acid or vitamin B_{12} deficiency include jaundice, angular cheilosis, brittle ridged concave nails, and sore red beefy tongue. Some patients may experience GI symptoms such as weight loss, loss of appetite, nausea, constipation, or diarrhea.

Neurological symptoms present in vitamin B_{12} deficiency include confusion, problems concentrating, loss of balance, numbness and tingling in hands and feet, hallucinations, and psychosis.

Assessment. Subjective data include the patient's complaints of palpitations, nausea, flatulence, constipation, diarrhea, and indigestion. The patient may complain that the tongue is tender and burning. Weakness and difficulty in swallowing (dysphagia) may occur. Neurologic symptoms include tingling of the hands and feet and loss of the sense of body position (impaired proprioception).

Collection of objective data includes observation of a smooth and erythematous tongue, brittle ridged concave nails, palpitations, and angular cheilosis. Cerebral signs include mental disorientation, personality changes, and behavior problems. Severe neurologic impairments can result, including partial or total paralysis from destruction of the nerve fibers of the spinal cord. If not treated promptly, the neurological symptoms of vitamin B_{12} deficiency may become permanent.

Diagnostic tests. In addition to the patient's signs and symptoms, several laboratory tests are used to diagnose megaloblastic anemia. The CBC is the most common test and helps in the preliminary diagnosis with the result of low RBC, Hgb, and Hct levels. An examination of the MCV will reveal a value greater than 100 fL (femtoliters). Further testing is required for an accurate diagnosis. These tests include reticulocyte count, which measures the number of RBCs in the blood, indicating if the bone marrow is producing RBCs; serum folate, serum megaloblastic anemia profile (discussed under laboratory and diagnostic tests section); intrinsic factor antibody test (its presence indicates pernicious anemia); and bone marrow aspiration and biopsy if other tests are not conclusive. Patients may also need further testing to determine the cause of the vitamin deficiency if it is not related to diet.

Medical management. Folic acid deficiency is treated with oral supplements of folic acid as well as a folate enriched diet. For patients with folic acid deficiency related to malabsorption, folic acid is administered intramuscularly and can also be administered intravenously. The recommended daily supplementation for folic acid is 1 mg per day. Patients who drink alcohol may need to ingest higher dosages of folic acid if they continue to keep drinking. It takes approximately 2 to 3 months to replace the depleted folic acid stores in the liver.

Vitamin B_{12} deficiency is treated with oral supplementation and changes in diet regimen. Strict vegans need to consume foods such as almond milk, soy milk, plant-based meats, and fortified cereals as sources of vitamin B_{12}. If the presence of vitamin B_{12} deficiency is due to lack of intrinsic factor or malabsorption issues, the patient is given intramuscular vitamin B_{12} injections on a monthly basis. A resolution of malabsorption derived vitamin B_{12} deficiency may allow the patient to ingest oral vitamin B_{12} after the cause of malabsorption is identified and treated. However, vitamin B_{12} deficiency arising from a lack of intrinsic factor will require intramuscular vitamin B_{12} injections for life.

Nursing interventions and patient teaching. The nursing interventions depend to some extent on the stage of the disease. A symptomatic approach is appropriate. When the patient is confined to the hospital, the nurse checks vital signs every 4 hours and performs special mouth care several times daily. The diet should be high in protein, vitamins, and minerals. Anemic patients are especially sensitive to cold, so additional lightweight, warm blankets may be needed. Interventions should conserve energy and prevent injury. The room

temperature may have to be increased for the patient's comfort.

Patient problems and interventions for the patient with megaloblastic anemia include but are not limited to the following:

PATIENT PROBLEM	NURSING INTERVENTIONS
Insufficient Nutrition, related to: • Sore mouth and tongue • Diarrhea • Constipation	Administer folic acid prescribed to promote the production of erythrocytes Administer vitamin B_{12} and other medications prescribed to promote production of erythrocytes Instruct patient on balanced diet high in protein, vitamins, and iron, such as red meat, dairy products, and eggs, to increase intake of vitamin B_{12} Instruct patient to eat uncooked vegetables and liver to increase folate levels Provide meticulous and frequent oral hygiene to promote improved appetite and prevent infection Provide six to eight small meals daily to conserve energy and decrease gastrointestinal distress Monitor patient's bowel movements, noting color, consistency, and amount

Emphasize the importance of continued supplementation of the missing vitamin and adequate diet intake containing the vitamin. Help patients understand that pernicious anemia will require the patient to take monthly vitamin B_{12} injections for life. Patients with neurological deficits due to vitamin B_{12} deficiency may need help with ADLs, frequent rest periods, and are taught to avoid excessive heat or cold.

Prognosis. This condition, if untreated, can be considered terminal in 1 to 3 years. With treatment, folic acid deficiency results in cessation of symptoms. Patients with vitamin B_{12} deficiency who have been left untreated for a while may never fully recover from the neurological manifestations.

Hemolytic anemias. Hemolytic anemias occur when erythrocytes are destroyed faster than they can be produced. Sickle cell anemia is a type of hemolytic anemia.

Sickle Cell

Sickle cell trait. Sickle cell trait is a term given to an individual that has a genetic mutation for hemoglobin that gives rise to the production of an abnormal hemoglobin. The normally occurring hemoglobin is referred to as HbA, and it remains soluble in water and does not precipitate in the presence of hypoxia. This aspect allows RBCs to remain in solution and maintain their biconcave shape. The hemoglobin caused by the gene mutation is referred to as HbS, and in the presence of hypoxia, all the hemoglobin S contained in a RBCs starts to polymerize or link up, causing the RBC to become sickle shaped. This sickle-shaped RBC then falls out of solution and starts to clump with other RBCs (Mangla, Ehsan, & Maruvada, 2020). Patients with sickle cell trait inherit the normal gene for hemoglobin from one parent and an abnormal hemoglobin gene from the other parent. Therefore, genetically speaking, a patient with sickle cell trait is heterozygous for hemoglobin. The presence of a normal hemoglobin (HbA) gene offsets many of the effects of the abnormal hemoglobin gene, therefore these patients do not have sickle cell disease and are not susceptible to vaso-occlusive crisis. However, some sickle cell trait patients when exposed to favorable conditions such as severe hypoxia, dehydration, hypothermia, hyperthermia, and release of inflammatory cells experience sickling of RBCs. The sickled RBCs clog tiny capillaries most especially in the bones and attract inflammatory cells and platelets that cause RBCs to adhere even more. Any organ may be affected, and multiple attacks could cause damage due to ischemia. The occurrence of sickle cell trait is 9% among the African American population and 0.2% among Caucasians. It is estimated that there are approximately 300 million people worldwide with sickle cell trait, and migration patterns will cause the number of people with sickle cell trait in the Western part of the world to rise. In all 50 US states, babies are tested for sickle cell trait before discharge (Ashorobi, Ramsey, Yarrarapu, et al., 2020).

Sickle Cell Anemia

Etiology and pathophysiology. Sickle cell disease is the most common genetic disorder in the United States, predominantly affecting those of African or Eastern Mediterranean heritage. It is estimated that sickle cell disease affects approximately 100,000 Americans or 1 out of every 365 African Americans (Mangla, Ehsan, & Maruvada, 2020). Sickle cell disease occurs when an individual inherits an abnormal hemoglobin S gene from both parents. In the presence of hypoxia, hemoglobin S polymerizes to form a sickle shape that then causes the RBC to fall out of solution and clump with other sickled RBCs. As the disease is inherited, patients with sickle cell disease manifest symptoms after 6 months of age, as the presence of remaining fetal hemoglobin provides protection against sickling (Mangla, Ehsan, & Maruvada, 2020). The most common symptom experienced is a vaso-occlusive crisis, which occurs when sickled RBCs clump together and get trapped in microcirculation along with trapping other cells such as leukocytes. The entrapment causes tissue hypoxia, inflammation, and necrosis to the tissue or organ being perfused. When circulation is restored, the clumped cells have lysed, which releases substances that cause further damage to the vessels in the area. The patient experiences severe pain and symptoms of the tissue or organ experiencing ischemia. Patients may also experience sequestration crisis, which occurs when sickled cells pool in an organ. The most common site for this occurrence is the spleen, and many children experience splenic infarction. In adults, the organs most likely involved in sequestration include the liver and the lungs. In addition, the hemolysis of RBCs causes a decrease in RBCs, Hgb, and HCT levels, and the patient experiences the signs and symptoms of anemia. Sickling of RBCs occurs during times of physical and emotional stress. As the sickling process takes time, quick administration of oxygen reverses the sickling process thus decreasing or arresting crisis.

Clinical manifestations. Symptoms of sickle cell anemia vary over time and can be multifactorial. Most patients with sickle cell anemia suffer from chronic anemia due to the hemolysis of sickled cells, which have a lifespan of 10 to 20 days. The chronic anemia leads to decreased oxygen levels and constant fatigue. Patients experience pain crisis brought on by ischemia secondary to sickled cells. The pain varies and can last from a few hours to weeks. Severe pain may require hospitalization. Infections and the signs and symptoms of infection are common due to a damaged spleen unable to perform its immune functions. Sickled cells may also damage the retina, leading to vision problems (Mayo Clinic, 2020).

Assessment. Collection of subjective data begins with assessing the patient's knowledge and feelings about the disease and factors that appear to precipitate crisis or exacerbate signs and symptoms. Fatigue may be reported when anemia is severe. The primary symptom associated with sickling is pain in the joints, especially those of the hands and feet. Abdominal pain is common with swelling of the spleen and engorgement of vital organs. Hypoxia occurs as fever and pain increase, causing the patient to breathe rapidly. A male patient may have a continuous painful erection (priapism) from impaired blood flow out of the erect penis. The pain associated with these attacks often is described as deep, gnawing, and throbbing.

Further collection of objective data includes observing for abdominal enlargement and jaundice, edema of the extremities, and signs of hemorrhage. As a result of the accelerated RBC breakdown, the patient has a characteristic clinical finding of hemolysis (jaundice, elevated serum bilirubin levels).

Diagnostic tests. Electrophoresis of Hgb from a patient with sickle cell anemia is specific for detecting sickle cell crisis or anemia. More than 80% of sickle cell Hgb as shown by electrophoresis is Hb-S, not Hb-A. A stained blood smear detects anemia only. The RBC, Hct, and Hgb levels are below normal values. WBCs are increased with infection. Skeletal x-rays demonstrate bone and joint deformities and flattening. MRI may be used to diagnose a stroke caused by occluded cerebral vessels from sickled cells.

Medical management. Sickle cell anemia has no specific treatment. Treatment is symptomatic, alleviating the symptoms that result from complications. Treatment should include adequate hydration, antibiotics for infections, and nonsteroidal anti-inflammatory (NSAIDs) medications for pain. *Haemophilus influenzae*, pneumococcal conjugate, meningococcal, and hepatitis immunizations should be administered to prevent infections. A bone marrow transplant, which infuses healthy stem cells into the bone marrow, may be performed in select patients to treat severe cases of the disease. The challenge is finding a match for transplantation (Mayo Clinic, 2020). Sickle cell crisis may require hospitalization. Oxygen may be administered to alter hypoxia and control sickling. Encourage rest and administer fluids and electrolytes intravenously to reduce blood viscosity and maintain renal function. Use analgesics to treat pain. Sickle cell crisis pain often is undertreated. The nurse needs a clear understanding of the disease process and of current approaches to pain management.

Opioid pain management is often necessary when NSAIDs are no longer effective. Patient-controlled analgesia may be used during an acute crisis. After discharge, patients may continue taking oral opioid analgesics for a period of time. Blood transfusion of packed RBCs may be necessary to treat severe anemia. However, frequent transfusions can cause high levels of iron to build up in the body. *Chelation* therapy, a medicine to reduce the amount of iron in the body and the problems that iron overload causes, may be prescribed (NHLBI, 2017). These patients have an increased need for folic acid, so it is important that they take daily supplements. Iron therapy generally is not suggested.

Another medication, hydroxyurea, currently is being prescribed as maintenance therapy to help prevent anemia and to prevent acute episodes of pain (Mayo Clinic, 2020). This medication boosts the levels of fetal Hgb (Hb-F). This lowers the concentration of Hb-S within a cell, resulting in less polymerization of the abnormal Hgb.

Nursing interventions and patient teaching. Supportive treatment depends on the signs and symptoms: hydration and analgesia during crises, and dilution of blood with increased fluid intake to reverse sickling. Monitoring the transfusion therapy for evidence of transfusion reaction is vital. Attention to fever and infection is important. Genetic counseling is indicated.

A patient problem and interventions for the patient with sickle cell anemia include but are not limited to the following:

PATIENT PROBLEM	NURSING INTERVENTIONS
Recent Onset of Pain, related to thrombotic crisis	Place patient in proper anatomic alignment, and protect joints
	Position patient by slow, gentle handling
	Apply warmth with soaks or compresses to relieve discomfort
	Give analgesics on a fixed time schedule to maintain a steady serum drug level, which improves pain control, minimizes complications, and decreases anxiety
	Medications may be administered by the nurse or a patient-controlled analgesic infusion pump provides a constant, low-dose infusion of an opioid for excellent pain control

Alert the patient to the need for family testing to determine the presence of Hb-S; genetic counseling is available for carriers. Explain how to avoid sickle cell crises: avoid high altitudes, flying in unpressurized planes, dehydration, extreme temperatures, iced liquids, alcohol, and vigorous exercise; use stress reduction methods. Patients should not smoke and should protect extremities from injury because of impaired circulation. Patients with sickle cell disease have frequent problems with infections. It is important for the patient to remain current with vaccinations and take prophylactic antibiotics to protect against these infections. Explain that young pregnant women with sickle cell anemia have a high risk for developing pulmonary and/or renal complications. Alert the patient to the signs and symptoms of increased intracranial pressure and to the need to blow the nose gently, avoid coughing, and avoid straining on elimination.

Practice ROM exercises with the patient and encourage regular physical activity to prevent bone demineralization. Instruct the patient in the need for a balance between rest (physical and mental) and activity, such as ROM and isometric exercises. Also discuss the principles of good nutrition, such as the importance of protein, calcium, vitamins, and adequate fluids. Provide patient education on how to monitor oral intake, urinary output, and urine protein.

Prognosis. The prognosis for sickle cell disease is guarded with treatment aimed at ensuring a good quality of life. Vaso-occlusive crisis, sequestration, and chronic anemia cause pain disability, depression, economic loss, infections, and joint damage. Patients are disabled for life, and premature death is common (Mangla, Ehsan, & Maruvada, 2020).

Hypovolemic anemia (anemia resulting from blood loss)

Etiology and pathophysiology. Secondary anemia occurs when deficiencies in RBCs and other components are caused by an abnormally low circulating blood volume resulting from acute or chronic blood loss. Loss of blood decreases the amount of circulating fluid and Hgb and thus decreases the amount of oxygen carried to the body tissues. The tissues must have oxygen to survive. The average adult has an approximate total blood volume of 6000 mL (6 L [12 pints]) and can tolerate a loss of up to 500 mL. Blood loss of 1000 mL or more in an adult can have severe consequences. This level of reduction in total blood volume can lead to hypovolemic shock. Such a loss usually is related to internal or external hemorrhage caused by a surgical procedure, GI bleeding, menorrhagia (abnormally prolonged menstrual bleeding), trauma, or severe burns. The rapidity of blood loss is related to the severity and number of signs and symptoms.

Clinical manifestations. Signs and symptoms include restlessness; a subtle rise in respiratory rate; weakness; stupor; irritability; a pale, cool, moist skin; and a rapid, thready pulse (see Box 7.1). Excessive blood loss results in shock. Shock occurs when there is a deprivation of oxygen and nutrients to organs. Hemorrhagic blood loss results in a decrease in blood volume. In shock, vasoconstriction occurs in blood vessels to noncritical organs such as skin, muscles, and intestines. This decreases the blood flow to these organs and shunts blood to the vital organs such as the heart and the brain.

The greater the amount of blood loss, the more the heart rate and blood pressure are affected. The body is able to compensate for blood loss less than 15% or 750 mL. The initial symptom may be only tachycardia, although there can be an initial rise in systolic blood pressure, then a fall to below 80 mm Hg. At 20% to 25% blood loss, tachycardia and mild to moderate hypotension are present. With a loss of 40% or greater (2000 mL), all clinical signs and symptoms of shock are present.

Hypovolemic anemia in a child often results in differing signs and symptoms initially than in adults. The child may be alert and have normal blood pressure, pulse, and perfusion initially. Signs and symptoms may progress to cool and clammy skin, hypotension, tachycardia, tachypnea, and reduced urine output. Treatment is similar to adults. IV fluid administration is the first treatment. If fluid administration is not effective, blood administration may be necessary.

The patient's clinical signs and symptoms of hypovolemic anemia are equally as important as the laboratory values. Be alert to the patient's expression of pain. Internal hemorrhage may cause pain because of tissue distention, organ displacement, and nerve compression. Pain may be localized or referred (*referred pain* is felt at a place other than where the damage actually is).

Decreased RBC, Hgb, and Hct levels decrease for 24 to 48 hours after blood loss until the plasma volume is replaced with blood or blood components (Maakaron, 2019). The severity of the patient's signs and symptoms correlates with the severity of the blood loss.

Assessment. Subjective data commonly include complaints of thirst, weakness, irritability, and restlessness.

Objective data include decreased blood pressure; rapid, weak, thready pulse; and rapid respirations. Cold, clammy skin with pallor is noted. Oliguria (urine output less than 400 mL in 24 hours) is often evident. Mental disorientation and physical collapse with prostration can occur.

Diagnostic tests. When blood loss is sudden and plasma volume has not yet had a chance to increase, the loss of RBCs is not reflected in laboratory data, and values may seem normal or high for 2 to 3 days. However, once the plasma is replaced, the RBC mass is less concentrated. RBC, Hgb, and Hct levels are severely decreased, often to half the normal values.

Medical management. In the case of massive hemorrhage, measures are taken to stop the blood loss and treat for shock and lost volume. Severe hemorrhaging often results in the need for mechanical ventilation. Oxygen therapy restores oxygen that is less available because of decreased Hgb in the blood. To replace fluid volume, IV saline is administered. In severe fluid volume depletion, a bolus of 2 L of normal saline (i.e., a 0.9% NaCl solution) is given. Current guidelines from the American Association of Blood Banks (AABB) recommend transfusing packed RBCs when the Hgb falls below 7 g/dL for the patient in an acute care setting or in the intensive care setting (ICU), and when the Hgb falls below 8 g/dL for the patient who is symptomatic for anemia, for the preoperative and postoperative cardiac and orthopedic patient, and the patient with cardiovascular disease. Often platelets, fresh frozen plasma (FFP), or cryoprecipitate is included in the treatment to control hemorrhage (Maerz, 2019).

Monitor the Hgb level to note the effectiveness of the treatment. One unit of packed RBCs should increase the Hgb level by 1 g/dL or raise the Hct by 3%. The patient also may need supplemental iron because the availability of iron affects the marrow production of erythrocytes. Oral or parenteral iron preparations often are administered.

Nursing interventions and patient teaching. Monitor blood and fluid restoration and identify blood loss sites to control the bleeding. Keep the patient flat and warm. Take vital signs at frequent intervals (every 15 minutes or more frequently) until the systolic blood pressure is above 90 mm Hg. Take precautions to prevent injury to a restless or disoriented patient. Measure intake and output (I&O), with careful monitoring of urinary output for oliguria caused by decreased renal perfusion. The decrease in urinary output correlates to the amount of blood lost.

If hemorrhage is caused by a chronic problem, teach the patient to monitor bleeding amounts and associated factors and to report to the health care provider immediately for treatment.

Prognosis. Without treatment, death results. With aggressive treatment, the prognosis is favorable.

Polycythemia (Erythrocytosis)

Etiology and pathophysiology. The two types of polycythemia are *primary polycythemia (polycythemia vera)* and *secondary polycythemia.* Their causes and pathophysiology differ, although their complications and clinical manifestations are similar and yet at times different.

Polycythemia vera is a rare blood disorder that occurs due to an acquired, not inherited, mutation in the JAK2 gene (Accurso, Santoro, & Mancuso, 2020) that affects a precursor blood forming cell in the bone marrow. The mutation results in an overproduction of particularly RBCs but also WBCs and platelets because a precursor cell in the myeloid line is affected. The cause of the genetic mutation is unknown, and even though there is no line of direct inheritance, oftentimes more than one family member is afflicted with the disease. Polycythemia vera occurs more commonly in men aged 60 years and older and has a slow progression and symptom onset. An overproduction of cells from the bone marrow results in increased blood viscosity and volume.

Secondary polycythemia can occur at any age and is caused by chronic hypoxia. Chronic hypoxemia occurs in patients for multiple reasons including living in high altitudes where atmospheric oxygen is lower, pulmonary disease, cardiovascular disease, and patients with obstructive sleep apnea. Chronic hypoxemic blood filters through the kidney, which senses low oxygen saturation. In response, the kidney releases erythropoietin, which stimulates the bone marrow to produce more RBCs. Secondary polycythemia occurs due to a physiological response where the body compensates for lower oxygen levels by producing more erythrocytes; no pathological process is in evidence.

Clinical manifestations. *Polycythemia vera* leads to an increased number of erythrocytes within the bloodstream. These extra RBCs cause the blood to be thicker or have an increased viscosity. Blood that is more viscous tends to be more sluggish, which affects multiple organs within the body. A sluggish circulatory process results in hypercoagulability. High platelet counts also contribute to the formation of thrombi. Patients are at an increased risk for blood clots in the deep veins of the arms and legs (deep vein thrombosis [DVT]), the lungs (pulmonary embolism [PE]), the heart (MI), and the brain (cerebrovascular accident [CVA]) (NIH, 2017a). In addition, the viscosity or stickiness of blood results in congestion of tissues all over the body. Viscous blood is harder to pump and therefore results in elevated blood pressure and left ventricular hypertrophy. Angina or congestive heart failure may also result due to thicker blood and tendency for platelets to clump in coronary vessels. The increase in RBCs causes blood to become a hypertonic solution whereby fluid is pulled from cells into the arteries and veins resulting in chronic hypervolemia. Hepatomegaly and splenomegaly, the result of organ engorgement, may contribute to patient complaints of satiety and fullness.

Secondary polycythemia results in an excess of erythrocytes only. Like polycythemia vera, patients are at risk for blood clots, left ventricular hypertrophy, congestive heart failure, and chronic hypervolemia. Hepatomegaly and splenomegaly are also common.

Assessment. Subjective symptoms may include largely asymptomatic patients to those presenting with a host of symptoms. Patient with either polycythemia vera or secondary polycythemia may complain of fatigue, abdominal fullness or discomfort, headaches, ringing in the ears, blurred vision, burning or pins-and-needles sensations in the feet, and difficulty breathing. Patients with polycythemia vera may complain of itchy skin or pruritus due to the high basophil count, gout, and bleeding or bruising.

Objective data for patients with polycythemia vera includes high blood pressure, shortness of breath, signs of clots, and an erythemic appearance to the skin. An ultrasound of the abdomen may reveal hepatomegaly and/or splenomegaly.

Diagnostic tests. CBC for patients with polycythemia vera reveals high levels of RBCs, Hgb, HCT, WBCs, and thrombocytes. Bone marrow examination reveals hypercellularity in WBCs, RBCs, and platelets. A genetic test reveals a mutation in the JAK2 gene for patients with polycythemia vera. However, erythropoietin levels in plasma are low in patients with polycythemia vera but high in patients with secondary polycythemia or erythrocytosis. The high erythropoietin level in secondary polycythemia is a distinguishing factor. The RBC, Hgb, and HCT levels will also be high in secondary polycythemia.

Medical management. In both polycythemia vera and secondary polycythemia, the mainstay of therapy includes decreasing blood viscosity. In secondary polycythemia, this is accomplished by prescribing low-dose aspirin and repeated phlebotomy. In phlebotomy, roughly 500 mL of blood is removed at a time until the hematocrit level in the body is maintained between 45% and 48%. Phlebotomy immediately relieves certain symptoms such as headaches, ringing of the ears, and dizziness. Patients with polycythemia vera may be managed with phlebotomy alone for many years.

Nursing interventions and patient teaching. Patients with secondary polycythemia are educated to control and avoid situations that lead to low oxygen levels. Therefore, patients are educated on smoking cessation, controlling chronic pulmonary disease, and being compliant with treatment for cardiovascular diseases. In addition, it is important for patients with secondary polycythemia and polycythemia vera to be compliant with taking aspirin as prescribed and attending all appointments for phlebotomy treatments.

The nurse monitors patients with polycythemia for signs and symptoms of fluid overload and dehydration. Intake and output are strictly monitored. A dietitian may assess the patient for nutritional deficiencies due to abdominal discomfort and feelings of fullness. Patients are encouraged to conduct passive or active leg exercises and ambulate as much as tolerated. Patients taking myelosuppressive drugs need to be monitored regularly for side effects. Laboratory studies such as CBC are also conducted regularly. The nurse needs to educate patients regarding symptoms of potential complications such as those associated with DVTs, strokes, PE, and MI.

Patient problems and interventions for the patient with polycythemia vera include but are not limited to the following:

PATIENT PROBLEM	NURSING INTERVENTIONS
Compromised Blood Flow to Tissue (cardiopulmonary, cerebral, gastrointestinal, and peripheral), related to: • Hyperviscosity of fluid • Potential bleeding	Keep patient in a comfortable position, turning frequently to relieve pressure Elevate head of bed, keeping legs in a nondependent position Use range-of-motion exercises to stimulate circulation Assess peripheral pulses and color and temperature of extremities every 4–6 h Assess for blood in urine and stools Assess for thrombus formation Monitor laboratory studies If patient has a bleeding tendency, avoid invasive procedures when possible Avoid trauma; provide education related to activities of daily living Monitor blood pressure Monitor for signs of dehydration such as skin turgor, dry mucus membranes

Prognosis. Polycythemia vera is a chronic, life-shortening disorder. Although the incidence is small, leukemia and lymphomas develop in some patients with polycythemia vera. This may occur as a result of the chemotherapeutic drugs used to treat the disease or may be secondary to a disorder in the stem cells that progresses to leukemia. The major cause of morbidity and mortality from polycythemia vera is thrombosis.

DISORDERS ASSOCIATED WITH LEUKOCYTES

Agranulocytosis
Etiology and pathophysiology. Agranulocytosis is a potentially life threatening and fatal condition that occurs when there is a severe reduction in the number of granulocytes, particularly neutrophils, circulating in blood. The absolute neutrophil count (ANC) is normally 3000

to 7000 cells/mm³. In agranulocytosis, the neutrophil count may be as low as 100 cells/mm³. This decrease in neutrophils is also represented in the WBC count, as 60% to 70% of WBCs are neutrophils. Therefore, a reduction in neutrophils causes a concomitant reduction in leukocytes. The patients' CBC results indicate neutropenia as well as leukopenia.

Agranulocytosis can be inherited or acquired. The inherited form manifests in infancy due to genetic abnormality and causes infantile genetic agranulocytosis. The acquired form of agranulocytosis is rare and occurs in 6 to 8 per million population per year. It also occurs more commonly in women than in men. Of these cases, 70% of agranulocytosis occurs due to medications. Common medications implicated in the cause of agranulocytosis include naproxen, propylthiouracil, procainamide, captopril, clozapine, amitrypiline, chloroquine, phenytoin, penicillin, cephalosporin, cimetidine, ranitidine, chemotherapeutics, and zidovudine, to name a few (Sedhai, Lamichhane, & Gupta, 2020). These medications cause bone marrow suppression, which reduces production of immune cells. Viral and bacterial infections have also been implicated as a cause of agranulocytosis. Other disease processes such as aplastic anemia, leukemia, and myelodysplastic syndrome may also result in this disease.

Clinical manifestations. Fever, chills, headache, and fatigue are symptoms associated with infection and the inflammatory process. Patients present with sores in their mouth, throat, or gums and recurrent chronic infections of the throat and skin. Bronchial pneumonia and urinary tract infections are complications that occur in the later stages.

Assessment. Subjective data include common complaints of fever, extreme fatigue, and infections that last for long periods of time. All medications taken, whether prescription or over-the-counter, are considered as possible causes of the condition. A thorough history may provide relevant cues to the cause of agranulocytosis.

Objective data include fever over 100.6°F (38.1°C). Erythema and pain from ulcerations may occur. Ulcerations are cultured for microorganisms. Lung and bronchial auscultation reveals crackles and rhonchi (course rattling sounds) because of trapped exudates.

Diagnostic tests. The initial workup requires a CBC with differential count that shows an ANC of 100 cells/m³ or less. A peripheral blood smear will reveal a marked decrease or absence of neutrophils. An examination of bone marrow will reveal a presence of large numbers of promyelocytes that, if matured, would have become granulocytes. For patients exhibiting infections, cultures can be obtained to determine the causative agent.

Medical management. The main objective of treatment is to alleviate the factors responsible for bone marrow depression and to prevent or treat infection. Medications contributing to the disease are immediately stopped. It takes roughly 1 to 3 weeks for medication-induced agranulocytosis to resolve (Sedhai, Lamichhane, & Gupta, 2020). Pathogens causing infections are promptly treated. Hematopoietic growth factors are used to stimulate production of granulocytes from the bone marrow. Granulocyte colony-stimulating factor (G-CSF) (filgrastim), pegfilgrastim, and granulocyte-macrophage colony-stimulating factor (GM-CSF) (sargramostim) are given subcutaneously or intravenously. Precautions to prevent infection in the neutropenic (immunocompromised) patient also may be instituted.

Nursing interventions and patient teaching. A patient with a compromised WBC system is highly susceptible to life-threatening infections. Nursing interventions are directed toward protecting the patient from potential sources of infection. Monitor the patient conscientiously to detect the earliest signs of infection so that therapy may be initiated promptly. Restrict visitors and prevent personnel with colds from caring for the patient. Meticulous hand hygiene and universal precautions by medical and nursing personnel and strict asepsis are mandatory.

A patient problem and interventions for the patient with agranulocytosis include but are not limited to the following:

PATIENT PROBLEM	NURSING INTERVENTIONS
Potential for Infection, related to depressed white blood cell (leukocyte) production	Institute neutropenic precautions
	Restrict visitors or medical personnel with bacterial or viral infections
	Provide instruction on handwashing to patient and visitors
	Monitor for signs and symptoms of infection
	Maintain standard precautions
	Use strict asepsis for procedures
	Avoid fresh flowers and plants
	Provide high-protein, high-vitamin, high-calorie soft diet to maintain nutritional status
	Avoid raw foods, such as sushi, Caesar salad dressing (may have raw eggs), blue cheese, and fruits that cannot be peeled or vegetables that cannot be well cleaned
	Encourage increased fluid intake to prevent dehydration
	Monitor vital signs to assess for signs of infection
	Observe the patient for extreme fatigue, sore throat or mouth, and fever as signs of infection
	Monitor laboratory values
	Relieve fever with tepid bath or cooling blanket
	Administer antibiotics as prescribed
	Provide hygiene with adequate rest periods

In patient teaching, discuss the use of frequent and meticulous oral hygiene to treat or prevent mouth and pharyngeal infection. Explain the need to avoid crowds, people with infectious diseases, and cold or hot environments; also teach signs and symptoms of infection and appropriate interventions. Explain the need for a soft, bland diet (if mouth ulcers are present) high in protein, vitamins, and calories. Encourage a balance between rest and activity to prevent fatigue and generalized weakness. Teach the patient to consult a medical provider before taking any over-the-counter medications.

Prognosis. Patients older than 65 years of age, ANC count of less than 100 µL, and pre-existing comorbidities such as renal, cardiac, respiratory, and systemic inflammatory diseases have poorer outcomes and a grim prognosis. Complications including worsening infections and sepsis contribute to adverse prognosis as well.

Leukemia

Etiology and pathophysiology. Leukemia is a malignant disorder of the hematopoietic system in which excessive numbers of abnormal leukocytes accumulate in the bone marrow and lymph nodes. Risk factors include genetics, viral infection, previous treatment with or exposure to radiation, chemotherapeutic agents, smoking, family history, and exposure to certain chemicals such as benzene (Mayo Clinic, 2018).

In leukemia, normal WBCs in the bone marrow are replaced with abnormal numbers and forms of rapidly dividing cells, which then spread to the circulation and infiltrate the lymph nodes, spleen, and other organs, including those of the central nervous system. Leukemic infiltration leads to problems such as hepatomegaly, splenomegaly, lymphadenopathy, bone pain, meningeal irritation, and oral lesions. Hematopoietic function is disrupted by incompetent bone marrow. Increased susceptibility to infection results.

Classification. Leukemia comes in multiple forms and is classified by identifying whether it is acute or chronic and what type of blood cell is involved. There are four common types of leukemia (ACS, 2018):

- *Acute lymphocytic (lymphoblastic) leukemia (ALL):* ALL affects lymphoid cells and grows quickly. Nearly 6000 new cases will be diagnosed annually. The majority of cases are in children under the age of 5 years and in males. After children, the next age group impacted are those over the age of 50 years.
- *Acute myeloid leukemia (AML):* AML affects myeloid cells and grows quickly. More than 19,000 new cases will be diagnosed annually. While it occurs in both adults and children, the majority of cases will be in adults.

- *Chronic lymphocytic leukemia (CLL):* CLL affects *lymphoid cells* (cells that become lymphocytes, often B cells) and usually grows slowly. Approximately 21,000 Americans will be diagnosed each year. The incidence is rare in children and young adults. Diagnosis is most commonly made in the seventh decade of life.
- *Chronic myeloid leukemia (CML):* CML affects *myeloid cells* (cells that become any type of blood cell other than lymphocytes) and usually grows slowly at first. Approximately 8500 cases are diagnosed each year. Most cases involve older adults.

Clinical manifestations. The clinical manifestations of leukemia vary. They relate to problems caused by bone marrow failure and the formation of leukemic infiltrates. Bone marrow failure results from (1) bone marrow overcrowding by abnormal cells and (2) inadequate production of normal marrow elements. The patient is predisposed to anemia and thrombocytopenia.

As leukemia progresses, fewer normal blood cells are produced. The abnormal WBCs continue to accumulate. The leukemic cells infiltrate the patient's organs, leading to problems such as splenomegaly, hepatomegaly, lymphadenopathy, bone pain, meningeal irritation, and oral lesions. Enlarged lymph nodes and painless splenomegaly may be the first signs of the disease in some patients.

Diagnostic tests. A CBC is a test to check the number of WBCs, RBCs, and platelets. Leukemia also may cause low levels of platelets and Hgb, which is found inside RBCs. It can cause the WBC count to be low, elevated, or excessively elevated. Anemia and thrombocytopenia are noted. Bone marrow biopsy shows immature leukocytes. Chest radiographic examination may show mediastinal lymph node and lung involvement and bone changes. Lymph node biopsy reveals excessive blasts (immature cells). Peripheral blood evaluation and bone marrow examination are the primary methods of diagnosing and classifying the type of leukemia. Further studies such as lumbar puncture and CT scan can be performed to determine the presence of leukemic cells outside of the blood and bone marrow.

Assessment. Subjective data include patient history and physical assessment. Patients often have pain in bones or joints, fatigue, malaise, decreased activity tolerance, and irritability.

Objective data include those signs listed in clinical manifestations. Data include laboratory studies of WBCs with differential. Cultures of throat, urine, stool, and blood are obtained to determine which organisms are present. Abnormalities of skin (petechiae, ecchymoses) and mucous membranes (bleeding) may be present.

Medical management. The goal of treatment is to achieve remission or to control the symptoms. Treatment is aimed at eradicating the leukemia with chemotherapy or bone marrow transplant. Combination chemotherapy is the mainstay for treating leukemia. Multiple drugs are used to (1) decrease drug resistance, (2) minimize the drug toxicity by using multiple drugs with varying toxicities (with lower dosages of each), and (3) interrupt cell growth at multiple points in the cell cycle. Observation for drug toxicity is imperative (Table 7.2).

Tremendous progress in the treatment of leukemia has been made in recent years with the use of a complex combination of chemotherapeutic drugs and radiation therapy. Bone marrow transplantation and HSCT may be the treatment of choice in patients with suitable donors and initial remission of the acute leukemia.

In chronic leukemia, which occurs almost exclusively in adults and develops slowly, the desired objectives of treatment depend on the kind of cells involved. Medications commonly used include chlorambucil, hydroxyurea, corticosteroids, and cyclophosphamide. Lymph nodes often are irradiated, and a blood transfusion may be given if anemia is severe. Although medications are not curative in chronic leukemia, they help to prolong life (see Table 7.2).

Nursing interventions and patient teaching. Prevent infection by teaching the patient and family the appropriate precautions for the neutropenic patient and the avoidance of infectious agents. Leukopenia (an abnormal decrease in the number of WBCs to less than 5000 cells/mm^3) can be fatal. The usual inflammatory process to control infection is decreased; thus frequent observation for signs and symptoms of infection is necessary. Thrombocytopenia-induced hemorrhage may be life threatening; prevent this condition through safe, gentle care. Control pain through pharmacologic and nonpharmacologic measures. Coping mechanisms may be strained because of pain, complexities of treatment, side effects and toxicities, change in body image, or fear of death. Support the patient and family by developing a positive nurse-patient-family relationship and referring them to community support groups.

Palliative care of the dying child should allow the child and family to experience the best quality of life possible. The child's illness and palliative care affect the whole family. Therefore the pediatric nurse needs to establish and develop effective communication with the family and between the dying child, parents, and siblings to help allay unnecessary fears and distress about imminent death and to support anticipatory grieving. Varied communication methods should be used to enable the nurse to understand the dying child and siblings' thoughts and feelings. Drawings

Table 7.2   Medications for Blood and Lymphatic Disorders

GENERIC NAME	ACTION	SIDE EFFECTS	NURSING IMPLICATIONS
cyanocobalamin, vitamin B$_{12}$	Needed for adequate nerve functioning, protein and carbohydrate metabolism, normal growth, RBC development, and cell reproduction	Flushing, diarrhea, itching, rash, hypokalemia	Assess GI functions and potassium levels at beginning of treatment; stress need for patients with pernicious anemia to return for monthly injections; give intramuscularly only
desmopressin acetate	Promotes reabsorption of water by kidneys and increase in plasma factor VIII levels, which increases platelet aggregation, resulting in vasopressor effect	Nasal irritation, congestion, drowsiness, headache, flushing, nausea, abdominal cramps, heartburn, vulval pain, hypertension	Avoid overhydration; assess pulse and blood pressure when giving drug subcutaneously; monitor factor VIII antigen levels and aPTT
ferrous sulfate	Replaces iron stores needed for RBC development	Nausea, constipation, epigastric pain, black and red tarry stools, vomiting, diarrhea, discolored urine, staining of teeth	Between-meal dosing is preferable but can be given with some foods, although absorption may be decreased; give tablets with orange juice to promote iron absorption; to avoid staining teeth, give elixir iron preparations through straw; oral iron may turn stools black
filgrastim, G-CSF	Stimulates proliferation and differentiation of neutrophils	Fever, alopecia, skeletal pain, nausea, vomiting, diarrhea, mucositis, anorexia	Monitor CBC and platelet count before treatment and twice weekly; refrigerate but do not freeze; avoid shaking; store at room temperature for at least 6 h; discard any vial that has been at room temperature for more than 6 h
folic acid, B complex vitamin	Needed for erythropoiesis; increases RBC, WBC, and platelet formation in megaloblastic anemias	Pruritus, rash, general malaise, bronchospasm, slight flushing	Drug may be administered by deep intramuscular, subcutaneous, or intravenous route; do not mix with other medications in same syringe for intramuscular injections
iron dextran	Released into the plasma and carried by transferrin to the bone marrow, where it is incorporated into Hgb	Stained skin at site of injection, fever, chills, headache, sweating, discolored urine, diarrhea	Administer 0.5-mL test dose by preferred route before therapy; wait at least 1 h before giving remaining portion

aPTT, Activated partial thromboplastin time; *CBC,* complete blood count; *G-CSF,* granulocyte colony-stimulating factor; *GI,* gastrointestinal; *RBC,* red blood cell; *WBC,* white blood cell.

can communicate perceptions and emotions about death and dying. These can relate to anger, fear, loss, hope, and acceptance of dying and can assist the nurse in providing holistic care for the child and family. Facilitating creative activity satisfies a basic need and gives the dying child the chance to do something while respecting individual autonomy, choice, and control (National Cancer Institute, 2020).

Palliative care supports the patient and family's goals for the future (including their hopes for cure or life prolongation) as well as their hopes for peace and dignity throughout the course of illness, the dying process, and death. The aims of palliative care include guiding the patient and family in making decisions that enable them to work toward their goals during their remaining time. Nurses facilitate shared decision making between health care professionals and patient/family, management of pain and symptoms, recognition and support of grief, and appropriate hospice referrals.

From a physical care perspective, it is challenging to make astute assessments and plan care to help the patient survive the severe side effects of chemotherapy. The life-threatening results of bone marrow suppression (anemia, thrombocytopenia, neutropenia) require aggressive nursing interventions. Additional complications of chemotherapy may affect the patient's GI tract, nutritional status, skin and mucosa, cardiopulmonary status, liver, kidneys, and neurologic system.

Understand all drugs being administered, including the mechanism of action, purpose, routes of administration, usual doses, potential side effects, safe handling considerations, and toxic effects. In addition, recognize laboratory data reflecting the effects of the drugs. Patient survival and comfort during aggressive chemotherapy are affected significantly by the quality of nursing intervention.

Include the patient and family by discussing procedures, meaning of treatments, and care plans. Be certain to cover the nature of the disease and previous information given to the patient. Community resources for support and information are invaluable for educating the patient and the family. Examine expectations of physical abilities, remission, and future plans. Encourage continuation of the medical regimen and avoidance of situations in which infection can be transmitted. Most patients should receive the pneumococcal vaccine at diagnosis and every 5 years and an annual influenza vaccine (Lyengar & Shimanovsky, 2020). Encourage six to eight small meals a day that consist of a diet high in calories, protein, and vitamins, as well as soft, bland food to reduce irritation to the mouth. Inform patient about the common side effects of their antileukemic therapy and the importance of taking these and other medications on schedule.

Prognosis. The prognosis for patients with AML is dependent on the age of the onset of the disease. The 5-year survival rate for adults is approximately 25%, and 65% for children and adolescents younger than 15 years of age (Nursing Care Plan 7.1). The prognosis for patients with acute lymphocytic leukemia (ALL) is about a 92% chance of experiencing remission in children, whereas adults have about a 69% 5-year survival rate. Adult patients with CLL generally have a 5-year survival rate of 83%. For adult patients with CML, the prognosis depends on the age of the patient, the stage of the disease, and the treatments used. The overall 5-year survival rate is approximately 59% (Lyengar & Shimanovsky, 2020).

DISORDERS ASSOCIATED WITH PLATELETS

Thrombocytopenia

Etiology and pathophysiology. Thrombocytopenia is an abnormal hematologic condition in which the number of platelets is reduced to fewer than $150,000/mm^3$. Platelets help maintain a homeostatic balance between bleeding and clotting. When platelet numbers start to fall, this homeostatic balance is disturbed, causing bleeding to occur. The lower the platelet counts, the higher the risk of spontaneous bleeding. The circulating volume of platelets may be affected because there is decreased production, increased destruction, or increased consumption of platelets. Multiple disorders can result in decreased production, including aplastic anemia, leukemia, tumors, and chemotherapy. Platelet destruction can occur as a result of diseases such as Hepatitis B and C, HIV, viral infections, and medications (Box 7.4). Platelets can also be destroyed in the spleen when the spleen is enlarged and traps too many blood cells. Immune disorders such

Box 7.4	Medications With Thrombocytopenic Effects
• Aspirin • Digitalis derivatives • Furosemide • Nonsteroidal anti-inflammatory agents (azathioprine, D-penicillamine, ibuprofen, indomethacin)	• Oral hypoglycemics • Penicillins • Quinidine • Rifampicin • Sulfonamides • Thiazides

as lupus and arthritis can also result in a destruction of platelets. Increased platelet consumption is caused by disseminated intravascular coagulation (DIC; discussed later). Thrombocytopenia commonly occurs due to a defined cause such as any number of diseases and medications. It may even occur in the presence of ethylenediaminetetraacetic acid (EDTA), which is a preservative used when collecting blood for a CBC, in which case it is pseudothrombocytopenia, and the blood test needs to be repeated in a tube containing citrate instead of EDTA. Thrombocytopenia can rarely occur in isolation from any of the causes mentioned and unrelated to any other immune disorders. This is termed *ITP* and occurs in the spleen, which is the site of antiplatelet antibody production and platelet clearance (Chaturvedi, Arnold, & McCrae, 2018). ITP is characterized by a destruction of platelets due to an antibody-antigen reaction where antiplatelet antibodies bind platelets. The antibody-bound platelets are then destroyed. The body attempts to replace the destroyed platelets by producing more, but often supply cannot keep up with demand. In addition, the antibodies enter the bone marrow and destroy platelets in the marrow, further reducing supply.

Clinical manifestations. Often patients with thrombocytopenia have no symptoms, and a low platelet finding occurs incidentally. Symptoms rarely occur at platelet counts greater than $50,000/mm^3$. Patients experiencing platelet counts less than $50,000/mm^3$ may present with petechiae and purpura. As the count drops even lower, the risk for bleeding from mucous membranes and in cutaneous sites and internal organs increases. Significant risk for serious bleeding occurs once the count is less than $20,000/mm^3$. Patients exhibit nasal and gingival bleeding, excessive menstrual bleeding, and any injury causes severe bleeding. When the platelet count is less than $5000/mm^3$, spontaneous, potentially fatal CNS or GI hemorrhage can occur.

Case studies have documented cyclic thrombocytopenia wherein platelet counts cycle from low to high in sync with the menstrual cycle causing menorrhagia (Dogara, Sani, Waziri, et al., 2016).

Assessment. Collection of subjective data includes questioning the patient about recent viral infections (which

Nursing Care Plan 7.1   The Patient With Leukemia

Ms. M. is a 26-year-old patient diagnosed with acute lymphocytic leukemia. She is married and the mother of a 3-year-old daughter. Ms. M. has been receiving chemotherapy and is immunocompromised, with a differential white blood cell (WBC) count revealing a neutrophil count of 22%. Her Hgb is 8.8 g/dL, and her platelets are 55,000/mm³. Her mouth appears edematous, and she complains of oral tenderness.

PATIENT PROBLEM

Potential for Infection, related to leukopenia

Patient Goals and Expected Outcomes	Nursing Interventions	Evaluation
Patient or caregiver will identify measures to prevent or control infection	Inspect all body sites for infection at least daily; note and report fever, sore throat, purulent exudate, chills, cough, burning with urination, erythema, edema, tenderness, and pain.	Patient will remain free of infection.
Patient or caregiver will verbalize and report signs and symptoms of infection	Monitor vital signs. Obtain cultures as ordered. Monitor WBC counts and culture reports. Administer antibiotics on time as ordered. Promote and maintain hygiene integrity of skin and mucous membranes. Use aseptic technique in treatments. Teach the patient and family: • Necessity of avoiding crowds or people with infections while WBC count is decreased. • Personal hygiene measures. • Signs and symptoms of infection.	Patient demonstrates no signs or symptoms of infection; temperature and WBC count are within normal range.

PATIENT PROBLEM

Impaired Coping, related to diagnosis and disease process

Patient Goals and Expected Outcomes	Nursing Intervention	Evaluation
Patient and family will demonstrate measures to effectively cope by verbalizing role of family, significant others, and support groups in therapeutic coping	Assess coping capabilities of patient and significant others. Discuss disease process and expectations. Alleviate knowledge deficit. Encourage questions and self-expression; listen actively, demonstrate compassion, reassure with touch and personal contact. Assess fear of threat of death; allow time for personal expression and provide one-on-one discussion opportunity.	Patient and family express factors that are causing anxiety and powerlessness.

CRITICAL THINKING QUESTIONS

1. What should the nurse do if a visitor with an obvious upper respiratory tract infection is seen approaching Ms. M.'s room?
2. What nursing interventions would be most appropriate in providing therapeutic oral hygiene for Ms. M.?
3. What personal hygiene and activities of daily living would be most beneficial for Ms. M.?

may produce a transient thrombocytopenia), medications in current use, and the extent of alcohol ingestion.

Collection of objective data includes observing the patient's skin for petechiae and ecchymoses, or possibly hematoma. Epistaxis and gingival bleeding are common. Signs of increased intracranial pressure caused by cerebral hemorrhage may be detected. If bleeding occurs in the GI tract, the patient may vomit blood (hematemesis) or may pass blood in the stool, resulting in bright red blood in the stools from bleeding in the lower GI tract, or dark, tarry stools (melena) from bleeding higher in the GI tract.

Diagnostic tests. To ascertain the characteristics of all blood cells, laboratory studies include platelet count, peripheral blood smear, and bleeding time (BT). In addition, a bone marrow analysis is performed to determine the presence of immature platelets. Examination also reveals the presence or absence of primary bone marrow abnormalities, such as neoplastic invasion or aplastic anemia.

Medical management. By treating the underlying cause of the thrombocytopenia, the patient's signs and symptoms may improve. Corticosteroids may help if the disorder is related to an autoimmune problem. Packed RBC or platelet transfusions are sometimes necessary. Other medical treatments for ITP include monoclonal antibodies such as Rituximab (Chaturvedi, Arnold, & McCrae, 2018) and thrombopoietin receptor agonists such as eltrombopag and romiplostim (Ghanima, Cooper, Rodeghiero, et al., 2019). Splenectomy is a treatment of last resort if the patient doesn't respond to monoclonal antibodies or thrombopoietin receptor agonist or if the patient is in the advanced stages of disease (Chaturvedi, Arnold, & McCrae, 2018).

Nursing interventions and patient teaching. Support the medical treatment regimen using specific interventions for specific disease causes. If medication toxicity is the cause, the medication is discontinued. Prevent infections by meticulous asepsis, universal precautions, and gentle handling of the patient. Closely monitor plasma and platelet infusion and whole blood transfusions for reaction and effects on the patient's condition.

A patient problem and interventions for the patient with thrombocytopenia include but are not limited to the following:

PATIENT PROBLEM	NURSING INTERVENTIONS
Compromised Blood Flow to Tissues (cerebral, cardiopulmonary, renal, gastrointestinal, peripheral), related to bleeding	Monitor vital signs and neurologic status
	Monitor platelet count and abnormal bleeding times
	Check for bleeding in urine, stool, and emesis
	Monitor invasive diagnostic procedure sites for bleeding
	Reduce medical interventions requiring punctures
	Maintain comfort measures and bed rest
	Avoid trauma and infection
	Monitor intake and output for untoward signs
	Monitor potential sites of hemorrhage

The patient must understand the disease process and causative agents to provide self-care and to prevent trauma or infection. Provide instructions on signs, symptoms, and preventive measures: avoid trauma, use stool softeners, maintain a high-fiber diet to prevent constipation, check for the presence of blood, use a soft toothbrush, and blow the nose gently. Stress the importance of notifying the health care provider of signs and symptoms of bleeding.

Prognosis. The prognosis is variable, depending on the underlying cause. Medication-induced thrombocytopenia usually resolves in 1 to 2 weeks after the medication has been stopped. In ITP, treatment may be necessary for 3 to 4 weeks before a complete response is seen. More than 80% of children with immune ITP require no treatment and have a spontaneous recovery from the disorder within weeks after diagnosis. In chronic ITP, transient remissions occur. Approximately 80% of patients benefit from splenectomy immediately after surgery, and 50%-70% experience a complete

or partial remission (Chaturvedi, Arnold, & McCrae, 2018).

DISORDERS ASSOCIATED WITH CLOTTING FACTOR DEFECTS

Hemophilia

Etiology and pathophysiology. Hemophilia is a coagulation disorder that occurs due to a reduction or deficiency in clotting factors VIII, IX, and XI. Patients missing clotting factor VIII are diagnosed with hemophilia A, those missing clotting factor IX are diagnosed with hemophilia B, and a deficiency in clotting factor XI is diagnosed as hemophilia C. Hemophilia A is the most prevalent, occurring in 80% to 85% of the hemophilia patient population. Hemophilia C is rare and occurs in 1 in 100,000 live births. Worldwide, the number of people living with hemophilia is 400,000 with a higher prevalence in cultures that marry within the family (Mehta & Reddivari, 2020).

Hemophilia is a disease that occurs due to genetic mutations occurring on over 1000 genes that code for clotting factors that exist on chromosome X (Mehta & Reddivari, 2020). As the mutation occurs on chromosome X and the disease is recessive, females are usually asymptomatic carriers for hemophilia while males manifest the disease. It is possible for females to manifest the disease if they inherit an affected X chromosome from the father and asymptomatic carrier X chromosome from the mother, but these instances are rare. In addition, it is estimated that 30% of hemophilia cases occur due to spontaneous genetic mutations (Mehta & Reddivari, 2020). The reduction or absence of clotting factors results in a disruption in the clotting mechanisms of the body, which then leads to prolonged bleeding. The severity of bleeding is dependent on the percentage of normal factor activity present.

Clinical manifestations. The overarching symptom of hemophilia is prolonged bleeding. Hemophilia can be distinguished into mild, moderate, and severe. Patients that retain 5% to 40% of normal factor activity have mild hemophilia and often present with significant bleeding after trauma or surgery. Spontaneous bleeding is generally not present in patients with mild hemophilia. Moderate hemophilia occurs when patients retain 1% to 5% of normal factor activity. These patients experience bleeding after trauma, injury, dental work, or surgery. Though bleeding in joint spaces occurs with severe hemophilia, it does also occur in 25% of the cases in patients with moderate hemophilia. Severe hemophilia occurs when patients retain less than 1% of normal factor activity (Mehta & Reddivari, 2020). These patients bleed spontaneously with extensive, deep bruising (ecchymosis) of muscle tissue, which may show deformity; hemorrhage also occurs into joints, which eventually become ankylosed (i.e., fused or obliterated). Hemarthrosis, or bleeding into a joint space, is a hallmark of severe disease and usually occurs in the knees, ankles, elbows, shoulders, and hips. Pain, edema, erythema, and fever accompany hemarthrosis. Small cuts can prove fatal; blood loss from simple dental procedures may be significant. Urine and stool may reveal bleeding along with unusual bleeding from something as simple as vaccinations (Mayo Clinic, 2020a). Any organ may exhibit bleeding and patients will manifest symptoms accordingly. Patients with mild or moderate hemophilia may not be diagnosed until later, and the age of diagnosis may coincide with the level of precipitating trauma. Patients with severe hemophilia may experience recurrent bleeding even in utero (Mehta & Reddivari, 2020).

Assessment. Subjective data include reports by patient and family of incidents of ecchymosis and hemorrhage from even the slightest trauma. Pain is associated with joint motion.

Collection of objective data includes noting blood in subcutaneous tissues, urine, or stool and noting edematous or immobile joints.

Diagnostic tests. Families with known hemophiliacs may opt to genetically test by chorionic villous sampling, amniocentesis, or obtaining a sample of umbilical cord blood at birth. Patients with high suspicion due to history and physical can diagnose using blood tests including CBC, PT, PTT, and BT. In patients with hemophilia A and B, PTT will be prolonged by two to three times the normal range, whereas PT and BT will be normal. Next, a mixing study will be conducted that will normalize PTT time by contributing clotting factors to correct the deficiency. This test is followed by a factor VIII and IX assay and then genetic testing as confirmation (Mehta & Reddivari, 2020).

Medical management. The treatment of a patient with hemophilia revolves around prophylaxis and management of acute bleeds. Patients can be placed on a prophylactic treatment of factor replacement, which has the advantage of reducing bleeding episodes, which reduces the need for hospitalizations, improves quality of life, and requires less frequent monitoring. Prophylactic treatments significantly reduce the amount of bleeding in joints and therefore reduce hemarthrosis, chronic pain, ankylosis, and the need for joint surgeries. Prophylactic treatments also reduce the risk of developing antibodies to factor replacement. Patients can opt for continuous or intermittent prophylactic treatment. Continuous treatment is defined by infusions of weekly factor replacement for 45 out of the 52 weeks in a year. Prophylactic treatment is also defined as primary, secondary, or tertiary based on the level of disease progress. Prophylactic treatment involves factor VIII or IX replacement two to three times a week.

Management of acute bleeding episodes needs simultaneous management of the location and severity of the bleed and immediate initiation of high-dose

clotting factor concentrate (CFC) with factor VIII or IX. For example, intracranial bleeding would require surgical intervention for the cranial bleed as well as CFC. Pain is managed with acetaminophen, Cox-2 inhibitors, and opioids. Aspirin and all NSAIDs are avoided to prevent further bleeding. All venipunctures and injections must be avoided if possible. Desmopressin (DDVAP), a synthetic analog of vasopressin, is given intranasally and induces the release of von Willebrand factor (vWF), which increases endogenous levels of factor VIII three- to fivefold. It can only be used for hemophilia A, as it has no effect on factor IX (Mehta & Reddivari, 2020).

Nursing interventions and patient teaching. Assess the patient's level of understanding of the clinical course of the disease and prevention of complications. Educate the patient and the entire family because many people may be involved in the patient care. Control hemorrhages in emergency situations by applying pressure and cold to the site. Support and reassurance are imperative. Monitor transfusions of factor VIII concentrate. Supportive care measures include pain management and genetic counseling. Do not give hemophilia patients aspirin or aspirin products, because they can further complicate the bleeding tendency.

Patient problems and interventions for the patient with hemophilia include but are not limited to the following:

PATIENT PROBLEM	NURSING INTERVENTIONS
Knowledge deficit, related to long-term illness	Educate patient and family about disease process
	Promote healthier life choices such as participation in noncontact sports such as swimming, cycling, or table tennis
	Wear protective gear when exercising
	Take warm baths to promote relaxation and mobility
	Wear a medical bracelet
Inadequate Fluid Volume, related to bleeding	Assess for extent of hemorrhage
	Prevent further hemorrhage or extension
Compromised Blood Flow to Tissue, related to blood loss from coagulation deficit	Monitor vital signs and laboratory reports
	Apply cold compresses to bleeding areas
	Assess for anxiety, shock, disorientation
	Assess for decreased urinary output
	Teach safety precautions to prevent trauma
	Administer analgesia as ordered
	Move patient gently and slowly, supporting joints
	Prevent deformity through support, splints, and physical therapy

Discuss with the patient ways to avoid injury and control bleeding. Also discuss physical activity within limits. Encourage the patient to wear a medical-alert tag. Emergency care teaching includes immobilizing the affected part, applying ice, and notifying the health care provider. Discuss diet to prevent obesity, which puts excess pressure on joints. Regular dental care and preventive dental and medical measures are important aspects. Overprotection is sometimes a factor to discuss. Neither aspirin nor any other medication, including over-the-counter medications, should be taken except with the health care provider's knowledge (see the Home Care Considerations box).

🏠 Home Care Considerations

Hemophilia

- Home management is a primary consideration for a patient with hemophilia because the disease follows a chronic, progressive course.
- The quantity and length of life may be affected significantly by the patient's knowledge of the illness and understanding of how to live with it.
- Refer the patient and family to the local chapter of the National Hemophilia Foundation to encourage association with other individuals who are dealing with the problems associated with hemophilia.
- Teach the patient with hemophilia to recognize disease-related problems and to learn which problems can be resolved at home and which require hospitalization.
- Immediate medical attention is required for severe pain or edema of a muscle or joint that restricts movement or inhibits sleep and for a head injury, edema in the neck or mouth, abdominal pain, hematuria, melena, and skin wounds in need of suturing.
- Oral hygiene must be performed gently, without trauma.
- Aspirin and aspirin products should not be taken, because they decrease platelet aggregation.
- Understanding how to prevent injuries is an important consideration. The patient can learn to participate in noncontact sports (e.g., golf) and wear gloves when doing household chores to prevent cuts or abrasions from knives, hammers, and other tools.
- The patient should wear a medical-alert tag to ensure that health care providers know about the hemophilia in case of an accident.
- A person with hemophilia who is mature enough, or a family member, can be taught to administer some of the factor replacement therapies at home.

Prognosis. Prior to factor replacement therapies, hemophiliacs had a life expectancy of 11 years and usually died in adolescence. The advent of factor replacement therapy has significantly changed the course of hemophilia in patients. Most patients with hemophilia live normal lives in the absence of co-morbid conditions.

von Willebrand Disease

Etiology and pathophysiology. von Willebrand disease (vWD) is an inherited genetic bleeding disorder passed down by either parent or both. In rare cases, vWF can occur due to a spontaneous genetic mutation and even rarer is the possibility of acquired vWF that occurs later in life. The acquired vWF usually occurs due to some other underlying medical condition. It is characterized by abnormally slow coagulation of blood and spontaneous episodes of GI bleeding, epistaxis, and gingival bleeding. The disease is caused by a deficiency of vWF, which is a protein that is critical for platelet adhesion (one of the earliest steps in blood coagulation). Because vWF is bound to factor VIII, protecting it from rapid breakdown in the blood, a patient with vWD also has low factor VIII levels. vWD is the most common bleeding disorder, occurring in 1 out of every 100 people. It occurs equally in men and women, though women tend to notice the symptoms caused by vWD due to heavier than normal menstrual periods and increased bleeding after giving birth (CDC, 2020).

Researchers have identified many variations of vWD, but most fall into three types (CDC.gov, 2020):

- *Type 1:* Most common and mildest form occurring in 85% of vWD cases. Patient has low levels of vWF and may also have low levels of factor VIII (which is different from hemophilia where factor VIII is very low or absent and vWF levels are normal)
- *Type 2:* The body produces enough vWF but it is somehow deficient in construction and thus unable to attach to platelet cells. Depending on the abnormality, patients may be classified as having type 2a or type 2b, type 2M, and 2N.
- *Type 3:* Rarest type occurring in about 3% of cases. Patients have very little or no vWF and have low levels of factor VIII.

Clinical manifestations. The symptoms experienced by patients vary in degree and severity based on the type of vWD. Common symptoms include frequent and hard-to-stop nose bleeds, easy bruising with very little or no trauma, heavy menstrual bleeding that often leads to a diagnosis of anemia, longer than normal bleeding after dental work or giving birth, blood in urine or stool, and painful joints due to bleeding in joint spaces.

Assessment. Subjective data includes history of easy bruising and bleeding, nose bleeds five or more times a year, and reports of blood clotting taking longer than usual.

Objective data includes physical evidence of bruising and bleeding, painful and swollen joints, and signs of anemia.

Diagnostic tests. A CBC will indicate decrease in RBCs, Hgb, and HCT. Prothrombin time (PT) and activated partial thromboplastin time (aPTT) results will be abnormally high as clotting is taking longer. Blood tests for clotting factors will help diagnose vWD and include vWF antigen, vWF activity, Factor VIII clotting activity, and vWF multimers (Mayo Clinic, 2019a).

Medical management. Patients with mild forms of vWD are treated with nasal or IV desmopressin acetate.

This drug is a synthetic form of the human antidiuretic hormone, vasopressin. It causes an increase in vWF release from storage sites in the body and of factor VIII. Desmopressin is often administered prophylactically to patients with mild vWD who require surgery or dental extractions. For patients with more severe forms of vWD or those that don't respond to desmopressin treatment includes IV transfusions of **Recombinant** (an organism, cell or genetic material formed by recombining things) VWF and medicines that contain both vWF and factor VIII such as Humate, Wilate, Alphanate, and Koate. Antifibrinolytic drugs such as Amicar and Lysteda can be prescribed to help slow the breakdown of clots and women with vWD can be prescribed birth control pills as it increases the levels of vWF and factor VIII while having the benefit of decreasing heavy menstrual flow (CDC, 2020).

Observation and nursing interventions for hemophilia A and B can be adapted easily to vWD.

Prognosis. The prognosis is usually good for patients with early diagnosis and effective treatment. Most people who have type 1 vWD are able to live normal lives with only mild bleeding issues. Individuals with type 2 are at an increased risk of experiencing mild to moderate bleeding and complications. During times of infection, surgery, or pregnancy the patient often has increased bleeding. Type 3 poses an increased risk for severe bleeding, externally and internally. These patients have a normal life expectancy (Pollak, 2017).

Disseminated Intravascular Coagulation

Etiology and pathophysiology. **Disseminated intravascular coagulation (DIC)** is a grave but rare coagulopathy resulting from the overstimulation of clotting and anticlotting processes that always occur due to an underlying medical condition involving some type of infection, inflammation, or cancer. Examples of medical conditions that cause DIC include septicemia, obstetric complications (abruptio placentae and preeclampsia or HELLP syndrome), malignancies, tissue trauma, transfusion reaction, burns, shock, and snake bites (Box 7.5). In DIC, widespread clotting

Box 7.5	Disorders Usually Associated With Disseminated Intravascular Coagulation

ACUTE DISSEMINATED INTRAVASCULAR COAGULATION
- Acute liver failure
- Gram negative
- Gram positive
- Organ destruction
- Organ destruction (e.g., pancreatitis)
  - Severe tissue damage (burns, crushing)
  - Head trauma
  - Obstetric complications (e.g., abruptio placenta, low platelets [HELLP] syndrome), amniotic embolism, abruptio placenta, eclampsia
  - Abortion
  - Intravascular hemolysis
  - Severe blood transfusion reaction
- Sepsis (most common)
- Toxins
- Trauma

CHRONIC DISSEMINATED INTRAVASCULAR COAGULATION
- Autoimmune disorders (transplant rejection)
- Cardiovascular diseases (e.g., valve stents, myocardial infarction, aneurysms)
- Hematologic disorders
- Inflammatory disorders
- Malignancy (especially solid tumors)
- Renal vascular disorders
- Retained fetal syndrome

(thrombosis) within small vessels occurs, with subsequent damage to multiple organs. Due to widespread coagulation, clotting factors are depleted from other parts of the body thus resulting in an imbalance between clotting and bleeding. The imbalance results in widespread bleeding. Thus, patients in DIC could be clotting and bleeding simultaneously. DIC can be acute or chronic and may develop slowly, over hours or days, or quickly.

Clinical Manifestations. Clinical manifestations include those of the underlying disorder that causes DIC as well as signs of clotting and bleeding. Blood clots resulting in DVT would cause pain, redness, swelling; blood clots in the microvasculature of the kidney would result in kidney failure and anuria, pain, and hypertension; neurological clots could cause obtunded mental status, coma, and paresthesias; pulmonary system blood clots would result in dyspnea, central cyanosis, palpitations and chest pain; and GI blood clots result in swelling and passing of clots in stool. Bleeding would occur from mucous membranes, venipuncture sites, surgical sites, and all orifices leading to circulatory collapse (hypotension, tachycardia) and acute respiratory distress (central cyanosis, air hunger). The patient exhibits petechiae on the soft palate, trunk, and extremities and bruising especially from venipuncture sites.

Assessment. Subjective data include patient complaints based on sites of bleeding and clotting.

Collection of objective data includes observing for occult or obvious bleeding. Purpura on the chest and abdomen, reflecting fibrin deposits in capillaries, is a common first sign of DIC. Note the color of skin and mucosa and the presence of petechiae. Abdominal tenderness may be present. GI bleeding, hematuria, pulmonary edema, PE, hypotension, tachycardia, absence of peripheral pulses, decreased blood pressure, restlessness, confusion, seizures, or coma may be present.

Diagnostic tests. DIC can be difficult to diagnose especially in chronic cases. Diagnosis is made by reviewing the clinical picture along with laboratory results. The coagulation profile shows prolonged prothrombin and aPTTs, as well as prolonged BT. The platelet count is low, showing marked thrombocytopenia. Other tests show fibrinogen deficiency (hypofibrinogenemia; reflecting the consumption of fibrinogen in DIC) and deficits of factors V, VII, VIII, X, and XII.

D-dimer test results are elevated as d-dimer is a breakdown of fibrinogen and therefore an indirect measure of clotting.

Medical management. The underlying cause of DIC must be addressed and corrected and the symptoms of DIC are treated with supportive medications. Hypovolemia (Box 7.1) caused due to hemorrhage is treated with transfusions of packed RBCs and fluids. Administration of platelet transfusion and factor replacement therapy is initiated when extensive bleeding occurs. FFP may be transfused to replace clotting factors to stop bleeding. Heparin therapy may be ordered if the patient has widespread fibrin deposition without significant bleeding; it is mostly used in cases of chronic DIC.

Nursing Interventions and patient teaching. Protection from bleeding and trauma and application of pressure to sites of hemorrhage are essential nursing measures. Support and reassurance of the patient may aid in relieving high stress levels. Monitor the patient in a quiet, nonstressful environment. Make sure the patient's bed has padded side rails and use foam or cotton swabs for mouth care. Monitor vital signs and administer heparin, blood and FFP transfusions, and factor replacement therapy as ordered. Use the blood pressure cuff infrequently to avoid subcutaneous bleeding.

Patient problems and interventions for the patient with DIC include but are not limited to the following:

PATIENT PROBLEM	NURSING INTERVENTIONS
Potential for Injury, Bleeding, and Fluid Deficit, related to: • Depleted coagulation factors • Adverse effect of heparin (excess heparin, insufficient heparin)	Monitor Hct and Hgb Assess skin surface for signs of bleeding; note petechiae; purpura; hematomas; oozing of blood from IV sites, drains, and wounds; and bleeding from mucous membranes Observe for signs of bleeding from GI and genitourinary tracts Note any hemoptysis or blood obtained during suctioning Monitor level of consciousness (LOC); institute neurologic checklist (mental status changes may occur with the decreased fluid volume or with decreasing Hgb) Monitor vital signs for signs of hemorrhage Observe for signs of orthostatic hypotension (drop of >15 mm Hg when changing from supine to sitting position indicates reduced circulating fluids) Avoid intramuscular injections; any needlestick is a potential bleeding site Apply pressure to bleeding site Prevent trauma to catheter and tubes by proper taping, minimum pulling

GI, Gastrointestinal; *Hct,* hematocrit; *Hgb,* hemoglobin; *IV,* intravenous.

Discuss with the patient and family the signs and symptoms of DIC and have them repeat this information to the nurse or health care provider. Teach the patient to self-administer heparin therapy subcutaneously if prescribed. Instruct the patient and family to avoid mechanical trauma, such as from a hard toothbrush, blade razor, rough nose blowing, or contact sports.

Prognosis. Mortality rates from DIC vary, depending on severity. Death is usually a result of either uncontrolled hemorrhage, irreversible end-organ damage, or both.

DISORDERS ASSOCIATED WITH PLASMA CELLS

Multiple Myeloma

Etiology and pathophysiology. Multiple myeloma, or plasma cell myeloma, is a malignant neoplastic disease of the bone marrow. Neoplastic plasma cells build up in the bone marrow and produce one or more tumors. The tumors destroy bone (osseous) tissue, especially in flat bones, causing pain, fractures, and skeletal deformities.

The specific immunoglobulin produced by the myeloma cells is present in the blood and/or urine and is referred to as *monoclonal protein, M protein,* or *paraprotein.* This protein is a helpful marker to monitor the extent of the disease and the patient's response to treatment. It is measured by serum or urine protein electrophoresis.

The older adult patient whose chief complaint is back pain and who has elevated total serum protein should be evaluated for possible multiple myeloma. It most frequently occurs in patients at a median age of 70 years and the male to female ratio for occurrence is three to two (Albagoush & Azevedo, 2020). Onset is gradual and insidious; the disease often goes unrecognized for years while the individual experiences frequent, recurrent bacterial infections (the result of immune dysfunction: there is too much of a particular nonfunctional immunoglobulin and not enough normal immunoglobulin). Early detection can decrease the amount of pain and disability resulting from bone destruction and pathologic fractures (Herget, Wäsch, Klein, et al., 2020). 1.8% of all new cancer cases in the United States is diagnosed as multiple myeloma (Albagoush & Azevedo, 2020).

Clinical manifestations. The disease process shows a proliferation of malignant plasma cells and development of single or multiple bone marrow tumors. This is followed by bone destruction with dissemination into lymph nodes, liver, spleen, and kidneys.

The skeletal system symptoms typically involve the ribs, spine, and pelvis. Osteolytic lesions are seen in the skull, vertebrae, and ribs. Vertebral destruction can lead to collapse of vertebrae with ensuing compression of the spinal cord. Patients complain of bone pain that increases with movement. About 30% develop pathologic fractures accompanied by severe pain.

In an individual with multiple myeloma, production of erythrocytes, platelets, and leukocytes is disrupted because the marrow is crowded by the abnormal proliferation of plasma cells. This leads to infection, anemia, and increased potential for bleeding. Calcium and phosphorus drain from bones, leading to hypercalcemia and renal problems. In addition, cell destruction contributes to the development of hyperuricemia (high uric acid in the blood), which, along with the high protein levels caused by the myeloma protein, can result in renal failure.

Assessment. Collection of subjective data includes assessment of the patient's complaints of pain, especially skeletal pain in the back, pelvis, the spine, and the ribs.

Collection of objective data includes assessing the patient's facial expression for signs of increased pain with movement, the ability to perform ADLs, increased body temperature, increased potential for bleeding, changes in urine characteristics, and effectiveness of medication administration.

Diagnostic tests. Diagnosis of multiple myeloma is made with radiographic skeletal studies, bone marrow biopsy, and laboratory examination of blood and urine. A monoclonal antibody (M protein) may be present, as evidenced in serum or urine electrophoresis. Bony degeneration also causes loss of calcium in the bones,

eventually causing hypercalcemia. Pancytopenia, hypercalcemia, hyperuricemia, and elevated creatinine may be found. In addition, an abnormal globulin known as Bence Jones protein is found in the urine and can result in renal failure.

Radiographic skeletal examinations reveal widespread demineralization, lytic lesions, and osteoporosis. Lytic lesions (destruction of an area of bone due to a disease process) may be seen on bone roentgenograms but are not well visualized on bone scans. Bone marrow studies reveal large numbers of immature plasma cells, which normally account for only 5% of marrow population.

Medical management. Treatments for multiple myeloma can be placed in two categories: patients eligible for bone marrow transplants and patients ineligible for bone marrow transplants. Transplant eligibility is determined based on disease progress and patient functional status. Those patients who are eligible undergo chemotherapy to decrease the size of the tumor, followed by harvesting of stem cells via PBSC transplant and autologous transplant. Patients ineligible for bone marrow transplants receive drug therapies including lenalidomide and dexamethasone, bortezomib and dexamethasone, melphalan/prednisone/bortezomib, or other bortezomib-based regimens. They can also be treated with proteasome inhibitors (stop enzyme complexes, proteasomes, in cells from breaking down proteins important for keeping cell division under control) and monoclonal antibodies (Albagoush & Azevedo, 2020).

Hypercalcemia (resulting from bone destruction) and pain also should be addressed. Analgesics, orthopedic supports, and localized radiation help reduce the skeletal pain. Hospitalization to administer chemotherapy, corticosteroids, and fluids may be required.

Nursing interventions and patient teaching. Care of the patient with multiple myeloma focuses on relieving pain, preventing infection and bone injury, administering chemotherapy and radiation, and maintaining hydration (Box 7.6). Encourage ambulation and adequate hydration to treat hypercalcemia, dehydration, and potential renal damage. Fluid intake of 3 to 4 L/day is encouraged to prevent dehydration and maintain a urinary output of 1.5 to 2 L/day. Patients with multiple myeloma with high tumor burdens (the total

Box 7.6	Chemotherapy Side Effects
• Alopecia (hair loss) • Appetite changes • Bleeding problems • Constipation/diarrhea • Fatigue • Infection • Mouth and throat changes • Nausea and vomiting	• Nerve changes • Pain • Sexual and fertility changes in women • Skin and nail changes • Swelling (fluid retention) • Urination changes

mass of tumor tissue carried by a patient with a malignancy) who receive chemotherapy have increased cell lysis and release of uric acid, resulting in hyperuricemia. Weight-bearing helps the bones reabsorb some calcium, and fluids dilute calcium and prevent protein precipitates from causing renal tubular obstruction.

Because of the potential for pathologic fractures, be careful when moving and ambulating the patient. A slight twist or strain on the bones may be sufficient to cause a fracture. Attention to the psychosocial, emotional, and spiritual needs is also extremely important.

Patient problems and interventions for the patient with multiple myeloma include but are not limited to the following:

PATIENT PROBLEM	NURSING INTERVENTIONS
Potential for Injury, related to: • Osteoporosis • Lytic lesions	Protect from bone injury; use logroll, turning sheet Use pillows to support bony prominences
Recent Onset of Pain, related to disease process	Administer analgesics as ordered (such as nonsteroidal anti-inflammatory drugs, acetaminophen, or an acetaminophen-opioid combination). Combination drugs may be more effective than opioids alone in diminishing bone pain Provide comfort measures Assess contributing factors

Teach the patient how to avoid traumatic bone injury and infection. Discuss the importance of adequate hydration and review the pain control modalities available. It is also important to identify spiritual resources. Address the patient's understanding of the disease, verbalization of discouragement and hopelessness, and desires for emotional and spiritual support.

Prognosis. The prognosis for multiple myeloma is dependent on several factors, including stage when diagnosed, effectiveness of medical treatment, comorbidities, and age of the patient. Generally, older patients with comorbid conditions have poorer survival rates than younger patients. Overall 5-year survival rate is around 35% (Albagoush & Azevedo, 2020).

DISORDERS OF THE LYMPHATIC SYSTEM

LYMPHANGITIS

Etiology and Pathophysiology
Lymphangitis can occur due to inflammation or infection. Infection typically results in one or more lymphatic vessels or channels from an acute streptococcal infection of the skin and less often staphylococcal infection.

The appearance of lymphangitis signals a worsening skin infection that could result in complications such as septicemia. Lymphangitis from inflammatory processes usually occur due to the presence of malignancy.

Clinical Manifestations
Lymphangitis is characterized by tender red streaks that radiate from the site of the infection toward the closest lymph glands. The lymph nodes in the surrounding area are enlarged and tender. Patients experience systemic symptoms such as malaise, fever, chills, headache, muscle aches, loss of appetite, and pain the infected area.

Assessment and diagnostic test. Subjective data includes presence of red streaks, reports of pain and tenderness in the affected area, complaints of headache and muscle pain.

Objective data includes fever, chills, red streaks, swollen and tender lymph nodes. Diagnosis is based on symptoms, presence of skin infections, inflammation due to malignancy, and possible biopsy of the lymph node. Blood cultures may be conducted as sepsis is a complication of lymphangitis.

Medical Management
Administration of antimicrobial drugs by oral or IV route controls the infection. Anti-inflammatory medications may be ordered to reduce inflammation and anti-pyretics for fever. Warm moist compresses may be used to reduce inflammation and pain. In certain cases, surgical management may be needed to remove obstructed or abscessed nodes.

Nursing Interventions
The affected area should be kept clean to promote healing. Rest and extremity elevation may relieve the pressure and reduce any swelling that may have occurred. Patients are taught to report increasing pain, growing streaks, or pus or fluid coming out of the lymph node.

Prognosis
With treatment, the prognosis is usually good.

LYMPHEDEMA
Etiology and Pathophysiology
Lymphedema is a primary or secondary disorder characterized by the accumulation of protein rich fluid in the soft tissue that leads to subsequent inflammation, fibrosis, and hypertrophy of adipose tissue (Kim, Hwang, Bae, et al., 2019). The accumulation of lymph fluid in soft tissue can be caused by various conditions. Obstruction of a lymph vessel could occur due to the presence of a cancerous tumor that blocks the movement of fluid into the lymph vessels. Often during cancer treatment, the cancerous tumor plus surrounding affected lymph nodes and vessels are removed which results in a buildup of fluid in soft tissue. Infections occurring in the surrounding tissues

can cause lymphedema by damaging lymph vessels. Lymphedema can also occur due to genetic mutations. Lymphedema typically occurs in the arms and legs though it can occur anywhere in the body including face, neck, trunk, abdomen, and genitals. Patients need to understand that lymphedema is a chronic condition that can become severe and cause serious problems.

Clinical Manifestations

Edema experienced by patients can range from mild to severe. Mild edema may cause achy pain, slight heaviness, and restlessness in the extremity. As the edema worsens, the limb feels heavier, patients experience tingling, the skin feels tight and looks thicker and more leathery. As the condition worsens, the patient experiences more restricted range of motion, constant aching and discomfort, and recurring infections. Wounds in the swollen extremity heal slower and joints of the affected extremity are stiff and sore.

Assessment and Diagnostic Test

Subjective data include history of cancer treatment, trauma or damage to the area, and complaints of pain, pressure, and presence of edema.

Collection of objective data includes observation of the extremities for edema, palpation of peripheral pulses, restricted range of motion, and infections in the affected extremity. Patients with recent history of tumor removals are diagnosed based on signs and symptoms. Patients with lymphedema without obvious cause undergo a procedure known as lymphoscintigraphy. This test involves injection of a radioactive substance under the skin between the first and second fingers or toes. If the affected extremity is the left arm, then the right arm is also injected with radioactive dye and studied as a comparison. The patients are then asked to squeeze a rubber ball to allow for transport of the radioactive substances (Kim, Hwang, Bae, et al., 2019). Blockages then can be detected by scanning the flow of the dye through the lymph system.

Medical Management

Treatment for lymphedema focuses on reducing swelling and controlling the pain. A lymphedema therapist can teach patients gentle exercises that encourage fluid drainage. Wrapping or compression bandages compress the affected extremity and move fluid away from the digits. The bandaging should be tightest at the fingers and looser moving up the affected extremity. Manual lymph massage conducted by a specially trained therapist may encourage the movement of lymph fluid. A pneumatic compression sleeve worn over the affected extremity inflates and deflates intermittently helping the fluid to move away from the digits. Mechanical management includes special massage techniques referred to as manual lymph drainage. These techniques should be performed only by specially trained individuals (Mayo Clinic, 2017).

Nursing Interventions and Patient Teaching

The primary goal of care is to increase lymphatic drainage and avoid trauma. Elevation of the extremities while asleep and periodically during the day facilitates drainage. Massage techniques previously discussed help improve lymph drainage. If the patient tolerates light exercise, it should be encouraged. Advise patients to avoid constrictive clothing, shoes, or stockings (except elastic stockings). Patients with lymphedema are at risk for infection in the affected extremity. Good skin care, avoiding injury, inspecting the skin daily for cuts or cracks in the skin, is important. Lotions can be applied to prevent dryness of the skin.

Emotional support for the patient is also important. Address body image disturbance related to the appearance of the lymphedematous extremity. Emphasize that lymphedema need not prevent the individual from engaging in routine activity.

A patient problem and interventions for lymphedema include but are not limited to the following:

PATIENT PROBLEM	NURSING INTERVENTIONS
Potential for infection, related to altered lymphatic drainage causing stasis of fluid	Elevate affected extremity Consider physical therapy or range-of-motion exercises (aids lymphatic flow) Assess skin for signs of infection (redness, warmth) Teach application of supportive stockings or elastic sleeves Monitor patient for systemic signs of infection (elevated white blood cell count, increased body temperature, increased erythrocyte sedimentation rate)

Make certain the patient is aware of the condition's progression and cause. If the disorder is long term and ongoing, discuss how to cope with its effects. Explain the rationale behind nursing interventions to enhance the ongoing medical regimen. Encourage the patient to maintain interests and socialize to enhance feelings of well-being.

Prognosis

Lymphedema has no cure, but signs and symptoms of the condition can be controlled by compliance with treatment. The goal of care is to prevent lymphedema when possible and to initiate prompt treatment when it does occur. Compliance with suggested treatment modalities can prevent complications of the disorder which include lymphangitis, cellulitis, and lymphangiosarcoma (Kim, Hwang, Bae, et al., 2019).

HODGKIN LYMPHOMA

Etiology and Pathophysiology

Hodgkin lymphoma, previously known as Hodgkin disease, is characterized by painless, progressive enlargement of lymphoid tissue. It is slightly more common in men than in women and accounts for 0.5% of newly diagnosed cancer cases in the United States with a death rate of 0.2% (Shanbhag & Ambinder, 2018). The age of incidence curve is bimodal (two separate populations), with a peak early in life at 15 to 35 years, and a peak later in life at 50 years. The two peaks in incidence may represent separate diseases. The first incident peak suggests a viral cause. Beginning as an inflammatory or infectious process, the condition develops into a neoplasm.

Hodgkin lymphoma has no major risk factors, but the disease occurs more frequently in people who have had mononucleosis (an infection caused by Epstein-Barr virus), have acquired or congenital immunodeficiency syndromes, are taking immunosuppressive drugs after organ transplantation, have been exposed to occupational toxins, or have a genetic predisposition. The presence of HIV increases the incidence of Hodgkin lymphoma.

Lymphoid tissue enlargement usually is noticed first in the cervical nodes and is characterized by abnormal or atypical cells. Reed-Sternberg cells are atypical histiocytes consisting of large, abnormal, multinucleated cells in the lymph nodes found in Hodgkin lymphoma. These cells increase in number, replacing normal cells. The main diagnostic feature of Hodgkin lymphoma is the presence of Reed-Sternberg cells in lymph node biopsy specimens.

The disease is believed to arise in a single location (the lymph nodes in most patients) and then spread along adjacent lymphatics. It eventually infiltrates other organs, especially the lungs, spleen, and liver. In the majority of patients, the cervical lymph nodes are affected first. Unless they exert pressure on adjacent nerves, the enlarged nodes are not painful. When the disease begins above the diaphragm, it remains confined to lymph nodes for a variable period. Disease originating below the diaphragm frequently spreads to extralymphoid sites such as the liver.

Clinical Manifestations

Painless enlargement of the cervical, axillary, or inguinal lymph nodes is most often the initial development. Anorexia, unexplained rapid weight loss, fever, night sweats, fatigue, and pruritus are complaints associated with this condition. One other unusual symptom is pain in the lymph nodes after ingesting alcohol (Mayo Clinic, 2019b). Night sweats, weight loss, and fever, which are referred to as "B" symptoms, are associated with a worse prognosis (Box 7.7). Low-grade fever may occur. Anemia and leukocytosis follow, with development of respiratory tract infections.

Assessment

Subjective data include the common complaints of fatigue and appetite loss. Pruritus is often severe. After the ingestion of even small amounts of alcohol,

---

Box 7.7   Cotswold-Modified Ann Arbor Staging System for Hodgkin Lymphoma

Stage I: Disease affecting a single lymph node region or lymphoid structure (e.g., spleen, thymus, Waldeyer ring).
Stage II: Disease affecting two or more discrete lymph node regions confined to the same side of the diaphragm.
Stage III: Disease affecting two or more discrete lymph node regions or lymphoid structures on both sides of the diaphragm.
Stage IV: Disease that has spread to one or more extranodal sites (that does not meet the criteria for E) or an extralymphatic structure including involvement of the bone marrow, liver, or lungs.

DESIGNATIONS
A: Absence of B symptoms[a]
B: Presence of B symptoms[a]
S: Involvement of the spleen
E: Single extranodal site or involvement of an extranodal site that is contiguous to an involved nodal region.
X: Bulky disease as defined as >1/3 mediastinum at its widest part or a nodal mass >10 cm at its greatest diameter.

[a] B symptoms: constitutional symptoms including night sweats, fevers, or weight loss (>10% over 6 months).
From Hoffman R, Anastasi J, Weitz J, et al: *Hematology: Basic principles and practice*, ed 7, St. Louis, 2018, Elsevier.

---

individuals with Hodgkin lymphoma may complain of a rapid onset of pain at the site of the disease. The cause for the alcohol-induced pain is unknown. Bone pain occurs later in the disease's course.

Collection of objective data includes palpating enlarged cervical and supraclavicular lymph nodes. Splenomegaly, hepatomegaly, and abdominal tenderness are found. Excoriation of skin and evidence of scratching from pruritus are noted. Clinical signs and symptoms vary depending on where the enlarged lymph nodes are located. If Hodgkin lymphoma affects lymph nodes inside the chest, the swelling of these nodes may press on the trachea, stimulating a cough reflex or dyspnea. Some patients may complain of pain behind the sternum and difficulty swallowing (ACS, 2018a).

Diagnostic Tests

Peripheral blood studies show anemia (normocytic, normochromic), WBC increase, and an abnormal erythrocyte sedimentation rate. Other blood studies may show hypoferremia (low iron level in the blood) caused by excessive iron intake by the liver and the spleen, elevated leukocyte alkaline phosphatase from liver and bone involvement, hypercalcemia from bone involvement, and hypoalbuminemia from liver involvement. Chest radiographic examination may reveal a mediastinal mass. CT or MRI can detect retroperitoneal node involvement. Lymph node biopsy that includes laparoscopy for retroperitoneal nodes is performed. Bone marrow biopsy is an important aspect of staging. A CT scan and an ultrasound examination can indicate an enlarged spleen or liver. The presence of Reed-Sternberg cells remains a hallmark of Hodgkin lymphoma.

Positron emission tomography (PET), CT scans, bone scans, and bone marrow biopsy aid in the staging of the disease by determining the extent of any metastasis (ACS, 2018a). The liver, lungs, and bone are common areas of metastasis.

Medical Management

Treatment depends on the staging process (see Box 7.7). The stage of Hodgkin lymphoma must be established before selecting an appropriate treatment plan.

Combination chemotherapy is used in some early stages in patients believed to have resistant disease or to be at high risk for relapse. Chemotherapy and radiation therapy are used against the generalized forms (stages III and IV). Advances in treatment now enable some stage IIIB and stage IV diseases to be cured with high-dose chemotherapy and bone marrow or peripheral stem cell transplantation (SCT). The site of the disease and the amount of resistant disease after chemotherapy determine the role of radiation in supplementing chemotherapy.

Treatment of early-stage Hodgkin lymphoma consists of two to four cycles of ABVD (doxorubicin, bleomycin, vinblastine, and dacarbazine) chemotherapy.

For advanced-stage Hodgkin lymphoma some people have ABVD for up to eight cycles. Other possible combinations include Stanford V (mechlorethamine, doxorubicin, vinblastine, vincristine, bleomycin, etoposide, and prednisone), and BEACOPP (bleomycin, etoposide, doxorubicin, cyclophosphamide, vincristine, procarbazine, and prednisone) (ACS, 2017a). If chemotherapy does not work well or the lymphoma comes back, some people have high-dose chemotherapy with SCT (ACS, 2018a).

Nursing Interventions and Patient Teaching

Plan care according to the staging level. Awareness of side effects of radiation therapy or chemotherapy is important in preparing the patient to deal effectively with the treatment. Because the survival of patients with Hodgkin lymphoma depends on their response to treatment, helping the patient deal with the consequences of treatment is extremely important. Comfort measures focus on skin integrity. Soothing baths with an antipruritic medication (as prescribed) can be effective. Control fever and moisture with medication (with attention to increased fluid intake) and linen changes as necessary to prevent further skin problems. Explain extensive tests to the patient to aid in reduction of anxiety and difficulty coping.

Patient problems include *Anxiousness* and *Fearfulness*, related to unknown outcome, and *Potential for Infection*, related to compromised immune system.

An additional patient problem and interventions for the patient with Hodgkin lymphoma include but are not limited to the following:

PATIENT PROBLEM	NURSING INTERVENTIONS
Compromised Skin Integrity, related to: • Pruritus • Jaundice • Diaphoresis	Assess skin and level of discomfort Administer skin care by baths and keep patient clean and dry Apply calamine lotion, cornstarch, sodium bicarbonate, and medicated powders to relieve pruritus Maintain adequate humidity and a cool room to decrease pruritus Monitor vital signs for fever; assess for perspiration and change linen, keeping it wrinkle free

Understanding the disease through education and teaching is important for the patient to perform self-care and retain independence. Fertility issues may be of particular concern because this disease frequently is seen in adolescents and young adults. Help ensure that these issues are addressed soon after diagnosis. The effect on the patient's life, as well as on significant others, is a prime consideration in patient attitude and adjustment. Realistic approaches to the illness and therapies are imperative. Referrals for patients seeking counseling for stress management can be helpful. Discuss special nutritional considerations concerning excess weight loss or an undernourished condition.

Prognosis

The staging of the disease is important in the prognosis. The disease is classified as stage I if the cancer is found in only one lymph node area or lymphoid organ, such as the thymus, or the cancer is found only in one area of a single organ outside the lymph system. Stage II is characterized by cancer being found in two or more lymph node areas on the same side of the diaphragm, or the cancer extends locally from one lymph node area into a nearby organ. Stage III is determined by the presence of cancer in lymph node areas on both sides of the diaphragm, or the cancer is in lymph nodes above the diaphragm and in the spleen. Cancer that has spread widely into at least one organ outside of the lymph system, such as the liver, bone marrow, or lungs is classified as stage IV Hodgkin lymphoma (ACS, 2018a). In general, the earlier the stage of the cancer, the higher the survival rate and chance for a cure. The 5-year survival rate for Hodgkin lymphoma is not based on staging directly but on whether the cancer is localized, reginal, or distant. Patients with localized Hodgkin lymphoma have a 5-year survival rate of 92%, regional Hodgkin lymphoma has a 5-year survival rate of 94%, and distant has a 5-year survival rate of 78% (ACS, 2018a).

NON-HODGKIN LYMPHOMA

Etiology and Pathophysiology

Non-Hodgkin lymphoma (NHL) is a neoplasm originating in lymphoid tissues of the body. Neoplasms are of B-cell or T-cell origin and give rise to cancerous cells that are varied in terms of epidemiology, etiology, clinical features, and response to therapy (Sapkota & Shaikh, 2020). NHL can also be classified as indolent or aggressive. Indolent NHL tends to grow and spread slowly, and patients with this type of NHL may be treated with a "watch and wait" approach. Aggressive NHL tends to grow and spread quickly and requires immediate treatment. The risk factors for getting NHL include the following: individuals over the age of 60; men more than women; more common in Caucasians than African Americans and Asians; occurs in developed countries more so than third-world countries; more common in people exposed to chemicals such as benzene, herbicides, insecticides, and chemotherapy drugs; immunosuppressed and HIV; autoimmune diseases; and infections such as Epstein Barr virus and herpes (ACS, 2018b).

Clinical Manifestations

Common symptoms of NHL include enlarged lymph nodes, fever, sweating and chills, weight loss, pruritus, fatigue, and susceptibility to infection. Abdominal distension may result if lymph nodes of the abdomen, liver, or spleen are enlarged as a result of the disease process. If NHL is in the chest, the patient may experience pain in the chest, pressure, a cough, and shortness of breath (ACS, 2018b). There is no hallmark pathologic feature in NHL that parallels the Reed-Sternberg cell of Hodgkin lymphoma. However, all NHLs involve lymphocytes arrested in various stages of development.

Assessment

Subjective data include frequent patient complaints of fatigue, malaise, and anorexia.

Collection of objective data includes examination of the abdomen for splenomegaly. Enlarged lymph nodes are also evident. Fever, night sweats, and weight loss are usually present.

Diagnostic Tests

Biopsies of lymph nodes, liver, and bone marrow are performed to establish the cell type and pattern. A bone scan may reveal fractures, lesions, and tumor infiltration. PET scans, CT, MRI, and chest x-ray are common tests for diagnosing NHL. Common serum lab tests include the CBC, immunohistochemistry (detects specific antibodies), flow cytometry (identifies specific types of cells), and DNA/genetic testing. Diagnostic studies used for NHL resemble those used for Hodgkin lymphoma (ACS, 2018b).

Staging, as described for Hodgkin lymphoma, is used to guide therapy. The four-stage system used with Hodgkin lymphoma is the same system used for NHL.

Medical Management

Once the diagnosis is made, the extent of the disease (staging) is determined. Accurate staging is crucial to determine the treatment regimen. The therapeutic regimen for NHLs includes chemotherapy and radiation. Indolent (slow-growing) lymphomas have a naturally long course but are difficult to treat effectively. In contrast, more aggressive lymphomas are more likely to be cured because they are more responsive to treatment. Some chemotherapy agents used are cyclophosphamide, vincristine, prednisone, doxorubicin, bleomycin, and methotrexate. The monoclonal antibody rituximab was approved for the treatment of follicular lymphoma. Ibritumomab is another monoclonal antibody that can be used in patients who are refractory to rituximab, or in conjunction with it. Conventional chemotherapy used to treat patients with relapsed, aggressive NHL, who are still responding to salvage chemotherapy, is not as effective as high-dose chemotherapy with autologous (tissue derived from the same individual) HSCT (ACS, 2018b).

Patients with lymphoma commonly receive radiation to the chest wall, mediastinum, axillae, and neck—the region known as the "mantle field." Some patients also need radiation to the abdomen; paraaortic area; spleen; and, less commonly, the pelvis.

Chemotherapy remains the traditional method of treatment of NHLs that are not localized. High-dose chemotherapy with PBSC or bone marrow transplantation may be indicated. Interferon is being used to help in boosting the immune system. Monoclonal antibodies are being designed to attack a specific target, such as a substance on the surface of lymphocytes, and destroy cancer cells. Targeted cancer therapies such as the use of monoclonal antibodies promise to be more selective for cancer cells than normal cells, thus harming fewer normal cells, reducing side effects, and improving quality of life (ACS, 2018b).

Nursing Interventions and Patient Teaching

Supportive care of the patient during radiation and chemotherapy is primary in nursing management. Observation for complications follows. Further intervention is similar to that for Hodgkin lymphoma.

Explanations of the extensive diagnostic workup and its importance for staging the disease and determining the treatment plan are an important focus of patient teaching during the diagnostic period.

Prognosis

The 5-year survival rate for NHL is 73% if local, 72% if regional, and 55% if distant (ACS, 2018a). Patients with aggressive lymphomas have worse prognosis, whereas patients with low-grade lymphomas survive 6 to 10 years. Low-grade lymphomas can turn into aggressive lymphomas (Sapkota & Shaikh, 2020).

NURSING PROCESS FOR THE PATIENT WITH A BLOOD OR LYMPHATIC DISORDER

ASSESSMENT

Collect data from diverse sources: patient and family observation, physical examination, and diagnostic evaluation results (see Table 7.1).

The subjective data collected at the onset of the disease process are generally vague and nonspecific: malaise, fatigue, and weakness. The patient may relate a history of illness, easy bruising, bleeding tendencies with petechiae, and ecchymoses. Integumentary

Lifespan Considerations

Older Adults

Blood or Lymphatic Disorder

- The subjective symptoms of hematologic disorders (e.g., fatigue, weakness, dizziness, and dyspnea) may be mistaken for normal changes of aging or attributed to other disease processes commonly seen in older adults.
- The most common blood disorders are forms of anemia.
- Decreased production of intrinsic factor in an aging gastric mucosa results in increased incidence of pernicious anemia.
- Many older adults suffer from conditions such as colonic diverticula, hiatal hernia, or ulcerations that can cause occult bleeding. Older adults with these conditions should be observed for iron deficiency anemia.
- Age-related problems such as altered dentition, limited financial resources, difficulty in food preparation, and poor appetite resulting from emotional upset or depression can cause an increased incidence of iron deficiency anemia.
- Severe or persistent anemia can place additional stress on the aging or diseased heart.
- Administer blood products with caution because older adults are at increased risk of developing congestive heart failure. Careful assessment of cardiopulmonary function and intake and output is essential.
- Oral administration of iron preparations increases the risk of gastrointestinal (GI) irritation and constipation in older adults.
- Ingestion of large amounts of aspirin and other anti-inflammatory medications commonly taken by older adults increases the risk of GI bleeding and can lead to alteration in clotting.
- Chronic lymphocytic leukemia is the most common form seen among older patients. This form of leukemia usually progresses slowly in older adults and rarely is treated.

Collection of objective data follows a system-by-system approach to confirm patient complaints. Manipulation of joints can reveal stiffness and hematoma and may produce pain. Examination of the oral cavity can reveal lesions, ulcers, signs of bleeding, or gingivitis. Cardiovascular and respiratory assessments include breath and heart sound variations. Note any patient anxiety, and observe for diminished comprehension. Listening and an unhurried interview may reveal many symptoms not previously mentioned.

changes (including pruritus, nonhealing cuts and bruises, draining lesions, jaundice, and palpable subcutaneous nodules) may be reported. Edema and tenderness in lymph node regions may be accompanied by pain, sometimes severe. GI complaints are noted, as well as cardiovascular and respiratory changes. Neurologic complaints include headache, numbness, tingling, paresthesias, and behavioral alteration (see the Lifespan Considerations box).

PATIENT PROBLEM

Patient problems are determined from the assessment, which provides data for identifying the patient's problems, strengths, potential complications, and learning needs. Patient problems for the patient with a blood or lymphatic disorder include but are not limited to the following:

- Compromised Blood Flow to Tissue
- Compromised Skin Integrity
- Impaired Coping
- Inability to Tolerate Activity
- Insufficient Knowledge of Condition and Disease Management
- Insufficient Oxygenation
- Lethargy or Malaise
- Potential for Harm or Damage to the Body, Potential for (Bleeding, Falls)
- Potential for Infection
- Prolonged Pain
- Recent Onset of Pain

EXPECTED OUTCOMES AND PLANNING

Most patients have more than one patient problem. Therefore, the planning step in the nursing process involves determining the priority for nursing interventions from the list of patient problems. Use Maslow's hierarchy of needs to prioritize needs. Life-threatening needs such as *Insufficient Oxygenation* would have a higher priority than *Ineffective Coping*.

Planning includes developing realistic goals and outcomes that stem from the identified nursing diagnosis. Examples of expected patient outcomes for the patient with a blood or lymphatic disorder may include but are not limited to the following:

Goal 1: Patient is free of signs and symptoms of an infection.

Goal 2: Patient has no evidence of bleeding (any bleeding is quickly controlled).

IMPLEMENTATION

The implementation of the nursing process is the actual initiation of the nursing care plan. Patient outcomes and goals are achieved by performance of the nursing interventions. Nursing interventions for the patient with a blood or lymphatic disorder may include the following:

- Place patient in private room; avoid contact with visitors or staff members who have an infection (for the immunocompromised patient).

- Stress careful hand hygiene to patient, significant others, and all caregivers.
- Assist in planning daily activities to include rest periods to decrease fatigue and weakness.
- Provide oxygen for dyspnea or excessive fatigue with exertion.
- Explain the disease process, and stress the importance of continued medical follow-up. Most important is the patient's ability to identify the body's signals that blood abnormalities are present. Petechiae, ecchymoses, and gingival bleeding are the warning signs to seek medical attention promptly.

EVALUATION

To evaluate the effectiveness of nursing interventions, compare the patient's behaviors with those stated in the expected patient outcomes. Successful achievement of patient outcomes for the patient with a blood or lymphatic disorder is indicated by the following evaluative measures:

- Patient shows no sign of infection; temperature and WBC count are within normal limits.
- Patient has not fallen.
- Patient shows no signs of bleeding (e.g., petechiae, hemorrhage); any bleeding is controlled quickly.
- Patient is able to bathe self in 30 minutes without becoming fatigued.
- Patient is able to correctly explain measures to prevent infection by good hand hygiene techniques and avoidance of people with infectious conditions.
- Patient is able to explain measures to prevent hemorrhage by avoiding traumatic injury and intramuscular injections.
- Patient reports no shortness of breath with activity.

Get Ready for the NCLEX® Examination!

Key Points

- Blood is a thick, red fluid composed of plasma, a light-yellow fluid; albumin, the most abundant protein in human blood plasma; RBCs; WBCs; platelets; and electrolytes, which regulate our nerve and muscle function, our body's hydration, blood pH, blood pressure, and the rebuilding of damaged tissue.
- The blood performs several critical functions: It transports oxygen and nutrients to the cells and waste products away from the cells; it regulates acid-base balance (pH) with buffers; and it protects the body against infection and prevents blood loss with special clotting mechanisms.
- Every person's blood is one of the following blood types in the ABO system of typing: A, B, AB, or O.
- The lymphatic system is a vast, complex network of capillaries, thin vessels, valves, ducts, nodes, and organs that helps to protect and maintain the internal fluid environment of the entire body by producing, filtering, and conveying lymph and by storing and releasing various immune cells.
- The tonsils are composed of lymphoid tissue and are responsible for filtering bacteria.
- The thymus gland is composed of lymphoid tissue in utero (before birth) and the early years of life. It aids in the development of the immune system.
- The spleen also is composed of lymphoid tissue and has many functions, such as filtering out old RBCs, storing a pint of blood, producing antibodies, and phagocytosing bacteria.
- Anemia may be caused by blood loss, impaired RBC production, increased RBC destruction, or nutritional deficiency.
- Shock occurs when organs are deprived of oxygen and nutrients. Shock is characterized by inadequate circulatory provision of oxygen, which causes vital organs and tissues to shut down. Blood pressure falls to a life-threatening low, either from reduced cardiac output or from reduced effective circulating blood volume.

- Hypotension, defined as a systolic blood pressure of less than 90 mm Hg and tachycardia of more than 120 bpm, occurs with blood loss of 1500 to 2000 mL. By the time blood pressure reaches this point, about 30% to 40% of the blood volume may have been lost, and end-organ damage may be irreversible.
- Weakness and fatigue are major symptoms of anemia. They result from decreased oxygenation from decreased levels of Hgb and increased energy needs required by increased RBC production.
- Ingestion of iron compounds or intramuscular Z-track administration of iron dextran is part of the therapy for iron deficiency anemia.
- Sickle cell anemia is a hemolytic anemia with a genetic basis; a sickle cell crisis occurs when the RBCs become deoxygenated and sickle shaped, thus causing stasis and obstruction of the microvasculature, leading to organ infarction and necrosis.
- Polycythemia vera is characterized by excessive bone marrow production that manifests with an increase in circulating erythrocytes, granulocytes, and platelets. Secondary polycythemia is caused by hypoxia rather than a defect in the development of the blood cells.
- Thrombocytopenia is a decrease in the number of circulating platelets and leads to bleeding; people with thrombocytopenia need to learn how to prevent injury and hemorrhage.
- Hemophilia is a hereditary coagulation disorder; hemophilia A is a lack of coagulation factor VIII, and hemophilia B is a lack of factor IX. Maintenance therapy consists of blood factor replacement therapy and prevention of injury.
- DIC is a coagulation disorder characterized initially by clotting and secondarily by hemorrhage. It results from an alteration in the balance between clotting factors and fibrinolytic factors; the person is usually critically ill.
- People with alterations of WBCs are at high risk of infection because leukocytes are a major factor in the body's defense against invading microorganisms.

- The leukemias are malignant disorders characterized by uncontrolled proliferation of WBCs and their precursors; the cause is unknown, but several theories have been proposed.
- Leukemias may be lymphocytic, or myelogenous, and acute or chronic. Acute leukemias have a rapid onset and a short course, if untreated; chronic leukemias have a more insidious onset and longer course. The major therapies for leukemias are chemotherapy and bone marrow transplantation.
- Multiple myeloma is a malignant neoplastic immunodeficiency disease of the bone marrow that affects the plasma cells. The specific immunoglobulin produced by the myeloma cells is present in the blood and urine and is referred to as the monoclonal protein.
- Lymphomas are malignant disorders of the lymphatic system. People with Hodgkin lymphoma have defective cellular immunity and are therefore at high risk for infection. NHL is a group of lymphoid malignancies. Chemotherapy and radiation are the primary medical treatment for lymphomas.

Additional Learning Resources

SG Go to your Study Guide for additional learning activities to help you master this chapter content.

Be sure to visit the Evolve site at http://evolve.elsevier.com/Cooper/adult/ for additional online resources.

Review Questions for the NCLEX® Examination

1. What compound in the blood carries oxygen to the cells from the lungs and carbon dioxide away from the cells to the lungs?

   1. Leukocyte
   2. Thrombocyte
   3. Hemoglobin
   4. Erythrocyte

2. A universal donor has which blood type?

   1. Type A
   2. Type B
   3. Type AB
   4. Type O

3. The spleen is located in which quadrant of the abdominal cavity?

   1. Upper right
   2. Upper left
   3. Lower left
   4. Lower right

4. A patient's platelet count is 18,000/mm³. What is the most appropriate nursing intervention?

   1. Provide oral hygiene four times per day.
   2. Institute bleeding precautions.
   3. Order a high-protein diet.
   4. Request an order for oxygen per nasal cannula.

5. A patient's spouse tells the nurse that her husband, who has been admitted to the hospital with advanced leukemia, is talking about dying and expresses fears of death. She asks for suggestions for helping her husband. Which response is best?

   1. "Your husband will probably die of another disease before he dies of leukemia."
   2. "Your husband is expressing a readiness to be admitted to a hospice."
   3. "Talk of death is natural at this time but will diminish as he feels better."
   4. "It's normal to want to talk about death; what we can do is be supportive by listening."

6. A 28-year-old man is admitted with fatigue; discomfort; enlarged, painless cervical lymph nodes; and pruritus. A lymph node biopsy leads to the diagnosis of Hodgkin lymphoma. What are the abnormal cells noted by the pathologist in Hodgkin lymphoma called?

   1. Rodem-Lee cells
   2. Bullus-Frendelenburg cells
   3. Reed-Sternberg cells
   4. Steven-Johnson cells

7. An adult patient is seen by the nurse at a health maintenance organization for signs of fatigue. The patient has a history of iron deficiency anemia. What data from the nursing history indicate that the anemia is not currently managed effectively?

   1. Pallor
   2. Poor skin turgor
   3. Heart rate of 68 bpm, weak pulse
   4. Respiration at 18 breaths/min and regular

8. What is an important teaching point for a patient who has iron deficiency anemia?

   1. Use birth control to avoid pregnancy.
   2. Increase fluids to stimulate erythropoiesis.
   3. Decrease fluids to prevent sickling of RBCs.
   4. Alternate periods of rest and activity to balance oxygen supply and demand.

9. The nurse instructs a patient about foods rich in iron. Which foods should be included in the diet?

   1. Fresh fruit and milk
   2. Cheeses and processed lunch meats
   3. Dark green, leafy vegetables and organ meats
   4. Fruit juices and cornmeal bread

10. Which statement by the patient with pernicious anemia would indicate that she understood the teaching?

    1. "I'll be glad when I can stop the injections and take only oral medicine."
    2. "I'll have to take B_{12} shots for the rest of my life."
    3. "After a while I'll no longer need to take shots, just the pills."
    4. "I was glad to hear that pills are available to treat me."

11. A patient is admitted with polycythemia vera. The patient's Hgb value is 20 g/dL. Which treatment will be ordered?

    1. Whole blood transfusion
    2. Platelet transfusion
    3. Phlebotomy with removal of 800 mL of blood
    4. Vitamin B_{12} injection

12. Which laboratory finding is a strong indicator of disseminated intravascular coagulation (DIC)?

    1. An elevated platelet count
    2. An elevated D-dimer test result
    3. A normal prothrombin time
    4. An elevated fibrinogen level

13. The nurse is teaching the patient with pernicious anemia about the disease. The nurse explains that pernicious anemia results from the lack of:

    1. folic acid.
    2. intrinsic factor.
    3. extrinsic factor.
    4. an RBC enzyme.

14. A patient with sickle cell anemia asks the nurse why the sickling crisis does not stop when oxygen therapy is started. Which statement by the nurse is the most accurate answer?

    1. "Sickling occurs in response to decreased blood viscosity, which is not affected by oxygen therapy."
    2. "When red cells sickle, they occlude small vessels, which cause more local hypoxia and more sickling."
    3. "The primary problem during a sickle cell crisis is destruction of the abnormal cells, resulting in fewer RBCs to carry oxygen."
    4. "Oxygen therapy does not alter the shape of the abnormal erythrocytes but only allows for increased oxygen concentration in Hgb."

15. What nursing interventions are indicated for a patient during a sickle cell crisis? *(Select all that apply.)*

    1. Frequent ambulation
    2. Apply antiembolism hose
    3. Restrict sodium intake
    4. Increase the oral fluid intake
    5. Administer therapeutic doses of continuous opioid analgesics

16. Hodgkin lymphoma occurs more frequently in individuals with which risk factor?

    1. A history of cancer treated with radiation
    2. Exposure to nuclear explosions
    3. Infection with the Epstein-Barr virus
    4. Infection with *Helicobacter pylori*

17. Which statement concerning Hodgkin lymphoma is correct?

    1. The 10-year survival rate for stage I or II Hodgkin lymphoma is more than 90%.
    2. Hodgkin lymphoma commonly occurs between the ages of 15 and 35 years.
    3. Hodgkin lymphoma is not a curable disease.
    4. The incidence of Hodgkin lymphoma in the female population has increased.

18. What is an appropriate nursing intervention for a patient with hemophilia who is hospitalized with acute knee pain and edema?

    1. Wrapping the knee with an elastic bandage
    2. Placing the patient on bed rest and applying ice to the joint

    3. Gently performing ROM exercises to the knee to prevent adhesions
    4. Administering nonsteroidal anti-inflammatory drugs as needed for pain

19. During a physical assessment of a patient with thrombocytopenia, the nurse would expect to find:

    1. petechiae and purpura.
    2. jaundiced sclera and skin.
    3. tender, enlarged lymph nodes.
    4. splenomegaly.

20. Which nursing interventions are necessary when caring for a patient who has a WBC count of 1800/mm³? *(Select all that apply.)*

    1. Prevent patient contact with people who have respiratory tract infections or influenza.
    2. Perform hand hygiene before and after patient contact.
    3. Report temperature elevation.
    4. Monitor Hgb.
    5. Assess for signs of bleeding.

21. Which are necessary for the maturation of a red blood cell? *(Select all that apply.)*

    1. Vitamin B$_{12}$
    2. Folic acid
    3. Renal erythropoietic factor
    4. Capric acid
    5. Iron

22. Which represents the correct medical management for the patient with DIC? *(Select all that apply.)*

    1. Addressing and correcting underlying cause
    2. Transfusion replacement
    3. Cryoprecipitate
    4. Administering colony-stimulating factor (filgrastim [Neupogen])
    5. Heparin therapy

23. A boy, 3, who is usually very easygoing and playful, lies down on the floor at his preschool and begins to cry uncontrollably. He does not answer when asked what's wrong but says, "My bones bite." One of the two classroom teachers takes his temperature, but it is normal. She asks, "Did you have trouble sleeping last night, sweetie?" He seems too tired even to answer her. He continues to lie on the floor during music, his favorite activity, and seems so exhausted that the teachers put a pillow beneath his head and invite him to lie on a mat. He doesn't move but blinks at them listlessly, eyes filling with tears. He tries to rally at snack time, but when he bites into an orange slice, he screams and drops it. A teacher looks in his mouth and sees very red sores. His mother is called from work, and she takes him straight to his pediatrician. There he presents with the oral lesions, as well as suspected anemia. His mother reports that he complained in the car of joint or bone pain (she is unsure which he means), as well as fatigue, malaise, decreased activity tolerance, and irritability. Examination reveals suspected painless splenomegaly and enlarged lymph nodes. The pediatrician also suspects possible hepatomegaly. The provider immediately ordered lab tests that include throat and urine cultures, chest radiography and peripheral blood CBC,

including evaluation of WBCs with differential. Test results indicate a diagnosis of ALL. The patient is hospitalized for bone marrow biopsy and lymph node biopsy to confirm, and as the treatment team awaits these results, he is scheduled for a combination therapy of chemo and radiation, but the oncologist investigates the possibility of either bone marrow transplantation or HSCT.

Place a check mark to indicate each test result that supports a diagnosis of ALL. Check all that apply.

TEST RESULT	SUPPORTS A DIAGNOSIS OF ALL
Total WBC count >10,000 cells/mm^3	
Total WBC count <5000 cells/mm^3	

TEST RESULT	SUPPORTS A DIAGNOSIS OF ALL
Total WBC count with >70% neutrophils	
Total WBC count with <20% lymphocytes	
Total WBC count with >40% lymphocytes	
Low levels of platelets and RBC Hgb	

Care of the Patient With a Cardiovascular or a Peripheral Vascular Disorder

8

Objectives

Anatomy and Physiology

1. Discuss the location, size, and position of the heart.
2. Identify the chambers and valves of the heart and their functions.
3. Discuss the electrical conduction system that causes the cardiac muscle fibers to contract.
4. Explain what produces the two main heart sounds.
5. Trace the path of blood through the coronary circulation.

Medico-Surgical

6. List diagnostic tests used to evaluate cardiovascular function.
7. For coronary artery disease, compare nonmodifiable risk factors with factors that are modifiable in lifestyle and health management.
8. Describe five cardiac dysrhythmias.
9. Compare the etiology and pathophysiology, clinical manifestations, assessment, diagnostic tests, medical management, nursing interventions, and prognosis for patients with angina pectoris, myocardial infarction, or heart failure.
10. Specify patient teaching for patients with cardiac dysrhythmias, angina pectoris, myocardial infarction, heart failure, and valvular heart disease.
11. Discuss the purposes of cardiac rehabilitation.
12. Discuss the etiology and pathophysiology, clinical manifestations, assessment, diagnostic tests, medical management, nursing interventions, and prognosis for the patient with pulmonary edema.
13. Compare and contrast the etiology and pathophysiology, clinical manifestations, assessment, diagnostic tests,

medical management, nursing interventions, and prognosis for the patient with rheumatic heart disease, pericarditis, and endocarditis.
14. Identify 10 conditions that may result in the development of secondary cardiomyopathy.
15. Discuss the indication for cardiac transplant.
16. Identify risk factors and the effects of aging associated with peripheral vascular disorders.
17. Compare and contrast signs and symptoms and discuss nursing interventions associated with arterial and venous disorders.
18. Compare essential (primary) hypertension, secondary hypertension, and malignant hypertension.
19. Discuss the etiology and pathophysiology, clinical manifestations, assessment, diagnostic tests, medical management, and nursing interventions and the importance of patient education for the patient with hypertension.
20. Compare and contrast the etiology and pathophysiology, clinical manifestations, assessment, diagnostic tests, medical management, nursing interventions, and prognosis for patients with arterial aneurysm, Buerger disease, and Raynaud disease.
21. Discuss the etiology and pathophysiology, clinical manifestations, assessment, diagnostic tests, medical management, nursing interventions, and prognosis and appropriate patient education for patients with thrombophlebitis, varicose veins, and stasis ulcer.

Key Terms

aneurysm (ĂN-ŭr-ĭ-zĭm, p. 360)

angina pectoris (ăn-JĪ-nă PĔK-tŏr-ĭs, p. 321)

arteriosclerosis (ăr-tē-rē-ō-sklĕ-RŌ-sĭs, p. 356)

atherosclerosis (ăth-ĕr-ō-sklĕ-RŌ-sĭs, p. 357)

bradycardia (brăd-ĕ-KĂR-dē-ă, p. 314)

B-type natriuretic peptide (BNP) (nā-trĕ-yū-RĔT-ĭk, p. 310)

cardioversion (kăr-dē-ō-VĔR-zhŭn, p. 309)

coronary artery disease (CAD) (p. 321)

defibrillation (dē-fĭb-rĭ-LĀ-shŭn, p. 318)

dysrhythmia (dĭs-RĬTH-mē-ă, p. 313)

embolus (ĔM-bō-lŭs, p. 326)

endarterectomy (ĕnd-ăr-tĕr-ĔK-tō-mē, p. 358)

heart failure (HF) (p. 333)

hypoxemia (hī-pŏk-SĒ-mē-ă, p. 309)

intermittent claudication (klăw-dĕ-KĀ-shŭn, p. 351)

ischemia (ĭs-KĒ-mē-ă, p. 322)

multigated acquisition (MUGA) scan (p. 328)

myocardial infarction (MI) (mī-ō-KĂR-dē-ăl ĭn-FĂRK-shŭn, p. 309)

orthopnea (ŏr-THŎP-nē-ă, p. 336)

peripheral (pĕ-RĬF-ĕr-ăl, p. 350)

pleural effusion (PLŪR-ăl ĕ-FŪ-zhŭn, p. 299)

polycythemia (pŏl-ē-sī-THĒ-mē-ă, p. 309)

pulmonary edema (PŪL-mō-nă-rē ĕ-DĒ-mă, p. 340)

rubor (p. 363)

tachycardia (tăk-ĕ-KĂR-dē-ă, p. 314)

ANATOMY AND PHYSIOLOGY OF THE CARDIOVASCULAR SYSTEM

The cardiovascular (circulatory) system is the transportation system of the body. It delivers oxygen and nutrients to the cells to support their individual activities and transports the cells' waste products to the appropriate organs for disposal. This chapter discusses the structure and function of the blood vessels and the heart.

HEART

The heart is a remarkable organ, not much bigger than a fist (Fig. 8.1). It pumps 1000 gallons of blood every day through the closed circuit of blood vessels. It beats 100,000 times a day and transports the blood 60,000 miles through a network of blood vessels. The heart is a hollow organ composed mainly of muscle tissue with a series of one-way valves.

   The heart is located in the chest cavity between the lungs in a region called the *mediastinum* (the organs and tissues separating the lungs; in addition to the heart and its greater vessels, the mediastinum contains the trachea and the esophagus). Two-thirds of the heart lies left of the midline. The wider *base* of the heart lies superior to and beneath the second rib. The *apex,* or narrow part, of the heart lies inferiorly, slightly to the left between the fifth and sixth ribs near the diaphragm.

Heart Wall

The heart wall is composed of three layers: pericardium, myocardium, and endocardium. The *pericardium* is a double-layered, serous membrane that covers the entire structure. Between the two thin membranes is a serous fluid that allows friction-free movement of the heart as it contracts and relaxes. The pericardium is the outermost layer of the heart. The *myocardium* forms the bulk of the heart wall and is the thickest and strongest layer of the heart. It is composed of cardiac muscle tissue. Contraction of this tissue is responsible for pumping blood. The *endocardium* (innermost layer) is composed of a layer of endothelial cells and a layer of subendocardial connective tissue. This structure lines the interior of the heart, the valves, and the larger vessels of the heart.

Heart Chambers

The heart is divided into right and left halves by a muscular partition called the interventricular *septum* (Fig. 8.2). The heart has the following four chambers:
1. The *right atrium* is the upper right chamber. It receives deoxygenated blood from the entire body. The superior vena cava returns blood from the head, the neck, and the arms. The inferior vena cava returns blood from the lower body. The coronary vein returns blood from the heart muscle to the coronary sinus.
2. The *right ventricle* is the lower right chamber. It receives deoxygenated blood from the right atrium. The right ventricle pumps deoxygenated blood to the lungs via the *pulmonary artery.*
3. The *left atrium* is the upper left chamber. It receives oxygenated blood from the lungs via the *pulmonary veins.*
4. The *left ventricle* is the lower left chamber. It receives oxygenated blood from the left atrium. It is the thickest, most muscular section of the heart and pumps oxygenated blood out through the aorta to all parts of the body.

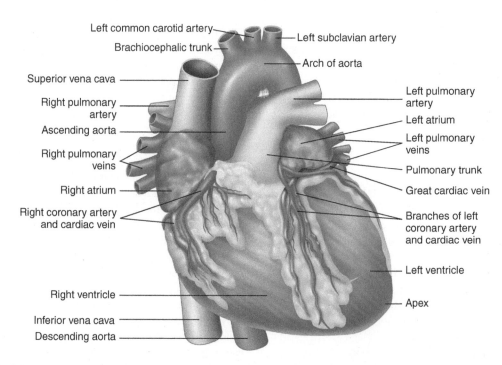

Fig. 8.1 Heart and major blood vessels viewed from the front (anterior). (From Patton KT, Thibodeau GA, Douglas MM: *Essentials of anatomy and physiology*, St. Louis, 2012, Mosby.)

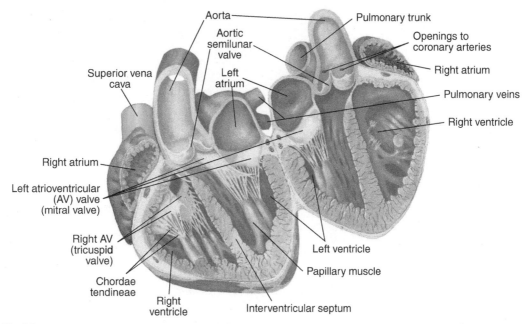

Fig. 8.2 Interior of the heart. This illustration shows the heart as it would appear if it were cut along a frontal plane and opened like a book. The front portion of the heart lies to the reader's right; the back portion of the heart lies to the reader's left. The four chambers of the heart—two atria and two ventricles—are easily seen. (From Patton KT, Thibodeau GA, Douglas MM: *Essentials of anatomy and physiology*, St. Louis, 2012, Mosby.)

Heart Valves

Located within the heart are four valves that keep the blood moving forward and prevent backflow. The heart has two *atrioventricular (AV) valves.* They are located between the atrium and the ventricles. The right AV valve, located between the right atrium and the right ventricle, is called the *tricuspid valve* because it contains three flaps, or cusps. The left AV valve is composed of two cusps (bicuspid) and is commonly called the *mitral valve.* It is located between the left atrium and the left ventricle. The AV valves are open during diastole (relaxation phase of the heart) and atrial contraction. During the ventricular contraction phase of the heart, the forceful beating of the ventricles forces the AV valves closed. A structure in the heart known as *chordae tendineae* are instrumental in keeping the AV valves closed and approximated. The chordae tendineae are thin fibrous bands made up of collagen, elastin, and endothelial cells. The chordae tendineae are attached to the AV valve cusps at one end and papillary muscles embedded in the ventricles at the other end. During ventricular contraction, papillary muscles contract which pull on the chordae tendineae which keeps the AV valves from inverting into the atrium and keeps them approximated. This prevents the back flow of blood from the ventricle into the atria.

The two remaining valves, the *semilunar valves,* have three cusps in the shape of a half moon, hence the name semilunar (see Fig. 8.2). The *pulmonary semilunar valve* or pulmonic valve is located between the right ventricle and the pulmonary artery and the aortic semilunar valve (see Fig. 8.2) or aortic valve is located between the left ventricle and the aorta. During diastole and atrial contraction, the semilunar valves are closed. They are forced open during ventricular contraction which moves blood from the right ventricle into the pulmonary artery, and from the left ventricle into the aorta. Upon cessation of ventricular contraction, a small amount of blood back flows from the pulmonary artery and aorta. This blood fills the cusps of the AV valves. The weight of the blood sitting in the cusps of the AV valves is what causes the AV valves to close.

Electrical Conduction System

The heart contains cells known as nodal cells and Purkinje cells. These are specialized cells in the heart that have three characteristics which include *automaticity*, *excitability*, and *conductivity*:

Automaticity—refers to the ability of these cells to generate an electrical impulse without any external stimuli.

Excitability—refers to the ability of these cells to respond to an electrical impulse.

Conductivity—refers to the ability of these cells to transmit an electrical impulse from one cell to another.

These properties are essential as they allow for synchronous beating of the atria and ventricles. Nodal cells are located in the **sinoatrial (SA)** node and the **atrioventricular** node. The SA node resides at the junction of the superior vena cava and the right atrium (Fig. 8.3). The SA node in normal healthy people

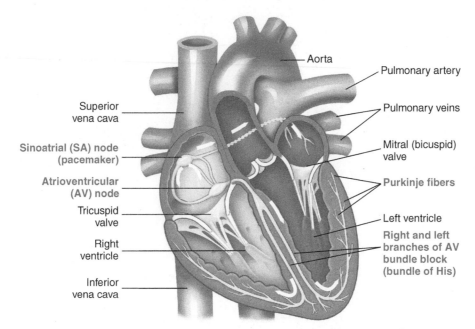

Fig. 8.3 Conduction system of the heart. Specialized cardiac muscle cells in the wall of the heart rapidly initiate or conduct an electrical impulse throughout the myocardium. The signal is initiated by the sinoatrial (SA) node (pacemaker) and spreads to the rest of the right atrial myocardium directly, to the left atrial myocardium by way of a bundle of interatrial conducting fibers, and to the atrioventricular (AV) node by way of three internodal bundles. The AV node then initiates a signal that is conducted through conduction fibers called the *bundle of His,* which breaks into right and left bundle branches to travel to smaller branches called the *Purkinje fibers,* which surround the ventricles. (From Thibodeau GA, Patton KT: *Structure and function of the body,* ed 14, St. Louis, 2012, Mosby.)

generates an electrical impulse at a rate of 60 to 100 impulses per minute. The electrical impulses initiated by the SA node are conducted to the other cells of the atria via internodal pathways. The conduction of the electrical impulses throughout the atria cause the myocardial cells of the atria to simultaneously contract. Once the electrical impulse transmits from the SA node to internodal pathways, it is conducted to the AV node. The AV node is located in the wall of the right atria near the tricuspid valve (see Fig. 8.3). The AV node manages the electrical impulse coming from the atria, and after a slight delay, relays the impulse to allow for ventricular contraction. The delay experienced at the AV node in impulse conduction is instrumental to heart function. The delay gives the atria time to contract and allows for maximum ventricular filling. The delay also preserves heart function in cases where disease causes the atria to beat out of control. The AV node then passes the electrical impulse to the *bundle of his* which is located in the interventricular septum (heart wall between the ventricles). The bundle of his divides into the right bundle branch and the left bundle branch. The right bundle branch relays the electrical impulse to the Purkinje fibers located in the right ventricle. The left bundle branch divides further into the anterior left bundle branch and posterior left bundle branch and then each division transmits the impulse into the Purkinje fibers of the left ventricle. The Purkinje fibers is the terminal point of impulse conduction and they conduct the electrical impulses to the myocardial cells of the heart causing

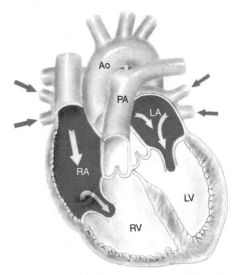

Fig. 8.4 Blood flow during diastole. *Ao,* Aorta; *LA,* left atrium; *LV,* left ventricle; *PA,* pulmonary artery; *RA,* right atrium; *RV,* right ventricle. (From Canobbio M: *Mosby's clinical nursing series: Cardiovascular disorders,* St. Louis, 1990, Mosby.)

rapid and synchronous contraction of both the right and left ventricle.

Since the SA and AV nodes are composed of nodal cells, they are able to initiate their own electrical impulses or demonstrate automaticity. As mentioned earlier, the SA node will automatically transmit impulses 60 to 100 times per minute. The AV node is also capable of automaticity, but in healthy people, it follows the impulse generation of the SA node as it is faster at initiating impulses. In the absence of the SA node, the AV

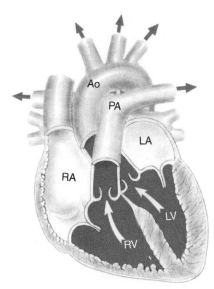

Fig. 8.5 Blood flow during systole. *Ao,* Aorta; *LA,* left atrium; *LV,* left ventricle; *PA,* pulmonary artery; *RA,* right atrium; *RV,* right ventricle. (From Canobbio M: *Mosby's clinical nursing series: Cardiovascular disorders,* St. Louis, 1990, Mosby.)

node becomes the main impulse generator and sends out 40 to 60 electrical impulses per minute. Should there be a malfunction in both the SA and the AV nodes, the Purkinje fibers, which also demonstrate automaticity, will set the rate of the heart. However, the rate set by the Purkinje fibers is 3 to 40 impulses per minute.

Cardiac Cycle

The cardiac cycle refers to the events that occur from one heartbeat to the next. There are three phases to the cardiac cycle: diastole, atrial systole, and ventricular systole. Diastole (Fig. 8.4) is a phase in which all four chambers of the heart are in a state of relaxation, the AV valves are open, and the semilunar valves are closed. Systole is the contraction phase of the heart. Atrial systole is a separate event from ventricular systole; the four chambers of the heart do not contract at the same time. During diastole, blood flows from the inferior and superior vena cava into the right atrium, and then passively flows from the right atrium into the right ventricle. At the same time, oxygenated blood flows from the lungs via the pulmonary veins into the left atrium, and then passively flows from the left atrium into the left ventricle. About 70% to 80% of the blood pumped out of the ventricles during ventricular systole is passively directed into the ventricles during the diastolic phase of the heart cycle (Namana, Gupta, Sabharwal et al., 2018). At the end of the diastolic period, the SA node generates an electrical impulse that transmits to both atria via the internodal pathways. This causes the myocardial cells of both the right and left atrium to contract simultaneously, thus signaling the next phase of the cardiac cycle which is atrial systole. Atrial systole contributes the remaining 20% to 30% of the blood that will be ejected out of the ventricles during ventricular systole. This volume of blood that is ejected due to

atrial contraction is referred to as atrial kick (Namana, Gupta, Sabharwal et al., 2018). Following atrial systole, ventricular systole begins. During ventricular systole (Fig. 8.5), the pressure in the ventricles rises dramatically which causes the AV valves to close and the semilunar valves to open. The ventricles contract and force blood to move from the right ventricle into the pulmonary artery and from the left ventricle into the aorta. The entire series of events—diastole, atrial systole, and ventricular systole—constitutes a complete cardiac cycle and takes an average of 0.8 seconds.

The heart sounds heard on auscultation are created by the closure of the AV and semilunar valves. The closure of AV valves during the beginning of ventricular systole creates the "lub" sound which is medically described as S1. The closure of the semilunar valves at the end of ventricular systole creates the "dub" sound which is medically described as S2. The S1 sound is heard loudest over the apical area and is described as a low pitch sound. The S2 sound is heard loudest over the aortic and pulmonic areas and can be described as a sharp sound.

CARDIAC OUTPUT

The cardiac cycle described above constitutes one beat of the heart from beginning to end. With every beat of the heart, a volume of blood measured in milliliters is ejected from the ventricles into the systemic and pulmonary circulation. This volume that is ejected per heartbeat is known as the stroke volume (SV). The average SV for a 70 kg male adult is 70 milliliters per beat of the heart (Bruss and Raja, 2020). The amount of blood that is ejected from the heart per minute can then be calculated using the SV and the number of times the heart beats per minute (bpm). Normal heart rates (HR) are 60 to 100 bpm. Therefore, if a patient ejects 70 mL of blood per heartbeat then in 60 beats the amount of blood ejected out of the heart is 4200 mL. This calculation that gives us the amount of blood ejected out of the heart per minute is known as cardiac output. Cardiac output is therefore a calculation of SV × HR. On the face of it, the equation to calculate cardiac output seems simple. You may have already thought that at 70 mL of blood ejected per heartbeat and 100 bpm, the cardiac output calculated would be 7000 mL. This linear computation does not always hold true as SV is affected by three factors: preload, afterload, and contractility. Preload is a measure of the amount of blood that fills each ventricle just before contraction. If the blood returning from the venous circulation or the lungs is decreased, then preload is reduced, which will reduce the amount of blood that will be ejected from the heart. Afterload is a function of the force the ventricle has to push against to pump the blood into the pulmonary and systemic circulation. If the blood pressure in the systemic or pulmonary circulation is high, the ventricle will have to push harder to pump out the same volume of blood. If the pressure or afterload is too high, then the SV will be decreased which will affect cardiac output. Lastly, contractility refers to the force generated by the myocardium. If preload, afterload, or contractility are affected, then the SV is affected which in turn affects cardiac output. Heart rate also affects cardiac output. At very slow heart rates, there is not enough blood circulation to sustain life. At very high heart rates, the diastolic time is reduced which means less blood fills in the ventricles and therefore the cardiac output is reduced. For this reason, a heart rate of 100 bpm does not necessarily yield a cardiac output of 7000 mL per minute.

BLOOD VESSELS

Three main types of blood vessels are organized to carry blood to and from the heart: arteries, veins, and capillaries. The heart delivers the blood to large vessels called *arteries,* which carry blood away from the heart. The arteries branch into smaller vessels called *arterioles,* which deliver the blood to the tissues. Within the tissues, the arterioles divide into microscopic vessels called *capillaries,* which form an extensive (50,000-mile) network that allows exchange of products and by-products between the tissues and blood. The capillaries then join to form tiny veins, or *venules,* that link with larger *veins,* which carry the blood toward the heart. The pattern is as follows:

Artery → Arteriole → Capillary → Venule → Vein

CIRCULATION

Coronary Blood Supply

To sustain life, the heart must pump blood throughout the body on a continuous basis. As a result, the heart muscle (or myocardium) requires a constant supply of blood containing nutrients and oxygen to function effectively. The delivery of oxygen and nutrient-rich arterial blood to cardiac muscle tissue and the return of oxygen-poor blood from this active tissue to the venous system are called the *coronary circulation* (Fig. 8.6).

Blood flows into the heart muscle by way of two small vessels, the right and left coronary arteries. The

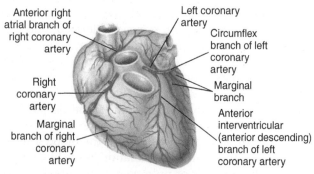

Fig. 8.6 Arterial coronary circulation (anterior). (From Canobbio M: *Mosby's clinical nursing series: Cardiovascular disorders,* St. Louis, 1990, Mosby.)

Anterior right atrial branch of right coronary artery
Left coronary artery
Circumflex branch of left coronary artery
Right coronary artery
Marginal branch
Marginal branch of right coronary artery
Anterior interventricular (anterior descending) branch of left coronary artery

right coronary artery (RCA) originates above the right cusp of the aortic valve while the left coronary artery (LCA) originates above the left posterior cusp of the aortic valve. The RCA branches into small arteries and supplies blood to the right atrium, right ventricle, and the SA node while the LCA branches into small arteries and supplies blood to the left atrium, left ventricle, the left bundle branch and a portion of the right bundle branch. The coronary arteries are located on the outside of the heart and wrap around the myocardium to supply the heart with oxygen and nutrients (see Figs. 8.1 and 8.6). The coronary arteries receive blood during the diastolic phase of the heart. Diseases that affect the length of time the heart is in diastole could potentially affect blood flow to the coronary arteries and the heart. Deoxygenated blood returns via cardiac veins to the coronary sinus which is located in the right atrium.

Systemic Circulation

Systemic circulation occurs when blood is pumped from the left ventricle of the heart through all parts of the body and returns to the right atrium. When the oxygenated blood leaves the left ventricle, it enters the largest artery (1 inch [2.5 cm] in diameter) of the body, the *aorta*. This is the main trunk of the systemic arterial circulation and is composed of four parts: the ascending aorta, the arch, the thoracic portion of the descending aorta, and the abdominal portion of the descending aorta. As the blood flows through the artery branches, the branches become smaller in diameter (arterioles). The blood continues to flow into the capillaries. The capillaries surround the cells and exchange oxygen and nutrients for carbon dioxide and other waste products. The blood flows to the tiny venules, then to the larger veins, and finally returns to the right atrium via the largest vein, the *vena cava* (one of two large veins returning blood from the peripheral circulation to the right atrium of the heart).

The blood is now deoxygenated and must be replenished with oxygen. In addition, the blood is carrying a high concentration of carbon dioxide. Note that the upper portion of the vena cava (superior vena cava) returns deoxygenated blood from the head, neck, chest, and upper extremities. The inferior vena cava returns deoxygenated blood from parts of the body below the diaphragm.

Pulmonary Circulation

The deoxygenated blood now passes through the pulmonary circulation to pick up the needed oxygen. Blood is pumped from the right atrium to the right ventricle, where it leaves the heart to travel via the pulmonary artery to the lungs. Once the blood reaches the lungs, it travels through arterioles to microscopic capillaries surrounding the *alveoli* (air sacs), where oxygen diffuses into the bloodstream and carbon dioxide diffuses into the alveoli and is exhaled. The capillaries then connect with the venules and finally with the four pulmonary veins, which return the oxygenated blood to the left atrium of the heart. It then is pumped to the left ventricle and to the aorta, and the systemic circulation then is repeated. The blood circulation pattern is as follows:

Superior or inferior vena cava → Right atrium

Tricuspid valve → Right ventricle

Pulmonary semilunar valve → Pulmonary artery

Capillaries in the lungs → Pulmonary veins

Left atrium → Bicuspid valve → Left ventricle

Aortic semilunar valve → Aorta

LABORATORY AND DIAGNOSTIC EXAMINATIONS

Many diagnostic tests are used to evaluate cardiovascular function. The nursing responsibilities are to prepare the patient physically for diagnostic procedures and to explain the examination to the patient.

Diagnostic Imaging

Chest x-ray. A chest x-ray is a two-dimensional image that is produced by using small amounts of ionizing radiation. It records the size, shape, and position of the heart and gives outlines of shadows. The size and position of the heart can reveal information regarding cardiomegaly. The chest x-ray also outlines the large vessels near the heart such as the aorta, pulmonary arteries, and pulmonary veins. It may reveal an aneurysm in these large vessels. Calcified areas of the heart are also visible in a chest x-ray. A chest x-ray can be used to verify placement of medical devices such as pacemakers, defibrillators, and central venous catheters (Mayo Clinic, 2020). Patients are asked to remove all jewelry prior to a chest x-ray. Pregnant women may need to wear extra protection if taking a chest x-ray or delay it if possible until after birth. Chest x-rays are usually taken from the front view and side view and the technician may take additionally x-rays as needed.

Fluoroscopy. Using a fluoroscope, the motion of internal structures such as the heart is examined with a device that emits x-rays that pass through the patient and fluoresce on a special screen, producing a sort of x-ray–based motion picture. Intravenous (IV) contrast dye may be injected to better visualize the organ or structure being studied. Patients undergoing procedures with contrast dye may have blood urea nitrogen (BUN) and creatinine labs done prior to the test. Fluoroscopy is used in cardiology to study the coronary arteries, during pacemaker or intracardial catheter placement.

Angiogram is a series of radiographs taken after a contrast medium (dye) is injected into an artery. Picturing the circulatory process aids in diagnosis of vessel occlusion, pooling in various heart chambers, and congenital anomalies. Angiography allows x-ray

visualization of the heart, aorta, inferior vena cava, pulmonary artery and vein, and coronary arteries.

In an **Aortogram**, the abdominal aorta and the major leg arteries are examined by x-ray visualization after a contrast medium is injected via a catheter (a thin, flexible tube) passed through the femoral artery and into the aorta. Aneurysms (abnormal bulges in the wall of a blood vessel) and many other abnormalities can be diagnosed. Contrast media also may be used to visualize the aortic arch and branches.

The nurse's role in preparing the patient for an angiogram and aortogram is to explain the procedure. Because dye is involved, it is very important to make sure the patient does not have an allergy to ingredients in the dye. This type of procedure requires the patient's informed consent. After the procedure, check the site of catheter insertion (usually the groin area) for excess bleeding, ensure that a compression device is in place, and alert the health care provider if excess bleeding is noted. Check for circulation in the periphery below the catheter insertion site, monitor vital signs, and ensure that the patient remains supine (lying face up) for the recommended amount of time.

Coronary Artery Calcium Score (CACS), also known as the coronary calcium scan, utilizes specialized x-ray technology called multidetector row or multi-slice computerized tomography (CT) to visualize plaque deposits in the heart. Research reveals that atherosclerotic plaques are not just made up of fats and cholesterol but contain deposits of calcium as well (Mayo Clinic, 2019e). The specialized CT scan is able to identify these calcium deposits in coronary arteries that help providers ascertain the risk of cardiovascular disease in asymptomatic populations (Greenland, Blaha, Budoff et al., 2018). The results obtained for this test include risk scores as follows (Mayo Clinic, 2019e):

0—no evidence of CAD, low chance of developing a heart attack in the future

10–300—moderate evidence of CAD, high risk of heart attack or other heart disease over the next 3 to 5 years

Over 300—very high to severe disease and heart attack risk

The risk scores are used to identify patients at risk and modify lifestyle choices to help decrease the risk of a heart attack. This test does expose patients to a small amount of radiation, but in most cases the risk outweighs the benefit of the test. This test is not recommended for patients who already have symptoms, have been diagnosed with coronary artery disease (CAD), or have known risk factors for heart disease such as smoking, diabetes, and hyperlipidemia. Patients can be recommended for a heart scan by a provider or can walk-in to clinics that offer the heart scan. Preparation includes avoiding caffeine and smoking 4 hours before the test and leaving jewelry such as necklaces and earrings at home. During the test, a technician applies electrodes to the chest to monitor the ECG rhythm. The ECG rhythm is used to take x-ray pictures when the heart is at rest. The technician may also ask the patient to hold their breath for a few seconds while taking pictures. The entire test takes 10 to 15 minutes (Mayo Clinic, 2019e).

Cardiac Catheterization and Angiography

Cardiac catheterization is an invasive procedure used to visualize the heart's chambers, valves, great vessels, and coronary arteries. This procedure aids in diagnosis, helps institute prevention measures for cardiac disease, and allows for accurate evaluation and treatment of the critically ill patients. A cardiac catheterization may be conducted to visualize the right or left side of the heart. Right sided cardiac catheterizations are usually performed prior to the left side and involve the use of a vein, either an antecubital or femoral vein. A right sided cardiac catheterization is performed to assess the function of the right ventricle, tricuspid and pulmonic valves, pulmonary artery pressures, or myocardial biopsies. A left sided heart catheterization involves the feeding of a flexible catheter through either the femoral or radial artery. It is used to evaluate the aorta and its arch, right and left coronary arteries, the valves on the left side of the heart, or the left ventricle and atrium. The study of the left side of the heart requires the instillation of a contrast agent, usually iodine based. Prior to use of contrast agents, kidney function and allergies to contrast dye need to be evaluated. Proper medical management with antihistamines or corticosteroids may allow the use of contrast dyes despite the presence of allergies. Patients with poor kidney function needing this procedure may be managed with IV hydration pre- and post-procedure. Both a left- and right-sided heart catheterization is conducted via the use of fluoroscopy which helps guide the placement of catheters. Patients undergoing this procedure are monitored via ECG and the use of continuous vitals monitoring. Placement of catheters inside the heart may result in chest pain, dyspnea, myocardial ischemia, dysrhythmias, and hemodynamic instability. The room in which this procedure is performed is equipped with emergency equipment in case resuscitation is required.

A cardiac catheterization is an invasive procedure that requires consent. Patients need instruction to fast for 8 to 12 hours prior to the procedure and may be instructed to hold certain medications. The nurse explains that the procedure usually takes 1 to 2 hours and that the patient will be awake but under moderate sedation during the procedure. Patients are instructed regarding the placement of 1 to 2 IV lines for infusion of fluids, medications, and anticoagulants. During the procedure, the patient may feel palpitations as the catheter is advanced and is informed ahead of time that the cardiologist may ask the patient to cough or breathe deeply to help clear the contrast agent. In addition, patients are informed that instilling of the contrast agent produces a flushed feeling

and may elicit the sensation of needing to void. After the procedure, depending on the site used for catheterization and the device used to secure clotting, the patient may be on bed rest for 2 to 6 hours. The site of catheterization is observed for the formation of hematoma and the extremity is monitored for pulse, color, capillary refill, and warmth. These checks along with vital signs are taken every 15 minutes for the first hour, every 30 minutes for the next hour, and every hour for the next 4 hours until discharge. In the presence of complications, checks may need to be conducted more often. This procedure is performed under sterile conditions either outpatient or in the hospital. Inform the patient that complications such as dysrhythmias, chest pain, hematomas etc. may require inpatient hospital care. It is advisable for the patient to have a ride home after the procedure and to avoid strenuous activity with the extremity used for the procedure.

Electrocardiography

The electrocardiogram (ECG or EKG) is a graphic study of the electrical activities of the myocardium to determine transmission of cardiac impulses through the muscles and conduction tissue. Each ECG has three distinct waves, or deflections: the *P wave,* the *QRS complex,* and the *T wave. Depolarization* refers to the electrical activity when the heart contracts. *Repolarization* is the relaxation phase. The P wave represents the depolarization of the atria. The QRS complex represents the depolarization of the ventricles. The T wave represents the repolarization of the ventricles. Atrial repolarization is not represented but does occur; the electrical recording of the atrial repolarization is covered by the large QRS complex and cannot be seen on the ECG tracing.

A standard ECG has 12 electrodes attached to the skin surface to measure the total electrical activity of the heart. Each lead records the electrical potential between the limbs or between the heart and limbs. A conductive gel enhances the contact and transmission. The patient typically is placed in the supine position; ambulatory ECGs and exercise stress test ECGs require position variation. The machine, an electrocardiograph or galvanometer, records the energy wave of each heartbeat through a vibrating needle on graph paper, which feeds through the machine at a standard rate. Each ECG waveform represents a single electrical impulse as it travels through the heart (Fig. 8.7).

The ECG tracing is read or interpreted by a cardiac specialist (cardiologist) or by internal medicine specialists, family practitioners, pediatricians, and emergency department practitioners. The reading also may be displayed on the fluorescent screen (oscilloscope) of a cardiac monitor. A graphic tracing may be printed out by the monitor.

Ambulatory ECGs can be used to monitor heart rhythm over prolonged periods—12, 24, or 48 hours—and compared with various activities or symptoms

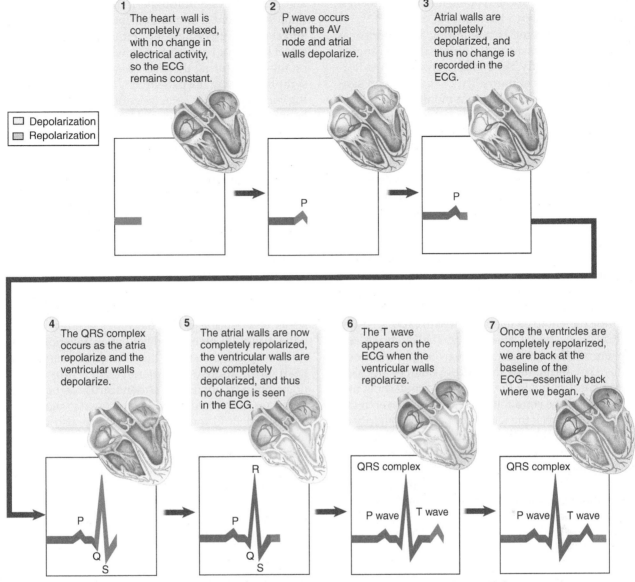

Fig. 8.7 Normal electrocardiographic (ECG) waves, or deflections. (From Thibodeau GA, Patton KT: *Structure and function of the body*, ed 14, St. Louis, 2012, Mosby.)

recorded in a diary kept by the patient. A Holter monitor (small portable recorder) is attached to the patient by leads, with a 2-pound tape recorder carried on a belt or shoulder strap. The monitor operates continuously to record the patterns and rhythms of the patient's heartbeat. In conjunction with the diary, the health care provider can note various events, times, and medication peaks that affect or precipitate dysrhythmias. An ambulatory ECG is particularly useful for patients whose clinical symptoms indicate heart disorders but who may have normal ECG tracings on a resting test. Thorough explanation by the health care provider is essential to ensure proper recordings by the patient, because this is an outpatient procedure.

Cardiac Monitors

It is common practice to assess continuously the cardiac electrical activity of patients who are known or suspected to have dysrhythmias or who are prone to develop dysrhythmias or acute cardiovascular symptoms. A cardiac monitor displays information on the electrical activity of the heart transferred via conductive electrodes placed on the chest.

Most monitors provide a visual display of cardiac electrical activity and the patient's heart rate. Preset alarms warn of heart rates that exceed or drop below limits considered acceptable for each patient and also warn of dysrhythmias.

Ambulatory patients (i.e., patients who are able to walk) are monitored more often by battery-powered ECG transmitters that do not connect the patient directly to an oscilloscope. This monitoring is called *telemetry*, which is the electronic transmission of data to a distant location. The electrodes placed on the patient's chest are attached to a transmitter the patient carries in a pocket or pouch. The transmitter sends a radio signal to a receiver, usually located at the nurses' station or a remote location within a hospital.

Patients need telemetry monitoring for various reasons, including a history of cardiac disease, angina pectoris, suspected dysrhythmias, a change in medications, an electrolyte abnormality, or unexplained syncope. Many of these patients are monitored in a centralized area such as an intermediate care or step-down unit (with monitors at the nurses' station). By remote telemetry, a patient on a medical-surgical unit may be monitored at a separate location, called the *home unit,* which is usually on a critical care unit. Remote telemetry patients are usually stable; but a stable patient's condition can change rapidly, and telemetry allows continuous heart monitoring to detect abnormalities.

Attachment to a cardiac monitor does not change a patient's need for nursing interventions. Ambulatory ECGs are conducted via a 5-lead tracing rather than 12-lead. The monitoring electrodes are placed on the anterior thorax (chest) rather than the extremities, enabling the patient to be relatively free to carry on usual activities. Pay special attention to the electrode site to ensure a constant tight seal between the electrode and the skin and to note the development of any skin impairment. Changing the electrodes regularly is recommended as the conduction gel dries out, even if the pad is sealed. Check the telemetry pack for integrity of the lead wires and test the monitoring device's battery with a battery tester. Inform the monitoring area whenever the patient is moved off the unit for a diagnostic test, because the patient may go outside the monitor's range. Another important safety measure is *never* to remove the telemetry device and allow the patient to shower unless the health care provider has written the order to allow a shower. The patient could be subject to severe dysrhythmia, which would not be detected with the telemetry device removed.

Exercise-stress. Patients often experience heart problems in a place where continuous monitoring of their ECG rhythms may not be occurring. In addition, patients wearing telemonitors on an outpatient basis may not perform the types of activities that stress the heart or it may just not occur. This is problematic as heart issues often become evident when the heart is experiencing emotional or physical stress. Cardiac stress testing is a test that is conducted in a controlled environment with the presence of medical personnel and monitoring equipment that is geared towards stressing the heart and catching any possible dysrhythmias or ischemia that may be occurring. There are two types of cardiac stress tests—exercise stress test and pharmacological stress test.

Exercise stress test. During an exercise stress test, patients are asked to walk/run on a treadmill, stationary bike or some other exercise machine that causes an increase in heart rate and oxygen demand. The patient is monitored using continuous vital signs monitoring

and ECG recording throughout the entire test. In addition, the patient is monitored for dyspnea, dizziness, and chest pain. The goal is to either reach the patient's target heart rate or reach a point where the stress placed on the heart during the test leads to symptomology. If symptoms occur, the patient may undergo further testing such as a cardiac catheterization. The patient is given instructions to fast for at least 3 hours prior to the test and wear comfortable clothing and tennis shoes. The patient is also asked to avoid any stimulants prior to the test and to refrain from applying any lotion as it will make it harder for the electrodes to adhere to the skin. An IV line will be inserted into the patient's arm in case medications need to be administered. Once the test is done, the patient is monitored to assure a return to baseline vitals.

Pharmacological stress test. Patients who are unable to participate by walking on a treadmill or any type of physical activity or are disabled will undergo a pharmacological stress test rather than an exercise stress test. During a pharmacological stress test, the patient will be given medications intravenously that cause vasodilation and thus simulate stress on the heart. Medications administered include dipyridamole (Persantne) or adenosine (Adenocard). As before, patients are monitored via continuous vital signs monitoring and ECG monitoring. They are also observed for symptoms such as chest pain, nausea, and dyspnea. The patient is instructed to be nil per os (NPO) for 3 hours before the test and not to intake any stimulants. The patient is informed to anticipate a flushed feeling upon infusion of medications and report any symptoms. The test takes 1 to 3 hours to complete and the patient is discharged after vitals return to baseline.

Nuclear Stress Test
A nuclear stress test involves the IV infusion of a radioactive dye. The dye is infused while the patient is at rest and then either with exercise or pharmacological stressors. The radioactive dye used is usually thallium 201. It is transported actively into normal cells. If the cells are ischemic or infarcted, the thallium will not be picked up. Thallium concentrates in tissues with normal blood flow; tissues with inadequate perfusion appear as dark areas on scanning—a "cold spot." Prior to the procedure, patients need to be NPO for 3 hours and refrain from stimulants including caffeine and smoking. Patients are informed to expect to feel cold as the radioactive dye is injected. It takes about 20 to 40 minutes for the radioactive dye to be absorbed by the heart after which images of the heart will be taken at rest and then during exercise or use of pharmacological drugs. The patient will be monitored during the entire test via continuous vital signs monitors and ECG monitors. Patients are again asked to report any symptoms. The test takes 2 to 3 hours after which patients are to avoid driving for the next 4 hours and to stand slowly from a sitting or lying position to avoid

orthostatic hypotension during that time. Based on test results, further testing may be necessary.

Echocardiography

Echocardiography uses a hand-held wand that directs high-frequency ultrasound waves toward the heart. These waves bounce off tissues and produce a graphic picture known as a sonogram. The sonogram provides information on the size, shape, and position of the heart. This test is used to detect pericardial effusion (collection of blood or other fluid in the pericardial sac), ventricular function, cardiac chamber size and contents, ventricular muscle and septal motion and thickness, cardiac output (ejection fraction [EF]), cardiac tumors, valvular function, and congenital heart disorders. An important diagnostic percentage ascertained from this test is the EF. The EF is the percentage of blood pumped out by the ventricle (left) during each heartbeat. Normal EF is 55% or above. This value may be given as left ventricular ejection fraction (LVEF) on an echocardiogram report. An EF of 40% to 55% represents a moderate EF and may indicate damage, perhaps from a previous heart attack but not necessarily heart failure. EFs less than 40% indicate severe heart disease. No preparation is required prior to this test. Patients do not have to undergo any preparation for this test. It takes approximately 20 to 30 minutes and can be done at outpatient or inpatient.

Positron Emission Tomography

Positron emission tomography (PET) is a computerized radiographic technique that uses radioactive substances to examine structures of the heart. It can be used to diagnose CAD, damage to the heart post myocardial infarct, and help select appropriate candidates for percutaneous coronary intervention (PCI) or coronary artery bypass graft (CABG). A radioactive tracer is injected intravenously and is taken up by the heart muscle. A special gamma detector picks up signals from the radiotracer and produces images.

Laboratory Tests

The history, physical examination, and blood studies help the health care provider diagnose and monitor the cardiovascular disease process. The nurse's responsibility is to prepare the patient by explaining the purpose behind the test and the preparation required for each test.

Blood cultures to detect growth of bacteria in the blood are crucial to the diagnosis of infectious endocarditis.

A *complete blood count (CBC)* is a determination of the number of red blood cells (erythrocytes) and white blood cells (WBCs; leukocytes) per cubic millimeter, as well as the proportions of the various kinds of white blood cells (the WBC differential), platelets, hemoglobin, and hematocrit (the volume percentage of red blood cells in whole blood). Lower hemoglobin levels reduce the ability of the blood to carry oxygen to the cells, resulting in anemia. An elevated WBC count indicates infection or inflammation. An elevated red blood cell count indicates that the body is compensating for chronic hypoxemia (an abnormal deficiency of oxygen in the arterial blood) by stimulating red blood cell production by the bone marrow, leading to secondary polycythemia (an abnormal increase in the number of red blood cells in the blood). Chronic hypoxemia is often found in heart failure.

Coagulation studies include prothrombin time (PT), international normalized ratio (INR), and partial thromboplastin time (PTT). These studies are used to monitor the patient receiving anticoagulant drug therapy, which is prescribed for patients after a myocardial infarction (MI) to dissolve the thrombus. Coagulation studies are also used in patients with chronic atrial fibrillation or those with atrial fibrillation who are undergoing electrical cardioversion (restoring the heart's normal sinus rhythm by delivering a synchronized electric shock through two metal paddles placed on the patient's chest).

Serum electrolyte tests focus on the body's balance of sodium, potassium, calcium, and magnesium, which are necessary for myocardial muscle function. Sodium (Na^+) does not directly impact the heart but sodium levels influence fluid balance which directly impacts heart function. The heart is very sensitive to potassium (K^+) levels in the body. High or low potassium levels can cause life threatening heart dysrhythmias such as ventricular tachycardia (VT), ventricular fibrillation, heart block, and asystole. Calcium is an electrolyte that is instrumental in blood coagulation, neuromuscular activity, and automaticity of the nodal cells in the heart. Changes in calcium levels affect heart electrophysiology (electrical conduction) and heart contractility. Magnesium (Mg^{2+}) helps maintain the correct level of electric excitability in the nerves and the muscles, including the myocardium and the cardiac conduction system. Low magnesium levels predispose patients to atrial or VTs, whereas high magnesium levels depress the contractibility and excitability of myocardial cells. ECG changes should provoke an order for blood chemistries especially potassium and magnesium and correction of electrolyte imbalances must be made promptly to preserve normal heart function.

Serum lipids are associated with vascular disease, particularly CAD. Cholesterol and triglycerides bound to plasma proteins are found in the blood as lipoproteins. Density levels vary according to the protein-to-fat ratio. An elevated level of high-density lipoprotein (HDL) is desired, but an elevated level of low-density lipoprotein (LDL) or very-low–density lipoprotein (VLDL) increases the risk for cardiovascular disease (Box 8.1).

Serum cardiac markers are certain proteins released into the circulation as a result of damage to the cardiac cells. These markers, specifically serum cardiac

Box 8.1   Cholesterol Numbers: What Do They Mean?

YOUR TOTAL CHOLESTEROL NUMBER	TOTAL CHOLESTEROL LEVEL
A total cholesterol level less than 200 mg/dL is considered desirable.	*Desirable:* Less than 200 mg/dL *Borderline:* 200 mg/dL to 239 mg/dL *High:* 240 mg/dL or greater
HDL CHOLESTEROL NUMBER	**HDL CHOLESTEROL LEVEL**
The higher the HDL cholesterol level, the better, because this means that there are more good lipoproteins to decrease the buildup of cholesterol from the arteries.	*Low:* Less than 40 mg/dL in men and less than 50 mg/dL in women *High:* Greater than 60 mg/dL
LDL CHOLESTEROL NUMBER	**LDL CHOLESTEROL LEVEL**
The higher the number of bad lipoproteins, or LDLs, in the blood, the risk of heart disease goes up.	*Optimal:* Less than 100 mg/dL *Near to above optimal:* 100 to 129 mg/dL *Borderline high:* 130 to 159 mg/dL *High:* 160 to 189 mg/dL *Very high:* Greater than 190 mg/dL
TRIGLYCERIDES	**LDL CHOLESTEROL LEVEL**
Fat build up in the arteries leading to narrowing of the vessel.	Less than 150 mg/dL: normal 150 to 199 mg/dL: borderline to high 200 to 499 mg/dL: high Above 500 mg/dL: very high
LDL CHOLESTEROL NUMBER	**TRIGLYCERIDE LEVEL**
The higher the number of bad lipoproteins, or LDLs, in the blood, the risk of heart disease goes up.	Less than 150 mg/dL: normal 150 to 199 mg/dL: borderline to high 200 to 499 mg/dL: high Above 500 mg/dL: very high

HDL, High-density lipoprotein; *LDL,* low-density lipoprotein.
Data from Wedro B: *Cholesterol charts (what the numbers mean),* n.d. Retrieved from http://www.emedicinehealth.com/understanding_your_cholesterol_level/page2_em.htm.

enzymes and troponin I, are important screening diagnostic criteria for an acute MI. The increase in serum cardiac enzymes that occurs after cell death can show whether cardiac damage is present and the approximate extent of the damage. The levels of cardiac enzyme creatine kinase (CK) and its isoenzyme, creatine phosphokinase (CK-MB), start to rise within 2 to 3 hours after the beginning of an MI, peak in 24 hours, and return to normal within 24 to 40 hours. CK and CK-MB have been the gold standard for years, but they have been replaced with troponins I and T. CK-MB is also found in skeletal muscle, and its blood level can be elevated by surgery, muscle trauma, and muscle diseases, making the differential diagnosis more difficult, so it is not a specific indicator for MI.

Troponins are myocardial muscle proteins released into the circulation after a myocardial injury. In the heart there are two subtypes: cardiac-specific troponin T and troponin I. These sensitive markers can indicate a very small amount of myocardial damage. Troponin T appears in the blood 3 to 5 hours after an MI, and its level may remain elevated for up to 21 days. Like CK-MB, the level of troponin T is affected by skeletal muscle injury and renal disease. Troponin I is a sensitive and specific cardiac marker, not influenced by skeletal muscle trauma or renal failure. The troponin I level rises 3 hours after MI, peaks at 14 to 18 hours,

and may remain elevated for 1 to 2 weeks after MI. Troponin I is most useful in diagnosing an MI because it is cardiac muscle specific. The ability to measure the myocardial contractile proteins (troponins) in serum, which are often present in very small amounts, is a major advance in the diagnosis of acute MI and acute myocardial damage.

Myoglobin is released into circulation within a few hours after an MI. Although it is one of the first serum cardiac markers that increase after an MI, myoglobin is also present in skeletal muscle, so an increase can be associated with noncardiac causes. In addition, it is excreted rapidly in urine, and blood levels return to normal range within 24 hours after an MI.

B-type natriuretic peptide (BNP) is a hormone secreted by the ventricles of the heart in response to ventricular expansion and pressure overload. A BNP level above 100 pg/mL indicates HF. The higher the BNP level, the more severe the HF.

Homocysteine is an amino acid produced during protein digestion. Normal values range from 4 to 14 μmol/L. Elevated blood levels of homocysteine may be an independent risk factor for ischemic heart disease, cerebrovascular disease, peripheral arterial disease (PAD), and venous thrombosis. Homocysteine appears to promote the progression of atherosclerosis by causing endothelial damage, promoting LDL deposits, and stimulating vascular smooth muscle growth. Homocysteine plays an important role in blood clotting. An elevated level results in increased platelet aggregation. Screening for elevated homocysteine levels (greater than 14 μmol/L) should be considered in patients with progressive and unexplained atherosclerosis despite normal levels of lipoproteins and those who have no other risk factors. It also is recommended in patients with an unusual family history of atherosclerosis, especially at a young age.

Dietary deficiency of vitamins B_6 (pyridoxine), B_{12} (cobalamin), or folate is the most common cause of elevated homocysteine. Some researchers believe that an elevated level of homocysteine can be treated by giving vitamins B_6, B_{12}, and folate. Whether this treatment will reduce the incidence of MI remains to be proven (MedlnePlus, 2018).

The liver produces *C-reactive protein (CRP)* during periods of systemic inflammation. As inflammation plays a role in atherosclerotic disease, high sensitivity CRP (hs-CRP) may be a predictor of cardiac disease risk. The test is administered via a simple blood draw. Patients with a low risk have a hs-CRP level of less than 2 mg/L while patient at high risk for cardiac disease have a level of greater than 2 mg/L. This test is not a definite predictor of cardiac disease but should be taken into consideration with the patient's health status (Mayo Clinic, 2017).

DISORDERS OF THE CARDIOVASCULAR SYSTEM

Cardiovascular disorders are a major health care problem in the United States. Public awareness, modifications in lifestyle, and improvements in medical treatment have contributed to a decline in overall deaths. The nurse's role in caring for patients with cardiovascular disorders includes being aware of the prevalence of cardiac disease, risk factors, and the disease process; implementing nursing interventions; and patient teaching.

EFFECTS OF NORMAL AGING ON THE CARDIOVASCULAR SYSTEM

By the time an individual reaches the age of 65 years, physiologic changes have reduced the heart's efficiency as a pump. However, the heart still is capable of functioning adequately unless there is underlying cardiac disease (see the Lifespan Considerations box). According to the American Heart Association (2020), all adults over the age of 20 should have their cholesterol levels checked once every 4 to 6 years. Older adults with high cholesterol should take steps to lower their cholesterol levels, including taking cholesterol-lowering medications, stopping smoking, increasing their activity levels, continuing their blood pressure medications, decreasing their weight, and, if they have diabetes, continuing to control their blood glucose level (CDC, 2020).

Lifespan Considerations
Older Adults

Cardiac Disease

- Changes in the cardiac musculature lead to reduced efficiency and strength, resulting in decreased cardiac output.
- Disorientation, syncope, and decreased tissue perfusion to organs and other body tissues can occur as a result of decreased cardiac output.
- Aging causes sclerotic changes in blood vessels and leads to decreased elasticity and narrowing of the lumen. Arterial disease resulting from the aging process causes hypertension because of the increased cardiac effort needed to pump blood through the circulatory system.
- Progressive coronary artery changes can lead to the development of collateral coronary circulation. This can modify the severity of signs and symptoms seen in MI. Angina symptoms may be less pronounced, and dyspnea may replace angina as a key symptom of acute infarction.
- Heart failure can result from rapid intravenous infusion.
- Edema secondary to heart failure may cause tissue impairment in the immobile older adult. Immobility leads to venous stasis (i.e., a slowing or stoppage of venous blood flow), venous ulcer, and poor wound healing. It also increases the risk of venous thrombosis and embolus formation.
- Older adults with cardiac disease often receive several medications, which often are prescribed at lower doses than for younger adults. Even with lower doses of medications, observe the older adult closely for signs of toxicity, because the rate of drug metabolism and excretion decreases with age.
- Independent older adults with cardiac conditions should receive adequate teaching regarding medication, diet, and warning signs of complications. Encourage them to maintain regular contact with the health care provider and to seek care at the first sign of problems.

RISK FACTORS

Risk factors indicate predispositions for developing cardiovascular disease. The presence of more than one risk factor is associated with an increased risk for developing cardiovascular disease. Risk factors are classified as *nonmodifiable* and *modifiable*.

Nonmodifiable Factors

An important aspect of caring for the patient with a cardiovascular disorder is understanding the risk factors for cardiovascular disease and incorporating them into patient teaching. The nonmodifiable risk factors (risk factors that cannot be changed) associated with cardiovascular disorders include age, genetics, and heredity.

Family history. A family member may be at a higher risk for heart disease due to genetics which play some role in hypertension and heart disease. Heart disease also tends to run in families; they may share common environmental factors (CDC, 2019).

Age. Normal physiologic changes that occur with aging and past lifestyle habits increase the patient's risk for developing cardiovascular disease with advancing age. CAD and MI occur most frequently among white, middle-aged men.

Gender. Middle-aged men are at greater risk of developing cardiovascular disease than middle-aged women. Although the incidence in men and women equalizes after age 65, cardiovascular disease is a more common cause of death in women than in men. Women develop CAD about 10 years later than men, because natural estrogen may have a cardioprotective effect before menopause. Despite this, the incidence of cardiovascular disease in women 50 years of age and older is increasing. Factors possibly responsible are increased social and economic pressures on women and changes in lifestyle. Ten times more women die from heart disease than die from breast cancer. The mortality rate for women with CAD has remained relatively constant even though cardiovascular disease remains the leading cause of death. Despite this statistic, only 15% of women consider CAD their greatest health risk. Recent research on CAD has shown that women often do not have the same signs and symptoms of an acute coronary event as those that are commonly seen in men (American Heart Association, 2017b).

Cultural and ethnic considerations. Heart disease is the leading cause of death for African Americans, American Indians, Native Alaskans, and Caucasians (CDC, 2019). Between 1999 and 2017, twice as many African Americans died of heart disease than Asians or Pacific Islanders (CDC, 2019) and out of those patients diagnosed with high blood pressure, African Americans are 40% more likely to have uncontrolled hypertension (HHS, 2020).

Modifiable Factors

Smoking. Individuals who smoke cigarettes have a two to three times greater risk of developing cardiovascular disease than nonsmokers. The degree of risk is proportional to the number of cigarettes smoked. Individuals who quit smoking decrease their risk. Tobacco smoke contains nicotine, which causes the release of catecholamine (i.e., epinephrine, norepinephrine). Catecholamine causes tachycardia, hypertension, and vasoconstriction of the peripheral arteries. This increases the workload of the heart, thus reducing the amount of available oxygen to the heart muscle. The other chemicals in cigarettes, including tar and carbon monoxide, also contribute to heart disease. These chemicals cause atherosclerosis because of the buildup of fatty plaque in the vessels. Fibrinogen levels also rise as a result of these chemicals, leading to clot formation, which can cause MI or stroke (Texas Heart Institute, n.d.).

With the increased use of marijuana because of legalization in some states, studies are being conducted regarding the potential harm to various organs. A recent study estimates that the explosion in the use of marijuana will add significantly to the cardiovascular disease burden as already events such as sudden cardiac death, arrythmias, and stress cardiomyopathy have been documented in healthy patients with no cardiac risk factors (Singh, Saluja, Kumar et al., 2018).

Hyperlipidemia. Hyperlipidemia is elevated concentrations of any or all lipids in the plasma. The ratio of HDL to LDL is the best predictor for the development of cardiovascular disease. Density levels vary according to the protein-to-fat ratio:

- VLDL contains more fat than protein (primarily triglycerides); triglycerides are the main storage form of lipids and constitute approximately 95% of fatty tissue.
- LDL contains an equal amount of fat and protein (approximately 50%) with moderate amounts of phospholipid cholesterol (see Box 8.1).
- HDL contains more protein than fat (which serves a protective function, removing cholesterol from tissues). It is suspected that HDL also removes cholesterol from the peripheral tissues and transports it to the liver for excretion. HDL may have a protective effect by preventing cellular uptake of cholesterol and lipids. Low levels (less than 40 mg/dL) are believed to increase a person's risk for CAD, whereas high levels (more than 60 mg/dL) are considered protective (see Box 8.1).

A diet high in saturated fat, cholesterol, and calories contributes to hyperlipidemia. Therefore, dietary control is an important aspect in modifying this risk factor. An overall serum cholesterol level of less than 200 mg/dL is desirable, 200 to 239 mg/dL is borderline high, and more than 239 mg/dL is high.

Change in diet is probably the most important method of lowering the cholesterol level. Weight reduction in overweight patients with abnormal lipid profiles is an essential element of dietary intervention. In addition to lowering LDL levels, weight reduction leads to decreases in triglyceride level and blood pressure. A combination of weight reduction and physical exercise improves the lipid profile, with a decrease in LDL level, an increase in HDL level, and a decrease in triglyceride levels. Low HDL levels are often familial and only somewhat modifiable.

Cholesterol-lowering drugs often are included in treatment of hyperlipidemia. Cholesterol-lowering drugs are divided into six classes: (1) bile acid sequestrants; (2) nicotinic acid (niacin); (3) statins such as atorvastatin (Lipitor), simvastatin (Zocor), pravastatin (Pravachol), and rosuvastatin (Crestor); (4) fibric acid derivatives such as gemfibrozil (Lopid) and probucol; (5) the cholesterol absorption inhibitor ezetimibe (Zetia); and (6) combination drugs such as ezetimibe and simvastatin (Vytorin). Pravastatin reduces the risk of a first MI by about one-third in hypercholesterolemic patients with no history of coronary disease. Simvastatin now is allowed by the US Food and Drug Administration (FDA) to add a label statement that the drug can reduce deaths by lowering cholesterol.

Hypertension. Hypertension is called the "silent killer" because a patient with elevated blood pressure does not display signs and symptoms of heart disease until damage has begun to develop. This damage increases the risks of heart disease, stroke, heart failure, or cardiovascular death. In 2017, the American College of Cardiology published definitions for high blood pressure and eliminated the prehypertension stage. New guidelines have normal blood pressure at less than 120/80 mm Hg; elevated blood pressure is a systolic of 120 to 129 mm Hg and a diastolic of less than 80 mm Hg; hypertension stage 1 occurs at systolic 130 to 139 mm Hg or diastolic 80 to 89 mm Hg; and hypertension stage 2 occurs at systolic equal to or greater than 140 mm Hg or diastolic equal to or greater than 90 mm Hg (CDC, 2020a).

Diabetes mellitus. Cardiac disease has been found to be more prevalent in individuals with diabetes mellitus. Diabetes poses a greater risk than other factors, possibly because an elevated blood glucose level damages the arterial intima (the innermost layer of an artery) and contributes to atherosclerosis. Patients with diabetes also have alterations in lipid metabolism and tend to have high levels of bad cholesterol and low levels of good cholesterol. This is known as diabetic dyslipidemia. Other contributing risk factors include poorly managed diabetes, high blood pressure, obesity, lack of physical activity, and smoking. According to the CDC (2020b), patients with diabetes are twice as likely to develop heart disease and the chances of heart disease due to diabetes increases based on the number of years since diagnosis. These risks can be mitigated with an active lifestyle and exercise, diet and weight control, managing stress, and keeping blood pressure under 140/90 mm Hg. It is also important to manage cholesterol levels and to stop smoking (CDC, 2020b).

Obesity. Excess body weight increases the workload of the heart. It also contributes to the severity of other risk factors. The CDC estimates that 35.7% of Americans are obese. This correlates to 97 million Americans with a body mass index (BMI) of 30 or above. As the BMI increases, so do the risk factors for developing diabetes, cardiovascular events, and stroke. A weight reduction program and maintaining an ideal body weight help modify the individual's risk.

Sedentary lifestyle. Lack of regular exercise has been correlated with an increased risk of developing cardiovascular disease. Regular aerobic exercise can improve the heart's efficiency and help lower the blood glucose level, improve the ratio of HDLs to LDLs, reduce weight, lower blood pressure, reduce stress, and improve overall feelings of well-being. Individuals with sedentary lifestyles should work with their health care provider to plan an exercise program that fits their lifestyle. Some health care providers define regular physical exercise as exercising at least three to five times a week for at least 30 minutes, causing perspiration and an increase in heart rate by 30 to 50 bpm. Yoga has been receiving increasing research as a form of exercise that increases musculoskeletal strengthening, flexibility, and relaxation. Yoga movements also have therapeutic cognitive effects of distraction and mindfulness, thereby reducing stress on the body. Another form of exercise receiving national attention is walking. Walking is one of the best forms of exercise, because it is the simplest and easiest way to exercise. Walking can strengthen bones, tune up the cardiovascular system, and clear a cluttered mind. Walking is a remedy for stress as well.

Stress. The body's stress response releases catecholamines that increase the heart rate. Catecholamines are hormones produced by the adrenal glands and released during times of physical and emotional stress. Catecholamines also affect myocardial cells and may cause cellular damage. The vasoconstriction that occurs may contribute to the development of cardiovascular disease. Stress reduction measures may help modify an individual's risk.

Psychosocial factors. In the early 1970s, health care providers used the term "type A personality" to describe a person who is always in a hurry, impatient, and irritable, or always angry or hostile. Recent studies have found that the term *type A* does not always fit the person with cardiovascular risks. More recent studies have found that the type D personality is more likely to suffer from increased cardiovascular symptoms. The person with a type D personality has chronic negative emotions, is pessimistic, and socially inhibited. Type D personalities tend to have increased levels of anxiety, irritation, and depressed mood across most situations and times. Type D people do not share their feelings because they fear disapproval, thereby increasing their chance of a cardiovascular event.

CARDIAC DYSRHYTHMIAS

A cardiac dysrhythmia (or arrhythmia) occurs when there is a change in the electrical conduction of the heart that affects the heart rate, rhythm of the heart, or both. To understand dysrhythmias, it is important to first understand the heart's normal electrophysiology. The normal electrophysiology of the heart causes a person to be in what is described as normal sinus rhythm. In a normal sinus rhythm, the primary functioning pacemaker of the heart is the sinus or SA node which depolarizes and send out depolarizing signals via the internodal system to affect the contraction of myocardial cells of the atrium. The SA node depolarizes at a regular rate and rhythm after which the electrical impulse follows the normal conduction system of going to the AV node, bundle of his, down the left/right bundle branch, and into the Purkinje fibers to then cause ventricular muscle contraction. When the SA node paces the heart at a regular rate and rhythm, the following characteristics are evident:

- *Rate:* 60 to 100 bpm
- *P waves (caused by atrial depolarization):* Precede each QRS complex, are upright, and have a consistent shape and size
- *P-R interval:* Time between the start of atrial contraction to the beginning of ventricular contraction; normal interval is between 0.12 and 0.2 seconds
- *QRS complex:* represents the time from the beginning of ventricular contraction to the end of ventricular contraction; normal interval is less than 0.12 seconds
- *T wave:* Ventricular repolarization
- *Rhythm:* Regular

A dysrhythmia is the result of an alteration in the formation of impulses through the SA node to the rest of the myocardium. It also results from irritation of the myocardial cells that generate impulses, independent of the conduction system. Signs and symptoms of dysrhythmia vary, as do treatment options, depending on the type and severity of the dysrhythmia. A short overview of each dysrhythmia follows.

Types of Cardiac Dysrhythmias

Sinus tachycardia. Sinus tachycardia is a rapid, regular rhythm originating in the SA node. It is characterized by the following: heartbeat of 100 to 120 bpm; P wave precedes each QRS complex though it may not be seen as it may be buried in the T wave; 1 P-wave for every QRS complex; PR interval is 0.12 to 0.2 seconds. Essentially, the only variable from normal sinus rhythm is an increase in rate above 100 bpm.

Causes of sinus tachycardia include exercise, anxiety, fever, shock, medications, HF, excessive caffeine, recreational drugs, sympathetic influence on the SA node, and tobacco use. Patient maybe asymptomatic or manifest symptoms such as palpitations, hypotension, dizziness, anxiety, headaches, shortness of breath, and chest pain. Treatment goals include slowing the heart rate when it occurs, figuring out the underlying cause and treating it, and preventing future episodes. The heart rate can be slowed down by doing vagal maneuvers which involves coughing, bearing down as if having a bowel movement, or placing an ice pack on the face. All of these actions stimulate the vagus nerve which stimulates the parasympathetic system and slows the heart rate. If vagal maneuvers are unsuccessful, anti-arrhythmic medications such as adenosine (Adenocard) is administered intravenously followed by the potential use of synchronized cardioversion. Future episodes of sinus tachycardia can be prevented by treating the underlying cause. Sometimes, sinus tachycardia occurs without an identifiable cause. In

these situations, a catheter ablation may be conducted which ablates a part of the sinus node thus decreasing the conduction of electrical impulses.

Sinus bradycardia. Sinus bradycardia is a slower than normal rhythm originating in the SA node. It is characterized by: a pulse rate of less than 60 bpm; ventricular and atrial rhythms occur at regular frequencies; P wave is preceded by a QRS complex; the PR interval is 0.12 to 0.2 seconds; and P to QRS complex ratio is 1:1. Essentially, the only difference between sinus rhythm and sinus bradycardia is the rate is slower than 60 bpm.

Causes of sinus bradycardia include lower metabolic rate, advancing age, inflammatory heart conditions, increased intracranial pressure, vagal nerve stimulation, carotid sinus massage, idiopathic sinus node dysfunction, athletic training, hypothyroidism, myocardial infarct, and medication (especially overuse of digitalis, beta-adrenergic blockers, or calcium channel blockers). Patients such as athletes in training may have sinus bradycardia without symptoms. In these patients, conditioning causes more efficient heart contractions such that the cardiac output is unchanged at lower heart rates. Symptomatic patients experience fainting, dizziness, shortness of breath, fatigue, activity intolerance, and chest pain. Treatments for sinus bradycardia include treating the underlying medical condition, changing medications, and preventing future episodes. If medication induced, a change in medication management is warranted. Patients stimulating the vagal nerve are taught to avoid bearing down during defecation. Hypothyroidism is treated with levothyroxine (Synthroid) and maintained at therapeutic levels. Patients experiencing hemodynamic instability with sinus bradycardia can be administered 0.5 mg of atropine IV every 3 to 5 minutes with a maximum dose of 3 mg. If this fails, a transcutaneous pacemaker is instituted with surgery scheduled for a permanent pacemaker. A pacemaker is a battery-operated device which contains 2 leads, one implanted in the atrium and one in the ventricle, that serves as the primary

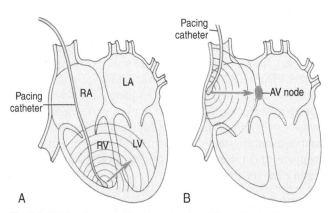

Fig. 8.8 (A) Ventricular pacing. Impulses are initiated in the right ventricle. (B) Atrial pacing. Impulses are initiated in the right atrium and travel to the ventricles via the normal conduction system through the atrioventricular (AV) node. *LA,* Left atrium; *LV,* left ventricle; *RA,* right atrium; *RV,* right ventricle.

pacemaker of the heart (Figs. 8.8 and 8.9.). A prescribed heart rate is set which serves as the rate at which a patient's heart beats.

Supraventricular tachycardia. Supraventricular tachycardia (SVT) is the onset of a heart rate greater than 100 bpm that originates either from the atria or from the AV node which is above the ventricles hence the name SVT. SVT originating from the atria is known is atrial tachycardia and is the less common form of SVT, usually manifests in children, and begins slowly with a gradual heart rate increase of more than 100 bpm. SVT originating from the AV node is called atrioventricular nodal reentry tachycardia (AVNRT) and is the most common form of SVT (Mayo Clinic, 2019). Since AVNRT is most common it is the subject of discussion here and will be referred to as SVT as is common practice.

SVT occurs due to an accessory pathway located in or near the AV node. This accessory pathway sends electrical impulses to the AV node that causes the impulse to be rerouted back to the AV node again and again at a very fast rate. Each time the impulse is rerouted to the AV node, it causes the AV node to propagate the impulse down the bundle of His, into right and left bundle branches, and to the Purkinjie fibers which causes fast ventricular myocardial contraction.

SVT has an abrupt onset and an abrupt cessation. It is characterized by an atrial rate of 150 to 250 bpm; ventricular rate of 120 to 200 bpm; regular rhythm of P and R waves; P wave that may be seen but is mostly hidden in the T wave (ventricular repolarization); and a P to QRS complex ratio of 1:1 or 2:1.

Causes of SVT include heart failure, thyroid disease, smoking, caffeine, drugs such as amphetamines and cocaine, surgery, anxiety and emotional stress, and pregnancy. Some patients may experience SVT with no identifiable cause. Clinical symptoms experienced vary depending on the rate, duration of occurrence, and the patient's underlying conditions. SVT is usually of short duration and causes palpitations. Other symptoms experienced include a fluttering in the chest, rapid heartbeat, shortness of breath, lightheadedness, sweating, syncope, and a pounding sensation in the neck (Mayo Clinic, 2019a).

Medical management first looks at how well the patient tolerates the dysrhythmia and at the overall clinical picture. Patients with minimum symptoms and quick termination of SVT may require no treatment and just be self-monitored and treated. Patients experiencing significant symptoms requiring emergency room visits to terminate SVT are treated with a focus of preventing future episodes (Hinkle and Cheever, 2018). In the immediacy, SVT is terminated using vagal maneuvers, one or more doses of adenosine with a calcium channel blocker, or cardioversion. Catheter ablation is the treatment of choice as it destroys the tissue in the AV node that allows for rerouting of the impulse back into the AV node.

Atrial fibrillation. Atrial fibrillation is one of the most common types of heart arrythmias occurring in the United States with one in four people over the age of 40 at risk for being diagnosed with atrial fibrillation (Xie, Yu, Ambale-Venkatesh et al., 2020). It occurs when structural or electrophysiological abnormalities alter atrial tissue and then the altered atrial tissue forms abnormal impulses resulting in rapid and uncoordinated twitching of the atria (Hinkle and Cheever, 2018). The atria quiver or fibrillate instead of all the myocardial cells of the atria contracting as a unit. This disorganized quivering can be likened to a disorganized orchestra where the cacophony of sounds created produce a broken piece of music and in the case of the atria loss of coordinated contraction of all myocardial cells in the left and right atrium. Since the atria quiver rather than contract, the atrial kick is lost which results in decreased cardiac output. In addition, the quivering atria are no longer moving blood along and thus this allows blood to stagnate within the atria making the blood susceptible to clots. These clots can break off, flow into the ventricles, and then be pumped into pulmonary and systemic circulation causing pulmonary embolism or stroke. In normal heartbeats, atrial contraction is followed by ventricular contraction. In atrial fibrillation, atrial and ventricular contraction do not follow each other and are out of sync. The ventricles contract irregularly which decreases ventricular filling time and further decreases the cardiac output. Atrial fibrillation is characterized by atrial rate of 300 to 600

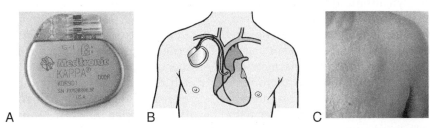

Fig. 8.9 (A) A dual-chamber, rate-responsive pacemaker from Medtronic, Inc., is designed to detect body movement and automatically increase or decrease paced heart rates based on the level of physical activity. (B) Cardiac leads, in the atrium and the ventricle, enable a dual-chamber pacemaker to sense and pace in both heart chambers. (C) Pacemaker in subcutaneous tissue.

bpm; ventricular rate of 120 to 200 bpm; a highly irregular atrial and ventricular rhythm; no discernible P waves but irregular and undulating waves that vary in amplitude and shape; the PR interval is unmeasurable; and the P to QRS complex ratio is many to 1.

Causes of atrial fibrillation include advancing age, high blood pressure, drinking alcohol, sleep apnea, any chronic condition such as diabetes, asthma, and hyperthyroidism, and underlying heart disease such as high blood pressure, valvular disease, cardiomyopathy, MI and cardiac surgery. Other not-so-obvious causes of atrial fibrillation can be energy drinks, high ingestion of caffeine, over-the-counter medications for colds such as Actifed, Sudafed, or Contact, and even some herbs, such as St. John's wort, which can interfere with clotting. In addition, atrial fibrillation can increase the risk of heart disease. This occurs in part due to the fact that the heart is contracting irregularly and faster which decreases the amount of time the heart spends in diastole. As a result, blood and oxygen supply to the coronary arteries is reduced leading to a risk for myocardial ischemia.

Patients with atrial fibrillation may be asymptomatic despite the loss in atrial kick and incomplete ventricular filling resulting in decreased cardiac output. Other patients may experience clinical symptoms such as palpitations, hypotension, shortness of breath, dyspnea on exertion, fatigue, syncope, chest pain, and a pulse deficit. Patients may also have signs and symptoms of emboli which vary based on the site of the embolization. Risk of stroke increases fivefold with atrial fibrillation. Risk of stroke is even higher in patients who have structural heart disease and hypertension and are over 65 years of age.

Medical management of atrial fibrillation is based on multiple factors including duration of the dysrhythmia and symptoms experienced by the patient. Patients with time identified new onset atrial fibrillation are treated with the goal of restoring normal sinus rhythm as soon as possible. When atrial fibrillation is identified within 24 to 48 hours of onset, the restoration to normal sinus rhythm may be achieved with administration of anti-rhythmics such as flecainide, dofetilide, propafenone, amiodarone, and IV ibutilide. If anti-arrhythmic medications are unsuccessful at converting atrial fibrillation to normal sinus rhythm, then synchronized cardioversion is used to convert the patient to normal sinus rhythm. If atrial fibrillation is discovered post 48 hours of onset or the duration is unknown, a transesophageal echocardiogram (TEE) is performed to determine the presence of thrombus in the atria prior to attempting conversion to a normal sinus rhythm. If no thrombi are present, conversion can be attempted either with medications or via electrical cardioversion. If the TEE images show thrombus in the atria, then anticoagulant therapy is initiated first as conversion to normal

sinus will dislodge clots from the atria and cause embolic events. Immediate anticoagulant therapy used includes use of low molecular weight heparin and IV heparin. Symptomatic patients are managed with beta blockers or calcium channel blockers to help decrease the heart rate to below 80 bpm. When anti-arrhythmic medications and electrical cardioversion are unsuccessful, catheter ablation is considered. Catheter ablation destroys the cells in the atria that are giving rise to abnormal electrical impulses. Maze or mini-maze procedures are used for patients with refractory atrial fibrillation and only conducted if patients are already scheduled for other cardiac surgeries (Hinkle and Cheever, 2018).

In some patients, atrial fibrillation occurs with other comorbid conditions or comorbid conditions do not allow the patient to undergo more invasive treatment options. In these cases, the atrial fibrillation is considered to be "permanent" and the patient is managed symptomatically. These patients take beta blockers, calcium channel blockers, and anticoagulants to control symptoms and prevent the risks of emboli.

Anticoagulant therapy used to occur with warfarin, but it required monitoring of PT/INR and is susceptible to vitamin K ingestion in diet. Novel oral anticoagulants (NOACs) such as dabigatran, rivaroxaban, and apixaban are now commonly prescribed for patients with atrial fibrillation. The NOACs do not require laboratory monitoring, have fewer drug-drug interactions, have a rapid onset and offset and do not require bridging therapy, and are better at reducing the risk of thromboembolic events. In addition, as of 2018 (Harvard Health Publishing), rivaroxaban and apixaban effects can be reversed by the antidote andexanet alfa and dabigatran can be reversed with the administration of idarucizumab.

Atrioventricular block. AV block occurs when a defect in the AV junction slows or impairs conduction of impulses from the SA node to the ventricles. Three types of blocks are seen: first degree, second degree, and third degree. A third-degree block indicates worsening of the impairment at the AV junction and a complete heart block.

Common causes of AV block include atherosclerotic heart disease (ASHD), MI, and HF. Other causes may be digitalis toxicity, congenital abnormality, drugs, and hypokalemia (low potassium in the blood).

First-degree heart block is often asymptomatic. Vertigo, weakness, and irregular pulse are seen with second-degree block. Disease that is progressing, as with third-degree block, will be accompanied by hypotension, angina, and bradycardia. The heart rate is often low, often between 30 and 40 bpm.

Medical management involves evaluating the patient's response and determining the cause of the dysrhythmia. Atropine and isoproterenol may be prescribed. A pacemaker frequently is needed with third-degree block (see Fig. 8.8).

Premature ventricular contractions. Premature ventricular contractions (PVCs) are abnormal heartbeats that arise from the right or left ventricle and cause ventricular contraction before the next normal sinus impulse. PVCs are early ventricular beats that occur in conjunction with the underlying rhythm, which is unchanged except for the PVC itself. PVC occurrences can be random or occur in patterns of bigeminy, trigeminy, or quadrigeminy meaning every other ventricular beat is a PVC, every third is a PVC, or every fourth is a PVC, respectively.

PVCs may originate from more than one location in the ventricles and be caused by irritability of the ventricular musculature, exercise, stress, electrolyte imbalance, digitalis toxicity, hypoxia, and MI.

Clinical manifestations depend on the frequency of PVCs and their effect on the heart's ability to pump blood effectively. Some patients are asymptomatic; others may experience palpitations, weakness, and lightheadedness. Other symptoms are associated with decreased cardiac output.

Medical management focuses on treating the underlying cause of PVCs such as eliminating caffeine or alcohol, managing stress, and correcting electrolyte imbalances. Symptomatic PVCs can be treated with beta-adrenergic blockers such as carvedilol, antianginals, propranolol (Inderal), and anti-dysrhythmics such as procainamide and amiodarone.

Ventricular tachycardia. VT is a heart rhythm that originates from the ventricles itself. It is most commonly caused by ischemic heart disease. Heart ischemia results in electrolyte derangement in myocardial cells, in this case potassium, which partially depolarizes the myocardial cells. This partial depolarization creates currents between infarcted tissue and healthy myocardium which triggers spontaneous electrical impulses causing the ventricles to contract. Other causes of VT include hypertrophic cardiomyopathy, long QT syndrome, and congenital coronary artery anomalies, cocaine, drugs, and digitalis toxicity (Foth, Gangwani, and Alvey, 2020). VT is distinguished from PVCs as VT is defined as the occurrence of three or more PVCs in a row occurring at a rate exceeding 100 bpm. It is further characterized by ventricular rate of 100 to 200 bpm; QRS complex duration 0.12 seconds or greater of bizarre or abnormal shape; PR interval and P to QRS ratio cannot be determined. It is further classified as non-sustained (occurring for less than 30 seconds and causing no symptoms) and sustained (occurring for 30 or more seconds or causing hemodynamic instability in less than 30 seconds). VT is also classified based on the shape of the QRS complex: monomorphic as QRS morphology is stable and polymorphic where each QRS complex from beat to beat looks different. These classifications are important as they guide treatment decisions.

Patients with stable VT are monitored with ECG and given anti-arrhythmic medications such as procainamide or sotalol for monomorphic VT without acute MI or severe heart failure and IV amiodarone if cardiac function is impaired due to other heart disease (Hinkle and Cheever, 2018). Patients with no underlying heart disease are started on a beta blocker or a calcium channel blocker (Foth, Gangwani, and Alvey, 2020). Patients in monomorphic VT who are symptomatic are cardioverted. Patients with VT who are pulseless are defibrillated. Treatment for VT also considers the EF. Patients with an EF of less than 35% are candidates for the placement of an implantable cardioverter defibrillator while patients with EFs above 35% are managed with oral amiodarone. Catheter ablation is also a treatment of choice (Hinkle and Cheever, 2018). Ongoing VT suppression is obtained with oral beta-adrenergic blockers or calcium channel blockers.

Ventricular fibrillation. Ventricular fibrillation occurs when part of the ventricular myocardium depolarizes erratically in an uncoordinated fashion. The result is quivering of the ventricles rather than a coordinated forceful contraction. The quivering of ventricles constitutes a medical emergency as cardiac output is essentially nil to all organs of the body including the coronary arteries of the heart. A continuance in ventricular fibrillation will result in more myocardial ischemia and eventual death. Patients in ventricular fibrillation are always without a pulse, an audible heartbeat, and respirations. Ventricular fibrillation is also characterized by a ventricular rate greater than 300 bpm, extremely irregular rhythm, no discernible P waves or QRS complexes, and the presence of irregular undulating QRS waves with changing amplitudes (Hinkle and Cheever, 2018).

The most common cause of ventricular fibrillation is CAD resulting in a myocardial infarct. Other causes of ventricular fibrillation include untreated VT, previous ventricular fibrillation episodes, previous MI, cardiomyopathy, illegal drugs (Ludhwani, Goyal, and Jagtap, 2020), electrolyte imbalances, digitalis or quinidine toxicity, and hypothermia.

Most patients in ventricular fibrillation suffer sudden collapses due to cardiac arrest. Patients may demonstrate some signs previous to the occurrence of ventricular fibrillation that may avert this dysrhythmia. These signs include chest pain, shortness of breath, nausea, and vomiting. Patients with chronic cardiac issues may also experience worsening of symptoms prior to the onset of ventricular fibrillation.

Medical management focuses on providing emergency treatment, including cardiopulmonary resuscitation (CPR), defibrillation (the termination of ventricular fibrillation by delivering a direct electrical countershock to the patient's precordium, i.e., that part of the patient's body surface covering the heart and stomach), and medications such as amiodarone and epinephrine. Defibrillation is the most effective method of ending ventricular fibrillation and ideally should be performed within 15 to 20 seconds of onset to avoid brain damage from the lack of blood flow.

Assessment and Diagnostic Tests of All Cardiac Dysrhythmias

Subjective data for the patient with a cardiac dysrhythmia include the patient's report of symptoms associated with the specific dysrhythmia. Symptoms may include palpitations, nausea, light headedness, vertigo, anxiety, dyspnea, fatigue, and chest discomfort.

Collection of objective data includes immediate visual observation of the patient. Signs may include syncope, irregular pulse, tachycardia, bradycardia, and tachypnea. Noting patient response to the dysrhythmia is essential as it guides treatment management.

Cardiac dysrhythmias are assessed by using electrocardiography. A 12 lead is preferred. Patients may also be diagnosed after wearing telemetry or Holter monitors for 24 hours or more. Laboratory work is also done to detect a medication toxicity.

Cardiac Dysrhythmias—Medical Management

Table 8.1 outlines medication treatments for various cardiac dysrhythmias.

Nursing Interventions and Patient Teaching for Cardiac Dysrhythmias

Nursing interventions focus on symptomatic relief, promotion of comfort, relief of anxiety, emergency action as needed, and patient teaching.

Assess the patient's apical pulse to obtain an accurate pulse rate when dysrhythmias are present. Because the rhythm is irregular, take the apical pulse for 1 minute. Assess the patient's anxiety and degree of understanding, noting verbal and nonverbal expressions regarding diagnosis, procedures, and treatments.

Explain the diagnostic and monitoring devices in use. Monitor heart rate and rhythm. Administer antidysrhythmic agents as ordered and monitor response. Maintain a quiet environment; administer sedation or analgesic medication as ordered. Administer oxygen per protocol.

Patient problems and interventions for the patient with a cardiac dysrhythmia include but are not limited to the following:

PATIENT PROBLEM	NURSING INTERVENTIONS
Discomfort, related to ischemia	Administer medications as ordered
	Teach relaxation techniques
	Institute position change and support
	Administer prescribed oxygen

PATIENT PROBLEM	NURSING INTERVENTIONS
Insufficient Cardiac Output, related to cardiovascular disease	Monitor heart rate and rhythm
	Reduce cardiac workload by encouraging bed rest
	Elevate head of bed 30–45 degrees for comfort
	Restrict activities as ordered; plan care to avoid fatigue
	Administer antidysrhythmic agents as ordered
	Monitor for signs of drug toxicity
Impaired Coping, related to fear of and uncertainty about disease process	Assist patient in identifying strengths and coping skills
	Supply emotional support
	Teach relaxation techniques
	Assess coping ability and level of family support
	Explain purpose of care as related to specific dysrhythmia

Teach the patient the importance of lifestyle changes such as avoiding or stopping smoking or use of nicotine products. Teach the patient about medication therapy and its purposes, desired effects, and dosage and the side effects to report to the health care provider. Explain the reason for and method of taking pulse rate and rhythm. Explain the need to avoid exercising beyond the tolerance level, to avoid strenuous or isometric activity, and to check with the health care provider regarding limitations and allowances. Instruct the patient regarding conserving energy for activities of daily living (ADLs): taking regular rest periods between activities and for 1 hour after meals; when possible, sitting rather than standing while performing a task; and stopping an activity or task if symptoms such as fatigue, dyspnea, or palpitations begin. Stress management is important to promote healing and prevent further cardiac events.

Cardiac Arrest

The sudden cessation of cardiac output and circulatory process is termed *cardiac arrest*. Conditions leading to cardiac arrest are severe VT, ventricular fibrillation, and ventricular asystole. The absence of oxygen–carbon dioxide exchange leads to symptoms of anaerobic tissue cell metabolism and respiratory and metabolic acidosis. Immediate CPR is necessary to prevent major organ damage. Signs and symptoms of cardiac arrest include abrupt loss of consciousness with no response to stimuli, gasping respirations followed by apnea, absence of pulse (radial, carotid, femoral, and apical), absence of blood pressure, pupil dilation, and pallor and cyanosis.

CPR is initiated by the first person to discover the condition. The aim is to reestablish circulation and ventilation. Prevention of severe damage to the brain, heart, liver, and kidneys as a result of anoxia (lack of oxygen) is of primary concern. Remember the CAB of CPR: *C*, circulation; *A*, restore airway; and *B*, restore

Table 8.1   Medications for Cardiac Dysrhythmias

GENERIC NAME	ACTION	NURSING INTERVENTIONS
Cardiac Glycoside		
digoxin	Used to control rapid ventricular rate in atrial fibrillation and to convert paroxysmal supraventricular tachycardia to normal sinus rhythm Increases cardiac force and efficiency, slows heart rate, increases cardiac output	Monitor apical pulse to ensure rate is above 60 bpm (call health care provider if digoxin withheld) Monitor for digitalis toxicity (nausea, vomiting, anorexia, dysrhythmias, bradycardia, tachycardia, headache, fatigue, visual disturbance)
Antidysrhythmic Agents		
procainamide	IV solutions given for severe ventricular dysrhythmias Depresses excitability of cardiac muscle to electrical stimulation and slows conduction in atrium, bundle of His, and ventricle, thus increasing refractory period	Observe for new dysrhythmias, dry mouth, blurred vision, bradycardia, hypotension, nausea, anorexia, dizziness, visual disturbances
lidocaine (IV)	Suppresses the impulse that triggers dysrhythmias	Monitor heart rate and BP closely
disopyramide	Provides long-term treatment of premature ventricular contractions, ventricular tachycardia, and atrial fibrillation	Monitor BP and apical pulse
adenosine	Slows conduction through AV node, can interrupt reentry pathways through AV node, and can restore normal sinus rhythm in patients with paroxysmal supraventricular tachycardia (PSVT)	Monitor BP, pulse rate, and respirations Assess patient for headache, dizziness, gastrointestinal complaints, new dysrhythmias Do not give caffeine within 4 to 6 h of adenosine because caffeine inhibits the effect of the drug
amiodarone	Prolongs duration of action potential and effective refractory period; provides noncompetitive alpha- and beta-adrenergic inhibition; increases P-R and Q-T intervals; decreases sinus rate; decreases peripheral vascular resistance. Used for severe ventricular tachycardia, supraventricular tachycardia, atrial fibrillation, ventricular fibrillation not controlled by first-line agents, cardiac arrest	Observe for headache, dizziness, hypotension, bradycardia, sinus arrest, heart failure, dysrhythmia Assess BP continuously for hypotension or hypertension Report dysrhythmia or bradycardia Monitor for dyspnea, chest pain
mexiletine propafenone	Decrease excitability of cardiac muscle	Monitor pulse, BP Monitor for diarrhea, visual disturbances, respiratory distress
tocainide	Suppresses automaticity of conduction tissue	Notify health care provider if cough, wheezing, or shortness of breath occurs
Beta-Adrenergic Blockers		
propranolol sotalol acebutolol esmolol metoprolol carvedilol	Used to treat supraventricular and ventricular dysrhythmias, persistent sinus tachycardia Decrease myocardial oxygen demand, decrease workload of the heart, decrease heart rate	Monitor heart rate and BP carefully. Use caution with patient with bronchospastic disease Monitor for bradycardia, hypotension, new dysrhythmias, dizziness, headache, nausea, diarrhea, sleep disturbances
Calcium Channel Blockers		
verapamil diltiazem	Treat supraventricular tachycardia and control rapid rates in atrial tachycardia Produce relaxation of coronary vascular smooth muscle, dilate coronary arteries	Use caution in patients with CHF Monitor apical pulse and BP Watch for fatigue, headache, dizziness, peripheral edema, nausea, tachycardia Verapamil and diltiazem increase the toxicity of digoxin
Inotropic Agent		
dobutamine (IV) dopamine (IV)	Used in severe CHF with pulmonary edema Increase myocardial contractility Increase cardiac output, increase BP, and improve renal blood flow	Monitor BP, heart rate, and urinary output continuously during the administration Palpate peripheral pulses; notify health care provider if extremities become cold or mottled

Continued

Table 8.1   Medications for Cardiac Dysrhythmias—cont'd

GENERIC NAME	ACTION	NURSING INTERVENTIONS
Anticoagulant		
warfarin	Used in treatment of atrial fibrillation with embolization to prevent complication of stroke	Assess patient for signs of bleeding and hemorrhage Monitor prothrombin time and international normalized ratio (PT/INR) frequently during therapy Review foods high in vitamin K. Patient should have consistently limited intake of these foods because these foods will cause levels to fluctuate

AV, Atrioventricular; *BP,* blood pressure; *bpm,* beats per minute; *CHF,* congestive heart failure; *HCl,* hydrochloride; *IV,* intravenous.

breathing. Resuscitation measures are divided into two components: basic cardiac life support in the form of CPR and advanced cardiac life support (ACLS).

ACLS is a systematic approach to provide early treatment of cardiac emergencies. ACLS includes (1) basic life support, (2) the use of adjunctive equipment and special techniques for establishing and maintaining effective ventilation and circulation, (3) ECG monitoring and dysrhythmia recognition, (4) therapies for emergency treatment of patient with cardiac or respiratory arrest, and (5) treatment of patient with suspected acute MI.

Artificial Cardiac Pacemakers

A pacemaker is made of titanium with computer circuits that control the pacing system; one or more leads are placed into the heart and a lithium battery is used (American Heart Association, 2016b). It initiates and controls the heart rate by delivering an electrical impulse via an electrode to the myocardium. These catheter-like electrodes are placed within the area to be paced: right atrium, right ventricle, or both (see Figs. 8.8 and 8.9). A permanent pacemaker power source is placed subcutaneously, usually over the pectoral muscle on the patient's nondominant side. Most are demand pacemakers, which send electrical stimuli to pace the heart when the heartbeat decreases below a preset rate. Some pacemakers have a single-chamber device with one lead that paces the right atrium or right ventricle; other pacemakers are dual-chamber with separate leads that connect to both the right atrium and the right ventricle.

Another pacemaker, the biventricular pacemaker, has three leads, one lead for each ventricle and one lead for the right atrium. This device restores normal simultaneous contraction of the ventricles. A biventricular pacemaker significantly improves left ventricular EF and exercise tolerance. It improves the quality of life for patients with worsening HF (American Heart Association, 2016b).

A pacemaker maintains a regular cardiac rhythm by electrically stimulating the heart muscle. It is used when patients experience adverse symptoms because of dysrhythmias that cannot be managed by

medications alone. These include second- and third-degree AV block, *bradydysrhythmia* (slow and/or irregular heartbeat), and *tachydysrhythmia* (rapid heartbeat that can be regular or irregular).

An external pacemaker is used in emergency situations on a short-term basis. Temporary pacemakers are used for cardiac support after some MIs or open-heart surgery. A permanent pacemaker is placed when other measures have failed to convert the dysrhythmia or conduction problem. The batteries used in permanent pacemakers today are small, weighing less than 1 ounce, and can last 15 years or more.

Nursing Interventions and Patient Teaching

After placement of a pacemaker, closely monitor heart rate and rhythm by apical pulse and by ECG patterns. Check vital signs and level of consciousness frequently until stable. Observe the insertion site for erythema, edema, and tenderness, which could indicate infection. The patient may be on bed rest with the arm on the pacemaker side immobilized for the first few hours. Discharge teaching includes instructions not to lift the arm on the surgical side over the head for 6 to 8 weeks. The patient needs to refrain from swimming, golfing, and weightlifting until given permission by the health care provider (American Heart Association, 2016b).

Inform the patient of the necessity to continue medical management, and advise that he or she wear medical-alert identification and carry pacemaker information. Emphasize the importance of reporting signs and symptoms of pacemaker failure: weakness, vertigo, chest pain, and pulse changes.

Teach the patient to avoid potentially hazardous situations. Each pacemaker manufacturer can provide a list of devices that patients with pacemakers should avoid getting close to. In the past patients had to avoid objects such as high-output electrical generators or large magnets such as a MRI scanner because these objects could cause interference resulting in the pacemaker going into a fixed mode. Because of the grade of titanium metals used, patients who have pacemakers placed in the past several years can have MRI testing without difficulty. The patient always should report the use of a pacemaker before having an MRI.

The pacemaker's pulse generator is set to produce a heart rate appropriate to the patient's clinical condition and the desired therapeutic goal. With rare exceptions, the rate is set between 70 and 80 bpm. If the heart rate falls below the preset level, notify the health care provider.

Teach the patient how and when to take a radial pulse. The pulse should be taken at the same time each day and when symptoms of vertigo or weakness occur. During patient education, remember to (1) list symptoms to expect and to report to the health care provider, (2) promote understanding of medication administration, (3) explain treatment outcomes, (4) explain the importance of maintaining prescribed diet and fluid amounts, and (5) explain the importance of not smoking. Teach the patient that shortness of breath occurring with exercise or exertion can be significant, because of the heart's inability to provide enough oxygen to the cells.

Prognosis

The patient can expect to lead a reasonably normal life with full resumption of most activities as prescribed by the health care provider.

DISORDERS OF THE HEART

CORONARY ARTERY DISEASE

Coronary artery disease CAD refers to diseased or damaged arteries that supply blood to the heart. CAD is the number one cause of death in the United States. In 2017, 42.6% of all deaths attributed to cardiovascular disease occurred due to CAD and every 40 seconds an American will suffer a myocardial infarct due to CAD (American Heart Association, 2020b). CAD can occur due to obstructive or nonobstructive causes. The most common cause of obstructive CAD is atherosclerotic changes that occur within coronary arteries.

CORONARY ATHEROSCLEROSIS

The coronary arteries of the heart run along the outer surface of the heart on the epicardial layer and supply the heart muscle with oxygen rich blood and nutrients. They originate from the base of the aorta with the RCA originating above the right cusp of the aortic valve and the LCA originating above the left posterior cusp of the aortic valve (see Fig. 8.6). The RCA and LCA are largest in diameter at one eighth of an inch and they supply nutrients to the heart by curving around the heart muscle and bifurcating as they descend towards the apex of the heart. As these arteries bifurcate, they become smaller in diameter and the smallest bifurcations of the coronary arteries even curve inward in the epicardial layer. The shapes, contours, and arrangements of these arteries make them more susceptible to atherosclerotic changes.

Coronary Atherosclerosis is a common arterial disorder characterized by yellowish plaques of cholesterol,

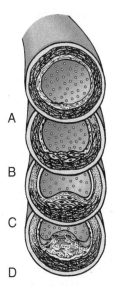

Fig. 8.10 Progressive development of coronary atherosclerosis. (A) Injury to intimal wall. (B) Lipoprotein invasion of smooth muscle cells. (C) Development of fatty streak and fibrous plaque. (D) Development of complicated lesion. (From Black JM, Hawks JH: *Medical-surgical nursing: Clinical management for positive outcomes*, ed 8, St. Louis, 2009, Mosby.)

lipids, and cellular debris affecting the coronary arteries of the heart and the most common cause of CAD. Multiple factors begin the process of atherosclerotic changes, all of which cause damage to the underlying endothelium such as high blood pressure that subjects arteries to continuous pounding, chemicals in tobacco smoke, insulin resistance, obesity, or diabetes, and inflammation occurring due to other diseases such as lupus and rheumatoid arthritis (Mayo Clinic, 2018). Once the endothelial layer is damaged, inflammatory responses occur which progresses to form plaques containing cholesterol lipids and other cells. These plaques progressively increase in size causing narrowing of the coronary artery which then progressively hinders blood flow. Plaques can also break off and travel deeper into the artery causing a block.

The symptoms experienced by patients with coronary atherosclerosis vary depending on the size and location of the plaque and the degree of obstructed blood flow (Fig. 8.10.). Since atherosclerosis is an insidious process, symptoms may not be felt until decreased blood flow results in myocardial ischemia. Myocardial ischemia results in chest pain or angina pectoris, the most common symptom of myocardial ischemia (see the Cultural Considerations box).

ANGINA PECTORIS

Etiology and Pathophysiology

Angina means a spasmodic, cramp-like, choking feeling. *Pectoris* refers to the breast or chest area. **Angina pectoris** refers to the paroxysmal (severe, usually episodic) thoracic pain and choking feeling caused by decreased oxygen flow to or lack of oxygen (anoxia) of the myocardium.

Angina pectoris occurs when the cardiac muscle is deprived of oxygen. Atherosclerosis of the coronary arteries is the most common cause. Due to atherosclerotic changes, narrowed lumina of the coronary arteries are unable to deliver enough oxygen-rich blood to the myocardium. When the myocardial oxygen demand exceeds the supply, ischemia (decreased blood supply to a body organ or part, often marked by pain and organ dysfunction) of the heart muscle occurs, resulting in chest pain or angina. In most cases, angina is attributed to demands for increased cardiac workload brought on by exposure to intense cold, exercise, unusually heavy meals, emotional stress, or any other strenuous activity. Stable angina pectoris occurs when the patient develops symptoms of chest pain during activity but goes away upon rest or taking medication such as nitroglycerin. Unstable angina pectoris occurs when the patient has an increase in the severity and frequency of chest pain that is not alleviated with rest or nitroglycerin. If unstable angina cannot be relieved, it may precipitate a MI. Prinzmetal or variant angina is rare and occurs mostly in younger patients. It is caused by spasms occurring in the coronary arteries that cuts off blood supply to the myocardium and occurs when the patient is at rest. It typically occurs between midnight and early morning and is very painful. An episode of prinzmetal angina can last up to 30 minutes and persistent spasms increase the chances of arrythmia or myocardial infarct (National Institutes of Health, 2018). Microvascular angina is chest pain that occurs due to the inability of the smallest coronary arteries to dilate in response to the need for increased blood flow or go into spasms thus decreasing blood flow to the myocardium. This type of angina is suspected when coronary angiography reveals no signs of obstructed arteries though it is to be noted that current techniques do not allow visualization of the smallest arteries. Microvascular angina is more common in women than in men (Aslan, Polat, Bozcali et al., 2020).

CAD is the number one killer in the United States. Many people who die from the disease, however, experience several episodes of unstable angina first. If unstable angina were diagnosed accurately and promptly managed, many deaths and much of the disability associated with CAD could be avoided.

Clinical Manifestations

An ischemic heart produces symptoms of pain (Fig. 8.11) that can range from mild discomfort to excruciating pain. Patients may describe the pain as pressure, burning, squeezing, or fullness. The pain is poorly localized and is often felt deep in the chest behind the sternum. Ischemic myocardial pain may radiate to the neck, jaw, and left arm. Besides pain, patients may have symptoms of mild indigestion, shortness of breath, nausea and vomiting, pallor, diaphoresis, and dizziness or lightheadedness. Symptoms of CAD in women vary and may be attributed to other disease

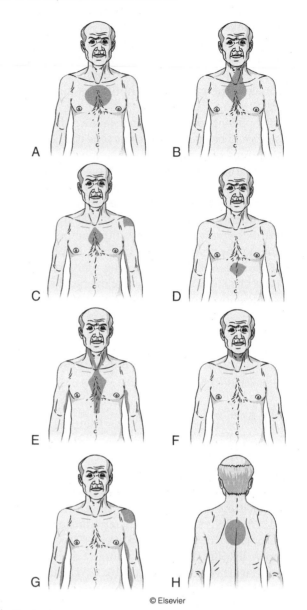

© Elsevier

Fig. 8.11 Sites to which ischemic myocardial pain may be referred. (A) Upper chest. (B) Beneath sternum, radiating to neck and jaw. (C) Beneath sternum, radiating down left arm. (D) Epigastric. (E) Epigastric, radiating to neck, jaw, and arms. (F) Neck and jaw. (G) Left shoulder and inner aspect of both arms. (H) Intrascapular.

🌐 Cultural Considerations

Cardiovascular Disorder

- White, middle-aged men have the highest incidence of coronary artery disease (CAD).
- African Americans and Hispanics have a higher incidence of hypertension than do white Americans.
- African Americans have an early age of onset of CAD.
- African American women have a higher incidence of CAD than do white American women.
- Native Americans younger than 35 years of age have a heart disease mortality rate twice as high as that of other Americans.
- Hispanics have a lower death rate from heart disease than do non-Hispanics.
- Major modifiable cardiovascular risk factors for Native Americans are obesity and diabetes mellitus.

processes as they tend to be vague. Women tend to experience symptoms that are unrelated to chest pain such as nausea, vomiting, fatigue, indigestion, shortness of breath, and upper back or abdominal discomfort (Mayo Clinic, 2019c).

It is also important to note that the symptoms of angina pectoris may be different in patients with diabetes. Diabetes can cause damage to nerves (neuropathy) that can make the usual signs and symptoms of chest pain harder to detect because of the decrease in sensation. The patient with neuropathy may have no pain with an MI. Patients with diabetes may experience chest discomfort, sweating, shortness of breath, or nausea and/or vomiting during an MI. These symptoms should be treated as a medical emergency.

Assessment

Subjective data include the patient's statements regarding the location, intensity, radiation, and duration of pain. The patient may express a feeling of impending death. Assess precipitating factors that led to the development of symptoms. Determine what relief measures have been used. Identify whether relief measures alleviated the symptoms in frequency or severity. Also ascertain previous incidences of angina pectoris.

Collection of objective data includes noting the patient's behavior, such as rubbing the left arm or pressing a fist against the sternum. Monitor vital signs and note changes or abnormalities. Increases in pulse rate, blood pressure, and respiratory rate may be noted. Identify the presence of diaphoresis or anxiety.

Diagnostic Tests

The diagnosis of angina pectoris frequently is based on the patient's history coupled with diagnostic tests and labs. The 12-lead ECG may reveal ischemia and rhythm changes. Laboratory studies include blood draw to check for the presence of cardiac biomarkers. The patient may undergo echocardiogram and cardiac catheterization (coronary angiography) to ascertain level and location of decreased arterial blood flow. The patient may also undergo an exercise stress test to determines ischemic changes in a controlled environment.

Medical Management

The focus of medical management is to control symptoms by reducing cardiac ischemia. Precipitating factors—such as exposure to intense cold, strenuous exercise, smoking, heavy meals, and emotional stress—are identified and avoided. Modifiable cardiovascular risk factors are identified and corrected if possible. Patients are encouraged to control and reduce cholesterol levels, hypertension, diabetes, and obesity. Over time, control of these factors in correspondence with physical activity as tolerated may decrease the incidence of precipitating factors resulting in ischemic episodes. Angina pectoris is treated on multiple fronts via medication

therapy. Nitroglycerin is standard treatment for angina pectoris, and it is a medication patients are encouraged to carry with them at all times to alleviate episodes of angina pectoris. Nitroglycerin works by vasodilating coronary arteries thereby increasing blood flow which brings oxygen and nutrients to the cardiac muscle, thus alleviating ischemia. Nitroglycerin also reduces the workload on the heart by dilating veins throughout the body. This causes blood pooling in the venous system and reduces the amount of blood returning back to the heart. Decreased return of blood to the heart decreases the amount of blood the heart must pump and therefore decreases cardiac workload. This can cause a markedly decreased cardiac output and hypotension so nitroglycerin therapy must be carefully managed. Patients arriving to the emergency room with angina pectoris may be treated with IV nitroglycerin. Use of IV nitroglycerin is contraindicated in patients with a systolic pressure of less than 90 mm Hg. IV nitroglycerin may be changed to sublingual or a nitroglycerin patch after the patient is symptom free. Anti-coagulants coronary artery bypass such as aspirin (acetylsalicylic acid, ASA) is administered immediately. This medication helps prevent platelet aggregation thus thinning the blood which makes it easier for the heart to pump. Along with aspirin, patients may be given clopidogrel which blocks another clotting cascade and thins blood. The stress on the heart is also reduced by prescribing beta blockers and calcium channel blockers. Oxygen therapy has traditionally been included in the treatment of angina pectoris. However, studies have been unable to document any positive or negative benefit in providing oxygen therapy to patients (Stub, 2017; Khoshnood, 2018). Beta blockers such as metoprolol block the stimulation the heart receives from the sympathetic system. By blocking this stimulation, the heart rate and force of cardiac muscle contraction is reduced. Beta blockers can be given intravenously in times of acute angina and are prescribed orally to prevent episodes of future angina. Calcium channel blockers reduce myocardial ischemia by decreasing SA node automaticity, impulse conduction through the AV node, and dilate coronary arteries. These actions reduce the workload on the heart and supply the heart muscle with more oxygen and nutrients.

Nursing Interventions and Patient Teaching

Nursing interventions are based on the patient's individual needs. They focus on achievement of five major patient outcomes.

1. *Ensure comfort.* Reduce or remove any known factors that are contributing to increased pain. Assess for causes of decreased pain tolerance, such as anxiety, fatigue, or lack of knowledge. Fatigue from increased oxygen demands with a decreased oxygen supply increases pain perception. Promote measures to reduce fatigue, such as providing rest periods. Provide a calm environment to decrease stress

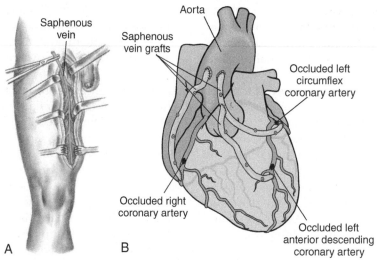

Fig. 8.12 (A) Saphenous vein. (B) Saphenous vein aortocoronary bypass or revascularization involves taking a piece of saphenous vein from the leg and creating a conduit for blood from the aorta to the area below the blockage in the coronary artery. A triple bypass is illustrated. (A, From Urden LD, Stacy KM, Lough ME: *Thelan's critical care nursing: Diagnosis and management*, ed 5, St. Louis, 2006, Mosby. B, From Lewis SL, Heitkemper MM, Dirksen SR, et al: *Medical-surgical nursing: Assessment and management of clinical problems*, ed 7, St. Louis, 2007, Mosby.)

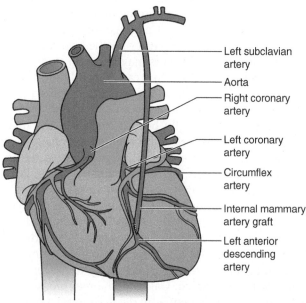

Fig. 8.13 Coronary artery bypass graft. Internal mammary artery is used; the distal end of this vessel is freed from the anterior chest wall and sutured in place distal to the occlusion in the coronary artery. (From Monahan FD, Sands JK, Neighbors M, et al: *Phipps' medical-surgical nursing: Health and illness perspectives*, ed 8, St. Louis, 2007, Mosby.)

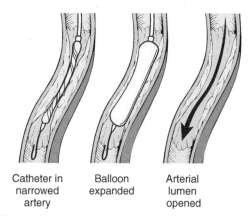

Fig. 8.14 Percutaneous transluminal coronary angioplasty. (From Frazier MS, Drzymkowski JW: *Essentials of human diseases and conditions*, ed 5, St. Louis, 2013, Saunders.)

and anxiety. Administer sublingual vasodilators, such as nitroglycerin, as ordered. Administer oxygen for high-risk patients with unstable angina and those with cyanosis or respiratory distress.

2. *Promote tissue perfusion.* Instruct the patient to avoid becoming overly fatigued and to stop activity immediately in the presence of chest pain, dyspnea, syncope, or vertigo, which indicate low tissue perfusion.

3. *Encourage activity and rest.* Increase the patient's activity tolerance by encouraging slower activity or shorter periods of activity with more rest periods.

Most people with angina pectoris are able to tolerate mild exercise such as walking or playing golf, but exertion such as running or climbing stairs rapidly causes pain. Nitroglycerin may be used prophylactically to prevent pain from strenuous activities. Isosorbide mononitrate and isosorbide dinitrate (Isordil) are nitrates used for acute treatment of angina attacks (sublingual only) or orally for prophylactic management of angina pectoris. Anginal pain occurs more easily in cold weather. The key is to avoid overexertion.

4. *Reduce anxiety and promote feelings of well-being.* Help the patient reduce the level of anxiety. The patient should minimize emotional outbursts, worry, and tension. People with angina may need continuing help in accepting situations. Supportive family members, a spiritual adviser, business associates, and friends can sometimes be of assistance. Relaxation techniques and music therapy may be beneficial. Peer support groups and behavioral

change programs are available. An optimistic outlook helps to relieve the work of the heart. Many people who learn to live within their limitations live out their expected lifespan despite the disease.

5. *Provide education to the patient and the family.* Delay teaching until the patient is ready (see the Communication box). The patient needs to be relatively free of pain and anxiety to learn. Promote a positive attitude and active participation of patient and family to encourage compliance. The teaching plan should include information on medications, ways to minimize the events that trigger angina pectoris, effects of exercise on reduction of myocardial oxygen needs, the need to stop smoking because of the vasoconstriction of nicotine, and the need for regular medical follow-up (see the Patient Teaching box).

Patient problems and interventions for the patient with angina pectoris include but are not limited to the following:

PATIENT PROBLEM	NURSING INTERVENTIONS
Discomfort, related to myocardial ischemia	Administer oxygen as ordered
	Administer prescribed nitroglycerin. Repeat q5min, three times. If pain is unrelieved, notify health care provider
	Monitor blood pressure and pulse before and after administration of nitroglycerin
	Promote rest
	Maintain diet as ordered; if chest pain occurs while eating or immediately after, advise small meals rather than two or three large meals
	Balance rest with activity
	Instruct patient to stop activity at the first sign of chest pain or other symptoms of cardiac ischemia

Communication

Methods to Decrease Angina Pectoris Attacks

Mrs. M., a patient with angina, has been admitted for further care, diagnosis, and treatment. After the initial nursing assessment, the nurse interviews the patient about the course of her anginal episodes. With the data gathered, the nurse participates in the development of a program to educate Mrs. M. how to minimize or control the attacks.

Nurse: I would like to ask you some questions about the anginal pain you are experiencing.

Patient: I already told the doctor about those attacks when I visited his office. Her nurse has all those records.

Nurse: Your health care provider asked us to help you plan a program for preventing or minimizing these attacks. With the information we gather, we can set goals for your care. We can also identify how angina relates to some of your activities.

Patient: OK, I would like to understand it better. Perhaps I would be less frightened when it happens. My friend told me about her aunt who had angina—she died. That really worries me.

Nurse: We hope to decrease some of your fears by helping you understand. First, when do your attacks usually occur?

Patient: Oh, mostly after a really busy day, you know—shopping or gardening or housecleaning. But a few times I had problems after my sister-in-law visited. She and my husband always seem to get into upsetting discussions. They never got along well. She upsets us both—she criticizes everything!

Nurse: Have you noticed if a big meal is related to the pain?

Patient: No, not really … well, only when my sister-in-law is there. We hardly ever eat big meals anymore, except when she comes. She expects to be fed well. My husband and I have cut down a lot. Big meals upset our systems—and then her, that harping on old problems, and how she thinks we should run our lives! She upsets me so!

Nurse: Mrs. M., I think we should talk about how to handle stressful situations like visits from your sister-in-law. But first, could you describe the pain for me? Does it come on suddenly? How long does it last? What does it feel like?

Patient: Oh, no, not all of a sudden. It is just dull at times, like an upset stomach. But then, it travels up in my chest and gets really heavy, like pressure. Sometimes it makes my face and teeth hurt … and my arm, too—this one [left]—all the way down to my little finger. If it's a really bad attack, I sometimes feel like I am going to vomit.

Nurse: On a scale of 0–10, how would you rate most of your angina attacks?

Patient: Probably 5–6 would be the average, but sometimes it's a 10.

Nurse: Does your heart beat faster?

Patient: Oh, yes, and I just have to sit down and be quiet or I can't catch my breath. That's when I take the nitroglycerin. I carry it with me all the time now, in this special little container.

Nurse: I see. And how long does it take for the pain to stop after you take the medicine?

Patient: I used to think it took forever, but my husband—he times it for me—says it lasts about 15–20 minutes. I relax a little, and it passes.

Nurse: What about the weather? Have you noticed that it affects your attacks in any way?

Patient: I don't know if it is all those clothes or the weather, but I get more pains if I get out in the cold.

Nurse: Do you or your husband smoke?

Patient: Not anymore. I gave up cigarettes when this angina started on me. I noticed the difference, too. Now I can't even stay in a room if people are smoking. I also cut down on coffee when I retired. My doctor said that too much caffeine isn't good for my heart. All the good things, they have to go when you get old!

Nurse: Maybe with some understanding of how certain activities and other factors affect your condition, you can find new "good things" that you'll enjoy just as much. We'll talk again soon. There are some effective coping methods we can explore to decrease your stress when your sister-in-law visits.

PATIENT PROBLEM	NURSING INTERVENTIONS
Compromised Blood Flow to Cardiac Tissue, related to narrowing of coronary arteries	Administer prescribed oxygen Instruct patient that nitroglycerin may need to be taken before exercise and sexual activity to prevent cardiac ischemia Encourage less strenuous or shorter periods of activity interspersed with rest Avoid exercise in cold weather Take prescribed nitroglycerin before activities that will increase the workload of the heart

Prognosis

The prognosis for the patient with angina pectoris is dependent on multiple conditions including age, comorbid conditions such as diabetes and chronic obstructive pulmonary disease, compliance with medication regimen, healthy alterations adopted into lifestyle, and the type of anginal pain. Based on these factors, some patients are stable for years experiencing episodes of stable angina while others experience fluctuations in symptoms and rapid progression over days or weeks.

MYOCARDIAL INFARCTION

Etiology and Pathophysiology

A **myocardial infarction (MI)**, or *heart attack,* is the necrosis (death) of heart muscle. It is caused by a severe reduction or cessation of blood flow through coronary arteries to the heart muscle. Lack of blood flow results in ischemia which results in cellular death. The extent to which a myocardial infarct impairs the heart's ability to pump blood volume depends on the location and severity of the ischemic episode (Fig. 8.15). For example, reduction or cessation of blood flow in the left anterior descending artery (LAD) would cause major problems in cardiac output as this artery supplies blood to the anterior ventricular septum and left ventricle. Patients presenting with this are normally referred to as having a "widow maker" as the mortality rates in this type of event are high.

Obstruction of major coronary arteries or one of its branches is one of the most common causes of a myocardial infarct. The obstruction is caused either by an atherosclerotic plaque, rupture of a atherosclerotic plaque, or by an **embolus** (a foreign object, a quantity of air or gas, a bit of tissue, or a piece of a thrombus that circulates in the bloodstream until it becomes lodged in a vessel) which cuts off blood flow and the affected part of the heart undergoes tissue ischemia. Seventy percent of all myocardial infarcts occur due to occlusions from atherosclerotic plaques. Researchers have found that 90% of men who suffered MIs had a modifiable risk factor while 94% of women had a modifiable risk factor that could have reduced the formation of atherosclerotic plaques. Other potential causes of myocardial infarct include drug use, coronary artery anomalies, and aortic dissection (Mechanic and Grossman, 2020).

An area of infarction can develop over minutes to hours. In response to reduced blood flow, cellular injury occurs that activates the inflammatory cascade. The inflammatory cascade includes the presence of monocytes and macrophages, thrombus formation, and platelet aggregation. This further reduces blood flow to the cells increasing myocardial cell damage, eventually leading to necrosis. The evolution of myocardial damage shows necrosis at the 12-hour mark, removal of dead cells by macrophages at the 3-day mark, appearance of granulation tissue and collagen deposition

Table 8.2	Signs and Symptoms of Myocardial Infarction
SUBJECTIVE DATA (SYMPTOMS)	**OBJECTIVE DATA (SIGNS)**
• Heavy pressure or squeezing in center of chest behind sternum • Pain, retrosternal and in heart region, often radiating down the left arm and to the neck, jaw, and teeth • Anxiety • Dyspnea • Weakness, faintness • Nausea	• Pallor • Erratic behavior • Hypotension, shock • Cardiac rhythm changes • Vomiting • Fever • Diaphoresis

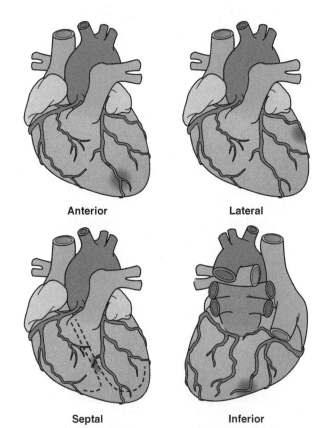

Anterior   **Lateral**

Septal   **Inferior**

Fig. 8.15 Four common locations where myocardial infarctions occur. (From Lewis SL, Heitkemper MM, Dirksen SR, et al: *Medical-surgical nursing: Assessment and management of clinical problems*, ed 7, St. Louis, 2007, Mosby.)

at the 10 day mark, and after 2 months the damaged myocardium is replaced by scar tissue.

Clinical Manifestations

Sometimes an asymptomatic MI or *silent MI* may occur. Many symptoms of MI are associated with irreversible ischemia, but they are similar to those of angina pectoris. In an MI, the symptoms are more severe and last longer than during an angina attack. Pain is the foremost symptom of MI (Table 8.2).

The pain location and radiation to other sites are depicted in Fig. 8.11. The pain often is described as crushing or viselike, an oppressive sensation as though a heavy object is sitting on the chest. The pain is retrosternal (behind the sternum) and in the heart region. In men, it often radiates down the left arm and to the neck, jaws, teeth, and epigastric area. It may occur suddenly, or it may build up over a few minutes. It may occur in conjunction with intense emotion, during exertion, or at rest. The pain is prolonged and more intense than anginal pain. It lasts 30 minutes to several hours or longer. It is not relieved by changes in body position, nitroglycerin, or rest. Health care providers often tell patients who call complaining of chest pain to take an aspirin (chewable if they have it) and report to the hospital emergency department. Other signs and symptoms that may occur with the pain include nausea, dyspnea, dizziness, weakness, diaphoresis, pallor, ashen color, and a sense of impending doom. Early signs and symptoms of an acute MI in women are unusual fatigue, sleep disturbances, shortness of breath, weakness, indigestion, and anxiety. Often, acute chest pain is not present in women, causing health care providers to fail to identify an MI. The health care provider may begin testing for other disorders such as gallbladder disease or anxiety. Table 8.3 provides a comparison of signs and symptoms and the medical management of angina pectoris and MI.

Assessment

Subjective data include the onset, location, quality, duration, and radiation of pain. The patient may complain of shortness of breath, dizziness, weakness, anxiety, fear, or unusual fatigue. Identify precipitating factors. Inquire about measures the patient has tried to relieve the pain.

Collection of objective data includes observation of the patient's behavior to detect apprehension and anxiety. Typical vital signs reveal hypotension, pulse abnormalities such as tachycardia or a barely perceptible pulse, and early temperature elevation. Note the presence of diaphoresis; vomiting; ashen color; cool,

Patient Teaching

Angina Pectoris

USING NITRATE MEDICATIONS
- Use nitroglycerin prophylactically to avoid pain known to occur with certain activities.
- A burning sensation on the tongue indicates nitroglycerin is activated.
- A throbbing sensation in the head and flushing may occur.
- When changing to a sitting or standing position, do it slowly after taking nitroglycerin. Postural hypotension is a side effect of nitroglycerin.
- Place a nitroglycerin tablet under the tongue at the onset of anginal pain; a second tablet can be taken after 5 min and a third tablet after another 5 min if pain is unrelieved.
- Call the health care provider if pain does not subside after the third nitroglycerin tablet; go to the nearest emergency department; do not drive yourself.
- Always carry nitroglycerin on your person.
- Store nitroglycerin in a dark bottle and keep it in a dry place.
- Replenish nitroglycerin supply every 6 months or before the expiration date.
- Remove all old nitrate ointment before application of new cream.
- Alter placement of nitrate ointment each morning to prevent skin irritation.
- Place nitroglycerin patches on skin in the morning and remove at bedtime. This prevents development of tolerance and maintains effectiveness.

MINIMIZING PRECIPITATING EVENTS
- Do not take medications for erectile dysfunction such as sildenafil (phosphodiesterase inhibitor) with nitroglycerin and nitrates. Nitrate medications may result in severe hypotension.
- Avoid overexertion. Take nitroglycerin before exercise.

- Try to reduce stress and anxiety, which cause blood vessels to constrict.
- Avoid overeating because it places an increased workload on the heart.
- Avoid cold weather (constricts coronary vessels to conserve body heat; hence anginal pain can develop more easily).
- Dress warmly in cold weather.
- Avoid hot, humid conditions (increases workload on the heart).
- Avoid walking uphill, in the cold, or against strong wind, because these activities increase the workload on the heart.
- Discontinue smoking. Nicotine causes vasoconstriction of the arteries.

EXERCISING TO REDUCE MYOCARDIAL OXYGEN NEEDS
- Engage in a regular exercise program, such as a walking program or yoga, to improve collateral circulation.
- Exercise conditions the heart muscle and can decrease oxygen demand during exertion.
- Space exercise period with rest periods.
- Take nitroglycerin before exertion.

MEDICATION MANAGEMENT TO REDUCE MYOCARDIAL OXYGEN NEEDS
- Beta blockers such as metoprolol need to be taken every day as prescribed.
- Do not abruptly stop beta blockers as it can worsen angina.
- Patients with diabetes taking beta blockers must check their blood glucose regularly as this medication will mask hypoglycemic symptoms.
- Use of non-cardioselective beta blockers is contraindicated in patients with pulmonary disorders such as asthma.
- Patients taking anti-coagulants may bruise easily.
- Report any bleeding from gums, nose, or any other area to the provider immediately.

Table 8.3   Coronary Artery Disorders

SIGNS AND SYMPTOMS	MEDICAL MANAGEMENT
Angina Pectoris	
Chest pain (substernal, retrosternal), may radiate to neck, jaw, left arm, and shoulder; great anxiety, fear of approaching death; face pale, ashen; pulse variable, usually tense and quick; blood pressure elevated during an attack; usually brought on by exertion, emotional upsets; relieved by rest, nitroglycerin	• Avoidance of precipitating factors • Reduction of modifiable risk factors • Medications: Nitrates, beta blockers, calcium channel blockers • Oxygen therapy • ECG monitoring • Aspirin for unstable angina
Myocardial Infarction	
Severe, crushing chest pain; prolonged heavy pressure or squeezing pain in center of chest; may spread to shoulder, neck, arm, fourth and fifth fingers on left hand, teeth, and jaw; may radiate as with angina; not relieved with rest or nitroglycerin; may be associated with dyspnea, diaphoresis, apprehension, nausea, and vomiting; signs and symptoms of cardiogenic shock (see Box 8.2) may develop; the pain is prolonged and more intense than anginal pain	• Relief of pain (oxygen), morphine, and other analgesics • ECG monitoring • Thrombolytic therapy to dissolve clot • Reduction of oxygen demand (rest) • Prevention of complications (through use of stool softeners, anticoagulants) • Treatment of complications (dysrhythmias, HF) • Anticoagulants to prevent further clotting
In women, these classic symptoms are far less common; most frequent early warning symptoms are unusual fatigue, sleep disturbances, shortness of breath, weakness, indigestion, and anxiety; in one study, only 30% of women reported chest pain, and acute chest pain was absent in 43%	

ECG, Electrocardiogram; *HF,* heart failure.

clammy skin; labored respirations; and cardiac dysrhythmias. If possible, find out about risk factors. A respiratory assessment also is necessary.

Diagnostic Tests

Diagnostic tests begin with an immediate 12-lead ECG. The ECG must be obtained within 10 minutes of arrival to the emergency rule and helps diagnose an acute MI Injured and ischemic cells experience a change in electrical impulse conduction and return to resting point (repolarization). An ECG that shows a myocardial infarct will have an elevation in the ST segment (seen in two leads), an inverted T wave, and the appearance

of an abnormal Q wave that develops over the course of 1 to 3 days. The presence of an elevation in the ST segment allows this to be classified as a STEMI—ST segment Elevation Myocardial Infarct. Further classifications of MI depend on additional testing. Serum cardiac markers (e.g., CK-MB, myoglobin) are released into the vascular system when infarcted myocardial muscle cells die. A sensitive cardiac marker present in serum, called *troponin I,* is the best indicator of myocardial infarct. Troponin I levels start to rise within 3 hours of injury, peak at 12 hours, and is detectable in blood for as long as 2 weeks post myocardial infarct. Patients presenting with no ST segment elevation but have elevated levels of troponin I are classified as having a non-STEMI—non-ST segment Elevation Myocardial Infarct. Patients presenting with no ST segment elevation, are negative for elevations in troponin levels, but have clinical manifestations of myocardial ischemia are classified as having unstable angina. Besides cardiac biomarkers, other laboratory tests conducted include CBC, lipid panel, renal function test, and a metabolic panel (CMP). An echocardiogram may be performed to visualize heart function and a cardiac angiography may be performed to determine the location and degree of blockages of coronary arteries.

In time the ST segment returns to normal and the T wave inverts. These ECG changes are important in confirming the diagnosis of MI. ECG findings are significantly different for men and women. A woman experiencing an MI is far less likely than a man to have concurrent ST-segment elevation, resulting in misdiagnosis and failure to receive the correct treatment. A chest x-ray is performed to note size and configuration of the heart. More complex tests occasionally are done, including cardiac fluoroscopy, myocardial imaging (thallium scan), echocardiogram, PET, and multigated acquisition (MUGA) scanning (a radioactive tracer is administered via a vein in order to determine the pumping ability of the ventricles). These tests may be done in conjunction with other tests to diagnose MI and determine the severity of CAD.

Medical Management

Medical management focuses on preventing further tissue injury and limiting the size of the infarction. It is extremely important that a patient with a suspected MI be diagnosed rapidly and treated to preserve cardiac muscle. Intervention is designed to restore cardiac tissue perfusion and reduce the workload of the heart. Promoting tissue oxygenation, relieving pain, preventing complications, improving tissue perfusion, and preventing further tissue damage are important medical considerations (Table 8.4).

Medical management for acute myocardial infarcts starts with immediate administration of chewable aspirin. The preferred dose is 160 to 325 mg. Aspirin inhibits platelet aggregation thus blood flows much more easily through all arteries but especially the coronary arteries. This allows for better perfusion of the

Box 8.2   Cardiogenic Shock

CLINICAL MANIFESTATIONS	SIGNS AND SYMPTOMS	MEDICAL MANAGEMENT	NURSING INTERVENTIONS
Decreased cardiac output Myocardial ischemia Cerebral hypoxia Impaired tissue perfusion Decreased renal circulation Anaerobic metabolism with lactic acidosis Peripheral vascular system collapse Shock	Dysrhythmias, chest pain Anxiety, agitation, restlessness, disorientation Urinary output diminished or absent Lactic acid accumulation in blood Tachycardia, thready pulse, tachypnea Decreased blood pressure Narrowed pulse pressure[a] Cyanosis; cold, moist, pale, clammy skin Decreased peripheral pulses Capillary refill time decreased Hypoactive bowel sounds	Recognition and control of life-threatening signs and symptoms Oxygenation to promote tissue perfusion Parenteral fluid as a volume expander Drug therapy: • Vasopressors: Raise arterial blood pressure • Cardiac glycoside: Digoxin increases cardiac contraction (inotropic) and strengthens and corrects dysrhythmias • Adrenergic drugs: Dopamine at therapeutic levels increases cardiac output and blood pressure • Sodium bicarbonate: Combats lactic acidosis (given sparingly because it causes fluid retention)	Monitor vital signs q5min during acute stage and q1h. when stabilized Administer oxygen as ordered Maintain bed rest to reduce myocardial workload and increase oxygenation Monitor acid-base balance Monitor urinary output hourly to determine adequate kidney perfusion Allow nothing by mouth Initiate bed rest to minimize energy expenditure Administer medications as ordered Provide comfort measures

[a]Pulse pressure is based on blood pressure: It is the numeric difference between the systolic and diastolic blood pressure. For example, if the blood pressure is 100/70 mm Hg, the pulse pressure is 30.

myocardium and an increase in oxygen and nutrient supply. Aspirin starts working within 20 to 30 minutes of administration and should be administered within 30 minutes of patient arrival to the emergency room. Patients experiencing decrease in oxygen saturation below 91% need supplemental oxygen. A medication instrumental in relieving pain and anxiety is morphine. Morphine also decreases blood pressure, heart rate, and venous return which reduces the workload of the heart. Nitroglycerin is administered intravenously but may also be given subcutaneously and via intradermal patch. Nitroglycerin and nitrates dilate both coronary arteries and veins thus increasing oxygen and nutrients to the heart and decreasing the workload on the heart. Both morphine and nitroglycerin may cause hypotension. Often the mnemonic MONA (Morphine, Oxygen, Nitroglycerin, and Aspirin) is used for this drug therapy regimen. Patients experiencing dysrhythmias may be treated with a beta blocker or other medications as indicated by the dysrhythmia.

Besides administration of MONA, Patients presenting with a STEMI are immediately taken to the cardiac catheterization lab for an emergent PCI. The PCI must be performed within 60 minutes of the patient's arrival in the emergency department. Emergency personnel may bypass a hospital that does not have a cardiac catheterization lab or the capabilities of performing a PCI for a hospital that is equipped with both. When availability of facilities does not permit a PCI within 60 minutes, patients are given thrombolytics (Mechanic and Grossman, 2020). Patients must meet the strict criteria prior to receiving thrombolytic therapy. The patient must present with a STEMI, have chest pain lasting longer than 20 minutes which is unrelieved by nitroglycerin, the time from pain onset must be less than 6 hours (Hinkle & Cheever, 2018), and PCI is unavailable. Before a thrombolytic is administered, obtain a thorough history. Thrombolytics are not used for patients with active internal bleeding, suspected aortic dissecting aneurysm, recent head trauma, history of hemorrhagic stroke within the past year, surgery within the past 10 days, pregnancy, uncontrolled hypertension, or intracranial vessel malformation. Labs must also be obtained especially coagulation studies. Fibrinolytic agents such as tissue plasminogen activator (tPA) (alteplase, Tenecteplase, and recteplase), streptokinase, and urokinase may be used to reperfuse coronary arteries.

Patients presenting with a non-STEMI are also administered morphine, oxygen (if less than 91%), nitroglycerin, and aspirin. Medical treatment varies based on patient clinical situation. Some patients may be admitted to the cardiac floor where they are placed on continuous telemetry and labs are drawn for serial troponins (every 3 hours). Clinicians are monitoring for potential changes in ECG to ST segment elevations or increase in troponin levels suggesting a continuation of myocardial infarct. A change to STEMI would warrant immediate PCI. Other patients may undergo echocardiogram, myocardial perfusion imaging tests, or a stress test within 72 hours of discharge from the hospital. Low risk patients presenting with a non-STEMI may be asked to follow up on an outpatient basis once medically stable (Basit, Malik, and Huecker, 2020).

Table 8.4   Medications for Myocardial Infarction

CLASSIFICATION	GENERIC NAME	ACTION
Vasopressor	dopamine	Raises systemic arterial pressure and cardiac output
Anticoagulants	heparin warfarin	Reduce incidence of clotting
Platelet aggregation inhibitor	ticlopidine	Decreases platelet release of thromboxane, so that vasoconstriction and platelet aggregation are decreased
	aspirin (acetylsalicylic acid; ASA)	Decreases platelet aggregation
Analgesic	morphine	Controls pain; reduces myocardial oxygen demand
Tranquilizer	diazepam	Decreases anxiety and restlessness
Thrombolytic agent	streptokinase	Thrombolytic (pertaining to dissolution of blood clots) agent used when acute MI symptoms have been present less than 6 h, preferably from 30 min to 1 h; restores blood flow and therefore limits infarct size in certain patients
Tissue plasminogen activator	alteplase	Dissolves blood clots and reduces blood viscosity
Nitrates	nitroglycerin isosorbide atenolol	Dilate blood vessels by reducing coronary artery spasm, increase coronary artery blood supply, and decrease oxygen demands
Beta-adrenergic blockers	propranolol nadolol metoprolol carvedilol	Block beta-adrenergic stimulation and decrease myocardial oxygen demands, thus decreasing myocardial damage; decrease mortality rate
Calcium channel blockers	nifedipine diltiazem verapamil amlodipine	Dilate blood vessels, increase coronary artery blood supply, and decrease myocardial oxygen demands
Angiotensin-converting enzyme (ACE) inhibitors	captopril enalapril	Can help prevent ventricular remodeling and prevent or slow the progression of HF Prevent conversion of angiotensin I to angiotensin II Decrease endothelial dysfunction
Salicylates	aspirin	Decrease platelet adhesion and thus decrease thrombosis formation
Antidysrhythmics	lidocaine IV	Treat ventricular dysrhythmias (rarely used except for ventricular tachycardia)
Stool softeners	docusate calcium docusate sodium	Reduce straining at stool; prevent constipation produced by decreased mobility and use of constipating narcotics
Diuretics	furosemide	Control edema
Electrolyte replacement	potassium chloride	May be necessary when diuretics are used
Inotropic agents	digoxin amrinone IV dobutamine	Increase the heart's pumping action (contractility) Indicated when left ventricle failure is present

HF, Heart failure; *IV,* intravenous; *MI,* myocardial infarction.

Patients with unstable angina are treated with the MONA drug regimen, may be given heparin or low molecular weight heparin, beta blockers, and statins (Goyal and Zeltser, 2020). They are discharged once medically stable. Follow-up care with a cardiology service is recommended.

Percutaneous coronary intervention. PCI also known as percutaneous transluminal coronary angioplasty (PTCA) is a surgical procedure for management of the patient with CAD. PTCA is an invasive procedure performed in the cardiac catheterization laboratory. In an *angioplasty,* the narrowing in a coronary artery is widened without open-heart surgery. *Percutaneous* indicates that the procedure is performed through the skin; *transluminal* means that it is done within the lumen of the artery. A signed informed consent is required for this procedure. This procedure also uses contrast dye, so it is important to ascertain kidney function and allergies to iodine or shellfish. The catheter in this procedure is inserted by puncturing either the femoral, radial, or brachial artery. The catheter is passed retrograde via the use of fluoroscopy up the artery punctured into the descending aorta, aortic arch, and the left/right coronary artery. Once in position, contrast dye is injected into the coronary artery. The areas with reduced or no blood flow will have little or no dye. A balloon catheter is inflated once it is positioned in the area of the blockage or stenosis (Fig. 8.14). The outward push of the balloon against the narrowed wall of the coronary artery breaks up the atherosclerotic plaque and reduces the constriction until it no longer interferes with blood flow to the heart muscle. The balloon may be inflated and deflated repeatedly to reestablish coronary artery patency.

Most PTCA procedures involve placement of a stent in the area of reestablished blood flow. Two types of stents are available: bare metal stents and drug eluting stents. Most people have drug eluting stents placed. A drug eluting stent is coated with medication that it releases slowly over time. The purpose of the drug is to prevent the growth of scar tissue in the artery lining. However, use of drug eluting stents requires the patient to take blood thinners for a longer period of time to prevent clotting around the stent. Patients with bare metal stents must also take blood thinners but the period is shorter. With a bare metal stent, the endothelial cells of the artery grow around the stent keeping it in place. Scar tissue formation is a problem with bare metal stents and the amount of scar tissue formed may end up occluding blood flow (Mayo Clinic, 2019d). PTCA with stent placement may take his procedure may take 30 minutes to 3 hours, with the patient usually awake but under conscious sedated. This procedure is widely performed, and major complications are rare. Possible complications include hematoma formation at the insertion site, infection of skin over the artery used, embolism, stroke, kidney injury from contrast dye, hypersensitivity to dye, vessel rupture, coronary artery dissection, and vasospasm. In addition, there is the long-term risk of possible re-stenosis of the stented vessel (Malik and Tivakaran, 2020).

Postprocedure nursing interventions are similar to those outlined after cardiac catheterization and angiography. In addition, the nurse monitors the patient for signs of bleeding as patients receive IV heparin during the procedure and are usually on an eptifibatide drip after the procedure. The sheath used to puncture the artery is usually removed after the procedure, but patients may also be admitted to a cardiac floor or intensive care unit with a vascular access sheath in the artery used for puncture. The sheaths are withdrawn once blood studies show that heparin is no longer active. Once the sheath is removed, hemostasis is achieved by the use of a device such as a FemoStop which applies pressure to the puncture site. Patients may go home the next day or may stay in the hospital for a few days.

PTCA is associated with lower rates of morbidity, mortality, shorter recovery, and lower cost.

Approximately 90% of patients that undergo PTCA express relief of anginal pain and symptoms and resumption or improvement in exercise capacity (Malik and Tivakaran, 2020).

CABG is heart surgery for patients who have experienced a myocardial infarct. Most patients undergo PTCA which helps diagnose the level and degree of blockage and to revascularize a blocked artery. However, patients who have multiple blocked arteries (especially blocks in RCA, left anterior descending artery, and left circumflex artery) have occlusions greater than 70%, have diabetes or heart failure, and poor left ventricular function are candidates for CABG.

A CABG is a procedure in which the blocked arteries of the heart are bypassed by grafting another vein or artery that acts as a "bridge" for the area above the block and below the block (Figs. 8.12 and 8.13). The vein or artery to be grafted is taken from the patient and includes the saphenous veins from one or both legs and the left internal mammary artery. If additional arteries are needed, then the right internal mammary artery, radial artery, and gastroepiploic artery may be grafted. The left internal mammary artery is used for grafts needed for the LAD as the LAD supplies blood to the left ventricle and the left internal mammary artery remains patent for a long period of time with 90% of grafts free of stenosis at ten years (Ahmed and Yandrapalli, 2020). In comparison, the saphenous veins start to show atherosclerotic changes within 5 to 10 years (Hinkle and Cheever, 2018) and are used to bypass other coronary arteries. During a CABG procedure, a number of grafts may be done at one time. In addition, CABG procedures can be done with the use of a cardiopulmonary bypass machine or without known as off pump CABG.

Patients post CABG are usually admitted to intensive care units. Nursing interventions include monitoring cardiopulmonary status, pain management, wound management, progressive activity, and nutrition. Nurses assess all body systems every four hours. Patients are kept on continuous vital signs monitors, input and output is strictly monitored and documented, lab studies are conducted and monitored for discrepancies, kidney function is monitored, and emotional and psychological status is assed. Patients undergo cardiac rehabilitation where they progressive in activity level gradually over time with the guidance of physical therapy.

Complications commonly associated with CABG include stroke, wound infection, graft failure, renal failure, postoperative atrial fibrillation, and death. 400,000 CABG procedures are performed on a yearly basis making CABG the most commonly performed major surgical procedure (Bachar and Manna, 2020).

Nursing Interventions and Patient Teaching
Patients with chest pain may present in the emergency room, may be admitted to the hospital through the

emergency room, or may be direct admits from outpatient clinics across the community. The nurse immediately decreases patient activity by encouraging bed rest and a reduction in all other activities to conserve oxygen for the heart. The following interventions occur almost simultaneously: raising the head of the bed to at least 30 degrees, attaching electrodes to get an electrocardiogram reading, inserting peripheral IV catheters, obtaining a history of previous heart conditions and the current incidence of chest pain, and taking vitals or placing the patient on continuous vitals monitoring if in the emergency room. Carrying out provider orders for medications such as morphine, aspirin, nitroglycerin and oxygen are also paramount to helping reduce the workload on the heart. Patients who may be constipated are prescribed stool softener to prevent rectal straining as an attempt to increase intra-abdominal pressure is conducted through the Valsalva maneuver. The Valsalva maneuver may cause severe changes in blood pressure and heart rate, which may trigger ischemia, dysrhythmias, or cardiac arrest. The institution of mechanical or chemical prophylaxis for deep vein thrombosis is essential as patients are encouraged to rest. It is also important for the nurse to get orders and make sure the patient remains nil per os (NPO) in case procedures such as cardiac catheterization need to be performed.

The following patient problem and interventions are relevant to the presentation of chest pain:

PATIENT PROBLEM	NURSING INTERVENTIONS
Pain, Recent Onset related to myocardial ischemia	Assess original pain and location, duration, radiation, and onset of new symptoms
	Administer prescribed analgesics (usually morphine sulfate, which relieves pain, reduces anxiety, causes vasodilation of vascular smooth muscle, and reduces myocardial workload)
	Maintain bed rest and reduced patient activity
	Administer oxygen as prescribed
	Record patient's response to pain relief measures
	Employ alternative methods of pain relief
	Provide calm, restful environment
Insufficient Cardiac Output, related to reduced myocardial pumping capacity	Assess and monitor vital signs q4h.
	Maintain bed rest with head of bed elevated 30 degrees
	Administer prescribed medications such as nitrates, anticoagulants, statins and beta blockers
	Auscultate breath sounds and heart rate q4h; increase activity level as prescribed
	Palpate for pedal pulses, assess capillary refill, auscultate bowel sounds, assess for pedal or dependent edema q4h, and strictly monitor intake and output (I&O)

Patients may be admitted for inpatient hospitalization post PTCA or CABG. Nursing interventions include continuous telemetry monitoring, vital signs monitoring, assessment of cardiac and respiratory function every four hours or as needed, maintaining IV lines, supporting oxygenation needs, and calculating strict intake and outputs. Post PTCA, nursing interventions include monitoring the puncture site for hematoma and assessing the extremity for pulse, color, temperature, sensation, and capillary refill. Vitals signs and assessment of extremity is done every 15 minutes for the first hour, every thirty minutes for the next hour, and every hour for the next four hours. These patients are usually on a blood thinner and need to be observed for bleeding. Patients receiving percutaneous intervention via femoral artery need to lay supine for up to 6 hours while patients with radial or brachial PTCA can be mobile within 2 to 3 hours. In addition, patients post PTCA may experience reperfusion ectopy as the myocardium lacking oxygen and nutrients releases chemicals into the blood. The most common reperfusion ectopy includes PVCs and VT.

Patients post CABG are admitted to the intensive care unit. Nursing interventions include maintaining hemodynamic monitoring, strict input and outputs, continuous vital signs monitoring, assessment of cardiac and respiratory function, and managing blood glucose levels if diabetic. These patients usually have chest tubes post CABG that need to be maintained. They may have had the saphenous vein harvested in one or both legs that need assessed for pulse, capillary refill, temperature, color, and sensation. Patients usually sit in a chair on post op day two, start walking with physical therapy after 3 days, and participate in a cardiac rehabilitation program. Once gag reflex has returned, diet is advanced as quickly as possible and patients are encouraged to eat foods high in protein to help healing.

Cardiac rehabilitation. The health care provider may prescribe cardiac rehabilitation after an MI. Before discharge from the hospital, discuss how participation in a monitored exercise program and continuing education as part of outpatient cardiac rehabilitation help the patient recover faster and return to a full and productive life. Cardiac rehabilitation has two major parts:

1. Exercise training to teach the patient how to exercise safely, strengthen muscles, and improve stamina. The exercise plan is based on the individual's ability, needs, and interests.
2. Education, counseling, and training to help the patient understand his or her heart condition and find ways to reduce the risk of future heart problems. The cardiac rehabilitation team assists the patient in adjusting to a new lifestyle and dealing with fears about the future. Cardiac rehabilitation may last 6 weeks, 6 months, or longer. Cardiac rehabilitation has lifelong favorable effects (see the Home Care Considerations box and Health Promotion box).

Home Care Considerations

Exercise Program After Myocardial Infarction

- After discharge from the hospital, many patients are encouraged to begin a 2- to 12-week walking program. This is a structured program designed to have the patient walking 2 miles in less than 60 min by the end of 12 weeks.
- Encourage patients to work through this program at their own rate until they achieve a pace below a slow jog and their heart rate is below the prescribed rate set by the cardiologist.
- Not all patients are physiologically capable of participating in a rigorous exercise program after an MI.
- Eventually, most patients are encouraged to participate in a maintenance (lifetime), unsupervised, home-based exercise program designed specifically for them.
- Almost everyone can benefit from some type of cardiac rehabilitation.

Prognosis

Medical care must be instituted without delay. Many patients with a MI who are not treated before reaching the hospital die. The prognosis also depends on the area and extent of the damage and the presence or absence of complications.

HEART FAILURE

Etiology and Pathophysiology

Heart failure is a chronic disease and the numbers of patients diagnosed with heart failure increases every year. The latest statistics from the American Heart Association (2017) show 5.7 million heart failure cases between 2009 and 2012 and 6.5 million cases between 2011 and 2014. It is projected that there will be a 46% rise in the number of heart failure cases by the year 2030 at a projected cost of $70 billion. Heart failure is a chronic condition that occurs when there is a structural or functional problem with heart. Structural and

Health Promotion

Myocardial Infarction

Teach the patient the following:
- The effects of MI, the healing process, and the treatment regimen.
- The effects of medications used to treat MI.
- The association between risk factors and coronary artery disease (CAD).
- How to identify nonmodifiable risk factors.
- How to identify modifiable risk factors (particularly cigarette smoking and stress). The patient should stop smoking and encourage family and significant others to stop.
- The effect of dietary restrictions on atherosclerotic heart disease or CAD. Recommended daily intake is 2 g of sodium, 1500 calories, low cholesterol, and fluid restrictions.
- To limit total fat intake to 25%–35% of total calories each day. Limit intake of saturated fats to less than 7% of total fat intake. Saturated fats (e.g., shortening, lard, or butter) are solid at room temperature; better sources of fat include vegetable, olive, and fish oils.
- To avoid foods high in sodium, saturated fats, and triglycerides. Review alternative ways of seasoning foods to avoid cooking with salt. Explain the need to limit intake of eggs, cream, butter, and foods high in animal fat. Teach the patient and family how to read labels on foods.
- To eat 20–30 g of soluble fiber every day. Foods such as bran, beans, and peas help lower bad cholesterol (low-density lipoprotein).
- The effect of activity on the heart and the need to participate in a progressive activity plan.
- Refer the patient to social support groups as indicated.
- Stress the importance of participating in cardiac rehabilitation services.
- Explain cardiac warning symptoms. Patients and their partners are often unsure which symptoms should be reported. If nitroglycerin has been prescribed, advise the patient to take it when experiencing chest pain and to notify the health care provider if the pain is not relieved within 15 min. Other signs to report include shortness of breath, rapid heart rate, dizziness, insomnia, a persistent increase in heart rate or blood pressure, and extreme fatigue after sexual activity.
- Most patients have concerns about resuming sexual activity after an MI but may not express them to the nurse. Initiate the conversation and include the topic of sexual activity when discussing other physical activities. Explain what is safe and when. The joint guidelines of the American College of Cardiology and the American Heart Association recommend that after an "uncomplicated MI" (i.e., the patient's condition was stable with no complications), sexual intercourse can be resumed in 7 to 10 days. However, many patients tend to resume sexual activity more gradually than this. A "complicated MI" means that the patient required CPR or had hypotension, serious dysrhythmia, or heart failure while hospitalized. Patients with complicated MIs should resume sexual activity more slowly, depending on their tolerance for exercise and activity. Encourage patients to talk to their health care providers about resuming sexual activity; the type and extent of damage from the MI may influence recommendations.
- Explain the importance of taking prescribed medications such as beta blockers. Patients who take beta-adrenergic blockers for 1 year after an MI have a reduced chance of reinfarction and increased survival. The patient should also continue to take lipid-lowering agents such as simvastatin (Zocor), atorvastatin (Lipitor), lovastatin, pravastatin (Pravachol), or rosuvastatin (Crestor).

functional problems arise due to multiple other diseases that can afflict the heart the most common being CAD. Atherosclerotic coronary arteries deprive the myocardial cells of the heart of oxygen and nutrients. These cells undergo necrosis and death which impairs their contractility. Impaired contractility places stress on the heart and leads to heart failure. The severity of the infarction caused by coronary atherosclerosis correlates with the severity of heart failure in patients. Valvular disorders cause structural changes that compromise the function of the heart as they allow blood to flow bidirectionally. This bidirectional blood flow places stress on the heart which eventually compromises the heart's pumping function. Changes in afterload such as high blood pressure in the systemic or pulmonary system places stress on the heart and makes it harder for the heart to pump blood. Examples of other disease processes that can cause heart failure include atrial fibrillation, renal failure, chronic obstructive pulmonary disease, and cardiomyopathy.

Heart failure can be classified in two different ways. The first classification involves systolic or diastolic heart failure. In systolic heart failure, the myocardial cells are too weak to contract optimally. As contraction is weak, cardiac output is reduced which causes blood congestion and symptoms. In diastolic heart failure, the ability of myocardial cells to stretch when filled with blood is reduced. As the stretching ability is reduced, the amount of blood that fills the ventricles is reduced which then compromises contractility (Frank Sterling Law). This too leads to a decrease in cardiac output and blood congestion which results in symptoms. Patients may have systolic heart failure, diastolic heart failure, or both. Systolic heart failure is differentiated from diastolic heart failure by measuring the EF. Patients with a normal EF of 55% to 65% have diastolic heart failure, whereas patients with reduced EFs have systolic heart failure. Heart failure can occur on the left, right, or both sides of the heart. Patients are therefore classified as having either right sided (ventricular) heart failure, left sided (ventricular) heart failure or both. This classification is discussed under clinical manifestations.

The pathophysiology of heart failure starts with a decrease in cardiac output that precipitates compensatory mechanisms within the body. Although these compensatory mechanisms are meant to help circulating blood volume, it results in decreases in contractile ability and increases the severity of heart failure. The pathophysiology of the compensatory mechanisms is explained in the following table:

METHODS TO INCREASE CARDIAC OUTPUT (CO)	RESULT
Sympathetic system releases epinephrine and norepinephrine	Causes vasoconstriction that increases blood pressure and therefore afterload which makes it harder for the heart to pump, results in decreased cardiac output

METHODS TO INCREASE CARDIAC OUTPUT (CO)	RESULT
Decrease in renal perfusion d/t low CO and vasoconstriction causes release of renin-angiotensin I-angiotensin II	Angiotensin II causes more vasoconstriction and therefore increases afterload even more, makes it harder for the heart to pump, and ends up decreasing CO Angiotensin II stimulates release of aldosterone which acts on the kidney by conserving sodium which conserves water. Absorption of more water from the kidney tubules increases blood pressure therefore afterload and makes it harder for the heart to pump and ends up decreasing CO Angiotensin II stimulates release of ADH which acts on the kidney to reabsorb water which increases blood pressure and afterload, thus making it harder for the heart to pump and decreasing CO

METHODS TO DECREASE AFTERLOAD AND PRELOAD	RESULT
Increase in preload and afterload caused by the compensatory mechanisms to increase cardiac output stretch the atria and ventricle which responds by secreting ANP and BNP	ANP (atrial natriuretic peptide) and BNP (beta natriuretic peptide) is released from the overstretched atria and ventricles, respectively, due to blood congestion; these two peptides promote vasodilation and diuresis, but their effect is not enough to overcome methods to increase cardiac output

The heart copes with the increase in workload by undergoing hypertrophic changes, whereas first the heart muscle cells get bigger, but this leads to ventricular remodeling that further impairs the hearts ability to pump blood.

According to the American Heart Association the most commonly used classification system used to express severity of HF is the New York Heart Association (NYHA) Functional Classification system (American Heart Association, 2017d). (Box 8.3.)

Clinical Manifestations

The clinical manifestations of heart failure are specific to the ventricle in the heart that is failing. Patients start out with either left sided or right sided heart failure and eventually the failure to pump blood on one side

Box 8.3   Classifying and Staging Heart Failure

NEW YORK HEART ASSOCIATION HEART FAILURE CLASSIFICATION
The New York Heart Association classification is a universal gauge of heart failure severity based on physical limitations.

CLASS I: MINIMAL
- No limitations.
- Ordinary physical activity does not cause undue fatigue, dyspnea, palpitations, or angina.

CLASS II: MILD
- Slightly limited physical activity.
- Comfortable at rest.
- Ordinary physical activity results in fatigue, palpitations, dyspnea, or angina.

CLASS III: MODERATE
- Markedly limited physical activity.
- Comfortable at rest.
- Less than ordinary activity causes fatigue, palpitations, dyspnea, or anginal pain.

CLASS IV: SEVERE
- Patient unable to perform any physical activity without discomfort.
- Angina or symptoms of cardiac inefficiency may develop at rest. Physical activity increases discomfort.

AMERICAN COLLEGE OF CARDIOLOGY AND AMERICAN HEART ASSOCIATION (ACC/AHA) HEART FAILURE STAGES
Stage A: Patient is at high risk for developing heart failure but has no structural disorder of the heart. The patient has a primary condition that is strongly associated with heart failure (such as diabetes mellitus, hypertension, substance abuse, or history of rheumatic fever) but no signs or symptoms of heart failure.
Stage B: Patient has a structural disorder of the heart, such as left ventricular remodeling, left ventricular hypertrophy, valvular heart disease, or previous myocardial infarction, but has never developed symptoms of heart failure.
Stage C: Patient has past or current symptoms of heart failure associated with underlying structural disease. The patient may display signs of dyspnea or fatigue but is responding to therapy.
Stage D: Patient has end-stage disease and requires specialized treatment strategies that may include mechanical circulatory support, continuous inotropic infusions, heart transplant, or hospice care. These patients are frequently hospitalized and cannot be discharged without symptom recurrence.

Data from American Heart Association: Classes of heart failure, 2017d. Retrieved from http://www.heart.org/HEARTORG/Conditions/HeartFailure/AboutHeartFailu re/Classes-of-Heart-Failure_UCM_306328_Article.jsp#.WajCAdEpD7M; and Graham KE: Heart Failure ACC/AHA Staging System for Patients, n.d. Retrieved from http://heartfailurecenter.com/HF-ACCAHA.htm.

of the heart places stress on the other side as well. As this chronic condition progresses, patients then exhibit symptoms of both left and right ventricular failure. (Box 8.4).

Left ventricular failure. In order to understand the signs and symptoms associated with left ventricular failure, it is important to have a clear understanding of normal physiology. In normal physiology, the flow of blood is continuous and constant within a closed circulatory system. Blood flows from chamber to chamber in the heart through the systemic and venous system and then back to the heart and lungs. Any breaks or hiccups in the constant flow affects blood that is moving forward and causes congestion of blood in the previous tract. The left ventricle is crucial in pumping blood out of the ventricle, into the aorta, and then throughout the systemic system. If the pumping ability of blood from the ventricle is compromised, the forward motion of blood decreases, more blood remains in the left ventricle at the end of systole, and blood backs up in the left atrium and lungs. A decrease in the forward motion of blood compromises cardiac output and leads to poor or low perfusion. The signs and symptoms manifested include oliguria, anorexia and nausea, dizziness or lightheadedness, weak peripheral pulses, decreased blood pressure, cooler extremities, nocturia, and palpitations and tachycardia. The excess blood left in the left ventricle after systole stretches the ventricle and causes more hypertrophic changes and decreased contractility. It is

Box 8.4   Signs and Symptoms of Heart Failure

DECREASED CARDIAC OUTPUT
- Fatigue
- Anginal pain
- Anxiety
- Oliguria
- Decreased gastrointestinal motility
- Pale, cool skin
- Weight gain
- Restlessness

LEFT VENTRICULAR FAILURE
- Dyspnea
- Paroxysmal nocturnal dyspnea
- Cough
- Frothy, blood-tinged sputum
- Orthopnea
- Pulmonary crackles (moist popping and cracking sounds heard most often at the end of inspiration)
- Radiographic evidence of pulmonary vascular congestion with pleural effusion

RIGHT VENTRICULAR FAILURE
- Distended jugular veins
- Anorexia, nausea, and abdominal distention
- Liver enlargement with right upper quadrant pain
- Ascites
- Edema in feet, ankles, sacrum; may progress up the legs into thighs, external genitalia, and lower trunk

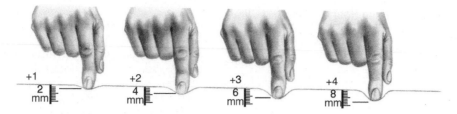

Fig. 8.16 Scale for pitting edema depth. (From Canobbio M: *Mosby's clinical nursing series: Cardiovascular disorders*, St. Louis, 1990, Mosby.)

Table 8.5   **Pitting Edema Scale**

SCALE	DEGREE	RESPONSE
+1: Trace	2 mm (0–{1/16} inch)	Rapid
+2: Mild	4 mm (0–¼ inch)	10–15 sec
+3: Moderate	6 mm (¼–½ inch)	1–2 min
+4: Severe	8 mm (½ inch)	2–5 min

this stretch that causes myocardial cells to release the peptide BNP. The amount of BNP detected signals the progression of heart failure. The congestion of blood in the left atrium stretches this chamber and causes the cells to secrete the peptide ANP. The congestion of blood in the lungs causes congestion of fluid in the capillary alveolar beds and leads to the following signs and symptoms: orthopnea, dyspnea on exertion, a dry hacking cough which is at first unproductive and then becomes moist over time, crackles auscultated in the lungs, decrease in oxygen saturation, pink frothy sputum, and decreased activity tolerance. Patients often find that over time the amount of activity they can participate in decreases as fatigue increases. Sleeping flat in bed becomes harder over time and patients may describe sleeping on one elevated pillow and then two elevated pillows and this may eventually graduate to patients sleeping in a recliner to assist with breathing.

Left ventricular heart failure can lead to right ventricular heart failure as the congestion of blood in the lungs causes the pressure in the capillary beds and arterioles in the lungs to increase. The right ventricle now must pump blood through the pulmonic valve and pulmonary artery into the lungs against higher pressure or afterload. This places stress on the right ventricle which starts to undergo hypertrophic changes and ventricular remodeling leading to the start of right ventricular heart failure. At this point, patients start to have symptoms of both left and right ventricular heart failure. Left ventricular heart failure is one of the most common causes of right ventricular heart failure after which is the presence of pulmonary diseases (Arrigo, Huber, Winnik et al., 2020).

Right ventricular failure. In order to understand the signs and symptoms associated with right ventricular failure, it is important to have a clear understanding of normal physiology as outlined under the left ventricular failure section. The right ventricle is a lower

pressure system than the left as it pumps blood into the pulmonary system where the pressure is typically lower than the systemic system. If the pumping ability of the right ventricle is compromised, the forward motion of blood (cardiac output from the right ventricle) decreases which causes congestion of blood in the right ventricle, right atrium, superior and inferior vena cava, and through the venous system. The backup of blood and its signs and symptoms evolve slowly over time as the right ventricle continues to fail. Increased venous volume and pressure causes engorgement of the spleen (splenomegaly) and liver (hepatomegaly). Hepatomegaly places pressure on the diaphragm which causes respiratory distress. Increased in venous volume and pressure causes the jugular vein to be distended known as jugular venous distension (JVD). Eventually the increase in volume and pressure force fluid out of the vasculature into interstitial tissues. This causes edema that settles in the lower legs, ankles, feet and only gets worse the longer the patient sits or stands and as the disease progresses. The edema may also progress up the legs into the thighs and genitalia. Edema in the peritoneal cavity is known as ascites which places pressure on the stomach and intestines causing gastrointestinal distress. Pitting edema occurs where the fluid in the tissues causes indentations in the skin (Fig. 8.16 and Table 8.5). The engorgement of the venous system and movement of fluid from the intravascular spaces into interstitial tissues causes weight gain.

Assessment
Subjective data include complaints of symptoms typical to either left sided heart failure, right sided heart failure, or both. Patients may describe dyspnea, orthopnea (an abnormal condition in which a person is able to breath better by leaning forward with arms extended on a table), paroxysmal nocturnal dyspnea (sudden awakening from sleep because of shortness of breath), and cough. The patient may report fatigue, anxiety, weight gain from fluid retention, and edema. Patients may also describe a decreased ability to conduct ADLs. Physical symptoms and impaired physical function may cause psychosocial stress.

Collection of objective data includes noting the presence of respiratory distress, the number of pillows required to breathe comfortably while attempting to rest (orthopnea), edema (site, degree of pitting), abdominal distention secondary to ascites, weight gain, adventitious breath sounds, abnormal heart sounds (gallop and murmurs), activity intolerance, and jugular vein distention. Oxygen deficit in tissues results in cyanosis and general debilitation.

Diagnostic Tests

Diagnosis is based on presenting signs and symptoms of HF and is confirmed by various diagnostic tests. A chest radiograph reveals pulmonary vascular congestion, **pleural effusion** (fluid in the pleural space surrounding the lungs), and cardiomegaly (cardiac enlargement). ECG shows either normal or dysrhythmias. In patients with normal rhythms, the ECG can rule out heart failure with an 89% sensitivity. Abnormal ECGs increase the likelihood of a heart failure diagnosis and also, at times, give clues to its etiology (Hajouli and Ludhwani, 2020). The most noninvasive diagnostic test for evaluating a patient with HF is an echocardiogram. Echocardiography helps to assess the valves and chambers of the heart and allows for calculation of the EF. This helps diagnose systolic or diastolic heart failure. It can also be used to identify the cause of heart failure such valvular heart disease and detect the presence of pericardial fluid.

Laboratory studies include electrolytes, sodium, calcium, magnesium, and potassium levels. Blood chemistry reveals elevated BUN and creatinine resulting from decreased glomerular filtration; liver function values (alanine aminotransferase, aspartate transaminase, gamma-glutamyltransferase, alkaline phosphatase) are mildly elevated.

Important laboratory study includes a BNP level in blood which is a hormone secreted by the heart in response to ventricular expansion and pressure overload. The laboratory may do a B-type natriuretic peptide (BNP) level or N-terminal pro-BNP level, either value gives similar information. Normal levels of BNP are less than 100 pg/mL. BNP levels above 100 pg/mL are suggestive of heart failure. As heart failure progresses, BNP is used to help mark disease progression and severity. Other important laboratory studies that are performed during initial workup, to help determine the underlying cause of heart failure, or to help monitor the effect of heart failure on other body systems include serum electrolytes, BUN, Creatinine, liver function tests, CBC, and urinalysis.

Exercise stress testing and cardiac catheterization may be performed to evaluate severity of disease and presence of other underlying heart conditions contributing to heart failure.

Medical Management

As heart failure is a chronic condition, the goals of treatment are not curative but rather to improve the functionality and quality of life. Medical management is tackled via lifestyle modifications, pharmacological treatments, nutritional therapy, oxygen therapy, and invasive interventions.

Lifestyle Modifications are an intricate part of treatment for heart failure. These modifications include smoking cessation, avoidance of any second or third hand smoke, institution of a regular exercise program that progresses as tolerated, reduction in alcohol intake and being aware of fluid intake and decrease in weight reduction. In addition, patients with comorbid disorders such as high blood pressure, diabetes, hyperlipidemia, and chronic obstructive pulmonary disease need to have strict adherence to treatment and control of lifestyle modifications that keep these diseases in check. These modifications help decrease the workload on the heart thereby improving cardiac output. An improved cardiac output will decrease blood congestion and therefore bring relief of symptoms.

Pharmacological treatments alleviate the symptoms of heart failure by working in multiple ways (Table 8.6). First line therapy for heart failure includes the use of a diuretic, angiotensin converting enzyme (ACE) inhibitor, and beta blockers. Diuretics help remove excess fluid from the extracellular spaces of the body through urination. Three common types of diuretics that may be prescribed help inhibit sodium and chloride reabsorption which in turn, decreases the amount of water reabsorbed in the kidney tubules. One of these diuretics, spironolactone (potassium sparing diuretic) is an aldosterone antagonist. It stops the action of aldosterone which conserves sodium and thereby water in the kidney thus halting this compensatory mechanism. The type of diuretic prescribed is based on the severity of heart failure symptoms. They are routinely given in oral doses but during acute heart failure they can be given intravenously. Ace inhibitors play a crucial role in halting one of the compensatory mechanisms that occur in heart failure that attempt to increase cardiac output. From the pathophysiology section, a decrease in renal perfusion causes the kidney to release renin which causes the release of angiotensin I which then converts to angiotensin II. The ACE inhibitor prevents the conversion of angiotensin I to angiotensin II (potent vasoconstrictor, causes release of aldosterone and ADH), which stops the body from conserving water to increase cardiac output. This essentially decreases afterload for the heart which improves cardiac output. Examples of ACE inhibitors include lisinopril and enalapril. Both medications can cause a dry persistent cough and hyperkalemia as side effects. Patients who are unable to tolerate ACE inhibitors may take angiotensin receptor blockers (ARBs). ARBs block the vasoconstrictive action of angiotensin II thus preventing a rise in blood pressure and afterload. Beta blockers prevent the progression of heart failure and help alleviate symptoms by blocking the effects of the sympathetic nervous system (which exerts its effects through the release of epinephrine and norepinephrine). Beta blockers relax blood vessels which lowers the blood pressure. This causes a decrease in afterload and reduces the blood return back to the heart which decreases

Table 8.6   Medications for Heart Failure

GENERIC NAME	ACTION	NURSING INTERVENTIONS
Cardiac Glycosides		
Digitalis preparations, such as digoxin	Strengthen cardiac force and efficiency Slow heart rate Increase circulation, effecting diuresis	Monitor apical pulse to ensure rate greater than 60 bpm; monitor for toxicity (nausea, vomiting, anorexia, dysrhythmia, bradycardia, tachycardia, headache, fatigue, and blurred or colored vision)
Diuretics		
Thiazides, such as chlorothiazide, hydrochlorothiazide	Increase renal secretion of sodium Are safe for long-term use Block sodium and water reabsorption in kidney tubules	Monitor electrolyte depletion; weigh daily to ascertain fluid loss
Sulfonamides (loop diuretic), such as furosemide, bumetanide	Act rapidly for less responsive edema	Administer in the morning to prevent nocturia Monitor for electrolyte depletion Consider sulfa allergy (furosemide)
Aldosterone antagonist (potassium-sparing), such as spironolactone	Relieves edema and ascites that do not respond to usual diuretics Blocks sodium-retaining and potassium-excreting properties of aldosterone	Monitor for gastrointestinal irritation and hyperkalemia
Potassium Supplements		
potassium	Restores electrolyte loss	Monitor blood potassium levels
Sedatives and Analgesics		
temazepam	Promotes rest and comfort	Monitor rest and sleep benefits
morphine	Relieves chest and abdominal pain, reduces anxiety, and decreases myocardial oxygen demands Lessens dyspnea	
Nitrates		
nitroglycerin	Dilates arteries, improves blood flow Reduces blood pressure	Monitor blood pressure for hypotension Monitor for headache and flushing
Angiotensin-Converting Enzyme (ACE) Inhibitors		
captopril enalapril ramipril benazepril lisinopril quinapril fosinopril moexipril perindopril trandolapril	Act as antihypertensives, reduce peripheral arterial resistance, and improve cardiac output	Observe patient closely for a precipitous drop in blood pressure within 3 h of initial dose; monitor blood pressure closely Monitor blood potassium levels
Beta-Adrenergic Blockers		
carvedilol	Directly blocks the sympathetic nervous system's negative effects on the failing heart	Start at a low dose, increasing the dose slowly every 2 weeks. as tolerated by the patient Monitor blood pressure and notify health care provider of significant change Monitor pulse: If <50 bpm, withhold drug and call health care provider
metoprolol	Blocks beta$_2$-adrenergic receptors in bronchial and vascular smooth muscle. Lowers blood pressure by beta-blocking effects; reduces elevated renin plasma levels	Monitor I&O, weigh daily Monitor apical or radial pulse before administration Notify health care provider of any significant changes, or if pulse <50 bpm

Table 8.6	Medications for Heart Failure—cont'd	
GENERIC NAME	ACTION	NURSING INTERVENTIONS
Inotropic Agents		
dobutamine dopamine	Low-dose dobutamine and low-dose dopamine are relatively safe on medical-surgical units; at low doses they dilate renal blood vessels, stimulating renal blood flow and glomerular filtration rate; this in turn promotes sodium excretion, often helping patients with CHF improve	Make certain patient is not taking monoamine oxidase (MAO) inhibitors, tricyclic antidepressants, phenytoin (Dilantin), or haloperidol (Haldol). Record accurate I&O; assess for dizziness, nausea, vomiting, headache. Assess vital signs carefully every 15 min for first 2 h, then every 2 h for the next 4 h, and finally once a shift. Observe carefully for extravasation, tachycardia, bradycardia, angina, palpitations, hypotension, hypertension, azotemia, and anxiety
Human B-Type Natriuretic Peptides		
nesiritide	New class of synthetic HF drugs; causes arterial and venous dilation, thereby decreasing systemic vascular resistance and pulmonary arterial pressures; decreases blood pressure, promotes better left ventricle ejection, and increases cardiac output; may also promote diuresis; an IV treatment for patients with acutely decompensated CHF	Observe carefully for hypotension. Natrecor should not be used for patients with cardiogenic shock or with a systolic blood pressure <90 mm Hg

ACE, Angiotensin-converting enzyme; *bpm,* beats per minute; *CHF,* congestive heart failure; *HF,* heart failure; *I&O,* intake and output.

preload. Beta blockers also cause the heart to beat with less force and therefore lowers blood pressure. Side effects of beta blockers include hypotension and bradycardia. Additional medications that may be prescribed for patients include hydralazine and isosorbide dinitrate (separately or as a combo pill) which helps decrease preload by relaxing veins and arteries making it easier for the heart to pump. Digitalis is a positive inotrope medication which was routinely used in heart failure treatment. It helps increase the force of myocardial contraction and slows conduction of the electrical impulse through the AV node thus decreasing the heart rate. Administration of digitalis requires the apical rate to be 60 bpm or above. It has serious side effects such as toxicity, anorexia, confusion, and visual disturbances. In acute cases of heart failure, patients may be given IV medications such as milrinone, dobutamine, and nitroprusside, nitroglycerin, or nesiritide. Milrinone and dobutamine increase the force of myocardial contraction thus improving cardiac output and nitrates help relax arteries and veins thus decreasing preload and afterload.

Nutritional therapy for heart failure consists of eating a low sodium diet, no more than 2 g/day, and avoiding excessive fluid intake. Sodium is restricted to 2 g/day as sodium holds water and eating a higher sodium diet would cause the body to retain more water which would impact preload. Patients are asked to weigh themselves daily as a way to gauge fluid retention.

Oxygen therapy is based on the severity of the patient's heart failure. As fluid congestion in the lungs increases, oxygen saturation falls and oxygen therapy is needed. Therapeutic oxygen management also includes lowering the oxygen requirements of body systems. This is done by elevating the head of the bed to 45 degrees or by having the patient sit on the edge of the bed with arms resting on the overbed table to reduce myocardial oxygen demand and decrease circulating volume returning to the heart.

Invasive interventions include placement of a biventricular pacemaker which can improve symptoms and function, improve quality of life, and decrease hospitalization for patients with HF who also have conduction system disorder. An implantable cardioverter-defibrillator can decrease the risk of sudden cardiac death for patients with a family history of sudden cardiac death, life-threatening dysrhythmias, or mild to moderate HF who have an EF of less than 35% (Hinkle and Cheever, 2018).

Nursing Interventions
Nursing interventions include measures to prevent disease progression and complications. Monitor vital signs for changes. Note any signs of respiratory distress or pulmonary edema. Carefully monitor signs and symptoms of left-sided versus right-sided HF. Urinary output is typically low, and edema is soft and pitting; legs are elevated to decrease edema.

Also note an increase in abdominal girth and total body weight as indicators of fluid retention, which is common in HF. Auscultate the lung fields to detect the presence of crackles and wheezes; also note coughing and complaints of dyspnea. Restful sleep may be possible only in the sitting position or with the aid of extra pillows. Teach patients to never stop their medications without speaking with their provider and teach patients to check pulse rate prior to taking medications such as digitalis. Activity intolerance is accompanied by extreme fatigue and anxiety. Assess patients for depression. Explain to patients with HF and depression that the depression is readily treatable and that several approaches can be used separately or in combination, including pharmacologic therapy, psychosocial and psychotherapeutic interventions, and cardiac rehabilitation.

Key components of care. The Institute for Healthcare Improvement recommends these components of care for all patients with HF (unless the patient cannot tolerate them or unless contraindicated):

- Assess left ventricular systolic function.
- At discharge from hospital (when left ventricular EF is less than 40%, indicating systolic dysfunction), administer ACE inhibitor or angiotensin.
- At discharge, administer an anticoagulant if the patient has chronic or recurrent atrial fibrillation.
- Encourage smoking cessation.
- Instruct the patient at discharge regarding activity, diet, medication, follow-up appointment, weight monitoring, and what to do if symptoms worsen.
- Provide influenza and pneumococcal immunization.
- At discharge, institute beta blocker therapy for stabilized patients with left ventricular systolic dysfunction who have no contraindications.

The new guidelines also recommend a discussion of end-of-life decisions with the patient and the family. Patients should talk with their health care providers about treatment preferences, advance directives, living wills, power of attorney for health care, and life support issues. HF is progressive, and patients should make decisions concerning health care wishes and plans while they are capable of expressing choices. Hospice services, originally developed to assist patients with cancer, are appropriate for the patient with end-stage HF (see the Patient Teaching box, Nursing Care Plan 8.1, and Box 8.5).

Prognosis

Approximately 10% of patients diagnosed with HF die in the first year, and 50% within 5 years. HF is a chronic condition. With treatment advances, many people now live for years with damaged hearts. With the advent of ACE inhibitors and new research on the benefits of prescribed exercise, improvement in the quality of life for patients with HF is being seen.

PULMONARY EDEMA

Etiology and Pathophysiology

Pulmonary edema (the accumulation of extravascular fluid in lung tissues and alveoli, most often caused by HF) is an acute and extensive, life-threatening complication of HF caused by severe left ventricular dysfunction. Fluid from the left side of the heart backs up into the pulmonary vasculature and results in extravascular fluid accumulation in the interstitial space and alveoli. This causes the patient to "drown" in the secretions.

Clinical Manifestations

The patient exhibits signs of severe respiratory distress when pulmonary edema occurs. Frothy sputum is produced from air mixing with the fluid in the alveoli; the sputum is blood-tinged from blood cells that have exuded into the alveoli.

Assessment

See Box 8.6 for signs and symptoms of pulmonary edema.

Box 8.5 **Guidelines for Nursing Interventions for the Patient With Heart Failure**

- Provide oxygenation.
- Administer oxygen by nasal cannula per protocol as prescribed for dyspnea.
- Patient should be well supported in semi-Fowler's or high Fowler's position.
- Reinforce importance of conservation of energy and planning for activities that avoid fatigue.
- Encourage activity within prescribed restrictions; monitor for intolerance to activity (dyspnea, fatigue, increased pulse rate that does not stabilize).
- Assist with activities of daily living as necessary; encourage independence within patient's limitations.
- Provide diversionary activity that will assist in conservation of energy.
- Monitor for signs of fluid and potassium imbalance; record daily weights, intake and output.
- Provide skin care, particularly over edematous areas; use prophylactic measures to prevent skin impairment.
- Assist in maintaining an adequate nutritional intake while observing prescribed dietary modifications (sodium restrictions).
- Monitor for constipation; give prescribed stool softeners.
- Give prescribed medications:
  - Digitalis (take apical pulse before administration)
  - Diuretics (assess for hypokalemia)
  - Vasodilators, angiotensin-converting enzyme inhibitors, beta blockers
  - Medications to reduce anxiety and promote sleep
- Provide the patient and the family opportunities to discuss their concerns.
- Teach the patient about the disorder and self-care.

Nursing Care Plan 8.1   **The Patient With Heart Failure**

Mr. D. is a 61-year-old clinical administrator. He was admitted to the hospital with the diagnosis of heart failure. He has a history of hypertension and coronary artery disease. Six months ago he had a myocardial infarction. He has felt tired for the past 3 weeks and has been experiencing increased dyspnea. He has noticed some edema in his ankles and is concerned about gaining 5 lb in the past week and having an increasing intolerance to exertion. The nursing admission history revealed:

- Mr. D. has not been taking his antihypertensive medication regularly. He did not like the side effects and stopped taking the medication, but he was too embarrassed to call his health care provider.
- Vital signs revealed an elevated blood pressure.
- He has shortness of breath during activities and when lying down.
- Pitting edema is seen on both ankles.
- Crackles are heard bilaterally in the lungs.

PATIENT PROBLEM

Insufficient Cardiac Output, related to cardiovascular disease

Patient Goals and Expected Outcomes	Nursing Intervention	Evaluation
Patient will have decreased adventitious lung sounds when lying in bed within 24 h Patient will have oxygen saturations at 91% with prescribed oxygen within 24 h Patient will have vital signs within acceptable levels within 72 h Patient will have decreased edema and weight loss of 5 lb within 72 h	Maintain initial bed rest with stress-free environment. Maintain semi-Fowler's to high Fowler's position. Explain and encourage gradual increases in activity to prevent a sudden increase in cardiac workload. Monitor respirations, lung sounds, heart sounds, and vital signs q4h. Palpate pedal pulses, and assess capillary refill q8h. Administer digitalis, diuretics, angiotensin-converting enzyme inhibitors, vasodilators, beta blockers, and antihypertensive medication as prescribed. Monitor intake and output and weigh daily. Monitor oxygen saturation with pulse oximetry q4h. Administer prescribed oxygen.	Patient has decreased crackles in lung fields within 24 h of admission. Patient has an oximetry reading of 91% oxygen saturation with oxygen prescribed within 24 h of admission. Patient has a heart rate of 80 bpm, respiratory rate of 22 breaths/min, and blood pressure of 148/86 mm Hg within 72 h of admission. Patient has a weight loss of 5 lb within 72 h of admission. Patient has pedal pitting edema decreased to 1+ within 2 days of admission.

PATIENT PROBLEM

Anxiousness, related to change in health status, lifestyle changes, fear of death, or threats to self-concept

Patient Goals and Expected Outcomes	Nursing Intervention	Evaluation
Patient will verbalize anxieties within 48 h of admission Patient will demonstrate reduction of anxiety by enjoying periods of rest and sleep undisturbed for 6 h within 48 h of admission	Identify coping techniques. Provide information to decrease fears. Identify support systems. Provide calm, relaxing environment. Administer antianxiety medications per health care provider's orders as needed. Help patient cope with lifestyle changes. He may feel anxious because of changes in body image, family and social roles, and finances. Focus on progress patient is making in managing his condition. Encourage patient to participate in health care decisions, and allow him to release anger and frustration. Allow patient to sleep undisturbed for 6 h when vital signs are stable.	Patient is verbalizing anger and frustration over current medical conditions within 48 h of admission. Patient is sleeping 5–6 h per night within 48 h of admission.

CRITICAL THINKING QUESTIONS

1. Mr. D. is experiencing severe dyspnea, with the presence of crackles bilaterally in all lung fields. His pulse is 108 bpm, and respirations are 33 breaths/min. When performing his morning ADLs, the nurse could perform which beneficial nursing interventions?
2. On assessing Mr. D.'s skin, the nurse notes 4+ pitting edema in his lower extremities. A weight gain of 6 lb in the past 24 h also is noted. For therapeutic diuresis to occur, what would the medical management likely include?
3. Mr. D. puts his call light on to request assistance to ambulate. The nurse notes subclavicular retractions and cyanosis of his nailbeds. What would be the most appropriate nursing actions?

Box 8.6   Signs and Symptoms of Pulmonary Edema

- Restlessness
- Vague uneasiness
- Agitation
- Disorientation
- Diaphoresis
- Severe dyspnea
- Tachypnea
- Tachycardia
- Pallor or cyanosis
- Cough; production of large quantities of blood-tinged, frothy sputum
- Audible wheezing, crackles
- Cold extremities

Table 8.7   Medical Management for Acute Pulmonary Edema

INTERVENTION	RATIONALE
Patient in high Fowler's position or over side of bed with arms supported on bedside table	Promotes expansion of lungs; legs in dependent position causes venous pooling and reduction in venous return (preload)
Morphine sulfate, 10–15 mg IV; titrated	Decreases patient anxiety; relieves pain; slows respirations; reduces venous return; decreases oxygen demand; dilates the pulmonary and systemic blood vessels
Oxygen at 40%–100%; nonrebreather face mask; intubation as needed	Promotes oxygenation; increased tidal volume also promotes removal of secretions from alveoli
Administer sublingual nitroglycerin	Increases myocardial blood flow
Diuretics: furosemide, bumetanide (IV)	Reduce pulmonary edema by decreasing the fluid in the lungs and increasing excretion through the kidneys
Insert indwelling catheter	Allows patient to rest and conserve energy; monitors urinary output after IV furosemide has been administered
Inotropic agents: dobutamine, amrinone	Increase myocardial contractility without increasing oxygen consumption; increase peripheral vasodilation; increase cardiac output
Nitroprusside	A potent vasodilator; improves myocardial contraction and reduces pulmonary congestion

IV, Intravenous.

Diagnostic Tests

Diagnosis is made by observing signs and symptoms and is supported by chest radiograph and arterial blood gas studies. PaO_2 and $PaCO_2$ (the partial

Patient Teaching

Heart Failure

- Monitor for signs and symptoms of recurring heart failure and report them to the health care provider or clinic. The following signs and symptoms indicate worsening heart failure:
  - Weight gain of 2–3 lb (1–1.5 kg) over a short period (about 2 days)
  - Shortness of breath
  - Orthopnea
  - Swelling of ankles, feet, or abdomen
  - Persistent cough
  - Frequent nighttime urination
- Avoid fatigue and plan activity to allow for rest periods.
- Plan and eat meals within prescribed sodium restrictions. Avoid salty foods.
- Avoid drugs with high sodium content (e.g., some laxatives and antacids, Alka-Seltzer); read the product labels. Ideally, limit sodium intake to 2 g/day.
- Maintain low-fat diet, with fat intake less than 30% of total calories.
- Eat several small meals rather than three large meals per day.
- Take medications as prescribed.
- If several medications are prescribed, develop a method to facilitate accurate administration.
- When taking digoxin, check own pulse rate daily; report a rate of less than 60 bpm to the health care provider. Do not take digoxin if pulse is less than 60 bpm.
- Take diuretics as prescribed.
- Weigh self daily at same time and in similar clothes.
- Eat foods high in potassium and low in sodium (such as oranges and bananas) if the patient is not taking a potassium-sparing diuretic.
- Take all prescribed medications.
- Report signs of hypotension (lightheadedness, rapid pulse, syncope) to the health care provider.
- Avoid alcohol when taking vasodilators.
- Reinforce the importance of regular exercise once heart failure is stabilized. A thorough treatment regimen may allow the patient to increase activity level over time. The health care provider may ultimately recommend 30–45 minutes of aerobic exercise three or four times a week to improve patient's well-being.
- Report to the health care provider for follow-up as directed.

pressures of oxygen and carbon dioxide, respectively, in the arterial blood) may reveal respiratory alkalosis or acidosis.

Medical Management

Medical management involves simultaneous interventions to promote oxygenation, improve cardiac output, and reduce pulmonary congestion. Respiratory failure may occur without prompt emergency treatment (Table 8.7).

Nursing Interventions

Interventions include administering oxygen. The patient should sit upright with legs in a dependent position to decrease venous return to the heart, relieving pulmonary congestion and dyspnea. Monitor arterial blood gases and administer drugs as ordered. Auscultate lung sounds often. Provide emotional support; remain with the patient. Explain all procedures. Monitor vital signs, fluid I&O, and serum electrolytes.

Patient problems and interventions for the patient with pulmonary edema include but are not limited to the following:

PATIENT PROBLEM	NURSING INTERVENTIONS
Fluid Volume Overload, related to fluid accumulation in pulmonary vessels	Administer medications as ordered
	Carefully monitor I&O
	Weigh patient at same time each day
	Assess for edema
Inefficient Oxygenation, related to fluid in lungs	Assess for signs of hypoxia, such as restlessness, disorientation, and irritability
	Monitor arterial blood gases per health care provider's order
	Administer oxygen per health care provider's order
	Position patient in high Fowler's position with legs in dependent position, or sitting and leaning forward on overbed table to facilitate breathing

Prognosis
Pulmonary edema is a grave, life-threatening condition that is usually responsive to aggressive interventions.

VALVULAR HEART DISEASE
Etiology and Pathophysiology
Valvular heart disease occurs when one or more valves in the heart is damaged or has a defect. Any of the four valves of the heart may be affected but the two most common valves affected are the mitral or aortic valve. Normally functioning heart valves allow blood to flow in one direction between chambers of the heart and into pulmonary and systemic circulation. It also involves complete closure of the AV heart valves at the beginning of ventricular systole and the closure of the semilunar valves at the end of ventricular systole. When valve closure is affected, the direction of blood flow is altered. Valve damage or defect leads to two problems: *stenosis*, where the valve itself thickens and becomes stiff causing a progressive narrowing of the opening of the involved valves; and incompetence of the valve where the leaflets of the valve do not close completely causing regurgitation of blood. Stenosis or regurgitation place stress on the heart and can eventually cause heart failure.

The risk factors for valvular disorders include advancing age, high blood pressure, coronary artery conditions, history of heart attack, heart failure or arrythmias, rheumatic fever or infective endocarditis, and congenital defects (American Heart Association, 2020a).

Clinical Manifestations
Signs and symptoms seen in valvular disorders are outlined in Table 8.8.

Table 8.8	Manifestations of Valvular Heart Disease
DIAGNOSIS	**MANIFESTATIONS**
Mitral valve stenosis	Dyspnea on exertion, hemoptysis; fatigue; atrial fibrillation on ECG, palpitations, stroke; loud, accentuated S_1; low-pitched, rumbling diastolic murmur
Mitral valve regurgitation	*Acute:* Generally poorly tolerated; new systolic murmur with pulmonary edema and cardiogenic shock developing rapidly *Chronic:* Weakness, fatigue, exertional dyspnea, palpitations; an S_3 gallop, holosystolic murmur
Mitral valve prolapse	Palpitations, dyspnea, chest pain, activity intolerance, syncope; holosystolic murmur
Aortic valve stenosis	Angina, syncope, dyspnea on exertion, heart failure; normal or soft S_1, diminished or absent S_2, systolic murmur, prominent S_4
Aortic valve regurgitation	*Acute:* Abrupt onset of profound dyspnea, chest pain, left ventricular failure, and cardiogenic shock *Chronic:* Fatigue, exertional dyspnea, orthopnea, paroxysmal nocturnal dyspnea; water-hammer pulse; heaving precordial impulse; diminished or absent S_1, S_3, or S_4; soft, high-pitched diastolic murmur, Austin Flint murmur
Tricuspid and pulmonic stenosis	*Tricuspid:* Peripheral edema, ascites, hepatomegaly; diastolic low-pitched murmur with increased intensity during inspiration *Pulmonic:* Fatigue, loud midsystolic murmur

ECG, Electrocardiogram; S_1, first heart sound (*lub*), produced by atrioventricular valve closure; S_2, second heart sound (*dub*), produced by semilunar valve closure; S_3 and S_4, gallop rhythms.
Modified from Lewis SL, Dirksen SR, Heitkemper MM, et al: *Medical-surgical nursing: Assessment and management of clinical problems,* ed 9, St. Louis, 2014, Mosby.

Assessment

Subjective data include the patient's statement of a history of rheumatic fever or infective endocarditis, history of previous heart disease, and congenital defects. The patient may also report an inability to perform activities and ADLs without fatigue or weakness. Ask the patient about chest pain, including its quality, duration, onset, precipitating factors, and measures that provide relief. The patient may complain of heart palpitations, lightheadedness, dizziness, or fainting. The history may include a patient statement of weight gain. Dyspnea, exertional dyspnea, nocturnal (night-time) dyspnea, and orthopnea often are reported, depending on the degree of HF.

Collection of objective data includes observing for a heart murmur and noting the presence and character of any adventitious breath sounds (crackles, wheezes) and edema (pitting or non-pitting).

Diagnostic Tests

An echocardiogram is the test used to diagnose heart valvular disease. It may also be found incidentally when conducting other tests such as cardiac catheterization or cardiac MRI.

Medical Management

Medical management includes activity limitations, sodium-restricted diet, diuretics, digoxin, and antidysrhythmics.

When medical therapy no longer alleviates clinical symptoms or when diagnostic evidence exists of progressive myocardial failure, surgery often is performed. The surgery may include the following:
- *Open mitral commissurotomy:* A surgical splitting of the fused mitral valve leaflet for treating stenosis of the mitral valve.
- *Valve replacement:* Replacement of the stenosed or incompetent valve with a bioprosthetic or mechanical valve. Commonly used valves include tilting disks, porcine (pig) heterografts (tissue taken from one species and grafted onto another), homografts (a graft of human tissue), and ball-in-cage valves.

Nursing Interventions and Patient Teaching

Nursing interventions focus on assisting with ADLs, relieving specific symptoms associated with decreased cardiac output, promoting comfort, and administering prescribed medications (diuretics, digoxin, and antidysrhythmics). Assess and review vital signs, breath sounds, and heart sounds for changes from the baseline assessment. Pulse oximetry is reviewed and evaluated at regular intervals. Maintain oxygen therapy as prescribed. Monitor fluid balance by assessing and recording the presence of edema, daily weight, and intake and output. Check for capillary perfusion and pedal pulses. Have the patient consume a sodium-restricted diet for control of edema. Discuss with the patient a plan for rest

periods and identify those ADLs that produce fatigue and require assistance.

Patient problems and interventions for the patient with valvular heart disease include but are not limited to the following:

PATIENT PROBLEM	NURSING INTERVENTIONS
Inability to Tolerate Activity, related to: • Weakness • Fatigue • Dyspnea	Balance activities with rest periods Identify fatiguing activities and obtain assistance as needed Use oxygen as prescribed by health care provider
Fluid Volume Overload, related to decreased cardiac output	Administer prescribed oxygen, digoxin, diuretics, and antidysrhythmic Monitor I&O Weigh patient daily at same time Perform respiratory assessment Perform cardiovascular assessment Inspect for presence of edema Obtain vital signs routinely Maintain sodium-restricted diet

Patient teaching focuses on medications, dietary management, activity limitations, diagnostic tests, surgical interventions, and postoperative care as appropriate. Describe the disease process and associated symptoms to report to the health care provider. Explain antibiotic prophylaxis to prevent infective endocarditis. Explain the importance of notifying the dentist, urologist, and gynecologist of valvular heart disease. The nurse emphasizes the need to take anticoagulants; the time frame for therapy with anticoagulants is based on the surgical procedure or type of valve used. Explain the need to maintain good oral hygiene and make regular visits to the dentist.

Prognosis

The prognosis for the patient with valvular heart disease varies, depending on the specific disease. The prognosis after surgery for the affected valve is fair to good with improvement of signs and symptoms but often without resolution of all abnormalities.

INFLAMMATORY HEART DISORDERS

All cardiac tissues are susceptible to inflammation, and HF can be a serious and rapid result of the inflammatory process.

RHEUMATIC HEART DISEASE

Etiology and Pathophysiology

Rheumatic heart disease is the result of rheumatic fever and the clinical manifestation of carditis resulting from an inadequately treated childhood pharyngeal or upper respiratory tract infection (group A beta-hemolytic streptococci). By the 1980s, rheumatic fever had almost disappeared in developed countries such as the United States. However, it has remained common and severe in most developing countries. Antibiotics, especially penicillin, are responsible for the decline in rheumatic fever.

Ineffective treatment of infection results in delayed reaction and inflammation of the cardiac tissues and the central nervous system, joints, skin, and subcutaneous tissues. Children between the ages of 5 and 15 years are most susceptible to rheumatic fever while children under age 3 and adults rarely get rheumatic fever (CDC, 2018). The onset of rheumatic fever is usually sudden, often occurring within 1 to 5 symptom-free weeks after recovery from pharyngitis (sore throat) or from scarlet fever. In some patients the rheumatic fever may progress without symptoms and go undiagnosed and untreated. Years later the patient may develop clinical manifestations of valvular heart disease.

Rheumatic heart disease can affect the pericardium, myocardium, or endocardium. The affected tissue develops small areas of necrosis, which heal, leaving scar tissue. The heart valves are typically the most affected by Aschoff's nodules (vegetative growth; in this context a "vegetative growth" refers to a growth of pathologic tissue), and they become fibrous and incompetent. With healing, the valves become thickened and deformed. These changes result in valvular stenosis and insufficiency, varying in extent and severity.

Clinical Manifestations

Fever, increased pulse, epistaxis, anemia, joint involvement, and nodules on joints and subcutaneous tissue may be noted. Carditis (inflammation of heart tissues) can develop. When valvular involvement occurs, signs and symptoms are specific to each valve condition.

Assessment

Collection of subjective data may reveal joint pain (polyarthritis) and chest pain. Lethargy and fatigue are also present.

Objective data include skin manifestations of small erythematous circles and wavy lines on the trunk and abdomen that appear and disappear rapidly (erythema marginatum). The nurse may observe involuntary, purposeless movement of the muscles if Sydenham chorea (St. Vitus' dance), a disorder of the central nervous system, is present. Heart murmur may be auscultated if the patient has carditis with valve involvement. Rheumatic heart disease is characterized by heart murmurs resulting from stenosis or insufficiency of the valves.

Diagnostic Tests

Diagnosis is made through signs and symptoms and supported by laboratory study results. An echocardiogram is done to determine the extent of damage to the valves and myocardium. An ECG shows cardiac dysrhythmia. Cardiac murmurs or friction rub can be heard. No specific diagnostic test exists for rheumatic fever. The erythrocyte sedimentation rate and leukocyte count are elevated. The development of serum antibodies against streptococci (measured by antistreptolysin-O titer) may occur. CRP, elevated in a specimen of blood, is abnormally high.

Medical Management

Preventive measures are the most effective interventions. Rapid treatment for pharyngeal infection, usually with prolonged antibiotic therapy, is desired. Penicillin is the preferred antibiotic. Prolonged periods of bed rest were recommended, but now the patient without carditis may be ambulatory as soon as acute symptoms have subsided. When carditis is present, ambulation is postponed until HF is controlled. Symptomatic treatment and care are given. Nonsteroidal anti-inflammatory drugs (NSAIDs) for joint pain and inflammation are accompanied by application of gentle heat. A well-balanced diet, following the personalized daily food choices and number of servings recommended by the US Department of Agriculture's My Plate food planning tool, is supplemented by vitamins B and C and high-volume fluid intake. In some patients, surgical commissurotomy or valve replacement is necessary.

Nursing Interventions and Patient Teaching

Signs and symptoms largely determine the type of nursing interventions. Bed rest during the acute phase is recommended when carditis is present. If the patient has polyarthritis, minimize joint pain by proper positioning. After the acute stage, the child or the adult is treated at home. Review a schedule of daily events with the patient and the parents.

Perform nursing interventions quickly and skillfully to minimize discomfort and avoid tiring the patient. Throughout the course of the disease, the patient and the family benefit from emotional support and appropriate diversions. Teaching focuses on increasing understanding of the disease process, signs and symptoms, and gradually increasing activity levels. Emphasize the importance of eating a nutritional diet and keeping appointments for medical checkups. Patients with a history of rheumatic fever or evidence of rheumatic heart disease should receive daily prophylactic penicillin by mouth or monthly intramuscular injections of penicillin to prevent streptococcal infection, at least during childhood and adolescence. Patients with evidence of deformed heart valves should be given prophylactic antibiotics before surgery and all dental procedures.

Prognosis

Prognosis depends on involvement of the heart; carditis can result in a serious heart disease, including valvular disease.

PERICARDITIS

Etiology and Pathophysiology

Pericarditis is inflammation of the membranous sac surrounding the heart. It may be an acute or a chronic condition. Bacterial, viral, or fungal infection is associated with acute pericarditis. It may occur as a complication of noninfectious conditions such as azotemia (too much urea and other nitrogenous compounds in the blood); acute MI; neoplasms such as lung cancer, breast cancer, leukemia, Hodgkin disease, and lymphoma; scleroderma; trauma after thoracic surgery; systemic lupus erythematosus; radiation; and drug reactions (e.g., from procainamide and hydralazine). Pericarditis is further classified as adhesive which occurs when the layers of the pericardium adhere to each other thus decreasing ventricular stretching and therefore filling or it can be classified by what accumulates between these layers. The pericardial layers may accumulate serous fluid, pus, calcium deposits, or malignant cancer.

Adhesions and accumulations within the pericardial sac cause restrictions in the hearts ability to fill which then causes a decrease in cardiac output and impedes the forward motion of blood flow. The severity of restrictions dictates signs and symptoms and treatment.

Clinical Manifestations

Pericarditis differs clinically from other inflammatory conditions of the heart in that patients often have debilitating chest pain, much like that of an MI. The pain is aggravated by lying supine, deep breathing, coughing, swallowing, and moving the trunk and is alleviated by sitting up and leaning forward. Dyspnea, fever, chills, diaphoresis, and leukocytosis are observed. The hallmark finding in acute pericarditis is pericardial friction rub; grating, scratching, and leathery sounds are detected on auscultation caused by the rubbing of the pericardial sac layers, although this appears in only about half of cases.

Decreased heart function to the level of cardiac failure can occur when the heart is compressed by excess fluid in the pericardial sac. Normally 15 to 50 mL of fluid are found in the pericardial sac, but with pericarditis 150 to 200 mL or more may develop.

Assessment

Subjective data include the patient's description of muscle aches, fatigue, and dyspnea. Excruciating chest pain is said to originate precordially and radiate to the neck and shoulders with severe and sudden onset.

Collection of objective data includes noting expressed substernal chest pain that radiates to the shoulder and neck; such pain is evidenced by orthopneic positioning (i.e., sitting propped up in a bed or chair) and facial grimace on inspiration. Elevated temperature accompanies chills and may be followed by diaphoresis. A nonproductive cough is often present.

Patients commonly verbalize anxiety, anticipation of danger, or uneasiness. Vital sign changes include a rapid and forcible pulse and rapid, shallow breathing. Pericardial friction rub heart sounds become muffled, and the health care provider may note a dysrhythmia.

Diagnostic Tests

ECG changes (dysrhythmia) are noted. Echocardiography shows pericardial effusion or cardiac tamponade (compression of the heart). Laboratory studies show leukocytosis (10,000 to 20,000/mm^3), and the erythrocyte sedimentation rate is elevated. Blood cultures may be ordered to identify the specific pathogen present. To rule out an MI, cardiac enzyme levels are determined. A CRP blood level commonly is ordered to aid in diagnosis. Elevated CRP levels indicate inflammation, which occurs with an infectious process. Chest radiographic findings are generally normal or nonspecific in acute pericarditis unless the patient has a large pericardial effusion.

Medical Management

Treatment for pericarditis is based on severity and managing the underlying cause. Analgesia for comfort and relief of pain reassures the anxious patient. Oxygen and parenteral fluids usually are given. Antibiotics are used to treat bacterial pericarditis. The health care provider prescribes salicylates for increased temperature and anti-inflammatory agents (e.g., indomethacin) and corticosteroids for a persistent inflammatory process. Use of colchicine (Colcrys) with aspirin or NSAIDs is the first line of therapy for patients experiencing acute pericarditis; corticosteroids are not used as it is linked with recurrent pericarditis (Daskalov and Valova-Ilieva, 2017). When pericardial effusion restricts heart movement (cardiac tamponade), a pericardial tap (pericardiocentesis) may be performed to remove excess fluid and restore normal heart function. Surgical intervention—pericardial fenestration (pericardial window) or pericardiocentesis (pericardial tap)—may be performed to provide continuous drainage of pericardial fluid and restore normal heart function. Complications include atelectasis and introduction of infectious agents.

Nursing Interventions

Carefully evaluate vital signs and auscultate lung and heart sounds. Provide supportive measures and observe for complications. Maintain bed rest to promote healing and decrease the cardiac workload. Elevate the head of the bed to 45 degrees to decrease dyspnea. Hypothermia treatment may be necessary to reduce elevated temperature. Remain with the patient if he or she is anxious. Explain all procedures thoroughly.

Patient problems and interventions for the patient with inflammatory heart conditions include but are not limited to the following:

PATIENT PROBLEM	NURSING INTERVENTIONS
Insufficient Cardiac Output, related to inflammatory process	Maintain bed rest with head of bed elevated to 45 degrees
	Assess vital signs q2–4h. as indicated by patient's condition
	Administer medications as ordered
	Monitor I&O
	Provide planned rest periods
Discomfort, related to inflammatory process	Assess and record pain type and quality
	Administer analgesics according to need, as ordered. (Pain is what the patient says it is)
	Maintain the patient on bed rest with the head of the bed elevated to 45 degrees and provide a padded overbed table on which the patient may rest his or her arms
	Use comfort measures to provide physical and emotional support
Fluid Volume Overload, related to ineffective myocardial pumping action	Restrict sodium in diet as prescribed; monitor I&O
	Weigh daily; compare values
	Administer diuretic therapy as ordered; monitor electrolyte values
	Observe respiration and pulse quality
	Assess for dyspnea and peripheral edema

Prognosis

The prognosis is good in patients with acute or viral pericarditis. The complication of cardiac tamponade is rare and prognosis in those cases is fair.

INFECTIVE ENDOCARDITIS

Etiology and Pathophysiology

Infective endocarditis is an infection or inflammation of the endocardium which is the inner lining of the chambers and valves of the heart. 80% to 90% of all cases of infective endocarditis is due to bacterial infection with streptococci, staphylococci, and enterococci the culprit. Fungal endocarditis occurs in less than 1% of infective endocarditis cases and usually occurs as a complication of systemic candida or aspergillus infection in immunocompromised patients. Risk factors for endocarditis can be split into health care acquired and community acquired. Health care acquired infective endocarditis occurs in patients with prosthetic valve placements, hemodialysis, vascular catheterizations, pacemaker and defibrillator placements, etc. Risk factors for community acquired infective endocarditis include immunosuppression, IV drug users, rheumatic disease, poor dentition (allows bacteria to enter the body), and degenerative valve disease. The actual occurrence of infective endocarditis is rare occurring in 3 to 10 out of 100,000 people, with males twice as likely as females, and patient age greater than 65 years old (Yallowitz and Decker, 2020).

The intact endocardium is mostly resistant to invasion but a deformity or injury such as might occur with catheterization of the heart can allow the previously impervious endocardium to become susceptible to invasion. Damaged endocardium elicits the inflammatory response and aggregation of fibrin, platelets, and blood cells. The substances of inflammatory response provide a surface for attachment for invading pathogens. As pathogenic invasion continues, the vegetative cluster grows layered by organism and clot which conceals the pathogen from the immune system. Infective endocarditis causes problems in two ways. The infection itself damages or deforms the underlying endocardium structure of the valves, chambers, and chordae tendineae and secondly the vegetative growth on the endocardium may fragment and embolize. The embolus then spreads the pathogen into systemic or pulmonary circulation and also clogs arteries. Embolizing infective endocarditis from the left side of the heart is more common than from the right side of the heart (Yallowitz and Decker, 2020).

Clinical Manifestations

Initial presenting systemic symptoms include fever, chills, malaise, fatigue, anorexia, headache, and generalized weakness. Localized symptoms include chest pain, dyspnea, decreased exercise tolerance, and orthopnea. Acute onset caused by valvular incompetence may present with symptoms of heart failure along with a new or changed heart murmur. Patients experiencing embolic events may present with symptoms specific to the location of the embolus.

Assessment

Subjective data include patient complaints of influenza-like symptoms with recurrent fever, undue fatigue, chest pain, headaches, joint pain, and chills.

Collection of objective data may reveal shortness of breath, swelling in the legs, and changed or new heart murmur. Less commonly found symptoms maybe petechiae in the conjunctiva, oral mucosa, neck, anterior chest, abdomen, and legs. Splinter hemorrhages (black longitudinal streaks) may occur in the nailbeds. Other signs are nontender macular lesions (in this case, flat reddish spots) on the palms and soles, plus tender erythematous, elevated nodules on the pads of the fingers and toes. Microemboli, vasculitis, and embolism are responsible for the development of these signs. They also have the potential to cause serious complications such as stroke, renal or splenic damage, and splenomegaly (Mayo Clinic, 2020a).

Diagnostic Tests

A precursory echocardiogram provides images of the chambers of the heart and valves that rule in infective endocarditis. A TEE provides clearer images of the heart chambers and valves and allows visualization of vegetation, thrombi, and abscesses on valves. Blood cultures identify the pathogen and sensitivity testing identifies the antimicrobial agent to be used in treatment. MRI and or CT may be ordered to visualize embolic areas and determine how far the infection has spread. A CBC reveals leukocytosis.

Medical Management

The medical management of the patient with endocarditis includes support of cardiac function, destruction of the pathogen, and prevention of complications.

Embolization, a serious and common complication, can occur. An embolus may go to the brain, the lungs, the coronary arteries, the spleen, the bowel, and the extremities, with catastrophic results. The most frequent embolic events usually occur during the first 2 weeks of acute infective endocarditis. Anticoagulation is not recommended because of the risk of an intracerebral hemorrhage. A patient who was receiving anticoagulation therapy before developing endocarditis may continue therapy as long as neurologic function is monitored carefully (Mayo Clinic, 2017a).

Management relies on rest to decrease the heart's workload. Complete bed rest usually is not indicated unless the temperature remains elevated and there are signs of HF. After the blood cultures, massive doses of antibiotics are administered, usually parenterally, to combat the organism. Antibiotic therapy continues often as long as 1 to 2 months. Traditionally this has required a prolonged hospitalization for most patients, but with newer, more versatile antibiotics (and growing economic concerns), outpatient treatment of patients with infective endocarditis is more common.

Prophylactic antibiotic treatment is recommended for individuals who are considered at high risk for developing infective endocarditis. Patients at risk include those with previous valve surgery, preexisting valvular heart disease, or congenital abnormalities. Infective endocarditis precautions involve antibiotic therapy as prescribed by the health care provider before any invasive procedure such as dental work or minor surgery.

Surgical repair of diseased valves or prosthetic valve replacement may be necessary if the patient's condition is severe. Valve replacement has become an important adjunct procedure in the management of endocarditis (Mayo Clinic, 2020a).

Nursing Interventions and Patient Teaching

The nursing interventions are based primarily on the signs and symptoms. Observe for signs and symptoms of respiratory and cardiac distress. During the acute phase, maintain the patient on decreased activity and provide a calm, quiet environment. Take vital signs, including apical pulse, every 4 hours. When increased activity or ambulation begins, assess pulse before and after to determine the effects on the heart muscle.

Ensuring adequate nutrition is important. Frequently patients have a decreased appetite because of the disease process. Provide attractive meals with supplemental between-meal nourishment. Promote rest and comfort and prevent further inflammation and infection during hospitalization.

Patient teaching focuses on identifying causes, infective endocarditis precautions, dietary requirements, and gradually increasing activity levels. Advise the patient on the need for prophylactic antibiotics before any invasive procedure if the patient has preexisting valvular heart disease. Instruct the patient about signs and symptoms that may indicate recurrent infections such as fever, fatigue, malaise, and chills and the need to report any of these signs and symptoms to the health care provider.

Prognosis

Before the advent of antibiotics, patients with infective endocarditis had a poor prognosis with a high mortality rate. Prompt treatment with intensive antibiotic therapy now cures a majority of the patients with this condition.

MYOCARDITIS

Acute myocarditis is relatively rare. Inflammation of the myocardium may originate from rheumatic heart disease; viral, bacterial, or fungal infection; or endocarditis or pericarditis. In the United States, most significant cases of acute myocarditis are caused by coxsackie virus type B (Muller, 2017). However, sometimes the cause may be unknown.

Signs and symptoms vary. The patient may have upper respiratory tract symptoms such as fever, chills, and sore throat; abdominal pain and nausea; vomiting; diarrhea; and myalgia. These generally occur up to 6 weeks before the patient has signs and symptoms of myocarditis, such as chest pain and overt HF with dyspnea (Mayo Clinic, 2017b). Cardiac enlargement, murmur, gallop, and tachycardia typically are seen in myocarditis. Cardiomyopathy may develop as a complication. Enlargement of the myocardium may result in dysrhythmias.

Early detection can help in treating myocarditis before complications develop. Useful tests to help diagnose myocarditis are chest x-ray, ECG, echocardiography, MRI, and cardiac catheterization with endomyocardial biopsy (Mayo Clinic, 2017c).

Therapy is symptomatic and primarily follows the same approach as that of endocarditis: bed rest, oxygen, antibiotics, anti-inflammatory agents, careful assessments, and correction of dysrhythmias.

The goals of treatment are to preserve myocardial function and to prevent HF and other serious complications such as dilated cardiomyopathy. Patients may recover but may later develop cardiomyopathy. As a result, the disease may have a long, benign course, or it may result in sudden death during exercise.

CARDIOMYOPATHY

Etiology and Pathophysiology

Cardiomyopathy is a term used to describe a group of heart muscle diseases that primarily affect the structural or functional ability of the myocardium. This primary dysfunction is not associated with CAD, hypertension, vascular disease, or pulmonary disease.

When cardiomyopathies are classified by cause, two forms are recognized: primary and secondary. Primary cardiomyopathy consists of heart muscle disease of unknown cause and is classified as dilated, hypertrophic, or restrictive:

- *Dilated cardiomyopathy:* Characterized by ventricular dilation, dilated cardiomyopathy is the most common type of primary cardiomyopathy.
- *Hypertrophic cardiomyopathy:* Hypertrophic cardiomyopathy results in increased size and mass of the heart because of increased muscle thickness (especially of the septal wall) and decreased ventricular size.
- *Restrictive cardiomyopathy:* In restrictive cardiomyopathy the ventricular walls are rigid, thus limiting the ventricles' ability to expand and resulting in impaired diastolic filling (American Heart Association, 2016c).

Secondary cardiomyopathy has a number of types: (1) infective (viral, bacterial, fungal, or protozoal myocarditis); (2) metabolic; (3) severe nutritional deprivation such as in anorexia nervosa, a mental disorder in which people see themselves as severely overweight and starve themselves; (4) alcohol (large quantities consumed over many years leading to dilated cardiomyopathy); (5) peripartum (unexplained cause; may develop in the last month of pregnancy or within the first few months after delivery); (6) drugs (doxorubicin or other medications); (7) radiation therapy; (8) systemic lupus erythematosus; (9) rheumatoid arthritis; and (10) "crack" heart, caused by cocaine abuse.

Cardiomyopathy caused by cocaine abuse causes intense vasoconstriction of the coronary arteries and peripheral vasoconstriction, resulting in hypertension. This can result in increased myocardial oxygen needs and decreased oxygen supply to the myocardium and can lead to acute MI or ischemic cardiomyopathy. Cocaine also causes high circulating levels of catecholamines, which may damage further myocardial cells, leading to ischemic or dilated cardiomyopathy. The cardiomyopathy produced is difficult to treat. Interventions deal mainly with the HF that ensues. The prognosis is poor.

Clinical Manifestations

Angina, syncope, fatigue, and dyspnea on exertion are common signs and symptoms. The most common symptom is severe exercise intolerance. The patient may have signs and symptoms of left-sided and right-sided HF, including dyspnea, peripheral edema, ascites, and hepatic dysfunction.

Diagnostic Tests

Diagnosis of cardiomyopathy is made by the patient's clinical manifestations and noninvasive and invasive cardiac procedures to rule out other causes of dysfunction. Diagnostic studies include ECG, chest radiograph, echocardiogram, CT scan, nuclear imaging studies, MUGA scanning, cardiac catheterization, and endomyocardial biopsy.

Medical Management

Medical management consists of treatment of the underlying cause and HF management to slow the progression of the disease and symptoms. Medications may include diuretics, ACE inhibitors, antidysrhythmics, and beta-adrenergic blockers. An automatic internal defibrillator occasionally is implanted. In patients with advanced disease that is not responding to medical treatment, cardiac transplantation (Box 8.7) may be considered. Advise the patient to avoid strenuous exercise because of the risk of sudden death.

Nursing Interventions and Patient Teaching

Nursing interventions focus on relieving symptoms, observing for and preventing complications,

---

Box 8.7	Indications and Contraindications for Cardiac Transplantation

INDICATIONS
- Suitable physiologic and chronologic age
- End-stage heart disease that is not responding to medical therapy
- Dilated cardiomyopathy
- Inoperable coronary artery disease
- Vigorous and healthy individual (except for end-stage cardiac disease) who would benefit from procedure
- Compliance with medical regimens
- Demonstrated emotional stability and social support system
- Financial resources available

CONTRAINDICATIONS
- Systemic disease with poor prognosis
- Active infection
- Active or recent malignancy
- Type 1 diabetes mellitus with end-organ damage
- Recent or unresolved pulmonary infarction
- Severe pulmonary hypertension unrelieved with medication
- Severe cerebrovascular or peripheral vascular disease
- Irreversible renal or hepatic dysfunction
- Active peptic ulcer disease
- Severe osteoporosis
- Severe obesity
- History of drug or alcohol abuse or mental illness

and providing emotional and psychological support. Monitor the response to medications and monitor for dysrhythmias. Teach patients to adjust their lifestyle to avoid strenuous activity and dehydration. Advise patients to space activities and allow for rest periods.

Prognosis

Most patients have a severe, progressively deteriorating course, and the majority (particularly those older than 55 years of age) die within 2 years of the onset of signs and symptoms. However, improvement or stabilization occurs in a minority of patients. Death is due to either HF or ventricular dysrhythmia. Sudden death resulting from dysrhythmia is a constant threat. The survival rate for adults with cardiac transplantation is approximately 85% for 1-year post-transplantation, and a 5-year survival rate of 69% (Mayo Clinic, 2019). A growing number of recipients survive more than 10 years after the procedure.

DISORDERS OF THE PERIPHERAL VASCULAR SYSTEM

Peripheral vascular disease is any abnormal condition that affects the blood vessels outside the heart and the lymphatic vessels. The word peripheral means pertaining to those areas away from the center (in this context, the heart). The peripheral vascular system consists of arteries, capillaries, and veins. This system supplies oxygen-rich blood to the upper and lower extremities of the body, and returns blood and carbon dioxide from those areas to the heart and lungs. Disorders of the peripheral vascular system occur when circulation to the upper and lower extremities is compromised.

EFFECTS OF NORMAL AGING ON THE PERIPHERAL VASCULAR SYSTEM

Degenerative changes occur in the vascular system as part of the normal aging process. These changes affect the walls of the blood vessels and lead to problems in the transport of blood and nutrients to the tissues. The inner walls of the blood vessels (tunica interna) become thick and less flexible. The middle walls of the blood vessels (tunica media) become less elastic. With marked decreases in the elasticity and flexibility of the vessels, peripheral vascular resistance increases, causing a rise in blood pressure and increasing a person's susceptibility to peripheral vascular disease (see the Lifespan Considerations box in the section "Effects of Normal Aging on the Cardiovascular System").

RISK FACTORS

Risk factors for peripheral vascular disorders are similar to those for cardiovascular disorders. An important aspect of caring for the patient with a peripheral vascular disorder is understanding the risk factors and incorporating them into patient teaching.

Nonmodifiable Factors

- *Age:* As a person ages, arteriosclerotic changes in the peripheral vascular system lead to increased peripheral vascular resistance and decreased blood flow to the tissues.
- *Gender:* Men are more susceptible than women to arteriosclerotic changes. This gender difference decreases after menopause, when the protective effects of estrogen are no longer present in women.
- *Family history:* A family history of atherosclerosis increases an individual's risk.

Modifiable Factors

- *Smoking:* Smoking is one of the major contributing factors in the development of peripheral vascular problems. The nicotine in cigarettes causes vasoconstriction and spasms of the arteries, elevates blood pressure, and reduces circulation to the extremities. The carbon monoxide inhaled in cigarette smoke reduces oxygen transport to the tissues.
- *Hypertension:* Increased blood pressure causes wear and damage to the inner arterial walls, resulting in a buildup of fibrous tissue. This in turn leads to further narrowing of the vessel and increased resistance to blood flow.
- *Hyperlipidemia:* An elevation in serum cholesterol and triglycerides contributes to the buildup of plaque inside the blood vessels. The patient should maintain a diet with decreased saturated fat and cholesterol. If serum cholesterol remains elevated, drug therapy must be considered.
- *Obesity:* Excessive body weight and body fat contribute to the severity of other risk factors. Extra weight in relation to bone structure and height places an increased workload on the heart and blood vessels and may contribute to congestion in the venous system. The body mass index (BMI) is an indicator of whether the patient is overweight or obese. Use the following formula for calculation: 703 × Patient's weight in pounds ÷ Patient's height in inches squared. The CDC defines obesity as a BMI of 30 or above (CDC, 2016c).
- *Lack of exercise:* Decreased activity may compromise the peripheral vascular system because of a lack of muscle tone. The contraction and relaxation of muscles facilitate the return of blood in the veins to the heart and the lungs. A sedentary person does not realize the benefits of regular physical activity, such as weight and stress reduction and improved vascular tone.
- *Emotional stress:* Stress contributes to increased blood pressure, increased production of cholesterol, and increased vasoconstriction of the blood vessels. Emotional stress is different with each patient. Some patients deal with stress with appropriate coping mechanisms, whereas other patients have difficulty coping with stress. Family and financial concerns impose the most stress on individuals.

- *Diabetes mellitus:* Uncontrolled elevated serum glucose levels contribute to the atherosclerotic process, although the exact mechanism by which diabetes mellitus leads to peripheral vascular disorders is unknown. Elevated serum glucose levels result in circulatory disorders.

ASSESSMENT

Arterial Assessment

The first symptom of decreased arterial circulation is pain from arterial insufficiency and ischemia. Arterial insufficiency occurs when not enough blood is available or able to flow through the arteries to body tissues. Ischemia occurs when the tissue does not receive enough oxygen-rich blood to function normally. Ischemic pain in the lower extremities is usually a dull ache in the calf muscles. It is often accompanied by leg fatigue and cramping. The pain is brought on by exercise and relieved by rest. It is referred to as intermittent claudication (a weakness of the legs accompanied by cramp-like pains in the calves caused by poor circulation of the arterial blood to the leg muscles). Pain also may be felt in the thighs and buttocks. As arterial disease progresses and becomes chronic, pain occurs even at rest. Burning, tingling, and numbness of the legs may occur at night while the patient is lying down.

Other nursing assessments include palpating and comparing pulses in the extremities. Pulses may be weak, thready, or absent in the affected extremity because of decreased blood flow. Several scales are used to measure pulses. To ensure that the patient's pulses are graded the same way each time, all nurses should use the same scale, such as the following:

0 Absent

+1 Barely palpable, intermittent

+2 Weak, possibly thready, but constantly palpable and with consistent quality

+3 Normal strength and quality

+4 Bounding, easily palpable, may be visible

A Doppler ultrasound device may be needed to check the patient's pulses if pulmonary vascular disease (PVD), low blood pressure, edema, or large amounts of subcutaneous tissue impede the assessment. If a Doppler device is used, record pulsation as *present* or *absent* rather than using the numeric scale. Many nurses will mark the area with a skin marker where the pulse was found with the Doppler to allow for better accuracy and less time for assessing the pulse later. Assess the affected extremity and compare it with the unaffected extremity for color, temperature, skin characteristics, and capillary refill time (Box 8.8).

For a uniform assessment and documentation technique for *veins* and *arteries,* the following mnemonic device, PATCHES, is helpful:

P for *pulses:* Assess the patient's affected extremity first. Then assess the apical pulse and bilateral temporal, carotid, brachial, radial, femoral, popliteal, posterior tibial, and dorsalis pedis pulses. Absence of pulses is generally a medical emergency that requires immediate treatment, but in some cases it may be normal. Compare the findings with previous ones or correlate them with the patient's signs and symptoms. The use of a Doppler ultrasound probe to assess pulses must be documented. This allows all nursing staff assessing peripheral pulses to assess in the same way for continuity of assessments and care.

A for *appearance:* Note whether the extremity is pale, mottled, cyanotic, or discolored red, black, or brown. Document areas of necrosis or bleeding and the size, depth, and location of ulcers. When assessing ulcers, note whether the edges are jagged or smooth and whether the area is painful to touch. Shiny skin often indicates the presence of edema or presence or absence of hair; a dull appearance may signal inadequate arterial blood supply. Look for superficial veins, erythema, or inflammation anywhere on the affected extremity. Standing allows the saphenous veins to fill, so varicosities in the saphenous system are evaluated best with the patient standing. If a line of color change is present, mark it with a skin marker and monitor for changes in location.

T for *temperature:* If the patient has an arterial problem, the affected extremity feels cool; if the problem is venous, the extremity feels normal or abnormally warm. However, problems in arteries and veins are not the only reasons for temperature changes in an extremity; aortoiliac disease, HF, hypovolemia, pulmonary embolism, and other conditions can also affect skin temperature by interfering with peripheral blood flow.

C for *capillary refill:* Capillary refill is normally less than 2 seconds, but it may be extended when the patient has PVD. Press on a nail until the nailbed blanches, and then release and count how many seconds it takes for normal color to return. Other sites to check capillary refill are the pads of the toes and fingers, the heel, and the muscles at the base of the thumb. Although abnormal capillary refill is not diagnostic, it adds valuable data to the assessment (see Box 8.8).

H for *hardness:* Palpate the extremity to determine whether the tissues are supple or hard and inelastic. Hardness may indicate longstanding PVD, chronic venous insufficiency, lymphedema, or chronic edema. Hardened subcutaneous skin also increases the risk of stasis ulcers.

Box 8.8	Capillary Refill Time

1. Apply pressure to a toenail or fingernail for several seconds until it blanches (the area loses its color).
2. Relieve the pressure.
3. Note the amount of time it takes for the color to return.
   - The color should return almost instantly—in less than 2 s.
   - With an arterial disorder, it will take more than 2 s for the color to return.

E for *edema:* Pitting edema frequently indicates an acute process, and non-pitting edema may be seen with chronic conditions, such as venous insufficiency. Assess both extremities for edema and compare and document the findings. To assess for pitting edema, gently press the skin on the affected extremity for at least 5 seconds. Release and grade pitting as follows: +1, 2-mm indentation; +2, 4-mm indentation; +3, 6-mm indentation; and +4, 8-mm indentation (Fig. 8.17). The most accurate way to determine the degree of non-pitting edema is to measure the circumference of the extremity and compare measurements with the other extremity and subsequent measurements. Measure at the point of edema, and then mark the point with a skin marker so that everyone assesses the same area. Accuracy is greatest if the measurements are taken at the same time every day, preferably in the morning before the patient ambulates.

S for *sensation:* Vascular discomfort can originate in arteries, in veins, or in the microcirculation if the patient has diabetes mellitus. In addition to asking the patient about pain, ask if he or she has other abnormal sensations, such as numbness or tingling. Tingling or tenderness can result from peripheral tissue ischemia, and the patient may say the extremity feels abnormally hot or cold.

Venous Assessment

Decreased venous circulation leads to edema. When the venous system does not return sufficient blood from the tissues to the heart and the lungs (venous insufficiency), excess fluid is left in the tissues of the affected extremity (edema). Assess for edema in the affected extremity and compare it with the unaffected extremity.

Venous insufficiency may lead to changes in skin pigmentation. Assess the skin for darker pigmentation, dryness, and scaling in the affected extremity. Chronic edema and stasis of blood from venous insufficiency may lead to ulceration of the tissues. These ulcers are referred to as *stasis ulcers.* Peripheral pulses are usually present with venous insufficiency. Pain, aching, and cramping associated with venous disorders usually are relieved by activity and/or elevating the extremity. Refer to Table 8.9 for a comparison of signs and symptoms associated with arterial and venous disorders.

Diagnostic Tests

Diagnostic tests for peripheral vascular disorders include noninvasive procedures and invasive procedures.

Noninvasive procedures include the following:
- *Treadmill test:* This exercise test is used to determine blood flow in the extremities after exercising. It identifies pain associated with exercise such as claudication.
- *Plethysmography:* Plethysmography is used to assess changes in blood volume in the veins of the calf or other body extremities. The test can be done in either

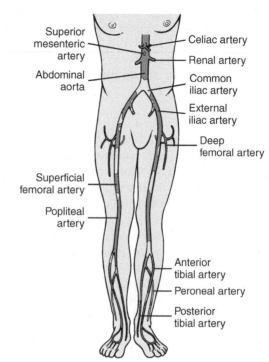

Fig. 8.17 Common anatomic locations of atherosclerotic lesions *(shown in yellow)* of the abdominal aorta and lower extremities. (From Lewis S, Dirksen SR, Heitkemper MM, et al: *Medical-surgical nursing: Assessment and management of clinical problems,* ed 8, St. Louis, 2011, Mosby.)

Table 8.9	Comparison of Signs and Symptoms Associated With Arterial and Venous Disorders	
SIGNS AND SYMPTOMS	**ARTERIAL DISORDER**	**VENOUS DISORDER**
Pain	Aching to sharp cramping; brought on by exercise; relieved by rest	Aching to cramping pain; relieved by activity or elevating extremity
Pulses	Diminished or absent	Usually present
Edema	Usually absent	Usually present; increases at the end of the day and when extremity is in a dependent position
Skin changes	Cool or cold Dry, shiny Hairless Pallor develops with elevation; becomes erythematous with dangling	Warm, thick, and toughened Darkened pigmentation Stasis ulcers

a health care provider's office or on an outpatient basis in the hospital. The patient is asked to recline in a semi-Fowler's position with the legs dangling. A blood pressure cuff in placed on the arm and leg of the affected side. The health care provider inflates the cuffs and a plethysmograph measures the pulses from each cuff.

- *Digital subtraction angiography:* Initially an IV contrast solution is administered. This allows blood vessels in the extremities to be visualized by radiography, using an image intensifier video system and a television monitor.
- *Doppler ultrasound:* A Doppler ultrasound flowmeter measures blood flow in arteries or veins to assess intermittent claudication, obstruction of deep veins, and other disorders of peripheral veins and arteries.

Invasive procedures include the following:

- *Venography:* A contrast medium is administered through a catheter placed in a foot vein. X-ray films are taken to detect filling defects. Venography is the gold standard by which to assess the condition of the deep leg veins and to diagnose DVT. Venography is invasive and costly, can be unpleasant, and may cause phlebitis. Before undergoing venography, the patient must sign an informed consent form, because the procedure involves the injection of a contrast medium. Because the contrast medium contains iodine, determine whether the patient is allergic to iodine or shellfish (the latter being an indication of sensitivity to iodine). Care after the procedure is similar to post-angiography care, including monitoring the pulse, assessing for edema, and monitoring sensation in the extremity.
- *Angiography:* This is done by injection of a contrast medium intravascularly and then visualizing the arteries by radiography.
- *D-dimer:* A serum venous blood test. D-dimer is a product of fibrin degradation (change to a less complex form). When a thrombus is present, plasma D-dimer concentrations are usually greater than 1591 ng/mL. The normal range for D-dimer is 68 to 494 ng/mL.
- *Duplex scanning:* This is a combination of ultrasound imaging techniques and Doppler capabilities to determine the location and extent of thrombi within veins (most widely used test to diagnose DVT).

HYPERTENSION

Hypertension is considered with peripheral vascular disorders because it is a risk factor in atherosclerosis, which leads to peripheral vascular disease.

Etiology and Pathophysiology

Normal blood pressure is a reading of less than 120 mm Hg systolic and 80 mm Hg diastolic. Per new CDC (2020a) guidelines, hypertension has been divided into the following categories:

Normal = Systolic less than 120 mm Hg and diastolic less than 80 mm Hg

Elevated = Systolic 120 to 129 mm Hg with a diastolic of less than 80 mm Hg

Hypertension Stage 1 = Systolic 130 to 139 mm Hg and diastolic 80 to 89 mm Hg

Hypertension Stage 2 = Systolic greater than 140 mm Hg and diastolic greater than or equal to 90 mm Hg

A diagnosis is not based on a one-time elevated blood pressure reading, but on an average of two or more elevated blood pressure readings taken on separate occasions.

Approximately 85 million Americans have hypertension, and an additional 25 million have prehypertension (American Heart Association, 2018b). It has been estimated that up to 30% of the adult population in the United States have undiagnosed hypertension. It is difficult to determine exact numbers, because most people are symptom free. Hypertension may not present with symptoms until it is too late which is why it is often called the "silent killer."

Arterial blood pressure is the pressure exerted by the blood on the walls of arteries. Systolic blood pressure is the greatest force caused by the contraction of the left ventricle of the heart. Diastolic blood pressure occurs during the relaxation phase between heartbeats and is the pressure on the arterial walls while the heart is at rest. Blood flow is determined by the amount of blood the heart pumps with each contraction and how fast the heart beats. Peripheral vascular resistance is affected by the diameter of the blood vessels and the viscosity of the blood. Blood flow and peripheral vascular resistance play an important role in regulating blood pressure. Increased peripheral vascular resistance resulting from *vasoconstriction,* or narrowing of peripheral blood vessels, is a common factor in hypertension.

Vasoconstriction and vasodilation are controlled by the sympathetic nervous system and the renin-angiotensin system of the kidney. Stimulation of the sympathetic nervous system and the release of epinephrine and/or norepinephrine cause blood vessel constriction and increased peripheral vascular resistance. The activation of the renin-angiotensin system occurs with decreased blood flow to the kidney. Renin leads to the formation of angiotensin, which is a potent vasoconstrictor. Angiotensin stimulates the secretion of aldosterone, leading to the retention of sodium and water. The result is an increase in blood pressure.

The two main types of hypertension are *essential (primary)* hypertension and *secondary* hypertension. The incidence of hypertension increases with age and other risk factors.

Essential (Primary) Hypertension

Essential (primary) hypertension makes up the majority of all diagnosed cases. Although there is no general agreement on the cause of essential hypertension, theories to explain the mechanisms involved include arteriolar changes, sympathetic nervous system activation, hormonal influence (renin-angiotensin-aldosterone system stimulation), genetic factors, greater-than-ideal body weight, sedentary lifestyle, increased

Box 8.9 Risk Factors for Essential Hypertension

NONMODIFIABLE RISK FACTORS
- *Age:* Risk increases as age advances above 30 years old
- *Gender:* Men are more at risk than women
- *Race:* Risk twice as high in African Americans as in white Americans
- *Family history:* Risk increased with a family history of hypertension

MODIFIABLE RISK FACTORS
- *Smoking:* Nicotine constricts blood vessels
- *Obesity:* Associated with increased blood volume
- *High-sodium diet:* Increases water retention, which increases blood volume
- *Elevated serum cholesterol:* Leads to atherosclerosis and narrowing of blood vessels
- *Oral contraceptives or estrogen therapy:* May contribute to elevated blood pressure
- *Alcohol:* Increases plasma catecholamines (biologically active amines, epinephrine, and norepinephrine), which leads to blood vessel constriction
- *Emotional stress:* Stimulates the sympathetic nervous system, which leads to blood vessel constriction
- *Sedentary lifestyle:* Regular exercise helps lower blood pressure over time

Table 8.10 Causes of Secondary Hypertension

CONDITION OR DISORDER	MECHANISM
Renal vascular disease	Kidney disease (glomerulonephritis, renal failure, renal artery stenosis, physiologic changes related to type of disease) affects renin and sodium and results in hypertension
Diseases of the adrenal cortex • Primary aldosteronism • Cushing syndrome • Pheochromocytoma	Atherosclerotic changes in renal arteries cause increase in peripheral vascular resistance Increase in aldosterone causes sodium and water retention and increases blood volume Increase in blood volume Excess secretion of catecholamines increases peripheral vascular resistance
Coarctation of the aorta (narrowing of the aorta)	Causes marked elevated blood pressure in upper extremities with decreased perfusion in lower extremities
Head trauma or cranial tumor	Increased intracranial pressure reduces cerebral blood flow and stimulates medulla oblongata to raise blood pressure
Pregnancy-induced hypertension	Cause unknown; generalized vasospasm may be a contributing factor

sodium intake, and excessive alcohol intake. For a long time, many experts believed that an increase in systolic blood pressure was a normal part of aging. In fact, some believed that "100 mm Hg plus the patient's age" was a tolerable systolic blood pressure in the older adult. Treatment for hypertension was based primarily on the diastolic reading, and isolated systolic hypertension (ISH) often was not treated.

Clinical trials have reemphasized that ISH is believed to raise the risk of cardiovascular disease and stroke (Mayo Clinic, 2018). ISH is actually a better overall predictor of cardiovascular morbidity and mortality than diastolic pressure. (Diastolic pressure remains the better predictor of CAD in people younger than 45 years.) ISH is defined as an elevated systolic blood pressure of 140 mm Hg or more with a diastolic blood pressure below 90 mm Hg. The value of treating ISH in older patients has been established only recently, but now those findings are widely circulated. The recommendations are now aimed at keeping systolic blood pressure at 140 mm Hg or less, with a diastolic blood pressure not less than 70 mm Hg.

Prognosis. With prolonged untreated essential hypertension, the elastic tissue in the arterioles is replaced by fibrous tissue. This process leads to decreased tissue perfusion and deterioration, especially in the target organs—the heart, kidney, and brain. CAD and cerebrovascular accident (stroke), the major causes of death and disability, are much more frequent in those who have elevated blood pressure than in those

who are normotensive. With treatment, the prognosis is usually good. Risk factors that contribute to the development of essential hypertension are listed in Box 8.9.

Secondary Hypertension
Secondary hypertension is attributed to an identifiable medical diagnosis. Conditions associated with secondary hypertension are given in Table 8.10.

Prognosis. In most instances, secondary hypertension subsides when the primary disease process is treated or corrected. Because of the varied conditions causing secondary hypertension, problems can be anywhere in the body. The results of untreated secondary hypertension can lead to atherosclerosis; aneurysms; heart failure; weakened or narrowed vessels in the kidneys; thickened, narrowed, or torn vessels in the eyes; metabolic syndrome; as well as trouble with memory or understanding.

Malignant Hypertension
Malignant hypertension is a severe, rapidly progressive elevation in blood pressure (diastolic pressure greater than 120 mm Hg) that causes damage

to the small arterioles in major organs (heart, kidneys, brain, eyes). A primary distinguishing finding is inflammation of arterioles (arteriolitis) in the eyes. This type of hypertension is most common in African American men younger than 40 years of age.

Prognosis. Unless medical treatment is successful, the course is rapidly fatal. The most common causes of death are MI, HF, stroke, and renal failure.

Clinical Manifestations
Hypertension is essentially a disease without symptoms until vascular changes occur in the heart, brain, eyes, or kidneys. Longstanding, untreated hypertension can cause target organ damage. Advanced target organ damage may account for left ventricular hypertrophy, angina pectoris, MI, HF, stroke or transient ischemic attack, nephropathy, PAD, or retinopathy. Signs and symptoms usually occur as a result of advanced hypertension. These signs and symptoms may include awakening with a headache, blurred vision, and spontaneous epistaxis (nosebleed).

Assessment
Collection of subjective data includes assessing for morning headache in the occipital area and blurred vision. Assess the patient for risk factors (see Box 8.9). Determine the patient's understanding of hypertension, including the definition, meaning of systolic and diastolic readings, complications of hypertension, and possible concerns regarding treatment.

Collection of objective data includes measuring the blood pressure in both arms with the patient in supine and sitting positions. Compare the reading with previous blood pressure results. Take two or more blood pressure measurements on two separate occasions. Also measure and record height and weight. Assess and record heart sounds, and palpate and record peripheral pulses.

Diagnostic Tests
Diagnostic tests associated with hypertension evaluate the functions of the brain, heart, and kidneys. The results indicate the effects of hypertension on these organs and provide baseline information for future reference. These tests include CBC; serum levels of sodium, potassium, calcium, and magnesium; lipid profile; fasting blood glucose level; creatinine, BUN, urinalysis, and IV pyelography (i.e., radiography of the kidneys and ureters); renal arteriography (the gold standard for confirming renal artery stenosis); and chest radiography, ECG, and possible echocardiography (to determine any effect on the heart).

Medical Management
Medical management is directed at controlling hypertension and preventing complications. The goal in older adults is to keep the blood pressure at less than 140/90 mm Hg. The general goal for younger adults with mild hypertension is to achieve blood pressure of less than 130/80 mm Hg. Treatment is based on the severity of the hypertension, associated risk factors, and damage to major organs. Antihypertensive medications and nonpharmacologic measures are used to lower blood pressure.

Drug therapy. For stage 1 or 2 hypertension, drug therapy may include the following (American Heart Association, 2017e):
- Diuretics (thiazides, loop diuretics, potassium-sparing drugs)
- Beta-adrenergic blockers such as metoprolol, nadolol, propranolol, acebutolol, atenolol, bisoprolol, timolol
- ACE inhibitors such as captopril, enalapril, lisinopril
- Angiotensin II receptor blockers such as valsartan, losartan, irbesartan, candesartan, telmisartan
- Calcium channel blockers such as diltiazem, amlodipine, nifedipine, felodipine, verapamil
- Alpha-agonists such as clonidine
- Drug combinations such as Caduet, which contain amlodipine and atorvastatin calcium; benazepril hydrochloride, which contains benazepril and hydrochlorothiazide; and others, in an attempt to lower the number of pills taken so that patients will be more compliant in taking blood pressure–lowering medications
- Aliskiren hemifumarate, the first antihypertensive drug that is a direct renin inhibitor, decreases plasma renin activity and inhibits the conversion of angiotensinogen to angiotensin I (NIH, 2016)

Special considerations include using ACE inhibitors for diabetes mellitus; using ACE inhibitors and diuretics for HF; using beta blockers and ACE inhibitors for MI; using calcium channel blockers and diuretics for African Americans; and using diuretics and long-acting calcium channel blockers for older adults with ISH.

Nonpharmacologic therapy. Nonpharmacologic therapy for hypertension includes the following:
- *Lose excess weight:* Being overweight is associated with increased blood pressure, abnormally high blood lipid levels, diabetes mellitus, and CAD. Limiting calorie intake and increasing physical exercise are the keys to losing weight.
- *Exercise regularly:* Thirty to 45 minutes of aerobic exercise, three or four times a week, helps decrease the risk of hypertension and cardiovascular disease.
- *Reduce saturated fat:* A patient with high blood lipid levels may require dietary modification or drug therapy to normalize them. A cardinal rule is to limit fat intake to less than 30% of total calories. According to the Dietary Approaches to Stop

Hypertension (DASH) study, a low-fat diet rich in fruits and vegetables is recommended.

- *Consume enough potassium, calcium, and magnesium:* Plenty of potassium in the diet helps decrease blood pressure, so eating potassium-rich fruits and vegetables may improve blood pressure control. Administering potassium supplements to a patient who is hypokalemic as a result of diuretic therapy also combats hypertension. A word of caution: Anyone receiving ACE inhibitors or potassium-sparing diuretics should receive potassium supplements only with extreme caution and close monitoring for hyperkalemia. Low dietary calcium and magnesium may contribute to hypertension (www.dashdiet.org); the National Heart, Lung, and Blood Institute suggests consuming adequate amounts of calcium and magnesium but does not recommend supplementation to combat hypertension.
- *Limit alcohol intake:* Excessive alcohol consumption may contribute to hypertension. A man of normal weight should not drink more than 1 ounce of ethanol per day (the equivalent of 24 ounces of beer, 10 ounces of wine, or 2 ounces of 100-proof whiskey). Women and lightweight men should restrict their intake to half this amount.
- *Reduce sodium intake:* High sodium intake can increase blood pressure, especially in African Americans, older adult patients with existing hypertension, and patients with diabetes mellitus. It is recommended that sodium intake be limited to 2.4 g/day. Encourage your patient to eat unsalted, unprocessed foods and to read labels when shopping.
- *Stop smoking:* Cigarette smoking is one of the leading risk factors for hypertension and heart disease. Smoking also inhibits the effect of antihypertensive medication, so techniques for stopping are an integral part of patient education. Counseling, support groups, and aids to stop smoking are effective. Individuals who discontinue smoking may gain weight. Provide information about weight management and exercise programs.
- *Use relaxation techniques and stress management:* Stress management and relaxation techniques have also been shown to offset hypertension and its symptoms.

Nursing Interventions and Patient Teaching

The main focus of nursing interventions is to maintain blood pressure management through patient teaching about hypertension, risk factors, and drug therapy. Patient compliance is improved with education about side effects of medications, dietary instruction, exercise, and stress-reduction techniques (Box 8.10).

Patient problems and interventions for the patient with hypertension include but are not limited to the following:

Box 8.10   Measures to Increase Compliance With Antihypertensive Therapy

- Be certain that patient understands that absence of symptoms does not indicate control of blood pressure; remind patient that symptoms do not occur until advanced stages of the disease.
- Advise patient against abrupt withdrawal of medication; rebound hypertension can occur.
- Encourage patient to discuss unpleasant side effects of medication with a health care professional.
- If remembering to take medications is a problem, discuss alternative ways to remember, such as taking them with certain meals or placing medication in separate containers labeled with times of day.
- Suggest patient participate in an exercise program with a friend or pay for the program (more likely to participate "to get money's worth").
- Include family and significant others in the teaching process to provide support and promote adherence to regimen.
- Explain reason for regular health care follow-up (high blood pressure is a chronic disorder).
- Contact patients who consistently cancel follow-up appointments.

PATIENT PROBLEM	NURSING INTERVENTIONS
Insufficient Knowledge, related to: • Disease process • Therapeutic management	Assess level of understanding Implement teaching plan for hypertension: • Disease process, risk factors • Prescribed medications and side effects; proper dosage and administration; necessity of taking medication, even when blood pressure readings are normal • Dietary restrictions • Exercise program • Relaxation techniques • Sexual dysfunction as a potential side effect of adrenergic inhibitors • Compliance with therapy and follow-up appointments • Encourage the patient to promptly report any problems to health care professionals for counseling

ARTERIAL DISORDERS

ARTERIOSCLEROSIS AND ATHEROSCLEROSIS

Arteriosclerosis is characterized by gradual thickening, loss of elasticity, and calcification of arterial walls, resulting in a decreased blood supply due to narrowing of the arterial lumen. Atherosclerosis is characterized by a gradual buildup of yellowish plaques of cholesterol, lipids, and cellular debris in the inner layers of the walls of large and medium-sized arteries. Arteriosclerosis and Atherosclerosis are often used interchangeably as even though the pathophysiology of each is different, the outcome is the same. Both results in narrowing of the arterial lumen. The narrowed lumen decreases the flow of blood, oxygen, and nutrients to areas of the body distal to the narrowing. As the narrowing of the arterial lumen is gradual, collateral circulation may be stimulated but it is often inadequate in meeting tissue needs. When the need for oxygen in the tissues exceeds the supply, ischemia occurs and may result in cell death and tissue necrosis. The degree of reduction in blood flow and oxygen determines the amount of ischemia and necrosis that occurs. Arteriosclerosis results in a loss of arterial wall elasticity. Loss of elasticity makes the artery less responsive to changes in blood volume and pressure. Thus, a complication of arteriosclerosis/atherosclerosis is aneurysm, ulceration, and rupture.

Atherosclerosis changes can occur anywhere in the body, but bifurcations of arteries are common sites of such changes. The risk factors for atherosclerosis include tobacco smoke, diabetes, high cholesterol levels, hypertension, and hyperchromocysteinemia. These conditions cause damage to the arteries over time and the damaged arteries undergo inflammatory processes. The inflammatory processes allow for plaque buildup which results in atherosclerosis. Prevention of atherosclerosis can be achieved maintaining a healthy diet, decreasing cholesterol levels by diet and/or medication, decreasing hypertension, and diabetes control. Specific peripheral vascular disorders that stem from arteriosclerosis and atherosclerosis are discussed individually in this chapter.

PERIPHERAL ARTERIAL DISEASE OF THE LOWER EXTREMITIES

Etiology and Pathophysiology

PAD of the lower extremities is a consequence of arteriosclerotic and atherosclerotic changes in the lumen of the artery. Plaque, as a result of the atherosclerotic process, forms on the internal wall of the blood vessel, causing partial or complete occlusion. The result is little or no blood flow to the affected extremity. The artery is progressively unable to supply blood and oxygen to the tissues, first while exercising and then even at rest. Thus, signs and symptoms associated with tissue ischemia appear.

PAD can occur in the upper extremities, but it mostly affects the lower extremities. The most common arteries affected in PAD of the lower extremities are the iliac, common femoral arteries, and superficial femoral arteries. Patients with diabetes mellitus are especially prone to develop PAD below the knees commonly in the anterior distal popliteal artery.

Clinical Manifestations

The severity of the signs and symptoms of PAD depends on the location and the extent of the atherosclerosis and on the amount of collateral circulation. Since the process of atherosclerosis is gradual, lumen narrowing is gradual too and patients may not have symptoms until the reduced blood flow is unable to keep up with demand.

Pain is the first symptom that occurs from tissue ischemia. The pain generally occurs in the affected extremity in conjunction with activity (see Table 8.9). When at rest, the pain subsides as muscle activity and demand for oxygen and nutrients has reduced therefore tissue ischemia reduces. This phenomenon of pain with activity and relief of pain at rest is known as *intermittent claudication*. Patients may notice that gradually over time the amount of activity they are able to do before pain occurs decreases while the amount of rest they require between activity increases. As the disease progresses, activity level keeps dropping and pain level with the slightest of activity keeps increasing. Eventually, the arterial lumen is so narrow that the patient experiences pain even at rest. The pain experienced by patients is a boring, aching, persistent pain. The pain is worse at night while sleeping. This is because blood flow to the lower extremity is not being helped by gravity. Patients soon realize that dangling their leg over the side of the bed reduces the pain while elevating the extremity makes it worse. Besides pain, patients may describe a coldness, numbness, or tingling sensation in their extremity.

Assessment

Collection of subjective data focuses on pain associated with intermittent claudication and the level of activity the patient can tolerate. Questions surrounding activity of daily living are appropriate to give insight into disease progression.

Collection of objective data includes assessment of pulses in the affected extremity, which may be weak or absent; comparison with pulses in the unaffected extremity; assessment of capillary refill (more than 3 seconds indicates PAD); ruddy and cyanotic extremity when placed in a dependent position; and shiny atrophic skin which may be dry and sparse of hair. The patient may also present with arterial or ischemic ulcers on the toes or feet. Arterial ulcers occur either when an injury causes a break in the skin that doesn't heal due to poor circulation or poor perfusion to the tissues causes the overlying skin to undergo necrosis thus causing the area to form an open wound. Once an open wound is present, poor circulation impedes healing. Arterial ulcers tend to be well defined having a characteristic "punched out" look; round and deep; and the base of the wound typically does not bleed and is yellow, brown, gray, or black in color. Arterial ulcers are extremely painful and may become gangrenous (Sudheendra, 2020).

Diagnostic Tests

A variety of tests are useful to diagnose PAD of the lower extremities. The ABI is a quick and noninvasive way to check for risk of peripheral artery disease. People who have a decreased ABI are at increased risk of developing a heart attack, stroke, poor circulation in the legs, and leg pain. The ABI is determined with the patient lying face up on a table while a technician measures the patient's blood pressure in both arms. Then the technician measures the patient's blood pressure in the two arteries in the left ankle, using an inflatable cuff and a hand-held Doppler ultrasound probe. The Doppler uses sound waves to produce images and lets the health care provider hear pulses in the ankle arteries after the blood pressure cuff is deflated. The test takes a few minutes, and no special precautions are necessary before or after the procedure. According to the American Heart Association and the American College of Cardiology, a borderline ABI of 0.91 to 0.99 puts the patient at minimal risk. An abnormal reading (anything below 0.9) puts the patient at higher risk of developing peripheral artery disease. The ABI can also be done after treadmill testing as it provides an indication of the severity of the narrowing (Mayo Clinic, 2020b). Additional testing includes duplex ultrasound which helps evaluate the extent of the disease, magnetic resonance angiography (MRA) which allows examination of large and small vessels, and computer tomography angiography (CTA) (Dominguez and Rowe, 2019).

Medical Management

Medical management involves a multifactorial approach. Patients are encouraged to make lifestyle modifications such as quit smoking if they do, gradual exercise to the point of pain followed by rest which helps establish collateral circulation, diet control especially a decrease in cholesterol containing foods, controlling diabetes for diabetic patients, and reducing blood pressure (Hinkle and Cheever, 2018). In conjunction with these, patients are prescribed antiplatelet medication that allow for easier blood flow at the narrowed artery. Aspirin and clopidogrel have the added benefit of preventing thromboembolism. Two medications specifically approved for use in PAD include pentoxifylline and cilostazol (Dominguez and Rowe, 2019). Pentoxifylline decreases the viscosity of blood (MedlinePlus, 2017) while cilostazol is a platelet-aggregation inhibitor (Hinkle and Cheever, 2018). Along with exercise and diet control, statins are also prescribed to help decrease values on the lipid profile.

Patients presenting with arterial ulcers should see a wound care specialist. Often, patients are taught how to dress the wound, clean it, and keep it free of infection. It is also important to keep the dressing dry.

Patients in the advanced stages of PAD may be managed via revascularization procedures. Revascularization procedures seek to restore as much blood flow as possible to the distal limb without conventional surgery. A balloon angioplasty with stent placement may help break the plaque, widen the artery, and leave a stent behind to keep the artery open and patent. An atherectomy may also be done which may involve the removal of plaque by clamping the affected artery at both ends of the blockage, dissecting the artery, and removing the plaque. A less invasive atherectomy involves the insertion of a catheter with a sharp blade at the end that allows the catheter to be threaded into an artery, the sharp blade cuts the plaque which is then retracted out of the artery with the catheter (Cleveland Clinic, 2019). For patients that have plaque blockage in their carotid arteries, the atherectomy procedure is called a carotid endarterectomy or simply **endarterectomy** and involves the dissection of the carotid artery with subsequent plaque removal.

Lastly, a conventional surgical procedure for PAD is a femoral-popliteal bypass graft (Fig. 8.18.). This procedure is performed for patients with severe disease who may be at risk of limb amputation. A femoral-popliteal or fem-pop bypass graft is further classified into an above the knee or below the knee referring to the site of the bypass graft. Under general anesthesia, a vein taken from the patient is grafted above and below the blocked artery. Once the graft is in place, an arteriogram is performed to confirm blood flow through the graft.

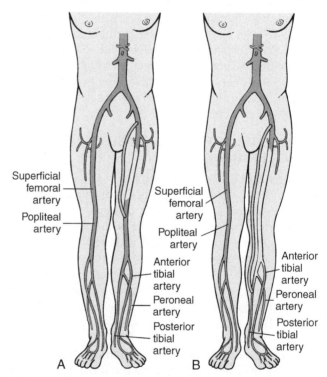

Fig. 8.18 (A) Femoral-popliteal bypass graft around an occluded superficial femoral artery. (B) Femoral posterior tibial bypass graft around occluded superficial femoral, popliteal, and proximal tibial arteries. (From Lewis S, Dirksen SR, Heitkemper MM, et al: *Medical-surgical nursing: Assessment and management of clinical problems*, ed 8, St. Louis, 2011, Mosby.)

Nursing Interventions and Patient Teaching

Nursing interventions are based on assessment findings and nursing diagnoses. Patient problems and nursing interventions for the patient with PAD of the lower extremities include but are not limited to the following:

PATIENT PROBLEM	NURSING INTERVENTIONS
Inability to Tolerate Activity, related to: • Ischemic pain • Immobility	Prevent hazards of immobility by turning, positioning, deep breathing, and performing isometric and range-of-motion exercises Encourage program of balanced exercise and rest to promote circulation Instruct the patient to use pain or intermittent claudication as a guide to limiting activity during exercise
Compromised Blood Flow to Tissue, peripheral, related to decreased arterial blood flow	Place patient's legs in a dependent position relative to the heart to improve peripheral blood flow Avoid raising feet above heart Promote vasodilation by providing warmth to extremities and keeping room warm Teach the patient to avoid vasoconstriction from nicotine, caffeine, stress, or chilling Teach the patient to avoid constrictive clothing such as garters, tight stockings, or belts Administer prescribed medications Teach the patient to avoid crossing the legs Teach the patient to examine lower extremities for injury Teach the patient to wear well-fitting shoes and socks and to avoid walking barefoot Teach the patient to avoid sitting or standing in one position for too long

Postsurgical nursing interventions include monitoring the affected extremity for pulse, amplitude, capillary refill time, pallor, coldness, and numbness. Disappearance of a pulse or abnormal capillary refill times may indicate graft occlusion.

Prognosis

In advanced disease, ischemia may lead to necrosis, ulceration, and gangrene (particularly of the toes and distal foot) because of the decreased circulation.

ARTERIAL EMBOLISM

Etiology and Pathophysiology

Arterial emboli are blood clots in the arterial bloodstream. They may originate in the heart from an atrial dysrhythmia, MI, valvular heart disease, or HF. Other foreign substances such as a detached atherosclerotic plaque or tissue may result in arterial emboli. An embolus becomes dangerous when it lodges within and occludes a blood vessel. Blood flow to the area distal to the lodged embolus is impaired, and ischemia occurs. Signs and symptoms depend on the site of the embolus, the size of the embolus, and the amount of circulation that is compromised. Pulmonary embolism are emboli that occur in the lungs and are discussed in Chapter 9. Cerebrovascular accidents are emboli that occur in the brain and are discussed in Chapter 14. Emboli that occur within coronary arteries cause angina and may lead to myocardial infarct and are discussed in CAD. The discussion henceforth is in regard to emboli in the peripheral extremities.

Clinical Manifestations

Sudden loss of blood flow to tissues causes severe pain. Distal pulses are absent, and the affected extremity may become pale, cool, and numb. Necrotic changes may occur. Shock may result if the embolus occludes a large artery.

Assessment

Collection of subjective data includes determining the onset of pain and numbness and the location, quality, and duration of these symptoms.

Collection of objective data includes assessing pulses in the affected extremity. Compare both extremities to determine skin temperature and color, in addition to pulse amplitude.

Diagnostic Tests

Doppler ultrasonography (see previously described studies on Doppler ultrasound) and angiography are indicated to obtain a diagnosis. An abnormal result may mean a blockage of an artery by a blood clot, fat embolism, or air embolism.

Medical Management

Medications used to treat obstructed arteries include anticoagulants such as coumadin (Warfarin) and antiplatelet medications such as aspirin or clopidogrel (Plavix). These medications prevent clots from forming. The patient may also be treated with thrombolytics such as streptokinase which dissolves the blood clot. Surgical interventions considered include those discussed under PAD.

Nursing Interventions and Patient Teaching

Nursing interventions are similar to those for PAD in terms of preventing further arterial problems. During the acute phase monitor the patient for changes in skin color and temperature of the extremity distal to the embolus. Increasing pallor, cyanosis, and coolness of the skin indicate worsening or occlusion of arterial circulation to the extremity. Keep the extremity warm, but do not apply direct heat.

Patient problems and postoperative nursing interventions for the patient requiring an artherectomy include but are not limited to the following:

PATIENT PROBLEM	NURSING INTERVENTIONS
Compromised Blood Flow to Tissue, related to decreased arterial blood flow	Monitor skin color and temperature of affected extremity every hour Assess sensation and movement in the distal extremity Assess peripheral pulses and capillary refill in the involved extremity: • Sudden absence of pulse may indicate thrombosis • Mark location of peripheral pulse with a skin pen to facilitate frequent assessment • Use a Doppler probe to verify whether pulses of the involved extremity are palpable or not, and compare with pulses of the uninvolved extremity Monitor extremity for edema Check incision for erythema, edema, and exudates Monitor and immediately report signs of complications, such as increasing pain, fever, changes in drainage, absent or weakening pulse, changes in skin color, limitation of movement, or paresthesia Promote circulation: • Reposition patient q2h. • Tell patient not to cross legs • Use a footboard and overbed cradle to keep linens off extremity • Encourage progressive activity when permitted • Avoid sharp flexion in area of graft • Monitor for signs of bleeding secondary to anticoagulation therapy

PATIENT PROBLEM	NURSING INTERVENTIONS
Insufficient Knowledge, related to anticoagulant therapy	Teach patient general action and side effects of prescribed drug; instruct patient to avoid taking anticoagulant medications with aspirin, which also has anticoagulant effect Instruct patient to take anticoagulant at same time every day and to not stop taking it until advised by health care provider Have patient check for signs of bleeding (gums, epistaxis [nosebleed], ecchymosis [bruising], cuts that do not stop bleeding with direct pressure, blood in urine or stool); report promptly to health care professional Encourage patient to wear a medical-alert bracelet or to carry an identification card containing the drug name, drug dosage, and health care provider's name in case of emergency Have patient report for prescribed blood tests (PTT, PT, INR) used to adjust drug dosage Tell patient not to add dark green and yellow vegetables to diet (these contain vitamin K, which counteracts the anticoagulant drug effect) Instruct patient to restrict alcohol intake (increases anticoagulant effect)

Patient teaching is the same as for PAD, with an emphasis on anticoagulant therapy.

Prognosis
Prognosis depends on the size of the embolus, the presence of collateral circulation, and the proximity to a major organ.

ARTERIAL ANEURYSM
Etiology and Pathophysiology
An aneurysm occurs when the wall of an artery weakens, resulting in bulging of the artery when it fills with blood. Aneurysms may be the result of arteriosclerosis, trauma, or a congenital defect. The force of blood

pushing against walls of the artery combined with damage or injury to the artery's walls have caused the aneurysm. Aneurysms of the lower extremities commonly affect the popliteal artery. Other areas predominantly affected are the thoracic and abdominal aorta and the coronary and cerebral arteries. The aorta is especially prone to aneurysm and rupture, because it is continuously exposed to high pressures. Aortic aneurysms are most common in men in their 60s and 70s, especially if they have ever smoked. Other risk factors are smoking, hypertension, atherosclerosis, and hyperlipidemia (CDC, 2020d). Dissections (separations and tears) and ruptures are more likely in the thoracic portion of the aorta than in the abdominal portion. An aneurysm starts with a weakened arterial wall that becomes dilated from blood flow and pressure in the area. The pathologic effect of this condition is differentiated according to shape and site of presentation (Fig. 8.19).

Clinical Manifestations
A large pulsating mass may be the only identifiable factor. Clinical signs and symptoms of a thoracic aortic aneurysm depend on its location. If it compresses adjacent structures, it can cause chest pain, shortness of breath, cough, hoarseness, or dysphagia. If it compresses the superior vena cava, the patient may have edema of the face, the neck, and the arms. In the early stages an abdominal aneurysm is unlikely to cause symptoms. As it expands, however, it may cause pain in the chest, the lower back, or, in men, the scrotum. A pulsatile, nontender upper abdominal mass may be palpated.

Assessment
Collection of subjective data may reveal no subjective symptoms unless the aneurysm is large and impinges on other structures, causing pain and inequality of pulses. A thoracic aortic aneurysm can result in chest pain, shortness of breath, or dysphagia.

Collection of objective data includes palpation of a large, nontender, pulsating mass at the site of the aneurysm.

Diagnostic Tests
Fluoroscopy, chest radiographic studies, CT scan, ultrasound, contrast aortography, arteriography, MRI, and TEE are used to diagnose an aneurysm (Mayo Clinic, 2020c).

Medical Management
Aneurysms are monitored for complications such as dissection, rupture, formation of thrombi, and ischemia. Control of hypertension is the priority of care. An oral beta blocker reduces blood pressure, heart rate, and myocardial contractility. Surgical intervention may be necessary but often aneurysms are treated with a watch and wait approach based on the size. The blood vessel may be ligated or grafts used to replace the section of the artery that contains the aneurysm or to bypass the aneurysm.

A fusiform or circumferential aneurysm (in which all the walls of the blood vessel dilate more or less equally, creating a tubular swelling) can be removed and repaired with a graft of synthetic fiber, such as Dacron or Teflon, or with a vessel taken from another region of the patient's body. Saccular aneurysms (an aneurysm, usually caused by trauma, that consists of a weak area on only one side of the vessel, causing an outpouching of the vessel wall that is attached to the artery by a narrow neck) can be removed and the vessel then sutured, or a patch graft can be used to replace the deformity (Figs. 8.20 and 8.21).

In repair of a popliteal aneurysm, popliteal blood flow is enhanced when a homograft (or *allograft*, tissue transferred between two genetically dissimilar individuals of the same species, such as two humans who are not identical twins) is used.

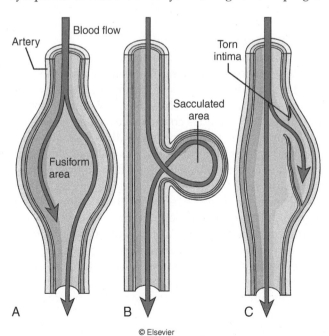

© Elsevier

Fig. 8.19 Types of aneurysms. (A) Fusiform. (B) Saccular. (C) Dissecting.

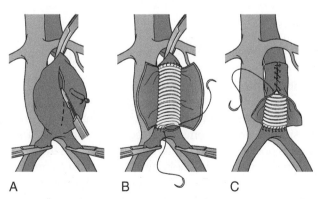

Fig. 8.20 Surgical repair of an abdominal aortic aneurysm. (A) Incising the aneurysmal sac. (B) Insertion of synthetic graft. (C) Suturing native aortic wall over synthetic graft.

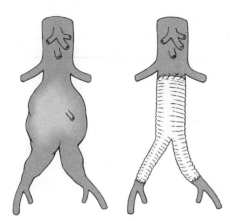

Fig. 8.21 Replacement of aortoiliac aneurysm with a bifurcated synthetic graft.

Nursing Interventions and Patient Teaching

Initial nursing interventions include monitoring the status of an existing aneurysm. Monitor the patient for signs of rupture of the aneurysm, such as paleness, weakness, tachycardia, hypotension, sudden onset of abdominal or chest pain, back pain, or groin pain and a pulsating mass in the abdomen.

Postoperative patient problems and interventions for the patient with arterial aneurysm include but are not limited to the following:

PATIENT PROBLEM	NURSING INTERVENTIONS
Compromised Blood Flow to Tissue, related to decreased arterial blood flow	Assess circulation (especially in extremities) by pedal pulse checks and capillary refill assessments
	Be alert for complications

Because aneurysm formation is associated most commonly with atherosclerosis, patient teaching focuses on managing risk factors, including control of hypertension, promotion of tissue perfusion, maintenance of skin integrity, and prevention of infection and injury.

Prognosis

An aneurysm may rupture and cause hemorrhage, resulting in death, unless emergency surgical intervention occurs. With surgical intervention, the prognosis is often good.

THROMBOANGIITIS OBLITERANS (BUERGER DISEASE)

Etiology and Pathophysiology

Thromboangiitis obliterans (Buerger disease) is an occlusive vascular condition in which the small and medium-sized arteries become inflamed and thrombotic. The cause is not understood fully, but men between the ages of 25 and 40 years who smoke are affected most commonly by the disorder. Women, however, make up as much as 40% of patients with Buerger disease. The disorder develops in the small arteries and veins of the feet and hands. Buerger disease causes inflammation and damage to the arterial walls and is a type of arteritis (Mayo Clinic,

2017d). The wrists and lower legs also may be involved. Occlusion of the arteries leads to ischemia; pain; and, in later stages, infection and ulceration. There is a strong relationship between Buerger disease and tobacco use. It is thought that the disease occurs only in smokers, and when smoking is stopped, the disease improves.

Clinical Manifestations

The inflammation of vessel walls causes occlusion of the vessel resulting in pain which is the most common symptom. Pain occurs with exercise affecting the arch of the foot, also called *instep claudication*. When the hands are involved, the pain is usually bilaterally symmetric (equal). Pain may occur at rest and be frequent and persistent, particularly when the patient also has atherosclerosis. The skin on the affected extremity may be cold and pale, and ulcers and gangrene may be present. Sensitivity to cold is an outstanding clinical manifestation.

Assessment

Subjective data include information about pain, claudication, and sensitivity to cold in affected extremities and risk factor assessment.

Objective data include presence of pulses, skin color, and temperature in the affected extremities.

Diagnostic Tests

No diagnostic tests are specific to Buerger disease. Diagnosis is based on age of onset; history of tobacco use; clinical symptoms; involvement of distal vessels; presence of ischemic ulcerations; and exclusion of diabetes mellitus, autoimmune disease, and proximal source of emboli. Diagnostic tests are done to rule out other diagnosis. An angiogram may help provide some insight and is conducted on more than one limb including a limb with no signs or symptoms (Mayo Clinic, 2019b).

Medical Management

Medical management is directed at preventing disease progression. Modifying risk factors and smoking cessation are the major focus. Smoking causes vasoconstriction and decreases blood supply to the extremities. Treatment includes complete cessation of tobacco use in any form (including secondhand smoke and nicotine-replacement products). Continued smoking can lead to complete lack of blood flow to extremities. Medications may be prescribed to dissolve clots dilate blood vessels and improve blood flow. Trauma to the extremities must be avoided. Exercise to develop collateral circulation is encouraged. Surgical intervention, such as amputation of gangrenous fingers and toes, may be indicated. A sympathectomy (a surgical interruption of part of the sympathetic nerve pathways) to alleviate pain and vasospasm also may be performed.

Nursing Interventions and Patient Teaching

The hazards of cigarette smoking and its relationship to Buerger disease are the primary focus of patient teaching. None of the palliative treatments are effective if the patient does not stop smoking. The patient is also educated to avoid secondhand smoke (Mayo Clinic, 2019b). Nowhere are the consequences of smoking so dramatically seen as with Buerger disease.

Other nursing interventions focus on managing risk factors, promoting tissue perfusion, providing comfort measures, and patient teaching. Care of the extremities to prevent necrosis and gangrene includes hydration and cleanliness. Well-fitting shoes and socks alleviate pressure. Wearing gloves in the winter helps protect hands from cold and decreases vasoconstriction. Exercise helps ease some of the pain of this disease therefore 30 minutes of moderate aerobic exercise on most days of the week is recommended (Mayo Clinic, 2019b).

Prognosis
Buerger disease is a chronic condition. Amputation may be necessary if the condition progresses to gangrene with chronic infection and extensive tissue destruction. The prognosis improves if the patient stops smoking. When patients are compliant with therapy, 94% of patients avoid amputation. The 8-year amputation rate for patients who continue to smoke is 43% (Nassiri, 2017).

RAYNAUD DISEASE
Etiology and Pathophysiology
Raynaud disease is caused by intermittent arterial spasms. Intermittent attacks of ischemia, especially of the fingers, toes, ears, and nose, are caused by exposure to cold or by emotional stimuli. Raynaud disease is either primary or secondary. The cause of primary Raynaud's is unknown, and the condition is usually mild. When symptoms occur in association with autoimmune diseases, a diagnosis of secondary Raynaud disease is made. Primary Raynaud disease usually occurs before 30 years of age, whereas secondary Raynaud disease usually occurs after age 30. Secondary Raynaud disease is associated with other conditions such as scleroderma (a relatively rare autoimmune disease affecting blood vessels and connective tissue), rheumatoid arthritis, systemic lupus erythematosus, drug intoxication, and occupational trauma. It usually affects women and is more prevalent during the winter months. The exact cause is unknown, but emotional stress, alterations in the nervous system and immunologic system, and hypersensitivity to cold may play a role in the development of signs and symptoms. Few arterial changes occur initially, but as the disease progresses, the intimal wall thickens and the medial wall hypertrophies.

Clinical Manifestations
The patient typically complains of chronically cold hands and feet. During arterial spasms, pallor, coldness, numbness, cutaneous cyanosis, and burning, throbbing pain occur. Chronic Raynaud disease may result in ulcerations on the fingers and toes.

Assessment
Collection of subjective data includes determining underlying disease processes and evaluating risk factors. The patient may complain of cold hands or feet and a throbbing, aching pain with a tingling sensation (Mayo Clinic, 2017e).

Collection of objective data includes assessment of pallor; edema; coldness; blanching; cyanosis; and reactive hyperemia (increased blood in part of the body, caused by increased blood flow), which instigates **rubor** (redness), after an arterial spasm. Inspect the fingers and toes for ulceration because of circulatory inadequacy and residual waste products.

Diagnostic Tests
A cold stimulation test is used to diagnose Raynaud disease. Skin temperature changes are recorded by a thermistor attached to each finger. Submerge the patient's hand in an ice water bath for 20 seconds and record ongoing temperatures. A comparison is made for baseline data.

Medical Management
Medical therapy is aimed at prevention. Drug therapy may be prescribed to reduce pain and promote circulation. At present, first-line drug therapy involves calcium channel blockers, such as nifedipine and diltiazem, to relax smooth muscles of the arterioles. Nifedipine is preferred over diltiazem, because it has a stronger vasodilating effect and less effect on the calcium channels in the conduction system in the heart (Mayo Clinic, 2017e). Biofeedback techniques have been used to increase skin temperature and thereby prevent spasms. Relaxation training and stress management are effective for some patients. Temperature extremes should be avoided. The patient should stop using all tobacco products and avoid caffeine and other drugs with vasoconstrictive effects such as amphetamines and cocaine. Possible surgical interventions include sympathectomy for symptomatic relief. If the disease is advanced, with ulcerations and gangrene, the involved area may have to be amputated.

Nursing Interventions and Patient Teaching
Nursing interventions are similar to those for other arterial disorders: promoting tissue perfusion, maintaining comfort, and preventing injury and infection. Risk factor management includes stress reduction techniques and smoking cessation as well as decreasing the amount of alcohol consumption. Patients should be cautioned to avoid drastic temperature changes. Exercise is encouraged to increase blood flow. Stress reduction techniques help in preventing triggers for attacks. Patients should be educated on what to do if an attack occurs. Gentle warming of extremities is stressed. If patients are outdoors, they should get indoors or to a warmer environment. Moving the fingers, hands, and arms can increase circulation as well

as placing the hands under the axilla and massaging hands and feet (Mayo Clinic, 2017e).

Patient problem statements and interventions stress patient teaching for the patient with Raynaud disease, including but not limited to the following:

PATIENT PROBLEM	NURSING INTERVENTIONS
Insufficient Knowledge, related to: • Effects of cigarette smoking • Stress reduction • Avoidance of exposure to cold	Develop teaching plan to include the following: • Effects of smoking on vasoconstriction and arterial blood flow • Techniques for smoking cessation: Stop-smoking programs, biofeedback, hypnosis • Techniques for stress reduction: Massage, imagery, music, exercise, lifestyle changes • Ways to avoid exposure to cold: Layer clothing, wear mittens and warm socks during winter, use caution when cleaning the refrigerator and freezer, wear gloves when handling frozen food, and avoid occupations requiring constant exposure to cold

Prognosis

Raynaud disease persists but may be controlled by protecting the body and extremities from the cold and using mild sedatives and vasodilators. No serious disability develops, but this condition sometimes is associated with rheumatoid arthritis or scleroderma.

VENOUS DISORDERS

Venous disorders occur when the blood flow is interrupted in returning from the tissues to the heart. Changes in smooth muscle and connective tissue make the veins less distensible. The valves in the veins may malfunction, causing backflow of blood. The major venous disorders are thrombophlebitis and varicose veins (Table 8.11).

THROMBOPHLEBITIS

Etiology and Pathophysiology

Thrombophlebitis is the inflammation of a vein in conjunction with the formation of a thrombus. It occurs more frequently in women and affects people of all races. The incidence increases with aging. Other factors associated with thrombophlebitis include venous stasis, hypercoagulability (excessive clotting) of the blood, and trauma to the blood vessel wall. Immobilized patients who have had surgical procedures involving pelvic blood vessel manipulation, such as total hip replacement or pelvic surgery, or patients with MI are prone to thrombophlebitis.

Table 8.11   Venous Disorders

SIGNS AND SYMPTOMS	MEDICAL MANAGEMENT AND NURSING INTERVENTIONS
Thrombophlebitis	
Entire extremity may be pale, cold, and edematous Area along vein may be erythematous and warm to touch Patient may have Homan sign: Pain in calf on dorsiflexion Superficial veins feel indurated (hard) and thready or cordlike and are sensitive to pressure Extremities have difference in circumference	Maintain bed rest during acute phase Apply warm, moist heat to reduce discomfort and pain per health care provider's orders Elevate extremity, but do not use pillows under the knees, and never bend the knees Assess circulation of the affected extremity, and skin condition and pulses in all extremities Measure calf circumference daily and record Use antiembolism stocking on unaffected extremity Administer heparin or enoxaparin and warfarin per health care provider's orders Administer fibrinolytics (streptokinase) to resolve the thrombus per health care provider's orders Begin exercise program after acute phase per health care provider's orders
Varicose Veins	
Veins appear as darkened, tortuous, raised blood vessels; more pronounced on prolonged standing Legs feel heavy Patient has fatigue Patient has pain and muscle cramps Legs are edematous Ulcers are seen on skin	Conservative treatment: • Elevate legs 10–15 min at least q2–3h. • Wear elastic stockings. • Unna's paste boot is recommended for the older or debilitated person with cutaneous ulcers. • Avoid standing for long periods. • Avoid anything that impedes venous flow, such as garters, tight girdles, crossing the legs, and prolonged sitting. • Reduce weight if obese. • Inject sclerosing solutions for small varicosities. Surgery: • Venous ligation and stripping

Thrombophlebitis develops in deep veins (DVT) (Fig. 8.22) or in superficial veins (superficial thrombophlebitis). Thrombophlebitis usually occurs in an extremity, most frequently a leg. Superficial thrombophlebitis is often minor and is treated with elevation, anti-inflammatory agents, and warm compresses. DVT is a condition involving a thrombus in a deep vein

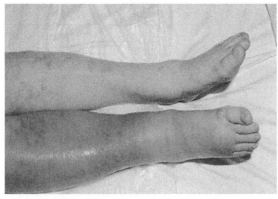

Fig. 8.22 Deep vein thrombosis. (From Lewis SL, Heitkemper MM, Dirksen SR, et al: *Medical-surgical nursing: Assessment and management of clinical problems*, ed 7, St. Louis, 2007, Mosby.)

such as the iliac or femoral veins. It is of greater significance and the thrombus can prevent blood flow to an area or it can become dislodged, carried to the lungs via the bloodstream, and cause a pulmonary embolus. Pulmonary embolism is a life-threatening complication. The CDC (2017) estimates that 900,000 people could be affected by DVT (1 to 2 per 1000) each year in the United States, and 60,000 to 100,000 Americans die of DVT/PE (pulmonary embolism). The CDC also estimates that 10% to 30% of people will die within 1 month of diagnosis, and sudden death is the first symptom in about one-fourth (25%) of people who have a PE.

Clinical Manifestations

Pain and edema commonly occur when the vein is obstructed; however, some patients do not experience pain. The circumference of the calf or thigh may increase. In the past it was believed that active dorsiflexion of the foot may result in calf pain when thrombophlebitis is present. This is referred to as a positive Homans sign. *Homans sign* has been found to be an unreliable sign, because it is not specific for DVT and appears in only 10% of patients with DVT. Superficial thrombophlebitis may show signs of inflammation such as erythema, warmth, and tenderness along the course of the vein.

Assessment

Subjective data include characteristics of pain in the affected extremity, noting onset and duration and any history of venous disorders.

Collection of objective data includes inspecting the extremity and determining color and temperature (pale and cold if vein is occluded; erythematous and warm if a superficial vein is inflamed). Measure both legs for circumference and comparison and to detect edema. Signs of decreased circulation may occur distal to the area of the clot. The degree of blockage determines the severity of the symptoms.

Diagnostic Tests

Diagnostic tests for DVT include venous Doppler, duplex scanning (the most widely used test), and

venography (phlebography). The results of a serum D-dimer test are elevated in DVT. D-dimer is a fibrin degradation fragment, the result of fibrinolysis. When a thrombus is undergoing lysis (destruction), it results in increased D-dimer fragments.

Medical Management

Anticoagulant therapy is used for DVT prevention and treatment. For an existing DVT, anticoagulant therapy prevents extension of the clot, development of a new clot, or embolization (embolus traveling through the bloodstream). Anticoagulants do not dissolve a clot, but they help the clot from growing in size. Warfarin can be given subcutaneously or intravenously. Other common anticoagulants that are administered subcutaneously include enoxaparin, dalteparin, or fondaparinux. Lysis (destruction) of the clot begins immediately by the body's own fibrinolytic system, but for more serious thrombi, thrombolytics such as streptokinase and tissue-type plasminogen activator (tPA) may be

---

⚠ Safety Alert

Patient on Anticoagulant Therapy

1. Teach patient receiving oral warfarin about the requirements for frequent follow-up with blood tests (PT, INR) to assess blood clotting and whether a change in drug dosage is required.
2. Teach patient side effects and adverse effects of anticoagulant therapy requiring medical attention.
   - Any bleeding that does not stop after a reasonable time (usually 10–15 min)
   - Blood in urine or stool or black, tarry stools
   - Unusual bleeding from gums, throat, skin, or nose, or heavy menstrual bleeding
   - Severe headaches or stomach pains
   - Weakness, dizziness, mental status changes
   - Vomiting blood
   - Cold, blue, or painful feet
3. Avoid any trauma or injury that may cause bleeding (e.g., vigorous brushing of teeth, contact sports, inline roller skating).
4. Do not take aspirin-containing drugs or NSAIDs because of the blood-thinning effects these drugs contribute.
5. Limit alcohol intake to small amounts. Alcohol interferes with metabolism of the drug.
6. Wear a medical-alert bracelet or necklace indicating what anticoagulant is being taken.
7. Avoid marked changes in eating habits, such as dramatically increasing foods high in vitamin K (e.g., broccoli, spinach, kale, greens). Do not take supplemental vitamin K.
8. Inform all health care providers, including dentist, of anticoagulant therapy.
9. Correct dosing is essential, and supervision may be required (e.g., for patients experiencing confusion).
10. Do not use herbal products that may alter coagulation.

administered intravenously or via a catheter placed with a cardiac catheterization. Venous filters may be necessary to prevent PE by blocking a moving clot if clots are large or if the patient cannot tolerate medications (Mayo Clinic, 2017f).

Low-molecular-weight heparin (LMWH) is effective for the prevention of venous thrombosis and any extension or recurrence. Enoxaparin and dalteparin are two types of LMWH. LMWH is administered subcutaneously in fixed doses, once or twice daily. LMWH has the practical advantage that it does not require anticoagulant monitoring and dose adjustment. LMWH has greater bioavailability, a more predictable dose response, and a longer half-life than heparin with less risk of bleeding complications.

The affected extremity is elevated periodically above heart level to prevent venous stasis and to reduce edema. Specific orders depend on the health care provider's preference. When the patient ambulates, elastic stockings (antiembolism stockings) are used to compress the superficial veins, increase blood flow through the deep veins, and prevent venous stasis. Warm compresses may be ordered if the thrombus is superficial.

Surgery is indicated only when conservative measures have been unsuccessful. A thrombectomy (removal of a clot from a blood vessel) or the transvenous placement of a grid or umbrella in the vena cava may be done to prevent the flow of emboli into the lungs. The inferior vena caval interruption device can be inserted percutaneously through the superficial femoral or internal jugular vein. When the filter device is opened, the spokes penetrate the vessel walls. The device creates a "sieve-type" obstruction, filtrating clots without interrupting blood flow.

Nursing Interventions and Patient Teaching
Early mobilization is the easiest and most cost-effective method to decrease the risk of DVT. Patients on bed rest must be instructed to change position, dorsiflex their feet, and rotate their ankles every 2 to 4 hours. Ambulatory patients should ambulate at least three times per day. Elastic compression stockings (e.g., thromboembolic disease hose) and/or an intermittent compression device are used for hospitalized patients at risk for DVT. The major emphasis for the patient with thrombophlebitis is to prevent complications, promote comfort, and teach about the disease and how to prevent a recurrence. Patients should avoid extended periods of inactivity. When traveling, the patient must wear antiembolism stockings and take frequent breaks to ambulate.

Patient problems and interventions for the patient with thrombophlebitis include but are not limited to the following:

NURSING DIAGNOSIS	NURSING INTERVENTIONS
Compromised Blood Flow to Tissue, related to decreased venous blood flow	Confine patient to bed in acute phase
	Elevate affected extremity according to health care provider's orders
	Check circulation frequently (monitor pedal pulses, capillary refill)
	Administer prescribed anticoagulants, and fibrinolytics
	Measure calf or thigh circumference daily
	Assess site for signs of inflammation and edema
	Have patient wear elastic stockings when ambulatory
	Implement graded exercise program as ordered
Insufficient Knowledge, related to disease process and risk factors	Develop a teaching plan to prevent venous stasis, including the following:
	• Avoid prolonged sitting or standing; begin weight reduction if obese
	• Avoid crossing the legs at the knee and wearing tight stockings or garters
	• Elevate legs when sitting
	• Do flexion-extension exercises of feet and legs when sitting or lying down to promote circulation and venous return
	• Do not massage extremities because of danger of embolization of clots (thrombus breaking off and becoming an embolus)
	• Take prescribed medication

Prognosis
A major risk during the acute phase of DVT is dislodgment of the thrombus, which can migrate to the lungs, causing a pulmonary embolus. Postphlebetic syndrome also may develop after a DVT. Inflammation of the vein at the site of the thrombus may be temporary or may be a long-term complication. Postphlebetic syndrome results in swelling of the extremity. Elevation and antiembolism stockings generally are prescribed.

VARICOSE VEINS

Etiology and Pathophysiology
A varicose vein is a tortuous, dilated vein with incompetent valves. The highest incidence of varicose veins occurs in women ages 40 to 60 years. Approximately 15% of the adult population is affected. Causes of

varicose veins include congenitally defective valves, an absent valve, or a valve that becomes incompetent. External pressure on the legs from pregnancy or obesity can place a strain on the vessels, and they become elongated and dilated. Poor posture, prolonged standing, and constrictive clothing also may contribute to this problem. The great and small saphenous veins of the legs are affected most often. The vessel wall weakens and dilates, stretching the valves and leaving the vessel unable to support a column of blood. Pooling of blood in the veins or varicosities is the result. Chronic blood pooling in the veins is referred to as *venous stasis.* Hemorrhage can occur if a varicose vein suffers trauma.

Clinical Manifestations
Varicose veins may be primary or secondary. Primary varicosities have a gradual onset and occur in superficial veins. Secondary varicosities affect the deep veins and result from chronic venous insufficiency or venous thrombosis. Often the only symptom is the appearance of darkened veins on the patient's legs. Symptoms include fatigue, dull aches, cramping of muscles, and a feeling of heaviness or pressure arising from decreased blood flow to the tissues. Signs and symptoms such as edema, pain, changes in skin color, and ulceration may occur as a result of venous stasis.

Assessment
Collection of subjective data includes gathering information about predisposing factors: a family history of varicose veins, pregnancy, or other conditions that could cause pressure on the veins. Also include symptoms the patient is experiencing such as aches, fatigue, cramping, heaviness, and pain.

Collection of objective data includes inspecting the legs for varicosities, edema, color, and temperature of the skin and observing for ulceration.

Diagnostic Tests
Trendelenburg test is done to diagnose the ability of the venous valves to support a column of blood by measuring venous filling time. The patient lies down with the affected leg raised to allow for venous emptying. A tourniquet is applied above the knee, and the patient stands. The direction and filling time of the veins are recorded before and after the tourniquet is removed. When the veins fill rapidly from a backward blood flow, the veins are determined to be incompetent.

Medical Management
Mild signs and symptoms may be controlled with elastic stockings, rest periods, and leg elevation. Sclerotherapy consists of injection of a sclerosing solution at the sites of the varicosities. It is done as an outpatient procedure and produces permanent obliteration (complete occlusion of a part) of collapsed veins and good cosmetic results. Elastic bandages are applied for continuous

pressure for 1 to 2 weeks. Surgical intervention is indicated for pain, progression of varicosities, edema, and stasis ulcers, and for cosmetic reasons. Surgery consists of vein ligation and stripping. The great saphenous vein is ligated (tied) close to the femoral junction. The great and small saphenous veins are stripped out through small incisions made in the inguinal area, above and below the knee and the ankle. The incisions are covered with sterile dressings, and an elastic bandage is applied and worn for at least 1 week. Newer, laser treatments are available for smaller varicosities.

Nursing Interventions and Patient Teaching
Nursing interventions focus on care of the patient after a surgical procedure, including maintaining comfort, maintaining peripheral circulation and venous return, and teaching the patient about varicose vein prevention and maintenance.

Patient problems and interventions for the patient with varicose veins include but are not limited to the following:

PATIENT PROBLEM	NURSING INTERVENTIONS
Compromised Blood Flow to Tissue, related to impaired venous blood return	Monitor for signs and symptoms of bleeding postoperatively. If bleeding occurs, apply pressure to the wound, elevate the leg, and notify the health care provider
	Keep elastic bandage snug and wrinkle free; do not remove bandage for daily dressing change
	Encourage deep breathing exercises and early ambulation to facilitate venous return
	Encourage dorsiflexion exercises while in bed or sitting to facilitate venous return
Insufficient Knowledge, related to disease process and measures to avoid venous stasis and promote venous return	Develop teaching plan to include the following: • Avoid anything that can increase pressure above the knees (crossing the legs, sitting in chairs that are too high, wearing garters and knee-high stockings) • Begin regular exercise to promote venous return by contraction of leg muscles • Avoid prolonged sitting or standing • Elevate legs when sitting • Maintain ideal weight • Wear elastic stockings for support for activities that require prolonged standing or when pregnant. These measures are aimed at those people who are at greater risk, to decrease occurrences

Prognosis

Varicosities are chronic conditions if not treated surgically; the affected person must know how to prevent venous stasis and encourage venous return. Prevention is the key to preventing complications. Patients should avoid prolonged sitting with regular exercise and weight reduction. Noncompliance can result in chronic swelling, pain, decreased circulation, and possibly ulcerations.

VENOUS STASIS ULCERS

Etiology and Pathophysiology

Venous stasis ulcers or leg ulcers occur from chronic deep vein insufficiency and stasis of blood in the venous system of the legs. Other causes include severe varicose veins, burns, trauma, sickle cell anemia, diabetes mellitus, neurogenic disorders, and hereditary factors. A leg ulcer is an open, necrotic lesion that results when an inadequate supply of oxygen-rich blood and nutrients reaches the tissue (Fig. 8.23). The results are cell death, tissue sloughing, and skin impairment. Decreased circulation to the area contributes to the development of infection and prolonged healing.

Clinical Manifestations

Patients may report varying degrees of pain, from mild discomfort to a dull, aching pain relieved by elevation of the extremity. The skin is visibly ulcerated and has a leathery appearance and dark pigmentation. Edema

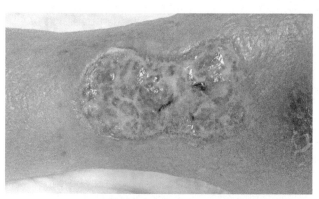

Fig. 8.23 Venous leg ulcer.

may be present. Ulcerations often occur around the medial aspect of the ankle. Pedal pulses are present.

Assessment

Subjective data include onset and duration of pain and successful relief measures. Predisposing factors such as thrombophlebitis, venous insufficiency, and diabetes mellitus are noted.

Collection of objective data includes inspection of ulcerated areas: size, location, and condition of skin; color; and temperature. Palpate pedal pulses and observe for edema.

Diagnostic Tests

Venography and Doppler ultrasonography are used to confirm venous insufficiency and stasis. See the section "Diagnostic Tests" under "Venous Assessment" for a description of what is included in these tests. They show slow progression of blood to the extremities.

Medical Management

Management focuses on promoting wound healing and preventing infection. Diet is important to ensure adequate protein intake, because large amounts of protein in the form of albumin are lost through the ulcers. Also, vitamins A and C and the mineral zinc are administered to promote tissue healing. Debridement of necrotic tissue, antibiotic therapy, and protection of the ulcerated area are usual treatments. Debridement can be mechanical with a debriding instrument. Debridement also may be chemical; enzyme ointments such as fibrinolysin with DNase (deoxyribonuclease, Elase) are placed over the ulcer to break down necrotic tissue. Medihoney is currently a common treatment. It is a medical-grade honey product that promotes healing by providing a low pH-balanced moisture environment. Therapy for a venous stasis ulcer also may consist of saline irrigation with ultrasound therapy called MIST therapy. Surgical debridement using a scalpel is done when other measures are not successful.

Applying compression to the affected area is essential to promote venous ulcer healing and to prevent

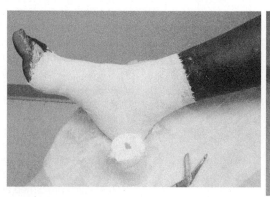
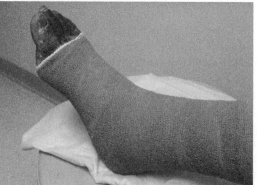

Fig. 8.24 The stages of application of the Unna's paste boot, using specially impregnated gauze. Most ulcers are on the inferior aspect of the patient's foot. (From Cameron MH, Monroe LG: *Physical rehabilitation for physical therapist assistant*, St. Louis, 2011, Saunders.)

ulcer recurrence. Compression options include elastic wraps, custom-fitted compression stockings, and intermittent compression devices. Coban can be used to apply compression. Compression therapy is usually maintained for an average of 3 days; therefore, circulation must be assessed to prevent decreased circulation from the extremity swelling or from the compression being applied too tightly. If copious amounts of drainage occur, compression therapy may be challenging. An Unna's paste boot can be used to protect the ulcer and provide constant and even support to the area (Fig. 8.24). Moist, impregnated gauze is wrapped around the patient's foot and leg. It hardens into a "boot" that may be left on for 1 to 2 weeks, although it may be changed more often if there is copious drainage. This treatment is not used as commonly today. Balanced nutrition to promote healing is important with an emphasis on increasing protein.

Nursing Interventions and Patient Teaching

Nursing interventions focus on promoting wound healing, promoting comfort, maintaining peripheral tissue perfusion, preventing infection, and patient teaching.

Patient problems and interventions for the patient with venous stasis ulcers include but are not limited to the following:

PATIENT PROBLEM	NURSING INTERVENTIONS
Compromised Skin Integrity, related to venous insufficiency as evidenced by open ulceration	Perform dressing changes per health care provider's order, using gauze, moistened with saline, topical drug treatments, and Unna's boot therapy
	Assess wound for signs and symptoms of infection
	Provide antibiotic therapy as prescribed
	Encourage nutritional intake to promote wound healing
Compromised Blood Flow to Tissue, related to insufficient venous circulation	Elevate extremities when sitting or lying down to promote venous return and decrease risk of edema and venous stasis
	Use overbed cradle to protect extremities from pressure of bed linens
	Use cotton between toes to prevent pressure on a toe ulcer
	Assess level of discomfort

Patient teaching focuses on preventing infection, maintaining peripheral tissue circulation, avoiding venous stasis, and providing proper wound care and dressing changes. See previous nursing diagnoses and interventions.

Prognosis

Venous stasis ulcers are a chronic condition caused by chronic venous insufficiency and delayed healing. Most venous ulcers heal with therapy.

❖ NURSING PROCESS FOR THE PATIENT WITH A CARDIOVASCULAR DISORDER

The role of the licensed practical nurse/licensed vocational nurse (LPN/LVN) in the nursing process as stated is that the LPN/LVN will:
- Participate in planning care for patients based on patient needs
- Review patient's care plan and recommend revisions as needed
- Review and follow defined prioritization for patient care
- Use clinical pathways, care maps, or care plans to guide and review patient care

Systemic cardiac assessment provides baseline data useful for identifying the patient's physiologic and psychosocial needs.

◆ ASSESSMENT

Begin assessment of the patient with a cardiovascular disorder by performing a complete health history and physical assessment. The physical assessment includes level of consciousness, vital signs, lung sounds (crackles, wheezes), bowel sounds, apical heart sounds (strength, regularity of rhythm), pedal pulses, capillary refill, skin color (pallor, cyanosis), turgor, temperature and moisture, and presence of edema. The history includes a description of symptoms, when they occurred, their course and duration, location, precipitating factors, and relief measures. Specific signs and symptoms to be aware of include the following:
- *Pain:* Note the character, quality, radiation, and associated symptoms. Ask the patient to rate pain on a scale of 0 to 10. Determine what, if anything, relieved the pain, such as rest or medication (e.g., nitroglycerin sublingually). Chest pain is the primary complaint when patients have symptoms of heart disease. Some patients with ischemia have pain in the jaw and left shoulder. The patient may describe the pain as dull, sharp, pressure, squeezing, crushing, viselike, grinding, or radiating. Note any factors precipitating the onset. Pain originating from cardiac muscle ischemia (decreased blood supply to a body organ or part) produces anxiety. It may lead to other signs and symptoms such as nausea, vertigo, or diaphoresis. Chest pain is significant in indicating cardiac ischemia or damage.
- *Palpitations:* Characterized by rapid, irregular, or pounding heartbeat, palpitations may be associated with cardiac dysrhythmias (any disturbance or abnormality in a normal rhythmic pattern) or cardiac ischemia. Patients may begin to notice the heartbeat

and describe it as "pounding" or "racing." This can be frightening for the patient.

- *Cyanosis:* A bluish discoloration of the skin and mucous membranes caused by an excess of deoxygenated hemoglobin in the blood. Cyanosis results from decreased cardiac output and poor peripheral perfusion.
- *Dyspnea:* Dyspnea is characterized by difficulty in breathing or shortness of breath. Observe for dyspnea with activity, referred to as *exertional dyspnea,* which commonly is associated with decreased cardiac function.
- *Orthopnea:* Orthopnea is an abnormal condition in which a person must sit or stand to breathe deeply or comfortably.
- *Cough:* The cough may be dry or productive and results from a fluid accumulation in the lungs. The patient may describe it as irritating or spasmodic. Dyspnea may be associated with it. The production of sputum should be observed for frothiness or hemoptysis (see the section "Pulmonary Edema").
- *Fatigue:* Exhaustion and activity intolerance are associated with decreased cardiac output. The patient may be unable to perform ADLs. Depression may accompany this or be a result of it.
- *Syncope:* Syncope or fainting is a brief lapse of consciousness caused by transient cerebral hypoxia. It usually is preceded by a sensation of lightheadedness. It can result from a sudden decrease in cardiac output to the brain as a result of dysrhythmia (bradycardia or tachycardia) or decreased pumping action of the heart.
- *Diaphoresis:* Sweating, especially profuse sweating, is associated with clamminess. Diaphoresis is a result of decreased cardiac output and poor peripheral perfusion.
- *Edema:* Weight gain of more than 3 pounds in 24 hours may be indicative of HF. The mechanism leading to edema in HF is the inability of the heart to pump efficiently or accept venous return, causing retrograde blood flow and an excessive amount of circulating blood volume. This increased blood volume results in increased hydrostatic pressure and an increase in fluid in the interstitial spaces.

◆ PATIENT PROBLEM

Assess the patient's cardiovascular system and identify characteristics that reveal a patient problem. Patient problems for cardiovascular problems may include the following:
- Anxiousness
- Compromised Blood Flow to Cardiac Tissue
- Discomfort
- Fluid Volume Overload
- Inability to Tolerate Activity
- Inefficient Oxygenation
- Insufficient Cardiac Output
- Insufficient Knowledge (specify)

◆ EXPECTED OUTCOMES AND PLANNING

Plan appropriate interventions to meet the needs of patients with cardiovascular problems. The nurse is uniquely qualified for ongoing patient monitoring and is able to participate in the development of nursing diagnoses, help select appropriate interventions, and document the care plan. Teaching throughout the hospital stay and when preparing for discharge is important. Reinforcement of good health habits improves the likelihood for compliance with the care plan.

◆ IMPLEMENTATION

Nursing interventions for the patient with a cardiovascular disorder include enhancing cardiac output, promoting tissue perfusion, promoting adequate gas exchange, improving activity tolerance, and promoting comfort. Patient teaching emphasizes adherence to diet and exercise and medication protocols and strategies for balancing activity, getting rest, and reducing stress.

◆ EVALUATION

Evaluate the expected outcomes as the final step of the nursing process and determine their effectiveness. Participate in the revision of the plan and nursing interventions when necessary.

Get Ready for the NCLEX® Examination!

Key Points

- The cardiovascular system is composed of the heart, blood vessels, and lymphatic structures.
- The functions of the cardiovascular system are to deliver oxygen and nutrients to the cells and to remove carbon dioxide and waste products from the cells.
- The heart is a large pump (the size of a human fist) that propels blood through the circulatory system.
- The heart is composed of four chambers: two atria and two ventricles.
- There are two coronary arteries; they supply the heart with nutrition and oxygen.
- The electrical impulse pathway starts at the SA node, which is the pacemaker of the heart; it initiates the heartbeat. The impulse travels to the AV node. From here the impulse travels to a bundle of fibers called the bundle of His, which divides into right and left bundle branches and finally to the Purkinje fibers.
- Three kinds of blood vessels are organized for carrying blood to and from the heart: the arteries, the veins, and the capillaries.

- Risk factors for developing CAD are classified as nonmodifiable and modifiable.
- Nonmodifiable risk factors for CAD include advancing age, male gender, black race, and a positive family history of CAD.
- Major modifiable risk factors for CAD include cigarette smoking, hyperlipidemia, stress, obesity, sedentary lifestyle, and hypertension. A diet high in cholesterol and saturated fats contributes to risk.
- An important aspect of caring for the patient with a cardiovascular disorder is understanding the risk factors and incorporating them into patient teaching.
- Major diagnostic tests to evaluate cardiovascular function include chest radiograph, arteriography, cardiac catheterization, ECG, echocardiogram, telemetry, stress test, PET, and thallium scanning.
- Common laboratory examinations to evaluate cardiovascular function are blood cultures, CBC, PT, INR, PTT, ESR, serum electrolytes, lipids (VLDL, LDL, HDL), triglycerides, arterial blood gases, BNP, and serum cardiac markers. Troponin I is a myocardial muscle protein released into the circulation after myocardial injury and is useful in diagnosing an MI.
- CAD includes a variety of conditions that obstruct blood flow in the coronary arteries.
- When the myocardial oxygen demand exceeds the myocardial oxygen supply, ischemia of the heart muscle occurs, resulting in chest pain or angina.
- Patient teaching to minimize the pain of angina pectoris includes taking nitroglycerin before exertion, eating small amounts more frequently rather than two or three larger meals in a day, balancing exercise periods with rest, stopping activity at the first sign of chest pain, avoiding exposure to extreme weather conditions, quitting smoking, and seeking a calm environment.
- Subjective data for the patient with MI may include heavy pressure or squeezing pressure in the chest, retrosternal pain radiating to left arm and jaw, anxiety, nausea, and dyspnea.
- Objective data for the patient with MI include pallor, hypertension, cardiac rhythm changes, vomiting, fever, and diaphoresis.
- Possible nursing diagnoses for the patient with MI include pain (acute), tissue perfusion (ineffective), activity intolerance, decreased cardiac output, anxiety, and constipation.
- Cardiac rehabilitation services are designed to help patients with heart disease recover faster and return to full and productive lives. Cardiac rehabilitation improves patient compliance.
- HF leads to the congested state of the heart, lungs, and systemic circulation as a result of the heart's inability to act as an effective pump. The most recent definition is that HF should be viewed as a neurohormonal problem that progresses as a result of chronic release in the body of substances such as catecholamines (epinephrine and norepinephrine). These substances may have toxic effects on the heart.
- It is important to realize that 1 L of fluid equals 1 kg (2.2 lb); so, a weight gain of 2.2 lb signifies a gain of 1 L of body fluid.
- Signs and symptoms of HF with left ventricular failure include dyspnea; cough; frothy, blood-tinged sputum;

pulmonary crackles; and evidence of pulmonary vascular congestion with pleural effusion.
- Signs and symptoms of HF with right ventricular failure include edema in feet, ankles, and sacrum, which may progress into the thigh and external genitalia; liver congestion; ascites; and distended jugular veins.
- Medical management of HF includes increasing cardiac efficiency with digitalis, vasodilators, and ACE inhibitors; administering a beta blocker (carvedilol) for mild to moderate HF; lowering oxygen requirements through bed rest; providing oxygen to the tissues through oxygen therapy if the patient is hypoxic; treating edema and pulmonary congestion with a diuretic and a sodium-restricted diet; and weighing daily to monitor fluid retention.
- Nursing interventions for the patient with valvular heart disease include administering the prescribed medications (diuretics, digoxin, and antidysrhythmics); monitoring I&O and daily weight; auscultating breath sounds and heart sounds; taking blood pressure; and assessing capillary perfusion, pedal pulses, and presence of edema.
- Teaching for the patient with valvular heart disease includes dietary management, activity limitations, and the importance of antibiotic prophylaxis before invasive procedures.
- Most patients with cardiomyopathy have a severe, progressively deteriorating course, and the majority older than age 55 years die within 2 years of the onset of signs and symptoms.
- PVD is any abnormal condition that affects the blood vessels outside the heart and the lymphatic vessels.
- Arteriosclerosis is the underlying problem associated with PVD.
- Hypertension occurs when there is a sustained elevated systolic blood pressure greater than 140 mm Hg and/or sustained elevated diastolic blood pressure of greater than 90 mm Hg on two or more readings.
- Nursing interventions for hypertension primarily focus on blood pressure management through patient teaching, risk factor recognition, drug therapy, dietary management, exercise, and stress-reduction techniques.
- An aneurysm is an enlarged, dilated portion of an artery and may be the result of arteriosclerosis, trauma, or a congenital defect.
- The hazards of cigarette smoking and its relationship to thromboangiitis obliterans (Buerger disease) are the primary focuses of teaching the patient with Buerger disease.
- The two major venous disorders are thrombophlebitis and varicose veins.
- Thrombophlebitis may result in calf pain on dorsiflexion of the foot, which is referred to as a positive Homans sign. However, a positive Homans sign appears in only 10% of patients with DVT.
- The patient with thrombophlebitis should be taught to avoid prolonged sitting or standing, avoid dehydration, reduce weight if obese, perform dorsiflexion-extension exercises of the feet and legs, not cross the legs at the knees, and to elevate legs when sitting.

Additional Learning Resources

SG Go to your Study Guide for additional learning activities to help you master this chapter content.

Be sure to visit the Evolve site at http://evolve.elsevier.com/Cooper/adult/ for additional online resources.

Review Questions for the NCLEX® Examination

1. A patient is admitted to the hospital with a diagnosis of heart failure. Recently the patient's symptoms have been getting worse as a result of arteriosclerosis. In establishing a patient care plan, what is the primary goal of treatment?

   1. Reduce the workload of the heart.
   2. Promote rest for the heart.
   3. Reduce fluid retention.
   4. Reduce circulating blood volume.

2. What is the best nursing action that will lessen the severity of a patient's orthostatic hypotension?

   1. Turn him from side to side every 2 hours.
   2. Limit times he will have to get in and out of the bed.
   3. Change his position routinely, especially from horizontal to vertical.
   4. Encourage him to move very slowly.

3. When caring for a patient whose health care provider has ordered furosemide (Lasix), what will the nurse recognize when the medication is having the desired effect? (Select all that apply.)

   1. The patient becomes very thirsty.
   2. The patient's resting heart rate slows.
   3. The patient's blood pressure is reduced.
   4. Production of urine is increased.
   5. The patient's weight decreases

4. A patient receives a diagnosis of angina pectoris, with no subsequent cardiac involvement. The health care provider prescribes nitroglycerin. What explanation would the nurse give to this patient about why this medication is given sublingually?

   1. Superficial blood vessels promote rapid absorption of the medication.
   2. Stomach acids destroy the medication.
   3. Saliva helps break down the medication for absorption.
   4. The medication is too rapidly absorbed in the stomach.

5. Before administering a dose of digoxin to an assigned patient, the nurse observes that the patient's pulse rate is 52. What is the most appropriate nursing action?

   1. Notify the charge nurse.
   2. Recognize that these are signs of digoxin toxicity and withhold the dose.
   3. Administer the medication.
   4. Hold the medication and notify the health care provider.

6. The nurse is assessing a patient and suspects the patient is experiencing thrombophlebitis in the lower leg. What symptoms would the nurse assess? (Select all that apply.)

   1. Numbness along a vein
   2. Severe cramping
   3. Edema of the extremity
   4. Calf is warm to the touch
   5. Pain in the effected extremity

7. When a patient is receiving heparin therapy, what would be the nurse's most appropriate action?

   1. Observe him for cyanosis.
   2. Assess degree of edema in all extremities.
   3. Give the injection intramuscularly.
   4. Observe emesis, urine, and stools for blood.

8. A patient is admitted to the medical floor with a diagnosis of HF. Which assessment findings are consistent with the medical diagnosis? (Select all that apply.)

   1. Increase in abdominal girth
   2. Weight loss of 6 pounds in the past 2 weeks
   3. Pitting edema
   4. Nervous tremors
   5. Night sweats

9. A 10-year-old patient is diagnosed with rheumatic fever. Of all the manifestations seen in rheumatic fever, which is most likely to lead to permanent complications?

   1. Sydenham chorea
   2. Erythema marginatum
   3. Subcutaneous nodules
   4. Carditis

10. A patient has a diagnosis of hypertension. When providing discharge teaching what should the nurse include? (Select all that apply.)

    1. Instruction in consuming a bland diet
    2. Instruction to limit sodium intake to 2 g/day
    3. Encouragement to begin a vigorous exercise program
    4. Monitoring and keeping a record of blood pressure measurements at home
    5. Education on continuing to take antihypertensive medications as prescribed

11. An 86-year-old patient is receiving an intravenous infusion at 83 mL/h via an electronic infusion pump. Why is it so vital that the IV lines of older adult patients be monitored carefully?

    1. These patients do not become dehydrated very easily.
    2. These patients are at an increased risk for developing fluid overload of the circulatory system.
    3. These patients are at an increased risk for developing a venous infection.
    4. Aging patients present an increased risk for developing thrombophlebitis in the peripheral system.

12. A patient with a history of IV drug use is diagnosed with acute infective endocarditis. Which nursing intervention for this patient is most appropriate?

    1. Early ambulation
    2. Restricted activity for several weeks
    3. Low-calorie diet
    4. Dilution of blood by increased fluid intake

13. A patient has a history of angina pectoris. To decrease the pain from angina pectoris, what should the patient do?

    1. Take a cardiac glycoside at the first symptom of cardiac pain.
    2. Avoid taking more than three or four nitroglycerin pills daily.
    3. Take nitroglycerin sublingually three times daily.

4. Take nitroglycerin sublingually prophylactically before strenuous exercise.

14. A 75-year-old patient is diagnosed with heart failure. The nursing diagnosis of *Activity Intolerance, related to dyspnea and fatigue,* would be appropriate. What nursing intervention would be most appropriate for this diagnosis?

    1. Plan frequent rest periods.
    2. Allow the patient to shower.
    3. Encourage the patient to perform all ADLs.
    4. Encourage fluid intake of 3000 mL/day.

15. A patient presents with dependent edema of the extremities, enlargement of the liver, oliguria, jugular vein distention, and abdominal distention. What does the nurse suspect the patient is experiencing?

    1. Right-sided heart failure
    2. Left-sided heart failure
    3. Cardiac dysrhythmias
    4. Valvular heart disease

16. What is the primary goal of patient teaching after a myocardial infarction?

    1. Explaining the disease process
    2. Assisting the patient in developing a healthy lifestyle
    3. Describing the precipitating causes and onset of pain
    4. Educating the patient on causative factors that initiate cardiac vasoconstriction

17. A patient experienced intense chest pain, anxiety, and nausea. The admitting diagnosis is suspected myocardial infarction. When providing care for the patient in the emergency department, the nurse must understand what about a myocardial infarction?

    1. It involves a critical reduction in blood supply to the myocardium.
    2. There is a marked increase in cardiac output.
    3. A sudden irregularity of cardiac contraction occurs.
    4. There is a marked decrease in cardiac output.

18. When providing patient teaching regarding coronary artery disease, the nurse can include which of the following when advising the patient about modifiable risk factors? *(Select all that apply.)*

    1. Family history
    2. Smoking
    3. Cholesterol level
    4. Obesity
    5. Ethnicity

19. When a patient returns to the unit following cardiac catheterization, which nursing activity should follow immediately after taking of vital signs?

    1. Placing the patient in a warm bed and encouraging sleep
    2. Providing the patient with fluids

3. Assessing the patient's peripheral pulses
4. Reapplying the patient's dressing where the dye was injected

20. What is the most useful noninvasive diagnostic tool for evaluating the patient with heart failure?

    1. Coronary angiography
    2. Echocardiogram
    3. Electrocardiogram
    4. Thallium scanning

21. What actions would the nurse expect to be used to treat heart failure? *(Select all that apply.)*

    1. Cardiotonic drugs (digitalis)
    2. Diuretic agents
    3. Generous fluid intake
    4. ACE inhibitors, beta-adrenergic blockers (carvedilol), nitrates
    5. Oxygen therapy

22. The nurse is aware that the patient will benefit from the administration of streptokinase and tissue plasminogen activators when administered how long after admission for acute MI signs and symptoms?

    1. In the first 24 hours
    2. In the first 30 minutes to 1 hour
    3. In the first 72 hours
    4. In the second 6 hours after an MI

23. A patient is admitted with a diagnosis of possible aortic abdominal aneurysm. What is the most important factor to monitor as a possible complication?

    1. Body temperature
    2. Skin turgor
    3. Respiratory rate
    4. Blood pressure

24. A patient has Buerger disease. What is the most important aspect of patient compliance to decrease signs and symptoms of Buerger disease?

    1. Low-fat diet
    2. Weight loss
    3. Cessation of tobacco use
    4. Keeping extremities warm

25. The nurse is providing patient teaching for a patient with Raynaud disease. Which information should be included? *(Select all that apply.)*

    1. Avoid cold.
    2. Warm hands and feet with heating pad.
    3. Practice stress reduction techniques.
    4. Comply with smoking cessation.
    5. Limit caffeine intake.

26. A man, 34, collapses at a local gym while lying on his back lifting weights. One of the trainers at the gym heard him gasp and drop his weights and turned towards him just in time to see him slide off the weight-lifting bench. Two trainers rushed over to the man, who was gasping for breath and complaining of severe weakness. One trainer took his pulse and found that it was rapid. When the man struggled harder to breathe and grabbed his chest, the trainers called for an ambulance. In the ED, the patient says that he has always struggled with his weight. "I thought I'd join a new gym," he says, "thinking no one would know me there and I could make a fresh start." The patient, who weighs 343 lb, says he has gained 5 pounds just in the last week, which is why he immediately joined a gym. Further questioning reveals that he is frequently short of breath with exertion or when lying on his back and frequently experiences fatigue "just trying to do the simplest, easiest things. It's very depressing, but it sure impresses the ladies." He says he suspects he needs a CPAP machine just like his dad had. With further questioning, he admits he was once diagnosed with heart failure, but says he resisted accepting that diagnosis. "It's what my grandpa died of," he says. He starts coughing again and coughs up pink, foamy mucus. The attending physician asks him if he knows what kind of heart failure he was diagnosed with earlier, but the patient shakes his head and says, "I didn't know there was more than one kind."

Use an X to indicate which potential assessment finding is associated with each possible client health problem. All should be used and can be used only once.

ASSESSMENT FINDINGS	LEFT VENTRICULAR FAILURE	RIGHT VENTRICULAR FAILURE
Ascites		
Distended jugular veins		
Frothy, blood-tinged sputum		
Liver enlargement with right upper quadrant pain		
Orthopnea		
Paroxysmal nocturnal dyspnea		
Pulmonary crackles		

Care of the Patient With a Respiratory Disorder

9

Objectives

Anatomy and Physiology

1. Differentiate between external and internal respiration.
2. Describe the purpose of the respiratory system and discuss the parts of the upper and lower respiratory tracts.
3. List the ways in which oxygen and carbon dioxide are transported in the blood.
4. Discuss the mechanisms that regulate respirations.

Medical-Surgical

5. Identify signs and symptoms that indicate a patient is experiencing hypoxia.
6. Differentiate among sonorous wheezes, sibilant wheezes, crackles, and pleural friction rub.
7. Describe the purpose, significance of results, and nursing interventions related to diagnostic examinations of the respiratory system.
8. Describe the significance of arterial blood gas values and differentiate between arterial oxygen tension (PaO_2) and arterial oxygen saturation (SaO_2).
9. Discuss the etiology and pathophysiology, clinical manifestations, assessment, diagnostic tests, medical management, nursing interventions, and prognosis of the patient with disorders of the upper airway.
10. Discuss nursing interventions for the patient with a laryngectomy.
11. Discuss the etiology and pathophysiology, clinical manifestations, assessment, diagnostic tests, medical management, nursing interventions, and prognosis of the patient with disorders of the lower airway.
12. Differentiate between tuberculosis infection and tuberculosis disease.
13. List nursing assessments and interventions pertaining to the care of the patient with closed-chest drainage.
14. Compare and contrast the etiology and pathophysiology, clinical manifestations, assessment, diagnostic tests, medical management, nursing interventions, and prognosis for the patient with chronic obstructive pulmonary disease, including emphysema, chronic bronchitis, asthma, and bronchiectasis.
15. State three possible nursing diagnoses for the patient with altered respiratory function.

Key Terms

adventitious (ăd-věn-TĬ-shŭs, p. 381)
atelectasis (ă-tě-LĔK-tă-sĭs, p. 413)
bronchoscopy (brŏn-KŎS-kō-pē, p. 383)
cor pulmonale (kŏr pŭl-mō-NĂ-lē, p. 423)
coryza (kō-RĬ-ză, p. 393)
crackles (KRĂK-ŭlz, p. 381)
cyanosis (sī-ă-NŌ-sĭs, p. 391)
dyspnea (DĬSP-nē-ă, p. 380)
embolism (ĔM-bō-lĭz-ŭm, p. 419)
empyema (ĕm-pī-Ē-mă, p. 408)
epistaxis (ĕp-ĭ-STĂK-sĭs, p. 386)
exacerbation (ĕg-zăs-ĕr-BĂ-shŭn, p. 427)
extrinsic (ĕk-STRĬN-zĭk, p. 428)
hypercapnia (hī-pĕr-KĂP-nē-ă, p. 427)

hypoventilation (hī-pō-věn-tĭ-LĂ-shŭn, p. 413)
hypoxia (hī-PŎK-sē-ă, p. 381)
intrinsic (ĭn-TRĬN-zĭk, p. 428)
orthopnea (ŏr-THŎP-nē-ă, p. 381)
pleural friction rubs (PLŪ-răl FRĬK-shŭn rŭbz, p. 381)
pneumothorax (nū-mō-THŎ-răks, p. 414)
proning- (p. 400)
sibilant wheezes (SĬB-ĭ-lănt wēz-ĕz, p. 381)
sonorous wheezes (sŏ-NŌR-ŭs wēz-ĕz, p. 381)
stertorous (STĔR-tĕr-ŭs, p. 388)
tachypnea (tăk-ĬP-nē-ă, p. 413)
thoracentesis (thŏ-ră-sĕn-TĒ-sĭs, p. 380)
vapotherm (p. 400)
virulent (VĬR-ū-lĕnt, p. 401)

ANATOMY AND PHYSIOLOGY OF THE RESPIRATORY SYSTEM

All cells require a continuous supply of oxygen to carry out their specialized activities. *External respiration*, or breathing, is the exchange of oxygen and carbon dioxide between the lungs and the environment. The respiratory system works with the cardiovascular system to deliver oxygen to the cells, where it provides energy to carry out metabolism. *Internal respiration* is the exchange of oxygen and carbon dioxide at the cellular level. Oxygen enters the cells while carbon dioxide leaves them. The gases diffuse across the cell

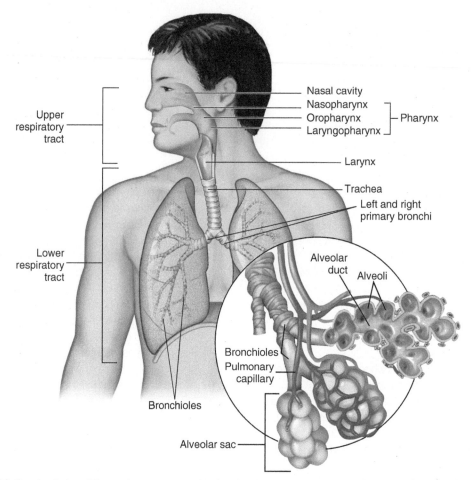

Fig. 9.1 Structural plan of the respiratory organs, showing the pharynx, trachea, bronchi, and lungs. The *inset* shows the grapelike alveolar sacs where the interchange of oxygen and carbon dioxide takes place through the thin walls of the alveoli. Capillaries surround the alveoli. (From Patton KT, Thibodeau GA: *Anatomy and physiology,* ed 8, St. Louis, 2013, Mosby.)

membrane into the bloodstream, which plays the role of transporter. Failure of the respiratory system or cardiovascular system has the same result: rapid cell death from oxygen starvation. Fig. 9.1 shows the structure of the respiratory organs.

UPPER RESPIRATORY TRACT

Nose

Air enters the respiratory tract through the nose. The air is filtered, moistened, and warmed as it enters the two nasal openings (nares) and travels to the nasal cavity. The nasal septum separates the nares. This entire area is lined with mucous membrane, which is vascular. The mucous membrane provides warmth and moisture and secretes 1 L of moisture every day.

Lateral to the nasal cavities are three scroll-like bones called *turbinates* or *conchae* (Fig. 9.2), which cause the air to move over a larger surface area. This increase in surface area provides more time for warming and moisturizing the air. Lining the nasal cavities are tiny hairs, which trap dust and other foreign particles and prevent them from entering the lower respiratory tract.

Communicating with the nasal structures are paranasal sinuses (Fig. 9.3). They are called the *frontal,*

maxillary, sphenoid, and *ethmoid cavities.* These are hollow areas that make the skull lighter and are believed to give resonance to the voice. They are lined with mucous membranes that are continuous with the nasal cavity. Because of this, nasal infections can cause sinusitis.

The receptors for the sense of smell are located in the mucosa of the nasal cavities. They are the nerve endings of the olfactory nerve, the first cranial nerve. The nasolacrimal ducts, or tear ducts, communicate with the upper nasal chamber. Therefore, crying is accompanied by copious nasal secretions.

Pharynx

The *pharynx,* or throat (a tubular structure about 5 inches [13 cm] long extending from the base of the skull to the esophagus and situated just in front of the vertebrae), is the passageway for air and food. At the distal end of the pharynx are three subdivisions: (1) the *nasopharynx* (superior portion), (2) the *oropharynx* (posterior to the mouth), and (3) the *laryngopharynx* (directly superior to the larynx) (see Fig. 9.2).

The eustachian tubes enter on either side of the nasopharynx, connecting it to the middle ear. Because the

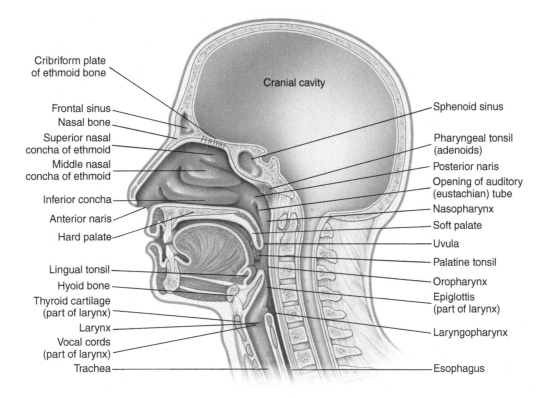

Fig. 9.2 Sagittal section through the face and the neck. (From Patton KT, Thibodeau GA: *The human body in health and disease,* ed 6, St. Louis, 2014, Mosby.)

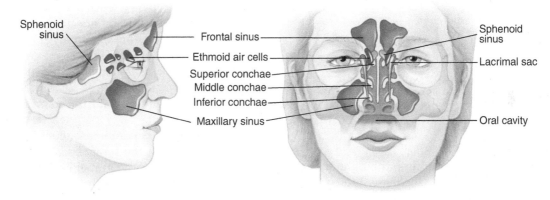

Fig. 9.3 Projections of paranasal sinuses and oral nasal cavities of the skull and the face. Note the connection between the sinuses and the nasal cavity. (From Patton KT, Thibodeau GA: *Anthonys textbook of anatomy and physiology,* ed 20, St. Louis, 2013, Mosby.)

inner linings of the pharynx and the eustachian tube are continuous, an infection of the pharynx can spread easily to the ear. This is common in children. The adenoids (pharyngeal tonsils) are in the nasopharynx, whereas the palatine tonsils are in the oropharynx.

Larynx

The *larynx* (Fig. 9.4A), or the voice box, is supported by nine areas of cartilage and connects the pharynx with the trachea. The largest area of cartilage is composed of two fused plates and is called the *thyroid cartilage,* or *Adam's apple.* It is the same size in girls and boys until puberty, when it enlarges in boys and produces a

projection in the neck. The *epiglottis,* a large leaf-shaped area of cartilage, protects the larynx when swallowing. It covers the larynx tightly to prevent food from entering the trachea and directs the food to the esophagus (see Fig. 9.4B).

The larynx contains the vocal cords. During expiration, air rushes over the vocal cords, causing them to vibrate. This enables speech to occur. The opening between the vocal cords is the glottis.

Trachea

The *trachea* (Fig. 9.5), or windpipe, is a tubelike structure that extends approximately 4⅓ inches (11 cm) to

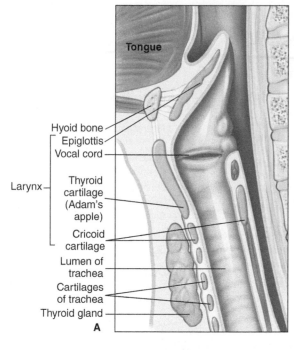

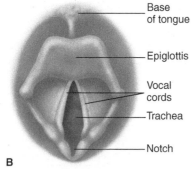

Fig. 9.4 (A) Sagittal section through the larynx. (B) Larynx and vocal cords as viewed from above, with a laryngeal mirror. (From Thibodeau GA, Patton KT: *Structure and function of the body*, ed 14, St. Louis, 2012, Mosby.)

the mid-chest, where it divides into the right and left bronchi. It lies anterior to the esophagus and connects the larynx with the bronchi. The ventral (anterior) surface of the tube is covered in the neck by the isthmus (narrow connection) of the thyroid gland. It contains C-shaped cartilaginous rings that keep it from collapsing. The open part of the C-shaped rings lies posterior to the column anterior to the esophagus, which allows the esophagus to expand during swallowing while maintaining patency of the trachea. This is necessary for uninterrupted breathing.

The entire structure is lined with mucous membranes and tiny *cilia* (small, hairlike processes on the outer surfaces of small cells, which produce motion or current in a fluid) that sweep dust or debris upward toward the nasal cavity. Any large particles initiate the cough reflex, which aids in the evacuation of foreign material. Sometimes, because of an airway obstruction, a health care provider performs a tracheotomy (i.e., creates a surgical opening, or tracheostomy, into

the trachea through which an indwelling tube may be inserted). Once this procedure is completed, the individual breathes through the tracheal opening rather than the nose or mouth. The opening is below the larynx, so air cannot pass over the vocal cords. The vocal cords cannot vibrate, and speech becomes physiologically impossible.

LOWER RESPIRATORY TRACT

Bronchial Tree

As the trachea enters the lungs, it divides into the right and left bronchi. The left bronchus enters the left lung. It is smaller in diameter and slightly more horizontal in position than the right bronchus. The right bronchus enters the right lung. It is larger in diameter and more vertical in descent than the left bronchus. Because of this positioning, foreign objects that are aspirated generally enter the right bronchus.

The bronchi divide into smaller structures called *bronchioles*. These structures divide into smaller, tubelike structures called *terminal bronchioles* or *alveolar ducts*. All these structures are lined with ciliated mucous membrane, as is the trachea. The end structures of the bronchial tree are called *alveoli*. These saclike structures resemble a bunch of grapes. A single grapelike structure is called an *alveolus* (Fig. 9.6; see Fig. 9.1). In this terminal structure of the bronchial tree, gas exchange takes place. Each alveolus is surrounded by a blood capillary, where diffusion of carbon dioxide and oxygen occurs. Alveoli are effective in gas exchange, mainly because they are extremely thin walled; each alveolus lies in contact with a blood capillary. In addition, each alveolus is coated with a thin covering of surfactant. Surfactant reduces the surface tension of the alveolus and prevents it from collapsing after each breath (see Fig. 9.6).

The lungs contain millions of alveoli; these give shape and form to the lungs and are filled with air. Alveoli, which are tiny, grapelike structures, are the most important feature of the respiratory system. In the alveoli, oxygen diffuses into the cardiovascular system.

MECHANICS OF BREATHING

Thoracic Cavity

The thoracic cavity is enclosed by the sternum, ribs, and thoracic vertebrae. The space within the cavity is occupied primarily by the lungs. The centermost area is referred to as the mediastinum or interpleural space and contains the heart and great vessels.

Lungs. The lungs are large, paired, spongy, cone-shaped organs (see Fig. 9.5). The right lung weighs approximately 625 g; the left lung weighs approximately 570 g. The right lung has three lobes; the left lung has two lobes. Located approximately 1 inch (2.5 cm) above the first rib is the narrow part (the apex) of each lung. The broad, inferior part (the base) lies on the diaphragm.

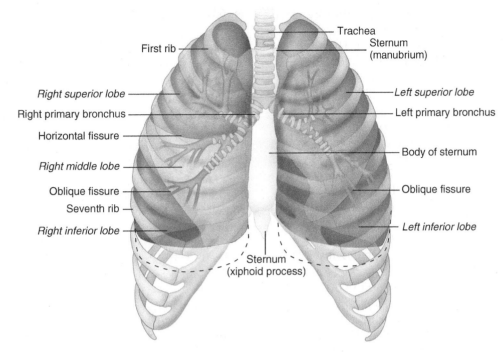

Fig. 9.5 Projection of the lungs and trachea in relation to ribcage and clavicles. *Dotted line* shows location of dome-shaped diaphragm at the end of expiration and before inspiration. Note that the apex of each lung projects above the clavicle. Ribs 11 and 12 are not visible in this view. (From Patton KT, Thibodeau GA: *Anatomy and physiology,* ed 8, St. Louis, 2013, Mosby.)

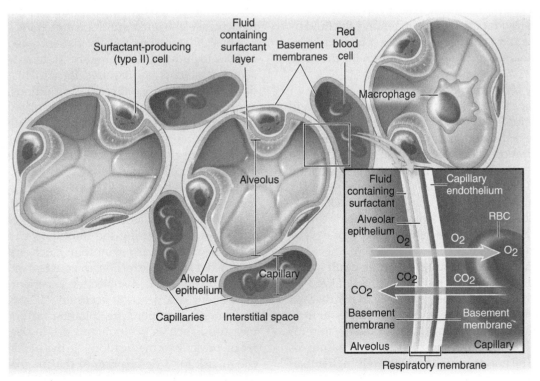

Fig. 9.6 Each alveolus is ventilated continuously with fresh air. *Inset* shows a magnified view of the respiratory membrane composed of the alveolar wall (surfactant, epithelial cells, and basement membrane), interstitial fluid, and the wall of a pulmonary capillary (basement membrane and endothelial cells). Carbon dioxide and oxygen diffuse across the respiratory membrane. (From Patton KT, Thibodeau GA: *The human body in health and disease,* ed 6, St. Louis, 2014, Mosby.)

The lungs receive their blood supply directly from the heart through the pulmonary arteries. Blood in the lung capillaries has little oxygen content. The air in the alveoli is rich in oxygen. Oxygen diffuses from the area of high concentration (alveolar air) to the area of low concentration (the lung capillaries). Blood in the lung capillaries is high in carbon dioxide, a waste product from the cells. Carbon dioxide also diffuses from the blood in the lung capillaries into the alveoli. After carbon dioxide has diffused into the alveoli and oxygen has diffused into the blood, carbon dioxide leaves the body by expiration of air from the lungs. The blood, now rich in oxygen and cleansed of its carbon dioxide, returns by the pulmonary veins to the left atrium of the heart for circulation to the rest of the body.

The surface of each lung is covered with a thin, moist, serous membrane called the *visceral pleura.* The walls of the thoracic cavity are covered with the same type of membrane, called the *parietal pleura.* The pleural cavity around the lungs is an airtight vacuum that contains negative pressure. The air in the lungs is at atmospheric pressure—higher than in the pleural cavity. The negative pressure assists in keeping the lungs inflated. The visceral and parietal pleura produce a serous secretion, which allows the lungs to slide over the walls of the thorax while breathing. Usually the body produces the exact amount of serous secretion needed. If too much serous secretion is produced, fluid accumulates in the pleural space; this is called *pleural effusion.* The pleural space becomes distended and puts pressure on the lungs, making it difficult to breathe. The health care provider may decide to remove the fluid by performing a thoracentesis—inserting a needlelike instrument into the pleural space and removing the fluid.

Respiratory Movements and Ranges

The rhythmic movements of the chest walls, ribs, and associated muscles when air is inhaled and exhaled make up the respiratory movements. The combination of one inspiration and one expiration equals one respiration. At rest the normal inspiration lasts about 2 seconds and expiration about 3 seconds.

Room air, when inhaled, contains about 21% oxygen; exhaled air contains 16% oxygen and 3.5% carbon dioxide. This represents the actual amount of oxygen used in a single breath.

The normal range of respiration for an adult at rest is 14 to 20 breaths/min. This rate can be affected by many variables, including age, sex, activity, disease, and body temperature. The respiratory rate is 40 to 60 breaths/min for a newborn, 22 to 24 breaths/min for an early school-age child, and 20 to 22 breaths/min for a teenager. The normal range for women is higher than that for men.

Members of the health care team should assess all factors influencing the patient's respiration and should count the respirations without the patient's awareness to prevent alterations in the breathing pattern.

REGULATION OF RESPIRATION

Nervous Control

The medulla oblongata and pons of the brain are responsible for the basic rhythm and depth of respiration. The body's demands can modify the rhythm. Other parts of the nervous system help coordinate the transfer from inspiration to expiration. Chemoreceptors clustered in areas of the carotid artery and aorta, called the carotid and aortic bodies, are specialized receptors. When stimulated by increasing levels of blood carbon dioxide, decreasing levels of blood oxygen, or increasing blood acidity, these receptors send nerve impulses to the respiratory centers, which in turn modify respiratory rates.

Carbon dioxide, which is present in the blood as carbonic acid, is considered the chemical stimulant for regulation of respiration. The normal pH of the blood is 7.35 to 7.45—a narrow range. If the blood pH goes outside this range, the patient develops either *acidosis* (too much acid, such as carbon dioxide, in the blood) or *alkalosis* (not enough carbon dioxide, or too much base, in the blood). After exhalation the blood becomes more alkaline.

ASSESSMENT OF THE RESPIRATORY SYSTEM

The function of the respiratory system is gas exchange (oxygen and carbon dioxide) at the alveolus-capillary level. This function depends on the lungs' ability to contract and expand, which in turn is influenced by musculoskeletal and neurologic functions.

Physical assessment of the patient's general health always includes the respiratory system. More extensive assessments are required for patients with acute or chronic respiratory or cardiac conditions, those with a history of respiratory impairment related to trauma or allergic reactions, or those who recently have undergone surgery or anesthesia. Because physical and emotional responses often are correlated, also inquire about any accompanying anxiety or stress. This information should be obtained in an unhurried, matter-of-fact manner.

The respiratory assessment includes collection of subjective data. During the interview, encourage the patient to describe any symptoms, such as shortness of breath, dyspnea on exertion, or cough. Dyspnea, or difficulty breathing, is a subjective experience that only the patient can describe accurately. Data should include onset; duration; precipitating factors; and relief measures, such as position and use of over-the-counter or prescribed medications. If the patient reports a cough, ask for a description of the cough: productive or nonproductive; harsh, dry, or hacking; and color and amount of mucus expectorated. Record this information as direct quotes from the patient when possible.

Next, gather objective data. Begin the assessment with observation. Assess respiratory rate and oxygen saturation. The patient's expression, chest movement, and respirations provide valuable visual clues. At times the patient cannot verbalize distress but has a wide-eyed, anxious look that reflects the fear of suffocating. Flaring nostrils indicate the patient is struggling to breathe, which is usually a late sign of respiratory distress. Initial observation yields information on the patient's skin color and turgor. Note any obvious respiratory distress, wheezes, or orthopnea (an abnormal condition in which a person must sit or stand to breathe deeply or comfortably).

To continue the assessment, auscultate all lung fields, anteriorly and posteriorly, comparing bilaterally. Note the presence of adventitious sounds (abnormal sounds superimposed on breath sounds, including sibilant wheezes [formerly called *wheezes*], sonorous wheezes [formerly called *rhonchi*], crackles [formerly called *rales*], and pleural friction rubs) (Table 9.1). Sibilant wheezes are musical, high-pitched, squeaking or whistling sounds caused by the rapid movement of air through narrowed bronchioles. Sonorous wheezes are low-pitched, loud, coarse, snoring sounds. They often are heard on expiration. Crackles are short, discrete, interrupted crackling or bubbling sounds that are heard most commonly during inspiration.

Crackles sound like hairs being rolled between the fingers close to the ear. They are thought to occur when air is forced through respiratory passages narrowed by fluid, mucus, or pus. They are associated with inflammation or infection of the small bronchi, bronchioles, and alveoli. Pleural friction rubs are low-pitched, grating, or creaking lung sounds that occur when inflamed pleural surfaces rub together during respiration.

Assess chest movement. Note whether the chest expands equally on both sides; chest expansion on one side only may indicate serious pulmonary complications, such as a collapsed lung. Look for retraction of the chest wall between the ribs and under the clavicle during inspiration. This can signal late-stage respiratory distress. Be alert for signs and symptoms of hypoxia (oxygen deficiency in the cellular tissues) (Box 9.1).

LABORATORY AND DIAGNOSTIC EXAMINATIONS

Diagnostic imaging, laboratory work, and more invasive measures are used to evaluate respiratory status and to identify respiratory conditions. Nurses should be familiar with these tests so they can prepare the patient adequately.

Table 9.1 Adventitious Breath Sounds

TYPE	CHARACTERISTICS	COMMENTS
Crackles (rales)	Brief, not continuous; more common in inspiration; interrupted crackling or bubbling sounds, similar to those produced by hairs being rolled between the fingers close to the ear	Caused by fluid, mucus, or pus in the small airways and alveoli
Fine crackles	As described above; high-pitched, sibilant crackling at end of inspiration	Found in diseases affecting bronchioles and alveoli
Medium crackles	As described above; medium pitch, more sonorous, moisture sound during mid-inspiration	Associated with diseases of small bronchi
Coarse crackles	As described above; loud, bubbly sound in early inspiration	Associated with diseases of small bronchi
Sonorous wheezes (rhonchi)	Deep, running sound that may be continuous; loud, low, coarse sound (like a snore) heard at any point of inspiration or expiration	Caused by air moving through narrowed tracheobronchial passages (caused by secretions, tumor, spasm); cough may alter sound if caused by mucus in trachea or large bronchi
Sibilant wheezes (wheezes)	High-pitched, musical, whistle-like sound during inspiration or expiration; sound may be several notes or one, and may vary from one minute to the next	Caused by narrowed bronchioles; bilateral wheeze is often the result of bronchospasm; unilateral, sharply localized wheeze may result from foreign matter or tumor compression
Pleural friction rub	Dry, creaking, grating, low-pitched sound with a machinelike quality during both inspiration and expiration; loudest over anterior chest	Sound originates outside respiratory tree, usually caused by inflammation; over the lung fields it suggests pleurisy; over the pericardium it suggests pericarditis with a pericardial friction rub. To distinguish the two, ask the patient to hold the breath briefly. If the rubbing sound persists, it is a pericardial friction rub because the inflamed pericardial layers continue rubbing together with each heartbeat; a pleural rub would stop when breathing stops

Box 9.1	Signs and Symptoms of Hypoxia

- Apprehension, anxiety, restlessness
- Decreased ability to concentrate
- Disorientation
- Decreased level of consciousness
- Increased fatigue
- Vertigo
- Behavioral changes
- Increased pulse rate; bradycardia as hypoxia advances
- Increased rate and depth of respiration; shallow, slow respirations as hypoxia progresses
- Elevated blood pressure; with continuing oxygen deficiency, decreased blood pressure
- Cardiac dysrhythmias
- Pallor
- Cyanosis (may not be present until hypoxia is severe)
- Clubbing
- Dyspnea

CHEST X-RAY

Sometimes called radiographs, x-rays are an essential diagnostic tool for evaluating disorders of the chest. A chest x-ray allows visualization of the thoracic cavity, lungs, heart, and major thoracic vessels. X-rays show changes in size and location of the pulmonary structures and blood flow and enable identification of lesions, infiltrates, foreign bodies, or fluid. A chest x-ray also shows whether a disorder involves the lung parenchyma (the tissue of an organ, as distinguished from supporting or connective tissue) or the interstitial spaces. Chest x-rays can confirm pneumothorax, pneumonia, pleural effusion, and pulmonary edema.

COMPUTED TOMOGRAPHY

Chest CT Scan

Computed tomography (CT) scans of the lungs take pictures of small layers of pulmonary tissue, usually to identify a pulmonary lesion. These views can be diagonal or cross-sectional, with a scanner rotating at various angles. Although this test is painless and noninvasive, patient teaching is necessary before the procedure to offer explanations and decrease anxiety.

Helical or spiral CT chest scan. *Helical* (also called *spiral* or *volume-averaging*) *CT scanning* is a marked improvement over standard CT scanning. The helical CT scan obtains images continuously. This produces faster and more accurate images than a traditional CT scan. Because the helical CT can scan the abdomen and chest in less than 30 seconds, the entire study can be performed with one breath-hold. Injection or swallowing of the contrast dye helps the organs or tissues show up more clearly.

Pulmonary angiography (pulmonary arteriography). *Pulmonary angiography (pulmonary arteriography)* uses a radiographic contrast material injected into the pulmonary arteries to visualize the pulmonary vasculature. Angiography is used to detect pulmonary embolism (PE) and a variety of congenital and acquired lesions of the pulmonary vessels.

When PE is suspected, typically a CT scan is performed first. If the lung scan is normal, PE is ruled out. If the scan is uncertain, the diagnosis of PE is questionable because pathologic processes (e.g., emphysema, pneumonia) also may cause abnormalities on the lung scan. Definitive diagnosis for PE may require pulmonary angiography.

Ventilation-perfusion scan (V/Q scan). *Ventilation-perfusion (V/Q) scanning* is used primarily to check for a PE. Ventilation *(V)* refers to the air reaching the alveoli; perfusion *(Q)* refers to the blood that reaches the alveoli. A radioisotope is given intravenously for the perfusion portion of the test, and an image of the pulmonary vasculature is obtained. For the ventilation portion of the test, the patient inhales a radioactive gas, and an image of the outlines of the alveoli is obtained. Normal scans show homogeneous radioactivity of both sorts; a high V/Q, however, indicates impaired blood circulation to the alveoli, suggesting the presence of a PE (Medline Plus, 2020a).

PULMONARY FUNCTION TESTING

Pulmonary function tests (PFTs) are performed to assess the presence and severity of disease in the large and small airways. PFTs include various procedures to obtain information on lung volume, ventilation, pulmonary spirometry, and gas exchange. Lung volume tests refer to the volume of air that can be exhaled completely and slowly after a maximum inhalation *(vital capacity)*. *Inspiratory capacity* is the largest amount of air that can be inhaled in one breath from the resting expiratory level. *Total lung capacity* is calculated to determine the volume of air in the lung after a maximal inhalation. Ventilation tests evaluate the volume of air inhaled or exhaled in each respiratory cycle. Pulmonary spirometry tests evaluate the amount of air that can be exhaled forcefully after maximum inhalation. These tests require the use of a spirometer.

Determining gas exchange is one of the most important PFTs done to diagnose respiratory diseases. The DLCO (diffusing capacity of the lungs for carbon monoxide) test determines how well oxygen diffusing from the alveoli is taken up by blood in the pulmonary capillary bed. Strangely enough, oxygen is not used in the test; carbon monoxide is used instead of oxygen. Because such a small amount of carbon monoxide is used, the test is not dangerous. After the DLCO test is completed, the patient's rate of oxygen transfer can be determined accurately.

Mediastinoscopy

Mediastinoscopy is a surgical endoscopic procedure in which an incision is created in the suprasternal notch (the base of the neck), allowing the endoscope to be passed into the upper mediastinum. A *biopsy* then is

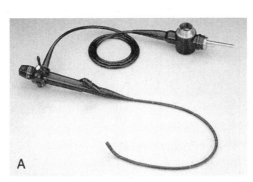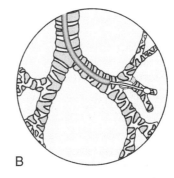

Fig. 9.7 Fiberoptic bronchoscope. (A) The transbronchoscopic balloon-tipped catheter and the flexible fiberoptic bronchoscope. (B) The catheter is introduced into a small airway and the balloon is inflated with 1.5 to 2 mL of air to occlude the airway. Bronchial alveolar lavage is performed by injecting and withdrawing 30-mL aliquots of sterile saline solution, gently aspirating after each instillation. Specimens are sent to the laboratory for analysis. (A, Courtesy Olympus America, Inc., Melville, New York. B, Reprinted with permission of the American Thoracic Society. Copyright 2013 American Thoracic Society. Meduri GU, Beals DH, Maijub AG, Baselski V: Protected bronchoalveolar lavage. A new bronchoscopic technique to retrieve uncontaminated distal airway secretions, *Am Rev Respir Dis* 143:855, 1991. Official journal of the American Thoracic Society.)

performed, in which a sample of lymph nodes is gathered and subsequently examined for the presence of a tumor. These lymph nodes receive lymphatic drainage from the lungs, so they are valuable in the diagnosis of malignant tumors. Tumors in the mediastinum (e.g., thymoma or lymphoma) also can be biopsied through the mediastinoscope. This procedure is performed in the operating room with the patient under general anesthesia.

Laryngoscopy

Laryngoscopy can be performed for either direct or indirect visualization of the larynx. Indirect laryngoscopy is probably the most common procedure for assessing respiratory difficulties. With the patient awake, a laryngeal mirror is positioned in the mouth for visualization. Direct laryngoscopy with a laryngoscope can be used for biopsy or polyp excision. It requires local or general anesthesia and exposes the vocal cords as the laryngoscope is passed down over the tongue.

Bronchoscopy

Bronchoscopy is performed by passing a bronchoscope into the trachea and bronchi. Using either a rigid bronchoscope or a flexible fiberoptic bronchoscope (the instrument of choice in most cases) allows visualization of the larynx, the trachea, and the bronchi (Fig. 9.7). Diagnostic bronchoscopic examination includes observation of the tracheobronchial tree for (1) abnormalities, (2) tissue biopsy, and (3) collection of secretions for cytologic (cell) or bacteriologic examination. A local anesthetic agent may be used, but an intravenous (IV) general anesthetic agent usually is given. The patient is treated as a surgical patient.

Nursing interventions for the patient after bronchoscopy include (1) keeping the patient on NPO (nothing by mouth) status until the gag reflex returns,

usually about 2 hours after the procedure; (2) keeping the patient in a semi-Fowler's position and turning on either side to facilitate removal of secretions (unless the health care provider specifies another position); (3) monitoring the patient for signs of laryngeal edema or laryngospasms, such as stridor or increasing dyspnea; and (4) if lung tissue biopsy is taken, monitoring sputum for signs of hemorrhage (blood-streaked sputum is expected for a few days after biopsy).

SPUTUM SPECIMEN

Sputum samples frequently are obtained for microscopic evaluation, such as Gram stain and culture and sensitivity (Box 9.2). For the range of sputum characteristics, see Box 9.3. When collecting sputum specimens, early morning, before the client has had anything to eat or drink is the best time to collect the specimen. If the client is unable to expel a specimen it may be collected via inducing coughing with a nebulizer or suctioning. Once the specimen has been collected, it should be labeled and sent to the laboratory as soon as possible.

CYTOLOGIC STUDIES

Cytologic tests can be performed on any body secretion, such as sputum or pleural fluid, to detect abnormal or malignant cells.

LUNG BIOPSY

Lung biopsy may be done transbronchially or as an open-lung biopsy. The purpose is to obtain tissue, cells, or secretions for evaluation. Transbronchial lung biopsy involves passing a forceps or needle through the bronchoscope to obtain a specimen. Specimens can be cultured or examined for malignant cells. Nursing interventions are the same as for fiberoptic bronchoscopy. Open-lung biopsy is used when pulmonary disease cannot be diagnosed by other procedures. The patient

Box 9.2   Guidelines for Sputum Specimen Collection

1. Explain to the patient that the sputum must be brought up from the lungs. Patients who have difficulty producing sputum or who have tenacious sputum may be dehydrated. Encourage fluid intake.
2. Collect the sputum specimen before prescribed antibiotics are started.
3. Collect specimens before meals to avoid possible emesis from coughing.
4. Instruct the patient to inhale and exhale deeply three times, then inhale swiftly, cough forcefully, and expectorate into the sterile sputum container. Usually early morning samples are collected on 3 consecutive days.
5. If the patient cannot raise sputum spontaneously, a hypertonic saline aerosol mist may help produce a good specimen. Instruct the patient to take several normal breaths of the mist, inhale deeply, cough, and expectorate.
6. Instruct the patient to rinse the mouth with water before expectorating into a sterile specimen bottle to decrease sputum contamination.
7. Properly label the sample and send it to the laboratory without delay.
8. Sputum samples also can be obtained indirectly, such as by nasotracheal suctioning with a catheter or by transtracheal aspiration. Take care to ensure that the suction catheters remain sterile. A health care provider's order must be obtained for endotracheal suctioning.

Box 9.3   Range of Sputum Characteristics

COLOR
- Clear
- White
- Yellow
- Green
- Brown
- Red
- Pink tinged
- Streaked with blood

ODOR
- None
- Malodorous

CONSISTENCY
- Frothy
- Watery
- Tenacious

BLOOD
- All the time
- Occasionally
- Early morning

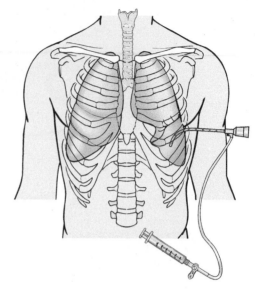

Fig. 9.8 Thoracentesis. The needle has penetrated the fluid-filled pleural space to remove fluid. (From Lewis S, Dirksen SR, Heitkemper MM, et al: *Medical-surgical nursing: assessment and management of clinical problems*, ed 8, St. Louis, 2011, Mosby.)

space for therapeutic purposes or for the removal of a specimen for biopsy (Fig. 9.8). Diagnostic indications for fluid removal include (1) examining the pleural fluid for specific gravity, white blood cell count, red blood cell count, protein, and glucose and (2) culturing the fluid for pathogens and checking for abnormal or malignant cells. Record the gross appearance of the fluid, the quantity obtained, and the site of the thoracentesis.

Therapeutic indications for thoracentesis include removal of fluid when it is a threat to the patient's safety or comfort and instillation of medication into the pleural space.

Nursing interventions for the patient undergoing thoracentesis include explaining the procedure and obtaining written consent. Try to relieve the patient's anxiety. The procedure usually is carried out in the patient's room. The patient sits on the edge of the bed with the head and arms resting on a pillow placed on an overbed table. If the patient cannot sit up, turn him or her to the unaffected side with the head of the bed elevated 30 degrees.

Monitor vital signs, general appearance, and respiratory status throughout the procedure. Because of the risk of intravascular fluid shift and resultant pulmonary edema, fluid removal is traditionally limited to 1300 mL. After thoracentesis, position the patient on the unaffected side. Label the specimen and send it immediately to the laboratory.

Arterial Blood Gases
Blood gas analysis is essential in diagnosing and monitoring patients with respiratory disorders. The lungs' ability to oxygenate arterial blood adequately

is anesthetized, the chest is opened with a thoracotomy incision, and a biopsy specimen is obtained.

THORACENTESIS

In thoracentesis the chest wall is pierced with a needle to withdraw (aspirate) fluid from the pleural

is determined by examination of the arterial oxygen tension (PaO_2) and arterial oxygen saturation (SaO_2). Oxygen is carried in the blood and dissolves in the plasma. After dissolving in the plasma oxygen attaches to hemoglobin to be carried to tissues and cells. The PaO_2 is expressed as millimeters of mercury (mm Hg). Oxygen *saturation* (SaO_2) is the measurement of the amount of oxygen bound to hemoglobin binding sites, compared with the amount of oxygen the hemoglobin could carry, and is expressed as a percentage. For example, if the SaO_2 is 92%, then 92% of the hemoglobin attachment sites for oxygen have oxygen bound to them. Note that oxygen first must dissolve in blood (PaO_2) before it can bind to hemoglobin (SaO_2) (Box 9.4).

The $PaCO_2$ is a measure of the partial pressure of carbon dioxide in the blood. $PaCO_2$ is referred to as the respiratory component in acid-base determination because this value is controlled primarily by the lungs. As the carbon dioxide level increases, the pH decreases. Therefore, the carbon dioxide level and pH are inversely proportional. The $PaCO_2$ level is elevated in primary respiratory acidosis and decreased in primary respiratory alkalosis. Because the lungs compensate for primary metabolic acid-based derangements, $PaCO_2$ levels are affected by metabolic disturbances as well. In metabolic acidosis the lungs attempt to compensate by "blowing off" carbon dioxide to raise the pH. In metabolic alkalosis the lungs attempt to compensate by retaining carbon dioxide to lower the pH.

The bicarbonate ion (HCO_3^-) is a measure of the metabolic (renal) component of the acid-base equilibrium. This ion can be measured directly by the bicarbonate value or indirectly by the carbon dioxide content. As the HCO_3^- level increases, the pH also increases; the relationship of bicarbonate to pH is directly proportional. HCO_3^- is elevated in metabolic alkalosis and decreased in metabolic acidosis. The kidneys also compensate for primary respiratory acid-base derangements. In respiratory acidosis, the kidneys attempt to compensate by reabsorbing increased amounts of HCO_3^-. In respiratory alkalosis the kidneys excrete HCO_3^- in increased amounts in an attempt to lower pH through compensation (Table 9.2).

Arterial blood gas (ABG) testing yields definitive information on the patient's respiratory status and metabolic balance. The procedure is performed at the bedside. A heparinized syringe and needle are used to withdraw 3 to 5 mL of arterial blood, usually from the radial artery. Other possible sites include femoral or brachial arteries. After the sample is obtained, place direct pressure on the puncture site for a minimum of 5 minutes to prevent hematoma formation and blood loss. If the patient is taking anticoagulants, maintain pressure for 20 minutes or longer, until the bleeding stops. Place the capped syringe in a basin of crushed ice and water to preserve the gas and pH levels of the specimen. Send the properly labeled specimen to the laboratory immediately.

Box 9.4	Guidelines for Interpreting Arterial Blood Gas Values

1. Examine each value by itself.
   - Normal arterial blood gas values (ABGs):
   - pH: 7.35–7.45
   - $PaCO_2$: 35–45 mm Hg
   - PaO_2: 80–100 mm Hg
   - HCO_3^-: 21–28 mEq/L
   - SaO_2: 95%–100%
2. Determine whether the pH reflects acidity or alkalinity.
   - pH ≤ 7.35 = acidity
   - pH ≥ 7.45 = alkalinity
3. Which other value corresponds with that condition?
   NOTE: $PaCO_2$ reflects respiratory factors; HCO_3^- reflects metabolic factors.
   - Carbon dioxide is a potential acid, so carbon dioxide greater than 45 mm Hg reflects acidity.
   - HCO_3^- is a basic (alkaline) substance, so HCO_3^- greater than 28 mEq/L reflects alkalinity.

Example 1: A patient with acute exacerbation of chronic obstructive pulmonary disease has the following ABGs:
- pH: 7.42
- $PaCO_2$: 49 mm Hg
- PaO_2: 50 mm Hg
- HCO_3^-: 31 mEq/L
- SaO_2: 84%

Because the pH is within the normal range, this is a compensated respiratory problem. The kidneys have increased the amount of bicarbonate they put into the blood to bring the pH to a normal level. The PaO_2 and the SaO_2 are low, indicating hypoxemia.

Example 2:
- pH: 7.21
- $PaCO_2$: 58 mm Hg
- PaO_2: 70 mm Hg
- HCO_3^-: 24 mEq/L
- • SaO_2: 84%

The pH is less than 7.35, indicating acidosis. The $PaCO_2$ is higher than 45 mm Hg, indicating acidosis. The $PaCO_2$ matches the pH, making it a respiratory acidosis. The HCO_3^- is normal, indicating there is no compensation. The PaO_2 and the SaO_2 are low, indicating hypoxemia. The full diagnosis for a patient with these ABG results is uncompensated respiratory acidosis with hypoxemia.

Woodruff D: Take these 6 easy steps to ABG analysis, *Nursing Made Incredibly Easy!* 41:4–7, 2006.

The blood gas values (see Box 9.4) assess the patient's metabolic (acid-base) status by measuring the pH. Carbon dioxide tension is measured by $PaCO_2$ and indicates the patient's ventilation. Oxygen saturation (PaO_2 and SaO_2) also is measured.

PULSE OXIMETRY

Pulse oximetry is a noninvasive way to monitor SaO_2 (saturation of oxygen) for assessment of gas exchange. The system consists of a probe that looks like a large clothespin, which is clipped to a finger, a toe, an earlobe, or the bridge of the nose. The noninvasive probe has a sensor that emits narrow beams of red and infrared light through the tissue and measures the amount of light being absorbed by oxygenated

Table 9.2	Acid-Base Disturbances and Compensatory Mechanisms
ACID-BASE DISTURBANCE	**MODE OF COMPENSATION**
Respiratory acidosis	Kidneys retain increased amounts of HCO_3^- to increase pH
Respiratory alkalosis	Kidneys excrete increased amounts of HCO_3^- to lower pH
Metabolic acidosis	Lungs "blow off" carbon dioxide to raise pH
Metabolic alkalosis	Lungs retain carbon dioxide to lower pH

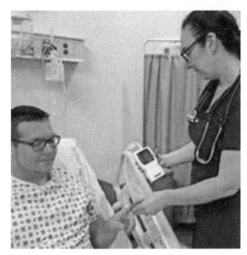

Fig. 9.9 Portable pulse oximeter with spring-tension digit probe displays oxygen saturation and pulse rate.

and deoxygenated hemoglobin in pulsating arterial blood. The probe is connected to a computer with a monitor that displays hemoglobin oxygen saturation and pulse rates (Fig. 9.9). A pulse oximeter beeps if the patient's SaO_2 registers outside of the limits set according to the health care provider's order. Pulse oximetry monitoring can be continuous or intermittent.

ABG results reflect a patient's oxygenation status at only one moment in time. Pulse oximetry permits continuous, noninvasive monitoring of SaO_2. Oximetry technology allows the nurse to assess changes in arterial saturation as they happen, intervene before hypoxemia (reduced oxygen in the blood) produces obvious and serious signs and symptoms, and evaluate the patient's response to treatment. Pulse oximetry alone does not provide data about PaO_2 and acid-base balance. In addition, pulse oximetry can result in inaccurate results if the area the probe is attached to is cold, if nail polish or artificial nails are present when the fingertip is used, or if the patient's heart rate is irregular. For these reasons, thorough assessment of the patient for signs of hypoxia is essential. ABG levels may be needed periodically as well.

An SaO_2 of 90% to 100% is needed to replenish tissues adequately with oxygen, with 95% to 100% desired. The ability of hemoglobin to feed oxygen to the tissues weakens significantly when the SaO_2 drops below 85%.

> ⚠ **Safety Alert**
>
> **An SaO_2 of Less Than 70% Is Considered Life Threatening**
>
> Arterial oxygen saturation can be determined quickly and noninvasively through pulse oximetry. Severe circulatory problems may diminish the accuracy of the reading. If oximetry results seem questionable, the health care provider usually orders ABG tests. A pulse oximeter can detect a change within 6 seconds. To get optimal results, remember these points:
> - Do not attach the probe to an extremity that has a blood pressure cuff or arterial catheter in place; these devices reduce blood flow.
> - Place the probe over a pulsating vascular bed.
> - While the probe is on the patient, protect it from strong light (such as direct sunlight), which can affect the reading.
> - Avoid excess patient movement to ensure accuracy.
> - Remember that hypothermia, hypotension, and vasoconstriction can affect readings.
>
> (For more information on the pulse oximeter refer to Chapter 14 in Foundations of Nursing)

DISORDERS OF THE UPPER AIRWAY

EPISTAXIS

Etiology and Pathophysiology

The underlying cause of epistaxis (bleeding from the nose) is congestion of the nasal membranes, leading to capillary rupture. This condition frequently is caused by injury and occurs more frequently in men.

Epistaxis can be either a primary disorder or secondary to other conditions. It can be related to menstrual flow in women or to hypertension. Other causes include local irritation of nasal mucosa, such as dryness, chronic infection, trauma (e.g., injury, vigorous nose blowing, or nose picking), topical corticosteroid use, nasal spray abuse, or street drug use. Epistaxis often results if the patient has a disorder that results in prolonged bleeding time or reduction in platelet counts. Bleeding also may be prolonged if the patient takes aspirin or nonsteroidal anti-inflammatory drugs (NSAIDs). A major factor in epistaxis is the many capillaries in the nasal passages.

> ⚠ **Safety Alert**
>
> If the patient has an episode of epistaxis or complains of frequent episodes of epistaxis, check his or her blood pressure!

Clinical Manifestations

The primary observation is bright red blood draining from one or both nostrils. With a severe nasal hemorrhage, adults can lose as much as 1 L of blood per hour, but this rate of loss is not prolonged. Exsanguination (loss of blood to the point at which life can no longer be sustained) from epistaxis is rare.

Assessment

Collection of subjective data includes asking the patient to relate the duration and severity of bleeding and identifying precipitating factors, if possible.

Collection of objective data involves assessing the presence of bleeding from one or both nostrils. If possible, determine whether the bleeding is occurring in the anterior or posterior portion of the nasal passageway. Assess the patient's blood pressure for hypotension, temperature, pulse, respirations, and any evidence of hypovolemic shock. Hypotension is a late sign of shock.

Diagnostic Tests

A hemoglobin and hematocrit determination aids in establishing an estimate of the blood loss. Prothrombin time (PT), international normalized ratio (INR), and partial thromboplastin time (PTT) assist in identifying contributing factors, such as a bleeding tendency and clotting abnormalities. A rhinoscopy may be performed to locate the bleeding site and possible causes and treatment. This procedure involves inserting a lighted nasal speculum into the nasal cavity.

Medical Management

Epistaxis has many possible treatments, including nasal packing with cotton saturated with 1:1000 epinephrine to promote local vasoconstriction. Cautery can be either electrical (burning [cauterizing] the bleeding vessel) or chemical (applying a silver nitrate stick to the site of the bleeding). Posterior packing of the nasal cavity may be needed. A balloon tampon may be done by inserting a Foley-like catheter into the nose and inflating the balloon after it is placed posteriorly. Traction then is placed on the catheter to compress the vessel in the area. Also, some health care providers prescribe antibiotics (penicillin) after the bleeding is controlled to minimize risk of infection.

Nursing Interventions and Patient Teaching

Nursing interventions include keeping the patient calm. Place the patient in a sitting position, leaning forward, or in a reclining position with head and shoulders elevated. Be aware that the patient may vomit if sitting in this position and have an emesis basin ready. Apply direct pressure by pinching the entire soft lower portion of the nose for 10 to 15 minutes. Apply ice compresses to the nose and have the patient suck on ice. Partially insert a small gauze pad into the bleeding nostril, and apply digital pressure if bleeding

continues. Monitor for signs and symptoms of hypovolemic shock.

Patient problems and interventions for the patient with epistaxis include but are not limited to the following:

PATIENT PROBLEM	NURSING INTERVENTIONS
Compromised Blood Flow to Cerebral and/or Cardiopulmonary Tissue, related to blood loss	Assess vital signs and level of consciousness q 15 min and report any changes Document estimated blood loss
Potential for Aspiration Into Airway, related to bleeding	Elevate head of bed; place patient in Fowler's position with the head forward; encourage patient to let the blood drain from the nose Pinch nostrils; have the patient breathe through the mouth; apply ice compresses over the nose (however, the primary benefit of the application of ice is that it requires the patient to remain still); assist patient in clearing secretions Maintain airway patency Instruct patient to expectorate any blood or clots rather than swallow them, which could cause nausea and vomiting

Instruct the patient (and the family, if possible) not to pick, scratch, or otherwise irritate the nares. To prevent recurrent hemorrhage, warn the patient not to blow the nose vigorously and to avoid dryness of the nose. Instruct the patient and the family regarding the risks of foreign objects inserted in the nose (this is especially important in pediatric patients). Encourage the patient to use a vaporizer and saline or nasal lubricants to keep nasal mucous membranes moist. Advise the patient to avoid using aspirin-containing products or NSAIDs and teach him or her to sneeze with the mouth open.

Prognosis

With treatment, the prognosis is good.

DEVIATED SEPTUM AND NASAL POLYPS

Etiology and Pathophysiology

Common conditions that cause nasal obstruction include nasal polyps or a deviated septum caused by congenital abnormality or, more likely, injury. The septum deviates from the midline and can obstruct the nasal passageway partially. Nasal polyps are tissue growths on the nasal tissues that frequently are caused by prolonged sinus inflammation; allergies are often the underlying cause.

Clinical Manifestations

The major manifestations of nasal septal deviations and polyps are stertorous (characterized by a harsh snoring sound) respirations, dyspnea, and sometimes postnasal drip.

Assessment

Collection of subjective data includes establishing the presence of previous injuries or infections, allergies, and sinus congestion. The patient complains of dyspnea.

Collection of objective data involves identifying the condition and its location. Note the rate and character of the patient's respirations.

Diagnostic Tests

Sinus radiographic studies depict the presence of shadowy sinuses when nasal polyps are present. A shift of the nasal septum is evident with a septal defect. A deviated septum also may be seen on visual examination.

Medical Management

These conditions frequently require surgical correction. Nasoseptoplasty is the operation of choice to reconstruct, align, and straighten the deviated nasal septum. A nasal polypectomy is performed to remove the polyps. Actions include nasal packing to control bleeding for 24 hours, and then maintaining nasal mucosa hydration with nasal irrigation of saline or application of a light layer of petroleum jelly to the external nares to prevent drying. Medications include (1) corticosteroids (prednisone), which cause polyps to decrease or disappear; and (2) antihistamines for allergy signs and symptoms and to decrease congestion in septal deviations and polyps. Antibiotic agents (penicillin) may be used in both conditions to prevent infection. Analgesics (acetaminophen) may be given to relieve the headache that occurs with septal deviation.

Nursing Interventions and Patient Teaching

Nursing interventions generally are aimed at maintaining airway patency and preventing infection. Postoperative interventions for nasal surgery include monitoring closely for infection or hemorrhage and maintaining patient comfort.

Patient problems and interventions for the patient with deviated septum or nasal polyps include but are not limited to the following:

PATIENT PROBLEM	NURSING INTERVENTIONS
Inability to Clear Airway, related to nasal exudates	Document patient's ability to clear secretions, and note respiratory status
	Elevate head of bed, and apply ice compresses to the nose to decrease edema, discoloration, discomfort, and bleeding
	Change nasal drip pad as needed, documenting color, consistency, and amount of exudates

PATIENT PROBLEM	NURSING INTERVENTIONS
Potential for Injury, related to trauma to bleeding site associated with vigorous nose blowing	Assess and report exudates (as stated above)
	Instruct patient against blowing nose in immediate postoperative period, because this could increase bleeding, edema, and ecchymosis

Instruct the patient to contact the health care provider if bleeding or signs of infection develops. The patient should use nasal sprays and drops judiciously because of the possible rebound effect on nasal mucous membranes. Remind the patient to avoid nose blowing, vigorous coughing, or Valsalva's maneuver (holding the breath and bearing down as if straining during a bowel movement) for 2 days postoperatively. Instruct the patient that facial ecchymosis and edema may persist for several days after surgery.

Prognosis

With surgical correction, the prognosis is excellent.

ANTIGEN-ANTIBODY ALLERGIC RHINITIS AND ALLERGIC CONJUNCTIVITIS (HAY FEVER)

Etiology and Pathophysiology

Allergic rhinitis and allergic conjunctivitis (hay fever) are atopic allergic conditions that result from antigen-antibody reactions in the nasal membranes, nasopharynx, and conjunctiva from inhaled or contact allergens. Many infants, children, and adults have these seasonal or perennial conditions, which often result in absences from school and work.

During the antigen-antibody reaction of rhinitis and conjunctivitis, ciliary action slows; mucosal gland secretion increases; leukocyte (eosinophil) infiltration occurs; and, because of increased capillary permeability and vasodilation, local tissue edema results. Common allergens are tree, grass, and weed pollens; mold spores; fungi; house dusts; mites; and animal dander. Some foods, drugs, and insect stings also may cause these reactions.

Clinical Manifestations

Acute ocular manifestations include edema, photophobia, excessive tearing, blurring of vision, and pruritus. Individuals with rhinitis complain of excessive secretions or inability to breathe through the nose because of congestion and/or edema. Otitis media symptoms can occur if the eustachian tubes are occluded. These symptoms occur more in childhood, with the individual complaining of ear fullness, ear popping, or decreased hearing.

Assessment

The initial complaints of seasonal rhinitis and conjunctivitis include severe sneezing, congestion, pruritus, and lacrimation (watery eyes). Cough, epistaxis, and headache also may occur. More chronic signs and symptoms include headache, severe nasal congestion, postnasal drip, and cough. If these are not treated, chronic sufferers eventually develop secondary infections, such as otitis media, bronchitis, sinusitis, and pneumonia.

Diagnostic Tests
In allergic rhinitis, the mucosa of the turbinates is usually pale because of venous engorgement, which is in contrast to the erythema of viral rhinitis.

Skin testing can be done in a health care provider's office. A site, usually an adult's forearm or a child's back, is cleaned with alcohol, and the nurse draws small marks on the skin with a special pen. Next to each mark the nurse uses a lancet to prick the skin with various allergens. A new lancet is used for each allergen. Some allergens react quickly, whereas others may take up to 15 minutes. If an allergic reaction is present, the patient has a raised, red, itchy bump, or *wheal,* that may look like a mosquito bite. The nurse then measures the size of the wheal and records the results.

Serum allergy testing may be done to identify the amount of immunoglobulin E present. The amount present of this antibody may indicate that a client has an allergy. Total or specific IgE tests may be done (Medline Plus, 2020b).

Medical Management
Treatment goals are to relieve signs and symptoms and prevent infections and other complaints, such as malaise, extreme fatigue, and severe headaches. Avoiding the allergen is effective. Perennial use of antihistamines, intranasal corticosteroids, and leukotriene receptor antagonists such as zafirlukast or montelukast is recommended. Changing from one antihistamine to another seasonally may help impede tolerance to any one medication.

Decongestants may be added and used intermittently for 3 to 5 days if congestion occurs. Common over-the-counter decongestants—such as phenylephrine, pseudoephedrine, chlorpheniramine, and phenylpropanolamine—are contained in may be used. These products may produce a "rebound" effect, causing the patient to feel more uncomfortable and congested if used for more than 3 to 5 days.

Lodoxamide four times a day is the recommended treatment for mild to moderately severe allergic conjunctivitis.

Although long-term, consistent use of topical or nasal corticosteroids once was considered appropriate treatment, they are no longer recommended because of the tolerance that is built up with continuous use. Medications included in this category are beclomethasone, dexamethasone, flunisolide, fluticasone , and budesonide .

Pressure headaches may require analgesics until signs and symptoms are relieved. Hot packs over facial sinuses offer relief if the headache is related to sinus congestion.

Nursing Interventions and Patient Teaching
These illnesses are self-limiting, so focus on health promotion and maintenance teaching to provide for self-care management. Include ways to avoid allergens, self-care management through symptom control, and medication action and usage.

OBSTRUCTIVE SLEEP APNEA
Etiology and Pathophysiology
Obstructive sleep apnea (OSA) is characterized by partial or complete upper airway obstruction during sleep, causing apnea and hypopnea. *Apnea* is the cessation of spontaneous respirations; *hypopnea* is abnormally shallow and slow respirations. Airflow obstruction occurs when the tongue and the soft palate fall backward and partially or completely obstruct the pharynx. The obstruction may last from 15 to 90 seconds. During the apneic period, the patient experiences severe hypoxemia (decreased PaO_2) and hypercapnia (increased $PaCO_2$). These changes are ventilatory stimulants and cause the patient to awaken partially. The patient has a generalized startle response, snorts, and gasps, which cause the tongue and soft palate to move forward and the airway to open. Apnea and arousal cycles occur repeatedly, as many as 200 to 400 times during 6 to 8 hours of sleep.

Sleep apnea occurs in an estimated 22 million adults in the United States, but as many as 80% of them are undiagnosed (American Sleep Apnea Association, 2021). Often patients are unaware of sleep apnea until pulmonary edema develops or when the patient needs general anesthesia, which can cause a serious complication. General anesthesia suppresses upper airway activity and allows the airway to close. Anesthesia may increase the number of episodes and the duration of episodes, thereby decreasing arterial oxygenation. Anesthesia inhibits the arousals that occur during sleep, making it harder to bring the patient out of anesthesia.

Clinical Manifestations and Assessment
Clinical manifestations of sleep apnea include frequent awakening at night, insomnia, excessive daytime sleepiness, and witnessed apneic episodes. The patient's bed partner may complain about loud snoring, sometimes so loud that both people cannot sleep in the same room. Other symptoms include morning headaches (from hypercapnia, which causes vasodilation of cerebral blood vessels), personality changes, and irritability. Systemic hypertension, cardiac dysrhythmias, right-sided heart failure from pulmonary hypertension caused by nocturnal hypoxemia, and stroke are serious complications that may occur.

Symptoms of sleep apnea alter many aspects of a patient's lifestyle. With chronic sleep loss, the patient may have diminished ability to concentrate, impaired memory, failure to accomplish daily tasks, and interpersonal difficulties. Men may experience impotence. Driving accidents are more common in habitually sleepy people. Family life and the patient's ability to maintain employment also often are compromised. As a result, the patient may experience severe depression. Risk factors for OSA include the following (Mayo Clinic, 2020e):

- *Male gender:* About twice as many men as women have OSA.
- *Older age:* Although younger patients can develop OSA, the incidence increases with age over 60 years, probably because of weight gain and loss of pharyngeal muscle strength.
- *Obesity:* An obese person's pharynx may be infiltrated with fat, and the tongue and soft palate may be enlarged, crowding the air passages. An obese individual also may have a short, thick neck increasing susceptibility to obstruction.
- *Nasal conditions:* Nasal allergies, polyps, or septal deviation decrease the diameter of the pharynx.
- *Neck circumference.* People with thicker necks might have narrower airways
- *Pharyngeal structural abnormalities:* A person with OSA may have enlarged tonsils, an elongated uvula, an especially long tongue, or a soft palate that rests on the base of the tongue. Any of these structural abnormalities can impinge on the airway.

Appropriate referral should be made if problems are identified. Cessation of breathing reported by the bed partner is usually a source of great anxiety because of fear that breathing may not resume.

Diagnostic Tests

Diagnosis of sleep apnea is made during sleep with the use of polysomnography. Electrodes are placed on the patient's scalp, mandibular area, and lateral area of the eyelids. A nasal cannula measures airflow, and pulse oximetry measures SpO_2 (Mayo Clinic, 2020e. The patient's chest and abdominal movements, oral airflow, nasal airflow, SpO_2, ocular movement, muscle activity, brain activity, and heart rate and rhythm are monitored, and time in each sleep stage is determined. A diagnosis of sleep apnea requires documentation of multiple episodes of apnea (no airflow with respiratory effort) or hypopnea (airflow diminished 30% to 50% with respiratory effort). Polysomnography may be carried out in a sleep laboratory, or the patient may be taught to attach monitoring leads for a home sleep study.

Medical Management and Nursing Interventions

Mild sleep apnea may respond to simple measures. Instruct the patient to avoid sedatives and alcoholic beverages for 3 to 4 hours before sleep. Referral to a weight loss program may help, because excessive weight exacerbates symptoms. Symptoms resolve in

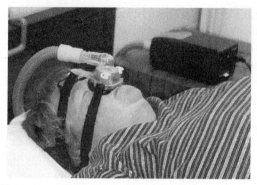

Fig. 9.10 Nasal continuous positive airway pressure (nCPAP). The patient applies a nasal mask attached to a blower to maintain positive pressure.

half of the patients with OSA who use an oral appliance during sleep that brings the mandible and tongue forward to enlarge the airway space, thereby preventing airway occlusion. Some individuals find a support group beneficial so that they can express concerns and feelings and discuss strategies for resolving problems.

In patients with more severe symptoms, nasal continuous positive airway pressure (nCPAP) may be used. With nCPAP the patient applies a nasal mask that is attached to a high-flow blower (Fig. 9.10). The blower is adjusted to maintain sufficient positive pressure (5 to 15 cm H_2O) in the airway during inspiration and expiration to prevent airway collapse. Some patients cannot adjust to exhaling against the high pressure. A technologically more sophisticated therapy, bilevel positive airway pressure (BiPAP), capable of delivering higher pressure during inspiration (when the airway is most likely to be occluded) and lower pressure during expiration, may be helpful and is better tolerated. Although CPAP is highly effective, compliance is poor even if symptoms of sleep apnea are relieved.

UPPER AIRWAY OBSTRUCTION

Etiology and Pathophysiology

Upper airway obstruction is precipitated by a recent respiratory event, such as traumatic injury to the airway or surrounding tissues. Common airway obstructions include choking on food; dentures; aspiration (inhalation) of vomitus or secretions; and, the most common airway obstruction in an unconscious person, the tongue.

Altered physiology includes any condition that could produce airway obstruction, such as laryngeal spasm caused by tetany resulting from hypocalcemia. Another cause may be laryngeal edema caused by injury.

Clinical Manifestations

The main signs are stertorous respirations, altered respiratory rate and character, and apneic periods. Severe obstructions are accompanied by cyanosis, choking, and difficulty in breathing. Behavioral signs of upper airway obstruction include agitation, changes in level of consciousness, and confusion.

Assessment

Subjective data are limited because a patient is unable to talk when the airway is obstructed. The nurse therefore must make a prompt and accurate assessment of objective data.

Collection of objective data includes prompt assessment for the classic sign of choking, in which the patient places a hand over his or her throat. Also monitor for signs of hypoxia (an inadequate, reduced tension of cellular oxygen) (see Box 9.1), cyanosis (slightly bluish, grayish, slate-like, or dark purple discoloration of the skin resulting from excessive amounts of deoxygenated hemoglobin in the blood), stertorous respirations, and wheezing or stridor (harsh, high-pitched sounds during respiration, caused by obstruction). As hypoxia progresses, the respiratory centers in the brain (medulla oblongata and pons) are depressed, resulting in bradycardia and shallow, slow respirations.

Diagnostic Tests

This is a medical emergency; the focus is on prompt management of the condition. This condition is diagnosed by prompt and accurate assessment. Foreign bodies may be identified by radiographic studies.

Medical Management

The patient may require abdominal thrusts (Heimlich maneuver) or an emergency tracheostomy to remove the obstruction. Depending on the cause of the obstruction, an artificial airway may be inserted to maintain patency. A pharyngeal, endotracheal, or tracheal artificial airway may be used.

Nursing Interventions and Patient Teaching

The most immediate nursing intervention is to open the airway and restore patency. This may be accomplished by properly repositioning the patient's head and neck, or it may require further maneuvers. The head-tilt/chin-lift technique recommended by the American Heart Association minimizes further damage in the presence of a suspected cervical neck fracture. With a foreign body airway obstruction, the Heimlich maneuver is used.

Patient problems and interventions for the patient with an airway obstruction include but are not limited to the following:

PATIENT PROBLEM	NURSING INTERVENTIONS
Inability to Clear Airway, related to obstruction in airway	Reestablish and maintain secure airway
	Administer oxygen as ordered
	Suction as needed and assess patient's ability to mobilize secretions
	Monitor vital signs and breath sounds closely

PATIENT PROBLEM	NURSING INTERVENTIONS
Potential for Aspiration Into Airway, related to partial airway obstruction	Monitor respiratory rate, rhythm, and effort
	Assess patient's ability to swallow secretions by elevating the head of the bed
	Assess and document breath sounds
	Facilitate optimal airway and functional swallowing by elevating head of bed
	Note amount, color, and characteristics of secretions
	Suction as needed

The goal of education is prevention. Teach the patient and the family how to assess for airway patency. Describe appropriate use of the Heimlich maneuver. Explain the rationale for all treatments and procedures.

PROGNOSIS

With immediate medical and nursing intervention, the prognosis is good; without emergency intervention, the condition is life threatening.

CANCER OF THE LARYNX

Etiology and Pathophysiology

The National Cancer Institute estimated that about 12,3700 new cases of laryngeal cancer and about 3750 deaths resulting from this disease would occur in 2020. There has been a decrease in the number of cases of larynx cancer since 2009 (National Cancer Institute, 2021).

Laryngeal cancers occur most often in people older than age 65. The incidence appears to be correlated to prolonged tobacco use (cigarettes, pipes, cigars, chewing tobacco, smokeless tobacco) and heavy alcohol use, chronic laryngitis, vocal abuse, gastroesophageal reflux disease (GERD), and family history. Because of the increase in the number of women who are heavy smokers, their incidence of carcinoma of the larynx is increasing.

Laryngeal cancer limited to the true vocal cords is slow growing because of decreased lymphatic supply; however, elsewhere in the larynx there is an abundance of lymph tissue, and cancer in these tissues spreads rapidly and metastasizes early to the deep lymph nodes of the neck.

Clinical Manifestations

Progressive or persistent hoarseness is an early sign. Any person who is hoarse longer than 2 weeks should seek medical treatment. Signs of metastasis to other areas include pain in the larynx radiating to the ear, difficulty in swallowing (dysphagia), a feeling of a lump in the throat, and enlarged cervical lymph nodes.

Assessment

Collection of subjective data includes assessing the onset and duration of symptoms. Complaints of referred pain to the ear (otalgia) and difficulty breathing (dyspnea) or swallowing should be noted.

Collection of objective data includes examining sputum for blood (*hemoptysis,* or blood expectorated from the respiratory tract).

Diagnostic Tests

Visual examination of the larynx by direct laryngoscopy, with a fiberoptic scope, is done to determine the presence of laryngeal cancer. Other diagnostic tests to detect local and regional spread of laryngeal cancer include CT scan, magnetic resonance imaging (MRI), and positron emission tomography (PET). The patient also may have a chest x-ray study and a CT scan to determine whether there is lung or liver metastasis (National Cancer Institute, 2021). A health history helps in making the diagnosis, and a biopsy and microscopic study of the lesion are definitive.

Medical Management

Treatment is determined by the extent of tumor growth. If the tumor is confined to the true vocal cord without limitation of cord movement, then radiation therapy is the best course of treatment. Surgical intervention is considered when extension of the tumor becomes affixed to one of the cords or extends upward or downward from the larynx; surgical options include a total or partial laryngectomy or a radical neck dissection. A partial laryngectomy is done to remove the diseased vocal cord and possibly a portion of thyroid cartilage. This requires placement of a temporary tracheostomy, which is closed when the edema has decreased. A total laryngectomy is performed when the cancer of the larynx is advanced; this requires placement of a permanent tracheostomy. Because the patient can no longer breathe through the nose, usually the sense of smell is lost and the sense of taste is affected. The voice is also absent once the larynx is removed. There is no connection between the patient's mouth and trachea.

A radical neck dissection to remove cervical lymph nodes is done often in conjunction with a total laryngectomy in patients who have a high risk of metastasis to the neck from carcinoma of the larynx. This surgery entails removal of the submandibular salivary gland, the sternocleidomastoid muscle, the spinal accessory nerve, and the internal jugular vein, which results in one-sided shoulder droop. This surgery results in a very large tracheostomy opening, and no tracheostomy tube is used. The opening narrows as the patient heals from chemotherapy.

Chemotherapy using cisplatin and 5-fluorouracil (5-FU) before and after surgery or radiation has achieved a positive response in many cases (American Cancer Society, 2021.).

Nursing Interventions and Patient Teaching

If a tracheostomy is created, then airway maintenance through proper suctioning techniques is important. Assess skin integrity surrounding the tracheal opening; be alert for signs of infection.

Monitor intake and output (I&O) balance and assist with tube feedings as ordered. Explain to the patient that the tube feedings are temporary and that normal eating may begin again when healing occurs in a few weeks. Weigh the patient daily and assess hydration status to determine the need for additional fluids; note skin turgor and observe for diarrhea.

Because of neck and facial disfigurement and loss of voice, a thorough psychosocial assessment and resultant interventions are beneficial. Encourage communication through writing and facial and hand gestures. Often no one can reassure a patient that speech can be regained as well as a fellow patient who has undergone the same surgical intervention. Many cities have a Lost Chord Club or a New Voice Club, whose members are willing to visit hospitalized patients. A speech therapist should meet with the patient after a total laryngectomy to discuss voice restoration options, including a voice prosthesis, esophageal speech, and an electrolarynx.

Patient problems and interventions for the patient with a tracheostomy include but are not limited to the following:

PATIENT PROBLEM	NURSING INTERVENTIONS
Inability to Clear Airway, related to secretions or obstruction	Suction secretions as needed
	Provide tracheostomy care according to protocol; ensure the availability of emergency equipment (oxygen and tracheostomy tray)
	Offer small, frequent feedings, and give liquid or pureed food as tolerated to avoid choking
	Teach patient stoma protection
	Assess respiratory rate and characteristics q 1–2 h.
	Auscultate lung sounds, monitor SaO_2 q 4 h.
	Elevate head of bed 30 degrees or higher
	Turn patient and encourage coughing and deep breathing q 2–4 h.
	Provide constant humidity
	Suction tracheostomy tube as needed, using aseptic technique; instruct patient to inhale as catheter is advanced
	Clean inner cannula of tracheostomy tube q 2–4 h and as needed, using a solution of ½ normal saline and {½} hydrogen peroxide

PATIENT PROBLEM	NURSING INTERVENTIONS
Compromised Verbal Communication	Provide patient with implements for communication, including pencil, paper, Magic Slate, picture books, or electronic voice device
	Anesthesia interferes with the patient's memory, so providing a notebook for the family to include relevant events can help orient the patient
	Keep call signal by patient's hand at all times
	If possible, ask patient questions that require only a yes or no response to avoid fatigue and frustration
	Refer patient to local support groups and the local chapter of the American Cancer Society
	Assist with speech rehabilitation
	Review instructions about esophageal and electroesophageal speech
	Reinforce need for regular follow-up with speech pathologist and surgeon after discharge

Explain techniques of airway maintenance, such as oxygen usage, deep breathing, and coughing. Discuss the importance of dietary management in relationship to airway maintenance. Encourage optimal fluid intake for the patient: an uncovered tracheostomy can dehydrate the patient. Promote optimal communication through speech rehabilitation and community support groups.

Prognosis

If the tumor is limited to the true cord, the cure rate is 80% to 90% for stage I, decreasing to 42% at stage IV. The prognosis in primary supraglottic and subglottic cancer is poorer. The 5-year survival rate is 60% for stage I, decreasing to 45% for stage IV (American Cancer Society, 2021).

RESPIRATORY INFECTIONS

ACUTE RHINITIS
Etiology and Pathophysiology

Acute rhinitis (or acute coryza), known as the *common cold,* is an inflammatory condition of the mucous membranes of the nose and accessory sinuses. It typically is characterized by edema of the nasal mucous membrane. The common cold usually is caused by one or more viruses; however, it may become complicated by a bacterial infection. Signs and symptoms usually are evident within 24 to 48 hours after exposure. Sinus congestion causes increased sinus drainage, leading to postnasal drip. The postnasal drip causes throat irritation, headache, and earache. Most people with colds contaminate their hands when coughing or sneezing, thus contaminating everything they touch. Others become infected when touching the telephone, computer, or anything else that has been touched by the person with a cold. Also, many colds are believed to be spread by shaking hands with a person who has a cold.

Clinical Manifestations

An increased amount of thin, serous nasal exudate and a productive cough are two of the most common signs. Sore throat and fever are often present. If the infection remains uncomplicated, it generally subsides in a week. In addition, the patient may report aches, pains, fatigue, and loss of appetite.

Assessment

Subjective data include the patient's complaints of sore throat, dyspnea, and congestion of varying duration.

Collection of objective data includes noting the color and consistency of the nasal exudate. A visual examination of the throat may reveal erythema, edema, and local irritation. Also document the presence and duration of fever.

Diagnostic Tests

Throat and sputum cultures indicate the presence and nature of microorganisms.

Medical Management

Medical management is aimed at accurate diagnosis and prevention of complications. No specific treatment is available for the common cold. Among the medications used are (1) aspirin or acetaminophen for analgesia and reduction of temperature (aspirin is not used in infants, children, and adolescents because of the danger of developing Reye syndrome); and either (2) a cough suppressant for a dry, nonproductive cough or (3) an expectorant to help dislodge mucus for a productive cough. If a secondary bacterial infection is confirmed, an antibiotic agent (e.g., erythromycin) is prescribed (see the Complementary and Alternative Therapies box).

Nursing Interventions and Patient Teaching

Nursing interventions are aimed at promoting comfort. Such measures include encouraging fluids and applying warm, moist packs to sinuses.

Patient problems and interventions for the patient with acute rhinitis include but are not limited to the following:

PATIENT PROBLEM	NURSING INTERVENTIONS
Inability to Clear Airway, related to nasal exudates	Encourage fluids to liquefy secretions and aid in their expectoration
	Use vaporizer to moisten mucous membranes and prevent further irritation

PATIENT PROBLEM	NURSING INTERVENTIONS
Willingness for Improved Health Management	Remind patient and family of health maintenance behaviors to decrease risk of illness, such as adequate fluid and nutritional management and sufficient rest Teach importance of hygiene measures to decrease spread of infection

Complementary and Alternative Therapies

Respiratory Disorders

- Herbal medicines for respiratory problems include remedies for nasal discharge and congestion, cough, sore throat, fever and headache, and immunostimulant effects. Ephedra (Ephedra sinica, Ephedra vulgaris) is a stimulant and is illegal in some areas. Expectorants include anise (Pimpinella anisum), coltsfoot (Tussilago farfara), and horehound (Marrubium vulgare). Coltsfoot and horehound also are believed to have antitussive action.
- Sore throat remedies include mint (Mentha piperita [peppermint], Mentha spicata [spearmint]), and slippery elm (Ulmus rubra). Remedies for the fever and headache that may accompany colds and influenza include boneset (Eupatorium perfoliatum), feverfew (Tanacetum parthenium), and willow (Salix purpurea, S. fragilis, S. daphnoides).
- Stimulants of the immune system, believed to help ward off colds and flu, include echinacea (Echinacea angustifolia, E. pallida, E. purpurea) and goldenseal (Hydrastis canadensis).
- Some interventions that contribute to comfort in patients experiencing dyspnea include the following:
  - Breathing exercises
  - Relaxation therapy
  - Massage
  - Acupuncture
  - Hypnosis
  - Visualization
- Some people believe that reflexology helps relieve congestion.
- Facial massage with diluted aromatic oils is believed by some to open occluded sinuses and relieve congestion. These essential oils include lavender, eucalyptus, peppermint, and tea tree oil.

Teach the patient the correct handwashing technique and proper disposal of tissues used for nasal secretions. Instruct the patient to limit exposure to others during the first 48 hours and to check his or her temperature every 4 hours.

A small ceramic pot, called a neti pot, is used to flush out the nasal passages with a saltwater solution—a process known as nasal irrigation. Some patients do not tolerate neti pot irrigations, but for those who do, the result is thinner mucus that drains more easily and less congestion.

Prognosis

Signs and symptoms resolve in 2 to 10 days. Even though the common cold does not cause death, its economic importance is vast, because it is the greatest cause of absenteeism in industry and schools.

ACUTE FOLLICULAR TONSILLITIS

Etiology and Pathophysiology

Acute follicular tonsillitis can be an acute inflammation of the tonsils. It is the result of an airborne or foodborne bacterial infection, often streptococci. Less frequently, it also often may be viral. If it is caused by group A beta-hemolytic streptococci, sequelae such as rheumatic fever, carditis, and nephritis must be considered. It appears to be most common in school-age children. Signs and symptoms of tonsillitis include sore throat, fever, chills, and anorexia. The tonsils become enlarged and often contain purulent exudate.

Clinical Manifestations

Acute follicular tonsillitis is manifest clinically with enlarged, tender cervical lymph nodes. Fever may be present with chills, general muscle aching, and malaise. Laboratory data reveal an elevated white blood cell count.

Assessment

Collection of subjective data includes monitoring the severity of throat pain and the possibility of referred pain to the ears. Note headache or joint pain.

Collection of objective data includes a visual examination that shows increased throat secretions and enlarged, erythematous tonsils.

Diagnostic Tests

Throat cultures identify the causative microorganism, most commonly beta-hemolytic streptococci. A complete blood count (CBC) is done to determine whether the white blood cell count is elevated. Commonly, the abnormal white blood cell count is 10,000 to 20,000/mm^3.

Medical Management

If antibiotics to which the offending organism is sensitive are administered early, infection subsides. An elective tonsillectomy and adenoidectomy (T&A), in which the tonsils and adenoids are excised surgically, is performed in people who have recurrent attacks of tonsillitis. The procedure usually is performed from 4 to 6 weeks after an acute attack has subsided. Either general or local anesthesia is used. Post-T&A hemostasis (i.e., the stoppage of bleeding) is paramount, because the patient can lose a large amount of blood through hemorrhage without demonstrating any signs of bleeding. The health care provider may be able to control minor postoperative bleeding by applying a sponge soaked in a solution of epinephrine to the site.

The patient who is bleeding excessively often is returned to the operating room for surgical treatment to stop the hemorrhage.

Medications used in tonsillitis include analgesics and antipyretics (e.g., acetaminophen) and antibiotic agents (e.g., penicillin). Warm saline gargles are also beneficial.

Nursing Interventions and Patient Teaching

One of the primary nursing goals for acute tonsillitis is to provide meticulous oral care, which promotes comfort and assists in combating infection. Observe and report if the patient swallows frequently, because this is often a subtle but reliable indication of excessive bleeding.

Postoperative care for tonsillectomy includes maintaining IV fluids until the nausea subsides, at which time the patient may begin drinking ice-cold clear liquids. The diet is advanced to custard and ice cream and then to a normal diet as soon as possible. Spicy foods should be avoided because they often irritate the throat after surgery. Hot liquids and food are avoided because these cause vasodilation, leading to bleeding. Apply an ice collar to the neck for comfort and to reduce bleeding by vasoconstriction. Monitor vital signs to assess for hemorrhage, postoperative fever, or other complications. Comfort measures are important, and emotional support is essential.

Patient problems and interventions for the patient with acute follicular tonsillitis include but are not limited to the following:

PATIENT PROBLEM	NURSING INTERVENTIONS
Discomfort, related to inflammation and irritation of the pharynx	Assess degree of pain and need for analgesics Document effectiveness of medication and offer analgesic as ordered Maintain bed rest and promote rest Offer warm saline gargles, ice chips, and ice collar as needed
Potential for Inadequate Fluid Volume, related to inability to maintain usual oral intake because of painful swallowing	Assess hydration status by noting mucous membranes, skin turgor, and urinary output Encourage ice pops, ice chips, and increased oral intake; cold liquids, sherbet, and ice cream are best tolerated; carbonated drinks may be taken if patient tolerates; avoid offering citrus juices because they may burn the throat
Potential for Aspiration Into Airway, related to postoperative bleeding	Maintain patent airway; keep patient lying on side as much as possible to prevent aspiration Observe for vomiting of dark brown fluid; patient may have "swallowed" blood during surgery

PATIENT PROBLEM	NURSING INTERVENTIONS
	Watch for frequent swallowing, which may indicate bleeding; check frequently with flashlight to see if blood is trickling down posterior pharynx

Instruct the patient (or the family for a child) that the patient should complete the entire course of the prescribed antibiotic. If the patient had surgery (T&A), offer dietary instruction regarding appropriate foods and liquids. Advise the patient to avoid attempting to clear the throat immediately after surgery (may initiate bleeding) and to avoid coughing, sneezing, or vigorous nose blowing for 1 to 2 weeks. Most surgeons no longer prescribe aspirin for pain after tonsillectomy, because it increases the tendency to bleed; acetaminophen or another aspirin substitute usually is ordered. Analgesics usually are given orally in liquid form. Remind the patient to avoid overexertion and make certain that the patient and the family know how to reach the health care provider in case of increased pain, fever, or bleeding.

Prognosis

Tonsillitis is usually self-limiting but may have serious complications, such as sinusitis, otitis media, mastoiditis, rheumatic fever, nephritis, or peritonsillar abscess.

LARYNGITIS

Etiology and Pathophysiology

Laryngitis often occurs secondary to other respiratory infections. Laryngeal inflammation is a common disorder that can be either chronic or acute. Acute laryngitis may cause severe respiratory distress in children younger than 5 years of age because the relatively small larynx is subject to spasm when irritated or infected and readily becomes partially or totally obstructed.

Acute laryngitis often accompanies viral or bacterial infections. Other causes include excessive use of the voice or inhalation of irritating fumes. Chronic laryngitis usually is associated with inflammation of the laryngeal mucosa or edematous vocal cords.

Clinical Manifestations

Laryngitis often produces hoarseness to some degree, or even complete voice loss. The throat feels scratchy and irritated, and the patient may have a persistent cough.

Assessment

Subjective data include the patient reporting progressive hoarseness and a cough that may be productive or may be dry and nonproductive. Attempt to identify any precipitating factors such as excessive voice use or exposure to inhaled irritants.

Collection of objective data includes evaluating the patient's voice quality and the characteristics (color, consistency, and amount) of sputum produced.

Diagnostic Tests

Laryngoscopy reveals abnormalities (edema, drainage) of vocal cords and erythematous laryngeal mucosa.

Medical Management

If the laryngitis is due to a virus, there is no specific therapy; if it is bacterial, medications include antibiotics (such as erythromycin or levofloxacin). Analgesics or antipyretics for comfort, antitussives to relieve cough (such as promethazine with codeine), and throat lozenges to promote comfort and decrease irritation are useful.

Nursing Interventions and Patient Teaching

General interventions include use of warm or cool mist inhalation via a vaporizer. Encourage the patient to rest the voice by limiting verbal communication.

Patient problems and interventions for the patient with laryngitis include but are not limited to the following:

PATIENT PROBLEM	NURSING INTERVENTIONS
Discomfort, related to pharyngeal irritation	Assess level of pain, and offer medications to promote comfort
	Use steam inhalation as ordered
	Instruct patient on the importance of resting the voice
Compromised Verbal Communication, related to edematous vocal cords	Instruct patient on the importance of resting the voice
	Provide other means for communication (written word, gestures)
	Anticipate patient's needs whenever possible

If the patient receives antibiotic agents, instruct him or her to finish the entire prescribed course. Remind the patient of the need to limit use of the voice. Encourage patients who are smokers to quit and to limit exposure to irritating fumes.

Prognosis

The prognosis is good in adults. In the infant and the young child, respiratory edema can result in respiratory distress.

PHARYNGITIS

Etiology and Pathophysiology

Pharyngitis may be either chronic or acute. It is the most common throat inflammation and frequently accompanies the common cold. Pharyngitis is usually viral but can be caused by beta-hemolytic streptococci, staphylococci, or other bacteria. There is increased evidence of gonococcal pharyngitis caused by the gram-negative diplococcus *Neisseria gonorrhoeae*. A severe form of acute pharyngitis often is referred to as *strep throat* because the *Streptococcus* organism is commonly the cause. This disorder is contagious for 2 or 3 days after the onset of signs and symptoms.

Clinical Manifestations

Pharyngitis is manifest clinically by a dry cough, tender tonsils, and enlarged cervical lymph glands. The throat appears erythematous, and soreness may range from slight scratchiness to severe pain with difficulty in swallowing.

Assessment

Subjective data include any reported pharyngeal discomfort, fever, or difficulty in swallowing.

Collection of objective data includes palpating for enlarged, edematous glands and associated tenderness and noting elevated temperature.

Diagnostic Tests

A rapid strep screen test is performed to determine the presence of beta-hemolytic streptococci. This is only a preliminary diagnosis. A culture is obtained at the same time in case the rapid strep screen yields a false-negative result. Obtain a specimen from the pharynx and make sure the swab does not touch the tongue or gums during insertion. The patient often gags if the specimen is obtained correctly.

Medical Management

Commonly ordered medications include antibiotics, such as penicillin or erythromycin, to (1) treat severe infections or (2) prevent superimposed infections, particularly in people who have a history of rheumatic fever or bacterial endocarditis. Analgesics and antipyretics, such as acetaminophen, are used to promote comfort.

Nursing Interventions and Patient Teaching

Offer saline throat rinses or gargles and encourage oral intake. Emphasize the importance of adequate rest and use of a vaporizer to increase humidity.

Patient problems and interventions for the patient with pharyngitis include but are not limited to the following:

PATIENT PROBLEM	NURSING INTERVENTIONS
Compromised Oral Mucous Membrane, related to edema	Provide warm saline gargles to promote comfort
	Assess level of pain and provide medications as ordered
	Encourage oral intake of fluids
	Offer frequent oral care
Potential for Inadequate Fluid Volume, related to decreased oral intake as a result of painful swallowing	Observe and record patient's hydration status
	Monitor I&O and patient's temperature
	Maintain IV therapy if indicated

Perform and document medication teaching, including the importance of completing the entire prescribed course of antibiotics and any side effects of medications. Instruct the patient to avoid exposure to inhaled irritants and to apply preventive measures, such as using a vaporizer and maintaining adequate fluid intake.

Prognosis
Signs and symptoms usually resolve in 4 to 6 days unless secondary complications develop.

SINUSITIS

Etiology and Pathophysiology
Sinusitis can be chronic or acute, involving any sinus area, such as the maxillary or frontal sinuses. This infection can be either viral or bacterial and often is a complication of pneumonia or nasal polyps. The underlying pathophysiology begins with an upper respiratory tract infection that leads to a sinus infection.

Clinical Manifestations
The patient with sinusitis often complains of a constant, severe headache with pain and tenderness in the particular sinus region and often has purulent exudate.

Assessment
Subjective data include patient reporting decreased appetite or nausea. The patient also may complain of generalized malaise, headache, diminished sense of smell, and increased pain in the sinus region when bending forward or when gentle pressure is applied over the infected sinus region.

Collection of objective data involves assessing vital signs, particularly temperature, and also assessing the character and amount of drainage. Headache, facial pain (with and/or without palpation), thick nasal secretions, congestion, edema of the eyelids, fatigue, and elevated temperature are common symptoms.

Diagnostic Tests
Sinus radiographic studies frequently are done to depict cloudy or fluid-filled sinus cavities. A simple way to diagnose sinusitis is with transillumination. This procedure involves shining a light in the mouth with the lips closed around it; infected sinuses look dark, whereas normal sinuses transilluminate. To confirm the diagnosis, a sinus CT scan may be performed.

Medical Management
Nasal windows or other surgical incisions can be created to allow better drainage and removal of diseased mucosal tissue. A common surgical procedure to relieve chronic maxillary sinusitis, the Caldwell-Luc operation (or radical antrum operation), involves making an incision between the gum and upper lip, allowing access to the floor of the maxillary sinus. This is followed by removal of a small piece of maxillary bone. This opening allows the infected maxillary sinus to drain.

Medications used to treat sinusitis include the following:
- *Saline nasal irrigation:* A saline solution is sprayed into the nose to rinse the nasal passages.
- *Nasal corticosteroids:* These nasal sprays help prevent and treat inflammation. Examples include fluticasone, budesonide, triamcinolone, mometasone, and beclomethasone.
- *Oral or injected corticosteroids:* These medications are used to relieve inflammation from severe sinusitis, especially if the patient also has nasal polyps. Examples include prednisone and methylprednisolone. Oral corticosteroids can cause serious side effects when used long term, so they are used only to treat severe symptoms.
- *Decongestants:* These medications are available as over-the-counter (OTC) and prescription liquids, tablets, and nasal sprays. An examples of OTC oral decongestants include pseudoephedrine. An example of an OTC nasal spray is oxymetazoline. These medications generally are taken for a few days at most; otherwise they can cause the return of more severe congestion (rebound congestion).
- *Over-the-counter pain relievers:* Over-the-counter pain relievers include aspirin, acetaminophen, and ibuprofen. Because of the risk of Reye syndrome—a potentially life-threatening illness—never give aspirin to anyone younger than age 18 years.
- *Antibiotics:* Antibiotics are prescribed only if the health care provider determines that the cause of the sinusitis is bacterial.

Nursing Interventions and Patient Teaching
Steam inhalation and warm, moist packs facilitate drainage and promote comfort.

Neti pots have been used for irrigation of the sinus cavities, using a salt and warm water solution. Care must be taken when making your own solution. Using filtered water or distilled water is recommended by the Centers for Disease Control and Prevention (CDC).

Patient problems and interventions for the patient with sinusitis include but are not limited to the following:

PATIENT PROBLEM	NURSING INTERVENTIONS
Inability to Maintain Adequate Breathing Pattern, related to nasal congestion	Assess respiratory status frequently, noting any changes; mouth breathing may be necessary because of nasal airway and sinus discomfort
Discomfort, related to sinus congestion	Document comfort level Assess need for analgesics and document patient response Elevate head of bed to promote drainage of secretions Apply warm, moist packs four times a day to promote secretion drainage and provide relief

The aim of patient education is to prevent recurrence or complications of sinus infection. Instruct the patient to be alert to signs and symptoms of sinusitis so that early treatment can be obtained.

Prognosis

Prognosis for uncomplicated sinusitis is good; complications include cavernous sinus thrombosis and spread of infection to bone, brain, or meninges, which can result in meningitis, osteomyelitis, or septicemia.

DISORDERS OF THE LOWER AIRWAY

ACUTE BRONCHITIS

Etiology and Pathophysiology

Usually acute bronchitis is secondary to an upper respiratory tract infection, but it can be related to exposure to inhaled irritants. Inflammation of the trachea and bronchial tree causes congestion of the mucous membranes, which results in retention of tenacious secretions. These secretions can become a culture medium for bacterial growth.

Clinical Manifestations

Acute bronchitis manifests itself with symptoms such as a productive cough, diffuse rhonchi and wheezes, dyspnea, chest pain, and low-grade fever. Generalized malaise and headache are also common symptoms.

Assessment

Subjective data include the patient's complaints of feeling poorly and experiencing headache and aching tightness in the chest.

Collection of objective data includes monitoring vital signs frequently, checking breath sounds, and noting the presence of wheezes or basilar crackles.

Diagnostic Tests

The usual diagnostic aids include a chest radiographic examination to ensure clear lung fields and a sputum specimen to determine the presence of associated bacterial infections.

Medical Management

A quick recovery is promoted by preventing further infectious complications. The health care provider may order sputum cultures periodically to ensure that there is no secondary infection.

Medication regimens include cough suppressants such as codeine and dextromethorphan, antipyretics (acetaminophen), and bronchodilators (albuterol). Antibiotics such as ampicillin may be ordered to combat or prevent an infectious process.

Nursing Interventions and Patient Teaching

The goal of nursing interventions is to facilitate recovery and prevent secondary infections. Such actions include placing the patient on bed rest to conserve energy, using a vaporizer to add humidity to inhaled air, and increasing fluid intake.

Patient problems and interventions for the patient with acute bronchitis include but are not limited to the following:

PATIENT PROBLEM	NURSING INTERVENTIONS
Potential for Infection, related to retained pulmonary secretions	Assess for signs and symptoms of infection: fever, dyspnea, mucopurulent (yellow-green) sputum, and amount of sputum production Administer antipyretics and antibiotics as ordered
Inability to Clear Airway, related to tenacious pulmonary secretions	Assess patient's ability to move secretions; also note any increase in retained pulmonary secretions Facilitate airway clearance by elevating head of bed and liquefying secretions by use of humidifier and adequate fluid intake (3000–4000 mL/day) Suction as needed When offering fluids, avoid dairy products, which tend to produce more tenacious secretions

Instruct the patient in measures that prevent exacerbation or recurrence of infection. Such measures include increasing oral fluid intake, incorporating rest periods between activities, and recognizing the signs that may indicate worsening infection (purulent sputum and increased dyspnea). Emphasize the importance of adhering to the prescribed medication regimen and using analgesics and antipyretics to reduce fever and malaise. Advise the patient to limit exposure to others reduce potential transmission of the infection. Avoid irritants such as smoking or fumes.

Prognosis

The prognosis for acute bronchitis is good.

LEGIONNAIRES' DISEASE

Etiology and Pathophysiology

The causative microorganism of legionnaires' disease is *Legionella pneumophila,* first identified in 1976 when it caused a pneumonia outbreak at a convention of the American Legion in Philadelphia. *L. pneumophila* is a gram-negative bacillus not previously recognized as an agent of human disease. This organism thrives in water reservoirs, such as in air conditioners, humidifiers, and whirlpool spas. It is transmitted through airborne routes. The *Legionella* microbe can progress in two different forms: influenza or legionnaires' disease. The latter characteristically results in life-threatening pneumonia that causes lung consolidation and alveolar necrosis. The disease progresses rapidly (less than 1 week) and can result in respiratory failure, renal failure, bacteremic shock, and ultimately death.

Clinical Manifestations
Clinical manifestations include significantly elevated temperature, headache, nonproductive cough, diarrhea, and general malaise.

Assessment
Collection of subjective data includes noting the patient's complaints of dyspnea, headache, and chest pain on inspiration.

Objective data include many significant signs associated with this infectious process. A significantly elevated temperature (102°F to 105°F [38.8°C to 40.5°C]) bears close watching and may require immediate interventions. The patient also has a nonproductive cough with difficult and rapid breathing. Auscultation of lungs reveals crackles or wheezes. Because of the high fever and extreme respiratory effort, tachycardia and signs of shock may be present. Hematuria may develop, indicative of renal impairment.

Diagnostic Tests
Urine testing is relatively inexpensive and may be used to confirm the diagnosis. Additional diagnostic tests may include blood, sputum, or pulmonary tissue or fluid cultures (CDC,2021d).

Medical Management
To control and compensate for impaired and ineffective respiratory function, the patient with legionnaires' disease needs oxygen therapy, possibly even mechanical ventilation. The patient placed on mechanical ventilation requires intubation via the mouth or nose, or directly via a tracheostomy tube. Close observation for disease progression is required. The patient needs adequate IV fluid therapy to maintain hydration and electrolyte status and may require temporary renal dialysis because of acute kidney failure.

Antibiotic agents (erythromycin) are given intravenously early in the disease and then orally for a prolonged period to treat the infection. Rifampin is also beneficial. Antipyretics are administered to reduce the patient's temperature. The patient also may require vasopressors (dopamine or dobutamine) and analgesics to treat shock and promote comfort.

Nursing Interventions and Patient Teaching
Maintain the patient on bed rest, with the head of the bed elevated at least 30 degrees for ease of respiratory effort, and monitor I&O.

Patient problems and interventions for the patient with legionnaires' disease include but are not limited to the following:

PATIENT PROBLEM	NURSING INTERVENTIONS
Compromised Blood Flow to Cardiopulmonary or Renal Tissue, related to lack of oxygen	Monitor and report signs and symptoms of impending shock (decreased blood pressure and increased pulse) Administer vasopressor drugs as ordered Maintain hydration status and urinary output Assess changes in level of consciousness Assist with acute hemodialysis if indicated
Inability to Maintain Adequate Breathing Pattern, related to respiratory failure	Assess signs and symptoms of respiratory failure Note respiratory rate, rhythm, and effort Be alert for cyanosis and dyspnea Assist with oxygen therapy or mechanical ventilation as ordered Facilitate optimal ventilation; place patient in semi-Fowler's position if tolerated; suction as needed Have patient cough and deep breathe q 2 h. if able Identify associated factors, such as ineffective airway clearance, pain, and altered level of consciousness

Because of the many alarming actions necessary to treat this disease and its complications, patient and family education is important. Instruct the patient and family on the purpose of respiratory support (oxygen therapy or ventilator assistance) and how to use these procedures for the greatest benefit. Before their implementation, explain all procedures, including the purpose of hemodialysis and why it is required. Stress the importance of controlling the patient's temperature and fluid and electrolyte status. Offer emotional support to the patient and the family as needed.

Prognosis
Usually the disease is self-limiting, but legionnaires' disease can be severe and fatal. The mortality rate is 1 out of 10 patients with the infection (CDC, 2021d).

COVID-19 (CORONAVIRUS DISEASE)
Etiology and Pathophysiology
Coronavirus disease (COVID-19) is caused by infection with severe acute respiratory syndrome coronavirus 2 (SARS-CoV-2) (Martines, Ritter, Matkovic, 2020). This is a new virus that has caused a pandemic that started in 2019. Understanding of the etiology and pathophysiology is emerging with numerous current studies being performed. Preventing the spread of the

infection is critical. Steps like frequent handwashing, wearing masks, frequent cleaning and quarantining if a person has been exposed are key (CDC, 2021a).

Clinical Manifestations
COVID-19 causes a systemic inflammatory response. Infection with this virus has caused a wide range of symptoms being reported—ranging from mild symptoms to severe illness. Symptoms may appear 2 to 14 days after exposure to the virus. Symptoms may include fever, chills, cough, shortness of breath, fatigue, muscle or body aches, headache, loss of taste and/or smell, sore throat, nasal congestion, nausea, vomiting and diarrhea. Not all people will have all the symptoms and some may have no symptoms at all. Some people will develop more severe symptoms such as trouble breathing, hypoxia, pneumonia, and acute respiratory distress syndrome (ARDS) that will require the patient to be hospitalized (CDC, 2021b).

Diagnostic Tests
Currently there are two types of COVID-19 tests, viral tests and antibody tests. Viral tests are done via an anterior nasal swab and can determine if the patient currently has a COVID-19 infection. Antibody testing can be done to determine if the patient has had a past infection.

If a patient has been hospitalized, diagnostic tests such as a chest radiograph may be done to determine the presence of an underlying pneumonia or the development of ARDS (CDC, 2021c).

Medical Management
Medical management is determined by the severity of symptoms. Less severe cases can be managed in an outpatient setting with rest, fluids, and over-the-counter medications such as acetaminophen to help reduce fever and treat body aches. Patients also need to quarantine along with any close contacts for up to 14 days. Unfortunately, due to adult respiratory distress many patients have required treatments such as Vapotherm (non-invasive, mask-free high-flow oxygen delivery device delivering up to 40L/min), proning (turning the patient to a prone position for better posterior lung field ventilation and clearing of secretions), and mechanical ventilation. The first vaccine was approved in December 2020.

Nursing Interventions and Patient Teaching
Notification of the local health department must be done. Infection control and isolation procedures must be followed such as wearing a N-95 respirator along with eye covering and a PAPR device (powered air purifying respirator) when caring for patients who are COVID-19 positive. If the patient is stable enough to be treated at home, education regarding increasing fluids, proper rest and the use of antipyretics such as acetaminophen will need to be provided. Information regarding quarantining of any close contacts will also need to be provided (CDC, 2020b).

Prognosis
Little is known regarding the long-term prognosis of those infected with the COVID-19 coronavirus. Some patient's recover in just a few days while others are still suffering symptoms months later. Hypoxia that requires the use of supplemental oxygen, blood clots, extreme fatigue are some of the lingering symptoms. As of December 2020, 17.5 million people have been infected by the virus and over 300,000 people in the US died (CDC, n.d.).

ANTHRAX
Etiology and Pathophysiology
Anthrax is an infectious disease caused by the spore-forming bacterium *Bacillus anthracis*. In nature, anthrax most commonly infects wild and domestic hoofed animals. It is spread through direct contact with the bacteria and its spores—dormant, encapsulated bacteria that become active when they enter a living host.

In humans, anthrax gains a foothold when spores enter the body via the skin, intestines, or lungs. It is not contagious by person-to-person contact, so treating family members and others in contact with an infected person is not recommended unless they were exposed to the same source of the spores that caused the infection.

Three types of anthrax. Anthrax symptoms depend on the initial site of infection. The three types of anthrax are as follows:

1. *Cutaneous anthrax,* the most common type, occurs after bacteria or spores enter the skin through a cut or abrasion. Within several days of exposure, a pruritic reddened macule or papule develops, followed by vesicle formation. The lesion resembles an insect bite at first, until black eschar (dead, sloughing tissue) appears at the center of the lesion, and the site becomes edematous. Although a patient may develop bacteremia if the organism enters his or her bloodstream, cutaneous anthrax is rarely fatal if it is treated with antibiotics.
2. *Gastrointestinal anthrax,* the least common type, occurs after ingestion of the organism in contaminated, undercooked food. Spores can germinate in the mouth, the esophagus, the stomach, or the small and large intestines, causing ulcers. Inflammation of the gastrointestinal tract can cause nausea, vomiting, fever, abdominal pain, and diarrhea. Unless treated early, a patient may die from sepsis.
3. *Inhalational anthrax,* seen in global germ warfare, is the most lethal type. It develops when spores are inhaled deeply into the lungs. Immune cells sent to fight the lung infection carry some bacteria back to the lymph system, which spreads the infection to other organs.

Initial symptoms of inhalational anthrax resemble those of the common cold or influenza, except that the patient usually does not develop an increased amount of thin, clear nasal exudate. Subsequent breathing problems may be mistaken for pneumonia, delaying diagnosis. Other severe symptoms, including hemorrhage, tissue necrosis, and lymphedema, are caused by bacterial toxins. Death usually results from blood loss and shock.

Diagnostic Tests

Initial testing for anthrax traditionally begins by ruling out other potential conditions. A chest x-ray helps differentiate inhalational anthrax from pneumonia. A widening mediastinum from lymphadenopathy is characteristic of inhalational anthrax infection; infiltrates characterize pneumonia.

Additional diagnostic tests for anthrax include blood and sputum cultures and lumbar punctures. When managing patients with symptoms consistent with inhalational anthrax, use standard precautions to obtain specimens for a blood smear and culture. A nasal swab is not recommended to diagnose anthrax infection. For a patient suspected of having cutaneous anthrax, obtain a culture specimen from the lesion's vesicular fluid. Obtain a stool specimen for culture if intestinal anthrax is suspected.

Medical Management

Antibiotic treatment is indicated for anyone diagnosed with anthrax or exposed to anthrax spores. For children and adults, ciprofloxacin has been considered the treatment of choice for all three forms of anthrax because of concerns that genetically engineered anthrax strains may resist older antibiotics. Most anthrax strains are susceptible to many other antibiotics, including penicillin and doxycycline. A 60-day therapy is prescribed. Because of concerns about drug resistance, health experts in the United States have urged health care providers to avoid prescribing antibiotics indiscriminately because of the danger of antimicrobial resistance (Mayo Clinic, 2020a).

The CDC recommends a 60-day course of therapy to ensure eradication of inactive spores and bacteria. An alternative treatment for postexposure prophylaxis is 30 days of antibiotics and three doses of the anthrax vaccine, if it is available. (The anthrax vaccine currently is not recommended for the general public in the absence of anthrax exposure.) Consult the US Food and Drug Administration (FDA) and CDC websites for prescribing information for children and other treatment updates (CDC, 2020a).

TUBERCULOSIS

Etiology and Pathophysiology

In 1882, Robert Koch identified the tubercle bacillus (*Mycobacterium tuberculosis*) as the causative agent for tuberculosis (TB). TB is a chronic pulmonary and extrapulmonary (outside of the lung) infectious disease acquired by inhalation of a dried droplet nucleus containing a tubercle bacillus, coughed or sneezed into the air by a person whose sputum contains virulent (capable of producing disease) tubercle bacilli, and inhaled into the alveolar structure of the lung. It is characterized by stages of early infection (frequently asymptomatic), latency, and a potential for recurrent postprimary disease. It most commonly affects the respiratory system, but other parts of the body such as the gastrointestinal and genitourinary tracts, bones, joints, nervous system, lymph nodes, and skin may become infected (see the Cultural Considerations box).

 Cultural Considerations

Tuberculosis

- Tuberculosis (TB) in the United States tends to be a disease of the older population, urban poor, minority groups, and patients with acquired immunodeficiency syndrome. All new admittances to nursing homes require a two-step TB test. Homeless patients admitted to the hospital also require a TB test. A total of 8916 TB cases (a rate of 2.7 cases per 100,000 persons) were reported in the United States in 2019 (CDC, 2020d).
- At all ages the incidence of TB among nonwhites is at least twice that of whites.
- TB is one of the top 10 causes of death worldwide (WHO, 2020).
- Ending the TB epidemic by 2030 is among the health targets of the newly adopted Sustainable Development Goals (WHO, 2020).
- Globally, the incidence of TB is falling about 2% per year. (WHO, 2020)
- In 2019, eight countries accounted for two-thirds of the new TB cases: India, Indonesia, China, Philippines, Pakistan, Nigeria, Bangladesh and South Africa (WHO, 2020).

It is important to differentiate *infection* with TB from *active disease*. Although infection always precedes the development of active disease, only about 10% of infections progress to active disease. TB infection is characterized by mycobacteria in the tissue of a host who is free of clinical signs and symptoms and who demonstrates the presence of antibodies against mycobacteria. TB disease is manifest as pathologic and functional signs and symptoms indicating destructive activity of mycobacteria in host tissue.

In the lung, pulmonary macrophages ingest TB bacteria. Macrophages engulf the organisms, but do not kill them. Instead they surround them and wall them off in tiny, hard capsules called *tubercles*. Macrophages activate lymphocytes, and within 2 to 10 weeks, activated lymphocytes usually control the initial infection in the lung and non-pulmonary sites. Non-multiplying tubercle bacilli can survive more than 50 years in human tissue.

Most people who become infected with the TB organism do not progress to the active disease stage. They remain asymptomatic and noninfectious. They have a positive tuberculin skin test, and chest radiographs are negative. These people still retain a lifelong risk of developing reactivation of TB if the immune system is compromised.

A common misconception about TB is that it is transmitted easily. In fact, most people exposed to TB do not become infected. The body's first line of defense, the upper airway, prevents most inhaled TB organisms from ever reaching the lungs. If the inhaled particles are small enough, the organisms can survive in the upper respiratory tract, reach the alveoli, and establish infection. Less commonly, transmission may occur by ingestion or by invasion of the skin or mucous membranes.

TB had been epidemic in the Western world. With the introduction of pharmacologic management in the late 1940s and early 1950s, the prevalence of TB decreased dramatically. TB had been responsible for one-third of the deaths of the young adults in Europe. After Koch's discovery, improvement in living conditions, sanitation, and the development of effective drug therapy and treatment brought about a steady decline in mortality attributable to TB. Shortly after the centennial of Koch's work, eradication of the disease in the United States by the year 2010 was considered a realistic goal.

TB has been particularly prevalent among people infected with human immunodeficiency virus (HIV). The status of the host's immune system is the major determinant for the development of active TB. The disease occurs most often in individuals with incompetent immune systems, such as HIV-infected people, older adults, people receiving immunosuppressive therapy, and the malnourished.

Hospitals are a high-risk setting for TB transmission, and health care workers are at high occupational risk for TB infection. Until recently the vulnerability of hospital workers to TB infection had not been emphasized. This complacency is changing with the wide publicity accompanying the increase in TB (Box 9.5).

Clinical Manifestations

The clinical manifestations are insidious. Generally, patients have fever, weight loss, weakness, and a productive cough. Later in the disease, daily recurring fever with chills, night sweats, and hemoptysis is seen.

Assessment

Subjective data include the patient reporting loss of muscle strength and weight loss.

Collection of objective data includes evaluating and recording the amount, color, and characteristics of sputum produced.

Box 9.5 | High-Risk Groups to Screen for Tuberculosis

- People infected with human immunodeficiency virus
- Close contacts (especially children and adolescents) of people with active infectious tuberculosis (TB)
- People with conditions that increase the risk of active TB after infection, such as silicosis, diabetes, chronic renal failure, history of gastrectomy, weight 10% below ideal body weight, prolonged corticosteroid or other immunosuppressive therapy, some hematologic disorders (e.g., leukemia and lymphomas), and other malignancies
- People born in countries with a high prevalence of TB
- Substance abusers, such as alcoholics, intravenous drug users, and cocaine or crack users
- Residents of long-term care facilities, nursing homes, prisons, mental institutions, homeless shelters, and other congregate housing settings
- Medically underserved low-income populations, including racial and ethnic minorities, homeless people, and migrant workers
- Health care workers and others who provide services to any high-risk group

---

Diagnostic Tests

Diagnostic evaluation includes the tuberculin skin test (Mantoux), using purified protein derivative (PPD), to identify people infected with the TB organism. A positive reaction indicates infection 2 to 10 weeks after exposure to the tubercle bacillus. To read the test 48 to 72 hours later, measure and record the subsequent induration (an area of hardened tissue); do not measure the erythema (redness). A negative reaction is based on the size of the induration. If the patient is infected with TB (whether active or dormant), lymphocytes recognize the PPD antigen in the skin test and cause a local indurated reaction. Generally, the larger the reaction, the greater the likelihood that the person is infected with the TB organism, unless of course the person has had a false-positive result in the past and does not have an active infection. However, a negative reaction does not rule out infection. An infected person whose immune system has been weakened by disease, drugs, or old age may have a limited or negative reaction. If the test is negative and the health care provider strongly suspects TB, a "second-strength" or two-step tuberculin test can be used. If this test is negative, the patient does not have TB.

Other diagnostic tests used to confirm the diagnosis of pulmonary TB are chest radiograph and evaluation of sputum specimens for mycobacterial organisms. Sputum specimens can be smeared, stained, and screened rapidly for the presence of acid-fast organisms, the definitive test for TB. Mycobacteria are one of the few organisms that are characteristically acid fast. Three positive acid-fast smears constitute a presumptive diagnosis of TB and indicate the need for treatment. The diagnosis of TB is confirmed if tubercle bacilli grow in culture, a process that may take 6 to 8 weeks.

QuantiFERON-TB Gold test. In May 2005 the FDA approved a blood test to aid in the diagnosis of latent TB. This blood test, the QuantiFERON-TB Gold (QFT-G), is more specific for *Mycobacterium* tubercle bacillus than the PPD skin test (WHO, 2011). The advantages of QFT-G are greater specificity and results 24 hours after blood is collected. The PPD skin test requires a 2- to 3-day wait and a return visit to the health care provider. Sputum smears and cultures are still done, but the QFT-G offers a quick and reliable diagnosis for the patient and health care provider.

All patients diagnosed with TB must be reported to the public health personnel for appropriate investigation and follow-up care (WHO, 2020).

Medical Management

Drug therapy is the mainstay of TB treatment. Infectiousness declines rapidly once drug therapy is initiated, even before sputum smears become negative. Cough frequently also declines with drug therapy.

Isolation is indicated for patients with pulmonary TB who have a positive sputum smear or a chest radiograph that strongly suggests current (active) TB. Laryngeal TB also is included in this isolation category. In general, infants and young children with pulmonary TB do not require isolation precautions because they rarely cough and their bronchial secretions contain few acid-fast bacilli (AFB), compared with adults with pulmonary TB. If there is a question of infectiousness in the adult patient with TB, hospitalized patients usually remain in respiratory isolation during their hospital stay.

Compared with most other infectious diseases, treatment for TB is lengthy, typically 6 to 9 months, and sometimes longer for extrapulmonary disease. If treatment is not continued for a long time, some of the TB organisms survive, and the patient is at risk for a relapse.

Treatment now involves multiple drugs to which the organisms are susceptible. If only one drug is given, the mycobacteria may become resistant to it. Treatment usually consists of a combination of at least four drugs, each of which helps prevent the emergence of organisms resistant to the others, thus increasing the therapeutic effectiveness. A series of medications that are often used to treat TB include isoniazid, rifampin, and pyrazinamide. Streptomycin or ethambutol is also used in the regimen. In the event the disease becomes resistant to the prescribed first-line therapy the second-line medications will be implemented. Second-line drugs are ethionamide, *para*-aminosalicylate sodium (PAS), cycloserine, capreomycin, kanamycin, amikacin, levofloxacin, ofloxacin, and ciprofloxacin (Table 9.3).

Table 9.3   Medications for Respiratory Disorders

GENERIC NAME	ACTION	SIDE EFFECTS	NURSING IMPLICATIONS
Acetylcysteine	Mucolytic agent; also used as antidote in acetaminophen overdose	Nausea, vomiting, rhinorrhea, mucorrhea, bronchospasm	Store product in refrigerator. Bad taste may be masked by mixing with soft drink when using as antidote.
Aminophylline	See entry for theophylline	See entry for theophylline	See entry for theophylline.
Azatadine; also available in numerous combination allergy and cold preparations	Antihistamine; blocks allergic response through histamine receptor blockade	Drowsiness, confusion, dry mouth, constipation, urinary retention, blurred vision, increased viscosity of respiratory secretions	Avoid use with alcohol or other CNS depressants. Avoid driving and other hazardous activities.
Short-acting beta$_2$-receptor agonists: albuterol , others	Beta$_2$-receptor agonists; cause bronchodilation, smooth muscle relaxation	Common: Anxiety, headache, insomnia, dizziness, restlessness, tachycardia Rare: Cardiac palpitations, angina or chest pain, cardiac dysrhythmias	Use with caution in cardiac disease. Teach patient that paradoxic bronchospasm may occur, and if so to stop drug immediately and call health care provider. Teach proper use of metered dose inhaler to achieve an appropriate therapeutic response.

Continued

Table 9.3 Medications for Respiratory Disorders—cont'd

GENERIC NAME	ACTION	SIDE EFFECTS	NURSING IMPLICATIONS
Long-acting beta$_2$-receptor agonists: salmeterol	Causes bronchodilation; used in prevention of exercise-induced asthma	Tremors, anxiety, insomnia, headache, stimulation, tachycardia, dry mouth, bronchospasm	Avoid use of OTC medications; overstimulation may occur. Use with caution in cardiac disorders, hyperthyroidism, hypertension, and narrow-angle glaucoma.
Corticosteroids: prednisone, methylprednisolone, hydrocortisone	Anti-inflammatory agents	Short-term: Sodium and water retention, hypokalemia, hyperglycemia, euphoria	Do not discontinue medication abruptly; dosage must be tapered slowly. Have patient carry identification signaling steroid use. Take with food or milk to minimize stomach upset.
Fluticasone (inhaled corticosteroid)		Long-term: Osteoporosis, increased susceptibility to infection, poor wound healing, bruising, thinning of skin, Cushingoid weight distribution, cataracts, glaucoma, peptic ulcer disease, myopathy, muscle weakness, suppression of endogenous glucocorticoid production	
Epinephrine	Beta$_1$- and beta$_2$-receptor agonist; causes bronchodilation and cardiac stimulation; alpha$_1$-agonist activity may cause vasoconstriction	Tachycardia, palpitations, angina, chest pain, myocardial infarction, cardiac dysrhythmias, hypertension, restlessness, agitation, anxiety	Use with extreme caution in cardiac disease; do not use in conjunction with OTC cough or cold preparations; do not use discolored preparations.
Ethambutol	Antitubercular agent	Optic neuritis, blurred vision or decreased visual acuity, hyperuricemia, exacerbation of gout, drowsiness, confusion, GI effects, hepatotoxicity, thrombocytopenia	Patient should have baseline visual examination at start of therapy. Emphasize that long-term therapy is required for cure.
Isoniazid	Antitubercular agent	Peripheral neuropathy, hepatotoxicity, SLE-like syndrome, hyperglycemia, bone marrow suppression	Monitor liver function. Emphasize that long-term therapy is required. Instruct patient to report numbness or tingling of extremities.
Leukotriene modifiers; leukotriene receptor antagonists (zafirlukast, montelukast); leukotriene synthesis inhibitors (zileuton)	Interferes with the synthesis, or blocks the action, of leukotrienes, causing both bronchodilator and anti-inflammatory effects; for long-term treatment of asthma	Zafirlukast: Hepatic dysfunction, systemic eosinophilia, headache, infection, nausea, asthenia (abnormal weakness), abdominal pain Montelukast: Tiredness, fever, abdominal pain, dizziness Zileuton: Headache, abdominal pain, asthenia, dyspepsia	Monitor for eosinophilia, worsening pulmonary symptoms, cardiac complications, and neuropathy. Administer after meals for GI symptoms.
Oxymetazoline	Vasoconstrictor, used for nasal congestion	Local nasal irritation, dryness, rebound congestion	Do not use for more than 4 consecutive days to minimize rebound congestion.
para-Aminosalicylate sodium	Antitubercular agent	Nausea, vomiting, diarrhea, abdominal pain, hypersensitivity reactions, hepatotoxicity, leukopenia, thrombocytopenia	Take with food. Discard if discolored. Use with caution in peptic ulcer disease or congestive heart failure. Emphasize that long-term therapy is required.

Table 9.3   Medications for Respiratory Disorders—cont'd

GENERIC NAME	ACTION	SIDE EFFECTS	NURSING IMPLICATIONS
Potassium iodide (many; also available in numerous combination preparations)	Expectorant, mucokinetic agent	Hypersensitivity, rash, metallic taste, burning in mouth or throat, GI irritation, headache, parotitis, hyperkalemia	Should not be used by pregnant women. Mix with fruit juice to mask taste.
Pyrazinamide	Antitubercular agent	Hyperuricemia, exacerbation of gout, hepatotoxicity	Monitor liver function tests and serum uric acid levels. Instruct patient not to use alcohol. Emphasize that long-term therapy is required.
Rifampin	Antitubercular agent	Flulike syndrome, hematopoietic reactions, hepatotoxicity, rash, red-orange coloration of body fluids, shortness of breath, heartburn, sore mouth and tongue, dizziness, confusion	Give on empty stomach; emphasize that long-term therapy is required. May accelerate metabolism of other drugs, including theophylline, oral contraceptives, and warfarin. Instruct patient that body fluids may be discolored; may cause permanent staining of soft contact lenses.
Rifapentine	Antitubercular agent	Hepatotoxicity, hyperuricemia, neutropenia, pyuria, proteinuria, rash, anemia, leukopenia, arthralgias, nausea, vomiting, dyspepsia, pseudomembranous colitis	Monitor liver function tests and serum uric acid. Monitor WBC count. Tell the patient that rifapentine may produce red-orange discoloration of body tissues or fluids (e.g., skin, teeth, tongue, urine, feces, saliva, sputum, tears, cerebrospinal fluid). Emphasize importance of not missing any doses.
Theophylline (aminophylline is a salt of theophylline)	Bronchodilator	Anxiety, restlessness, insomnia, headache, seizures, tachycardia, cardiac dysrhythmias, nausea, epigastric pain, hematemesis, gastroesophageal reflux, tachypnea	Do not crush sustained-release preparations; contents of pellet-containing capsules may be sprinkled over food. Avoid caffeine; use with caution in peptic ulcer disease or cardiac dysrhythmias. Metabolism is affected by other medications (erythromycin, ciprofloxacin, cimetidine, rifampin); monitor serum concentrations.

GI, Gastrointestinal; *OTC,* over-the-counter; *SLE,* systemic lupus erythematosus; *WBC,* white blood cell.

Monitoring patients with TB is critical; failure to complete prescribed medication treatment is a major factor in the emergence of multidrug resistance and treatment failures (Mayo Clinic, 2021b). To ensure compliance and to help prevent the development of drug-resistant strains of the tubercle bacillus, in some cases the health care worker may need to watch the patient take the medications; this is referred to as *directly observed therapy.*

Nursing Interventions and Patient Teaching

If TB is suspected, immediately ask permission to place the patient under AFB isolation precautions. These precautions include the use of isolation rooms with negative air pressure so that air flows into, rather than out of, the room. Keep doors and windows closed to maintain airflow control. Room air should be exhausted directly to the outside and not recirculated to other rooms. Also included in AFB isolation precautions is the use of high-efficiency particulate respiration masks (because AFB particles pass through standard masks). Although TB is not transmitted easily, it is transmitted more easily in closed spaces and in areas with poor ventilation and no environmental controls.

Perhaps the simplest, most effective technique for stopping TB at the source is kindly insisting that patients cover their noses and mouths when coughing or sneezing. The CDC recommends the following for coughing:

- *Cover your mouth and nose* with a tissue when you cough or sneeze.
- Put your used tissue in a waste basket.
- If you do not have a tissue, cough or sneeze into your upper sleeve, not your hands.
- Remember to *wash your hands* after coughing or sneezing (CDC, 2020f).

To help the patient comply with the prescribed medication regimen, develop a supportive relationship. Nursing interventions focus on preventing complications and illness transmission.

Patient problems and interventions for the patient with TB include but are not limited to the following:

PATIENT PROBLEM	NURSING INTERVENTIONS
Inability to Maintain Adequate Breathing Pattern, related to pulmonary infection process	Monitor breathing for evidence of dyspnea or signs and symptoms of pneumothorax
	Evaluate degree of respiratory effort and assist as needed
	Assess expectorated sputum for hemoptysis
	Help immobile patient to turn, cough, and deep breathe q 2–4 h to prevent pooling of secretions
Potential for Infection (patient contacts), related to viable *M. tuberculosis* in respiratory secretions	Obtain specimen for culture (incorrect collection and handling may destroy or contaminate specimen, thus interfering with diagnostic results)
	Employ AFB isolation until antimicrobial therapy is initiated successfully for sputum-positive patients, to prevent transmission of organisms
	Employ drainage and secretion precautions until wounds from patient with extrapulmonary TB stop draining, to prevent transmission of organism
	Instruct the patient to cough and sneeze into tissue and properly dispose of it to prevent organism transmission

Teach the patient techniques of proper disposal and handwashing related to coughing and sneezing. These measures decrease the spread of infection. Explain the importance of adhering to the medication regimen as ordered, complying with prolonged treatment

(possibly 6 months or longer), and completing the regimen to avoid multidrug-resistant TB strains. Instruct the patient on medication, dosage, frequency, and possible side effects. Emphasize the need to report hemoptysis, dyspnea, vertigo, or chest pain. Remind the patient to maintain adequate fluid and nutritional intake. Patients with TB need follow-up appointments with their health care provider or their county Health Department to ensure that they are indeed taking the medications and to discuss any side effects they may be experiencing.

Prognosis

Active TB requires a long course of drug ingestion—6 to 9 months minimum, and often longer—to stop the disease. The length of treatment leads some patient to become noncompliant with therapy which increases the number of drug-resistant cases. Numerous drug-resistant TB cases have been reported in HIV-infected people (CDC, 2017).

PNEUMONIA

Etiology and Pathophysiology

Pneumonia is an inflammatory process of the respiratory bronchioles and the alveolar spaces that is caused by an infection. It also may be caused by oversedation, inadequate ventilation, or aspiration.

Pneumonia can occur in any season but is most common during winter and early spring. People of all ages are susceptible, but pneumonia is more common among infants and older adults. Pneumonia often is caused by aspiration of infected materials into the distal bronchioles and alveoli. High-risk people include those whose normal respiratory defense mechanisms are damaged or altered (those with COPD, influenza, or tracheostomy and those who have recently had anesthesia); people who have a disease affecting the antibody response; people with alcoholism, in whom there is increased danger of aspiration; and people with delayed white blood cell response to infection. Increasingly, nosocomial (hospital-acquired) pneumonia is a cause of morbidity and mortality (see the Health Promotion box).

Pneumonia is a communicable disease; the mode of transmission depends on the infecting organism. Pneumonia is classified according to the offending organism rather than the anatomic location (lobar or bronchial), as was the practice in the past. Pneumonia can be caused by bacteria, viruses, mycoplasma, fungi, and chemicals. Currently, about half of pneumonia cases are caused by bacteria and half by virus. Up to 96% of bacterial pneumonia is caused by four organisms: *Streptococcus pneumoniae* (pneumococcal), hemolytic *Streptococcus* type A, *Staphylococcus aureus,* and *Haemophilus influenzae* type B. Nonbacterial or atypical pneumonia is caused by *Mycoplasma pneumoniae, L. pneumophila* (legionnaires' disease), and *Pneumocystis jiroveci* (formerly *carinii*) pneumonia.

🏃 Health Promotion

Pneumonia

- A number of nursing interventions can help prevent the occurrence of, as well as the morbidity associated with, pneumonia.
- Teach the patient to practice good health habits, such as proper diet and hygiene, adequate rest, and regular exercise, to maintain the natural resistance to infecting organisms.
- Encourage the individual at risk for pneumonia (e.g., the chronically ill, older adult) to obtain influenza and pneumococcal vaccines.
- In the hospital, identify the patient at risk and take measures to prevent the development of pneumonia.
- Place the patient with altered consciousness in positions that will prevent or minimize the risk of aspiration (e.g., side lying, upright). Turn and reposition the patient at least every 2 hours to facilitate adequate lung expansion and to discourage pooling of secretions.
- The patient who has difficulty swallowing (e.g., stroke patient) needs assistance in eating, drinking, and taking medication to prevent aspiration.
- The patient who recently has had surgery and others who are immobile need assistance with turning and deep-breathing measures at frequent intervals and use of incentive spirometer.
- Aspiration pneumonia can occur as a result of nasogastric tube feedings. Always check for correct placement and keep the head of the bed elevated to 30 degrees.
- Be careful to avoid overmedication with opioids or sedatives, which can cause a depressed cough reflex and accumulation of fluid in the lungs.
- Before providing food or fluids, ensure the gag reflex has returned to the patient who had local anesthesia to the throat.
- Practice strict medical asepsis and adherence to infection control guidelines to reduce the incidence of nosocomial infections. Health care providers should wash their hands each time before they provide care to a patient. Comply with current Centers for Disease Control and Prevention (CDC) hand hygiene guidelines.
- The CDC (2020c) suggests vaccination with the pneumococcal conjugate vaccine for all babies and children younger than 2 years old, all adults 65 years or older, and people 2 through 64 years old with certain medical conditions. Pneumococcal polysaccharide vaccine is recommended for all adults 65 years or older, people 2 through 64 years old who are at increased risk for disease because of certain medical conditions, and adults 19 through 64 years old who smoke cigarettes.

Aspiration pneumonia is frequently called *necrotizing pneumonia* because of the pathologic changes in the lungs. Aspiration pneumonia occurs most commonly as a result of aspiration of vomitus when the patient is in an altered state of consciousness because of a seizure, drugs, alcohol, anesthesia, acute infection, or shock. Aspiration pneumonia may be acquired through foreign body aspiration, such as food or fluids, especially if the person has dysphagia, or may follow aspiration of toxic materials, such as gasoline or kerosene.

The causative agents of bacterial aspiration pneumonia include *S. aureus, Escherichia coli, Klebsiella pneumoniae, Pseudomonas aeruginosa,* and *Proteus* species.

The pathophysiology of pneumonia depends on the causative agent. Bacterial pneumonia is marked by an alveolar suppurative (process of pus formation) exudate with consolidation of infection. Mycoplasmal and viral pneumonia produce interstitial inflammation with no consolidation or exudate. Fungal and mycobacterial pneumonias are marked by patchy distribution that may undergo necrosis with the development of cavities. Aspiration pneumonia is manifest with various physiologic responses depending on the pH of the aspirated substance.

An overview of the pathophysiology is as follows: (1) pulmonary cilia cannot remove accumulating secretions from the respiratory tract; (2) these retained secretions then become infected; (3) inflammation of some part of the respiratory tract develops, leading to a localized edema; and (4) this causes decreased oxygen–carbon dioxide exchange. This process can begin in the bronchi or in the lobe of one lung, and it can become more extensive.

Clinical Manifestations

Many significant signs and symptoms are seen in pneumonia. A productive cough is common; color and consistency of sputum vary depending on the type of pneumonia present. Severe chills, elevated temperature, and increased heart and respiratory rates may accompany the painful, productive cough (see the Lifespan Considerations box).

Clinical manifestations depend on the type of pneumonia:

- *Streptococcal (pneumococcal):* Sudden onset; chest pain; chills; fever; headache; cough; rust-colored sputum; crackles and possibly friction rub; hypoxemia as blood is shunted away from area of consolidation; cyanosis; area of consolidation visible on chest radiograph; sputum culture needed to determine causative agent
- *Staphylococcal:* Many of the same signs as streptococcal; sputum copious and salmon-colored
- *Klebsiella:* Many of the same signs and symptoms as streptococcal; onset more gradual; more bronchopneumonia (inflammation of the terminal bronchioles and alveoli) visible on chest radiograph; if treatment is delayed beyond the second day after onset, the patient becomes critically ill and the mortality rate is high
- *Haemophilus:* Commonly follows upper respiratory tract infection; low-grade fever; croupy cough; malaise; arthralgias; yellow or green sputum
- *Mycoplasmal:* Gradual onset; headache; fever; malaise; chills; cough severe and nonproductive; decreased breath sounds and crackles; chest radiograph clear; white blood cell count normal
- *Viral:* Signs and symptoms generally mild; cold symptoms; headache; anorexia; myalgia (tenderness or pain in muscles); irritating cough that produces mucopurulent or bloody sputum; bronchopneumonic type of infiltration on chest radiograph; white blood cell count usually normal; rise in antibody titers

Lifespan Considerations

Older Adults

Respiratory Disorders

- Signs and symptoms of pneumonia are often atypical in older adults. Fever, cough, and purulent sputum may be absent. Generalized signs and symptoms such as lethargy, disorientation, dyspnea, tachypnea, chills, chest pain, and vomiting, as well as an unexpected exacerbation of coexisting conditions, should be viewed with suspicion because they may indicate pneumonia in the older adult.
- Adequate hydration is important for the older person with pneumonia. It helps liquefy secretions and promotes expectoration.
- Many older adults have difficulty expectorating. This slows resolution of congestion and increases the difficulty of obtaining sputum specimens. Because deep breathing and coughing are difficult, the older person may require suctioning to remove respiratory secretions. Perform this with caution, because too-frequent suctioning can stimulate increased production of secretions.
- Older adults, particularly those living in an institution, should have routine skin tests for tuberculosis. Many older adults were exposed to tuberculosis during their childhood and have positive results on skin tests. These individuals should receive routine chest radiographic studies. Older adults who have a history of inactive tuberculosis should be watched for recurrence of active tuberculosis. Signs and symptoms are often vague and include loss of appetite and weight loss.
- Closely watch older immigrants and immunosuppressed older adults for drug-resistant strains of tuberculosis.
- Provided that there is no serious disease of the respiratory tract, the older person is generally able to maintain adequate ventilation and oxygenation. However, changes of aging do have an effect on respiratory function.
- Drier mucous membranes and decreased number of cilia affect the older individual's ability to humidify inhaled air and trap debris. This increases the risk for inflammation and irritation of the upper respiratory tract.
- Kyphosis and calcification of costal cartilage are common changes. These restrict expansion of the thoracic cavity and lead to a barrel-chested appearance.
- Intercostal muscles and the diaphragm lose elasticity, resulting in a decreased ability to breathe deeply and cough.
- The elasticity of airways and alveoli decreases, alveoli thicken, and pulmonary blood flow decreases, resulting in an increased risk for impaired gas exchange.
- Years of exposure to air pollution, smoke, and mechanical irritants increase the risk for respiratory disease in older adults, particularly those who have emphysema or chronic bronchitis.
- Inactivity and immobility increase the risk of stasis pooling of respiratory secretions. This increases the risk of pneumonia.
- Neurologic damage as a result of strokes, Parkinson's disease, and other conditions is increasingly common in the older adult. Any neurologic disorder that decreases the gag or swallow reflexes increases the risk of aspiration of fluids and food, with resultant trauma to the respiratory tract.
- Cor pulmonale with right-sided heart failure, as well as left-sided heart failure with pulmonary congestion, are common complications of chronic obstructive pulmonary disease in the older adult.

Assessment

Subjective data include the patient's description of the onset and duration of cough. The patient may complain of fever and night sweats.

Collection of objective data includes checking the level of consciousness and vital signs, especially temperature and respirations, every 2 hours or as ordered. Note the color, consistency, and amount of sputum produced. Inspect the thorax to determine the patient's use of accessory muscles (abdominal or intercostal) in respiratory effort, and note any cyanosis or dyspnea. Perform auscultation; the patient will have crackles on inspiration and possibly a pleural effusion.

Diagnostic Tests

Blood and sputum cultures help identify organisms. Collect sputum for culture and sensitivity before starting antibiotic therapy. Chest radiographic studies reveal changes in density, primarily in the lower lobes. The white blood cell count is normal or even low in viral or mycoplasmal pneumonia, whereas it is elevated in bacterial pneumonia. Leukocytosis is found in the majority of patients with bacterial pneumonia, usually with a white blood cell count greater than $15,000/mm^3$.

PFTs may be done to determine whether lung volume is decreased, and ABG values are determined to identify altered gas exchange. Pulse oximetry is ordered to monitor oxygen saturation of arterial blood levels. Oximetry is invaluable for rapid and continuous assessment of oxygen needs.

Medical Management

If pus accumulates in the pleural space (empyema), the health care provider inserts a chest tube for drainage. The health care provider also prescribes oxygen therapy and physiotherapy (chest percussion and postural drainage). Encourage patients to cough and breathe deeply to maximize ventilatory capabilities.

Commonly prescribed medications include antibiotics (penicillin, erythromycin, cephalosporin, and tetracycline), depending on the causative organism and sensitivity. With prompt treatment and correct antibiotic therapy, patients with bacterial or mycoplasma pneumonia usually respond to therapy fairly quickly. Currently, viral pneumonia has no definitive treatment. Analgesics and antipyretics (acetaminophen or aspirin), expectorants, and bronchodilators often are prescribed. Humidification with a humidifier or nebulizer, if secretions are tenacious and copious, is useful. Oxygenation is prescribed if the patient has an oxygen saturation of less than 90% to 92%.

A vaccine is now available for the most common and important bacterial pneumonia, that is, streptococcal (or pneumococcal) pneumonia. The pneumococcal vaccine is indicated primarily for the individual considered at risk who (1) has chronic illnesses such as lung and heart disease and diabetes mellitus, (2) is recovering from a severe illness, (3) is 65 years of age or older, or (4) is in a nursing home or other long-term care facility. This is particularly important because the rate of drug-resistant streptococcal pneumonia is increasing. The vaccine is 50% to 80% effective in preventing pneumococcal disease. The current recommendation is that pneumococcal vaccine is good for the person's lifetime. However, in the immunosuppressed individual or the older adult at risk for development of fatal pneumococcal infection, revaccination should be considered every 5 years. When given in different arms, the influenza vaccine and the pneumococcal vaccine may be administered at the same time.

Nursing Interventions and Patient Teaching

Nursing strategies are aimed at helping the patient conserve energy. Allow rest periods and facilitate optimal air exchange by placing the patient in a high Fowler's position. Place the patient on the side with the "good lung down." This position benefits those with unilateral pulmonary disease, including unilateral pneumonia. In pneumonia and many other pulmonary problems, PaO_2 rises when the healthy lung is dependent (or "good lung down"). When the unimpaired lung is down, this better ventilated lung also is perfused much better. Studies have revealed that hypoxia worsened when patients were placed on their back or side with the affected (sick) lung down.

Assess the patient's ability to move secretions. If the patient is unable to expectorate secretions, assist with appropriate measures (such as coughing, positioning, suctioning, and liquefying secretions). Promptly administer bronchodilators, mucolytics, and expectorants as prescribed to dilate bronchioles and remove secretions. Carefully and frequently auscultate the chest for quality of breath sounds and adventitious sounds. Note cough and sputum characteristics and document. Provide hydration to liquefy secretions and replace fluids. Fluid intake of at least 3 L/day is important in the supportive treatment of pneumonia. If oral intake cannot be maintained, IV administration of fluids and electrolytes may be necessary for the acutely ill patient. Fluid intake must be individualized for patients with heart failure.

An intake of at least 1500 calories/day should be maintained to provide energy for the patient's increased metabolic processes. Small, frequent meals are better tolerated by the dyspneic patient.

Patient problems and interventions for the patient with pneumonia include but are not limited to the following:

PATIENT PROBLEM	NURSING INTERVENTIONS
Inability to Maintain Adequate Breathing Pattern, related to inflammatory process and pleuritic pain	Assess ventilation, including breathing rate, rhythm, and depth; chest expansion; and presence of respiratory distress such as dyspnea, shortness of breath, nasal flaring, pursed-lip breathing, or prolonged expiratory phase and use of accessory muscles
	Auscultate lungs for crackles, wheezes, and pleural friction rub
	Identify contributing factors such as airway clearance or obstruction problem or weakness
	Encourage increased fluid intake to 3 L/day, unless contraindicated, to liquefy secretions for easier expectoration
	Maintain patient in position that facilitates ventilation (head of bed in semi-Fowler's position or sitting and leaning forward on overbed table)
Inefficient Oxygenation, related to alveolar-capillary membrane changes secondary to inflammation	Assess patient to identify signs (e.g., restlessness, disorientation, and irritability) that may indicate the body's response to altered blood gas states (hypoxemia)
	If necessary and with health care provider consultation, administer oxygen by nasal cannula or Venturi mask to maintain oxygen saturations above 90%
	Carefully monitor body temperature, which may fluctuate because of alterations in metabolism or infection

Teach the patient and the family about (1) deep-breathing and coughing techniques and the use of an incentive spirometer; (2) the importance of handwashing to prevent the spread of the disease; (3) prescribed medications such as antibiotics, including the purpose, action, dosage, frequency of administration, and side effects; (4) the specific type of pneumonia the patient has, treatment, anticipated response, possible complications, and probable disease duration; (5) the importance of consuming large quantities of fluid; except in the patient with pulmonary edema, congestive heart failure, and/or renal failure; (6) adaptive exercise and rest techniques; and (7) the availability of pneumococcal vaccine. Also inform the patient about changes in health status that must be reported to the health care provider. These include a change in sputum characteristics or color, decreased activity tolerance, fever despite the antibiotics, increasing chest pain, or a feeling that things are not getting better.

Prognosis

Improvement occurs in 48 to 72 hours with appropriate antibiotics in uncomplicated cases (Mayo Clinic, 2020c). The disease usually resolves within 2 to 3 weeks with proper treatment. However, pneumonia is the most common cause of death from infectious disease in North America. It is also the major cause of disease and death in critically ill or older adult patients. Even with treatment with new antimicrobial agents, pneumonia and influenza still remain the ninth leading cause of death in the United States (CDC, 2019).

PLEURISY

Etiology and Pathophysiology

Pleurisy is an inflammation of the visceral and parietal pleura. Pleurisy can be caused by either a bacterial or viral infection. The underlying physiologic change is an inflammation of any portion of the pleura. It may occur spontaneously but more frequently is a complication of pneumonia; pulmonary infarctions; viral infections; trauma to the chest, ribs, or intercostal muscles; or early stages of TB or lung tumor.

Clinical Manifestations

One of the first symptoms of pleurisy may be a severe inspiratory pain, often radiating to the shoulder or abdomen of the affected side. The pain is caused by stretching of the inflamed pleura. If pleural effusion develops, pain subsides and fever and dry cough occur. Other signs and symptoms include dyspnea, cough, and elevated temperature.

Assessment

Subjective data include the patient's complaint of chest pain on inspiration. The patient also may report an elevated temperature.

Collection of objective data includes assessment of the inspiratory pain, noting its radiation points. Monitor vital signs, especially temperature, every 2 to 4 hours. Monitor and document respiratory rate and rhythm, including dyspnea. On auscultation of the lungs, a pleural friction rub is heard.

Diagnostic Tests

The presence of a pleural friction rub may be considered diagnostic. Chest radiographic examination is of limited value in diagnosing pleurisy unless pleural effusion is present and fluid accumulates.

Medical Management

The health care provider may inject an anesthetic around the vertebrae to block the intercostal nerves, thus relieving pain. Prescribed medications may include antibiotics (penicillin) to combat the infection

and analgesics to decrease pain when the patient takes deep breaths and coughs. Antipyretics (acetaminophen) are used for fever. Oxygen may be administered.

Nursing Interventions and Patient Teaching

Position the patient comfortably on the affected side to splint the chest, and apply heat to the area.

Patient problems and interventions for the patient with pleurisy include but are not limited to the following:

PATIENT PROBLEM	NURSING INTERVENTIONS
Discomfort, related to stretching of the pulmonary pleura as a result of fluid accumulation	Assess patient's pain level and need for analgesics; administer as needed, documenting effectiveness
	Assist with splinting affected side when patient coughs and takes deep breaths
Inefficient Oxygenation, related to pain on inspiration and expiration	Assess patient's level of consciousness, noting any increase in restlessness or disorientation, which may indicate ineffective breathing
	Auscultate lungs for wheezes, crackles, and pleural friction rub
	Reposition patient q 2 h to prevent pooling of secretions and to promote optimal lung expansion
	Elevate head of bed to facilitate optimal ventilation

Instruct the patient to be alert to signs and symptoms of exacerbation: purulent sputum production, further increase in temperature, and increased pain. Teach the patient to cough effectively every 2 hours and to splint the affected side.

Prognosis

The prognosis is usually excellent. Complications such as atelectasis (collapsed lung caused by airway blockage) or secondary infection such as pneumonia may develop.

PLEURAL EFFUSION/EMPYEMA

Etiology and Pathophysiology

Once the pleural lining is inflamed (as in pleurisy), fluid can accumulate in the pleural space. This accumulation of fluid is known as *pleural effusion*. Pleural effusion is rarely a disease by itself but occurs as a secondary problem when the physiologic pressure in the lungs and pleurae is disturbed. If the fluid becomes infected, it is called *empyema*, which is the accumulation of pus in a body cavity, especially the pleural space.

Pleural effusions happen when the normal flow of pleural fluid through the pleural space is disrupted, often leading to pleural empyema. Empyema may be acute or chronic. In acute empyema the affected area is inflamed with a thin layer of fluid. If this goes untreated, the fluid thickens and the pleura becomes scarred and fibrosed, losing its elasticity.

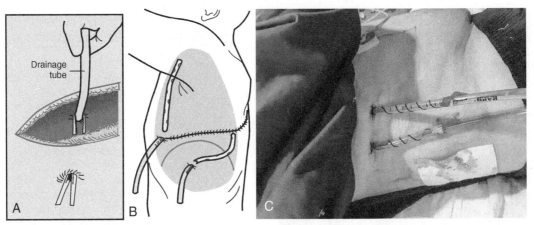

Fig. 9.11 A, Drainage tube inserted into pleural space. B, Note that anterior and posterior tubes are placed well into the pleural space. C, View of chest tubes in a patient

Clinical Manifestations

Pleural effusion generally is associated with other disease processes, such as pancreatitis, cirrhosis of the liver, pulmonary edema, congestive heart failure, kidney disease, or carcinoma involving altered capillary permeability. Empyema usually is seen as a result of bacterial infection, as in pneumonia, TB, or blunt chest trauma. The patient may have a persistent fever in spite of receiving antibiotics.

Assessment

Subjective data include patient complaints of dyspnea and air hunger. The patient also may report fear and anxiety related to decreased levels of oxygen.

Collection of objective data in pleural effusion and empyema includes assessment of signs and symptoms of respiratory distress, such as nasal flaring, tachypnea, and decreased breath sounds. Assess breath sounds and vital signs, especially temperature, frequently.

Diagnostic Tests

Effusions, or pleural fluid, will be evident on chest radiographic examination. Often a thoracentesis (needle inserted into the pleural space to aspirate excess fluid) is done to obtain a specimen for culture to identify the causative agent and to relieve dyspnea and discomfort.

Medical Management

Usually this condition requires a thoracentesis to remove fluid from the pleural space. A possible danger from this procedure is removing fluid too rapidly; less than 1300 to 1500 mL at one time is recommended.

A chest tube or tubes may be inserted for continuous drainage of fluid, blood, or air from the pleural cavity and for medication instillation. The tubes are sutured in place and covered with a sterile dressing. To prevent the lung from collapsing, a closed drainage system is used, which maintains the lung cavity's normal negative pressure. Under normal conditions, intrapleural pressure is below atmospheric pressure (approximately 4 to 5 cm H_2O below atmospheric pressure during

expiration and approximately 8 to 10 cm H_2O below atmospheric pressure during inspiration). If intrapleural pressure becomes equal to atmospheric pressure, the lungs will collapse. The chest tubes and attached closed drainage system restore normal intrapleural pressure and facilitate expansion of the lung.

With this procedure one or, more commonly, two thoracotomy tubes are inserted into the pleural space and are attached to a closed-drainage, water-seal system. One catheter is inserted through a stab wound in the anterior chest wall; this is referred to as the *anterior tube*. It removes air from the pleural space. The second tube, the *posterior tube*, is inserted through a stab wound in the posterior chest. It is primarily for the drainage of serosanguineous fluid or purulent exudate. The posterior (lower) tube may be larger in diameter than the anterior (upper) tube to prevent it from becoming occluded with exudate or clots (Fig. 9.11). Chest tubes connect to a pleural drainage system with a water-seal to reestablish negative pressure in the thoracic cavity. Suction applied to the drainage system may be ordered by the health care provider (Fig. 9.12).

Nursing Interventions and Patient Teaching

General nursing measures include placing the patient on bed rest. If the patient is receiving oxygen therapy, provide frequent oral care to keep mucous membranes moist. Also encourage effective coughing and deep-breathing techniques and respiratory treatments. If the patient has had a thoracentesis, apply a large sterile dressing and assess it for drainage, noting the color and amount.

Ensure that patency of the chest tube system is maintained so that it can drain fluid adequately. Areas of concern are the following:

- *Proper system function:* Ensure that the water in the water-seal chamber fluctuates when suction is applied. There should not be any bubbling in the water seal, because this indicates an air leak.
- *Potential atelectasis resulting from hypoventilation:* Assess for increased dyspnea; check chest

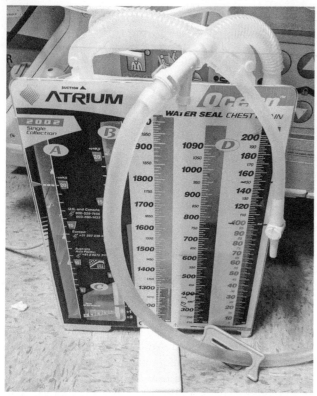

Fig. 9.12 Atrium chest tube drainage system with drainage in tubing and collection device, post lobectomy

radiographic studies frequently to compare degree of lung consolidation.

• *Increased air in the pleural space:* Note any air leaks in the system; ensure tubing is secure and remains patent.

• *Infection:* Note any increase in white blood cells, elevated temperature, and presence of purulent drainage.

A patient with a chest tube in place usually is positioned on the unaffected side to keep the tube from becoming kinked; however, the patient may assume any position of comfort in bed. There is no contraindication to ambulation with a chest tube in place, as long as the water-seal bottle remains below the level of the chest. Never elevate the drainage system to the level of the patient's chest, because this would cause fluid to drain back into the pleural cavity. Facilitate coughing and deep-breathing procedures at least every 2 hours and auscultate breath sounds frequently. Document the amount and characteristics of pleural fluid drainage by marking the drainage level on the container at the end of each shift, along with the date and the hour (Box 9.6). Prevent a chest tube from being removed accidentally by paying careful attention to securing connections and positioning drainage tubes. Be careful to keep tubing as straight as possible and coiled loosely. Do not let the patient lie on it. Tubing never should be placed over the side rails. Administer antibiotic agents as ordered.

Box 9.6 Guidelines for Care of Patient With Chest Tubes and Water-Seal Drainage

• Keep all tubing as straight as possible and coiled loosely below chest level. Do not let the patient lie on it.

• Keep all connections between chest tubes, drainage tubing, and the drainage collector tight, and apply tape at connections.

• Keep the water-seal and suction control chamber at the appropriate water levels by adding sterile water as needed, because water loss by evaporation may occur.

• Mark the time measurement and the fluid level with a black marker pen on the drainage chamber according to the prescribed orders. Marking intervals may range from every hour to every 8 hours. Any change in the quantity or characteristics of drainage (e.g., clear yellow to serosanguineous) should be reported to the health care provider and recorded. Record output on chart.

• Observe for air bubbling in the water-seal chamber and fluctuations (tidaling). If no tidaling is observed (rising with inspiration and falling with expiration in the spontaneously breathing patient; the opposite occurs during positive-pressure mechanical ventilation), the drainage system is occluded or the lungs are reexpanded. If bubbling increases, there may be an air leak.

• Bubbling in the water seal may occur intermittently. When bubbling is continuous and constant, the source of the air leak may be determined by momentarily clamping the tubing at successively distal points away from the patient until the bubbling ceases. Retaping tubing connections or replacing the drainage apparatus may be necessary to correct the air leak.

• Monitor the patient's clinical status. Take vital signs frequently, auscultate lungs, and observe the chest wall for any abnormal chest movements.

• Never elevate the drainage system to the level of the patient's chest, because this will cause fluid to drain back into the pleural space. Secure the drainage system to the metal drainage stand or racks. Do not empty the drainage chamber unless it is in danger of overflowing.

• Encourage the patient to breathe deeply periodically to facilitate lung expansion, and encourage range-of-motion exercises to the shoulder on the affected side.

• Check the position of the chest drainage system. If it is overturned and the water seal is disrupted, return the system to an upright position and encourage the patient to take a few deep breaths, followed by forced exhalations and cough maneuvers.

• Do not strip or milk chest tubes routinely because this increases pleural pressures.

• If the drainage system breaks, place the distal end of the chest tubing connection in a sterile water container at a 2-cm level as an emergency water seal.

• Chest tubes are not clamped routinely. Clamps with rubber protection are kept at the bedside for special procedures such as changing the chest drainage system and assessment before removal of chest tubes.

Patient problems and interventions for the patient with pleural effusion or empyema include but are not limited to the following:

PATIENT PROBLEM	NURSING INTERVENTIONS
Inefficient Oxygenation, related to ineffective breathing pattern	Assess for changes in level of consciousness, such as disorientation, restlessness, or irritability, because these may indicate increasing hypoxia as a result of ineffective breathing Monitor ABGs and pulse oximetry Encourage coughing and deep breathing to remove secretions and facilitate lung expansion Reposition patient q 2 h to prevent pooling of secretions Assess for atelectasis
Inability to Feed, Dress, and/or Bathe Self	Assess patient's ability to care for self, and assist when needed Encourage increasing activity level when fever is reduced

Explain all procedures before their implementation. Prepare the patient emotionally for chest tube insertion. Teach the patient and the family about this condition and the healing process. Instruct the patient on effective coughing and deep-breathing techniques.

Prognosis
The prognosis is variable, depending on the patient's overall health status.

ATELECTASIS
Etiology and Pathophysiology
Atelectasis (the collapse of alveoli, preventing the respiratory exchange of carbon dioxide and oxygen) occurs from occlusion of air (blockage) to a portion of the lung. Atelectasis is a common postoperative complication from a mucous plug resulting from shallow breathing, which interferes with coughing and effective clearance of secretions. All or part of the lung collapses, usually as a result of hypoventilation (the condition in which the amount of air that enters the alveoli and takes part in gas exchange is not adequate for the body's metabolic needs), which then leads to bronchial obstruction caused by mucus accumulation. Accumulation of secretions, a foreign body, or a tenacious plug of mucus may occlude a bronchus completely, closing off all air to a portion of the patient's lung. Atelectasis also can result from obstruction of the airway by aspiration of a foreign body or compression of lung tissue caused by emphysema, pneumothorax, or tumor.

The altered physiology depends on the site and degree of occlusion. If the mainstem bronchus is obstructed, severe ventilatory compromise occurs. When a small bronchiole becomes obstructed, as with secretion accumulation, fewer signs and symptoms are seen,

because the respiratory system tries to compensate. However, in either case, atelectasis can lead to stasis pneumonia (because the retained secretions are rich in nutrients for the growth of bacteria) and lung damage.

Clinical Manifestations
The patient displays dyspnea, tachypnea (an abnormally rapid rate of breathing), pleural friction rub, restlessness, hypertension, and elevated temperature.

Assessment
Subjective data include patient complaints of severe shortness of breath (dyspnea) requiring much effort, which results in fatigue. The patient also may verbalize a feeling of air hunger and resulting anxiety.

Objective data include decreased breath sounds and crackles on auscultation. Assess vital signs frequently because tachycardia and hypertension are present at first, followed by hypotension and bradycardia. Note respiration rate and amount of effort required for breathing. The patient may exhibit altered levels of consciousness caused by hypoxia.

Diagnostic Tests
Serial chest radiographic studies (repeated radiographic examinations of the same area, done for comparison) demonstrate atelectatic changes. A chest CT scan can detect compression in the airway and also may reveal the underlying pathologic condition contributing to the problem. ABGs reveal a PaO_2 of less than 80 mm Hg initially; this generally improves within the first 24 hours. Pulse oximetry reveals oxygen saturation levels below 90%. $PaCO_2$ is normal or low because of hypoventilation. Bronchoscopy with a flexible fiberoptic bronchoscope may reveal a bronchial obstruction; this procedure also can be used to remove a mucous plug or retained secretions.

Medical Management
Maintenance of ventilation by intubation often is required. Incentive spirometry 10 times every hour while the patient is awake helps provide visual feedback of respiratory effort. Respiratory therapy with oxygen is ordered. Chest physiotherapy with postural drainage is administered. The patient may require suctioning, encouragement to cough, and vigorous respiratory and physical therapy if a mechanical obstruction is present. Prescribed medications may include bronchodilators (e.g., albuterol) to facilitate secretion removal, antibiotics to prevent infection, and mucolytic agents (e.g., acetylcysteine) to reduce the viscosity of secretions. A bronchoscope can be used to remove a thick, tenacious secretion or a mucous plug.

Nursing Interventions and Patient Teaching
Postoperatively, remind patients to cough, breathe deeply, use their incentive spirometer, and change positions every 1 to 2 hours. Effective coughing is essential

in mobilizing secretions. If secretions are present in the respiratory passages, deep breathing and use of the incentive spirometer often move them up to stimulate the cough reflex, and then they can be expectorated. Administer analgesics to relieve pain and increase the patient's ability to carry out respiratory exercises and to clear airway passages. Provide emotional support. Encourage early ambulation.

Patient problems and interventions for the patient with atelectasis include but are not limited to the following:

PATIENT PROBLEM	NURSING INTERVENTIONS
Inability to Clear Airway, related to inability to clear secretions	Assess patient's ability to move secretions, and assist if needed Encourage use of incentive spirometer 10 times q h while awake Encourage coughing and deep breathing q 1–2 h while awake Encourage adequate hydration to liquefy secretions Auscultate breath sounds frequently, documenting and reporting any changes Assess color, consistency, and amount of secretions removed via either coughing or suction
Impaired Coping, related to invasive medical regimen	Assess the patient's ability to comply with the prescribed regimen and to cooperate with caregivers Identify patient's emotional support systems

Instruct the patient on proper techniques for effective coughing, deep breathing, and other measures to facilitate optimal air exchange, such as increasing movement and changing position. Medication teaching should address the rationale and side effects of prescribed medications.

Prognosis
The prognosis depends on the patient's age and any preexisting illness.

PNEUMOTHORAX
Etiology and Pathophysiology
Pneumothorax, like atelectasis, is a collapsed lung; but it is due to a collection of air or other gas in the pleural space, causing the lung to collapse. It can be secondary to a ruptured bleb on the lung surface (as in emphysema) or a severe coughing episode. It can be caused by a penetrating chest injury that punctures the pleural lining, fractured ribs, or injury to the pleura from insertion of a subclavian catheter. A spontaneous pneumothorax also may occur suddenly without any apparent cause (Fig. 9.13).

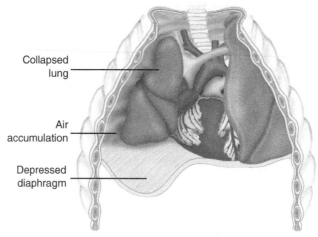

Fig. 9.13 Pneumothorax (complete collapse of the right lung). (From Seidel HM, Ball JW, Dains JE, et al: *Mosby's guide to physical examination*, ed 7, St. Louis, 2011, Mosby.)

When the pleural space is penetrated, air enters, thus interrupting the normal negative pressure. Consequently, the lung cannot remain fully inflated.

Clinical Manifestations
The patient may have had a recent chest injury. He or she will have decreased breath sounds on the affected side and a sudden, sharp, pleuritic chest pain with dyspnea. The patient may be diaphoretic (perspiring) and exhibit an increased heart rate, tachypnea, and dyspnea. Normal chest movements on the affected side cease. With a pneumothorax resulting from penetrating injury, a sucking sound is heard on inspiration.

As intrathoracic pressure increases in the pleural space, the lung collapses. Because lung tissue no longer expands, the mediastinum may shift to the unaffected side (mediastinal shift), which subsequently is compressed. As the intrathoracic pressure increases, cardiac output is altered because of decreased venous return and compression of the great vessels.

Assessment
Collection of subjective data includes reporting a precipitating respiratory condition, such as COPD, a recent penetrating chest injury, or severe coughing episode. The patient may complain of chest pain, shortness of breath of sudden onset, and feelings of anxiety associated with air hunger.

Collection of objective data involves taking frequent vital signs, noting any change in respiratory and cardiac rate and rhythm. A small pneumothorax usually manifests with mild tachycardia and dyspnea. A larger pneumothorax causes respiratory distress, including rapid shallow respirations, air hunger, dyspnea, and oxygen desaturation. Hemoptysis and cough may be present in some cases of pneumothorax, but this is not always present. Findings on auscultation are bilaterally unequal breath sounds, with no breath sounds over the affected area. Note color, characteristics, and amount of sputum.

Diagnostic Tests

Chest radiographic examination shows the presence of pneumothorax. ABGs show a decrease in pH and PaO_2, with an increased $PaCO_2$.

Medical Management

Cutting through the chest wall (a thoracotomy) may be needed, with insertion of a chest tube. The chest tube is inserted in the fifth or sixth intercostal space, under the patient's arm (i.e., at the midaxillary line). The chest tube is attached to a water-seal drainage system (see Figs. 9.11 and 9.12). The patient will require a follow-up chest x-ray to determine correct placement of the chest tube.

Another approach to correcting a pneumothorax is the use of a Heimlich valve, which typically is applied as a stopgap measure until chest tube therapy can be started. The one-way valve attaches to a catheter and is inserted into the chest. As the patient exhales, air and fluid drain through the valve into a plastic bag. When the patient inhales, however, the flexible tubing in the valve collapses, preventing secretions and air from re-entering the pleura.

Nursing Interventions and Patient Teaching

General measures include maintaining airway patency and providing adequate oxygenation. Assess and document patency of the chest tube system, keeping it free from kinks. Note the color and amount of drainage and assess integrity of the drainage system. Monitor blood pressure and place the patient in a high Fowler's position to promote airway clearance and lung expansion. Control pain by administering appropriate analgesics, but medications should be avoided if they cause respiratory depression.

Patient problems and interventions for the patient with pneumothorax include but are not limited to the following:

PATIENT PROBLEM	NURSING INTERVENTIONS
Inability to Maintain Adequate Breathing Pattern, related to nonfunctioning lung	Assess respiratory rate and rhythm, and note any signs of respiratory distress, such as dyspnea, use of accessory muscles, nasal flaring, and anxiety
	Provide chest tube care, maintaining secure placement
	Facilitate ventilation by elevating head of bed, and administer oxygen as ordered
	Suction as needed to remove secretions
	Encourage adaptive breathing techniques to decrease respiratory effort
	Encourage rest periods interspersed with activities

PATIENT PROBLEM	NURSING INTERVENTIONS
Discomfort, related to feeling of air hunger	Assess patient's feelings of fear related to health concerns and feeling of air hunger
	Identify positive coping methods, and support their use
	Determine support systems available to patient

Explain the rationale for treatments (oxygen therapy and chest tube drainage) before their implementation. Reinforce effective breathing techniques and the need for ongoing medical care. Instruct the patient to limit exposure to people who may have infections, such as upper respiratory tract infection or influenza. Advise the patient not to smoke but to drink plenty of fluids, to avoid fatigue and strenuous activity, and to report any signs and symptoms of recurrence (e.g., chest pain, difficulty breathing, or fever) to the health care provider.

Prognosis

The lung usually reexpands within several days. The health care provider removes the chest tube when a chest radiograph shows that the lungs are expanded completely. An occlusive dressing is placed over the chest area where the tube was removed, with a gauze pad taped in place to prevent air from reentering the pleural cavity. After removal of the chest tube, check the chest area for drainage and listen for complaints of pain by the patient. Monitor for shortness of breath, which would mean that air is once again entering the chest cavity.

CANCER OF THE LUNG

Etiology and Pathophysiology

The incidence of lung cancer has been increasing steadily over the past 50 years in men and women. In 1987, cancer of the lung surpassed breast cancer to become the number one cancer killer of women. Responsible for 25% of all cancer deaths, lung cancer is now the leading cause of death from cancer in men and women. The American Cancer Society estimates that about 228,820 new cases of lung cancer (116,300 in men and 112,520 in women) and about 135,720 deaths from lung cancer (72,500 in men and 63,220 in women) will occur in 2020 (American Cancer Society, 2021a).

Lung tumors may be primary tumors or may result from metastasis anywhere in the body; metastasis from the colon and kidney is common. Metastasis to the lungs may be discovered before the primary lesion is known, and sometimes the location of the primary lesion is not determined during the person's life. The majority of lung tumors are linked to cigarette smoking. A history of smoking, especially for 20 years or more, is considered to be a prime risk factor. The more cigarettes someone smokes each day, the higher the risk. "Passive smoking" (breathing in sidestream smoke) is qualitatively similar to mainstream smoking; involuntary (secondhand) smoking poses a risk for the development of lung cancer in nonsmokers. Occupational exposure, such as to asbestos, radon, and uranium, is also a risk factor. It is suspected that air pollutants may increase risk. Most people who develop the disease are older than 50 years of age.

Many studies suggest the importance of certain antioxidant vitamins, especially vitamins A and E, to reduce the risk of developing lung cancer. Studies report that an increased intake of fruits and vegetables can lower the risk for lung cancer development. Beta-carotene supplements have been shown to raise the risk of lung cancer in smokers. No changes to the rate of risk for nonsmokers has been demonstrated (American Lung Association, 2019).

The mortality of people with lung cancer depends primarily on the specific type of cancer and the size of the tumor when detected. Lung cancer is classified by microscopic study of the tumor. Treatment is based on the type and extent of the disease, using two major classifications. Small cell lung cancer (SCLC) (oat cell cancer) constitutes about 10% to 15% of lung cancers. This type of lung cancer tends to spread quickly; non-small lung cancer (NSCLC) is the most common type of lung cancer, comprising 85% of all lung cancers. Squamous cell, adenocarcinoma, and large cell carcinoma make up this group of lung cancer; lung carcinoid tumors make up less than 5% of lung cancers. They also are called neuroendocrine tumors, and they tend to grow slowly and seldom spread (American Cancer Society, 2019a).

Clinical Manifestations

Lung cancer is insidious, because it is usually asymptomatic in the early stages. If the lesion is located peripherally, it produces few symptoms and may not be discovered until visualized on a routine chest radiographic examination. If the peripheral lesion perforates the pleural space, pleural effusion and severe pain occur. Central lesions originate from a larger branch of the bronchial tree. These lesions cause obstruction and erosion of the bronchus. Signs and symptoms are cough, hemoptysis, dyspnea, fever, and chills. Auscultation may reveal wheezing on the affected side. Phrenic nerve involvement causes paralysis of the diaphragm.

As the disease progresses, metastasis may occur, along with weight loss, fatigue, decreased stamina, and changes in functional status. Pain is unlikely, unless the tumor is pressing on a nerve or the cancer has spread to the bones. Primary lung tumors usually metastasize to the liver or to nearby structures, such as the esophagus, the pericardium, skeletal bone, and the brain.

Assessment

Subjective data include the patient's complaints of a chronic cough and of hoarseness. The patient also may report weight loss and extreme fatigue. Interview the patient regarding a family history, especially a history of cigarette smoking and of exposure to occupational irritants.

Collection of objective data includes assessing the cough, noting color (especially blood streaks) and consistency of sputum, as well as frequency, duration, and precipitating factors. Also assess the characteristics of the cough (moist, dry, hacking) and effect of body position and identify with the patient what, if anything, helps to relieve the cough. Auscultate the lungs to determine if unilateral wheezing or crackles are present. Invasion of the superior vena cava causes edema of the neck and face and is called *superior vena cava syndrome.*

Diagnostic Tests

Initially, imaging studies such as x-rays and spiral CT scans of the chest are used to identify the location and size of the tumor. MRI may be used along with or instead of spiral CT scans and endobronchial ultrasound. PET may be used to differentiate between malignant and benign lung masses. When the lesion is on the lung periphery, the health care provider can obtain specimens via percutaneous fine-needle aspiration guided by fluoroscopy or CT. Bronchoscopy with biopsy or brushings for cytologic findings indicates the presence of malignant cells (American Cancer Society, 2021b)). A mediastinoscopy may be done to determine whether the tumor has spread to the lymph nodes. A scalene lymph node biopsy also may be done to identify metastasis. In this procedure, lymph node tissue is excised from supraclavicular lymph nodes in the neck, close to the scalene muscles.

Medical Management

The treatment of lung cancer depends on the type and stage. Unfortunately, most patients are not diagnosed early enough for curative surgical intervention. It is estimated that one-third of patients are inoperable when first seen because of the advanced stage of the disease, and that another one-third are found to be inoperable on exploratory thoracotomy. One in twenty patients has only a single tumor; patients with single tumors typically have the best surgical outcomes. The more advanced the stage of lung cancer, the less probable it is that surgery is a viable option (American Cancer Society, 2021c.). A pneumonectomy is the most common surgical treatment. This consists of removing the entire lung. Because there is no lung left to require reexpansion, drainage tubes are usually not necessary. The fluid remaining in that area consolidates eventually, which helps prevent a mediastinal shift. A lobectomy is performed when one lobe is involved rather than the entire lung. If only a portion of a lobe of a lung is involved, a segmental resection is done. Lobectomy and segmental resection require chest tube insertion with water-seal drainage to facilitate lung reexpansion (see Figs. 9.11 and 9.12). Video-assisted thoracoscopic surgery allows surgeons to remove tumors through a small keyhole incision in the chest cavity.

Radiation therapy and chemotherapy often are done in conjunction with surgery to enhance recovery for NSCLC. The oral drug gefitinib has been approved as monotherapy in patients with locally advanced or metastatic NSCLC after failure of first-line treatment with platinum-based and docetaxel chemotherapies (see the Home Care Considerations box). In small cell lung carcinoma (SCLC), chemotherapy alone or combined with radiation has replaced surgery as the treatment of choice because, regardless of staging, SCLC is considered to be metastatic at diagnosis. A large percentage of these patients experience remission; in a few cases the remission has been long lasting. At present about one-third of the patients who have surgery experience tumor spread.

Among the promising biological response modifiers are interferon-alpha, interleukin-2, interleukin-4, tumor necrosis factor, and monoclonal antibodies. The latter are being investigated alone and in combination with radioisotopes, toxins, and standard chemotherapeutic drugs to see if they can identify and destroy cancer cells with specific antigens (American Cancer Society, 2019b).

 Home Care Considerations

Lung Cancer

- If the patient with lung cancer smokes, teach her or him that stopping smoking can improve pulmonary function, minimize postoperative complications, decrease the risk of pneumonia, and improve appetite during treatment.
- The patient who has had a surgical resection of the lung with intent to cure should be followed up carefully after discharge for manifestations of metastasis.
- Instruct the patient and the family to contact the health care provider if symptoms such as hemoptysis, dysphagia, chest pain, and hoarseness develop.
- For many individuals who have lung cancer, little can be done to significantly prolong their lives.
- Many people with lung cancer require palliative and hospice care. Encourage the patient and his or her family to adjust their expectations and adapt their goals from controlling disease to improving symptom relief.
- Radiation therapy and chemotherapy can provide palliative relief from distressing symptoms.
- Constant pain usually becomes a major problem, requiring measures to relieve pain.

Nursing Interventions and Patient Teaching
Whether treatment offers comfort or cure, the patient needs comprehensive nursing interventions. From patient education to symptom management to emotional support, nursing care can improve the quality of life and help the patient and the family cope with a frightening diagnosis. Nursing interventions often are directed at postsurgical interventions, including facilitating recovery and preventing complications by promoting effective airway clearance through frequent repositioning, coughing, and deep breathing.

Encourage the use of incentive spirometry. Explain the importance of changing position (to prevent atelectasis) and exercising the legs and feet (to prevent deep vein thrombosis [DVT]). Administer supplemental oxygen and monitor oxygen saturation levels. If a patient has chest tubes to water-seal drainage system, assess for patency, and record the amount, color, and consistency of drainage. Carefully assess lung sounds and record findings. Assess vital signs frequently. After checking routine postoperative vital signs, check the patient every 2 hours until he or she is stable, and then every 4 hours.

Prescribed medications are primarily antineoplastic agents to prevent or reduce tumor growth. Medications are also given for symptomatic relief: opioid analgesics for pain control, antipyretics for fever, and antiemetics for nausea.

Patient problems and interventions for the patient with lung cancer include but are not limited to the following:

PATIENT PROBLEM	NURSING INTERVENTIONS
Inability to Clear Airway, related to lung surgery	Facilitate optimal breathing by placing patient in a sitting position Assist with position changes frequently Promote coughing and deep breathing, providing necessary splinting Encourage early ambulation to mobilize secretions Encourage use of an incentive spirometer
Fearfulness, related to cancer, treatment, and prognosis	Monitor changes in communication patterns with others Monitor expression of feelings, such as worthlessness, anxiety, powerlessness, abandonment, or exhaustion Listen and accept expressions of anger without taking it personally Encourage patient to identify problem, redefine the situation, obtain needed information, generate alternatives, and focus on solutions

Teach the patient effective coughing techniques. Instruct the patient and the family regarding nutritional needs and the importance of maintaining physical mobility. If the patient smokes, encourage him or her to quit; encourage family members to stop also. Encourage the patient to eat a diet high in protein and calories. Instruct the patient and the family regarding signs and symptoms that could indicate recurrence of metastasis, such as fatigue, weight loss, increased coughing or hemoptysis, central nervous system

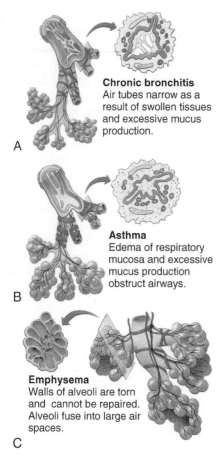

Chronic bronchitis
Air tubes narrow as a result of swollen tissues and excessive mucus production.

A

Asthma
Edema of respiratory mucosa and excessive mucus production obstruct airways.

B

Emphysema
Walls of alveoli are torn and cannot be repaired. Alveoli fuse into large air spaces.

C

Fig. 9.14 Disorders of the airways in patients with chronic bronchitis, asthma, and emphysema. (A) *Chronic bronchitis:* Excessive amounts of mucus accumulate in the airways, obstructing airflow and impairing ciliary function. (B) *Asthma:* Bronchial smooth muscle constricts in response to irritants, resulting in airflow obstruction and wheezing. (C) *Emphysema:* Alveoli become overinflated and destructive changes occur in alveolar walls. (From Lewis SL, Collier IC, Heitkemper MM: *Medical-surgical nursing: assessment and management of clinical problems,* ed 4, St. Louis, 1996, Mosby.)

changes, and arm or shoulder pain. Identify resources in the community, such as the American Cancer Society and the American Lung Association, that can assist the patient and the family with information, support groups, and equipment needed.

Prognosis

According to the American Lung Association the 5-year survival rate after diagnosis is 18.6% (American Lung Association, 2020a). For cancers diagnosed while still localized in the lung, the 5-year survival rate raises to 56%. Unfortunately, only about 16% of lung cancer cases are diagnosed at an early stage. For distant tumors (spread to other organs), the 5-year survival rate drops to 5%.

PULMONARY EDEMA

Etiology and Pathophysiology

Pulmonary edema is an accumulation of serous fluid in interstitial lung tissue and alveoli. Some causes include (Mayo Clinic, 2020d):

• Coronary artery disease

• As diseased vessels prevent effective circulation through the heart, blood begins backing up to the lungs. Fluid then begins passing through the capillary walls into the lung tissue and alveoli.
• Cardiomyopathy, resulting in left ventricular failure
   • This decreases the heart's ability to circulate blood throughout the body.
• Rapid administration of IV fluids (packed red blood cells, plasma, or fluids)
• Altered capillary permeability of lungs: inhaled toxins, inflammation (e.g., pneumonia), severe hypoxia, near-drowning
• PE, result on blockage of circulations through the lungs
• Opioid overdose causing depressed respirations
• Acute pulmonary edema found in patients with sleep apnea can be the initial feature in the diagnosis of sleep apnea

Cardiogenic pulmonary edema usually accompanies underlying cardiac disease in which the failure of the left ventricle causes pooling of fluid, which backs up into the left atrium and into the pulmonary veins and capillaries. The most common cause of pulmonary edema is increased capillary pressure from left ventricular failure. Because the pulmonary capillary pressure exceeds the intravascular pressure, serous fluid is forced rapidly into the alveoli. Fluid rapidly reaches the bronchioles and bronchi, and patients begin to drown in their own secretions. As oxygen decreases, the person shows signs of severe respiratory distress. Pulmonary edema is acute and extensive and may lead to death unless treated immediately.

Clinical Manifestations

The primary signs and symptoms of pulmonary edema are dyspnea and related breathing disturbances. Labored respirations; tachypnea; tachycardia; cyanosis; and, especially, pink (or blood-tinged), frothy sputum are the most obvious signs. The patient also may exhibit restlessness or agitation because of the altered tissue perfusion and resulting hypoxia and respiratory failure.

Assessment

Subjective data include the patient's complaints of severe dyspnea and a feeling of impending death.

Collection of objective data involves assessing for signs of respiratory distress, including nasal flaring and sternal retractions with inspiration; rapid, stertorous respirations; hypertension; tachycardia; restlessness; and disorientation. On auscultation the nurse will most likely hear wheezing and crackles. The patient may have a sudden weight gain because of fluid retention; decreased urinary output as a result of retained fluid in the pulmonary vasculature; and a productive cough of frothy, pink sputum.

Diagnostic Tests

Chest radiographic examination reveals fluid infiltrates, indicating alveolar edema, increased pleural space fluid (pleural effusion), and enlarged heart (cardiomegaly). ABGs are altered, with varying PaO_2 and $PaCO_2$ levels. The patient may have respiratory alkalosis or acidosis. Sputum cultures are done periodically to rule out a bronchopulmonary infection.

Medical Management

The health care provider orders oxygen therapy and may intubate the patient for adequate ventilation support. Medications include diuretics to reduce alveolar and systemic edema by increasing urinary output (furosemide). Patients also are given an opioid analgesic, usually morphine sulfate, to decrease the respiratory rate; lower the anxiety level; reduce venous return; and dilate the pulmonary and systemic blood vessels, thus improving the exchange of gases. IV nitroprusside is a potent vasodilator that improves myocardial contraction and reduces pulmonary congestion. Because of its effects on the vascular system, it is the drug of choice for the patient with pulmonary edema. Medications for the treatment of heart failure are used to address underlying cardiac conditions.

Nursing Interventions and Patient Teaching

An important nursing measure is accurate assessment and documentation to identify changes in the patient's condition. This includes assessment of respiratory status and frequent monitoring of cardiac status, I&O, vital signs, ABGs, pulse oximetry, and electrolyte values. Maintain oxygenation therapy as ordered—commonly delivered by Venturi mask at 40% to 70% concentration. Mechanical ventilation may be required; in this case provide the intubated patient with oral and tracheostomy care according to protocol. Facilitate optimal air exchange by placing the patient in a high Fowler's position. Maintain a patent IV line (saline lock) for administering prescribed IV medications. IV fluids usually are withheld to prevent adding even more fluid to the overloaded patient.

Patient problems and interventions for the patient with pulmonary edema include but are not limited to the following:

PATIENT PROBLEM	NURSING INTERVENTIONS
Inefficient Oxygenation, related to excess fluid in pulmonary vessels interfering with oxygen diffusion	Be alert for any signs indicating altered ventilation, such as restlessness, irritability, disorientation, or apprehension
	Monitor ABGs and notify health care provider of any change
	Frequently monitor vital signs, including cardiac rhythm
	Administer oxygen therapy as ordered and document patient response
	Administer diuretics, bronchodilators, morphine sulfate, cardiotonic glycosides, and other medications as ordered

PATIENT PROBLEM	NURSING INTERVENTIONS
Fluid Volume Overload, related to altered tissue permeability	Assess indicators of patient's fluid volume status, such as breath sounds and skin turgor
	Monitor I&O accurately
	Monitor electrolyte values closely, and notify health care provider of alterations
	Administer diuretics as ordered, and note patient response
	Weigh patient daily on same scale at same time of day with same amount of bed linen and patient clothing
	Provide low-sodium diet to prevent excess fluid retention

Teach the patient effective breathing techniques. Inform the patient and the family about actions, side effects, and dosage of prescribed medications. Instruct the patient and the family about a low-sodium diet and refer them to a dietitian for follow-up. Emphasize the signs and symptoms to observe that would indicate an alteration in health, such as a productive cough (noting the color and characteristics of sputum), activity intolerance, or dyspnea.

Prognosis

The prognosis for acute pulmonary edema is guarded; it may lead to death unless treated rapidly. The health care provider normally orders oxygen therapy at a lower dose, 2 to 3 L/min, via mask. A nasal cannula may be used, if the patient will leave it in place and the oxygen saturation stays above 90%.

PULMONARY EMBOLISM
Etiology and Pathophysiology

The most common pulmonary perfusion abnormality, pulmonary embolism, is caused by the passage of a foreign substance (blood clot, fat, air, tumor tissue, or amniotic fluid) into the pulmonary artery or its branches, with resulting obstruction of the blood supply to lung tissue and subsequent collapse. PE usually occurs in patients identified to be at risk, such as those with prior thrombophlebitis; those who have recently had surgery, been pregnant, or given birth; women who are taking contraceptives on a long-term basis; and those with a history of congestive heart failure, obesity, or immobilization from fracture. Immobilization appears to be a key consideration.

Venous stasis, venous wall injury, and increased coagulability of blood cause the formation of a venous thrombus. The thrombus (usually in the deep veins of the lower extremities) dislodges and travels through the venous circulation; it passes through the right side of the heart and enters the pulmonary artery, where it becomes lodged. NOTE: A thrombus that breaks loose and travels elsewhere in the body is referred to as an embolus.

Once an embolus obstructs pulmonary blood flow, a V/Q mismatch develops: an area of lung is ventilated but not perfused (for review, see the description of V/Q scans in the earlier section "Laboratory and Diagnostic Examinations"). The obstruction hinders oxygenation of the blood. Atelectasis develops, and pulmonary vascular resistance increases. Arterial hypoxia is the result.

Clinical Manifestations
The classic signs and symptoms of a PE are dyspnea, hemoptysis, and chest pain. Unfortunately, not all patients have all the classic symptoms. This can make diagnosis difficult. A PE may be manifest by a sudden, sharp, constant, non-radiating, pleuritic chest pain that worsens with inspiration. The impairment of gas exchange may result in the patient experiencing acute dyspnea. The respiratory rate is rapid. In small areas of infarction, presenting signs and symptoms include a small amount of hemoptysis, pleuritic chest pain, elevated temperature, and increased white blood cell count. In large areas of infarction, symptoms include hypoxia, hemoptysis, hypotension, tachycardia, diaphoresis, and tachypnea. Regional bronchoconstriction, atelectasis, and pulmonary edema develop, along with decreased surfactant production. Lung sounds are diminished, and wheezes may be present.

Assessment
Subjective data include the patient's report of dyspnea (presence and degree) and pleuritic chest pain. The patient may complain of a sense of impending doom. Nursing assessment also includes identifying associated risk factors.

Collection of objective data involves assessing for pleuritic pain and noting the nature of the patient's cough. Also assess breath sounds and vital signs, and be alert for tachycardia, hypotension, and tachypnea. Auscultation reveals crackles, decreased breath sounds over the affected area, and a pleural friction rub. In assessing the patient's psychological response, document the presence and degree of anxiety, which often is associated with air hunger. Other objective data may include hemoptysis, elevated temperature, increased white blood cell count, and diaphoresis.

Diagnostic Tests
ABGs are altered significantly, indicating hypoxia. The pH remains normal unless respiratory alkalosis develops early from hyperventilation as respiratory drive diminishes. Respiratory acidosis with hypoxemia often follows.

Initially, the chest radiograph is normal. After 24 hours the radiograph may reveal small infiltrates secondary to atelectasis. Chest radiographic examination also shows an enlarged main pulmonary artery. In most cases of PE, the chest radiograph is normal and is useful only to rule out pulmonary edema or pneumothorax.

A helical (or spiral) CT scan of the lung to visualize the pulmonary vasculature is ordered. This noninvasive scan can be performed in a few seconds and is replacing the V/Q scan, although the V/Q scan still is used in smaller facilities where spiral CT is not available. If the V/Q scan result, that is, the V/Q ratio, is intermediate or low, but the health care provider still suspects a PE based on the patient's signs, symptoms, and risk factors, he or she may order a pulmonary angiogram.

The pulmonary angiogram is considered a leading test for the detection of PE because it provides a direct anatomic view of the pulmonary vessels to assess perfusion defects. ABG analysis is important, as is a D-dimer serum test. D-dimer is a product of fibrin degradation (a change to a less complex form). When a thrombus or embolus is present, plasma D-dimer concentrations are usually greater than 1591 ng/mL. The normal range for D-dimer is 68 to 494 ng/L. If the D-dimer levels are elevated, a venous ultrasound is indicated to look for a DVT. Positive results from venous ultrasound are helpful in diagnosing DVT.

Medical Management
When multiple PEs are present, an umbrella filter may be placed in the inferior vena cava to retain the emboli, preventing their migration to other parts of the body.

The health care provider prescribes anticoagulant therapy, for example, oral warfarin or subcutaneous low-molecular-weight heparin (enoxaparin sodium, or dalteparin), to prevent clot formation. Initially heparin may be administered intravenously by a continuous pump infusion.

Heparin does not dissolve an existing thrombus; its role is to keep it from enlarging and to prevent more thrombi from forming while the body's natural fibrinolytic mechanism lyses (destroys) the existing clot. The effectiveness of heparin is determined by monitoring PTT values, which should be maintained at 1½ to 2 times the control (or normal) values. In the event of over-heparinization resulting in profound bleeding, the treatment is IV administration of protamine sulfate. Heparin therapy is tapered gradually (it may take several days). Oral anticoagulation (warfarin) then is initiated. The patient takes warfarin for up to 1 year. The effectiveness of warfarin therapy is determined by monitoring PT and INR values, with the goal being 1{¼} to 1{½} times the control (or normal) values. Vitamin K reverses the effects of warfarin. Fresh frozen plasma may be required in cases of severe bleeding.

A massive PE must be dissolved by administering thrombolytics such as the tissue plasminogen activator alteplase.

Nursing Interventions and Patient Teaching
General nursing interventions include applying anti-embolism stockings (e.g., TED [thromboembolism-deterrent] stockings) and elevating the lower extremities.

Check peripheral pulses and frequently measure bilateral calf circumference to monitor for occlusion caused by a clot. Slightly elevate the head of the bed, and administer oxygen by mask or nasal cannula to facilitate optimal gas exchange. Promote lung expansion by encouraging the patient to cough and breathe deeply.

Related nursing interventions include assessing for signs of bleeding: epistaxis, hemoptysis, bleeding from gums or rectum, and ecchymosis. Keep the patient adequately hydrated; place the patient on bed rest for the first few days, and gradually increase activity.

Patient problems and interventions for the patient with PE include but are not limited to the following:

PATIENT PROBLEM	NURSING INTERVENTIONS
Inefficient Oxygenation, related to alteration in pulmonary vasculature	Assess sensorium and vital signs q 2 h or as needed, noting any changes indicative of altered oxygenation or ventilation Elevate head of bed 30 degrees to improve ventilation Administer oxygen as ordered Monitor ABGs frequently, reporting any increase or decrease in $PaCO_2$ and PaO_2 of more than 10 mm Hg
Compromised Blood Flow to Tissue, related to risk of prolonged bleeding or hemorrhage secondary to anticoagulation therapy	Monitor vital signs for indicators of profuse bleeding or hemorrhage resulting from anticoagulant therapy: hypotension, tachycardia, and tachypnea At least once a shift, check stool, urine, sputum, and vomitus for occult blood, using agency-approved method for testing At least once a shift, inspect wounds, oral mucous membranes, any entry site of an invasive procedure, and nares for evidence of bleeding To prevent hematoma formation, avoid giving intramuscular injection unless it is unavoidable Teach patient the necessity of using sponge-tipped applicators and mouthwash for oral care to minimize the risk of gum bleeding Instruct patient to shave with an electric rather than a bladed razor

Medication teaching regarding long-term anticoagulant therapy is a major nursing concern. Patients with recurrent emboli are treated indefinitely; typical anticoagulant therapy continues for at least 3 to 6 months. Oral anticoagulation often becomes a lifelong regimen that bears close monitoring. Assess the patient's present knowledge base and expand on it. Preventive measures are also important, especially in the postoperative period. Teach the patient techniques to reduce venous pooling (which could precipitate thrombophlebitis),

such as changing positions and wearing nonrestrictive clothing. Tell the patient to avoid crossing the legs while sitting or lying down and to avoid standing in one place for a prolonged period, because these activities increase venous pooling. Teach the rationale and application procedure for TED hose. Explain that the patient should put them on in the morning before getting out of bed. Instruct the patient and the family about signs and symptoms of PE to report to the health care provider, such as chest pain, dyspnea, and blood-tinged sputum or blood in the urine, which could result from anticoagulant therapy.

Prognosis
Early diagnosis and appropriate treatment reduce mortality to under 5%. Untreated PE carries a 30% mortality rate. It is one of the most common causes of preventable death in hospitalized patients (CDC, 2020e). Although most PEs resolve completely and leave no residual deficits, some patients may be left with chronic pulmonary hypertension.

ACUTE RESPIRATORY DISTRESS SYNDROME
Etiology and Pathophysiology
ARDS is not a disease but a complication that occurs as a result of other disease processes. ARDS has many causes, which result from either a direct or an indirect pulmonary injury. Possible causes include viral or bacterial pneumonia, chest trauma, pulmonary contusion, aspiration, inhalation injury, near-drowning, fat emboli, sepsis, or any type of shock. Drug overdoses, renal failure, and pancreatitis also are known causative factors, as are COPD, neuromuscular defects with Guillain-Barré syndrome, and myasthenia gravis. Among these, sepsis is the most common precursor of ARDS.

Regardless of the cause of ARDS, the body's response follows a similar sequence. The surface of the alveolar capillary membrane is altered, causing increased permeability, which then allows fluid to leak into the interstitial spaces and alveoli. This creates pulmonary edema and hypoxia. The alveoli lose their elasticity and collapse, which causes the blood to be shunted through the impaired alveoli, interfering with oxygen transport. The damaged capillaries allow plasma and red blood cells to leak out, resulting in hemorrhage. ARDS is characterized by pulmonary artery hypertension, which results from vasoconstriction.

Clinical Manifestations
ARDS manifests 12 to 24 hours after injury, resulting in lung tissue damage or hypovolemic shock; 5 to 10 days after sepsis development, the patient experiences respiratory distress with altered breath sounds. There may be altered sensorium as a result of elevated $PaCO_2$ and decreased PaO_2. Additional signs include tachycardia, hypotension, and decreased urinary output.

Assessment

Subjective data include background information and a history of the present illness (obtained from family members, because the patient is usually too ill to give details).

Collection of objective data involves being an astute observer of any change in the patient's condition, no matter how small or gradual. Make an accurate and thorough initial assessment so that such changes are recognized quickly. Initial assessment includes identifying and documenting respiratory rate, rhythm, and effort. Note signs of dyspnea, such as nasal flaring, sternal and sub-clavicular retractions, or cyanosis. Auscultate the lungs and document the presence of crackles or wheezing. Closely observe vital signs. Frequent assessment of the level of consciousness, with particular attention to increased restlessness or lethargy, is necessary.

Diagnostic Tests

PFTs are done to determine the ease or difficulty with which oxygen crosses the alveolar capillary membrane. ABGs show definitive changes: PaO_2 is decreased (less than 70 mm Hg), $PaCO_2$ is increased (greater than 35 mm Hg), and HCO_3^- is decreased (less than 22 mEq/L). Initially, HCO_3^- increases to buffer the elevated $PaCO_2$ level, thereby maintaining pH in the normal range. The pH is elevated initially but steadily decreases as the patient's condition deteriorates. A chest radiographic examination depicts thickened bronchial margins and possibly diffuse infiltrates.

Medical Management

The medical plan focuses on supportive treatment by maintaining adequate oxygenation and treating the cause: drug overdose, infections, or inhaled toxins. Medications commonly used to treat associated conditions include corticosteroids, antibiotics, vasodilators such as nitroprusside, bronchodilators, mucolytics, and diuretics to treat pulmonary edema, aiding in restoring lung tissue to its normal structure and function. Morphine sulfate commonly is given to sedate restless patients and to decrease the respiratory rate. When the patient is intubated and ventilator dependent, a neurologic blocking agent, such as pancuronium, may be administered to suppress the patient's own respiratory effort, relying instead on controlled ventilator assistance. Positive end-expiratory pressure is the most important ventilator treatment component for the patient with ARDS (Mayo Clinic, 2018). Other medications may include cardiotonic glycosides (digoxin) to enhance cardiac function.

An experimental treatment involves the administration of nitric oxide gas, which, when inhaled, causes local vasodilation and maximizes perfusion in ventilated areas of the lungs, often significantly improving oxygenation. Nitric oxide usually is administered via a face mask; if the patient is ventilator dependent, however, the ventilator is the mode of delivery.

Nursing Interventions and Patient Teaching

The goal of nursing interventions is to provide adequate oxygenation and ventilation and to treat the multisystem responses caused by ARDS. Nurses must be knowledgeable about mechanical ventilator settings and effects. Care for intubated patients includes suctioning, providing oral care, and assessing for signs of inadequate ventilation. Closely monitor ABGs and pulse oximetry and report any changes.

To improve gas exchange, frequently reposition the patient from side to side, thus preventing one region of the lung from being in a dependent position for prolonged periods. Studies suggest some people with ARDS demonstrate a marked improvement in PaO_2 when turned from the supine to prone position (Scholten et al., 2017). Not all patients respond to prone positioning. Furthermore, an accurate, ongoing assessment of cardiac function is important. Be alert for and document any rate or rhythm changes. The registered nurse notifies the health care provider of any changes.

Assess vital signs and identify elevated temperatures so that cultures can be obtained to treat infections.

Patient problems and interventions for the patient with ARDS include but are not limited to the following:

PATIENT PROBLEM	NURSING INTERVENTIONS
Inefficient Oxygenation, related to tachypnea	Monitor ABGs and report any changes
	Address any factors that would contribute to restlessness and anxiety because they increase the body's oxygen demand and exacerbate the patient's already serious condition
	Administer oxygen as ordered, assessing and recording patient response
	Monitor electrocardiogram (ECG) changes
	Report any changes in vital signs and any change in patient's response, no matter how small or gradual
Inability to Maintain Adequate Breathing Pattern, related to respiratory distress	Assess respiratory rate, rhythm, and effort, being alert to signs of dyspnea
	Facilitate optimal ventilation by proper positioning
	Maintain airway patency by encouraging frequent coughing and deep breathing, if able, or suctioning as needed

Teach the patient effective breathing techniques, emphasizing the importance of frequent position changes, coughing, and deep breathing. If the patient is intubated, explain all procedures before their implementation and explain the importance of working with the ventilator and not trying to breathe independently. Reassure the patient that the ventilator will breathe for him or her and that those breaths will be more effective than his or her own. Explain to the patient and the family the importance of using rest and activity appropriately. Also explain the purpose and side effects of all medications.

Prognosis

ARDS affects an estimated 150,000 to 200,000 people each year. The complications that may arise from the condition include pneumothorax, lung scarring, infections, and blood clots. The disorder is associated with mortality rates of 40% with severe ARDS when trauma is the cause and 55% to 70% when the condition is associated with sepsis.

CHRONIC OBSTRUCTIVE PULMONARY DISEASE

COPD is a progressive and irreversible condition characterized by diminished inspiratory and expiratory capacity of the lungs. It is a chronic respiratory condition that obstructs the flow of air to or from the patient's bronchioles (Fig. 9.14). COPD includes emphysema and chronic bronchitis. These diseases are characterized by chronic airflow limitation.

EMPHYSEMA

Etiology and Pathophysiology

Emphysema symptoms usually develop when the patient is in his or her 40s, with disability increasing by age 50 to 60. This condition is characterized by changes in the alveolar walls and capillaries: thus emphysema is primarily an *alveolar disease* (see Fig. 9.14C).

Emphysema is an abnormal, permanent enlargement of the alveoli distal to the terminal bronchioles, accompanied by destruction of their walls. There is usually an overlap between chronic bronchitis and emphysema. The bronchi, bronchioles, and alveoli become inflamed as a result of chronic irritation. Because of bronchiole lumen narrowing, air becomes trapped in the alveoli during expiration, causing alveolar distention (Fig. 9.15). The alveoli then rupture and scar, losing their elasticity. Oxygen in the arterial blood decreases and carbon dioxide increases.

This process is worsened by cigarette smoking and other inhaled irritants. There is a lag of 30 to 35 years, on average, between taking up smoking and the onset of signs and symptoms. Cigarette smoking is by far the most common cause of emphysema and chronic bronchitis; 90% of COPD cases are caused by smoking, whereas as few as 25% of nonsmokers develop the disorder. This suggests that genetic susceptibility may play a role in the risk for COPD (American Lung Association, 2021). Risk factors for emphysema are the same as for chronic bronchitis, with one addition: heredity. An inherited form of emphysema is caused by a deficiency of alpha$_1$-antitrypsin (ATT), a

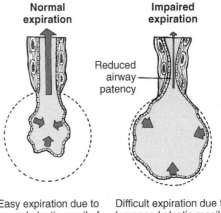

Normal expiration — **Impaired expiration**

Reduced airway patency

Easy expiration due to normal elastic recoil of alveolus and open bronchiole

Difficult expiration due to decreased elastic recoil of alveolus and narrowed bronchiole

Fig. 9.15 Mechanisms of air trapping in emphysema. Damaged or destroyed alveolar walls no longer support and hold airways open. Alveoli lose their property of passive elastic recoil. Both of these factors contribute to collapse during expiration. (From McCance KL, Huether SE: *Pathophysiology: the biologic basis for disease in adults and children*, ed 5, St. Louis, 2006, Mosby.)

lung-protective protein produced by the liver, which acts predominantly by inhibiting neutrophil elastase in the lungs. ATT deficiency accounts for less than 1% of emphysema in the United States.

The patient with emphysema is disabled because all available energy must be used for breathing. COPD can lead to cor pulmonale, an abnormal cardiac condition characterized by hypertrophy of the right ventricle of the heart as a result of hypertension of the pulmonary circulation. Cor pulmonale results in edema in the lower extremities and in the sacral and perineal areas, distended neck veins, and enlargement of the liver with ascites. Cor pulmonale is a late complication of emphysema.

Clinical Manifestations

The primary symptom of emphysema is dyspnea on exertion, which becomes progressively more severe. Over time the dyspnea worsens and becomes present even at rest. Initially there is little sputum production, but later it becomes copious. Many patients assume a barrel-chested appearance (an increased anteroposterior diameter caused by overinflation) and begin using accessory muscles for breathing (Fig. 9.16). Spontaneous pursed-lip breathing and chronic weight loss with emaciation ensue.

Assessment

Subjective data include a history of onset of symptoms. Note the duration and intensity of dyspnea, cough, and sputum production (documenting color and amount). Also determine the patient's reported history of smoking and exposure to inhalants and the family history of respiratory disorders.

Collection of objective data includes assessment of presenting signs, such as tachycardia, tachypnea,

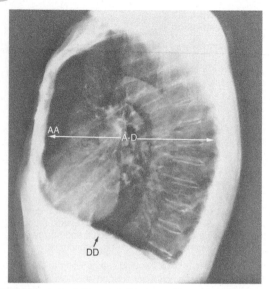

Fig. 9.16 Barrel chest. Hyperinflation is manifested by *AA*, increased anterior air space; *DD*, depressed diaphragm; and *A-D*, increased anteroposterior dimension. (From Heuer AJ, Scanlan CL: *Wilkins' clinical assessment in respiratory care*, ed 8, St. Louis, 2018, Elsevier.)

orthopnea, peripheral cyanosis, clubbing of fingers, and a barrel chest. The most outstanding feature of clubbing is a lateral and longitudinal curvature of the nails accompanied by soft tissue enlargement, presenting a bulbous (bulb-shaped), shiny appearance. A barrel chest, which occurs late in the disease, is more difficult to distinguish. Have the patient sit so that the health care provider will have a lateral view of the patient; this makes the assessment of a barrel chest easier. Hypoxemia (especially during exercise) may be present, but hypercapnia does not develop until late in the disease. The patient with COPD often begins to exhibit weight loss. The patient is in a hypermetabolic state with increased energy requirements that are due partly to the increased work of breathing. A therapeutic posture for the patient with COPD is the orthopneic position (leaning forward with the head forward and the arms resting on the patient's legs or a table). Expiration is prolonged as the patient forces his or her breath out through obstructed airways.

Diagnostic Tests

An important goal of the diagnostic workup is to determine the major disease component of COPD, the severity of the disease, and the impact of the disease on the patient's quality of life. A history and physical examination are extremely important.

PFTs measure total lung capacity, which is decreased with COPD. Residual volume is increased, as are compliance and airway resistance. Ventilatory response is decreased. Pulse oximetry is useful in assessing oxygen saturation in arterial blood.

ABGs usually are assessed in the severe stages and are monitored in hospitalized patients with acute exacerbations. ABGs reveal respiratory acidosis. A chest radiographic examination shows hyperinflation of the lungs, widened intercostal spaces, and flattened diaphragm with increased anteroposterior diameter (barrel chest). Hematologic studies determine whether the patient is positive for AAT deficiency (a deficiency that causes airway abnormalities, resulting in emphysema); this is present in an inherited form of emphysema. CBC reveals elevated erythrocytes and hemoglobin and hematocrit levels (secondary polycythemia, as a compensatory response to chronic hypoxia). This is also a late manifestation of emphysema.

Medical Management

The medical plan includes long-term management with home oxygen therapy and chest physiotherapy as needed. In an acute exacerbation the patient may require mechanical ventilation.

Prescribed medications include bronchodilators such as beta-adrenergic agonists (e.g., short-acting albuterol and long-acting inhaled salmeterol) or theophylline. Anticholinergics such as ipratropium are also effective bronchodilators. Bronchodilators enlarge the bronchioles for greater oxygenation and ease of secretion clearance, and corticosteroids decrease pulmonary inflammation and obstruction. Corticosteroids usually are prescribed only during an acute exacerbation because of the many side effects seen in long-term steroid therapy. Antibiotics frequently are ordered to reduce the risk of infection related to retained pulmonary secretions. Diuretics assist with fluid removal. Pulmonary therapy can help mobilize secretions and improve oxygenation.

Many health care providers prescribe pulmonary rehabilitation therapy that includes aerobic exercise such as walking. Prescribed exercise training improves aerobic capacity, endurance, and strength; improves and maintains functional performance in everyday life; and reduces breathlessness and fatigue during exertion.

During an acute exacerbation, severe dyspnea can produce considerable anxiety, restlessness, or irritability. Carefully monitor the patient with COPD because of the increased risk for respiratory failure from central nervous system depressants. Careful evaluation for hypoxemia is necessary before a central nervous system depressant is prescribed.

Nursing Interventions and Patient Teaching

Nursing interventions are directed toward decreasing the patient's anxiety and promoting optimal air exchange. Such measures include elevating the head of the bed and administering low-flow oxygen (1 to 2 L by nasal cannula) as ordered. This is extremely important for patients with COPD because a higher flow of oxygen delivery can be dangerous, because it diminishes the responsiveness of the brain's respiratory (regulatory) center, leading to decreased respiratory drive and respiratory failure. Avoid use of respiratory depressants to ensure adequate alveolar ventilation. Assist with chest physiotherapy, which includes percussion, vibration, and postural drainage. All three techniques help loosen secretions to be expectorated; sometimes it takes several hours after chest physiotherapy before the patient can expectorate loosened secretions. Increasing oral intake of fluids liquefies secretions, thus aiding in their removal. In addition, the use of a humidifier enhances this process. Allow sufficient rest periods and assist the patient in activities of daily living to prevent a decrease in oxygen saturation levels.

Assist the patient in maintaining nutritional intake by advising rest for 30 minutes before eating. This conserves energy and decreases dyspnea. The patient with emphysema has a markedly increased need for protein and calories to maintain an adequate nutritional status. A high-protein, high-calorie diet should be divided into five or six small meals a day. Oral fluid intake should be 2 to 3 L/day unless contraindicated (e.g., because of congestive heart failure). Instruct the patient to drink fluids between meals, rather than with meals, to reduce gastric distention and pressure on the diaphragm. Perform frequent oral hygiene to freshen the patient's mouth after coughing exercises and before meals.

Cessation of cigarette smoking in the early stages is probably the most significant factor in slowing the progression of the disease and improving pulmonary function. Use of nicotine replacement therapy or medications to assist with smoking cessation may be required. These therapies should be combined with other modalities such as support groups, education materials, and behavior modification programs.

The patient with COPD should receive an influenza virus vaccine yearly and a pneumococcal revaccination every 5 years.

Patient problems and interventions for the patient with emphysema include but are not limited to the following:

PATIENT PROBLEM	NURSING INTERVENTIONS
Inability to Clear Airway, related to narrowed bronchioles	Assess patient's ability to mobilize secretions, intervening as needed Encourage coughing and deep breathing, frequent position changes, and increased oral intake (up to 2–3 L/day) Elevate head of bed; suction as needed Assist with respiratory treatments Auscultate lungs, and report any changes in lung sounds

PATIENT PROBLEM	NURSING INTERVENTIONS
Inability to Tolerate Activity, related to imbalance between oxygen supply and demand, secondary to inefficient work of breathing	Organize care so that periods of activity are interspersed with at least 90 min of undisturbed rest Assist patient with active range-of-motion exercises to build stamina and prevent complications of decreased mobility Monitor patient's respiratory response to activity. Activity intolerance is indicated by excessively increased respiratory rate (e.g., increased more than 10 breaths/min above patient's baseline) and depth, dyspnea, and use of accessory muscles of respiration

Instruct the patient and the family on (1) the importance of not smoking and of reducing exposure to other inhaled irritants, (2) effective breathing techniques (such as pursed-lip breathing), and (3) relaxation exercises for anxiety control. Teach the patient about the dangers of increased oxygen intake for a patient dependent on hypoxic drive (stimulation of respiration by low PaO_2) for ventilation. Also teach the patient and the family how to prevent infection and symptoms that should be reported to the health care provider (see the Home Care Considerations box, the Communication box, and Nursing Care Plan 9.1).

Prognosis

Emphysema is usually irreversible. There are numerous complications associated with the condition. They include right-sided heart failure, frequent pulmonary infections, cardiac arrhythmias, pneumonia, and pneumothorax. COPD is the fourth leading cause of death in the United States. COPD affects about 13 million Americans with 159,486 deaths in 2018 (CDC/NCHS, 2021).

 Home Care Considerations

Chronic Oxygen Therapy at Home

- Improved prognosis has been noted in patients with chronic obstructive pulmonary disease who receive nocturnal or continuous oxygen to treat hypoxemia.
- The longer the continuous daily use of oxygen is maintained, the greater the improvement.
- Periodic reevaluations are necessary for the patient who is using chronic supplemental oxygen in the home.
- Home oxygen systems usually are rented from a company that sends a respiratory therapist or pulmonary nurse specialist to the patient's home.
- The therapist teaches the patient how to use the oxygen system, how to care for it, and how to recognize when the supply is running low and needs to be reordered.
- Post "No smoking" warning signs where they can be seen in the home.
- Do not use electric razors, portable radios, open flames, wool blankets, petroleum-based products, or mineral oils in the area where oxygen is in use.
- Do not allow smoking in the home.

Nursing Care Plan 9.1   **The Patient With Emphysema**

Mr. O. is a 91-year-old patient admitted with an exacerbation of chronic obstructive pulmonary disease (COPD). His respirations are 32 breaths/min and labored. He has nasal flaring, and his nailbeds are cyanotic. He has a barrel chest and digital clubbing. He states he has a productive cough and "can't get my air." It is noted he expectorates tenacious yellow mucus. He appears anxious during the assessment.

PATIENT PROBLEM
Inability to Clear Airway, related to tenacious secretions and expiratory airflow obstruction

Patient Goals and Expected Outcomes	Nursing Interventions	Evaluation
Patient will maintain patent airway as evidenced by decreased wheezes, tachypnea, dyspnea, and arterial blood gas (ABG) values within limits (for this patient)	Assess lung sounds q 2–4 h Encourage turning, coughing, and deep breathing q 2–4 h Suction as needed. Explain all medications used in inhalation therapy and assist with treatment. Monitor effectiveness. Ensure hydration: oral intake of 2–3 L/day to liquefy secretions for easier expectoration.	Patient's respiratory status remains within baseline for this patient. Patient has normal breath sounds on auscultation. Patient is able to expectorate sputum without difficulty.

PATIENT PROBLEM
Inability to Maintain Adequate Breathing Pattern, related to decreased lung expansion secondary to chronic airflow limitations

Patient Goals and Expected Outcomes	Nursing Interventions	Evaluation
After treatment intervention, patient's breathing pattern will improve as evidenced by patient maintaining respiratory rate within 5 breaths/min of baseline Patient will demonstrate relaxed appearance	Assess for indicators of respiratory distress (agitation, restlessness, decreased level of consciousness, and use of accessory muscles of respiration). Auscultate breath sounds; report a decrease in breath sounds or an increase in adventitious breath sounds. Instruct patient in the use of pursed-lip breathing, which provides internal stability to the airways and may prevent airway collapse during expiration. Administer bronchodilator therapy as prescribed. Monitor patient's response to prescribed oxygen therapy. Be aware that high concentrations of oxygen can depress the respiratory drive in individuals with chronic carbon dioxide retention. Avoid use of respiratory depressants to ensure adequate alveolar ventilation.	Patient's arterial blood gases are within normal values. Patient has absence of adventitious breath sounds. Patient is sleeping for 5–6 h without respiratory distress.

CRITICAL THINKING QUESTIONS
1. Mr. O. turns on his call light and states, "I'm unable to get my air." The nurse notes sub-clavicular retractions and a respiratory rate of 36 breaths/min. His oxygen is flowing at 1 L/min via nasal cannula. What nursing interventions would decrease his dyspnea?
2. While the nurse is performing an assessment on Mr. O., he states, "I'm so tired of fighting to breathe that I wish I could just go to sleep and never wake up." What is an appropriate response?
3. When performing the assessment, the nurse notes the following: temperature is 102°F (38.8°C), pulse rate is 110 bpm, and the respiratory rate is 44 breaths/min. What risk factors are increased as a result of Mr. O.'s COPD?

Communication

Mr. O., a 91-year-old, lives at home with his wife of 38 years. He was admitted to the hospital with an acute **exacerbation** (an increase in the seriousness of a disease or disorder as marked by greater intensity in the signs or symptoms) of emphysema. Mr. O. has a 24-year history of emphysema, with progression of signs and symptoms, including exertional dyspnea, expectoration of copious amounts of tenacious mucus, fatigue, and fear of suffocation.

Patient: Will it always be like this? I'm so short of air.

Nurse: Tell me how you are feeling.

Patient: I'm not afraid of dying, but it's the constant struggle to breathe.

Nurse: (gently touches Mr. Oden's arm) Try taking slow, deep breaths.

Patient: Sometimes I can't even get to the bathroom and do my business—much less help my wife with the dishes or even putter in the yard like I enjoy doing.

Nurse: Have you talked with your wife about your feelings?

Patient: I have to be good to my wife. I want to have something left to give her.

Nurse: I think sharing your feelings with your wife is a good thing to do.

Patient: Just having you listen to my concerns has been helpful. I feel like my breathing is getting a little better now.

Nurse: Yes, I can see that. I am going to let you rest now and will check on you soon.

CHRONIC BRONCHITIS

Etiology and Pathophysiology

Chronic bronchitis is characterized by a recurrent or chronic productive cough for a minimum of 3 months/year for at least 2 years. It is caused by physical or chemical irritants and recurrent lung infections. Cigarette smoking is by far the most common cause of chronic bronchitis. Workers exposed to dust, such as coal miners and grain handlers, also are at higher risk. The underlying process is an impairment of cilia, so they can no longer move secretions. Mucous gland hypertrophy causes hypersecretion, altering cilia function (see Fig. 9.14A). Excessive mucus is trapped in edematous airways, obstructing airflow. The lining of the bronchial tubes becomes inflamed and eventually scarred. The patient cannot clear tenacious mucus, and it becomes a medium for bacteria and infection. This increased airway resistance leads to bronchospasm. The condition results in altered oxygen–carbon dioxide exchange, hypoxia (an inadequate, reduced tension of cellular oxygen), and **hypercapnia** (greater than normal amounts of carbon dioxide in the blood).

Clinical Manifestations

Primary signs include a productive cough, most pronounced in the mornings (this often is overlooked by cigarette smokers). The patient also has increased dyspnea and use of accessory muscles. A complication of chronic bronchitis is cor pulmonale, which is hypertrophy of the right side of the heart resulting from pulmonary hypertension. Cyanosis develops, often accompanied by right ventricular failure. The patient with chronic bronchitis often has a characteristic reddish blue skin (resulting from chronic hypoxia, which stimulates erythropoiesis, thus resulting in polycythemia, cyanosis, and dependent edema).

Assessment

Subjective data include a detailed history of smoking or exposure to irritants and family history of respiratory disorders. Also determine the patient's current medication and treatment regimen.

Collection of objective data includes assessing the patient's productive cough, noting characteristics and amount of sputum. Assess the severity of dyspnea and presence of wheezing, and note the patient's level of restlessness. Obtain vital signs. Assess degree of tachycardia and tachypnea. Record any temperature elevation.

Diagnostic Tests

Chest radiographs taken early in the disease may not show abnormalities; later in the disease they will. An ECG may be normal or show signs indicative of right ventricular failure. An echocardiogram can be used to evaluate right and left ventricular function.

A CBC shows increased erythrocytes, hemoglobin, hematocrit, and white blood cell count. Polycythemia develops as a result of increased production of red blood cells as the body attempts to compensate for chronic hypoxemia. Hemoglobin concentrations may reach 20 g/dL or more. ABG values reveal respiratory acidosis, hypoxia, and hypercapnia. Pulse oximetry is valuable to assess oxygen saturation levels in arterial blood. PFTs reveal airflow limitation on expiration, increased airway resistance and residual volume, and often electrolyte abnormalities. Monitor oximetry levels on all patients with hypoxia.

Medical Management

The medical plan is aimed at slowing the disease progression and facilitating optimal air exchange by reducing spasms and secretions.

Three main classes of bronchodilators typically are used to treat COPD. To reverse bronchospasm, the health care provider may order beta-adrenergic agonists such as short-acting albuterol and long-acting salmeterol. Both theophylline as well as anticholinergic medications such as ipratropium are effective bronchodilators. Corticosteroids are helpful in reducing airway inflammation. Long-term use of systemic steroids can lead to many adverse reactions, including osteoporosis, diabetes, and eye problems. Inhaled steroids have fewer systemic effects and are preferred. Mucolytics such as guaifenesin to break up tenacious mucus may be helpful. Antibiotic agents (erythromycin) are commonly ordered.

Nursing Interventions and Patient Teaching

Provide adequate hydration to liquefy secretions and aid in their removal. Suction the patient as needed, and provide low-flow oxygen to maintain SaO_2 above 90%. Offer frequent oral hygiene and provide rest periods. The nutritional needs are similar to those of the patient with emphysema.

Patient problems and interventions for the patient with chronic bronchitis include but are not limited to the following:

PATIENT PROBLEM	NURSING INTERVENTIONS
Inability to Maintain Adequate Breathing Pattern, related to retained pulmonary secretions	Assess degree of dyspnea, noting nasal flaring, sternal retractions, and pursed-lip breathing Instruct on effective breathing techniques Suction as needed
Lethargy or Malaise, related to increased respiratory effort	Assess degree of fatigue, and use problem-solving techniques with patient to explore ways to decrease fatigue Provide treatments in calm, unhurried manner Identify support systems and provide referrals if needed Encourage adequate periods of rest

Teach the patient effective breathing techniques and instruct the patient and the family on avoidance of infection exposure. Instruct the patient to notify the health care provider at the first sign of a respiratory infection. Usually the best indication of such an infection is a change in the color, consistency, or amount of sputum. Provide medication teaching, including action, rationale, and side effects. Stress the importance of increasing fluid intake, unless contraindicated. Encourage the patient and the family not to smoke. Provide information concerning smoking cessation programs.

Prognosis

Chronic bronchitis is usually irreversible. COPD is the fourth leading cause of death in the United States. The chronic nature of the condition often leads to debilitating damage to the lung tissues and impacts the overall quality of life.

ASTHMA

Etiology and Pathophysiology

Asthma is a broad clinical syndrome and an airway pathologic condition. It involves episodic increased tracheal and bronchial responsiveness to various stimuli, resulting in widespread narrowing of the airways. Asthma usually improves either spontaneously or with treatment. It is classified as extrinsic or intrinsic.

Extrinsic means it is caused by external factors, such as environmental allergens (e.g., pollen, dust, feathers, animal dander, foods); *intrinsic* asthma is from internal causes, not fully understood but often triggered by respiratory tract infection. Recurrence of attacks is influenced strongly by secondary factors, by mental or physical fatigue, and by emotional factors.

Asthma can result from an altered immune response or increased airway resistance and altered air exchange. GERD can trigger an asthma attack. The actual course of GERD resulting in an asthma attack is unknown, but it is assumed that the gastric acid reflux in the esophagus is aspirated into the lungs, resulting in vagal stimulation and bronchoconstriction (Mayo Clinic, 2021a). An acute asthma attack may be caused by an antigen-antibody reaction in which histamine is released. There are three mechanisms involved (see Fig. 9.14B):

- Recurrent, reversible obstruction of airflow in the bronchioles and smaller bronchi secondary to bronchospasm. The muscles around the bronchioles tighten and narrow the air passages.
- Increased capillary permeability resulting in edema of mucous membranes with increased narrowing of airways and increased mucus secretion.
- An acute inflammatory response by mast cells in the lungs, caused by exposure to an asthma trigger. These cells release histamine and other inflammatory agents. Systemic immune system cells release substances that cause circulating inflammatory cells to migrate to the lungs.

Clinical Manifestations

Mild asthma is manifested by dyspnea on exertion and wheezing. Symptoms usually are controlled by medications. An acute asthma attack usually occurs at night and includes tachypnea, tachycardia, diaphoresis, chest tightness, cough, expiratory wheezing, use of accessory muscles, and nasal flaring. The wheezing sound characteristic of asthma is caused by air forcing its way through the narrowed bronchioles and by vibrating mucus. The patient also has increased anxiety; diaphoresis; and a productive cough of copious, thick mucus. Asthma can be triggered by external factors (e.g., dust, mold, or lint) or precipitated intrinsically by a respiratory tract infection or exercise.

Status asthmaticus is a severe, unrelenting, life-threatening attack that fails to respond to usual treatment and places the patient at risk for respiratory failure. Symptoms of an acute attack are present, and the trapped air leads to exhaustion and ultimately respiratory failure.

Assessment

Subjective data include complaints of anxiety, fear of suffocation, breathlessness, chest tightness, and cough, particularly at night and in the early morning (Mayo Clinic, 2020b)

Collection of objective data includes assessing for signs of hypoxia, which may include restlessness, inappropriate behavior, increased pulse and blood pressure, and tachypnea. The patient may assume a "hunched forward" position to get more air. Auscultate the lungs for inspiratory and expiratory wheezing as well as expectoration of mucus.

Diagnostic Tests

PFTs are performed to assess respiratory capacity. The spirometry test is performed to assess the amount of air that is exhaled during the expiratory phase of the respiratory process. Peak flow testing is used to determine the force exerted by the lungs with breathing. Normal values for these tests vary, depending on the patient's age, weight, and sex. In an acute asthma episode, the patient cannot perform a complete pulmonary function study, but the nurse can check the peak expiratory flow rate. ABGs may be ordered during an acute exacerbation of asthma. Pulse oximetry is used to monitor the patient's SaO_2.

Obtain a sputum culture from the patient to rule out any secondary infection. CBC and differential reveal an increased eosinophil count, which is indicative of an allergic response. If the patient has been taking theophylline, draw a blood sample to determine whether the prescribed dosage is maintained at a therapeutic level; the acceptable therapeutic range is 10 to 20 mcg/mL. This also reduces the risk of complications as a result of toxicity.

Medical Management

Medication management of asthma can be placed in two categories: maintenance therapy and acute (or rescue) therapy. *Maintenance therapy* prevents and minimizes symptoms; the medications are taken on a regular basis. These include the long-acting beta$_2$-agonist salmeterol and formoterol, which are used prophylactically only; inhaled corticosteroids, such as fluticasone; cromolyn; and theophylline. A combination of fluticasone and salmeterol sometimes is prescribed also.

A group of drugs called *leukotriene modifiers* is now available for the prophylaxis and chronic treatment of asthma. Leukotrienes are chemicals present in the body that are powerful bronchoconstrictors and vasodilators; some also cause airway edema and inflammation, thus contributing to the symptoms of asthma. The two types of leukotriene modifiers are leukotriene receptor antagonists (zafirlukast, montelukast) and leukotriene synthesis inhibitors (zileuton). These drugs interfere with the synthesis, or block the action, of leukotrienes. A major advantage is that they have bronchodilator and anti-inflammatory effects. These drugs are not recommended as the only treatment for persistent asthma. A broad range of patients, with mild to severe asthma, can benefit from leukotriene modifiers. Leukotriene modifiers are not indicated for use in the reversal of bronchospasms in acute asthma attacks. They are indicated for the chronic treatment of asthma (see Table 9.3).

Acute (or *rescue*) *therapy* works immediately to relieve the symptoms of an asthma attack. The drugs involved include short-acting inhaled beta$_2$-agonist albuterol and pirbuterol taken by means of a metered dose inhaler using spacer devices or by a nebulizer; oral or IV corticosteroids; and epinephrine. One study has shown that inhaled corticosteroids, given with short-acting beta$_2$-agonists, may be better and faster than IV corticosteroids at treating an acute exacerbation (Ortega and Genese, 2019). Short-acting beta$_2$-agonists quickly relax the muscles around the airway and are the most effective drugs for relieving acute bronchospasms (see Table 9.3). Epinephrine, given subcutaneously or intramuscularly, may be considered in an emergency when symptoms have not been relieved by the use of a beta$_2$-agonist. Epinephrine acts as a bronchodilator. Although the value of administering aminophylline in the treatment of acute asthma has been questioned, IV aminophylline may be considered if the asthma is severe or there is minimal or no response to short-acting inhaled beta$_2$-agonists.

In acute asthma, oxygen therapy should be started immediately and its administration monitored by pulse oximetry and, in severe cases, by measurement of ABGs.

Using a peak flowmeter can help the patient manage asthma. This device measures the peak expiratory flow rate—the flow of air in a forced exhalation in liters per minute, which is a good indicator of lung function. Peak flow monitoring measures how well air moves out of the lungs when blown out as hard and fast as possible. Peak flow measurement can help the patient detect early signs of asthma episodes before symptoms occur. Normal peak flow is 80% to 100% of the value predicted for the patient based on height, weight, age, and sex. Severe, persistent asthma is characterized by a peak flow of less than 60% of the predicted value. A severe, life-threatening exacerbation of asthma is characterized by a peak flow of less than 50% of the patient's predicted value.

Once the acute event is over, the medical plan includes identifying precipitating factors and promoting optimal health. Elimination of allergens or countermeasures, such as desensitization or hyposensitization, are desirable.

Nursing Interventions and Patient Teaching

Nursing interventions include administering prescribed medications and ensuring adequate fluid intake and optimal ventilation. To accomplish these goals, incorporate rest periods into activities and interventions; elevate the head of the bed; teach effective breathing techniques, such as pursed-lip breathing and correct use of the peak flowmeter; and provide oxygen therapy as ordered. Monitor vital signs and electrolytes. Kind and empathic emotional support is vital.

Patient problems and interventions for the patient with asthma include but are not limited to the following:

PATIENT PROBLEM	NURSING INTERVENTIONS
Inability to Maintain Adequate Breathing Pattern, related to narrowed airway	Assess ventilation, and be alert for signs of increasing dyspnea, such as using accessory muscles, nasal flaring, pursed-lip breathing, or prolonged expiration
	Maintain position to facilitate ventilation
	Administer prescribed medications
	Assist with administration of respiratory treatments
	Provide care in calm, unhurried manner
	Attempt to minimize exposure to dust and other irritants by maintaining clean environment and use of humidifier
	Maintain adequate hydration
Impaired Health Maintenance, related to possible allergens in the home	Implement mutual problem solving to explore with patient and family what stimulants may be in home environment, such as allergens
	Facilitate allergy testing if needed
	Teach the patient and the family importance of avoiding exposure to known irritants

Educate the patient and the family to identify signs and symptoms and recognize asthma "triggers" and avoid them or lessen their effects to prevent recurrent attacks. Instruct the patient on relaxation techniques to manage anxiety. Stress the importance of health maintenance measures, such as adequate fluid intake and effective breathing techniques. Teach the patient to take prescribed medications correctly and on time, to monitor peak flowmeter results to recognize the early signs of an asthma attack and begin treatment immediately, and to follow the program treatment steps during an attack. The goal is to provide good control of symptoms with the least possible medication.

Prognosis

The diagnosis of asthma can have a profound impact on the patient's quality of life. Some patients are unable to participate in activities they enjoy. Sleep may be impaired by the presentation of nighttime attacks. There can be permanent damage to the lungs as well as a nagging and persistent cough. Ongoing breathing problems can require the use of breathing machines. Although the incidence of asthma has increased steadily, the mortality and morbidity rates currently are decreasing. Current statistics from the CDC indicate 3518 deaths per year from asthma (CDC, 2018),

which is disheartening, because treatment and education can reduce or eliminate asthma attacks. If status asthmaticus is not reversed, death will ensue.

BRONCHIECTASIS

Etiology and Pathophysiology

Bronchiectasis is a disease characterized by abnormal permanent dilation of one or more large bronchi. This dilation eventually destroys muscular elements and bronchial elastic fibers that support the bronchial wall. Pulmonary muscle tone is lost gradually after one or, more often, repeated pulmonary infections in children and adults. Because of the disease, it is much more difficult to clear mucus from the lungs, and the lungs experience decreased expiratory airflow.

This condition is usually secondary to failure of normal lung tissue defenses (as caused by cystic fibrosis, foreign body, or tumor). It occurs as a complication of a recurrent inflammation and infection process that gradually alters the pulmonary structures.

Clinical Manifestations

Signs and symptoms occur after a respiratory tract infection. The late signs and symptoms usually seen are dyspnea, cyanosis, and clubbing of fingers. The patient has paroxysms of coughing when arising in the morning and when lying down. This severe coughing produces copious amounts of foul-smelling sputum. Fatigue, weakness, and a loss of appetite also are noted.

Assessment

Subjective data include the patient's report of difficulty breathing, weight loss, and fever.

Objective data include fine crackles and wheezes in the lower lobes on auscultation. The patient exhibits a prolonged expiratory phase and increased dyspnea. Hemoptysis is seen in 50% of the patients.

Diagnostic Tests

Chest radiographic examination is essentially normal, but inflammation and mediastinal shift may result from overinflation of specific lobes. High-resolution CT scan of the chest is the gold standard for diagnosing bronchiectasis. Sputum cultures can rule out a bacterial infection. PFTs show a decreased forced expiratory volume.

Medical Management

Medical management of bronchiectasis involves treatment of exacerbations with antibiotics, bronchodilators, and expectorants. A sputum culture is preferable before treatment with antibiotics, but if a culture is not obtainable, an antibiotic is still prescribed (American Lung Association, 2020b).

Oxygen may be ordered at low-flow volume. Hydration and chest physiotherapy also are included in the plan of care. If a patient does not respond to more conservative treatment modalities, he or she may benefit from a lobectomy.

Nursing Interventions and Patient Teaching

General nursing interventions include using a cool mist vaporizer to provide humidity and increasing oral intake of fluids to aid in secretion removal. Assess vital signs and lung sounds every 2 to 4 hours. Suction the patient as needed and provide assistance in turning, coughing, and deep breathing every 2 hours. Assist with chest physiotherapy.

Patient problems and interventions for the patient with bronchiectasis include but are not limited to the following:

PATIENT PROBLEM	NURSING INTERVENTIONS
Inability to Clear Airway, related to retained pulmonary secretions	Assess patient's ability to mobilize secretions, assisting as needed
Encourage postural drainage and coughing; suction if needed
Encourage frequent position changes to facilitate secretion mobility and removal
Maintain adequate hydration
Administer mucolytic agents as ordered, and note patient response
Compromised Physical Mobility, related to decreased exercise tolerance	Assess patient's activity tolerance, and promote adaptive techniques, such as incorporating rest periods into activities
Promote a gradual increase in activity, noting patient tolerance
Problem solve with patient and family to identify methods of energy conservation and ways to integrate them into lifestyle

Teach the patient and the family environmental awareness (avoidance of smoke, fumes, and irritating inhalants). Discourage smoking, and advise the patient on appropriate rest and exercise practices. Perform medication teaching, including dosage, rationale, and side effects. Instruct the patient and the family about signs and symptoms of a secondary infection, and make sure the patient knows how to reach the health care provider after discharge.

Prognosis

Bronchiectasis is a chronic disease. Surgical removal of a portion of the patient's lung is the only cure. Complications may include cor pulmonale, hypoxia, and recurrent respiratory infections.

❖ NURSING PROCESS FOR THE PATIENT WITH A RESPIRATORY DISORDER

The role of the licensed practical nurse/licensed vocational nurse (LPN/LVN) in the nursing process as stated is that the LPN/LVN will:

- Participate in planning care for patients based on patient needs
- Review patient's care plan and recommend revisions as needed

- Review and follow defined prioritization for patient care
- Use clinical pathways, care maps, or care plans to guide and review patient care

◆ ASSESSMENT

When a patient is admitted with a respiratory disorder, a thorough, immediate, and accurate nursing assessment is an essential first step. The assessment should include the patient's level of consciousness, vital signs, lung sounds (crackles, wheezes, pleural friction rub), and oximetry level. Ask if the patient has shortness of breath, dyspnea on exertion, or cough. If the patient has a cough, ask whether it is productive or nonproductive and the amount and the color of the sputum expectorated. Observe the patient's facial expressions and for signs of respiratory distress such as flaring nostrils, substernal or clavicular retractions, asymmetric chest wall expansion, and abdominal breathing.

◆ PATIENT PROBLEM

Assist in the development of nursing diagnoses. Patient problems specific to the patient with a respiratory disorder include but are not limited to the following:

- Anxiousness
- Inability to Clear Airway
- Inability to Maintain Adequate Breathing Pattern
- Inability to Tolerate Activity
- Inefficient Oxygenation
- Insufficient Nutrition

◆ EXPECTED OUTCOMES AND PLANNING

The overall goals are that the patient with a respiratory disorder will have (1) effective breathing patterns, (2) adequate airway clearance, (3) adequate oxygenation of tissues, and (4) a realistic attitude toward compliance to treatment. The care plan may include the following goals:
Goal 1: Patient will achieve improved activity tolerance.
Outcome: Patient reports lessened dyspnea with exercise.
Goal 2: Patient will maintain a patent airway.
Outcome: Patient clears airway by coughing.

◆ IMPLEMENTATION

Maintaining the patient's optimal health is important in reducing respiratory symptoms. Nursing interventions may include improving the patient's activity tolerance. This enables the patient to perform activities of daily living while not increasing dyspnea.

◆ EVALUATION

Evaluate the expected outcomes and determine their effectiveness. Notify the health care provider if the patient's respiratory status does not improve immediately. Examples of goals and evaluative measures are as follows:
Goal 1: Patient will achieve improved activity tolerance.
Evaluative measure: Assess patient's exercise tolerance.
Goal 2: Patient will maintain a patent airway.
Evaluative measure: Auscultate lungs after hearing patient cough.

Get Ready for the NCLEX® Examination!

Key Points

- The primary function of the respiratory system is to exchange oxygen and carbon dioxide at the alveolar-capillary level.
- The most important structure of the respiratory system is the alveolus, where oxygen and carbon dioxide exchange occurs.
- The combination of one inspiration plus one expiration equals one respiration.
- For breathing to occur, pressure changes must take place within the thoracic cavity.
- The lungs' ability to expand and contract depends on musculoskeletal and neurologic functions, as well as physiologic conditions affecting the respiratory system.
- When air is inhaled, it is warmed, moistened, and filtered to prepare it for use by the body.
- Activity tolerance frequently is altered as a result of decreased oxygenation-ventilation.
- Anxiety can exacerbate pulmonary disorders, increasing the body's need for oxygen.
- Breathing exercises can improve ventilation.
- Effective breathing techniques include elevating the head and chest to maintain airway patency; deep breathing and coughing exercises to facilitate lung expansion; and pursed-lip breathing to decrease the effort of breathing.
- Adequate fluid intake and humidity help moisten secretions, thus aiding in their clearance.
- A thorough psychosocial assessment and resultant interventions are necessary for the patient with a laryngectomy because of loss of voice and neck and facial disfigurement.
- In May 2005 the FDA approved a new version of a blood test to aid in diagnosing latent TB infection and active TB. It is called QuantiFERON-TB Gold (QFT-G), and it can be used in place of the traditional PPD skin test. The QFT-G may detect TB with greater specificity than the PPD test.
- COVID-19 Coronavirus caused a global pandemic in the year 2020
- COVID-19 Coronavirus infection rate in the U.S. was 17.5 million people with over 300,000 dying from the virus
- COVID-19 Coronavirus causes various symptoms that are either acute or long-lasting

- Clinical manifestations of sleep apnea include frequent awakening at night, insomnia, excessive daytime sleepiness, witnessed apneic episodes, morning headaches, personality changes, and irritability.
- Chest drainage serves a twofold purpose: (1) it drains air, blood, or fluid from the pleural space; and (2) restores negative pressure. It requires a water seal to prevent air from reentering the pleural space.
- Techniques used in chest physiotherapy include percussion, vibration, and postural drainage.
- Nursing interventions after thoracic surgery that assist in preventing complications by promoting effective airway clearance are (1) frequent repositioning, (2) coughing, and (3) deep breathing.
- Studies have revealed that hypoxia worsens when patients are placed on their backs or sides with the affected (sick) lung down.
- Low-flow oxygen therapy is required for patients with COPD because higher oxygen concentrations depress the body's own respiratory regulatory centers.
- Hospitals are a high-risk setting for TB transmission, and health care workers are at high occupational risk for TB infection.
- Because PE impairs gas exchange, its hallmark is acute, unexplained dyspnea with abrupt, constant, non-radiating pain that worsens with inspiration.
- Patients with respiratory disorders must reduce exposure to infection, which increases the body's oxygen demands.
- COPD disorders include emphysema, chronic bronchitis, asthma, and bronchiectasis.
- Transmission of TB is primarily by inhalation of minute droplet nuclei (each containing a single tubercle bacillus) coughed or sneezed by a person whose sputum contains tubercle bacilli.
- Pulse oximetry is a noninvasive method providing continuing monitoring of SaO_2 (saturation of oxygen).

Additional Learning Resources

SG Go to your Study Guide for additional learning activities to help you master this chapter content.

Be sure to visit the Evolve site at http://evolve.elsevier.com/Cooper/adult/ for additional online resources.

Review Questions for the NCLEX® Examination

1. When are rapid and deeper respirations stimulated by the respiratory center of the brain?

   1. When oxygen saturation levels are greater than 90%
   2. When carbon dioxide levels increase
   3. When the alveoli contract
   4. When the diaphragm contracts and lowers its dome

2. What is the most appropriate nursing intervention for a patient requiring finger probe pulse oximetry?

   1. Apply a sensor probe over a finger and cover lightly with gauze to prevent skin breakdown.
   2. Set alarms on the oximeter to at least 100%.
   3. Identify if the patient has had a recent diagnostic test using intravenous dye.
   4. Remove the sensor between oxygen saturation readings.

3. The walls of the thoracic cavity are lined with a serous membrane composed of tough endothelial cells; what is this membrane called?

   1. Visceral pleura
   2. Apneustic serosa
   3. Pneumotaxic serosa
   4. Parietal pleura

4. A patient is diagnosed with chronic bronchitis. He is very dyspneic and must sit up to breathe. What is the name of this abnormal condition, in which there is discomfort in breathing in any but an erect sitting position?

   1. Orthopnea
   2. Dyspnea
   3. Orthopsia
   4. Cheyne-Stokes

5. A patient is being evaluated to rule out pulmonary tuberculosis (TB). Which finding is most closely associated with TB?

   1. Leg cramps
   2. Night sweats
   3. Skin discoloration
   4. Green-colored sputum

6. The health care workers caring for a patient with active TB are instructed in methods of protecting themselves from contracting TB. What does the Centers for Disease Control and Prevention currently recommend for health care workers who care for TB-infected patients?

   1. Ask the patient to wear a mask while in isolation
   2. Wear a surgical mask
   3. Wear a small-micron, fitted filtration mask
   4. Receive the BCG vaccine

7. The health care provider ordered a blood culture and sputum specimen for a patient who has pneumonia. When should the nurse collect these specimens? *(Select all that apply.)*

   1. After initiation of antibiotic therapy
   2. The morning after admission
   3. Before initiation of antibiotic therapy
   4. At the first sign of elevated temperature
   5. After the patient has had breakfast

8. A patient has just returned to her room after a bronchoscopy. No food or fluids shall be given after the examination until which event has occurred?

   1. There is a total absence of blood-streaked sputum
   2. The head nurse gives the order
   3. The patient's gag reflex returns
   4. The patient is up and about and steady on her feet

9. A second-day postoperative patient is recovering from thoracic surgery. Which therapeutic nursing intervention would the nurse carry out first?

   1. Help the patient cough and deeply breathe by splinting the anterior and posterior chest
   2. Splint the anterior chest for coughing
   3. Place the patient in a supine position
   4. Allow the patient to sleep uninterrupted for 8 hours

10. Which patient problem for a client with an acute asthma attack has the highest priority?

    1. Anxiousness, related to difficulty in breathing
    2. Inability to Clear Airway, related to bronchoconstriction and increased mucus production.
    3. Inability to Maintain Adequate Breathing Pattern, related to anxiety
    4. Impaired Health Maintenance, related to lack of knowledge about attack triggers and appropriate use of medications

11. A patient had a laryngectomy because of cancer of the larynx. Discharge instructions are given to the patient and his family. Which response, by written communication from the patient or verbal response by the family, indicates that the instructions need to be clarified?

    1. Report swelling, pain, or excessive drainage
    2. The suctioning at home must be a clean procedure, not sterile
    3. Cleanse skin around stoma twice daily (bid), using hydrogen peroxide; rinse with water; pat dry
    4. It is acceptable to take over-the-counter medications now that the condition is stable

12. Where do most pulmonary embolisms (PEs) originate?

    1. Deep vein thrombosis (DVT)
    2. Ventilation/perfusion (V/Q) mismatch
    3. Increased pulmonary vascular resistance
    4. Right-sided heart failure

13. Which health promotion activities planned by a nurse working with a group of community-dwelling senior citizens would be most likely to prevent influenza and pneumonia? *(Select all that apply.)*

    1. Indoor exercise programs during the winter months
    2. Influenza vaccine clinics at the senior citizen centers
    3. Teaching effective handwashing
    4. Advising seniors to avoid crowds
    5. Encouraging seniors not to visit with children

14. A patient was seen in a clinic for an episode of epistaxis, which was controlled by placement of anterior nasal packing. During discharge teaching, what instructions will the nurse discuss with the patient?

    1. Avoid vigorous nose blowing and strenuous activity
    2. Use aspirin or aspirin-containing compounds for pain relief
    3. Apply ice compresses to the nose every 4 hours for the first 48 hours
    4. Leave the packing in place for 7 to 10 days until it is removed by the health care provider

15. How is TB spread?

    1. Contact with clothing, bedding, or food
    2. Eating from utensils used by an infected person
    3. Inhaling the TB bacteria after a person with TB coughs, speaks, or sneezes
    4. Talking with an individual with TB

16. A patient with TB has a patient problem statement of *Noncooperation or Nonconformity.* What does the nurse recognize as the most common etiologic factor?

    1. Fatigue and lack of energy to manage self-care
    2. Lack of knowledge about how the disease is transmitted
    3. Little or no motivation to adhere to a long-term drug regimen
    4. Feelings of shame and the response to the social stigma associated with TB

17. To obtain optimal results from pulse oximetry, which statements are correct? *(Select all that apply.)*

    1. Do not attach the transducer to an extremity that has a blood pressure cuff in place
    2. While the probe is in place, protect it from decreased light, which can affect the reading
    3. Place the probe over a pulsating vascular bed
    4. Hypothermia, hypotension, and vasoconstriction can affect readings
    5. Reduced body temperature will affect readings

18. Inability to Clear Airway, related to tracheobronchial obstruction or secretions, is a problem statement for a patient with COPD. Which nursing interventions are correct? (Select all that apply.)

    1. Offer small, frequent, high-calorie, high-protein feedings
    2. Encourage generous fluid intake
    3. Restrict fluid intake to decrease congestion
    4. Have the patient turn and cough every 2 hours
    5. Teach effective coughing technique

19. Inability to Maintain Adequate Breathing Pattern, related to decreased lung expansion during an acute attack of asthma, is an appropriate patient problem statement. Which nursing interventions are correct? *(Select all that apply.)*

    1. Place patient in a supine position
    2. Administer oxygen therapy as ordered
    3. Remain with patient during acute attack to decrease fear and anxiety
    4. Incorporate rest periods into activities and interventions
    5. Maintain semi-Fowler's position to facilitate ventilation

20. What does the patient with respiratory acidosis demonstrate? *(Select all that apply.)*

    1. Disorientation
    2. pH less than 7.35
    3. pH more than 7.44
    4. Rapid respirations
    5. Slow deep respirations

21. Patient teaching after a tonsillectomy and adenoidectomy would include which instruction(s)? *(Select all that apply.)*

    1. Avoid attempting to clear the throat, coughing, and sneezing
    2. Avoid vigorous nose blowing for 1 to 2 weeks
    3. Resume foods and fluids as tolerated
    4. Take aspirin, gr 10 (10 grains), every 4 hours
    5. Notify the health care provider in case of increased pain, fever, or bleeding

22. If the patient has an epistaxis, what is the correct nursing intervention(s)? *(Select all that apply.)*

    1. Place the patient in Fowler's position with the head forward
    2. Place the patient in Fowler's position with the head extended
    3. Compress the nostrils tightly below the bone and hold for 10 minutes or longer
    4. Place ice compresses over the nose
    5. Encourage slow, deep breathing through the mouth

23. In pulmonary edema, what is often included in medical management? *(Select all that apply.)*

    1. IV infusion fluid bolus
    2. Furosemide (Lasix) IV
    3. Oxygen therapy
    4. Orthopneic position
    5. Morphine sulfate to decrease respiratory rate

24. An appropriate problem statement for a patient with pulmonary edema is *Fluid Volume Overload, related to altered tissue permeability.* Which nursing intervention(s) for this patient problem statement are correct? *(Select all that apply.)*

    1. Assess indicators of patient's fluid volume status, such as breath sounds; skin turgor; and pedal, sacral, and periorbital edema
    2. Monitor intake and output accurately
    3. Administer diuretics as ordered
    4. Weigh daily
    5. Provide regular diet with normal sodium intake

25. The nurse should educate the patient in the proper techniques to use for the collection of a sputum specimen. Which guideline(s) are correct? *(Select all that apply.)*

    1. Explain to the patient the need to bring the sputum up from the lungs
    2. Encourage fluid intake
    3. Collect specimens after meals, when patient feels stronger
    4. Notify staff as soon as specimen is collected so that it can be sent to the laboratory without delay
    5. Place sputum specimen in sterile container

26. Medical management and nursing interventions for the patient with pulmonary embolism usually include: *(Select all that apply.)*

    1. bed rest
    2. administration of intravenous heparin per protocol
    3. semi-Fowler's position
    4. administration of vitamin K subcutaneously
    5. oxygen by mask or nasal cannula

27. A boy, 13, is skateboarding with friends when he tries to do a trick on his skateboard. He doesn't quite make it to the top when he flips with the skateboard, and rolls back down, the skateboard just ahead of him. He lands chest first near the base of the ramp, hitting his chest hard on the sharp toe of the board. He seems unhurt, except for a few scrapes, and his friends help him home, where his parents call their pediatrician. The nurse asks a few questions and then offers guidance in how to observe him for the evening to make sure he doesn't have a concussion. He eats a little dinner and is watching TV with his sister while his parents sit talking in the kitchen. They look up to find their son standing in the kitchen doorway, looking pale. His lips are slightly cyanotic, and they both stand. "I can't breathe very well," he whispers, holding himself in a stiff, careful posture. They take him to the ED where auscultation and chest radiography reveal a bruised rib and collapsed lung from where he fell against the tip of the skateboard. Vital signs are normal, except for shallow respirations. However, because he has mild signs of cyanosis, he is admitted for overnight, at least, and a chest tube is inserted to assist with lung re-expansion. The nurse checks in on him every half hour at first.

Choose the *Most Likely* Options to Complete the Statement Below

While checking on this patient, the nurse notices continuous and constant bubbling in the water-seal chamber, which could indicate that ____1____; thus, the nurse should ____2____, and then ***most likely*** ___3___.

OPTIONS FOR 1	OPTIONS FOR 2	OPTIONS FOR 3
The drainage system is occluded	Observe for tidaling in the water-seal chamber	Administer spirometry and document ease of respirations.
The patient is lying on the tubing	Shift patient to lie on the affected side	Encourage the patient to use forced exhalations
Water loss has occurred by evaporation	Remove the patient from all mechanical ventilation	Observe the chest wall for any abnormal chest movements.
There is an air leak	Empty the drainage chamber	Elevate the drainage system to the level of the patient's chest
The patient is breathing spontaneously	Switch to mechanical positive-pressure ventilation	Replace the drainage apparatus
Positive-pressure ventilation has kicked in	Raise the drainage system to the level of the patient's chest	Notify the physician and then stay with the patient
The lungs have re-expanded	Clamp the tubing at successively distal points	Refill the water-seal chamber and secure to metal rack

Care of the Patient With a Urinary Disorder

Objectives

Anatomy and Physiology

1. Describe the structures of the urinary system.
2. Describe the function of the urinary structures.
3. List the three processes involved in urine formation.
4. Compare the normal components of urine with the abnormal components.

Medical-Surgical

5. Identify the effects of aging on urinary system function.
6. Describe the changes in body image created when the patient experiences an alteration in urinary function.
7. Incorporate pharmacotherapeutic and nutritional considerations into the nursing care plan of the patient with a urinary disorder.

8. Prioritize the special needs of the patient with urinary dysfunction.
9. Describe the alterations in kidney function associated with disorders of the urinary tract.
10. Address patient concerns in teaching about altered sexuality secondary to urinary disorders and treatments.
11. Investigate community resources for support for the patient and significant others as they face lifestyle changes from chronic urinary disorders and treatments.
12. Select patient problem statements related to alterations in urinary function.

Key Terms

anasarca (ăn-ă-SĂR-kă, p. 471)
anuria (ă-NŪ-rē-ă, p. 475)
asthenia (ăs-THĒ-nē-ă, p. 454)
azotemia (ă-zō-TĒ-mē-ă, p. 458)
bacteriuria (băk-tēr-ē-Ū-rē-ŭh, p. 453)
costovertebral angle (CVA) (kŏs-tŏ-VĔR-tĕ-brăl ĂNG-gŭl, p. 458)
cytologic evaluation (sī-tŏ-LŎJ-ĭk ĕ-văl-ū-Ā-shŭn, p. 465)
dialysis (dī-ĂL-ĭ-sĭs, p. 476)
dysuria (dĭs-Ū-rē-ă, p. 443)
hematuria (hĕm-ă-TŪ-rē-ă, p. 439)
hydronephrosis (hī-drō-nĕ-FRŌ-sĭs, p. 459)
ileal conduit (ĭl-ē-ăl KŎN-dū-ĭt, p. 482)

Kegel exercises (p. 449)
micturition (mĭk-tū-RĬSH-ŭn, p. 460)
nephrotoxins (nĕf-rō-TŎK-sĭnz, p. 483)
nocturia (nŏk-TŪ-rē-ă, p. 454)
oliguria (ŏl-ĭ-GŪ-rē-ă, p. 465)
pessary (p. 451)
prostatodynia (prŏs-tĕ-tō-DĬN-ē-ă, p. 457)
pyuria (pĭ-Ū-rē-ă, p. 454)
renal colic (p. 459)
residual urine (rĕ-ZĬ-dū-ăl Ū-rĭn, p. 447)
urinary retention (rē-TĔN-shŭn, p. 449)
urolithiasis (ū-rō-lĭ-THĬ-ă-sĭs, p. 460)

ANATOMY AND PHYSIOLOGY OF THE URINARY SYSTEM

Each day, the cells throughout the body metabolize ingested nutrients. This process provides energy for the body and produces waste products. As proteins break down, nitrogenous waste—urea, ammonia, and *creatinine* (a nitrogenous compound produced by metabolic processes in the body's muscles)—is produced. The urinary system is largely responsible for maintenance of homeostasis in the body. The primary function of the kidneys is excretion of these waste products. The kidneys also assist in regulating the body's water, electrolytes, secretion of erythropoietin (which stimulates red blood cell [RBC] production), and acid-base balance.

The urinary system consists of two kidneys, two ureters, the bladder, and the urethra. The kidneys remove waste, excess water, and electrolytes from the blood and concentrate them into urine. The ureters transport urine from the kidneys to the bladder. The bladder collects and stores urine. The urethra transports urine from the bladder to the outside of the body during elimination (Fig. 10.1). This chapter explores the filtering process of the kidneys, the composition of urine, and the how urine is removed from the body.

KIDNEYS

The kidneys lie behind the parietal peritoneum (retroperitoneal), just below the diaphragm, on each side

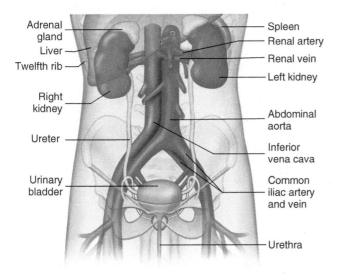

Fig. 10.1 Location of urinary system organs. (From Patton KT, Thibodeau GA: *Anatomy and physiology,* ed 8, St. Louis, 2013, Mosby.)

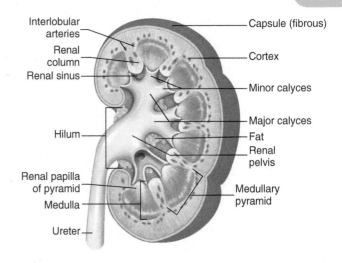

Fig. 10.2 Coronal section of the kidney. (From Patton KT, Thibodeau GA: *Anatomy and physiology,* ed 8, St. Louis, 2013, Mosby.)

of the vertebral column. Kidneys are dark red, bean-shaped organs that are 4 to 5 inches (10 to 12 cm) long, 2 to 3 inches (5 to 7.5 cm) wide, and about 1 inch (2.5 cm) thick. Because of the position of the liver, the right kidney lies slightly lower than the left. The kidneys are surrounded and anchored in place by a layer of adipose tissue. Near the center of each kidney's medial border is a notch or indentation called the *hilus,* where the renal artery enters and the renal vein and the ureter exit the kidney.

The adrenal glands, a part of the endocrine system, sit near the top of each kidney. The adrenal glands secrete hormones that help control blood pressure and heart rate, among other functions. The primary substance secreted by the adrenal cortex is a mineralocorticoid hormone called aldosterone. The level of potassium concentration in the plasma is the primary regulator of aldosterone. Changes evoked through the adrenal glands produce changes in kidney function (see Chapter 11).

Gross Anatomic Structure

The outer covering of the kidney is a strong layer of connective tissue called the *renal capsule.* Directly beneath the renal capsule is the renal *cortex.* It contains 1.25 million renal tubules, which are part of the microscopic filtration system. Immediately beneath the cortex is the *medulla,* which is a darker color. The medulla contains the triangular *pyramids.* Continuing inward, the narrow points of the pyramids *(papillae)* empty urine into the calyces. The *calyces* (singular, *calyx)* are cuplike extensions of the renal pelvis that guide urine into the main part of the renal pelvis. The *renal pelvis* is an expansion of the upper end of the ureter; the ureter in turn drains the finished product, urine, into the bladder (Fig. 10.2).

Microscopic Structure

Nephron. Each kidney contains more than 1 million nephrons. The *nephron* resembles a microscopic funnel with a long stem and two convoluted sections (Fig. 10.3). It filters the blood and processes the urine by: (1) controlling body fluid levels by selectively removing or retaining water, (2) helping to regulate the pH of the blood, and (3) removing toxic waste from the blood. Approximately 60 times a day, the body's entire volume of blood is filtered through the kidneys.

A nephron has two main structures: the renal corpuscle and renal tubule. The renal corpuscle is a tightly bound network of capillaries called *glomeruli* (singular, *glomerulus)* that are held inside a cuplike structure, the *Bowman capsule.* The renal arteries (right and left) branch off the abdominal aorta and enter each kidney at the hilus. The renal arteries continue branching inside the kidney until blood is delivered to the glomerulus by an afferent arteriole. The filtered blood leaves the glomerulus through an efferent arteriole and flows to a peritubular capillary. The cleansed blood finally reaches the renal veins and flows into the inferior vena cava.

The renal tubule becomes tightly coiled (at the proximal convoluted tubule), makes a sudden straight drop, and curves back upward like a hairpin (at Henle loop, or nephron loop) and becomes tightly coiled again (at the distal convoluted tubule). The convoluted tubule terminates at the collecting tubule or duct. Several collecting ducts unite in a pyramid and open at the papilla to empty urine into the associated calyx.

The juxtaglomerular apparatus is a microscopic structure in the kidney that regulates the function of each nephron. The juxtaglomerular apparatus is named for its proximity to the glomerulus; it is found between the vascular pole of the renal corpuscle and the returning distal convoluted tubule of the same nephron. This location is critical to its function in regulating renal

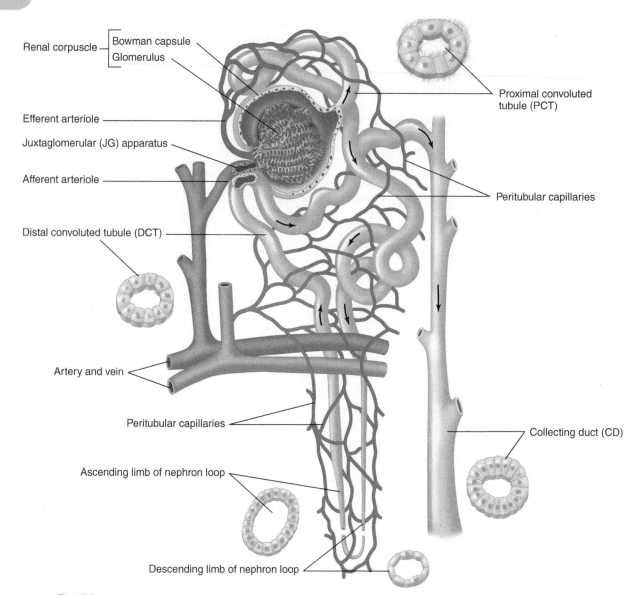

Renal corpuscle — ┌ Bowman capsule
                  └ Glomerulus

Efferent arteriole

Juxtaglomerular (JG) apparatus

Afferent arteriole

Distal convoluted tubule (DCT)

Artery and vein

Peritubular capillaries

Ascending limb of nephron loop

Descending limb of nephron loop

Proximal convoluted tubule (PCT)

Peritubular capillaries

Collecting duct (CD)

Fig. 10.3 The nephron unit. Cross-sections from the four segments of the renal tubule are shown. The differences in appearance in tubular cells seen in a cross-section reflect the differing functions of each nephron segment. (From Thibodeau GA, Patton KT: *Structure and function of the body*, ed 14, St. Louis, 2012, Mosby.)

blood flow and the glomerular filtration rate (GFR). The juxtaglomerular apparatus is where the afferent arterioles come into direct contact with the distal convoluted tubule. The juxtaglomerular apparatus regulates systemic blood pressure and filtrate formation.

The specialized cells of the afferent arteriole at this region are called *juxtaglomerular cells*. These cells contain the enzyme renin and sense blood pressure.

The specialized cells of the distal convoluted tubule at the point of contact with the afferent arteriole are the macula densa cells. These cells sense changes in the solute concentration and flow rate of the filtrate.

When systemic blood pressure decreases, the juxtaglomerular cells have a decreased stretch, which leads to their release of renin. Renin release activates the renin-angiotensin mechanism, which ultimately leads to increased blood pressure.

Reabsorption begins as soon as the filtrate reaches the tubule system. The filtrate contains important products needed by the body: water, glucose, and ions are absorbed. In fact, 99% of the filtrate returns to the body (see Fig. 10.3).

In summary, the three phases of urine formation (Table 10.1) and location of the processes are as follows:
1. *Filtration* of water and blood products occurs in the glomerulus of Bowman capsule.
2. *Reabsorption* of water, glucose, and necessary ions back into the blood occurs primarily in the proximal convoluted tubules, Henle loop, and the distal convoluted tubules.

Table 10.1 Functions of the Parts of the Nephron in Urine Formation

PART OF NEPHRON	PROCESS IN URINE FORMATION	SUBSTANCES MOVED AND DIRECTION OF MOVEMENT
Glomerulus	Filtration	Water and solutes (sodium and other ions, nitrogenous wastes [urea, uric acid, creatinine], glucose, and other nutrients) filter through the glomeruli into Bowman capsule
Proximal convoluted tubule	Reabsorption	Water and solutes
Loop of Henle	Reabsorption	Sodium and chloride ions
Distal convoluted and collecting tubules	Reabsorption	Water, sodium and other ions
	Secretion	Ammonia, potassium ions, urea, uric acid, creatinine, hydrogen ions, and some drugs

Box 10.1 Major Functions of the Kidneys

Urine formation: Glomerular filtration, tubular reabsorption, and secretion; 1000–2000 mL of urine formed each day
Fluid and electrolyte control: Maintain correct balance of fluid and electrolytes within a normal range by excretion, secretion, and reabsorption
Acid-base balance: Maintain pH of blood (7.35–7.45) at normal range by directly excreting hydrogen ions and forming bicarbonate for buffering
Excretion of waste products: Direct removal of metabolic waste products contained in the glomerular filtrate
Blood pressure regulation: Regulation of blood pressure by controlling the circulating volume and renin secretion
Red blood cell (RBC) production: Secretion of erythropoietin, which stimulates bone marrow to produce RBCs
Regulation of calcium-phosphate metabolism: Regulation of vitamin D activation

3. *Secretion* of certain ions, nitrogenous waste products, and drugs occurs primarily in the distal convoluted tubule. This process is the reverse of reabsorption; the substances move from the blood to the filtrate.

Hormonal influence on nephron function. When the body experiences increased fluid loss through hemorrhage, diaphoresis, vomiting, diarrhea, or other means, the blood pressure drops. These events decrease the amount of filtrate produced by the kidneys. The posterior pituitary gland releases antidiuretic hormone (ADH). ADH causes the cells of the distal convoluted tubules to increase their rate of water reabsorption. This action returns the water to the bloodstream, which raises the blood pressure to a more normal level and causes the urine to become concentrated. Box 10.1 for major functions of kidneys.

URINE COMPOSITION AND CHARACTERISTICS

The word *urine* comes from one of its components, uric acid. Each day, the body forms 1000 to 2000 mL of urine; this amount is influenced by several factors, including mental and physical health, oral intake, and blood pressure. Urine is 95% water; the remainder is nitrogenous waste and salts. It is usually a transparent yellow with a characteristic odor. Normal urine is yellow because of urochrome, a pigment resulting from the body's destruction of hemoglobin. Urine is slightly acidic, with a pH of 4.6 to 8 and a specific gravity of 1.005 to 1.030. Healthy urine is sterile, but at room temperature it rapidly decomposes and smells like ammonia as a result of the breakdown of urea.

URINE ABNORMALITIES

A urinalysis, which examines the physical, chemical, and microscopic properties of urine, can provide important diagnostic information. If the body's homeostasis has been compromised, certain substances may spill into the urine. Some of the more common substances include the following:

- *Albumin* in the urine (albuminuria) indicates possible renal disease, increased blood pressure, or toxicity of the kidney cells from heavy metals.
- *Glucose* (sugar) in the urine (glycosuria) most often indicates a high blood glucose level. When the blood glucose level rises above the renal threshold (the point at which the renal tubules can no longer reabsorb), the glucose spills into the urine.
- *Erythrocytes* in the urine (hematuria) may indicate infection, tumors, or renal disease. Occasionally an individual may have a renal calculus (kidney stone; plural, *calculi*), and irritation produces hematuria.
- *Ketone bodies* in the urine are called *ketoaciduria* (or ketonuria). It occurs when too many fatty acids are oxidized. This condition is seen with diabetes mellitus, starvation, or any other metabolic condition in which fats are catabolized rapidly.
- *Leukocytes* (white blood cells [WBCs]) are found in urine when there is an infection in the urinary tract.

URETERS

Once the urine has been formed in the nephrons, it passes to the paired ureters. Ureters are extensions of the renal pelvis and extend downward 10 to 12 inches (25 to 30 cm) to the lower part of the urinary bladder. As the ureters leave the kidneys, they remain in the retroperitoneal space and pass under the urinary bladder before entering it. As the ureters enter the bladder

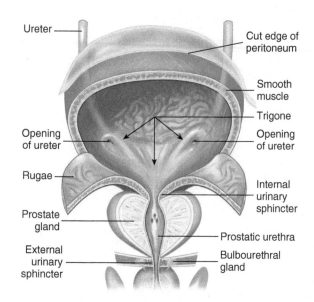

Fig. 10.4 The male urinary bladder, cut to show the interior. Note how the prostate gland surrounds the urethra as it exits the bladder. (From Thibodeau GA, Patton KT: *Structure and function of the body,* ed 14, St. Louis, 2012, Mosby.)

(at the ureterovesical junction), internal mucous membrane folds act as a valve to prevent backflow of urine.

URINARY BLADDER

The urinary bladder (Fig. 10.4) is a temporary storage pouch for urine. It is composed of collapsible muscle and is located anterior to the small intestine and posterior to the symphysis pubis (where the right and left pelvic bones join, just above the penis in men, and just above the vulva in women). As the bladder fills with urine, it rises into the abdominal cavity and can be palpated. The bladder can hold 750 to 1000 mL of urine. When the bladder contains approximately 250 mL of urine, the individual has a conscious desire to urinate. This is because the stretch receptors become activated and a message is sent to the spinal cord. A moderately full bladder holds 450 mL (1 pint) of urine.

Two sphincters control the release of urine. The internal sphincter, located at the bladder neck, is composed of involuntary muscle. As the bladder becomes full, the stretch receptors cause contractions, pushing the urine past the internal sphincter. The urine then presses on the external sphincter, which is composed of skeletal or voluntary muscle at the terminus of the urethra.

URETHRA

The *urethra* is the terminal portion of the urinary system. It is a small tube that carries urine by peristalsis from the bladder out of its external opening, the *urinary meatus.* In females it is embedded in the anterior wall of the vagina vestibule and exits between the clitoris and the vaginal opening. The female urethra

is approximately ¼ inch in diameter and 1½ inches long. In males the urethra is approximately 8 inches long, passing through the prostate gland and extending the length of the glans penis. In the male the urethra serves two functions: as a passageway for urine and semen.

EFFECTS OF NORMAL AGING ON THE URINARY SYSTEM

With aging the kidneys lose part of their normal functioning capacity. By age 70 the filtering mechanism is only 50% as efficient as at age 40. This occurs because of decreased blood supply and loss of nephrons.

In the aging woman the bladder loses tone and the perineal muscles may relax, resulting in stress incontinence. In the aging man the prostate gland may become enlarged, leading to constriction of the urethra. Incomplete emptying of the bladder in men and women increases the possibility of urinary tract infection (UTI) (see the Lifespan Considerations box).

 Lifespan Considerations

Older Adults

Urinary Disorders

- Urinary frequency, urgency, nocturia (excessive urination at night), retention, and incontinence are common with aging. These occur because of weakened musculature in the bladder and urethra, diminished neurologic sensation combined with decreased bladder capacity, and the effects of medications such as diuretics.
- Urinary incontinence can lead to a loss of self-esteem and result in decreased participation in social activities.
- Older women are at risk for stress incontinence because of hormonal changes and weakened pelvic musculature.
- Older men are at risk for urinary retention because of prostatic hypertrophy.
- Urinary tract infections in older adults often are associated with invasive procedures such as catheterization, diabetes mellitus, and neurologic disorders.
- Inadequate fluid intake, immobility, and conditions that lead to urinary stasis increase the risk of infection in the older adult.
- Frequent toileting and meticulous skin care can reduce the risk of skin impairment secondary to urinary incontinence.

LABORATORY AND DIAGNOSTIC EXAMINATIONS

Diagnostic tests for urinary tract conditions include laboratory tests, diagnostic imaging, and endoscopic procedures. Nursing responsibilities vary according to the studies performed. Be aware of specific patient variables that may influence test results: state of hydration, nutritional status, or trauma (see the Cultural Considerations box). Prepare patients for diagnostic testing by briefly describing the purpose of the procedure and what the patient can expect to happen.

🌐 **Cultural Considerations**

Urinary Disorders

A cultural assessment reflects a dynamic process in which the health care team seeks to gain insights concerning the patient's understanding of the meaning of care, health, and well-being. Integral components of a cultural assessment include communication, time orientation, personal space, pain, religious beliefs, taboos, customs, dietary practices, health practices, family roles, and views of death.

Professional discussion of urinary problems requires sensitivity because of the association of the urinary system with the reproductive system and the associated cultural taboos surrounding sexuality. Often the patient's self-image and sexual performance are affected by altered urinary function. Be sensitive to the patient's feelings, guiding the interview to ensure accurate assessment while maintaining the patient's dignity.

Table 10.2	**Urinalysis**	
CONSTITUENT	**NORMAL RANGE**	**INFLUENCING FACTORS**
Color	Pale yellow to amber	Diabetes insipidus, biliary obstruction, medications, diet
Turbidity	Clear to slightly cloudy	Phosphates, white blood cells, bacteria
Odor	Mildly aromatic	Medication, bacteria, diet
pH	4.6–8	Stale specimen, food intake, infection, homeostatic imbalance
Specific gravity	1.005–1.030	State of hydration, medications
Glucose	Negative	Diabetes mellitus, medications, diet
Protein	Negative	Renal disease, muscle exertion, dehydration
Bilirubin	Negative	Liver disease with obstruction or damage, medications
Hemoglobin	Negative	Trauma, renal disease
Ketones	Negative	Diabetes mellitus, diet, medications
Red blood cells	Up to 2 per LPF	Renal or bladder disease, trauma, medications
White blood cells	0–4 per LPF	Renal disease, urinary tract infection
Casts	Rare	Renal disease
Bacteria	Negative	Urinary tract infection

LPF, Low-power field.

URINALYSIS

The most common urinary diagnostic study is the urinalysis. Table 10.2 describes normal and abnormal constituents in the urine and possible factors that influence test results. A urinalysis may be done during assessments of other body systems because of the role of the kidneys in maintaining homeostasis. Urine culture and sensitivity may be done to confirm suspected infections, to identify causative organisms, and to determine appropriate antimicrobial therapy. Cultures also are obtained for periodic screening of urine when the threat of a UTI persists. Various reagent strips to test urine for abnormal substances are a quick reference that can be used in a clinical setting or at home. Common substances measured to monitor kidney function include total urine protein, creatinine, urea, uric acid levels, and catecholamines. Low levels of protein in the urine are normal. Elevated levels may be noted temporarily with illness. Chronically elevated levels are seen in renal damage and cardiac disease. Creatinine level abnormalities are nonspecific, but may be noted with a variety of conditions, including kidney failure, urinary obstruction, and infection. Uric acid results from the breakdown of purines. Low levels may be tied to alcohol use and glomerulonephritis. Catecholamines are made by nervous tissue and the adrenal glands. Their levels may be elevated with the ingestion of many medications, including tricyclic antidepressants and amphetamines. Levels are reduced with monoamine oxidase (MAO) inhibitors and salicylates. Elevated levels may be associated with metastatic cancers, bone marrow disorders, and gout.

Urinalysis is performed on a sample obtained using clean-catch technique or by catheterization. A sterile urine specimen can be obtained either by inserting a straight catheter into the urinary bladder and removing urine or by obtaining a specimen via the catheter port of an indwelling catheter, using sterile technique. Because the kidneys excrete substances in varying amounts and rates during a 24-hour period, a 24-hour urine sample may be collected. Discard the first voiding and note the time at the beginning of the 24-hour urine collection. For the next 24 hours all urine is collected and placed in a special laboratory container that is opaque to prevent light damage to substances in the urine. The collection container is stored on ice or in the refrigerator during the collection period.

URINE SPECIFIC GRAVITY

To determine the specific gravity of urine, the density of a urine sample is compared with that of water. It is only an approximation of the concentration of particles (i.e., solutes) in urine, but it indicates a patient's hydration status and gives information about the kidneys' ability to concentrate urine. Urine specific gravity is decreased by high fluid intake, reduced renal concentrating ability, diabetes insipidus (an endocrine disorder in which the kidneys are unable to conserve water when they purify blood), and diuretic use. It is increased in dehydration because of fever, diaphoresis, vomiting, diarrhea, and medical conditions such as diabetic ketoacidosis or hyperglycemic hyperosmolar nonketotic coma (complications of diabetes mellitus in which the kidneys are unable to excrete the high amounts of glucose in the blood) and inappropriate secretion of ADH. The normal value ranges between 1.005 and 1.030, with the lower values suggesting more dilute urine ().

BLOOD (SERUM) UREA NITROGEN

Blood urea nitrogen (BUN) is a laboratory test used to assist in determining the kidneys' ability to rid the blood of nonprotein nitrogenous (NPN) waste and urea, which result from protein breakdown (catabolism). The test may be performed to assess the overall function of the kidneys, to monitor the progression of kidney disease, or to evaluate the effectiveness of prescribed therapies. The acceptable serum range for BUN is 7 to 20 mg/dL. In addition to renal disease, elevated levels are associated with dehydration, heart disease, and a diet high in protein. If the BUN is elevated, institute preventive nursing measures to protect the patient from possible disorientation or seizures.

BLOOD (SERUM) CREATININE

Creatinine is a catabolic product of creatine, which is used in skeletal muscle contraction. The daily production of creatine, and subsequently creatinine, depends on muscle mass, which fluctuates little. Creatinine, as with BUN, is excreted entirely by the kidneys and is therefore directly proportional to renal excretory function. Thus, with normal renal excretory function, the serum creatinine level should remain constant and normal. Elevated levels may be caused by nonrenal factors such as dehydration, preeclampsia, and muscular dystrophy. Levels may be elevated as a result of renal causes, including acute tubular necrosis, glomerulonephritis (inflammation of the glomeruli), pyelonephritis (typically a bacterial infection of the kidneys and upper urinary tract), reduced kidney function, and renal failure. Lower levels may be noted with myasthenia gravis and late-stage muscular dystrophy.

The serum creatinine test, as with BUN, is used to diagnose impaired kidney function. However, unlike BUN, the creatinine level is affected little by dehydration, malnutrition, or hepatic function. The creatinine level is interpreted in conjunction with the BUN. The acceptable serum creatinine range is 0.6 to 1.2 mg/dL (female) and 0.6 to 1.4 mg/dL (male). The level in women is lower because they usually have less muscle mass (National Kidney Foundation, 2017).

CREATININE CLEARANCE

Creatinine, an NPN substance, is present in the blood and urine. Creatinine is generated during muscle contraction and then excreted by glomerular filtration. Levels are related directly to muscle mass and usually are measured for a 24-hour period. During the testing period, the patient avoids excessive physical activity. A fasting blood sample is drawn at the onset

of testing and another at the conclusion. Discard the initial urine specimen and start the 24-hour timing at that point. Collect all urine in the 24-hour period, because any deviation will alter test results. An elevated serum level with a decline in urine level indicates renal disease. Normal ranges are as follows: *serum*, 0.6 to 1.1 mg/dL (female), 0.7 to 1.3 mg/dL (male); *urine*, 88 to 128 mL/min (female), 97 to 137 mL/min (male) (National Library of Medicine, 2021b).

PROSTATE-SPECIFIC ANTIGEN

Prostate-specific antigen (PSA) is an organ-specific glycoprotein produced by normal prostatic tissue. Measurement of PSA has almost replaced that of prostatic acid phosphatase because it is a more accurate test. The normal range is less than 4 ng/mL. Older men normally have levels higher than those of younger men. It may be used to evaluate the prostate health of men being treated for cancer or as a diagnostic screening. Elevated levels may result from prostate cancer, inflammation or infection, UTI, or recent cystoscopy or prostatic biopsies. The test is not a specific determination of the presence of prostate cancer. Elevations in levels warrant additional studies.

URINE OSMOLALITY

Assessment of urine *osmolality*, which directly determines the number of particles (i.e., solute) per volume of water (i.e., solvent), is sometimes more informative than urine specific gravity but is a more difficult test to perform. Plasma osmolality may be determined in conjunction with the urine sampling when pituitary disorders are suspected. Results provide information on the concentrating ability of the kidneys.

KIDNEY-URETER-BLADDER RADIOGRAPHY

A kidney-ureter-bladder (KUB) radiograph assesses the general status of the abdomen and the size, structure, and position of the urinary tract structures. No special preparation is necessary. Explain to the patient that the procedure involves changing position on the radiography table, which may be uncomfortably firm. Abnormal findings related to the urinary system may indicate tumors, calculi, glomerulonephritis, cysts, and other conditions.

INTRAVENOUS PYELOGRAPHY OR INTRAVENOUS UROGRAPHY

Intravenous pyelography (IVP), also called intravenous urography (IVU), evaluates structures of the urinary tract, filling of the renal pelvis with urine, and transport of urine via the ureters to the bladder. Before performing this procedure, it is critical to determine whether the patient has an allergy to iodine (or iodine-containing foods such as iodized salt, saltwater fish, seaweed products, or vegetables grown in iodine-rich soils), because iodine is the basis of the radiopaque dye injected into the patient's vein for this and other radiologic examinations. If the patient is allergic to iodine, the health care provider may order administration of a corticosteroid or an antihistamine before testing or, alternatively, may order ultrasonography.

Because kidneys and ureters are positioned in the retroperitoneal space, gas and stool in the intestines interfere with radiographic visualization. Preparation usually includes eating a light evening meal, taking a non–gas-forming laxative, and remaining NPO for 8 hours before the test. If additional tests using barium-based studies are planned, the IVP is scheduled first. When the dye is injected, the patient experiences a warm, flushing sensation and a metallic taste. During the procedure, monitor vital signs frequently. Radiographs are taken at various intervals to monitor movement of the dye. Abnormal findings may indicate structural deviations, hydronephrosis (kidney swelling), calculi within the urinary tract, polycystic renal (kidney) disease (PKD), tumors, and other conditions.

RETROGRADE PYELOGRAPHY

Retrograde pyelography involves examination of the lower urinary tract with a cystoscope under aseptic conditions. The urologist injects radiopaque dye directly into the ureters to visualize the upper urinary tract. Urine samples can be obtained directly from the renal pelvis. Additional retrograde studies include the following:

- *Retrograde cystography:* Radiopaque dye is injected through an indwelling catheter into the urinary bladder to evaluate its structure or to determine the cause of recurrent infections.
- *Retrograde urethrography:* A catheter is inserted and dye injected as in retrograde cystography to assess the status of the urethral structure.

VOIDING CYSTOURETHROGRAPHY

Voiding cystourethrography is used in conjunction with other diagnostic studies to detect abnormalities of the urinary bladder and the urethra. Preparation includes administering an enema before the test. An indwelling catheter is inserted into the urinary bladder, and dye is injected to outline the lower urinary tract. Radiographs are taken, and the catheter is then removed. The patient is asked to void while radiographs are being taken. Some patients experience embarrassment or anxiety related to the procedure and should be given the opportunity to express their feelings. Structural abnormalities, diverticula, and reflux into the ureter may be detected.

ENDOSCOPIC PROCEDURES

Endoscopic procedures are visual examinations of hollow organs, done with a scope (typically a flexible tube equipped with a light and camera). Because of the invasive nature of the procedure, a signed written consent is necessary. The procedure may be done in the surgical suite; if so, the patient requires preoperative preparation (see Chapter 2). The procedure is performed by a urologist.

Cystoscopy is a visual examination done to inspect, treat, or diagnose disorders of the urinary bladder and proximal structures. As with all medical procedures, patient preparation includes a description of what is going to happen. Usually the procedure is carried out with a local anesthetic after the patient has been sedated. Patient safety is paramount when the patient is sedated. The patient is placed in a lithotomy position (i.e., supine, with the legs spread apart and the feet in stirrups) for the procedure, which may produce embarrassment and anxiety. The thought of a scope being inserted while the patient is awake may intensify these feelings. Provide an opportunity for the patient to verbalize feelings.

The scope is inserted under aseptic conditions after a local anesthetic has been instilled into the urethra. The patient experiences a feeling of pressure as the scope enters. Continuous fluid irrigation of the bladder is necessary to facilitate visualization. Care after the procedure includes hydration to dilute the urine. Monitor the first voiding after the procedure, assessing time, amount, color, and any dysuria (painful or difficult urination). The first voiding is occasionally blood tinged because of the trauma of the procedure.

The urologist can perform a brush biopsy via a ureteral catheter during a cystoscopy. A nylon brush is inserted through the catheter to obtain specimens from the renal pelvis or calyces. Nephroscopy (renal endoscopy) done via the percutaneous route (i.e., through the skin) provides direct visualization of the upper urinary structures. The urologist can obtain biopsy or urine specimens or remove calculi.

RENAL ANGIOGRAPHY

The use of renal angiography helps to evaluate blood supply to the kidneys, assesses masses, and detects possible complications after kidney transplantation. Withhold oral intake the night before the procedure. The procedure requires passing a small catheter into an artery (usually the femoral artery) to provide a port for the injection of radiopaque dye. Therefore, when the procedure is completed, the patient must lie flat in bed for several hours to minimize the risk of bleeding. Assess the puncture site for bleeding or hematoma and maintain the pressure dressing at the site. Assess the circulatory status of the involved extremity every 15 minutes for 1 hour and then every 2 hours for 24 hours.

RENAL VENOGRAPHY

Renal venography provides information about the kidneys' venous drainage. The catheter through which a radiopaque dye is injected is inserted into the femoral vein. Care after the procedure includes assessment of vital signs. Monitor the patient for bleeding at the puncture site. Assess for bruising and swelling at the site. Assess pulses distal to the puncture site. Potential complications after the procedure include allergic reaction to the dye, bleeding, clots, or injury to the vein.

COMPUTED TOMOGRAPHY

A computed tomography (CT) scan differentiates masses in the kidney. Images are obtained by a computer-controlled scanner. A radiopaque dye may be injected to enhance the images. Serum urea and creatinine levels are obtained before use of radiopaque dye. The dye is not used if inadequate kidney function is noted. Inform the patient that the table on which he or she is placed and the machine "taking pictures" will move at intervals and that it is important to lie still. The CT body-scanning unit takes multiple cross-sectional pictures at several different sites, creating a three-dimensional map of the renal structure. The adrenal glands, the bladder, and the prostate also may be visualized.

MAGNETIC RESONANCE IMAGING

Magnetic resonance imaging (MRI) uses nuclear magnetic resonance as its source of energy to obtain a visual assessment of body tissues. The patient requires no special preparation other than removal of all metal objects that may be attracted by the magnet. Patients with metal prostheses (such as heart valves, orthopedic screws, or cardiac pacemakers) cannot undergo MRI.

Emphasize that the examination area will be confining and that a repetitive "pounding" sound will be heard (somewhat like the sound of a muffled jackhammer). MRI can be used to diagnose pathologic conditions of the renal system.

RENAL SCAN

A radionuclide tracer substance that will be taken up by renal tubular cells or excreted by the glomerular filtrate is injected intravenously. A series of computer-generated images then is made. The scan provides data related to functional parenchyma (the essential parts of an organ that are concerned with its function). No special patient preparation is needed. Check facility policy concerning the disposal of the patient's urine for the first 24 hours. Pregnant nurses should refrain from caring for patients administered radioactive substances.

ULTRASONOGRAPHY

Ultrasonography is a diagnostic tool that uses the reflection of sound waves to produce images of deep body structures. Inform the patient that a conducting jelly will be applied on the skin over the area to be studied; this improves the transmission of sound waves. The sound waves are high frequency and inaudible to the human ear; the waves are converted into electrical impulses that are photographed for study.

Ultrasonography can visualize size, shape, and position of the kidney and delineate any irregularities in structure. Deviations from normal findings may indicate tumors, congenital anomalies, cysts, or obstructions. No special patient preparation is necessary.

TRANSRECTAL ULTRASOUND

Transrectal ultrasound instrumentation of the prostate gland provides clear images of prostatic tumors that otherwise may go undiagnosed. Transrectal ultrasound–guided biopsy is performed to obtain samples of prostatic tissue from various areas with minimal discomfort to the patient.

RENAL BIOPSY

The kidney can be biopsied by an open procedure similar to other surgical procedures on the kidney or by the less invasive method of needle biopsy, also called a *percutaneous biopsy*. Inform the patient that he or she may experience pain during the procedure and should follow instructions, such as holding the breath. The patient will need to rest for the next 4 to 6 hours to help prevent bleeding at the biopsy site in the kidney. After discharge from the hospital, the patient should limit activity for another 12 to 48 hours. Blood in the urine may occur for 1 to 2 days following the procedure, but gross hematuria should be reported. Potential complications associated with the procedure include infection, damage to the kidney, and bleeding. Teach the patient to report signs of complications including temperature elevations, unrelieved pain, and difficulty voiding.

URODYNAMIC STUDIES

Urodynamic studies are indicated when neurologic disease is thought to be the underlying cause of incontinence. These studies evaluate the activity level of the urinary bladder muscle (detrusor). This may cause the patient to be embarrassed and somewhat uncomfortable. A simple urodynamic study is cystometrography, in which a catheter is inserted into the bladder and then connected to a cystometer, which measures bladder capacity and pressure. The examiner asks the patient about sensations of heat, cold, and urge to void and instructs the patient at times to void and change position.

Cholinergic and anticholinergic medications may be administered during urodynamic studies to determine their effects on bladder function. A cholinergic drug, such as bethanechol (Urecholine), stimulates an atonic bladder; an anticholinergic drug, such as atropine, brings an overactive bladder to a more normal level or function.

Associated testing includes rectal electromyography, which involves placement of an electrode into the anal sphincter; and a urethral pressure profile, in which a special catheter connected to a transducer evaluates urethral pressures.

MEDICATION CONSIDERATIONS

The kidneys filter a wide range of water-soluble products from the blood, including medications. The kidneys' ability to remove certain medications from the blood may be affected by various conditions, such as renal disease, changes in the urine pH, and age. Patients with renal disease are given smaller doses of medications to minimize further damage or drug toxicity. Alteration in urinary pH affects the absorption rate of certain medications. Older patients may have decreased physiologic functioning, diminishing the kidneys' capacity to excrete drugs. Diminished kidney function interferes with the filtration of water-soluble medications.

The medications included in this discussion are representative of those that directly affect kidney function or are used to treat urinary disorders.

DIURETICS TO ENHANCE URINARY OUTPUT

Diuretics enhance urinary output by increasing the filtration of sodium, chloride, and water at various sites in the kidney. Diuretics are used in the management of a variety of disorders, such as heart failure and hypertension. Diuretics are classified by chemical structure and by the site and type of action in the kidney.

Thiazide Diuretics

Thiazide diuretics such as chlorothiazide act at the distal convoluted tubule to impair sodium and chloride reabsorption, leading to excretion of electrolytes and water. In addition to their intended effects, thiazide diuretics can cause hypokalemia (extreme potassium depletion in blood), hyponatremia (decreased sodium concentration in blood), and/or hypercalcemia (excessive amounts of calcium in blood). Hypochloremic alkalosis occurs from a deficiency of chloride. The primary indication for use is to manage systemic edema and control mild to moderate hypertension. It may take a month to achieve the full antihypertensive effect.

Loop Diuretics

Loop diuretics such as furosemide act primarily in the ascending loop of Henle to inhibit tubular reabsorption of sodium and chloride. This group is the most potent of all diuretics and may lead to significant electrolyte depletion. These diuretics are effective for use in patients with impaired kidney function.

In addition to their intended effects, loop diuretics can cause hypokalemia, hypochloremia, hyponatremia, hypocalcemia (abnormally low blood calcium), and/or hypomagnesemia (decreased magnesium in the blood). Their effect on the acid-base balance can lead to the development of hypochloremic alkalosis. Furosemide is used in nephrotic syndrome, heart failure, and pulmonary edema. Side effects are those associated with rapid fluid loss: vertigo, hypotension, and possible circulatory collapse.

Potassium-Sparing Diuretics

Potassium-sparing diuretics act on the distal convoluted tubule to inhibit sodium reabsorption and potassium secretion. Potassium-sparing diuretics decrease the sodium-potassium exchange. Although the actions of these medications vary, they all conserve potassium that usually is lost with sodium in diuresis. However, because they are weak, they usually are used in combination with other diuretics. Potassium-sparing diuretics are contraindicated in patients with hyperkalemia because further retention of potassium could cause a fatal cardiac dysrhythmia.

The aldosterone antagonist spironolactone blocks aldosterone in the distal tubule to promote potassium uptake in exchange for sodium secretion. Although it can be used in combination with other diuretics, primarily in the treatment of hypertension and edema, spironolactone is used most frequently for its potassium-sparing quality.

Osmotic Diuretics

Osmotic diuretics act at the proximal convoluted tubule to increase plasma osmotic pressure, causing redistribution of fluid toward the circulatory vessels. Osmotic diuretics are used to manage edema, promote systemic diuresis in cerebral edema, decrease intraocular pressure, and improve kidney function in acute renal failure (ARF). In ARF, osmotics are used to prevent irreversible failure, but they are contraindicated in advanced stages of renal failure.

An example of an osmotic diuretic is mannitol. It increases the osmolarity of glomerular filtrate; decreases reabsorption of water electrolytes; and increases urinary output, sodium excretion, and chloride excretion, while exerting only a minimal effect on the acid-base balance. Mannitol is used to prevent or treat the oliguric phase of ARF, promote systemic diuresis in cerebral edema, and decrease intraocular pressure. Careful assessment of the cardiovascular system before administering mannitol is essential because of the high risk of inducing heart failure. Avoid extravasation (escape of the medication from the blood vessel into the tissues), which may lead to tissue irritation or necrosis.

Carbonic Anhydrase Inhibitor Diuretics

The enzyme carbonic anhydrase (present in RBCs) converts water and carbon dioxide to bicarbonate, helping maintain the acid-base balance in the blood. In the proximal convoluted tubules of the kidneys, acetazolamide inhibits this enzyme, which leads to diuresis; therefore acetazolamide is called a *carbonic anhydrase inhibitor diuretic*. It has limited usefulness as a diuretic and is used to lower intraocular pressure.

Nursing Interventions

Because patients receiving diuretics often have complicated disease conditions such as heart failure and pulmonary edema, monitor for signs and symptoms of fluid overload: changes in pulse rate, respirations, cardiac sounds, and lung fields. Record daily morning weights for the patient receiving diuretics. Keep accurate intake and output (I&O) records, and document blood pressure, pulse, and respirations four times a day for the patient on diuretic therapy. Assess BUN, serum electrolytes, and urine as ordered. When instructing the patient and the family about diet, include a warning to avoid overuse of salt in cooking or as a table additive. Several salt substitutes are currently on the market; however, the long-term effects of those potassium preparations are not known and could complicate the renal patient's condition further. The use of most diuretics, with the exception of the potassium-sparing diuretics, requires adding daily potassium sources (e.g., baked potatoes with the skin, raw bananas, apricots, or navel oranges). In some cases the health care provider orders potassium supplements to be taken with the diuretic.

When a diuretic is effective, the serum concentration of other medications may increase as a result. Carefully monitor this potentiating effect to prevent toxicity from other medications. For example, as diuretics effectively decrease the volume of extracellular fluid, the serum level of digoxin may increase proportionately, resulting in digitoxicity. Special care is required in the selection and management of diuretics in the treatment of children, adolescents, and older adults.

MEDICATIONS FOR URINARY TRACT INFECTIONS

Certain antimicrobial agents are administered primarily to treat infections within the urinary tract. Culture and sensitivity testing are used to aid in the selection of the medication that will eradicate the identified pathogen. Urinary antiseptics inhibit bacterial growth and are used to prevent and treat urethritis and cystitis. The health history should include factors such as pregnancy and allergies to ensure the correct medications for the individual are selected.

Medications used to manage UTIs include several categories of medications. Representatives from classes frequently used are listed below.

Fluoroquinolones

Fluoroquinolones are used to treat UTIs caused by gram-negative microbes (e.g., *Escherichia coli* and *Proteus mirabilis*) and gram-negative bacteria (e.g., *E. coli, P. mirabilis, Pseudomonas* organisms, *Staphylococcus aureus,* and *Staphylococcus epidermidis*). The fluoroquinolones include ciprofloxacin, which works against gram-negative bacteria, and levofloxacin, which works against gram-positive and gram-negative bacteria. They are used in the treatment of UTIs, gonorrhea, and gonococcal urethritis. The drug is administered with a full glass of water 1 hour before or 2 hours after meals or with antacids.

The common side effects are headaches, nausea, vomiting, and diarrhea.

Nitrofurantoin

Nitrofurantoin is effective against gram-positive and gram-negative microbes (e.g., *Streptococcus faecalis, E. coli,* and *P. mirabilis*) in the urinary tract. Common side effects are loss of appetite, nausea, and vomiting.

Methenamine

Methenamine hippurate suppresses fungi and gram-negative and gram-positive organisms (e.g., *E. coli,* staphylococci, and enterococci). Acidification of the urine by means of an acid-ash diet (such as a diet high in meat, whole grains, eggs, cheese, cranberries, prunes, and plums) or other acidifiers to a pH of less than 5.5 is necessary for effective action. Methenamine mandelate is used for patients with chronic, recurrent UTIs as a preventive measure after antibiotics have cleared the infection. Although side effects are rare, they include nausea, vomiting, skin rash, and urticaria (hives).

NURSING INTERVENTIONS

Before administering antibiotics for UTIs, be certain to check all medications the patient is using for potential negative drug interactions. Instruct the patient to complete the full course of the medication, even though the symptoms may subside quickly. Hydrate the patient to produce a daily urinary output of 2000 mL, unless contraindicated. When indicated, teach the patient to consume an acid-ash diet to help maintain a urine pH of 5.5. Soothe skin irritations with cornstarch or a bath of bicarbonate of soda or dilute vinegar. Report continuing signs of infection.

Monitor the patient receiving nitrofurantoin for signs of allergic response such as erythema, chills, fever, and dyspnea. If these signs or symptoms develop, discontinue the medication and notify the health care provider. Trial doses of this medication may be used to detect a possible allergic reaction before administering the full dose.

NUTRITIONAL CONSIDERATIONS

The nutritional needs of the patient with a urinary tract disorder vary with each disease process. Some general guidelines include provision of food choices and number of servings as recommended by the US Department of Agriculture's MyPlate nutrition planning tool and a daily intake of 2000 mL of water, unless contraindicated. Unique nutritional requirements are discussed with each disorder. Box 10.2 gives an example of dietary modifications to prevent urolithiasis (calculi or stones formed anywhere in the urinary system). Patients with other systemic diseases, such as diabetes mellitus, require strict adherence to those restrictions as well.

Box 10.2 | Acid-Ash and Alkaline-Ash Foods

ACID-ASH FOODS
- Meat, whole grains, eggs, cheese, cranberries, prunes, and plums

ALKALINE-ASH FOODS
- Milk, vegetables, fruits (except cranberries, prunes, and plums)

MAINTAINING ADEQUATE URINARY DRAINAGE

Urine clears the body of waste materials and helps balance electrolytes. Conditions that interfere with urinary drainage may create a health crisis. It is important to reestablish urine flow as soon as possible to prevent the buildup of toxins in the bloodstream. Patients at risk for difficulty with urine elimination include those who have undergone surgical procedures of the bladder, the prostate, or the vagina; patients with primary urologic problems, such as urethral stricture (an abnormal narrowing of the urethra); and those who are critically ill with multisystem problems.

Urinary catheters are used to maintain urine flow, to divert urine flow to facilitate healing postoperatively, to introduce medications by irrigation, and to dilate or prevent narrowing of some portion of the urinary tract. Catheters may be used for intermittent or continuous urinary drainage. Urinary catheters may be introduced into the bladder, the ureter, or the kidney. The type and size of urinary catheter are determined by where it is to be placed and by the cause of the urinary tract problem. Catheter size is measured by the French (Fr) system: 1 Fr equals a diameter of 0.3 mm. Urethral catheters range from 14 to 24 Fr for adult patients. Ureteral catheters are usually 4 to 6 Fr. The health care provider always inserts ureteral catheters, whereas the nurse usually inserts indwelling urethral catheters.

TYPES OF CATHETERS

Catheter type varies by purpose (Fig. 10.5). The *coudé catheter* has a tapered tip and is selected for ease of insertion when enlargement of the prostate gland is suspected. The coudé catheter is less traumatic during insertion because it slides more easily past areas such as blockages, enlargement of the prostate, and a narrowed urethra. The *Foley catheter* has a balloon near its tip that may be inflated after insertion, holding the catheter in the urinary bladder for continuous drainage. *Malecot* and *de Pezzer*, or *mushroom, catheters* are used to drain urine from the renal pelvis of the kidney. The *Robinson catheter* has multiple openings in its tip to facilitate intermittent drainage.

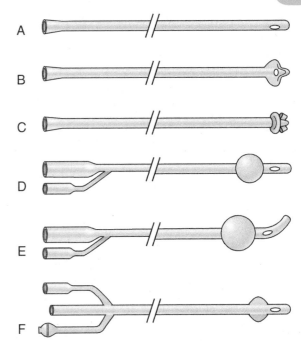

Fig. 10.5 Commonly used catheters. (A) Simple urethral catheter. (B) Mushroom or de Pezzer (can be used for suprapubic catheterization). (C) Winged-tip or Malecot. (D) Indwelling with inflated balloon. (E) Indwelling with coudé tip. (F) Three-way indwelling (the third lumen is used for irrigation of the bladder).

Ureteral catheters are long and slender to pass into the ureters. The *whistle-tip catheter* has a slanted, larger orifice at its tip to be used if there is blood in the urine. The *cystostomy, vesicostomy,* or *suprapubic catheter* is introduced by the health care provider through the abdominal wall above the symphysis pubis. This catheter diverts urine flow from the urethra as needed to treat injury to the bony pelvis, the urinary tract, or surrounding organs; strictures; or obstruction. The catheter is inserted via surgical incision or puncture of the abdominal and bladder walls with a trocar (a sharp-pointed instrument). The catheter is connected to a sterile closed drainage system and secured to avoid accidental removal; the wound is covered with a sterile dressing. When the lower urinary tract has healed, the patient's ability to void is tested by clamping the catheter so that the patient can try to void naturally. When the measured residual urine (the amount left in the bladder after urination) is consistently less than 50 mL, the catheter is usually removed and a sterile dressing is placed over the wound.

An *external (condom) catheter* is not actually a catheter but rather a drainage system connected to the external male genitalia. This noninvasive appliance is used for the incontinent male to minimize skin irritation from urine and to reduce risk of infection from an indwelling catheter. The appliance is removed daily for cleansing and inspection of the skin. Use of the external catheter allows the patient to have a more normal lifestyle.

An external catheter has been developed for women who are experiencing incontinence. The device places a wick between the labia and the gluteus. This is then attached to a low suction which pulls the urine away. The wick is changed two to three times per day or when soiled (BD, n.d.). Refer to Chapter 15 in Foundations of Nursing for more information about urinary elimination devices.

NURSING INTERVENTIONS AND PATIENT TEACHING

Problems of the urinary tract may be indicative of a primary disorder or may be one of multiple symptoms of complex, chronic disease. It is important to assess urinary elimination at the time of admission. Because of embarrassment and sociocultural taboos, some patients may be reluctant to share information with the nurse. Often the medical system intensifies this discomfort by repeatedly asking the patient to describe the problem to staff in the laboratory, radiology department, and other departments. Discretion during the admission interview and health assessment with strict adherence to Health Insurance Portability and Accountability Act standards enhance patient privacy and comfort.

Nursing interventions for the patient with a urinary drainage system involve considerations to prevent and detect infection and trauma:

1. Follow aseptic technique to avoid introducing microorganisms from the environment. Never rest the collecting bag on the floor.
2. Record I&O. For precision monitoring, such as hourly urinary output, add a urometer to the drainage system. If urinary output falls below 30 mL/h, check the drainage system for proper placement and function before contacting the health care provider.
3. Adequately hydrate the patient to flush the urinary tract.
4. Do not open the drainage system after it is in place except to irrigate the catheter, and then only with health care provider orders. It is important to maintain a closed system to prevent UTIs.
5. Perform catheter care twice daily and as needed, using standard precautions. Each institution has a specific protocol for catheter care. Cleanse the perineum (the region between the thighs, from the scrotum to the anus [in males] or vulva [in females]) with mild soap and warm water, from the front to the back; rinse well; and pat dry. At times an antiseptic solution may be ordered for catheter care.
6. Check the drainage system daily for leaks.
7. Avoid placement of the urinary drainage bag above the level of the catheter insertion, which would cause urine to reenter the drainage system and contaminate the urinary tract.
8. Prevent tension on the system or backflow of urine while transferring the patient.
9. Ambulate the patient, if possible, to facilitate urine flow. If the patient's activity must be restricted, turn and reposition every 2 hours.
10. Avoid kinks or compression of the drainage tube that may cause pooling of the urine within the urinary tract. Gently coil excess tubing, secure with a clamp or pin to avoid dislodging the catheter, and release the tubing before transferring or repositioning the patient.
11. Gently inspect the catheter entry site for blood or exudate that may indicate trauma or infection. Observe the color and composition of the urine for blood or sediment. During drainage of the collection bag, note the presence of odor that is not consistent with the normal smell of urine.
12. Collect specimens from the catheter by clamping the catheter for 30 minutes, cleansing the drainage port with alcohol and then withdrawing the urine with a sterile adapter and a sterile 10-mL syringe, using standard precautions. Send the urine specimen immediately to the laboratory.
13. Report and record assessment findings and interventions initiated.

Refer to Chapter 15 in Foundations of Nursing for further information regarding urinary drainage systems.

After the urinary catheter is removed, the patient may experience difficulty voiding until bladder tone and sensation return. If the patient complains of urinary retention, stimulate urination by running water, placing the patient's hands in water, using a warm compress on the perineum, or pouring water over the perineum. With the last method, subtract the amount of water used in calculating the correct amount voided. If the patient's condition and activity order permits, a woman can sit on a bathroom stool or commode with a urine specimen collector in place, and a male can stand to void using a urinal. Being in a normal voiding position assists the patient with urination.

The patient may experience some dribbling of urine after voiding as a result of dilation of the sphincter from the catheter. Record the time, amount, and color of the urinary output. Nursing care for patients who have had their indwelling catheter removed includes assessment of the volume voided, encouraging fluids (especially water) if no fluid restriction is present, review of intake with consideration to output, and bladder palpation to ensure urinary retention is not occurring.

Patient problem statements and interventions for the patient with a urinary catheter include but are not limited to the following:

PATIENT PROBLEM	NURSING INTERVENTIONS
Potential for Trauma, related to insertion and maintenance of the catheter	Maintain sterile technique during insertion Use smallest size catheter possible Lubricate catheter Secure catheter to leg, as appropriate Provide adequate fluids Administer urinary analgesic as ordered Allow enough slack in tubing for patient to move about freely while in bed Inspect insertion site to determine whether area is clean and without signs of possible infection or bleeding
Potential for Infection, related to invasive use of catheter	Use aseptic technique and meticulous catheter care Maintain closed urinary drainage system Avoid placement of drainage bag above level of catheter insertion (meatus) Avoid reflux of urine Encourage adequate fluid intake Administer antimicrobials as ordered Monitor patient's temperature and the color, odor, and clarity of urine

Instruct the patient about proper transfer from bed, chair, or stretcher and the principles of catheter care. Encourage fluid intake to flush the urinary system.

Self-Catheterization
Self-catheterization may be the intervention of choice for the patient who experiences spinal cord injury or other neurologic disorders that interfere with urinary elimination. Intermittent self-catheterization promotes independent function. At home there is less risk of cross-contamination than in the hospital, so the catheterization procedure can be modified safely as a clean technique. Nevertheless, instruct the patient in the use of strict surgical asepsis in the hospital because of the risk of infection there. Emphasize the need for the patient to be alert for signs and symptoms of infection and to undergo periodic evaluations by the health care provider. Follow institutional guidelines for catheter insertion.

Bladder Training
Bladder training involves developing the muscles of the perineum to improve voluntary control over voiding; bladder training may be modified for different problems. In preparation for removal of a urethral catheter, the health care provider may order a clamp-unclamp routine to improve bladder tone. This method was once widely used but is now less common. A patient with stress incontinence can learn to control leakage by performing Kegel exercises, or *pubococcygeal exercises*, that tighten the muscles of the perineal floor. The patient can develop awareness of the appropriate muscle group by trying to stop the flow of urine during voiding. Once the patient has identified the correct muscles and the feeling of their contraction, direct her to tighten the muscles of the perineum, hold that tension for 10 seconds, and then relax for 10 seconds. The exercises should be done initially in groups of 10, building to groups of 20, four times a day. Because muscle control develops gradually, it may take 4 to 6 weeks to learn to control leakage.

For habit training, establish a voiding schedule. Monitor the patient's voiding for a few days to identify patterns, or schedule voiding times to correlate with the patient's activities. Typical voiding times are on arising, before each meal, and at bedtime. Help the patient void as scheduled. After a few days, evaluate whether the scheduled voiding pattern keeps the patient continent. Modify the schedule until continence is established. Fluid intake and medications may influence voiding patterns (e.g., the patient may need to void 30 minutes after ingesting coffee or furosemide in response to the diuretic effect). Reduction of fluid intake before bedtime may help keep the patient dry during sleep.

PROGNOSIS
The outcome for patients with urinary disorders depends on many variables: age, preexisting health conditions, general health status, complications, compliance, and available family and community support.

DISORDERS OF THE URINARY SYSTEM
ALTERATIONS IN VOIDING PATTERNS

URINARY RETENTION
Etiology and Pathophysiology
Urinary retention is the inability to void even with an urge to void. The patient may not be able to empty the bladder, creating urinary stasis and increasing the possibility of infection. Bladder capacity may be exceeded, and the urine may overflow the bladder, causing incontinence. The incontinence may be partial or complete. The condition may be acute or chronic. Individuals experiencing acute urinary retention may be completely unable to void despite having a full bladder. Chronic retention is characterized by a sense of the need to void but being unable to completely empty the bladder. These patients often have excessive residual urine.

Urinary retention has a variety of causes that may be classified as obstructive, infectious/inflammatory, pharmacologic, neurologic, or other. Obstructions may include calculi or tumor. Infectious/inflammatory processes include UTIs and pyelonephritis. Medications implicated in urinary retention include antiarrhythmics such as disopyramide; antihistamines such as fexofenadine and diphenhydramine; antispasmodics/anticholinergics including oxybutynin; and tricyclic antidepressants including imipramine and amitriptyline (NIDDK, n.d.). The effects of anesthesia often lead to urinary retention during the early postoperative period. Damage to the nerves controlling bladder emptying may be the result of spinal cord injury, stroke, or postoperative complications resulting in interference with the sphincter muscles. Other potential causes may include childbirth or other trauma.

Clinical Manifestations
The signs and symptoms of urinary retention are sometimes vague and easily overlooked. The bladder becomes increasingly distended and may be palpated above the symphysis pubis. Urinary retention may cause the patient considerable discomfort and anxiety, as well as a feeling of restlessness.

Assessment
Subjective data include patient complaints of frequency with or without symptoms of burning, urgency, nocturia, and occasionally acute discomfort. Initial symptoms may not seem to be associated directly with urinary retention.

Collection of objective data includes assessing urinary bladder distention (palpable ovoid [egg-shaped] bladder arising suprapubically). The patient may void frequently, void small amounts, and have episodes of incontinence. Patients with diminished sensorium, as from spinal cord injury or organic brain disorder, may be restless and irritable without direct complaints about difficulty voiding.

Medical Management
Diagnostic studies used to confirm diagnosis and potential causes include laboratory studies such as urinalysis, serum BUN, and PSA and imaging studies including renal, bladder, and pelvic ultrasonography, and CT of the abdomen and pelvis.

Mechanical methods, such as the use of urinary catheters or the surgical release of obstructions, may be needed to treat urinary retention. Administer urinary analgesics and antispasmodics as prescribed to enhance patient relaxation and comfort. Continued medical treatments focus on alleviating the underlying cause.

Nursing Interventions
The primary goal of nursing interventions is the reinstitution of normal voiding patterns. Regardless of the pathologic findings and medical intervention, help the patient achieve adequate voiding by providing a private, relaxed environment. Bladder training approaches may assist the patient in emptying the bladder. Warm showers or sitz baths may promote relaxation of the abdominal, gluteal, and sphincter muscles. Provide warm beverages to help the patient relax. If possible, permit the patient whatever position is preferred for voiding: for women, sitting on a commode or bathroom stool is best; for men, standing may be more natural.

When continence is established, the patient may be catheterized intermittently to determine whether the bladder is emptying. Allow the patient to void and measure the amount. Residual urine amounts can be assessed by immediately after voiding the bladder is scanned with a bladder scanner (a portable handheld ultrasound device) to visualize any remaining urine in the bladder. If a scanner is not available, the patient can be catheterized and the amount of urine retained in the bladder can be measured. *Residual urine* amount should be less than 50 mL. If the underlying pathologic condition remains unchanged, this patient may be at risk for again developing retention. Urinary retention also can be the root cause of repeated urinary tract infections. Teach the patient or primary caretaker to observe for signs and symptoms of urinary retention and to notify the health care provider immediately if they return.

A patient problem statement and interventions for the patient with urinary retention include but are not limited to the following:

PATIENT PROBLEM	NURSING INTERVENTIONS
Retaining Urine or Inability to Urinate, related to: • Sensory or motor impairment • Neuromuscular impairment • Mechanical trauma	Establish urinary drainage Develop a voiding schedule Teach the patient Kegel exercises Assist with skin care Suggest use of protective clothing Engage patient in social activities Teach importance of adequate fluid intake Ensure that patient verbalizes an understanding of factors that alter urinary pattern

URINARY INCONTINENCE
Urinary incontinence (UI) refers to the loss of bladder control. It may range from leaking to full loss of the bladder's contents. An estimated 10 to 13 million Americans are affected by urinary continence; 75% of that total are women. Underreporting is likely, given the potential embarrassment related to the condition (Vasavada, 2019).

Etiology and Pathophysiology
UI is the involuntary loss of urine from the bladder. The patient may be totally incontinent, have dribbling, or experience leakage while lifting or sneezing (stress incontinence). Incontinence may arise as a complication of many disorders, such as UTI, loss of sphincter control, or sudden change of pressure within the abdomen. Incontinence may be permanent, as with spinal

cord trauma, or temporary, as with pregnancy. Women with weakened structures of the pelvic floor are prone to stress incontinence. Although incontinence may occur at any age, loss of control of urination is a particular problem for older adults.

Physical exertion such as heavy lifting, jobs that require long periods of standing, and high-impact sports may increase an individual's risk for UI. UI may also result from physiologic conditions such as obesity, chronic lung disease, smoking, pelvic floor injury, and surgery. Lack of estrogen in postmenopausal women contributes to atrophy of the vaginal and urethral walls with subsequent loss of muscle tone that may result in postvoiding urine retention and possible prolapse of the bladder.

There are various types of incontinence, which are classified according to their causes. Types of incontinence include the following:

- *Stress incontinence:* Results from the pressure or stressors on the bladder sphincter by events such as sneezing, laughing, coughing or heavy lifting
- *Urge incontinence:* Feelings of an urgency to void quickly followed by incontinence. It is associated with conditions such as Parkinson disease and Alzheimer disease, infections
- *Overflow incontinence:* Repeated inability to fully empty the bladder results in an overly full bladder, which leaks out unexpectedly. Partial rather than complete incontinence is common with this type of incontinence.
- *Mixed incontinence:* A mixture of stress and urge incontinence
- *Functional incontinence:* The influence of mental and physical impairments resulting in an inability to make it to the toilet in time to void. Conditions such as debilitating arthritis, confusion and/or disorientation, and orthopedic surgery or injuries that effect mobility are common causes.

Clinical Manifestations

The cardinal sign of UI is the involuntary loss of urine, which may or may not be the primary reason the patient seeks treatment. Incontinence may be partial or complete.

Assessment

Subjective data include information concerning the patient's inability to control the urine. Determine factors related to the episodes of incontinence. Review voiding patterns and behaviors.

Collection of objective data requires alertness for clues that the patient is experiencing difficulty controlling the flow of urine. Follow the assessment guidelines to clarify the patient's complaints. Although more common in women, UI is a common symptom for men who have benign prostatic hypertrophy (BPH) and should be included in the assessment.

Medical Management

The management of incontinence depends on the underlying cause. If the problem arises from a disorder within the neck of the bladder, surgical repair may be necessary. Incontinence related to sphincter or urethral weakness may be treated by injecting bulking materials into the tissue surrounding the urethra. This offers support and keeps it closed preventing loss of urine. Botulinum toxin type A (Botox) may be used to manage overactive bladder. The medication is injected into the bladder muscle. Temporary or permanent urinary diversion by an indwelling catheter may be indicated. A nerve stimulator may be implanted to emit an electrical stimulus to the nerves of the bladder. This is implanted under the skin in the buttock, providing access to the sacral nerves.

The pessary is a device that can be inserted into the vagina to support the bladder and to reduce pressure on the bladder from the uterus in cases of prolapse (Fig. 10.6). This option is beneficial to those patients who are not candidates for surgery or pharmacologic management. It also may be the first line of treatment before more aggressive management approaches are attempted.

Management of stress incontinence should include behavior modification, pelvic floor muscle therapies (Kegel exercises), medications, and mechanical devices before resorting to surgical procedures. If these strategies are not effective, surgical interventions offer other treatment options. One procedure is the transvaginal

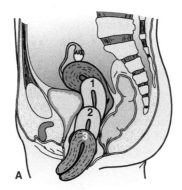 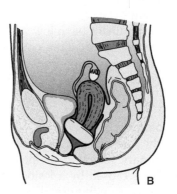

Fig. 10.6 (A) Uterine prolapse. (B) Donut pessary in place to correct uterine prolapse. (From Phillips NF: *Berry & Kohn's operating room technique,* ed 12, St. Louis, 2013, Mosby.)

tape sling procedure. The surgeon passes a permanent polypropylene mesh tape, covered by a protective plastic sheath with stainless steel needles attached at each end, through a small incision in the anterior vaginal wall. The U-shaped sling supports the urethra during stress and increased intra-abdominal pressure during routine activities. This procedure is not without difficulties. Careful patient teaching is important before any surgical treatment.

Estrogen replacement for the treatment of UI is controversial, and its reported effectiveness varies. Topical administration of prednisone and estrogen may help restore turgor and elasticity of the vaginal submucosa. Transdermal oxybutynin is effective in reducing the symptoms of an overactive bladder with few side effects. A self-catheterization system, the Self-Cath Closed System, is available for patients who must maintain intermittent self-catheterization. It is designed for patient convenience and minimization of bacterial contamination. An artificial urinary sphincter is a surgical option to reestablish continence, although there is controversy over its use.

Nursing Interventions

The incontinent patient may reduce fluid intake to decrease voiding, but without adequate fluids, urine may become more concentrated, irritating the bladder mucosa and increasing the urge to urinate. Therapeutic dietary modifications to assist in the management of UI include avoidance of alcohol, caffeine, and spicy foods, which may be sources of bladder irritation, resulting in urgency and ultimately incontinence. Discuss timing of intake to avoid late hours just before retiring. Bladder training exercises may be implemented to improve the tone of the perineal muscles. For the female patient, Kegel exercises are helpful; 10 repetitions, 5 to 10 times a day is suggested to improve muscle tone. Establish a 2-hour schedule for the patient to go to the bathroom. Once continence has been achieved, the goal may be raised to 3 hours or as needed.

Incontinence pads of various absorbencies are available in most grocery stores and pharmacies. They can increase the patient's confidence to participate in social activities. Use of protective undergarments may help keep the patient and the patient's clothing dry.

Many patients who are incontinent have low self-esteem. Be supportive by listening, encouraging the patient to express feelings, and providing kind reassurances. Never scold the patient.

NEUROGENIC BLADDER

Etiology and Pathophysiology

Neurogenic bladder means the loss of voluntary voiding control, resulting in urinary retention or incontinence. Neurogenic bladder is caused by a lesion of the nervous system that interferes with normal nerve conduction to the urinary bladder. The lesion may be caused by a congenital anomaly (e.g., spina bifida), a

neurologic disease (e.g., multiple sclerosis), or trauma (as in spinal cord injury). The two types of neurogenic bladder are *spastic* and *flaccid*.

Spastic (reflex or automatic) bladder is caused by an upper motor neuron lesion (above the voiding reflex arc) that results in a loss of the urge to void and a loss of motor control. The bladder wall atrophies, decreasing bladder capacity. Urine is released on reflex, with little or no conscious control.

A flaccid (atonic, nonreflex) bladder, caused by a lower motor neuron lesion (below the voiding reflex arc), continues to fill and distend, with pooling of urine and incomplete emptying. Because of the accompanying loss of sensation, the patient may not experience discomfort that would indicate retention.

Clinical Manifestations

Identification of the disease process is the first step in assessing the potential problem of neurogenic bladder. Prevention of complications is a major concern; infection occurs from urinary stasis and repeated catheterization. Retention of urine may lead to backup of urine (reflux) into the upper urinary tract and to distention of structures of the urinary tract.

Assessment

Subjective data include patient complaints of diaphoresis, flushing, and nausea before reflex incontinence, or infrequent voiding.

Collection of objective data involves investigating the urinary status of the patient at risk for neurogenic bladder; this includes patients with a congenital anomaly, a neurologic disease, or a spinal cord injury. The patient with a spastic bladder experiences UI, whereas the patient with a flaccid bladder describes infrequent voiding.

Diagnostic Tests

Bladder function tests are used to detect neurogenic bladder. These tests are referred to as urodynamic studies which test the nerve function using sensors placed on the skin near the urethra. Additional diagnostic tests include cystoscopy, x-rays to outline structural changes, urine culture, CT scans and MRIs (Urology Care Foundation, n.d.a.).

Medical Management

Closely monitor patients identified as at risk for neurogenic bladder. Assess urinary function early in the course of treatment and give antibiotics to treat signs of infection. The patient is aided by the use of parasympathomimetic medication (e.g., bethanechol) to increase the bladder's contractility. The patient may need to use intermittent self-catheterization or a urinary collection system if continence is not achieved.

Sacral nerve modulation (sacral neuromodulation) and stimulation. Electronic devices to modulate nerve impulses are used experimentally and in clinical practice for treating various bladder problems: urinary frequency, urgency, incontinence, chronic pain, and interstitial cystitis (IC).

Sacral nerve stimulation for urinary urge incontinence involves the use of a permanently implantable electrical stimulation device to change neuronal activity in the sacral efferent and afferent nerves to reduce urinary urge incontinence. The InterStim device, marketed by Medtronic Inc., delivers continuous low-level electrical impulses to the bladder and urethral sphincters via the sacral nerves. It corrects UI by modulating the neural reflexes, reducing stimulation to an overactive bladder, or by boosting stimulation to an underactive one. The mode of action of the impulses is unknown.

Four electrodes are connected to a battery-operated generator. The wire is inserted into the sacral foramen through a 2-cm incision. The end of the wire is tunneled across subcutaneous tissue, exits on the patient's back, and is connected to a temporary generator attached to the outside of the body. The patient tests this temporary implant for 1 to 2 weeks. If the patient achieves 50% continence, a permanent implant is put in place.

Nursing Interventions and Patient Teaching

The management goal for the patient with neurogenic bladder is to establish urinary elimination and prevent complications. Because neurologic function is disturbed, it may not be possible to reinstate normal voiding. The patient with a spastic bladder may be placed on a bladder training program, with scheduled voiding every 2 hours to empty the bladder: Diet changes such as limiting caffeine intake is often helpful in controlling symptoms. Anticholinergics drugs help control the overactivity of the bladder and botulinum toxin can be injected into the bladder wall to decrease contraction of the bladder (Urology Care Foundation, n.d.a.).

Management of the patient with a flaccid bladder is similar with scheduled voiding and dietary changes. Additional interventions include teaching the patient how to double void. The patient voids, waits a few minutes, then tries to void again (Urology Care Foundation, n.d.a.). Cholinergic medications may be used to stimulate the bladder in some patients. Catheterization may be necessary for some patients. Catheterization may be intermittent with a straight catheter or continuous with an indwelling catheter. Patients with continuous catheter drainage may use a traditional bedside bag or a leg bag. Residual urine may be measured by use of a bladder scanner or by catheterization when performing intermittent catheterization. Some patients may be able to become proficient in emptying the bladder, leading to the time between catheterizations to be increased until voiding independently is achieved. It is important to educate the patient to be alert for signs of the bladder becoming distended.

INFLAMMATORY AND INFECTIOUS DISORDERS OF THE URINARY SYSTEM

URINARY TRACT INFECTIONS

A UTI is caused by the multiplication of microorganisms in any urinary system structure. Infections may result from bacteria, viruses, or fungi. Bacteriuria (bacteria in the urine) is the most common of all nosocomial (hospital-acquired) infections. *E. coli* is the most common pathogen. Risk factors associated with UTIs include instrumentation (catheterization, surgical manipulation, and invasive diagnostic testing such as a cystoscopy), diaphragm use, condom use, and conditions causing urinary stasis or retention. Immobility, sensory impairment, and multiple organ impairment may increase the chances of infection in older adults. Women are more susceptible to UTIs than men because the urethra is short and proximal to the vagina and rectum.

Etiology and Pathophysiology

UTIs are caused by pathogens that enter the urinary tract and may or may not cause symptoms. Normally the flushing of the urinary tract with urine is sufficient to wash away pathogens. However, some conditions interfere with this process; urinary obstruction, neurogenic bladder, ureterovesical or urethrovesical reflux, sexual intercourse, and catheterization may introduce bacteria into the urinary system. Immunosuppressive medications or diseases may increase the chances of UTIs. Many chronic health problems predispose the patient to a UTI: diabetes mellitus, multiple sclerosis, spinal cord injuries, hypertension, and renal diseases.

Changes in urinary tract homeostasis allow the concentration of bacteria and increase the risk of infection. This happens when the urine, which should be acidic, becomes alkaline. Infections of the lower urinary tract increase the risk of infection of the upper urinary tract, especially if untreated.

Gram-negative microorganisms that commonly infect the urinary tract (e.g., *E. coli* and *Klebsiella, Proteus,* or *Pseudomonas* organisms) are usually from the gastrointestinal tract and ascend through the urinary meatus. Normally the body's defenses keep infections in check and clear them from the system before signs and symptoms appear. If there is incomplete emptying of the bladder or reflux of urine, the retained urine supports growth of bacteria.

Clinical Manifestations

The common signs and symptoms associated with UTI are urgency, frequency, burning on urination, and hematuria that is microscopic (visible without the aid of a microscope) to gross. UTIs are identified by the location of the infection: urethritis (urethra), cystitis (urinary bladder), pyelonephritis (kidney), and prostatitis (prostate gland). Infections of the bladder are said to be *lower* UTIs, whereas infections of the kidneys are *upper* UTIs.

Assessment

Subjective data include patient complaints of pain or burning on urination, urgency, frequency, and nocturia (excessive urination at night). The patient also may have related asthenia (a general feeling of tiredness and listlessness). Abdominal discomfort, perineal pain, or back pain (often in the flank area) may be present, depending on the extent of the disease process and site of infection.

Collection of objective data involves palpation of the lower abdomen, which may produce discomfort over the urinary bladder. Urine may be cloudy or blood tinged. Confusion and disorientation is a common sign of a UTI in the elderly patient who was previously oriented.

Diagnostic Tests

Urine culture and bacteriologic tests confirm the diagnosis. For patients with recurrent UTIs or systemic disease, more detailed urologic studies, such as an IVP and a voiding cystogram, are completed to assess the extent of involvement and damage to the structures of the urinary tract. Microscopic inspection of the urine often reveals bacteria, *hematuria* (blood in the urine), and pyuria (pus in the urine). Prostatitis is confirmed by patient history and culture of prostatic fluid or tissue.

Medical Management

The goal of medical management is to eliminate bacteria from the urinary tract, thereby relieving symptoms, preventing damage to renal structures, and preventing spread of infection to other body systems. The primary care provider prescribes anti-infective medications. Medications to treat uncomplicated UTIs often include a 3-day regimen of sulfamethoxazole-trimethoprim or ciprofloxacin. Longer therapies for 7 to 10 days of amoxicillin or ampicillin, nitrofurantoin, and levofloxacin may be prescribed for more complicated infections or those that do not respond to 3-day therapy. Most patients report symptom relief in 24 to 48 hours after treatment begins. It is important to instruct patients to complete the full prescribed therapy to aid in the prevention of recurrence. Many patients experience significant discomfort with voiding until the anti-infectives begin to take effect. Phenazopyridine, an over-the-counter medication, may be encouraged to manage the discomfort and to decrease the burning sensation that may occur with voiding. Its use should be limited to 2 days unless instructed otherwise by the provider. It is important to inform the patient that the medication will turn the urine's color to a bright orange.

Some individuals experience recurrent infections. They may be placed on longer-term prophylactic antibiotic therapies for up to an additional 6 months. If the infection is complicated by obstruction, that obstruction should be removed. For neurogenic bladder or other retention, intermittent catheterization permits urinary drainage (see the Complementary and Alternative Therapies box).

Complementary and Alternative Therapies

Urinary Disorders

- Cranberry has been used to manage urinary tract infections (UTIs), particularly in women prone to recurrent infection. Studies supporting its use are limited. It also has been used to treat acute UTIs. Monitor patients for lack of therapeutic effect.
- Echinacea stimulates the immune system and treats UTI. Patients with human immunodeficiency virus infections, including acquired immunodeficiency syndrome, tuberculosis, collagen disease, multiple sclerosis, or other autoimmune disease, should avoid its use. Echinacea should not be used in place of antibiotic therapy.
- Sea holly (*Eryngium campestre*), specifically the above-ground plant parts, have a mild diuretic effect. The roots have an antispasmodic effect. The above-ground parts are used in UTI and prostatitis treatments; the roots are used to treat kidney and bladder calculi, renal colic, kidney and urinary tract inflammation, and urinary retention.
- Nettle (*Urtica dioica*) currently is being investigated as an irrigation for the urinary tract and to treat benign prostatic hypertrophy. Patients with fluid retention caused by reduced cardiac or renal activity should not use this herb.
- Some believe that acupuncture applied to the abdominal meridian may help relieve cystitis.
- Some advocate massage with diluted rosemary, juniper, or lavender to aid in relieving pain associated with cystitis.

Nursing Interventions

Nursing interventions should be supportive, with patient education for adequate hydration and hygiene. Because these infections tend to recur or persist, patient education must include early detection. Comfort measures include a regimen of anti-infective agents, urinary analgesics (e.g., phenazopyridine), adequate fluid intake with non-caffeinated liquids, and perineal care. If treatment is effective, the patient should receive relief quickly. Infection may spread from the urinary system to other parts of the body. *Urosepsis* is infection in the blood stream resulting from infection in the urinary system. This may be a life-threatening condition.

Because of the high incidence of nosocomial UTIs, it is important that regular staff periodically review the basic procedures for catheter insertion and maintenance. Patient education for those who practice self-catheterization should include return demonstration to evaluate the success of maintaining clean technique.

URETHRITIS

Etiology and Pathophysiology

Urethritis, inflammation of the urethra, is classified by the presence or absence of gonorrhea. Nongonorrheal urethritis is called *nonspecific urethritis (NSU)*. NSU may be caused by bacteria such as *Chlamydia* or by the protozoan *Trichomonas*. Viral causes include herpes simplex virus. Sensitivity to contraceptive spermicides also may result in urethritis. Bacteria are normally present in the urethra but do not cause problems unless the integrity of the mucous membrane or tissues is interrupted, as when a catheter is in place or trauma has occurred.

Clinical Manifestations
The clinical manifestations include inflammation of the urethra with pus formation in the mucus-forming glands within the urethral lining. With gonorrheal urethritis, acute infection of the mucous membrane of the urethra causes a purulent exudate from the meatus; the patient feels discomfort, frequency, and burning on urination.

Assessment
Subjective data vary: the patient may be asymptomatic or may complain of dysuria, urethral pruritus, and urethral discharge. Women may complain of vaginal discharge or vulvar irritation.

Collection of objective data includes light palpation of the lower abdomen, which may produce discomfort over the urinary bladder. Inspection of the urethra may reveal purulent exudates or inflammation. Culture and sensitivity tests may be ordered to identify the microorganism and the antibiotics to which it is sensitive.

Diagnostic Tests
Diagnostic tests usually are limited to a Gram stain of the exudate to identify the pathogen. The urine sample for this test is obtained by a midstream clean catch specimen or by straight catheterization.

Medical Management
The first step in medical management is prevention of injury to the urethra during catheterization or sexual intercourse. Treatment is based on identifying and treating the cause and providing symptomatic relief. Drugs that may be prescribed are sulfamethoxazole-trimethoprim, metronidazole, clotrimazole, and nystatin. Comfort measures include antibiotics, adequate fluid intake to flush the system, warm sitz baths, and special care of the perineum using clean technique.

Nursing Interventions
Nursing interventions focus on patient education: avoid sexual activity until the infection clears; take all medications, especially antibiotics, to ensure the infection is resolved; and use condoms for protection from reinfection. Instruct patients with sexually transmitted urethritis to refer their sexual partners for evaluation and testing if they had sexual contact in the 60 days preceding onset of the patient's symptoms or diagnosis.

CYSTITIS
Etiology and Pathophysiology
Cystitis is an inflammation of the wall of the urinary bladder, usually caused by urethrovesical reflux, introduction of a catheter or similar instrument, or contamination from feces. The most common microorganism causing acute cystitis is *E. coli*. Cystitis is most common in women because of the ease of entrance of pathogens through the short urethra, even during voiding. Conflicting data exist about the role of bubble baths, clothing, and hygiene in increasing the risk of cystitis in women. Cystitis in men usually occurs secondary to another infection, such as prostatitis or epididymitis (see the Patient Teaching box).

 Patient Teaching

Cystitis

- Teach the patient to cleanse the perineal area from front to back to prevent contamination by spread of pathogens (especially *E. coli*) from the rectum to the short urethra.
- Encourage drinking 2000 mL of liquids per day unless contraindicated.
- Instruct the patient to take all prescribed medications even though symptoms may subside quickly.
- Remind the patient to empty the bladder as soon after intercourse as possible.
- If UTIs are associated with intercourse, recommend cleansing the genitalia with soap and water before having sexual relations.
- Encourage showers instead of tub baths.

Clinical Manifestations
The common signs and symptoms associated with cystitis are dysuria, urinary frequency, and pyuria.

Assessment
Collection of subjective data includes assessment of the lower abdomen, which may produce discomfort over the urinary bladder. Patient complaints include burning on urination, dysuria, frequency, urgency, and nocturia. The urine may be cloudy, strong-smelling, or have visible or occult hematuria. A low-grade fever may also be present.

Collection of objective data includes a clean-catch or catheterized urinalysis with culture and sensitivity tests to aid in confirming the diagnosis and in determining the appropriate treatment.

Diagnostic Tests
Microscopic inspection of the urine often reveals bacteria and hematuria. A voiding cystogram may be used to identify reflux of urine into the bladder. Diagnosis is confirmed by a clean-catch, midstream urinalysis that reveals a bacterial count greater than 100,000 organisms/mL.

Medical Management

For cystitis without the complications of obstruction or other underlying pathologic conditions, medical management consists of short-term therapy (usually 3 days) with an anti-infective agent. If the treatment is effective, the patient should receive relief quickly. A repeat urinalysis 1 to 3 days after initiation of the medication confirms the effectiveness of the intervention.

Nursing Interventions and Patient Teaching

Nursing interventions focus on teaching that these infections tend to recur by either reinfection or persistent infection. Encourage the patient to drink 2000 mL of caffeine-free fluid per day. Record accurate I&O. Include early detection in the teaching. Long-term prophylaxis with low doses of medication may be necessary. Encourage the patient to contact the provider when symptoms begin in order to prevent infections from becoming a complicated UTI.

Prognosis

Successful treatment depends on the patient's ability to adequately flush the urinary tract and complete the course of antibiotics prescribed.

INTERSTITIAL CYSTITIS

Etiology and Pathophysiology

IC is a chronic pelvic pain disorder with recurring discomfort or pain in the urinary bladder and surrounding region. Up to an estimated 8 million Americans have IC. It can affect any age and gender, but it most commonly strikes women at age 30 to 40 years. The pathophysiology is unknown. Bacterial infection does not trigger it. It seems to be caused by a breech in the bladder's protective mucosal lining that allows urine to seep through to the bladder wall, resulting in pain, inflammation, and small vessel bleeding. The bladder wall is infiltrated by inflammatory cells, resulting in ulceration and scarring of the mucosa, spasm of the detrusor muscle, hematuria, urgency, frequency, and pain on urination. Activities of daily living (ADLs) and personal relationships may be disrupted by voiding patterns; some patients report voiding 60 times a day (Mayo Clinic, 2019a).

Diagnosing the condition may be challenging. It is often mistaken for a UTI, prostatitis, or overactive bladder. The diagnostic workup involves eliminating other potential causes. The absence of bacteria in the urinalysis or a negative urine culture supports the diagnosis. Cystoscopy, biopsy, a bladder diary, and urine cytology are also used in diagnosing the condition.

Clinical Manifestations

The common signs and symptoms associated with IC are similar to those of cystitis: dysuria, urinary frequency, and microscopic bleeding. IC is characterized by urinary frequency, urgency, suprapubic pain, and dyspareunia (abnormal pain during sexual intercourse); it often is associated with fibromyalgia and irritable bowel syndrome. Autoimmune, allergic, and infectious causes are being studied.

Assessment

Subjective data include complaints of discomfort over the urinary bladder, dysuria, frequency, urgency, and nocturia.

Collection of objective data includes assessment of the lower abdomen, which may produce discomfort over the urinary bladder and the lower quadrants of the abdomen. A clean-catch midstream sample for urinalysis is used to rule out infection. Cystoscopy and tissue biopsy are used to establish a differential diagnosis.

Medical Management

IC is difficult to treat. Pharmacologic therapies are geared at symptom management. Antihistamines such as hydroxyzine pamoate help reduce urinary frequency. Amitriptyline and nortriptyline are two antidepressants that reduce the burning pain and frequency of urination. The only oral medication approved by the US Food and Drug Administration to treat the pain or discomfort of IC is pentosan polysulfate sodium. It improves the bladder's protective mucosal layer and relieves the pain of IC by decreasing the irritating effects of urine on the bladder wall. More invasive medication therapies may include dimethyl sulfoxide (DMA), heparin, or lidocaine instillation directly into the bladder. Nonpharmacologic management strategies include biofeedback and physical therapy to manage spasms of the pelvic floor. Dietary therapies also have received some attention. Patients may benefit from diets that avoid foods and beverages known to cause bladder irritation. These foods include aged cheeses, alcohol, artificial sweeteners, chocolate, citrus juices, onions, soy, caffeine, and tomatoes.

Relief of symptoms takes time: it may be 4 weeks to 3 months before significant improvement occurs. For immediate relief, a brief course of opioid analgesics may be prescribed.

Surgical interventions include studies of the effect of sacral nerve root stimulation via implantation of electrodes; cystectomy, with the creation of a urostomy; and urinary diversion. Some patients continue to experience pain even after surgery.

Nursing Interventions and Patient Teaching

Nursing interventions focus on pain control and comfort measures. Because all medications have side effects, patients must consult their health care provider before taking any prescription or over-the-counter medication. Pelvic floor exercise may help decrease urgency and nocturia. Patients may be asked to keep a daily bladder diary; this information can be used to make treatment decisions.

Teach the patient about dietary choices. A complete IC diet, self-management strategies, and other nonmedical management tools are available from the Interstitial Cystitis Association.

IC often is associated with a reduced quality of life. Embarrassment, pain, and inability to manage elimination may lead to withdrawal from business, social, and intimate relationships. The patient and significant others need psychosocial support to face an uncertain outcome.

Prognosis
Only about half of patients with IC recover fully. Until researchers find a cause and an effective treatment, symptoms continue.

PROSTATITIS
Etiology and Pathophysiology
Prostatitis, defined as inflammation and/or infection of the prostate gland, is a group of diseases. Bacterial prostatitis is caused by infectious organisms such as *Pseudomonas* organisms and *S. faecalis* traveling up the urethra. Nonbacterial prostatitis may result from a variety of conditions related to occlusion of the urethra, such as enlargement of the prostate gland.

Prostatodynia
Prostatodynia (pain in the prostate gland) manifests with neither inflammation nor infection but demonstrates the other symptoms typical of prostatitis.

Clinical Manifestations
The signs and symptoms vary in number and intensity. The patient may experience fever; chills; malaise; arthralgia; myalgia; perineal prostatic pain; dysuria; obstructive urinary tract symptoms, including frequency, urgency, dysuria, nocturia, hesitancy, weak stream, and incomplete voiding; low back pain; low abdominal pain; spontaneous urethral discharge; ejaculatory pain; and erectile dysfunction. Chronic bacterial prostatitis may be asymptomatic. Edema of the prostate gland may serve as an obstruction, causing urinary retention as a complication to the prostatitis. Pooling of urine also may foster stone formation. Other complications are epididymitis, pyelonephritis, and bacteremia (the presence of bacteria in the blood). The patient may be asymptomatic, but the symptoms of acute bacterial prostatitis are often the same as those of UTI, with pain in the low back, perineum, or rectum. The condition may become chronic.

Diagnostic Tests
Diagnostic tests include a transrectal ultrasound (transducer is inserted into the rectum) to provide a picture of the prostate, cystoscopy, and CT scan. Another diagnostic test the urologist may perform is testing of prostatic fluid or urine. The expressed prostatic secretion (EPS), including urine, is considered useful in the diagnosis of prostatitis. EPS is obtained using a premassage and postmassage test. Fluid is collected just after prostate massage via a digital rectal exam (DRE) (Urology Care Foundation, n.d.b.). Prostatic massage (for EPS) should be avoided if acute bacterial prostatitis is suspected, because compression is extremely painful and increases the risk of bacterial spread. A urinalysis and urine culture, WBC count, and blood cultures also may be performed.

Assessment
Subjective data include complaints of chills and low back and perineal pain. Chronic bacterial prostatitis causes dysuria; urgency; frequency; nocturia; and pain in the lower abdomen or back, perineum, or genitalia.

Collection of objective data involves assessing for elevated temperature and rectal palpation of the prostate gland by the health care provider, which may reveal it to be firm, edematous, and tender.

Medical Management
If the condition is infectious, management focuses on control of the infection and prevention of the complications of abscess formation or bacteremia. Patients with acute prostatitis who have a high fever or other signs consistent with impending sepsis will be hospitalized and prescribed intravenous antibiotics. Patients who are more stable are managed from home. Antibiotics commonly used for acute and chronic bacterial prostatitis include trimethoprim-sulfamethoxazole or fluoroquinolone. The course of therapy ranges from 2 to 4 weeks. Doxycycline or tetracycline may be prescribed for patients with multiple sex partners. Additional pharmacologic needs may include antipyretics, urinary analgesics, analgesics, and stool softeners. Anti-inflammatories are the most common agents used for pain control in prostatitis, but these provide only moderate pain relief. Opioid analgesics can be given, but cautiously, because this pain can be chronic. The pain resolves as the infection is treated.

Patients with chronic bacterial prostatitis are given oral antibiotic therapy for 4 to 16 weeks.

Nursing Interventions and Patient Teaching
Comfort measures used are analgesics, sitz baths, and stool softeners to reduce pain, edema, spasm, and straining pressure in the pelvis. Education is needed concerning the medication regimen.

Warn the patient with acute prostatitis to avoid sexual arousal and intercourse so that the prostate can rest; however, intercourse may be beneficial in the treatment of chronic prostatitis to relieve pressure from the prostate. Surgery to remove the prostate may be necessary in cases where chronic prostatitis does not respond to treatment. Follow-up with the health care provider is crucial because of the likelihood that the disorder will become chronic.

Prognosis

Prostatitis is difficult to cure and requires long periods of antibiotic treatment if bacteria is the cause. Stress the importance of taking all the antibiotics prescribed, even after the initial symptoms have subsided.

PYELONEPHRITIS

Etiology and Pathophysiology

Pyelonephritis is an inflammation of the structures of the kidney—the renal pelvis, renal tubules, and interstitial tissue. Pyelonephritis is usually caused by E. coli. The kidney becomes edematous and inflamed, and the blood vessels are congested. The urine may be cloudy and contain pus (pyuria), mucus, and blood. Small abscesses may form in the kidney.

Pyelonephritis is commonly seen in association with pregnancy, chronic health problems such as diabetes mellitus, or polycystic or hypertensive renal disease, insult to the urinary tract from catheterization, or infection, obstruction, or trauma. Reflux in the urinary system, and nerve damage involving the bladder are additional causes. Careful management of these disorders is important to prevent pyelonephritis.

Clinical Manifestations

Acute pyelonephritis may be unilateral or bilateral, causing chills, fever, prostration, and flank pain. Repeated episodes of pyelonephritis lead to a chronic disease pattern, with atrophy of the kidney as the nephrons are destroyed. Azotemia (the retention of excessive amounts of nitrogenous compounds in the blood) develops if enough nephrons are nonfunctional.

Assessment

Subjective data in acute pyelonephritis include a patient who is acutely ill, with malaise and pain in the costovertebral angle (CVA) (the angle formed on either side of the patient's back by the twelfth rib and spinal column; the patient's kidneys lie just under the CVA). CVA tenderness to percussion is a common finding in pyelonephritis. In the chronic phase the patient may only show unremarkable symptoms, such as nausea and general malaise.

Collection of objective data includes assessing the patient for signs of infection: elevated temperature, vomiting, and chills. The chronic disease results in systemic signs: elevated blood pressure and gastrointestinal irritation such as vomiting and diarrhea.

Diagnostic Tests

Diagnosis is confirmed by the presence of bacteria and pus in the urine, varying degrees of hematuria, WBCs and WBC casts in the urine (indicating involvement of the renal parenchyma), and leukocytosis. A clean-catch or catheterized urinalysis with culture and sensitivity tests identifies the pathogen and determines appropriate antimicrobial therapy. To prevent spread of infection in the early stages of acute pyelonephritis,

imaging examinations, such as an intravenous pyelogram (IVP) or CT scan requiring injection of contrast materials, usually are not performed. Ultrasound of the urinary system often is done to identify anatomic abnormalities such as renal abscesses, obstructing calculus, or hydronephrosis. BUN and creatinine levels of the blood and urine may be assessed to monitor kidney function.

Medical Management

The patient with mild signs and symptoms may be treated on an outpatient basis with antibiotics for 14 to 21 days. Parenteral (intravenous) antibiotics often are given initially in the hospital to establish high serum and urinary medication levels. When initial treatment resolves the acute symptoms and the patient can tolerate oral fluids and medications, he or she may be discharged on a regimen of oral antibiotics for an additional 14 to 21 days. Antibiotics are selected according to results of urine culture and sensitivity tests and may include broad-spectrum medications such as ampicillin or vancomycin combined with an aminoglycoside (e.g., tobramycin, gentamicin); other treatment options include trimethoprim-sulfamethoxazole and fluoroquinolones, such as ciprofloxacin and ofloxacin.

Adequate fluids (at least 2000 mL/day) are encouraged. Urinary analgesics such as phenazopyridine are helpful. Follow-up urine culture is indicated. In the case of chronic pyelonephritis the patient will have urine testing routinely performed at intervals of every 3 to 6 months since few symptoms are noted in this disorder. Untreated pyelonephritis can lead to urosepsis.

NURSING INTERVENTIONS AND PATIENT TEACHING

Patient problems and interventions for the patient with pyelonephritis include but are not limited to the following:

PATIENT PROBLEM	NURSING INTERVENTIONS
Potential for Infection, related to bacteria in the urinary tract	Monitor urine character and odor Encourage oral fluids Instruct patient to void when he or she feels the urge Encourage perineal hygiene
Willingness for Improved Health Management, related to desire for prevention of further renal disease	Assess knowledge level concerning measures to prevent recurrence of symptoms Discuss personal health habits (diet, exercise) Discuss treatment plan with patient and family

Teach the patient to identify the signs and symptoms of infection: elevated temperature, flank pain, chills, fever, nausea and vomiting, urgency, fatigue, and general malaise. Also teach the patient indications, dose, length of course, and side effects of the medications.

Emphasize the importance of follow-up care with the health care provider on a routine basis and when signs of infection arise.

Prognosis

Prognosis depends on early detection and successful treatment. Baseline assessment for every patient must include urinary assessment, because pyelonephritis can occur as a primary or secondary disorder (a condition resulting from complications of another disorder).

OBSTRUCTIVE DISORDERS OF THE URINARY TRACT

URINARY OBSTRUCTION
Etiology and Pathophysiology

Obstruction at any point within the urinary tract can affect function adversely and alter structure. Causes of obstruction include strictures, kinks, cysts, tumors, calculi, and prostatic hypertrophy. Obstruction may lead to alterations in blood chemistry; infection, which thrives as a result of urine stasis; ischemia resulting from compression; or atrophy of renal tissue.

Clinical Manifestations

The patient may be unaware of any problems at first if the obstruction is partial, allowing urine to drain and kidney function to remain within normal limits. With prostatic hypertrophy the obstructive process may be so gradual that the patient ignores the vague symptom of dull flank pain and seeks medical attention only when urination becomes acutely difficult. Acute pain occurs as the musculature is stretched by increasing pressure from urine accumulation and as muscular contractions increase to try to move urine past the obstruction. This acute pain is called renal colic and is a classic symptom of renal calculi.

Assessment

Subjective data include the patient's cardinal complaint of a sensation of needing to void but only being able to void small amounts. Pain may range from dull flank pain to acute, incapacitating pain. Nausea often accompanies acute pain.

Collection of objective data includes noting on physical assessment whether the bladder is palpable suprapubically because of urine retention. The affected kidney also may be palpable. Retention with overflow occurs when the patient is unable to completely empty the urinary bladder and it quickly refills, causing the urge to void again. Assess time and amount of voidings.

Diagnostic Tests

As a quick evaluation, the health care provider may order a KUB radiograph. Renal ultrasonography or IVP provides definitive information about structural changes. Other diagnostic tests may include visual examinations with the aid of endoscopy and a blood chemistry profile.

Medical Management

Initial intervention is aimed at establishing urine drainage and relieving discomfort. Conservative measures include inserting an indwelling catheter and administering an analgesic (usually opioid) and an anticholinergic agent (atropine) to decrease smooth muscle motility. It may be necessary to establish urine drainage surgically by inserting a catheter directly into the bladder through the abdominal wall (suprapubic cystostomy), into a ureter (ureterostomy), or into the kidney (nephrostomy).

Surgical correction of an obstruction in the urinary system may involve a tube, called a *stent*. Stent insertion is used for patients who are poor operative risks. A meshlike tube or coil-shaped device is inserted through an endoscope into the ureter. The stent holds the tubular structure open to facilitate drainage. Stents may be permanent or temporary. Closely monitor the patient for signs of infection, obstruction, and pain.

Nursing Interventions

After surgery, observe the patient for hemorrhage, provide aseptic care of the surgical site, and provide a safe environment to prevent injury and infection.

Prognosis

The prognosis varies, depending on the cause of the obstruction. If surgical correction is successful, the prognosis is excellent.

HYDRONEPHROSIS
Etiology and Pathophysiology

Hydronephrosis (dilation of the renal pelvis and calyces) may be congenital or may develop at any time. It can occur unilaterally or bilaterally. Hydronephrosis is caused by obstructions in the lower urinary tract, the ureters, or the kidneys. The location of the obstruction determines whether one or both kidneys are affected. Potential causes may include renal calculi, tumors, strictures, vesicoureteric reflux, and scarring (Fig. 10.7).

An obstruction generates pressure from accumulated urine that cannot flow past it. This pressure may cause functional and anatomic damage to the renal system. The renal pelvis and ureters dilate and hypertrophy. This pressure, if prolonged, causes fibrosis and loss of function in affected nephrons. If the condition is left untreated, the kidney may be destroyed.

Clinical Manifestations

Hydronephrosis can occur without any symptoms as long as kidney function is adequate and urine can drain. The amount of pain is proportional to the rate of stretching of urinary tract structures. Slowly developing hydronephrosis may cause only a dull flank pain, whereas a sudden occlusion of the ureter, such as from a calculus, causes a severe stabbing (colicky) pain in the flank. Nausea and vomiting, which often

HYDRONEPHROSIS   NORMAL KIDNEY

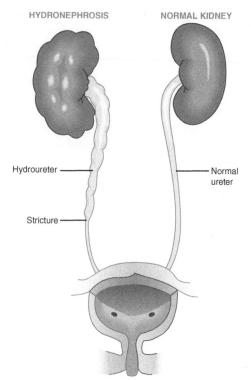

Hydroureter

Normal
ureter

Stricture

Fig. 10.7 Hydronephrosis. (From Adams AP, Proctor DB: *Kinn's
medical assistant: An applied learning approach*, ed 11, St. Louis,
2011, Saunders.)

accompany hydronephrosis, are a reflex reaction to the
pain and usually subside when the pain is controlled.

Assessment
Subjective data include patient reports of pain, including location, intensity, and character, and nausea.
Discuss the patient's voiding pattern: frequency, difficulty starting a stream of urine, dribbling at the end of
micturition (voiding), nocturia, and burning on urination. Note any history of obstructive disorders.

Collection of objective data includes assessing the
patient suspected of having hydronephrosis for vomiting, hematuria, urinary output, edema, a palpable
mass in the abdomen, bladder distention (detected on
palpation), and tenderness over the kidneys or bladder.

Diagnostic Tests
Urinalysis and serum kidney function studies that
include measurement of urea and creatinine are obtained. Cystoscopy may be performed with or without retrograde pyelogram. Radiographic examinations
may include IVP or IVU, KUB radiograph, CT scan,
or ultrasound evaluation. Sometimes a renal biopsy is
performed.

Medical Management
Management is usually conservative if the condition
is not severe. Surgery relieves the obstruction and
preserves kidney function. If the kidney is severely
damaged, a nephrectomy may be necessary. If infection is present, antibiotics are administered: penicillin

in combination with sulfamethoxazole-trimethoprim.
Opioids, such as morphine and meperidine, in combination with antispasmodic drugs, such as propantheline and belladonna preparations, are usually necessary to relieve severe, colicky pain.

Nursing Interventions and Patient Teaching
Nursing interventions for the patient with hydronephrosis include administering medications as ordered,
monitoring I&O, observing for signs and symptoms of
infection, and monitoring vital signs. Encourage the
patient to take fluids and assess the patient for pain.
Keep any drainage tubes open and anchored to avoid
inadvertent displacement. If a catheter is present, provide catheter care. If surgery has been performed, observe the dressing because drainage of urine may continue for some time. Keep the area clean and dry to
avoid excoriation of the skin. Explain all procedures to
the patient and the family.

Patient teaching includes explaining the abnormality and the signs and symptoms of infection or obstruction. Describe measures to prevent infection, such
as adequate fluid intake, perineal hygiene daily with
mild soap and water (drying thoroughly), and regular
emptying of the bladder.

Prognosis
Prognosis depends on the degree of urinary system
destruction and the need for surgical intervention. If
hydronephrosis is not treated unreversible kidney
damage can result. Rarely are both kidneys affected
by hydronephrosis, so kidney failure is not commonly
seen as a result of the damage to the kidney (Mayo
Clinic, 2020b).

UROLITHIASIS
Urolithiasis (formation of urinary calculi) can develop
in any area of the urinary tract. *Urolithiasis* is a general
term that encompasses all urinary calculi, but specific
names also are used to indicate where they are located
or formed: *nephrolithiasis* (formation of a kidney stone,
or *nephrolith*), *ureterolithiasis* (formation of a stone in
the ureter, or *ureterolith*), and *cystolithiasis* (a bladder
stone, or *cystolith*). Another descriptive term is *litho-
genesis* (the formation of stones).

Etiology and Pathophysiology
Urolithiasis occurs when minerals precipitate out of
solution and adhere, forming stones that vary in size
and shape. The event that initiates stone formation remains unknown. Factors predisposing individuals to
urolithiasis include immobility, obesity, family history,
male gender, hyperparathyroidism (in which calcium
leaves the bones and accumulates in the bloodstream),
or recurrent UTIs. Dietary influences may contribute to
stone development. Chronic use of medications such
as diuretics, calcium-based antacids, and topiramate
are linked to stone formation. Thorough assessment

and analysis of the composition of the stones guide medical and nursing management.

Clinical Manifestations
Symptoms depend on the stones' size and degree of mobility. The patient with renal colic seeks care immediately, whereas a person with a less mobile stone may not seek assistance until signs of infection or hydronephrosis occur.

Assessment
Subjective data include the patient with mobile calculi complaining of intractable pain (pain that is unrelieved by ordinary medical measures and usually is accompanied by nausea and vomiting). The patient describes the pain as starting in the flank and radiating into the groin, the genitalia, and the inner thigh. The patient with a less mobile stone may develop signs and symptoms associated with UTI secondary to hydronephrosis.

Collection of objective data includes assessing for hematuria and vomiting.

Diagnostic Tests
Diagnostic tests include KUB and IVP or IVU radiography, ultrasound, cystoscopy, and urinalysis. Other tests may be ordered to determine stone content, presence of infection, and alterations in blood chemistry that influence stone formation. Twenty-four-hour urine examination may detect abnormal excretion of calcium oxalate, phosphorus, or uric acid.

Medical Management
Stone removal and pain management are the primary goals of treatment. Antibiotics may be administered to treat infection or prophylactically. If stones are not passed, invasive techniques may be indicated (Fig. 10.8). Stones in the lower tract can be removed by cystoscopy with stone manipulation or by surgical incision. Terminology describes the location:

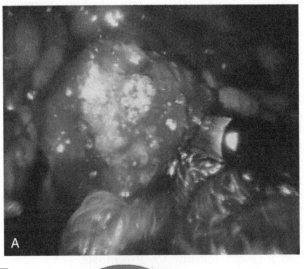

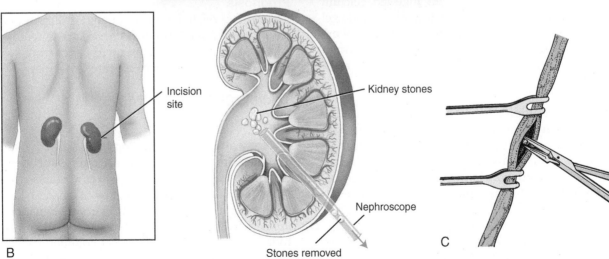

Fig. 10.8 Location and methods of removing renal calculi from upper urinary tract. (A) Pyelolithotomy, removal of stone through renal pelvis. (B) Nephrolithotomy, removal of staghorn calculus from renal parenchyma (kidney split). (C) Ureterolithotomy, removal of stone from ureter. (A., Bishoff JT, Kavoussi LR: *Atlas of laparoscopic and robotic urologic surgery*, ed 3, Philadelphia, 2017, Elsevier. B, Brooks DL, Brooks ML: *Exploring medical language*, ed 10, St. Louis, 2018, Elsevier. C, From Beare PG, Myers JL: *Adult health nursing*, ed 3, St. Louis, 1998, Mosby.)

ureterolithotomy, pyelolithotomy, and nephrolithotomy. Chemolytic agents, either alkylating or acidifying agents, may be instilled to dissolve stones.

Extracorporeal shock wave lithotripsy is an alternative to surgery that is frequently performed. With the assistance of fluoroscopy the stone/stones are precisely identified and shock waves are used to pulverize the stone. Following the procedure, the patient may be asked to strain the urine to collect the stone particles for testing to determine their composition. Renal colic may occur as the patient passes the stone fragments. The procedure is often uncomfortable, so some degree of sedation or anesthetic is advised.

Percutaneous nephrolithotomy may be used to manage larger stones that are not able to be passed. A nephroscope allows the stone to be visualized and removed through a small incision directly into the kidney through the back. Then, a small rubber catheter is placed into the kidney and the stone is removed. If the stone is large, it may be broken down using lasers before removal.

Long-term management may include dietary adjustments to alter urine pH or to decrease the availability of certain substances that cause stone formation. Moderate reduction of foods containing calcium, phosphorus, and purine may help when stones are caused by metabolic abnormalities. Foods to avoid include cheese, greens, whole grains, carbonated beverages, nuts, chocolate, shellfish, and organ meat. Daily fluid intake of 2000 mL (unless clinically contraindicated) helps cleanse the urinary tract. Additional dietary modifications may be implemented based upon the composition of the stones being experienced. Diets should only be altered if the composition of the stone warrants a change.

Drug therapy depends on stone composition. To prevent calcium stone formation, sodium cellulose phosphate is taken; it binds with ingested calcium and prevents its absorption. Aluminum hydroxide gel binds with excess phosphorus, allowing intestinal excretion rather than urinary excretion; and allopurinol reduces serum urate levels, thereby facilitating reabsorption of urate crystals.

Nursing Interventions and Patient Teaching

Physical activity and hydration facilitate stone passage. The patient may require opioid medications to manage the pain. If analgesics are given, provide assistance with ambulation. If the patient is unable to tolerate sufficient oral intake, intravenous fluids may be prescribed. All urine is strained. Any stones or "gravel" noted must be sent to the laboratory for analysis. Assess urine for possible hematuria. Monitor BUN and creatinine for indications of continuing urinary tract obstruction.

Patient problems and interventions for the patient with urolithiasis include but are not limited to the following:

PATIENT PROBLEM	NURSING INTERVENTIONS
Potential for Infection, related to bacteria in the urinary tract	Monitor urine character and odor Encourage oral fluids Instruct the patient to void when urge is felt Encourage perineal hygiene Encourage fluid intake
Willingness for Improved Health Management, related to desire for prevention of further renal disease	Assess knowledge level concerning measures to prevent recurrence of symptoms Discuss personal health habits (diet, exercise) Discuss treatment plan with patient and family

Discuss the prescribed diet, including fluid intake, and home medications (their purpose, dosage, refills, and side effects). The patient should avoid inactivity by walking frequently. Emphasize the need for follow-up with the health care provider, including keeping scheduled appointments and reporting difficulty with urination.

Although opinions vary greatly as to benefits of dietary restrictions, the nurse may be responsible for clarifying diet instructions. Encourage a fluid intake of at least 2000 mL in 24 hours, unless contraindicated. People who tend to form calcium stones may need to curtail their intake of dietary calcium (dairy products, antacids) to within minimum recommended dietary allowance guidelines. New research on the impact of diet on the development of calcium oxalate kidney stones concludes that restricting consumption of animal protein and salt in combination with normal calcium intake reduces the risk of kidney stones better than the traditional low-calcium diet.

Prognosis

Prognosis is related to the location of the stone and the extent of invasive procedures necessary to remove the stone. Some patients are prone to developing urinary calculi and will experience repeated episodes.

TUMORS OF THE URINARY SYSTEM

RENAL TUMORS
Etiology and Pathophysiology

The majority of renal tumors are malignant adenocarcinomas, also known as renal cell carcinomas, that develop unilaterally and are often large when first detected. Renal cell carcinoma as a primary malignant tumor appears to arise from cells of the proximal convoluted tubules. This is the eighth most common cancer, accounting for 4.1% of all cancers in adults, with a median age at diagnosis of 64 years. The estimated number of people having kidney cancer in 2020 is 73,750. Twice as many men as women are diagnosed with renal cancer (National Cancer Institute, n.d.).

Risk factors include a history of dialysis (filtration of the blood to remove excess water and waste products), family history, hypertension, horseshoe kidney (a developmental anomaly in which the kidneys are fused together), polycystic kidney disease (PKD), use of acetaminophen, and smoking. The strongest risk factors appear to be genetic; multifocal renal adenocarcinomas have a hereditary basis, which is being studied intensively. Several multiorgan syndromes are associated with a high risk for renal malignancies; the most prominent is von Hippel–Lindau disease, an autosomal dominant hereditary disease (American Cancer Society, 2020b).

Because of the isolated anatomic location of the kidney, renal adenocarcinomas can grow large while remaining clinically silent. Most demonstrate a characteristic hypervascularity. Renal adenocarcinomas tend to grow intravascularly, within the renal vein and into the inferior vena cava. These tumor thrombi may extend as far as the right atrium, presenting a unique surgical challenge. Although essentially every organ can be affected, the most common sites of metastases are the lungs, adrenal glands, liver, and bones.

Clinical Manifestations

The historic sign-and-symptom triad of renal adenocarcinoma is hematuria, flank pain, and a flank mass. Most cases with these symptoms are advanced and incurable. Other common signs and symptoms are hypercalcemia, fever, anemia, weakness, and erythrocytosis. Gross hematuria is rarely a sign of renal adenocarcinoma until the malignancy is advanced. Check the patient's home medications for anticoagulant therapy, because this may be the cause of hematuria.

Assessment

Subjective data include a patient history of blood in the urine, which "comes and goes." When the bleeding occurs, there is usually no associated pain. In advanced stages of the illness, the patient experiences weight loss, fatigue, and dull flank pain.

Collection of objective data involves a physical assessment that reveals a mass in the patient's flank in the advanced stages of the illness. Hematuria and signs related to systemic metastasis may be obvious.

Diagnostic Tests

Localized adenocarcinoma may be diagnosed in patients who have no signs and symptoms specifically related to the tumor; these tumors often are discovered incidentally during evaluation of other complaints. Patients with gross hematuria should be assessed by a urologist. A cystoscopy followed by an IVP with tomography should be performed.

The majority of solid masses are malignant and require definitive evaluation and treatment. Percutaneous biopsy of a solid renal mass assists with staging. A CT (with or without contrast), MRI, x-ray, and, in some cases, a bone scan are used to stage renal adenocarcinoma.

Medical Management

Surgery is the most common treatment for renal cancer. The standard procedure is radical nephrectomy along with removal of adjacent lymph nodes and tissue. In the patient with renal insufficiency, a small tumor, or having only one kidney, partial nephrectomy may be indicated. Other treatments include targeted chemotherapy and immunotherapy. For small tumors cryoablation or radiofrequency ablation may be indicated. These procedures involve using a needle passed through the skin into the kidney to instill either cold gas to freeze the tumor or an electrical current to burn the tumor. Radiation therapy is typically used to treat metastasis (Mayo Clinic, 2020a).

Nursing Interventions and Patient Teaching

Care of the patient with surgery of the urinary tract is addressed later in this chapter.

Patient problems and interventions for the patient with renal tumors include but are not limited to the following:

PATIENT PROBLEM	NURSING INTERVENTIONS
Impaired Coping, related to powerlessness	Encourage patient to express feelings Assist patient in identifying personal strengths and coping skills Actively listen Support realistic hope; answer questions honestly
Impaired Decision-Making Ability, with verbalized uncertainty about choice to have renal surgery	Assess patient's capacity to make decisions Assess knowledge of procedure Review outline of surgical procedure and what nursing interventions the patient and significant others can expect postoperatively
Compromised Physical Mobility, related to pain and discomfort	Plan activities when pain control is greatest Encourage active or passive range-of-motion exercises Assess need for assistive devices

Instruct the patient about community resources, support groups, and home health care. Emphasize the importance of follow-up care, including following discharge instructions and keeping return appointment.

Prognosis

Survival rates are tied closely to the staging of cancer at the time of diagnosis. Localized renal cancer has a 5-year survival rate of 93%. Regional metastasis survival rate is 70%, and distant metastasis has a 12% 5-year survival rate (American Cancer Society, 2020a). The natural history of renal adenocarcinoma is far more unpredictable than that of most solid tumors. Disease may recur more than 15 years after removal of the original primary lesion. Metastatic disease has a poor prognosis and is rarely curable. Metastatic recurrence at a remotely distant time is not uncommon.

RENAL CYSTS

Etiology and Pathophysiology

Simple renal cysts are round, fluid-filled sacs on the kidneys. Cysts increase in frequency with aging. Many cysts initially are observed during imaging diagnostic testing. Cysts must be evaluated to distinguish them from more causes of cystic disease such as renal cell carcinoma. Renal cell carcinoma is typically irregular or multiloculated with irregular walls and areas of unclear demarcation. Simple renal cysts do not usually cause the patient any problems. There is no increased risk for decreased kidney function with simple renal cysts and they do not alter the structure or size of the kidney (NIDDK, 2019).

Patients with renal cysts have a higher incidence of renal carcinoma. Some health care providers periodically screen patients with cysts for renal carcinoma, using ultrasonography or CT.

On rare occasions a renal cyst can cause discomfort, block urine flow, burst or become infected. Approximately 1 in 10 people have a simple kidney cysts. In people age 50 and older, the likelihood increases to a 1 in 5 chance (NIDDK, 2019).

The most significant problems arise with *polycystic kidney disease*. PKD is a genetic disorder characterized by the growth of numerous fluid-filled cysts, which can slowly replace much of the kidney. A patient with long-standing renal insufficiency or a dialysis patient may develop polycystic disease. Kidney function is compromised by the pressure of the cysts on renal structures, secondary infections, and tissue scarring caused by rupture of the cysts. The patient may progress to end-stage renal disease (ESKD).

Clinical Manifestations

Signs and symptoms for PKD are influenced by the degree of renal structure involvement. The most common site is the collecting ducts, which fill with urine and/or blood. As the disease progresses, fewer nephrons are available to maintain normal kidney function.

Assessment

Subjective data include the most common symptoms of abdominal and flank pain, followed by headache, gastrointestinal complaints, voiding disturbances, and a history of recurrent UTIs.

Collection of objective data involves observation for systemic changes. Closely monitor blood pressure, which usually is elevated, and hematuria. Document patient complaints and response to intervention.

Diagnostic Tests

For simple renal cysts, x-ray, ultrasound, MRI, and CT scan are the likely tests to be performed for diagnosis. With PKD, diagnosis is established by family history, physical examination, IVP, and imaging of cysts on radiographic examination or sonography. CT and MRI may also be performed. Blood chemistry results, such as urea and creatinine levels, are used to monitor the level of kidney function.

Medical Management

PKD has no specific treatment. Medical treatment is aimed at relief of pain and other symptoms. Heat and analgesics may relieve some of the discomfort caused by the enlarging kidneys. If the patient bleeds, discontinue heat and place the patient on bed rest. Hypertension is treated vigorously with antihypertensive agents, diuretics, and fluid and dietary modifications. Because infections are common, antibiotics often are prescribed. As the disease progresses, dialysis or kidney transplantation may be required.

Nursing Interventions

Individual complaints and the severity of the disease process influence nursing interventions. Provide information to patients and family members about the availability of genetic counseling. Emphasize the need to report any changes in health status to the health care provider.

Prognosis

The prognosis is favorable with a simple renal cyst. Monitoring the cyst is usually all that is necessary. PKD requires ongoing treatment and monitoring because of its chronic nature. Hypertension and UTIs are common. Approximately 75% of patients with PKD will require dialysis or a kidney transplant at some point (Fung, 2021).

TUMORS OF THE URINARY BLADDER

Etiology and Pathophysiology

The bladder is the most common site of cancer in the urinary tract. A bladder tumor is an excess growth of cells that line the inside of the bladder, in many cases because the cells were exposed to certain chemicals. Tumors of the urinary bladder range from benign papillomas to invasive carcinomas. Papillomas have the potential to become cancerous and are removed when detected. Benign tumors of the kidney can be problematic and traditionally are removed.

Bladder cancer is the sixth most common cancer diagnosed in the United States. It is four times more common in men than women and 90% of the people diagnosed with bladder cancer are over the age of 55. Risk factors include smoking, a family history of bladder cancer, and occupational exposures to chemicals in paint, dye, and petroleum products (Saginala et al., 2020).

Several types of carcinoma arise on the bladder surface. The most common type diagnosed in North America is transitional cell carcinoma (TCC), which can occur anywhere in the urinary tract but usually is found in the urinary bladder. TCC involves development of a papillary tumor that projects into the bladder lumen and, if untreated, continues into the bladder muscle, where it can metastasize.

Clinical Manifestations

The patient may delay seeking medical attention because the primary sign of bladder cancer is painless, intermittent hematuria.

Assessment

Subjective data include symptoms such as changes in voiding patterns, signs of urinary obstruction, or renal failure, depending on the extent of the disease process.

Collection of objective data includes assessing the patient's understanding of his or her current health status, which aids in planning teaching interventions. Accurately document the time and amount of voiding, including a urine description.

Diagnostic Tests

Diagnosing bladder cancer often begins with a urinalysis and culture. This identifies abnormalities in the urine such as blood or infection. Urine tumor marker testing may be completed. This allows the urine to be assessed for particles secreted by bladder cancer cells. The next level of diagnostic testing includes a urine cytologic evaluation (study of cells) and/or one of several available bladder cancer markers. Bladder biopsies are needed to confirm a diagnosis.

Bladder cancer tumors are staged most commonly according to the system developed by the American Joint Committee on Cancer. The stage of the tumor is the most important indicator of prognosis and overall survival for patients with invasive tumors. Staging is an assessment of how far the tumor has spread.

Medical Management

Local disease may be treated by fulguration (also called electrocautery): removing the tissue by burning it away with the tip of an electrically heated electrode. Laser treatment, instillation of chemotherapy agents, or radiation therapy also may be used. Closely monitor these patients with cytologic studies and cystoscopy, because the recurrence rate is as high as 70% (Levy and Jones, 2019). A partial or total cystectomy may be performed to remove invasive lesions. With complete removal of the urinary bladder, urinary diversion or a neobladder (i.e., a new bladder created from intestinal tissue) is necessary. (See the section "Urinary Diversion" regarding ileal conduits and sigmoid conduits.)

Nursing Interventions and Patient Teaching

Care of the patient with bladder cancer is influenced by the extent of the disease process, medical treatment, coincidental illness, and the patient's response to treatment. Observe voiding patterns and urine characteristics to monitor response to these therapies. Provide teaching and support so that the patient can return to optimum performance of ADLs. Emphasize the importance of follow-up care for the patient with papillomas.

Prognosis

The prognosis is related directly to the extent of the disease process when diagnosed. When the cancer is diagnosed and in only located only in the bladder, the 5-year survival rate is 96%. When there is metastasis is considered regional, 5-year survival rates drop to 36% and drop to 5% when the metastasis is considered distant. (American Cancer Society, 2021b) Another important aspect in recovery is the patient's adaptability to any changes in urinary elimination as a result of treatment.

CONDITIONS AFFECTING THE PROSTATE GLAND

BENIGN PROSTATIC HYPERTROPHY
Etiology and Pathophysiology

The prostate gland encircles the male urethra at the base of the urinary bladder. It secretes an alkaline fluid that helps neutralize seminal fluid and increases sperm motility. BPH, enlargement of the prostate gland, is common in men older than 50 years of age. The cause is unclear but may be influenced by hormonal changes. The prostate enlarges, exerting pressure on the urethra and vesicle neck of the urinary bladder, which prevents complete emptying.

Clinical Manifestations

The patient has symptoms associated with urinary obstruction. Other clinical manifestations include complications of urinary obstruction, such as UTI, hematuria, oliguria (decreased urinary output), and signs of renal insufficiency.

Assessment

Subjective data include the patient describing urination as painful, and the urine stream as difficult to start and to slow, with complaints of frequency and nocturia. Collectively, these symptoms may be referred to as *prostatism* (any condition of the prostate gland that causes retention of urine in the bladder).

Collection of objective data involves eliciting information about voiding patterns to aid in determining the severity of the obstruction.

Diagnostic Tests

On rectal examination the health care provider may palpate the enlarged prostate gland, which has an elastic consistency. The hypertrophied prostate is enlarged symmetrically with a uniform, boggy presentation. Severity of the process can be determined by detecting alterations in blood chemistry, by measuring residual urine, or by cystoscopy or IVP. Cytologic evaluation determines whether the process is benign or malignant.

Medical Management

Treatment is based on the degree of occlusion and on signs and symptoms. Pharmacologic agents include alpha blockers, which improve the ability to urinate by relaxing the bladder neck and the fibers of the prostate. These medications elicit improved voiding in only a few days. Examples include terazosin, doxazosin, and tamsulosin. To shrink the prostate, 5-alpha-reductase inhibitors are prescribed. Medications in this group include finasteride and dutasteride. The 5-alpha-reductase inhibitors take weeks or months before changes in condition are noted. The two therapies may be combined to manage the condition.

Pharmacologic options are investigated first. If the condition worsens, surgery may be necessary. Deciding which treatment intervention to choose is difficult. Transurethral resection of the prostate (TURP) still is considered the standard for surgical intervention. The newer, less invasive treatments still are being evaluated. In general, these treatments are considered to cause less morbidity, but the results are not considered as effective or long-lasting as those of TURP.

Transurethral microwave thermotherapy. Transurethral microwave thermotherapy (TUMT) is one of various procedures used for the treatment of lower urinary tract symptoms resulting from BPH. TUMT involves the insertion of a specially designed urinary catheter into the bladder, allowing a microwave antenna to be positioned within the prostate; there it heats and destroys hyperplastic prostate tissue. The goal of TUMT is to provide a one-time treatment. Candidates for TUMT include persons with moderate-to-severe voiding symptoms resulting from BPH: those with side effects to medical therapy, those in whom medical therapy has failed, and those who choose not to be treated medically. There are many exclusions to the use of TUMT, so all patients require a thorough history and physical examination (Mayo Clinic, 2019c).

Patients should return to the clinic for follow-up. If a catheter is placed, it can be removed at home or in the clinic. Instruct patients to watch for an inability to void, painful voiding, high fevers, abdominal pain, or other problems. Posttreatment convalescence is relatively rapid, with most patients able to void and recover in less than 5 days at home.

Transurethral needle ablation. Transurethral needle ablation (TUNA) of the prostate is another procedure used to treat BPH. It is performed by placing interstitial radiofrequency needles through the urethra and into the lateral lobes of the prostate, causing heat-induced coagulation necrosis. The tissue is heated to 230°F (110°C) for approximately 3 minutes per lesion. A coagulation defect is created. A comprehensive history and physical examination are necessary to determine the benefits of using this procedure. Urethrocystoscopy may be indicated to help select the optimal form of therapy (Mayo Clinic, 2019).

Photoselective vaporization of the prostate. Photoselective vaporization of the prostate (PVP), using a GreenLight laser, is another option for the treatment of BPH. PVP is a safe alternative for patients who are seriously ill, are taking anticoagulants, or have unfavorable anatomy (i.e., a large prostate). The technique employs a laser beam, which emits a visible green light at a wavelength that has shallow tissue penetration and is absorbed selectively by blood. A urologist delivers the laser's energy by way of a thin fiber inserted into the urethra through a cystoscope. The GreenLight laser vaporizes the prostate tissue (Mayo Clinic, 2019b).

Nursing Interventions

Initial management is aimed at relieving the obstruction, usually by insertion of a Foley catheter. Take care to avoid rapid decompression of the bladder to prevent rupture of mucosal blood vessels. Usually no more than 1000 mL of urine should be removed from a distended bladder initially. Follow the health care provider's orders for the individual patient.

Prostatectomy (removal of the prostate gland) is indicated to relieve or prevent further obstruction of the urethra. The health care provider chooses the surgical approach for the prostatectomy after thorough appraisal of the patient. Preoperatively, the health care provider may order an enema to reduce the possibility of the patient's straining to defecate after surgery, which could cause bleeding. Other preoperative preparations are standard, as noted in Chapter 2. A prostatectomy may be done using any of four surgical techniques (Box 10.3 and Fig. 10.9).

With BPH, TURP is the resection most often chosen because it is less invasive and less stressful for the patient, especially the older patient or the patient with coincidental illness. The tissue is removed through the urethra. With this procedure the outer capsule of the prostate gland is left in place, maintaining the continuity between the bladder and the lower urethra (see Fig. 10.9A). Care of this patient centers on observing urine characteristics and maintaining patency of the Foley catheter.

The patient who has a TURP may have continuous closed bladder irrigation or intermittent irrigation to

---

Box 10.3   Four Prostatectomy Techniques

1. *Transurethral prostatectomy* involves approaching the gland through the penis and bladder, using a resectoscope, a surgical instrument with an electric cutting wire for resection and cautery to resect the lobes away from the capsule (see Fig. 10.9A).
2. *Suprapubic prostatectomy* is accomplished by an incision through the abdomen; the bladder is opened, and the gland is removed from above with the finger (see Fig. 10.9B).
3. *Radical perineal prostatectomy* requires an incision through the perineum between the scrotum and the rectum (see Fig. 10.9C).
4. *Retropubic prostatectomy* requires a low abdominal incision, but the bladder is not opened. The gland is removed by making an incision into the capsule encasing the prostate gland (see Fig. 10.9D).

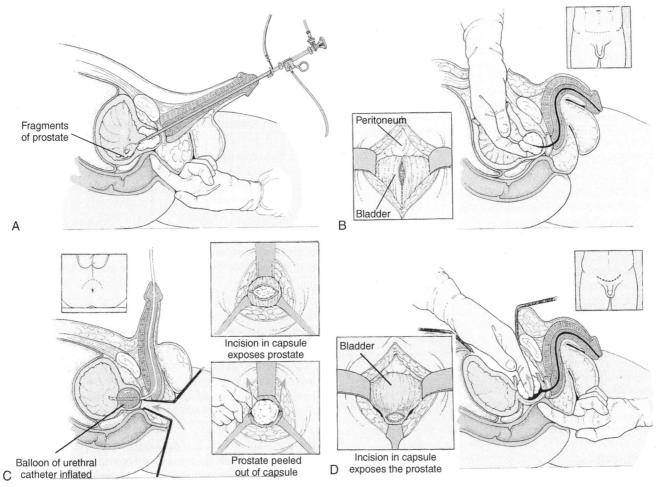

Fragments
of prostate

Peritoneum

Bladder

A   B

Incision in capsule
exposes prostate

Prostate peeled
out of capsule

Bladder

Balloon of urethral
C   catheter inflated

Incision in capsule
D   exposes the prostate

Fig. 10.9 Four types of prostatectomies. (A) Transurethral resection of prostate gland by means of resectoscope. Note the enlarged prostate gland surrounding the urethra and the tiny pieces of prostatic tissue that have been cut away. (B) Suprapubic. (C) Radical perineal. (D) Retropubic prostatectomy.

prevent occlusion of the catheter with blood clots, which would cause bladder spasms. Inform the patient and the family that hematuria is expected after prostatic surgery. Monitor vital signs and urine color every 2 hours for the first 24 hours to detect early signs of complications. With continuous bladder irrigation the urine will be light red to pink, and with intermittent irrigation the urine will be a clear, cherry red. Continuous irrigation is achieved with a three-way catheter (one lumen for irrigation fluid, one for urine drainage, and one to the retention balloon) or by using two catheters (Foley and suprapubic—one for irrigation fluid and one for urine drainage). The irrigant is an isotonic solution, frequently normal saline. To determine urinary output, subtract the amount of irrigation fluid used from the Foley catheter output. This is reported as "actual urinary output." Check catheter drainage tubes frequently for kinks that would occlude urine flow and cause bladder spasms. Advise the patient not to try to void around the catheter because this contributes to bladder spasms. Hemorrhage is always a possibility.

Belladonna and opium rectal suppositories are helpful to relieve bladder spasms but are not used in the retropubic approach because rectal stimulation is contraindicated.

Institute routine postoperative care. Have the patient avoid prolonged sitting because the increased intraabdominal pressure may cause the operative site to bleed. Remove the catheter when the urine becomes clear. Inform the patient that initially he may experience frequency, voiding small amounts with some dribbling. Instruct him to void with the first urge to prevent increased bladder pressure against the operative site.

Some health care providers may request that samples of the most recent voiding be saved for assessment. Record the time, the amount, and the color of each voiding.

A suprapubic or abdominal approach requires dressing observations and changes. When a suprapubic catheter is present, observe it for unobstructed flow and color of the urine and monitor it for total output (see the Patient Teaching box).

Patient Teaching

Postprostatectomy

ACTIVITY
- Light activity for 48 h to avoid postoperative bleeding.
- Do not drive for 48 h.
- No sexual activity for 2 weeks or as directed by health care provider.
- Avoid constipation. Maintain oral fluid intake and a diet high in fiber and roughage.
- Report signs of urinary track infection such as burning with urination.
- Do not take aspirin or other anticoagulant medications.
- Follow prescribed medication therapies as directed.

MANAGING URINARY INCONTINENCE
- It usually takes several weeks to achieve urinary continence. Continence may improve for up to 12 months.
- Maintain oral fluids between 2000 and 3000 mL/day (unless contraindicated).

ERECTILE DYSFUNCTION
- Sexual counseling and treatment options may be necessary if erectile dysfunction becomes a chronic or permanent problem.

INDWELLING CATHETER
- If the patient goes home with an indwelling catheter, send instructions for catheter care and local stores where supplies can be purchased.

Prognosis

Prognosis is favorable without residual effects. Problems with urine dribbling vary.

CANCER OF THE PROSTATE

Etiology and Pathophysiology

Prostatic cancer is common in men older than 50 years of age. This insidious cancer usually starts as a nodule on the posterior portion of the prostate without noticeable symptoms. When the tumor causes urinary symptoms, the cancer is in advanced stages. At this point, metastasis is common; frequent sites are the pelvic lymph nodes and bone. Regular rectal examinations and PSA measurement to detect abnormalities of the prostate gland lead to early treatment and an increased survival rate.

Clinical Manifestations

The patient has signs and symptoms related to urinary obstruction. Other signs and symptoms are determined by the presence or degree of metastasis.

Assessment

Collection of subjective data involves understanding that the patient with prostatic cancer may have no symptoms until the disease is advanced. The patient may seek medical intervention for BPH, which often accompanies prostate cancer, or when he experiences back pain or sciatica from metastatic changes in the bony pelvis. The patient may complain of dysuria, frequency, and nocturia.

Objective data include metastatic changes in the lymph glands of the pelvis and in the bones of the lower spine, the pelvis, and the hips with associated signs. Hematuria may or may not be present, depending on the stage of the malignancy.

Diagnostic Tests

On rectal examination by the health care provider, the involved area of the prostate gland feels firm and fixed with hardened nodules typically in the posterior lobe of the gland. Definitive diagnosis is made by cytologic examination. Prostate cells can be obtained by needle aspiration.

Men should consider a yearly PSA and digital rectal examination starting at age 50 or at age 45 if at high risk (African Americans or men with a father or brother diagnosed with prostate cancer at an early age). PSA test increases greatly the odds of early diagnosis. PSA, normally secreted and disposed of by the prostate, increases in the bloodstream in cancer of the prostate as well as in the harmless condition of BPH. The normal PSA level is 0 to 4 ng/mL. It is important to monitor even a slight increase in PSA levels. Elevated PSA levels mean further diagnostic evaluation is needed. When PSA levels are high, but a digital examination is normal, transrectal ultrasound is proving increasingly helpful in detecting cancer of the prostate gland too small to be palpated rectally. Other tests, such as a bone scan and serum alkaline phosphatase, are performed to assess the degree of metastasis.

The Gleason grading system is the most widely used system for grading prostate cancer. Based on microscopic identification of glandular differentiation in tumor cells, tumors are graded from 1 to 5. Grade 1 represents the most well differentiated (most like the original cells), and grade 5 represents the most poorly differentiated (undifferentiated). Gleason grades are given to the two most commonly occurring patterns of cells and added together. The Gleason score, a number from 2 to 10, is used to predict how quickly the cancer will progress. A score of 2 to 4 indicates a slow-growing tumor. Grades 5 to 7 are associated with a more aggressive tumor (Prostate Cancer Treatment Guide, n.d.).

Medical Management

Treatment is based on the stage of the cancer—whether it has spread beyond the wall of the prostate, and to what extent—and the patient's age. In an older man with an estimated remaining lifespan of 5 to 10 years, controlling the disease with radiation or hormone therapy may be enough. In many cases, particularly in men older than 70 years of age, prostate cancer grows slowly, and hormone therapy can hold the disease at bay for several years.

Localized prostate cancer can be cured by radiation therapy or surgery. A treatment in which radioactive seed implants are placed directly in the prostate gland while sparing the surrounding tissue (rectum and bladder) is called *brachytherapy*. The seeds are placed accurately with a needle through a grid template guided by transrectal ultrasound. Brachytherapy is a convenient, one-time outpatient procedure, whereas external radiation can take 5 to 6 weeks (American Cancer Society, 2019). The seeds remain in the body, but their radioactivity declines over a period of months. Patients are advised to refrain from having children (or adults) sit in their lap and to avoid intercourse during the first 2 months after therapy. Radiation therapy also is used in an attempt to destroy cancer cells and shrink the prostate when the cancer has spread to just outside the gland.

The operation to remove the prostate is a radical prostatectomy. Radical prostatectomy by the perineal approach is used in patients in the early stages of clinical disease and is considered one of the most effective ways of eradicating the tumor. This procedure involves removing the entire prostate, including the true prostatic capsule, seminal vesicles, and a portion of the bladder neck. The remaining portion of the bladder neck is reanastomosed (reconnected) to the urethra. The retropubic approach is often the first choice because it provides access to the pelvic lymph nodes (pelvic lymphadenectomy) and affords more urinary control and less stricture formation. A third, nerve-sparing prostatectomy procedure uses a retropubic and perineal approach to try to prevent impotence and reduce the likelihood of UI.

The three goals of a radical prostatectomy are (1) removal of the entire tumor, (2) preservation of urine control, and (3) maintenance of sexual function. Extent of sexual function may not be known for 6 to 12 months postoperatively. The patient needs emotional support related to the cancer and the possibility of impotence after surgery. Preoperative teaching should include an opportunity for the patient and his partner to discuss treatment options and mortality rate.

When the capsule of the prostate gland is removed, as with the perineal approach, the bladder and the lower urethra are no longer connected. The area where these two structures are reconnected usually is supported by placement of a Foley catheter. Extreme care must be taken to avoid placing tension on the catheter, which would disturb the surgical area. The catheter remains in place for several postoperative days.

Prostate cancer cells typically grow in response to testosterone making hormone deprivation therapy a potential method of treatment for cases of advanced prostatic cancer. The therapy alters tumor growth by blocking testosterone production. Hormone deprivation therapy can involve other hormones and drugs as well: estrogen, gonadotropin-releasing hormone analogues, antiandrogens, and luteinizing hormone–releasing hormone (LHRH) drugs:

- *LHRH agonists* act indirectly by causing an initial surge in luteinizing hormone and testosterone, rapidly followed by a decline in testosterone level similar to that achieved by castration. The primary forms of LHRH agonists are leuprolide (Lupron) and goserelin (Zoladex).
- *LHRH antagonists* act more directly, stopping the production of testosterone in the testes.

Degarelix is a second-generation LHRH antagonist. Alternatives to LHRH drugs include oral nonsteroidal antiandrogens, including bicalutamide flutamide, and nilutamide (American Cancer Society, 2021a) Palliative therapy for patients with metastatic disease also may include orchiectomy (removal of the testes). Bilateral orchiectomy eliminates 95% of testosterone production, a step that is useful in managing metastatic disease. The patient may receive relief from such symptoms as pain or obstruction but may experience feminization, increased incidence of cardiac disease, thrombophlebitis, pulmonary embolus, and stroke. Additional therapies are instituted to treat these side effects.

Radiation therapy may be used in advanced stages of the illness as primary or palliative treatment. Management of disseminated disease with cytotoxic drugs has been marginally successful.

Because a cure for cancer of the prostate is possible only when the tumor is discovered early, it is important to teach all male patients older than the age of 40 to have annual or biannual rectal examinations and yearly PSA serum level determinations.

Nursing Interventions and Patient Teaching

Postoperative nursing management for prostatectomy is similar to that for perineal surgery, with special attention to maintenance of bowel and bladder function while keeping the surgical wound clean and avoiding pressure on the perineum and wound. Adequate fluid intake, modification of dietary selections, and perineal exercises may be used to promote regulation of bowel and bladder function. Take extreme care to prevent further trauma to the perineum; one unintended sequela of prostatectomy is fistula formation, in which a channel forms between the urethra and rectum. Rectal temperature-taking, enemas, and use of rectal tubes therefore are forbidden. Also take care not to place tension on the Foley catheter, which would disturb the surgical area. Observe the color of the urine for signs of bleeding. The patient will also have a tissue drain inserted during surgery to promote drainage from the wound in the perineum. Initially there may be a small amount of urine from the drain, but this should cease in 1 or 2 days. Follow surgical asepsis during dressing changes. Irrigation of the perineum may be ordered to cleanse the wound and soothe the patient. Administer comfort measures and analgesics as ordered for pain control in the lower back, pelvis, upper thighs, and operative site.

Patient problems and interventions for the patient undergoing prostate surgery include but are not limited to the following:

PATIENT PROBLEM	NURSING INTERVENTIONS
Potential for Inadequate Fluid Volume, related to hemorrhage or decreased fluid intake	Monitor signs and symptoms of fluid deficit (decreasing or increasing blood pressure, dyspnea) Observe catheter for urine color and amount Avoid manipulation of rectum by thermometer or rectal tube
Impaired Sexual Expression, related to surgical trauma and altered body function	Encourage verbalization of sexual concerns Provide privacy with significant others to discuss concerns Inform health care provider of patient concerns Explore professional resources (clergy, sexual counselors)

Because UI may occur postoperatively, teach the patient how to keep himself clean. He may need to discuss feelings of depression about his altered body function. Modifying lifestyle and maintaining confidence are important for his return to preillness function. Discuss alternative expressions of sexuality, the value of sexual counseling, and the possibility of recovering some or all sexual function after the treatment is completed.

Emphasize the need for adequate fluid intake, exercise, and rest. Instruct the patient regarding pain-relieving measures such as exercise, warmth, and medication. Discuss new pharmacologic agents that act as adjuvants in the treatment of cancer and for pain relief during the postoperative recovery period.

Prognosis
The patient's prognosis is correlated directly to the extent of the disease process when diagnosed. Grading of the tumor (well, moderately, or poorly differentiated) correlates with the prognosis; the more poorly differentiated the tumor, the poorer the prognosis. Under the Gleason system discussed previously, a low score of 2 through 4 is good; a high score of 7 through 10 is not. The treatment goal for the localized disease process is a cure; palliation is used for the extended disease process.

DISORDERS OF THE URINARY TRACT

URETHRAL STRICTURES
Etiology and Pathophysiology
A *urethral stricture* is a narrowing of the lumen of the urethra that interferes with urine flow. Narrowing may be congenital or acquired. Acquired strictures may be caused by chronic infection, trauma, or tumor or occur as a complication of radiation treatment of the pelvis.

Clinical Manifestations
Signs and symptoms include dysuria, weak stream, splaying (spreading out) of the urine stream, nocturia, and increasing pain with bladder distention. In the presence of infection, fever and malaise may be apparent.

Assessment
Subjective data include patient complaints of difficulty initiating the urine stream and the stream seeming to splay more than usual or even seeming to "fork."

Collection of objective data includes assessing for signs that may indicate an infectious process and for information indicating the extent of the stricture and possible presence of an obstruction.

Diagnostic Tests
Diagnosis can be confirmed by a voiding cystourethrogram, which demonstrates stricture. Additional diagnostic studies help evaluate damage caused by the obstruction.

Medical Management
Correction of the stricture may be achieved by dilation with metal sounds (instruments designed to dilate the urethra) or surgical release (internal urethrotomy).

Nursing Interventions
Care includes adequate hydration to decrease discomfort when voiding and monitoring urinary output. Mild analgesics should relieve discomfort. Sitz baths may encourage voiding. Reconstruction of the urethra (urethroplasty) may require temporary urinary diversion. After the procedure a splinting catheter supports the suture line. Take care not to place tension on the catheter.

Prognosis
The prognosis after surgical correction or dilation is favorable.

URINARY TRACT TRAUMA
Etiology and Pathophysiology
Assess any patient with a history of traumatic injury for possible involvement of the urinary tract. Such injuries may include contusions or rupture of the urinary structures. Also observe a patient who has undergone abdominal surgery for possible incidental injury sustained during the operation. Traumatic invasion of the urinary tract may be evident in open wounds to the lower abdomen, such as gunshot or stab wounds. Trauma to the bladder can occur from a fractured pelvis. Contusion or laceration of the urethra may lead to urethral stricture and possible impotence in men secondary to soft tissue, blood vessel, and nerve damage.

Clinical Manifestations
Monitor urinary output hourly for amount and color. Report any evidence of hematuria. Assess the patient for abdominal pain and tenderness, which may

indicate internal hemorrhage, peritonitis, or seepage of urine into the tissues.

Assessment

Collection of subjective data involves understanding that the trauma patient may be unable to relate any symptoms that would aid in the assessment of urinary tract involvement. If the patient can respond, asking about signs of hematuria is extremely important.

Collection of objective data includes a comprehensive assessment of the trauma patient, reviewing all body systems. Assessment related to the urinary tract includes hourly measurement of I&O; observation of urine character or difficulty voiding; evaluation of complaints of abdominal, flank, or referred shoulder pain; and evaluation of abdominal distention and girth.

Diagnostic Tests

Diagnosis of traumatic involvement of the urinary tract may be aided by KUB radiography, IVP, urinalysis, excretory urography, and cystoscopy.

Medical Management

Surgical intervention is necessary for correction of tears or rupture of the urinary tract to reinstate urine flow. If damage is severe, removal of a kidney or the bladder may be necessary with the creation of urinary diversion, as discussed later in this chapter. Management of possible hemorrhage and prevention of infection are necessary before and after surgery.

Nursing Interventions

Document and report all findings.

Prognosis

The prognosis depends on the extent and location of the trauma.

IMMUNOLOGIC DISORDERS OF THE KIDNEY

NEPHROTIC SYNDROME

Etiology and Pathophysiology

Nephrotic syndrome (nephrosis) is a disorder characterized by marked proteinuria, hyperlipidemia, hypoalbuminemia, and edema. Several events may precipitate nephrotic syndrome; the primary form of nephrosis occurs in the absence of glomerulonephritis or systemic disease, with the inciting event being an upper respiratory tract infection or allergic reaction.

The most common sign is excess fluid in the body. This may take several forms: periorbital edema (around the eyes), characteristically in the morning; pitting edema over the legs; fluid in the pleural cavity (pleural effusion); or fluid in the peritoneal cavity (ascites).

In nephrotic syndrome, the glomeruli become damaged because of inflammation so that small proteins, such as albumins, immunoglobulins, and antithrombin, can pass through the kidneys into the urine. Physiologic changes in the glomeruli interfere with selective permeability. Blood protein is allowed to pass into the urine (proteinuria), causing a loss of serum protein (hypoalbuminemia). This decreases serum osmotic pressure, thus allowing fluid to seep into interstitial spaces, and edema occurs.

Immune responses, humoral and cellular, are altered in the patient with nephrotic syndrome; as a result, infection is an important cause of morbidity and mortality.

Clinical Manifestations

The patient has severe generalized edema (anasarca). Weight loss is evident. When questioned about his or her diet, the patient reports anorexia. Activity intolerance and fatigue are reported. Urine is foamy.

Assessment

Subjective data include patient complaints of loss of interest in eating, constant fatigue, foamy urine from the presence of protein, and decreased urinary output (oliguria), less than 500 mL in 24 hours.

Collection of objective data includes assessing the degree of fluid retention by monitoring daily weight, I&O, respiratory effort, and level of consciousness. The patient may relate problems with "swelling" of the face, hands, and feet. Assess skin integrity to determine special needs. Assess lung fields for the presence of crackles indicating fluid buildup. Assess for neck vein distention.

Diagnostic Tests

Blood chemistry findings include hypoalbuminemia and hyperlipidemia. The urinalysis reveals protein in the urine. A 24-hour urine collection is included in the diagnostic workup. Renal biopsy provides identification of the type and extent of tissue change. Other diagnostic testing is performed to identify the specific underlying cause.

Medical Management

Medical management depends on the extent of tissue involvement and may include the use of corticosteroids (prednisone); antineoplastic agents for immunosuppressive effect; loop diuretics; and a low-sodium, high-protein diet for therapeutic management of edema. Hypoproteinemia may be treated with normal serum albumin and protein-rich nutrition replacement therapy.

Nursing Interventions and Patient Teaching

Nursing interventions include monitoring fluid balance. Daily weight should be determined. The abdominal girth should be measured daily for changes. I&O should be recorded along with characteristics of urine passed. Other nursing interventions include maintaining bed rest in the presence of extreme edema (recumbent position may initiate diuresis) and assessing for electrolyte imbalance. Skin care is important, as is a gradual increase in activity as the edema is resolved.

Diet includes protein replacement, using foods that provide high biological value (meat, fish, poultry, cheese, eggs) and restriction of sodium to decrease edema. Blood pressure often is elevated and should be monitored closely for changes.

As the patient begins to convalesce, the teaching plan includes the medication regimen (type, dosage, side effects, and need to finish all prescriptions), nutrition (high protein, low sodium), self-assessment of fluid status (monitor weight, presence of edema), awareness of signs and symptoms indicating a need for medical attention (increase in edema, fatigue, headache, infection), and the need for follow-up care.

Prognosis

In approximately 25% of children and 50% to 75% of adults who develop nephrosis, the disease progresses to renal failure within 5 years. Other patients (particularly children) may have remissions or chronic nephrotic syndrome. Aside from treating the underlying illness, little can be done to prevent a recurrence of nephrosis.

NEPHRITIS

Nephritis encompasses renal disorders characterized by inflammation of the kidney—involving the glomeruli, tubules, or interstitial tissue—and abnormal function. Included in this group of disorders is acute and chronic glomerulonephritis.

Acute Glomerulonephritis

Etiology and pathophysiology. The health history commonly reveals that the onset of acute glomerulonephritis was preceded by an infection, such as a sore throat or skin infection (most commonly beta-hemolytic streptococci) 2 to 3 weeks earlier, or other preexisting multisystem diseases, such as systemic lupus erythematosus. The infectious disease process triggers an immune response that results in inflammation of glomeruli that allows excretion of RBCs and protein in the urine. This condition is common in children and young adults.

Clinical manifestations. Often family members first note that the individual has "swelling" of the face, especially around the eyes. Some patients may be acutely ill with a multitude of symptoms, whereas others may be diagnosed on routine examination with only vague symptoms.

Assessment. Subjective data include symptoms indicative of anorexia, nocturia, malaise, and exertional dyspnea.

Collection of objective data includes assessment of skin integrity and general condition of skin; the presence and degree of edema with associated difficulty in breathing on exertion, when recumbent, or as evidenced by changes in lung and heart sounds (unusual heart sounds, crackles over lung fields, distention of neck veins); hematuria with changes in urine color from "cola" to frankly sanguineous; or changes in voiding, a decrease in amount of urinary output, or dysuria.

Diagnostic tests. Diagnostic tests reveal elevation of BUN, serum creatinine, potassium, erythrocyte sedimentation rate, and antistreptolysin-O titer. Urinalysis shows RBCs, casts, and/or protein.

Medical management. Medical management includes treatment of primary symptoms while preventing complications to cerebral and cardiac function. Serum electrolyte levels (sodium and potassium) may indicate a need to adjust dietary intake of sodium and potassium. Level of consciousness should be monitored when the BUN is elevated. Bed rest and fluid intake adjustments are guided by urinary output until diuresis is adequate.

A prophylactic antimicrobial agent, such as penicillin, may be administered for several months after the acute phase of the illness to protect against recurrence of infection. Diuretics may be prescribed to control fluid retention and antihypertensives to reduce blood pressure.

Nursing interventions and patient teaching. Nursing interventions are guided by individual patient needs, focusing on control of symptoms and prevention of complications. Dietary intake includes protein restrictions (to decrease blood urea levels), with carbohydrates providing a source of energy.

Monitor I&O and vital signs. Determine the level of activity based on the degree of edema, hypertension, proteinuria, and hematuria, because excessive activity may increase these signs (see the Health Promotion box).

 Health Promotion

The Patient With Nephritis

ACTIVITY
- Keep patient on bed rest until edema and blood pressure are reduced.
- Encourage quiet diversional activities.
- Ambulate gradually with assistance.
- Space out activities to lessen fatigue.

FLUID BALANCE MAINTENANCE
- Implement dietary restrictions.
- Monitor intake and output.
- Document reactions to medication.

DIET THERAPY
- Restrict protein to decrease nitrogenous wastes.
- Restrict sodium to prevent further fluid retention.
- Increase calories for energy source.

DRUG THERAPY
- Prophylactic antibiotics
- Antihypertensives
- Diuretics
- Drug interactions, side effects to expect and report

HEALTH MAINTENANCE
- Recovery may be extended.
- Health care provider will monitor urine for albumin and red blood cells (RBCs).
- Teach early signs of fluid retention.
- Signs and symptoms may resolve and then become worse.
- Normal activities may be resumed after urine is free of albumin and RBCs for 1 month, although the patient is not considered cured until the urine is free of albumin and RBCs for 6 months.
- Report hematuria, headache, edema.

Because glomerulonephritis is long term, patient teaching is important. Proteinuria and hematuria may exist microscopically even when other symptoms subside. Although possibly fatigued, these patients usually feel well; they often must be convinced of the need to continue prescribed treatment and to return for follow-up care. Explain the nature of the illness and the effect of diet and fluids on fluid balance and sodium retention. Teach about prescribed sodium and fluid restrictions (provide written information regarding sodium content of foods, as necessary). Include information about protein restrictions and carbohydrate sources. Also discuss the medication regimen (dose, frequency, side effects, need to continue per health care provider instructions). Stress the need to pace activities with rest if fatigued; to avoid trauma and infection (which may exacerbate the illness); and to obtain follow-up health care. Teach the patient about the signs and symptoms indicating the need for medical attention (hematuria, headache, edema, hypertension).

Prognosis. The prognosis for patients with acute poststreptococcal glomerulonephritis is generally good; however, some patients develop chronic glomerulonephritis and ESKD, requiring dialysis or kidney transplantation.

Chronic Glomerulonephritis

Etiology and pathophysiology. With chronic glomerulonephritis there is usually no indication of an inciting event. Occasionally the patient with acute glomerulonephritis progresses to a chronic phase. Because other chronic illnesses (e.g., diabetes mellitus or systemic lupus erythematosus) may mask the symptoms of renal degeneration, many patients do not seek medical attention until kidney function is compromised. Chronic glomerulonephritis is characterized by slow, progressive destruction of glomeruli with related loss of function. The kidneys atrophy (actually decrease in size).

Clinical manifestations. Signs and symptoms may include malaise, morning headaches, dyspnea with exertion, visual and digestive disturbances, edema, and fatigue. Physical findings include hypertension, anemia, proteinuria, anasarca, and cardiac and cerebral manifestations.

Assessment. Subjective data include patient complaints of fatigue and a decreased ability to perform ADLs as a result of dyspnea and decreasing ability to concentrate. Investigate complaints of morning headaches (their location, pattern, and character), and note the presence of any visual disturbance.

Collection of objective data includes clarifying outward manifestations of the headache and respiratory effort that may interfere with daily task performance. Assess mental functioning, irritability, slurred speech, ataxia, or tremors. Carefully assess and document the degree of edema, noting specific location and response to pressure by pressing the fingers into the edematous

area and observing for pitting. Note skin color, ecchymoses (irregularly formed hemorrhagic areas of the skin) or rash, dry skin, and scratching. Observe urine color and amount. Monitor vital signs, including a chest assessment for cardiac and pulmonary signs of fluid retention: unusual heart sounds, crackles over lung fields, and distention of neck veins.

Diagnostic tests. Early disease shows albumin and RBCs in the urine, although kidney function test results are within normal limits. With advanced destruction of nephrons, the specific gravity becomes fixed and blood levels of NPN wastes (creatinine and urea) increase. Creatinine clearance may be as low as 5 to 10 mL/min, compared with the normal range of 107 to 139 mL/min in men and 87 to 107 mL/min in women.

Medical management. Medical management includes control of secondary side effects as discussed for acute glomerulonephritis, with renal dialysis and possible kidney transplantation to provide elimination of wastes from the body.

Nursing interventions and patient teaching. Nursing interventions for the patient with chronic glomerulonephritis represent a special challenge. This patient already has had major damage to the kidney filtration system. It is crucial that the patient's condition not be further compromised by infection or other complications. Monitor changes in vital signs and diagnostic tests to aid in choosing proper nursing interventions. Interventions parallel those noted with nephrotic syndrome and acute glomerulonephritis. Chronic glomerulonephritis may progress to ESKD, necessitating related nursing interventions (see the Health Promotion box: The Patient With Nephritis).

Patient problems and interventions for the patient with chronic glomerulonephritis include but are not limited to the following:

PATIENT PROBLEM	NURSING INTERVENTIONS
Fluid Volume Overload, related to decreased urinary output	Assess the patient's understanding of therapeutic interventions
	Note I&O q h (or more often)
	Monitor signs and symptoms of fluid excess (weight gain, hypertension, edema, dyspnea)
	Provide ice chips for thirst with prescribed diet
	Monitor and report abnormal laboratory results
Inability to Tolerate Activity, related to kidney dysfunction	Assess level of activity tolerance
	Encourage patient to report activities that increase fatigue
	Plan activities to minimize fatigue

Patient teaching focuses on preventive health maintenance, emphasizing a health-promoting lifestyle, with prevention and early treatment of infections.

Prognosis. Some people with minimal impairment in kidney function continue to feel well and show little progression of disease. With other patients the progression of renal deterioration may be slow but steady and end in renal failure. In still others the disease progresses rapidly.

RENAL FAILURE

Renal failure is characterized by the kidneys' inability to remove wastes, concentrate urine, and conserve or eliminate electrolytes. Diabetes mellitus is the most common cause of renal failure, with hypertension being the second most common cause (CDC, 2020). Other predisposing concurrent illnesses include burns, trauma, heart failure, volume depletion, and renal disease. Nursing interventions to prevent the development of renal failure include providing adequate hydration, preventing infections, monitoring for signs and symptoms of shock, and teaching drug side effects to report immediately.

ACUTE RENAL FAILURE (ACUTE KIDNEY INJURY)
Etiology and Pathophysiology
Kidney function may be altered by interference with the kidneys' ability to be selective in filtering blood or by an actual decrease in blood flow to the kidneys. ARF is also referred to as acute kidney injury (AKI) can be caused by many medical conditions, such as obstruction in the kidney, hemorrhage, trauma, infection, and decreased cardiac output. Certain medications also may be nephrotoxic. These include medications such as chemotherapy drugs, analgesics (ibuprofen), and antimicrobials (penicillin and cephalosporin).

The course of AKI is divided into phases (Hinkle and Cheever, 2018). Damage to the kidneys happens during the initiation phase. Once damage has occurred the next phase, *oliguric phase,* begins. BUN and serum creatinine levels rise while urinary output decreases to less than 400 mL in 24 hours. The oliguric phase may last from several days to 4 weeks to several months. During this phase hyperkalemia may develop. In the *diuretic phase,* blood chemistry levels begin to return to normal and urinary output increases to 1 to 2 L in 24 hours. The diuretic phase usually lasts 1 to 3 weeks. The patient still needs watched closely in case dehydration occurs. Return to normal or near-normal function occurs in the *recovery phase.* Recovery begins as the GFR rises. The GFR may permanently be 1% to 3% reduced, but this is usually not a significant issue. Recovery can take from 3 months up to 1 year.

Clinical Manifestations
The patient may experience anorexia, nausea, vomiting, edema, and associated signs and symptoms of diminished kidney function.

Assessment
Subjective data include patient reports of lethargy, loss of appetite, nausea, and headache.

Objective data involve physical findings of progression of the disease process. Assess for dry mucous membranes, poor skin turgor, urinary output of less than 400 mL in 24 hours, vomiting, diarrhea, and anasarca. Note skin color changes. Monitor daily weight and changes in body mass. Assessment findings may include central nervous system manifestations of drowsiness, muscle twitching, and seizures.

Diagnostic Tests
Physical assessment, history, and elevated blood chemistry tests such as GFR, BUN, and creatinine (azotemia) confirm the diagnosis. After the patient is stabilized, further studies may be done to assess for residual damage.

Medical Management
Measures include administration of fluids and osmotic preparations to prevent decreased renal perfusion, manage fluid volume, and treat electrolyte imbalances. Renal dialysis may be necessary to manage systemic fluid shifts, especially cardiac and respiratory, and may be effective in removing some nephrotoxins.

Diet should be protein sparing, high in carbohydrates, and low in potassium and sodium. Drug therapy may include diuretics to increase urinary output (e.g., furosemide, hydrochlorothiazide). Potassium-lowering agents are used to remove potassium through the gastrointestinal tract; sodium polystyrene sulfonate is administered orally, per nasogastric tube, or as a retention enema. Antibiotics that are not dependent on kidney excretion are used to eradicate or prevent infection. Whatever combination of drug therapy is used, dosage and administration times require adjustment according to the level of kidney function.

Nursing Interventions and Patient Teaching
Accurately document urinary output to identify the level of kidney function. Azotemia may be revealed by blood chemistry studies. Observe the patient with azotemia for changes in level of consciousness. Closely monitor fluid status, vital signs, and response to therapies. Frequent skin care with tepid water to remove urea crystals is comforting. Dialysis presents special nursing challenges, discussed later in this chapter.

Teaching includes identifying preventable environmental or health factors contributing to the illness (such as hypertension, nephrotoxic drugs). Teach the patient about activity restrictions, dietary restrictions, and the medication regimen. Provide nutritional support with specialized enteral formulas, which may contain essential amino acids and minerals, in addition to replacement of electrolytes (especially sodium to match insensible loss) and provision of caloric needs. Make a nutritional assessment with appropriate modifications daily.

Stress the need to report signs and symptoms of infection and of returning renal failure to the health care provider. Emphasize the need for ongoing follow-up care.

Prognosis

Recovery from an episode of ARF depends on the underlying illness, the patient's condition, and careful supportive management given during the period of kidney shutdown. The leading cause of death is infection, such as that of the urinary tract, lungs, and peritoneum. Mortality from fluid overload and acidosis has been reduced as a result of dialysis and other forms of therapy. Patients who survive the acute episode of tubular insufficiency have a chance of recovering kidney function. Although renal tissue may regenerate more completely after toxic injury than ischemia, both forms usually show a return to normal or near-normal kidney function.

For those in whom ARF has been caused by glomerular disease or severe infection of renal tissue, the prognosis may not be as favorable. Return of kidney function is determined by the extent of scarring and destruction of functional renal tissue that has occurred during the acute episode of renal failure.

CHRONIC RENAL FAILURE (END-STAGE KIDNEY DISEASE)

Etiology and Pathophysiology

Chronic renal failure, or ESKD, exists when the kidneys are unable to regain normal function. ESKD develops slowly over an extended period as a result of renal disease or other disease processes that compromise renal blood perfusion. As much as 80% of nephrons may be severely impaired before loss of kidney function is detected. The most common causes of ESKD are pyelonephritis, chronic glomerulonephritis, glomerulosclerosis, chronic urinary obstruction, severe hypertension, diabetes mellitus, gout, and PKD. Whatever the cause, dialysis or kidney transplantation is needed to maintain life.

ESKD represents a significant health problem worldwide. In 2016, there were more than 726,000 people in the United States that required dialysis or a kidney transplant to survive CDC, 2021). ESKD also may cause a financial crisis for patients and their families. For some, the government actively helps defray costs through the Medicare program.

Clinical Manifestations

The onset of signs and symptoms may be so gradual and so vague that the patient is unable to identify when the problems started. When questioned, the patient may be able to relate occurrences that seemed insignificant at the time. The clinical picture is usually unique to the individual. Common symptoms include headache; lethargy; asthenia (decreased strength or energy); anorexia; pruritus; elimination changes; anuria (less than 100 mL of urine production per day); muscle cramps or twitching; impotence; characteristic dusky yellow-tan or gray skin color from retained urochrome pigments; and signs and symptoms characteristic of central nervous system involvement, such as disorientation and mental lapses.

Other associated conditions are responsible for many of the symptoms. Azotemia develops as excessive amounts of nitrogenous compounds build up in the blood. Anemia occurs when the production of renal erythropoietin is decreased as a result of loss of kidney function. Acidosis, hypertension, and glucose intolerance may occur as a result of the insult to homeostasis.

Assessment

Subjective data include patient complaints of joint pain and edema; severe headaches; nausea; anorexia; intermittent chest pain; weakness; and in particular, fatigue, intractable singultus (hiccups), decreased libido, menstrual irregularities, and impaired concentration. The clinical consequences of renal failure are far-reaching, affecting nearly every body system.

Collection of objective data involves a nursing assessment that may yield unremarkable results, except for signs and symptoms that support the patient complaints. Uremic encephalopathy affects the central nervous system. Usually the first sign is a reduction in alertness and awareness. The patient exhibits Kussmaul's respirations (abnormally deep, very rapid sighing respirations), and coma develops. The accumulation of urates results in halitosis with a urine odor and "uremic frost" on the skin in the form of a white powder.

Diagnostic Tests

Diagnosis of ESKD is confirmed by elevated BUN of at least 50 mg/dL and serum creatinine levels greater than 5 mg/dL, electrolyte imbalance (including decreased bicarbonate and magnesium and increased potassium, sodium, and phosphate), and other indicators related to the underlying cause. Kidney function studies assess the degree of damage or level of kidney function.

Medical Management

Medical management is instituted to conserve kidney function as long as possible. Dialysis is initiated when necessary, and the patient may be prepared for kidney transplantation. Drug therapy may include anticonvulsants to control seizure activity (phenytoin [Dilantin], diazepam [Valium]), antianemics, vitamin supplements to counteract nutritional deficiencies, antiemetics (prochlorperazine), antipruritics (cyproheptadine), and biological response modifiers to stimulate red cell production (epoetin alfa [Epogen, EPO]) to treat anemia caused by a reduced production of erythropoietin. Iron deficiency anemia must be treated with ferrous sulfate orally or with iron dextran (DexFerrum by Z-track intramuscular injection) before epoetin alfa will be effective.

Nursing Interventions and Patient Teaching

Nursing interventions focus on restoring homeostasis. Measures to control fluid and electrolyte balance vary greatly, according to individual patient needs.

Nutritional therapy is aimed at preserving protein stores and preventing production of additional protein waste products that the kidney would have to clear. Patients on dialysis often need 8 to 10 g of protein daily.

The diet is high in calories from carbohydrates and fats from polyunsaturated sources (to maintain weight and spare protein), at least 2500 to 3000 calories daily. Other dietary restrictions are related to the patient's degree of acidosis. Potassium is retained, so foods high in potassium are restricted. Sodium is controlled at a level sufficient to replace sodium loss without causing fluid retention.

Nursing interventions for ARF also are instituted for ESKD. Provide emotional support for the patient who faces role changes and invasive treatments such as dialysis or kidney transplantation. As discussed in the Health Promotion box, fluid balance is of prime importance. The patient may have fluid equal to the amount excreted in the urine plus about 300 to 600 mL to compensate for *insensible* (imperceptible) *fluid loss* (fluid lost through the lungs, perspiration, and feces). Salt substitutes are not advised because most contain potassium. If seizure activity occurs, institute safety measures to protect the patient (Nursing Care Plan 10.1).

Patient teaching should emphasize food exchanges and fluid intake within restrictions prescribed for that patient. Encourage the patient to increase activity as tolerated; maintain impeccable skin care; prevent infection and injury; and develop coping behaviors to adapt to lifestyle changes for patient, family, and caregiver.

CARE OF THE PATIENT REQUIRING DIALYSIS

Dialysis is a medical procedure for the removal of certain elements from the blood; the process is based on differences in the rate of diffusion of these elements through an external semipermeable membrane or, in the case of peritoneal dialysis, through the peritoneal membrane. Dialysis mimics kidney function, helping to restore balance when normal kidney function is interrupted temporarily or permanently. Dialysis involves the *diffusion* of wastes, drugs, and/or excess electrolytes and *osmosis* of water across a semipermeable membrane into a dialysate fluid that is prescribed to meet individual needs. Dialysis is achieved by the process of hemodialysis or peritoneal dialysis.

HEMODIALYSIS

Hemodialysis is used for patients with acute or irreversible renal failure and fluid and electrolyte imbalances. Hemodialysis requires access to the patient's circulatory system to route blood through the artificial kidney (dialyzer) for removal of wastes, fluids, and electrolytes; the blood is then returned to the patient's body. Box 10.4 lists nursing intervention guidelines. Temporary methods include subclavian or femoral catheters or an external shunt placed in the nondominant forearm (Fig. 10.10A). In ESKD, access can be achieved by constructing a

 Health Promotion

The Patient With Renal Failure

FLUID AND ELECTROLYTE BALANCE
- Assess intake and output (hourly if indicated).
- Weigh daily (same time, same clothing, same scale).
- Assess overt (open to view) signs of hydration status: edema, turgor.
- Assess covert (hidden) signs of hydration status: breath sounds, laboratory studies, and so on.

NUTRITION
- Provide prescribed diet.
- Guide patient food selection.
- Plan fluid intake per shift within prescribed limits and according to patient preference.
- Reinforce diet instructions as indicated.

COMFORT AND SAFETY
- Provide quiet environment (sound and lighting).
- Space nursing interventions to conserve patient energy.
- Medicate as needed for comfort.
- Provide skin care to alleviate discomfort from pruritus.
- Provide mouth care as needed.
- Maintain asepsis during procedures.
- Prevent exposure to pathogens.

COPING BEHAVIORS
- Listen (to patient and significant others).
- Refer to pastoral care or religious support group.
- Provide private times with significant others.
- Offer interview with social services.

DOCUMENTATION AND REPORTING
- Document all relevant findings.
- Maintain open communications with supervisory staff.
- Adjust nursing care plan as indicated to meet changing patient needs.
- Maintain dietary restrictions: food exchange, measuring fluids, food diary.
- Take health promotion–illness prevention measures.

direct arteriovenous (AV) fistula (surgically connecting an artery to a vein) or a graft (placing a synthetic tubelike material between an artery and a vein) (see Fig. 10.10B). The AV fistula is preferred for permanent access because synthetic grafts frequently become clotted with blood ("clotting off"). Hemodialysis usually is scheduled three times a week. Each session lasts around 4 hours. Patients can be maintained on dialysis therapy indefinitely or while waiting for kidney transplantation. Hemodialysis while managing the condition does not cure or reverse it.

There are complications of hemodialysis. Cardiovascular complications include heart failure, stroke, angina, and peripheral vascular disease. The leading cause of disease of patients on hemodialysis is cardiovascular disease. Additional complications related to rapid changes in fluid and electrolyte levels include hypotension, muscle cramping, dysrhythmias, headaches, nausea, and vomiting (Hinkle and Cheever, 2018).

Nursing Care Plan 10.1 | **The Patient With End-Stage Renal Disease**

Mr. J., a 37-year-old high school basketball coach, visited his family health care provider with complaints of weight gain, decreasing strength, increasing inability to concentrate, and morning headaches. Physical examination revealed severe hypertension, yellow-gray skin color, and pale mucous membranes. After diagnostic studies reveal chronic glomerulonephritis with end-stage renal disease (ESKD), Mr. J. is admitted to the hospital to stabilize his condition.

PATIENT PROBLEM

Fluid Volume Overload, related to compromised renal regulatory mechanism, as evidenced by systemic edema

Patient Goals and Expected Outcomes	Nursing Interventions	Evaluation
The patient will be able to reduce fluid to precrisis level	Record baseline assessment data. Create chart for patient to monitor: • Daily weight • Intake and output • Edema	Patient is able to complete daily self-monitoring with 1-lb weight loss daily.
The patient will modify diet to exclude foods and fluids that foster sodium, potassium, and water retention	Teach nutritional guidelines for dietary and fluid parameters with scheduling. Evaluate daily or as needed for systemic edema: girth, skin turgor, respiratory rate and quality. Monitor for manifestations of electrolyte imbalance. Teach patient and significant other about the type, cause, and treatment for fluid and electrolyte imbalance, as appropriate.	Patient can order daily diet and fluids within prescribed parameters.

PATIENT PROBLEM

Helplessness, related to sudden onset of life-altering illness as evidenced by patient statements: "I've always tried to take care of myself—look where it got me. Nowhere! Now I have to face my own death!"

Patient Goals and Expected Outcomes	Nursing Interventions	Evaluation
The patient will be empowered to assist in planning own care and in goal achievement	Provide support for the patient. Explain plans and procedures before scheduled times, according to patient's ability to understand. Negotiate with patient when changes are necessary. Accept patient's expression of self and values. Include significant other in planning for the patient's maximum role in self-management. Communicate unique patient planning arrangements for continuity with all treatment team members.	Patient voices a sense that the staff is sensitive to his needs. Patient seems able to plan modifications in work and home schedules to accommodate health needs.

PATIENT PROBLEM

Insufficient Knowledge, related to health education and home maintenance for ESKD

Patient Goals and Expected Outcomes	Nursing Interventions	Evaluation
The patient will describe the fundamental characteristics of ESKD and treatment options	Assess the amount and depth of the patient's information about ESKD. Collaborate with health care provider and treatment team in individualizing established institutional protocol for care of the patient with ESKD: 1. What happens when kidneys fail? 2. Treatment options include hemodialysis, peritoneal dialysis, and kidney transplantation 3. Inpatient versus outpatient care 4. Financing treatment 5. Teaching aids 6. Organizations that can helpPlan time to listen to the patient's and family's concerns and fears. Allow time for questions and answers and teaching reinforcement each day. Arrange (with patient's permission) opportunity for patient and family to meet with a patient or family that is positively adapting to ESKD. Be consistent in scheduling treatments with primary health care providers. Participate in end-of-life planning, when and if appropriate.	Patient can correctly answer basic questions about treatment options. Patient can correctly answer questions from teaching and is open to pose new questions.

Nursing Care Plan 10.1   The Patient With End-Stage Renal Disease—cont'd

CRITICAL THINKING QUESTIONS

1. Mr. J. complains of loss of appetite and limited food choices. What would be some helpful suggestions to improve his nutritional status?
2. Mr. J. established a therapeutic nurse-patient relationship with the nurse and confided that he is having marital problems partly because of his inability to have a satisfactory sexual relationship with his wife. What would be an appropriate response?
3. The nurse notes Mr. J.'s lack of interest in his therapeutic regimen of diet, medications, and fluid restrictions. He states, "What's the use? I will never be well again." What would be some therapeutic interventions?

Medical Management

Medical management includes continuation of previously instituted therapies. Closely monitor blood levels of drugs excreted by the kidney to maintain therapeutic levels and prevent toxic accumulations. Dose adjustments are affected by the GFR, dialysis, vomiting, and doses missed during hospital treatments. Medication may include antihypertensives, cardiac glycosides, antibiotics, and antidysrhythmics. Instruct the patient not to take over-the-counter medications without consulting the health care provider.

Nursing Interventions

Nursing interventions are dictated by individual patient conditions, including other acute or chronic problems. Most patients are dialyzed on an outpatient basis. (General nursing intervention guidelines are noted in Box 10.4 and Nursing Care Plan 10.1.) Psychosocial aspects of care for patients receiving dialysis are illustrated in the Communication box.

Nurses have a key responsibility for maintaining access sites and preventing or managing infection. Use a structured teaching program, with individualized patient teaching strategies to accommodate culture and knowledge level.

PERITONEAL DIALYSIS

Peritoneal dialysis can be performed with a minimum of equipment and by an ambulatory patient. Unlike hemodialysis, peritoneal dialysis is performed three to four times a day, 7 days a week. One exchange cycle usually requires 30 to 40 minutes along with a longer overnight exchange (NIDDK, 2021). The principle of osmosis and diffusion through a semipermeable membrane is the same as in hemodialysis, but the peritoneal membrane lining the peritoneum is used as the semipermeable membrane instead of an artificial kidney. Peritoneal dialysis is contraindicated for patients with systemic inflammatory disease, previous abdominal surgery, and chronic back pain, among other conditions.

To facilitate peritoneal dialysis, the health care provider places a catheter into the peritoneal space under aseptic conditions (Fig. 10.11). The dialyzing fluid is instilled for a predetermined period; this fluid draws waste from blood vessels in the peritoneal lining and

---

Box 10.4   Nursing Intervention Guidelines for the Patient Undergoing Hemodialysis

PATIENT TEACHING
- Reinforce explanation of dialysis procedure.
- Inform of community resources.
- Explain dietary restrictions.
- Teach about self-care and provide general information.

MONITORING DURING DIALYSIS
- Maintain asepsis and universal precautions.
- Weigh before and after treatment.
- Obtain vital signs every 30–60 min (take blood pressure in arm without fistula).
- Maintain orientation (thought processes may be altered).
- Assess for hemorrhage resulting from heparin use during dialysis.
- Monitor equipment (interruption of procedure).

ACTIVITY
- Provide diversions (reading, television, sleep).
- Ensure patient comfort (reclining, sitting, lying).
- Monitor dietary intake (may be hungry or nauseated).

CARE AFTER DIALYSIS OR BETWEEN TREATMENTS
- Schedule fluid intake within restrictions.
- Monitor for signs of fluid and electrolyte imbalance.
- Assess the access site for signs of infection, adequate circulation.
- Post signs regarding location of access site; do not take blood pressure or perform a venipuncture on arm with access site.
- Auscultate arteriovenous fistula for bruit (adventitious sound of venous or arterial origin heard on auscultation); palpate arteriovenous fistula for thrill (abnormal tremor).
- Assess, document, and report changes in general status.
- Provide skin care: bathe with tepid water to remove urea deposits.

---

then is drained and replaced. The patient with ESKD may be maintained on peritoneal dialysis, continuous ambulatory peritoneal dialysis (CAPD), or continuous cycle peritoneal dialysis (CCPD). Nocturnal intermittent peritoneal dialysis can be done three to five times per week for 10 to 12 hours. The patient is taught how to do the dialysis, which allows for more freedom. Although hemodialysis also can be done at home using

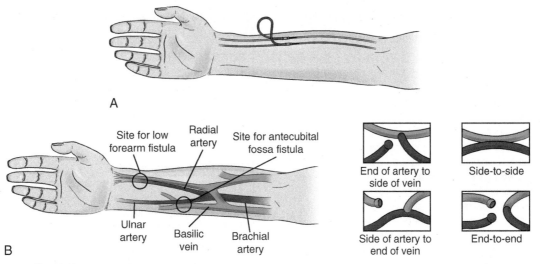

Fig. 10.10 (A) External arteriovenous shunt. (B) Internal arteriovenous fistula. Types of fistula construction.

strict aseptic technique, it is much more expensive and confining than CAPD.

Nursing Interventions
Common complications associated with peritoneal dialysis guide nursing interventions. Hypotension may occur with excessive sodium and fluid removal. Peritonitis may arise from sepsis. Pain and hemorrhage may accompany instillation of the dialysate. Box 10.5 lists nursing intervention guidelines for peritoneal dialysis.

Patient problems and interventions for the patient undergoing dialysis include but are not limited to the following:

PATIENT PROBLEM	NURSING INTERVENTIONS
Impaired Role Functioning, related to: • Chronic illness • Treatment side effects	Encourage verbalization of self-concept Assist in identifying personal strengths Assist patient and significant others with clarifying expected roles and those that must be relinquished or altered Support grief work if loss of role has occurred
Compromised Blood Flow to Tissue, Peripheral, related to: • Risk of disconnection • Clotting of vascular access	Avoid taking blood pressure and performing venipuncture in arm with fistula or graft Auscultate for bruits Observe access site for skin color and condition After dialysis, inspect needle puncture sites for bleeding

Prognosis
The patient with effective medical management can be maintained indefinitely on dialysis.

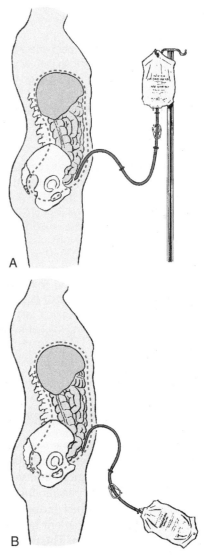

Fig. 10.11 Peritoneal dialysis. (A) Inflow. (B) Outflow. (From Tucker S, Canobbio MM, Paquette EV, et al: *Patient care standards: Collaborative practice planning guides,* ed 6, St. Louis, 1996, Mosby.)

Communication

Psychosocial Aspects of Care for Patients Receiving Dialysis

Mr. J., a student nurse, enters Mr. K.'s room to complete the initial morning assessment and finds him crying while struggling to get out of bed.

Nurse: Mr. K., what's wrong? (general lead, allows patient to describe)

Patient: Oh, nothing!

Nurse: (therapeutic silence, remains attentive, gives time)

Patient: Nothing is going right. I might as well be dead.

Nurse: What's wrong? (general lead, patient did not answer, encourages description)

Patient: I was trying to get up to take a shower, but I'm so weak I can't get myself out of bed.

Nurse: That must be frustrating. (voicing the implied)

Patient: That's an understatement! Look at me! I'm 37 years old—I should be in my prime but instead I'm gaining weight. I can't do my job because I can't concentrate. How am I supposed to feel?

Nurse: It must be frightening to experience all these changes. It would be understandable for you to be scared. (validating feelings)

Patient: I am scared! What if I never get better? I read this article about someone younger than I am who had the same thing, and he died when he had to go on dialysis.

Nurse: What do you think will happen to you? (general lead, encourages description without prescribing response)

Patient: Well, I don't know. The doctor keeps avoiding my questions and I see myself being less able to do anything. Maybe I am afraid—afraid of dying.

Nurse: (therapeutic silence, allows time for reflection)

Patient: Well, I never thought I'd say that—being afraid to die. It doesn't seem so frightening to say. I guess I didn't trust myself to be honest with myself or anyone else.

Nurse: Being honest with yourself is an important step to understanding. (pause) It seems, too, that you may not have accurate information about your illness. Let's plan to talk with your doctor about what you can reasonably expect—things you will be able to do, limitations, and things that you can do to enhance your physical and emotional health. (summarizing and goal setting for individualized patient teaching and discharge planning)

Patient: That sounds great, Mr. J. I really do want to do whatever I can to improve my chances of a better life. Would you help me get up to shower?

SURGICAL PROCEDURES FOR URINARY DYSFUNCTION

If damage to the urinary system cannot be corrected by medical management, surgical intervention may be necessary for temporary or permanent resection of the affected organ, such as when kidney function is lost. Dialysis is a viable management alternative, but a kidney transplant is preferable. The patient may require a kidney from a live or cadaver donor to replace the damaged kidney. Common surgical interventions and nursing intervention priorities are listed in Table 10.3. Preoperative and intraoperative management measures are the same as for major abdominal surgery

| Box 10.5 | Nursing Intervention Guidelines for the Patient Undergoing Peritoneal Dialysis |

PATIENT TEACHING
- Explanation of procedure
- Signs of complications
- Diet or fluid restrictions
- Medication (schedule in relation to dialysis time)
- Dialysate kept at body temperature to lessen discomfort

MONITORING DURING DIALYSIS
- Weight before and after procedure
- Hemorrhage (smoky, pink, or red-tinged dialysate)
- Type of dialysate (tailored to patient needs)
- Amount and timing of dialysate instillation
- Vital signs

CARE BETWEEN DIALYSES
- Signs of peritonitis (pain, fever, cloudy fluid)
- Strict aseptic care of catheter site
- Weigh daily

with general anesthesia (see Chapter 2). Suggested patient problem statements include those for abdominal surgery.

NEPHRECTOMY

Nephrectomy is the surgical removal of the kidney, either a small portion or the entire organ and surrounding tissues. In partial nephrectomy, only the diseased or infected portion of the kidney is removed. Radical nephrectomy involves removing the entire kidney, a section of the ureter, the adrenal gland, and the fatty tissue surrounding the kidney.

Postoperative management for surgical removal of the kidney is based on the prevention and detection of hemorrhage by monitoring vital signs, especially pulse and blood pressure; observation for restlessness and for gastrointestinal complications of nausea, vomiting, and abdominal distention; and establishment of adequate urinary drainage. Record I&O. If the thoracic cavity is opened during surgery, the patient will have chest tubes (see Chapter 9). Pain may compromise respiratory efficiency. Administer analgesics as ordered to facilitate lung expansion and the patient's activity level. Reposition the patient every 2 hours and ambulate as ordered. Change dressings according to the health care provider's order and record the amount and color of any drainage. Maintain close surveillance on the function of the remaining kidney.

Patient Teaching

Instruct the patient to avoid heavy lifting, drink 2000 mL of fluid each day (unless contraindicated), monitor output, avoid consumption of alcohol, and avoid respiratory tract infections and hazardous activities that could damage the remaining kidney.

Table 10.3 Surgical Procedures for Urinary Dysfunction	
SURGICAL INTERVENTION	**NURSING INTERVENTION PRIORITIES**
Nephrostomy: Surgical procedure in which an incision is made on the patient's flank so that a catheter can be inserted into the renal pelvis for drainage	Meticulous skin care, assessment for hemorrhage, accurate intake and output (I&O)
Nephrectomy: Surgical removal of the kidney	Assessment for hemorrhage, promotion of respiratory effort, accurate I&O
Cystectomy: Surgical removal of the bladder	Promotion of urinary drainage via ileal conduit, I&O
Ureterosigmoidostomy: Surgical procedure in which a ureter is implanted in the sigmoid colon of the intestinal tract	Meticulous skin care, monitoring of electrolyte imbalance, assessment of signs and symptoms of infection
Cutaneous ureterostomy: Surgical implantation of the terminal ends of the ureter under the skin	Meticulous skin care, assessment of urinary obstruction, accurate I&O

Prognosis

Complete recovery from nephrectomy is expected in the absence of any complication.

NEPHROSTOMY

A nephrostomy is an incision created between the kidney and the skin to drain urine directly from the renal pelvis. A nephrostomy is performed when an occlusion keeps urine from passing from the kidney, through the ureter, and into the urinary bladder. Without a way for urine to drain, pressure would rise within the urinary system and damage the kidneys. The most common cause of obstruction is cancer. This procedure also can be used to remove kidney stones.

Catheters are used to drain the wound. Take care to prevent obstruction of the catheters with blood clots postoperatively. Measure and record the amount and nature of drainage from the catheters, and change dressings frequently, keeping the skin clean by surgical asepsis. Turn the patient to position on the affected side as ordered to facilitate drainage and assist in respiratory ventilation. Never clamp a nephrostomy catheter (tube); acute pyelonephritis may result. If ordered by the health care provider, irrigate a nephrostomy catheter, using strict aseptic technique. Gentle instillation of no more than 5 mL of sterile saline solution at one time prevents renal damage.

KIDNEY TRANSPLANTATION

Kidney transplantation is performed as an intervention in irreversible renal failure. The donor kidney surgically is placed retroperitoneally in the iliac fossa. The nonfunctioning kidney is typically not removed. The donor renal artery is anastomosed to the recipient's internal or external iliac artery and the donor renal vein to the recipient's iliac vein. Usually, the kidney begins to function immediately.

Selection of a transplant recipient is based on careful evaluation of the patient's medical, immunologic, and psychosocial status. Usually a recipient is younger than age 70, has an estimated life expectancy of 2 years or more, and is expected to have improved quality of life after transplantation. Through conservative

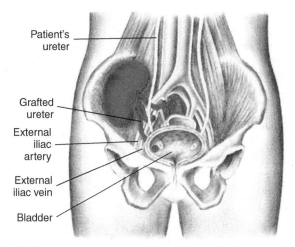

Fig. 10.12 Kidney transplantation. (From Belcher AE: *Cancer nursing*, St. Louis, 1992, Mosby.)

management and dialysis, the patient's state is as nontoxic as possible. Preoperative nursing intervention is complicated by the patient's fear and anxiety about transplantation and about possible rejection of the implanted organ. The patient is dialyzed until surgery can be completed satisfactorily. In surgery the nonfunctioning kidney remains in place and the donor kidney is positioned in the iliac fossa anterior to the crest of the ileum. The ureter is anastomosed into either the patient's ureter or bladder (Fig. 10.12). However, bilateral nephrectomy may be performed before the transplantation procedure for persistent or active bacterial pyelonephritis, uncontrolled renin-mediated hypertension, polycystic kidneys, or rapidly progressive glomerulonephritis.

Postoperatively, assess the patient for signs of rejection and infection: apprehension, generalized edema, fever, increased blood pressure, oliguria, edema, and tenderness over the graft site. An immunosuppressive agent, such as cyclosporine, is used alone or in conjunction with steroids. Cyclosporine is considered an effective drug in suppressing the immune system's efforts to reject tissue while leaving the recipient sufficient immune activity to combat infection. Mycophenolate (CellCept) and tacrolimus (Prograf) are drugs used to prevent rejection of kidney transplants; they are used in combination with corticosteroids. Immunosuppressive therapy increases the risk for infection and possible steroid-induced bleeding. Teaching the patient about the medications prescribed to prevent rejection is key to the patient's successful recovery.

Patient Teaching

Postoperative care includes special assessment of kidney function and electrolyte balance. The function of the transplanted kidney is the primary concern after surgery. Home follow-up becomes a life pattern for the transplantation patient. Patient education is extensive: diet, fluids, daily weights, strict I&O measurements, prevention of infection, and avoidance of activities that may compromise the integrity of the urinary tract. Community support groups, sponsored by the American Association of Kidney Patients, help the patient and the family adapt to living with dialysis and transplantation. The National Kidney Foundation has a written protocol for the procurement of organs for donation.

Prognosis

Success of kidney transplantation parallels the individual patient's general health status and compliance with the treatment plan. Transplantation offers the only possibility of return to a normal lifestyle for the patient with ESKD. Successful kidney transplantation prolongs and markedly improves quality of life, freeing the patient from the restrictions of dialysis.

URINARY DIVERSION

Several types of procedures are used to divert the flow of urine when required for treatment of bladder cancer, invasive cervical cancer, neurogenic bladder, and congenital anomalies. Often a cystectomy (the surgical removal of the bladder) is performed.

The cystectomy patient presents a unique challenge because of the need to create an artificial port for urine elimination. The most common urinary diversion procedure is the **ileal conduit** (Bricker's procedure or ileal loop); the ureters are implanted into a loop of the ileum that is isolated and brought to the surface of the abdominal wall (Fig. 10.13). On occasion, a segment of the sigmoid colon is isolated and used instead of the ileum to form a sigmoid conduit. Bowel function is maintained with anastomosis of the remaining intestine. A drainage bag (urostomy bag or appliance) is fitted over the stoma to contain the constant drainage of urine. Continuous urine drainage prevents increased pressure within the conduit that would cause backflow to the kidneys, compromise the circulatory integrity of the conduit, or rupture the surgical anastomosis. Decreased urinary output and low abdominal pain may signal the onset of such problems. Complications of this procedure are wound infection, dehiscence (unintended wound opening), urinary leakage, ureteral obstruction, small bowel obstruction, stomal gangrene

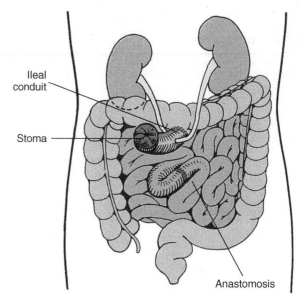

Fig. 10.13 Ileal conduit or ileal loop.

or atrophy, pyelonephritis, renal calculi, and compromised respiratory status secondary to incisional pain.

Postoperatively, measure urine flow hourly. Report output less than 30 mL/h to the health care provider immediately. A healthy stoma appears moist and pink and may even bleed slightly. Inspect the skin around the stoma daily for signs of bleeding, excoriation, and infection. Mucus is present in the urine from the intestinal secretions. The patient should ingest large quantities of water to flush the ileal conduit. Any odor of urine about the patient may indicate an infection or leak of urine from the drainage bag. Early signs of urinary leakage (indicating a leak in an anastomosis) include increased abdominal girth; fever; and drainage through the incision, tubes, or drains. Ureteral separation from the conduit may cause urine to seep into the peritoneal cavity; observe the patient for signs and symptoms of peritonitis such as fever, abdominal pain and rigidity, and absence of bowel sounds.

Care of the patient with an ileal conduit is a nursing challenge because of the continuous drainage of urine through the stoma.

To change the urostomy bag, remove and drain it. Cleanse the skin with water, and apply the new appliance as outlined in the institution's standards of care. When the peristomal skin is healed, the bag is emptied at 2- to 3-hour intervals. At night a straight drainage tube is connected to a drainage bag. A permanent urostomy bag can be left in place for 4 to 7 days if it remains sealed. Recommend that the patient have two bags so that one can be worn while the other is washed. Some patients prefer to use disposable bags. Odor is controlled by using deodorant drops or tablets in the urostomy bag; avoiding odor-producing foods, such as beans, onions, cabbage, asparagus, high-fiber wheat, simple sugars, and milk in the lactose-intolerant patient; and cleansing the urostomy bag with a vinegar-and-water rinse and thoroughly drying.

The *continent ileal urinary reservoir,* or *Kock pouch,* is created by implantation of the ureters into a segment of the small intestine that has been surgically removed from the rest of the bowel and anastomosed to the abdominal wall. Urine flow is controlled by a nipple-like valve that prevents leakage. To drain urine from the reservoir, the patient inserts a catheter through the valve at regular intervals, thus minimizing the reabsorption of waste materials from the urine and reflux into the ureters.

Patient Teaching

Patient teaching centers on the tasks of lifestyle adaptation: care of the stoma, nutrition, fluid intake, maintenance of self-esteem considering altered body image, modification of sexual activities, and early detection of complications. Patient teaching begins with selecting an appliance, sizing the stoma, and changing the appliances. The home health nurse can assist the patient in modifying care in the home environment and by providing support during this stressful adjustment period (see the Home Care Considerations box).

 Home Care Considerations

Urinary Diversion Warning Signs

Provide the patient and significant others with the following list of warning signs and symptoms that, if they occur at home, should be reported to the health care provider:

- Keep this list handy and call the health care provider (phone number: ___-___-____) if you notice any of the following signs or symptoms:
  - Decrease in urinary output
  - Change in urine color: bloody, cloudy
  - Fever greater than 101°F
  - Change in appearance of stoma: pale color, swelling, "drawing in" of stoma
  - Skin changes around stoma: redness, burning, breakdown
  - General feeling of weakness
  - Nausea and vomiting
  - Abdominal distention or pain
  - Any other health changes that are new or worse

Prognosis

Although the patient may recover fully without recurrence, the day-to-day challenges of managing a urinary diversion are permanent.

❖ NURSING PROCESS FOR THE PATIENT WITH A URINARY DISORDER

The role of the licensed practical nurse/licensed vocational nurse (LPN/LVN) in the nursing process as stated is that the LPN/LVN will:

- Participate in planning care for patients based on patient needs
- Review patient's care plan and recommend revisions as needed

- Review and follow defined prioritization for patient care
- Use clinical pathways, care maps, or care plans to guide and review patient care

◆ ASSESSMENT

Assessment of the urinary tract is included in baseline data for all patients. The assessment includes subjective data: the patient's description of urination patterns and associated sensations, such as complaints of burning or pain on urination or difficulty maintaining the urine stream. Supplement subjective data with objective data by assessing for signs of fluid overload or depletion. The skin provides easily assessed clues about the patient's state of hydration. For example, dryness and pruritus (itching) can occur as a result of electrolyte imbalance or the buildup of waste products.

Pay careful attention to assessment of high-risk populations. Urinary disorders are associated with systemic malformations and structural anomalies in newborns. Pediatric patients, especially girls, are susceptible to UTIs because of their short urethra. Geriatric patients may experience weakened musculature and sphincter tone, with resultant difficulty in bladder control. In male patients, enlargement of the prostate gland may interfere with initiating and maintaining an adequate urine stream.

Occupational and environmental factors also contribute to the development of renal disease. Nephrotoxins are substances with specific destructive properties for the kidneys. Sources include industrial exposure to heavy metals, such as lead and mercury, and medical treatment with cisplatin, aminoglycoside antibiotics (gentamicin or kanamycin), nonsteroidal anti-inflammatory drugs, or radiopaque contrast media.

Other vulnerable populations include patients experiencing systemic changes from altered health states, such as pregnancy, diabetes mellitus, or hypertension. Most susceptible are those with conditions that directly compromise kidney function: trauma, fluid depletion or retention, and active or suspected renal disease.

◆ PATIENT PROBLEM

The LPN/LVN assists in the development of patient problem statements. Patient problem statements for the patient with a urinary disorder include but are not limited to the following:

- Alteration in Urinary Elimination
- Compromised Blood Flow to Tissue: Renal
- Fluid Volume Overload
- Impaired Sexual Expression
- Insufficient Knowledge
- Potential for Inadequate Fluid Volume
- Potential for Infection
- Recent Onset of Pain; Prolonged Pain

◆ EXPECTED OUTCOMES AND PLANNING

For the patient with a urinary disorder, the nursing care priority is the short-term goal of reestablishing urinary flow and kidney function. Long-term planning for the patient and the family or significant other focuses on prevention of complications and quick response to recurrent problems. Goals are individualized for each patient and are modified to adapt to the patient's changing health status and urinary elimination management. The care plan may include the following goals and outcomes:

Goal 1: The patient will achieve control of the elimination of urine.

Outcome: Patient reports effective management of normal patterns of urination.

Goal 2: The patient will practice proper protocol such as drinking adequate fluids and correct methods of perineal cleansing for the female to prevent UTI.

Outcome: Patient reports no signs or symptoms of recurrent urinary difficulty.

◆ IMPLEMENTATION

Assist the patient in bladder training to promote normal patterns of urination. Educate the patient in the importance of drinking 2 to 3 L of water daily (unless contraindicated). Teach the female patient the importance of cleansing from anterior to posterior in the perineal area after a bowel movement to prevent contamination of the urethra with *E. coli*.

◆ EVALUATION

Evaluation of urinary status is determined by success in attaining expected outcomes. Monitoring urinary output and character is continual. Because some urinary disorders become chronic, patient involvement in the prevention of complications is vital. Avoidance of risk factors and early detection of symptoms are essential to limit damage to the urinary tract. Examples of goals and evaluative measures are as follows:

Goal 1: The patient will experience normal patterns of urinary elimination.

Evaluative measure: Patient reports return to own normal voiding.

Goal 2: The patient will monitor self for early signs and symptoms of recurrent UTI.

Evaluative measure: Patient can answer questions correctly about signs and symptoms and appropriate measures to take for treatment.

Get Ready for the NCLEX® Examination!

Key Points

- The kidneys lie retroperitoneally, just below the diaphragm.
- The functioning unit of the kidney is the nephron.
- The kidneys rid the body of wastes and excess electrolytes, maintain water and electrolyte balance, and maintain acid-base balance.
- Kidney function is achieved by the processes of filtration, secretion, and reabsorption.
- Assessment of the urinary tract is included in baseline data for all patients.
- The subject of urinary problems is an embarrassing topic for many patients. Be sensitive to the patient's feelings and be supportive.
- Aging may have a negative influence on urinary function, but many problems can be corrected.
- Hydration status is monitored by assessing weight daily, I&O, laboratory studies, skin and mucous membranes, and level of consciousness.
- A large percentage of nosocomial infections involve the urinary tract.
- Proper care of urinary catheters decreases the chance of UTIs.
- Surgical intervention may be indicated for urinary dysfunction that cannot be corrected by medical management.
- Dialysis, which mimics kidney function, may be used temporarily or as a long-term therapy.
- Dietary, fluid, and medication modifications may be necessary for the patient with urinary dysfunction.
- Sacral nerve stimulation for urinary urge incontinence is conducted with a permanently implanted electrical stimulation device that changes neuronal activity in the sacral efferent and afferent nerves.

Additional Learning Resources

SG Go to your Study Guide for additional learning activities to help you master this chapter content.

Be sure to visit the Evolve site at http://evolve.elsevier.com/Cooper/adult/ for additional online resources.

Review Questions for the NCLEX® Examination

1. The nurse is reviewing the urinalysis report on an assigned patient. The nurse recognizes which findings to be normal? *(Select all that apply.)*

   1. Turbidity clear
   2. pH 6.0
   3. Glucose negative
   4. Red blood cells, 15 to 20
   5. White blood cells, 1 to 3

2. The nurse is caring for a patient who has just had a renal angiography performed. What is the priority assessment?

   1. Blood pressure
   2. Respiratory effort
   3. Puncture site
   4. Urinary output

3. The nursing care plan includes teaching a patient Kegel exercises. What would be the best instruction when teaching this patient this type of exercise?

   1. "Tighten and relax the muscles in your pelvic floor several times a day in sets of 10."
   2. "Exercise the muscles around your urinary meatus several times a day."
   3. "A good way to learn how to do these exercises is to start urinating, then try to stop urinating."
   4. "The muscles in your pelvis should be exercised several times a day to tighten them."

4. The health care provider has talked to a patient and his wife about the treatment plan for his bladder cancer. Later, the patient tells the nurse he does not understand what the health care provider is going to do. What is the most appropriate initial response by the nurse?

   1. "Okay. I'll explain it to you again."
   2. "Make a list of questions for the doctor."
   3. "Try not to think about the treatment."
   4. "Tell me what you know about the treatment."

5. Which activity would be most harmful for the incontinent patient?

   1. Restricting fluid intake
   2. Drinking only water
   3. Fluid intake of 2000 mL/day
   4. Restricting acidic fruit juice intake

6. The nurse is reviewing the orders for a patient and finds that a culture and sensitivity test has been ordered. What instruction does the nurse provide to the patient regarding this diagnostic test?

   1. "You will need to urinate into a clean specimen container."
   2. "It is important that we obtain all of your urine for the next 24 hours in order for the test results to be accurate."
   3. "This test is ordered in order to determine the type of bacteria causing your infection and the antibiotic that will treat the infection."
   4. "The only way to obtain this specimen is through urinary catheterization."

7. Which factor will most likely promote patient compliance with the prescribed treatment plan?

   1. A set time schedule to follow
   2. Data on success rates
   3. Written information about the plan
   4. An active role in the planning

8. When scheduling the administration of furosemide (Lasix), it would be in a patient's best interest to schedule the medication to be given what time?

   1. 0900
   2. 1200
   3. 2100
   4. 2400

9. In discussing dietary needs with a patient with ESKD, the nurse indicates that potassium-rich foods should be limited in the diet. Which selections should be limited? *(Select all that apply.)*

   1. Baked potatoes
   2. Bananas
   3. Apricots
   4. Apples
   5. Pine nuts

10. Phenazopyridine hydrochloride has been prescribed for a patient. What information should be provided to the patient about this medication? *(Select all that apply.)*

    1. "This medication will result in experiencing reduced bladder discomfort."
    2. "Decrease in burning sensation will be experienced as a result of this medication therapy."
    3. "This medication will result in an increased urinary output."
    4. "The urine will have an orange hue as a result of this medication."
    5. "This medication should be taken during the entire 7-day period of treatment with the antibiotics prescribed."

11. When calculating actual urinary output during continuous bladder irrigations, the nurse would:

    1. Measure and record all fluid output in the drainage bag
    2. Measure the total output and deduct the amount of irrigation solution used
    3. Add the total of all intravenous and irrigation solutions and deduct output
    4. Measure total output and deduct the total intravenous solutions

12. What statement by a patient indicates the need for further teaching before renal angiography?

    1. "I will miss having breakfast."
    2. "I know the nurse will be checking my pulse after the test."
    3. "I'm glad I don't have to stay in bed after the test."
    4. "I had a test similar to this 3 years ago."

13. The nurse performs a bladder scan immediately after a patient voids and obtains 30 mL of residual urine. What action by the nurse should be taken next?

    1. Document the procedure with outcome data.
    2. Continue the bladder scan routine after each voiding.
    3. Restrict fluid intake after dinner.
    4. Immediately notify the health care provider of the results.

14. Which goal would have priority in planning care of the aging patient with urinary incontinence?

    1. Recognizes the urge to void
    2. Mobility necessary for toileting independently
    3. Episodes of incontinence decrease
    4. Drinks a minimum of 2000 mL of fluid per day

15. A patient with chronic kidney injury is starting peritoneal dialysis. Which statement to the patient best describes the purpose of this treatment?

1. "Since your kidneys no longer work efficiently, peritoneal dialysis will filter toxins from your blood in place of your kidneys."
2. "You have developed a great deal of swelling since diagnosed with chronic kidney injury so this treatment is prescribed to reduce your swelling."
3. "This treatment is prescribed to allow your kidneys to rest so that they can eventually work efficiently again."
4. "You will need to visit a dialysis clinic two to three times per week for your treatment."

16. The nurse is caring for a patient during the postoperative period after an arteriovenous shunt has been placed. What is the most important action to be taken?

1. Secure the shunt with an elastic bandage.
2. Notify the health care provider if a bruit or thrill is present.
3. Change the shunt if clotting occurs.
4. Use strict surgical asepsis for dressing changes.

17. What is the primary function of the kidney?

1. Regulation of enzymes
2. Filtration of water and blood products
3. Collection of urine from the body
4. Control of the adrenal glands

18. The priority short-term goal for disorders of the urinary system is:

1. Patient confidentiality
2. Privacy
3. Education for patient and family
4. Normal patterns of urinary elimination

19. The nurse making rounds discovers that there is no urine drainage from a postoperative patient's Foley catheter. What action by the nurse should be performed first?

1. Ensure patency.
2. Irrigate until clear.
3. Call the health care provider.
4. Insert larger lumen catheter.

20. Which problem constitutes a medical emergency?

1. Anuria
2. Polyuria
3. Dysuria
4. Dyspnea

21. The most common cause of renal failure is:

1. Trauma
2. Diabetes mellitus
3. Cancer
4. Heart failure

22. What clinical findings in the oliguric phase of acute renal failure will be noted?

1. BUN levels rise.
2. Urinary output may increase or decrease.
3. Signs of impending shock are present.
4. Blood flow to the kidneys increases.
5. Creatinine levels decrease.

23. What are correct patient teachings for a patient with cystitis? (Select all that apply.)

1. Teach the patient to drink apple juice to treat and prevent UTIs.
2. Teach the female patient to cleanse the perineal area from anterior to posterior to prevent rectal *E. coli* contamination of the urethra.
3. Encourage the patient to drink 2000 mL of fluid per day, unless contraindicated.
4. Instruct the patient that it is acceptable to stop taking prescribed medications when symptoms subside.
5. Instruct the patient to void as soon after sexual intercourse as possible.

24. The nurse is reviewing the health history of a patient suspected of having renal calculi. What factors in the patient's history increase the patient's risk for developing the condition? (Select all that apply.)

1. Stasis of urine caused by obstruction
2. Infections of urinary tract
3. Hypoparathyroidism
4. Diabetes mellitus
5. Immobility

25. The collection of subjective and objective data for a patient with acute glomerulonephritis could include which symptoms? (Select all that apply.)

1. Periorbital edema
2. Anorexia
3. Hypotension
4. Frankly sanguineous urine
5. Headaches

26. Careful preparation of a patient for an IVP is necessary. What nursing interventions would be included in the preparation? (Select all that apply.)

1. NPO for about 8 hours before examination
2. Ascertaining whether patient has allergy to magnesium
3. Giving prescribed bowel prep
4. Instructing patient concerning IVP
5. Discussing the anesthesia needed for the procedure

27. A patient diagnosed with ESKD is treated with conservative management, including erythropoietin injections. After teaching the patient about management of ESKD, the nurse determines teaching has been effective when the patient makes which statement?

1. "I will measure my urinary output each day to help calculate the amount I can drink."
2. "I need to take the erythropoietin to boost my immune system and help prevent infection."
3. "I need to try to get more protein from dairy products."
4. "I will try to increase my intake of fruits and vegetables."

28. As the nurse reviews a diet plan with a patient with diabetes mellitus and renal insufficiency, the patient states that with diabetes and renal failure there is nothing that is good to eat. The patient says, "I am going to eat what I want; I'm going to die anyway!" What is the best patient problem statement for this patient?

    1. Insufficient Nutrition, related to knowledge deficit about appropriate diet
    2. Potential for Noncompliance or Nonconformity, related to feelings of anger
    3. Grief, related to actual and perceived losses
    4. Potential for Impaired Health Maintenance, related to complexity of therapeutic regimen

29. The nurse has instructed a patient who is receiving hemodialysis about dietary management. Which diet choices by the patient indicate that the teaching has been successful?

    1. Scrambled eggs, English muffin, and apple juice
    2. Cheese sandwich, tomato soup, and cranberry juice
    3. Split-pea soup, whole-wheat toast, and nonfat milk
    4. Oatmeal with cream, half a banana, and herbal tea

30. A woman, 77, with well-controlled multiple sclerosis (MS) is referred to a urologist after asking her primary care physician for more help with urinary incontinence. "I don't pee that often," she says. "In fact, most of the time now I can't, but when I do, I get absolutely no warning. So I started buying maxi-pads at the supermarket—back on those things again after all these years!—then graduated to incontinence underwear. I've been using those for nearly a year now, but it's just getting worse." Subjective data include reports of diaphoresis, flushing, and infrequent voiding followed by "a feeling of just peeing with absolutely no warning at all." After further history, urine culture, urodynamic testing, and cystoscopy, the patient is diagnosed with flaccid (atonic) bladder. Unfortunately, insurance will not qualify her for a sacral nerve stimulation device, so she and her urologist develop a treatment plan that will combine medication with scheduled voiding and a few dietary changes. While the goal may be to establish urinary elimination and prevent complications, the nurse must ensure that the patient understands that it may not be possible to completely return to normal voiding. The nurse prepares instructions on how to use her prescribed medication.

What else should be included in this patient's education plan? Check all that apply:

    A. Teach her how to double void.
    B. Teach her to monitor for side effects when taking the cholinergic bethanechol.
    C. Guide her through the process and precautions used in botulinum toxin injections.
    D. Teach her that it is important not to use this medication beyond its 3-day regimen.
    E. Teach her the importance of learning to be alert for signs of bladder distention.
    F. Warn her that her medication will turn the urine bright orange and not to be alarmed by this.

11

Care of the Patient With an Endocrine Disorder

http://evolve.elsevier.com/Cooper/adult/

Objectives

Anatomy and Physiology

1. List and describe the endocrine glands and pertinent endocrine hormones.
2. Define *negative feedback*.
3. Explain the action of hormones and how they work on targeted organs.
4. Comprehend how the hypothalamus controls the anterior and posterior lobes of the pituitary gland.

Medical-Surgical

5. Discuss the etiology and pathophysiology, clinical manifestations, assessment, diagnostic tests, medical management, nursing interventions, patient teaching, and prognosis for patients with acromegaly, gigantism, dwarfism, diabetes insipidus, syndrome of inappropriate antidiuretic hormone, hyperthyroidism, hypothyroidism, goiter, thyroid cancer, hyperparathyroidism, hypoparathyroidism, Cushing syndrome, and Addison's disease.
6. Explain how to test for Chvostek sign, Trousseau sign, and carpopedal spasms.
7. List two significant complications that may occur after thyroidectomy.

8. Describe the etiology and pathophysiology, clinical manifestations, assessment, diagnostic tests, medical management, nursing interventions, patient teaching, and prognosis for the patient with diabetes mellitus.
9. Differentiate between the signs and symptoms of hyperglycemia and hypoglycemia.
10. Differentiate among the signs and symptoms of diabetic ketoacidosis, hyperglycemic hyperosmolar non-ketotic coma, and hypoglycemic reaction.
11. Explain the roles of nutrition, exercise, and medication in the control of diabetes mellitus.
12. Discuss how the various classes of oral hypoglycemic medications work to improve the mechanisms by which insulin and glucose are produced and used by the body.
13. Discuss the various insulin types and their characteristics.
14. Describe the correct way to draw up and administer insulin.
15. Discuss the acute and long-term complications of diabetes mellitus.

Key Terms

Chvostek sign (KHVŎS-tĕks sīn, p. 502)
Circadian rhythm (sĕr Kā dē ăn Rĭ thĕm, p. 492)
dysphagia (dĭs-FĀ-jē-ă, p. 501)
endocrinologist (ĕn-dō-krĭ-NŎL-ŏ-jĭst, p. 495)
glycosuria (glī-kōs-Ū-rē-ă, p. 515)
hirsutism (HĔR-sūt-ĭszm, p. 509)
hyperglycemia (hī-pĕr-glī-SĒ-mē-ă, p. 515)
hypocalcemia (hī-pō-kăl-SĒ-mē-ă, p. 491)
hypoglycemia (hī-pō-glī-SĒ-mē-ă, p. 522)
hypokalemia (hī-pō-kă-LĒ-mē-ă, p. 509)
idiopathic hyperplasia (ĭd-ē-ō-PĂTH-ĭk hī-pĕr-PLĀ-zhă, p. 492)

ketoacidosis (kē-tō-ă-sĭ-DŌ-sĭs, p. 515)
ketone bodies (KĒ-tōn BŎD-ēz, p. 509)
lipohypertrophy (lĭp-ō-HĪ-pĕr-trŏ-fē, p. 521)
neuropathy (nū-RŎP-ĕ-thē, p. 524)
polydipsia (pŏl-ē-DĬP-sē-ă, p. 496)
polyphagia (pŏl-ē-FĀ-jă, p. 515)
polyuria (pŏl-ē-Ū-rē-ă, p. 496)
Trousseau sign (trū-SŌZ sīn, p. 502)
turgor (TŬR-gŏr, p. 497)
Type 1 DM (tīp 1 dī-ă-BĒ-tēz MĔL-ĭ-tŭs, p. 514)
type 2 diabetes mellitus (tīp 2 dī-ă-BĒ-tēz MĔL-ĭ-tŭs, p. 530)

ANATOMY AND PHYSIOLOGY OF THE ENDOCRINE SYSTEM

ENDOCRINE GLANDS AND HORMONES

A *gland* is a specialized organ devised from a group of epithelial cells that form tissues that work together to produce and secrete hormones, enzymes, and other components that help regulate the body. There are two different types of glands, and each one regulates a reciprocal system. The *exocrine glands* secrete fluid products called enzymes. The enzymes are transported through a series of ducts and/or channels. The primary purpose of the exocrine ducts and channels is to move substances into the body or outside the body. The exocrine gland is responsible for the digestive system (gastric enzymes and saliva) as well as the sweat glands. The exocrine gland secretions are protective and functional.

Endocrine glands are ductless and release hormones directly into the bloodstream. The hormones control regulatory function such as cellular metabolism, human growth, fluid and electrolyte balance, and finally the production of energy. Endocrine and exocrine glands control homeostasis (constant balance) by communicating with other organs and tissues while regulating their assigned bodily functions. *Hormones* are chemical messengers that travel through the bloodstream to their target organs and work closely with the nervous system. Metabolic changes occur in response to the actions of hormones.

The slightest change in hormonal levels can disrupt the metabolic balance of the entire body. Hormones can increase or decrease a normal body process by affecting a target organ, and the actions are known to be interrelated. Interrelatedness refers to a fluctuation in a single hormone, which can significantly affect the actions of other hormones. The endocrine glands (Fig. 11.1) have a generalized effect on the patient's metabolism, growth, development, reproduction, and many other bodily activities such as temperature, fluid balance, and emotional responses as seen in the fight-or-flight response.

The amount of hormone released is controlled by *negative feedback inhibition*. The negative feedback inhibition process occurs when a gland releases a primary hormone, which stimulates target cells to release a secondary hormone; the gland slows the release of the primary hormone as it senses the rise of the secondary hormone. Information is exchanged constantly via the bloodstream between target organs and endocrine glands, which is described specifically later in this chapter.

Pituitary Gland

The pea-sized *pituitary gland* (hypophysis) is one of the most powerful glands in the body. It has been called the "master gland" because, through negative feedback, it controls the other endocrine glands. This gland is located beneath the hypothalamus of the brain in a cranial cavity in a small, saddle-like depression in the sphenoid bone. It is divided into two segments: the *anterior pituitary* (adenohypophysis) and the *posterior pituitary* (neurohypophysis). Each segment produces specialized hormones for specific targeted responses. The hypothalamus produces the hormones of the posterior pituitary and releases the hormones for storage in the posterior pituitary gland. The hormones are released from the posterior pituitary as a result of nerve impulses received from the hypothalamus.

Anterior pituitary gland. Six major hormones are secreted by the anterior pituitary gland:
1. Somatotropin, or growth hormone (GH)
2. Adrenocorticotropic hormone (ACTH)
3. Thyroid-stimulating hormone (TSH)
4 and 5. Gonadotropic hormones: Follicle-stimulating hormone (FSH) and luteinizing hormone (LH)
6. Prolactin (PRL)

The first five hormones in the list are known as *tropic* hormones. Tropic hormones are defined as ones that stimulate the activity of another endocrine gland. Prolactin is a non-tropic hormone and has a direct effect on the mammary glands, which in return are stimulated to *produce* milk. These hormones and their functions are shown in Fig. 11.2.

Posterior pituitary gland. Oxytocin and the *antidiuretic hormone* (ADH) are the only two hormones stored in the posterior pituitary and released by the posterior pituitary when the hypothalamus is stimulated (see Fig. 11.2). Oxytocin promotes the *release* of milk and stimulates uterine contractions during labor. ADH, also called *vasopressin*, causes the kidneys to conserve water by decreasing the amount of urine produced. ADH/vasopressin also causes constriction of the arterioles in the body, producing a systemic pressor effect, which results in increased blood pressure.

Thyroid Gland

The *thyroid gland* is butterfly shaped, with one lobe lying on either side of the trachea just below the larynx (Fig. 11.3). The lobes are connected by the *isthmus*. The thyroid gland is very vascular and receives approximately 80 to 120 mL of blood per minute.

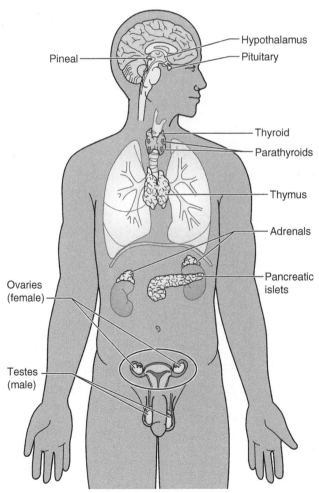

Fig. 11.1 Endocrine glands in the body.

Pineal — Hypothalamus — Pituitary — Thyroid — Parathyroids — Thymus — Adrenals — Pancreatic islets — Ovaries (female) — Testes (male)

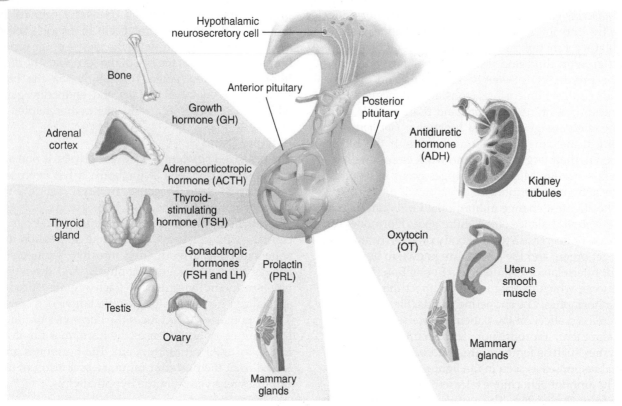

Fig. 11.2 Pituitary hormones. Shown are the principal anterior and posterior pituitary hormones and their target organs. *FSH,* Follicle-stimulating hormone; *LH,* luteinizing hormone. (From Patton KT, Thibodeau GA: *Anatomy and physiology,* ed 8, St. Louis, 2013, Mosby.)

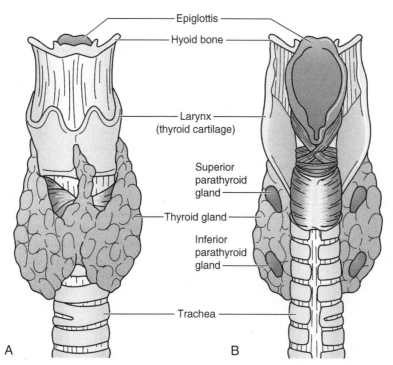

Fig. 11.3 Thyroid and parathyroid glands. Note their relations to each other and to the larynx and trachea. (A) Anteroposterior view. (B) Posteroanterior view.

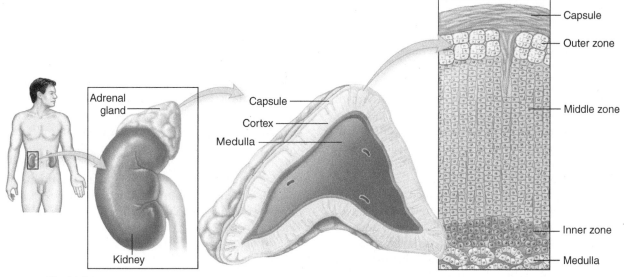

Fig. 11.4 Structure of the adrenal gland. The outer zone (zona glomerulosa) of the cortex secretes abundant amounts of glucocorticoids, chiefly aldosterone. The middle zone (zona fasciculata) secretes glucocorticoids, primarily cortisol, as well as small amounts of sex hormone. The inner zone (zona reticularis) secretes sex hormones. A portion of the medulla is visible at the bottom of the illustration. (From Patton KT, Thibodeau GA, Douglas MM: *Essentials of anatomy and physiology*, ed 1, St. Louis, 2012, Mosby.)

The thyroid gland secretes two main hormones: *triiodothyronine* (T_3) and *thyroxine* (T_4). Adequate oral intake of iodine is necessary for the formation of thyroid hormones. These two specific hormones regulate three functions: (1) growth and development, (2) metabolism, and (3) activity of the nervous system. Their function is controlled by the release of TSH from the pituitary gland.

Calcitonin is the third hormone released by the thyroid gland. It decreases blood calcium levels by causing calcium to be stored in the bones.

Parathyroid Glands

The four parathyroid glands are located on the posterior surface of the thyroid gland (see Fig. 11.3) and secrete *parathyroid hormone* (PTH, parathormone). As an antagonist to calcitonin from the thyroid, PTH tends to increase the concentration of calcium in the blood. It also regulates the amount of phosphorus in the blood.

The delicate balance of calcium in the blood is extremely important for normal body function. When calcium blood levels are low (hypocalcemia), the nerve cells become excited and stimulate the muscles with too many impulses, resulting in spasms *(tetany)*. Hypocalcemia also slows the heart rate, causing cardiac irritability and heart failure. When blood calcium levels are abnormally high (hypercalcemia), heart function becomes impaired and can result in death if not treated. Under the influence of PTH, two changes occur in the kidneys: increasing the reabsorption of calcium and magnesium from the kidney tubules, and accelerating the elimination of phosphorus in the urine.

Adrenal Glands

The two adrenal glands (suprarenal glands) are small, yellow masses that sit on top of the kidneys. Both glands contain the adrenal cortex (outer section) and the adrenal medulla (inner section) (Fig. 11.4).

Adrenal cortex. The adrenal cortex is divided into three separate layers. Each layer secretes a particular hormone, called a *steroid:*

- *Mineralocorticoids* are secreted by the outer zone (zona glomerulosa): These are involved primarily in water and electrolyte balance (homeostasis) and indirectly manage blood pressure. Aldosterone, the principal mineralocorticoid, regulates sodium and potassium levels by affecting the renal tubules. It decreases the level of potassium and increases the level of sodium in the bloodstream. The retention of sodium causes retention of water, which leads to an increase in blood volume and blood pressure.
- *Glucocorticoids* are secreted by the middle zone (zona fasciculata). The most important of these is cortisol, which is involved in glucose metabolism and provides extra reserve energy in times of stress. Glucocorticoids also exhibit anti-inflammatory properties.
- *Sex hormones* are secreted by the inner zone (zona reticularis): Androgen hormones are the primary hormones secreted and are needed early for the development of the male reproductive system and then create the testosterone hormone, which is stored and secreted in the male testes, and estrogen hormone in females. In the adult, the adrenal glands release a relatively small amount of these hormones, which have an insignificant impact on the system.

Adrenal medulla. The cells composing the adrenal medulla arise from the same type of cells as the sympathetic nervous system. Two hormones are released during times of stress: (1) *epinephrine* (adrenaline) and (2) *norepinephrine*. They cause the heart rate and blood pressure to increase, the blood vessels to constrict, and the liver to release glucose reserves for immediate energy. This is a systemic preparation of the body for a "fight-or-flight" response needed in times of crisis.

Pancreas

The pancreas is an elongated gland that lies posterior to the stomach. It is an active organ, composed of exocrine and endocrine tissue. The endocrine tissue of the pancreas contains more than a million tiny clusters of cells known collectively as the islets of Langerhans. These cells secrete two major hormones. The first, *insulin*, is secreted by the *beta cells* in response to increased levels of glucose in the blood. The secretion pattern of insulin is a physiologic example of negative feedback between insulin and glucose. Elevated blood glucose levels stimulate the pancreas to secrete insulin. The stimulus for insulin secretion decreases as blood glucose levels decrease. The homeostatic mechanism is considered negative feedback because it reverses the change in blood glucose level. The second pancreatic hormone is *glucagon*. Glucagon is secreted by *alpha cells* in response to decreased levels of glucose in the blood. Insulin and glucagon play a major role in carbohydrate, fat, and protein metabolism.

Female Sex Glands

Deep in the lower abdominal region, lying to the left and right of the uterus, are two almond-shaped *ovaries*, the major female sex glands. At puberty, the ovaries begin producing two hormones: *estrogen* (responsible for the development of secondary sex characteristics, such as axillary hair and pubic hair, and for maturation of the reproductive organs) and *progesterone*. Progesterone continues the preparation of the reproductive organs that was initiated by estrogen. (See Chapter 12 for more information.)

The *placenta* is a temporary endocrine gland that forms and functions during pregnancy. During this time the ovaries become inactive, and the placenta releases the estrogen and progesterone needed to maintain the pregnancy. (For a more in-depth discussion, see Chapter 12.)

Male Sex Glands

Suspended outside the body in the *scrotum*, a saclike structure, are the two oval sex glands called the *testes*. They release the hormone *testosterone*, which is responsible for the development of the male secondary sex characteristics, including axillary, pubic, and facial hair; maturation of the reproductive organs; deepening of the voice; and development of muscle and bone mass. Testosterone is necessary for sperm formation.

Thymus Gland

The thymus gland lies in the upper thorax, posterior to the sternum (see Fig. 11.1). It produces the hormone *thymosin*, which plays an active role in the immune system. T lymphocytes (a type of white blood cell) are stimulated to carry out immune reactions to certain types of antigens. The thymus gland programs this information into the T lymphocytes in utero and during the first few months of life.

Pineal Gland

The pineal gland is a small, cone-shaped gland located in the roof of the third ventricle of the brain (see Fig. 11.1). It secretes the hormone *melatonin*. This hormone is linked to sleep functions of the body and regulation of circadian rhythms. Circadian rhythms are physical, mental, and behavioral changes that follow a daily cycle. They respond primarily to light and darkness in an organism's environment (National Institute of General Medical Science [NIGMS], 2018).

DISORDERS OF THE PITUITARY GLAND (HYPOPHYSIS)

ACROMEGALY
Etiology and Pathophysiology

An overproduction of somatotropin (growth hormone-GH) after the onset of puberty and closure of the growth plates of the bones causes *acromegaly,* a condition that results in 3000 new diagnoses annually in the United States. The cause may be either (1) idiopathic hyperplasia (an increase in the number of cells, without a known cause) of the anterior lobe of the pituitary gland or (2) tumor growth. Unfortunately, growth changes that occur in acromegaly are irreversible, even with adequate medical or surgical intervention.

Clinical Manifestations

Manifestations of acromegaly begin gradually, usually in the third or fourth decade of life. Typically, an average of 7 to 9 years passes between the initial onset of signs and symptoms and final diagnosis. The subsequent overabundance of somatotropin produces many changes throughout the patient's body, including enlarged cranium and lower jaw, separated and maloccluded teeth, bulging forehead, bulbous nose, thick lips, enlarged tongue, and generalized coarsening of the facial features (Fig. 11.5). Enlargement of the tongue results in speech difficulties, and the voice deepens as a result of hypertrophy of the vocal cords. The hands and feet grow larger; the fingertips develop a tufted or clubbed appearance. There is enlargement of the heart, liver, and spleen. Muscle weakness usually develops. Joints may hypertrophy and become painful and stiff. Male patients may become impotent, and female patients may develop a deepened voice, increased facial hair, and amenorrhea (lack of menstrual cycles). If a tumor is present, pressure on the optic nerve may cause partial or complete blindness. Visual disturbances are often a first sign of acromegaly. Severe headaches are common.

Assessment

Subjective data include headaches or visual disturbances and painful, stiff joints. Evaluate muscle weakness

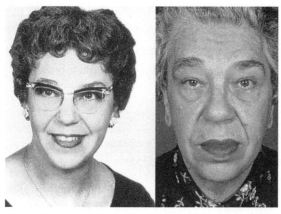

Fig. 11.5 *Left,* A patient's face before she developed a pituitary tumor. *Right,* The same patient, years later; her face shows the coarse features typical of acromegaly. (Courtesy the Group for Research in Pathology Education.)

and its effect on the patient's ability to perform activities. Encourage patients to share their emotional responses to sexual problems (such as impotence in men and masculinization in women). Particular attention should be paid to the psychological distress associated with the physical changes during the progression of acromegaly.

Collection of objective data includes ongoing assessment of bone enlargement and joint involvement, as evidenced by gait changes and decreasing ability to perform activities. Changes in vital signs that may herald the onset of early heart failure include dyspnea, tachycardia, weak pulse, and hypotension. The patient's fluid volume status should be assessed with each interaction. After surgical removal of the pituitary tumor, the patient is at risk for diabetes insipidus. If the posterior pituitary gland was damaged during surgery, it may cause a lack of ADH, resulting in diabetes insipidus. Diabetes insipidus is a condition in which the kidneys do not conserve water properly, and is discussed more in depth in this chapter. Hypertension, heart failure, and cardiomyopathy are possible complications secondary to enlargement of the heart and other organs.

Diagnostic Tests

Diagnosis of acromegaly is based on the history and clinical manifestations, computed tomography (CT) scan, magnetic resonance imaging (MRI), and cranial radiographic evaluation. A complete ophthalmologic examination, including visual fields, usually is performed because a large tumor of the pituitary gland potentially causes pressure on the optic nerves or optic chiasm (where the optic nerves cross, just in front of the pituitary gland). Laboratory tests confirm elevated levels of serum GH and plasma insulin-like growth factor-1. The definitive test for acromegaly is the GH suppression test (Mayo Clinic, 2021).). This test requires the patient to be NPO in the 10-12 hours preceding the test. A glucose solution is ingested. GH levels will fall in the normal patient. When the patient with acromegaly drinks the solution, the GH levels remain elevated (National Library of Medicine [NLM], 2019 (NLM, 2018).

Medical Management

Medical treatments include dopamine agonists, such as cabergoline, and somatostatin analogues (which inhibit GH), such as octreotide (Sandostatin) (Table 11.1), especially in patients who are not candidates for surgery or radiation therapy. These drugs are used in an attempt to suppress GH secretion. Surgical treatment to remove pituitary tumors associated with acromegaly is accomplished with the transsphenoidal removal of tumor tissue. The goal of transsphenoidal surgery is to remove only the tumor that is causing GH secretion. Irradiation procedures using proton beam therapy have been used to destroy GH-secreting tumors. Proton beam treatment uses very low doses of radiation and is much less destructive to adjacent tissues, such as the hypothalamus and temporal lobes, than conventional radiation therapy. This procedure is known as the *gamma knife radiosurgery.*

Nursing Interventions and Patient Teaching

Nursing interventions are primarily supportive and are geared toward relieving the discomforts of the patient. Muscle weakness, joint pain, and stiffness warrant assessment of the ability to perform activities of daily living (ADLs). Joint pain/discomfort should be assessed frequently. Headache may impair the patient's ability to socialize and also may impede education and employment. Worsening headaches may indicate tumor progression. Jaw muscles and the temporomandibular joint may be involved. The diet should be soft and easy to chew. Encourage the patient to chew thoroughly, and allow adequate time during meals, assisting when necessary. Non-opioid analgesics may be given for pain relief. Visual impairment may increase the risk of injury for these patients, so take care to prevent them from stumbling into furniture or dropping objects.

As the body changes, the patient may develop problems with self-esteem and may feel physically unattractive. The patient may have difficulty communicating with significant others, which can disrupt individual or family coping methods. Other complications of acromegaly are related to enlargement of the liver, spleen, and heart. Cardiac dysrhythmias may develop, and the patient may experience heart failure. Abdominal girth may increase as a result of weight gain and inactivity, and respiratory difficulty may occur.

A patient problem and interventions for the patient with acromegaly include but are not limited to the following:

PATIENT PROBLEM	NURSING INTERVENTIONS
Distorted Body Image, related to physical manifestations of the condition (may include enlargement of hands, feet, tongue, jaw, and soft tissue)	Convey respect and nonjudgmental acceptance of patient as a person
	Help the patient set achievable short-term goals

Table 11.1 Medications for Endocrine Disorders

GENERIC NAME (TRADE NAME)	ACTION	SIDE EFFECTS	NURSING IMPLICATIONS
Bromocriptine	Inhibits prolactin secretion; lowers serum levels of growth hormone, dopamine receptor agonist	Nausea, headache, dizziness, abdominal cramping, orthostatic hypotension	Give with meals to prevent GI effects; change positions carefully to prevent orthostatic hypotension; contraindicated with hypersensitivity to ergot derivatives
Calcium salts	Calcium electrolyte replacement	Hypercalcemia, phlebitis, necrosis, and burning at IV site; bradycardia, hypotension, and dysrhythmias with rapid IV administration	Monitor cardiac status and blood pressure and for extravasation when giving intravenously
Fludrocortisone	Adrenal corticosteroid with mineralocorticoid activity; promotes sodium and water retention	Hypertension, edema, sweating, rash, hypokalemia	Monitor for hypokalemia and fluid retention or depletion; do not discontinue abruptly; patient should carry identification signaling use
Levothyroxine Liothyronine Liotrix Thyroid	Thyroid hormone replacement	Most side effects are due to therapeutic overdose; include anxiety, insomnia, headache, hypertension, tremors, angina, dysrhythmias, tachycardia, menstrual irregularities, nervousness, irritability, nausea, diarrhea, appetite changes, leg cramps	Give in morning to minimize insomnia; use caution in older adults or patients with coronary artery disease; monitor for signs of overdose; do not switch brands unless instructed
Mitotane	Adrenal cytotoxic agent; reduces production of adrenal steroids	Anorexia, nausea, vomiting, diarrhea, lethargy, somnolence, vertigo, rash	Tell patient to use contraception; instruct patient to use caution when driving or performing tasks requiring alertness; monitor for dehydration
Potassium iodide	Blocks release of thyroid hormone in thyroid storm and hyperthyroidism; also used as an expectorant	Hypersensitivity reactions, rash, metallic taste, burning in mouth or throat, GI irritation, headache, parotitis, hyperkalemia	Do not use in pregnant women; mix with fruit juice to mask taste
Somatostatin analogues: octreotide	Inhibits growth hormone secretion; suppresses secretion of serotonin, gastroenteropancreatic peptides; enhances fluid and electrolyte absorption from the GI tract; used to treat carcinoid tumors, VIPomas,[a] and high-output fistulas[b]	Nausea, diarrhea, abdominal pain, headache, injection site discomfort, hyperglycemia, hypoglycemia	SubQ route of administration is preferred but also may be given IV
Antidiuretic hormone: vasopressin	Synthetic pituitary hormone with antidiuretic effects on the kidney (used to treat diabetes insipidus); also a potent vasoconstrictor (used to treat bleeding esophageal varices)	Nasal irritation and congestion with nasal preparations; hypertension; ischemia of heart, mesenteric organs, and kidneys; angina; myocardial infarction; water retention; hyponatremia	Use with caution in older adults or patients with coronary artery disease or heart failure; discontinue if chest pain develops; monitor urinary output and serum sodium

[a]VIPomas are neuroendocrine tumors of the pancreas that secrete vasoactive intestinal polypeptide (VIP) autonomously.
[b]A *fistula* is an abnormal passage from an internal organ through the skin to the outside of the body, and through which internal secretions and water pass. They often are triggered by surgery. A high-output fistula produces 500 mL/day or more.
GI, Gastrointestinal; *IV,* intravenous; *subQ,* subcutaneous.

The patient should remain under the supervision of a health care provider so that any complications can be diagnosed promptly and adequately treated. Teach the patient exercises that can be performed at home, such as active range of motion of joints of the extremities and of the neck, to help prevent muscle atrophy and loss of movement.

Prognosis
Even with adequate medical or surgical treatment, the physical changes are irreversible, and the patient is prone to developing complications such as diabetes, heart failure, hypertension, osteoarthritis, colon polyps, sleep apnea, and vision loss (Mayo Clinic, 2021).

GIGANTISM
Etiology and Pathophysiology
Gigantism usually results from an oversecretion of GH before the onset of puberty, as a result of hyperplasia of the anterior pituitary. The hyperplastic tissue may develop into a tumor. Another possible cause is a defect in the hypothalamus that directs the anterior pituitary to release excessive amounts of GH.

Clinical Manifestations
When overproduction of GH occurs in a child before the epiphyses (growth plates at each end of the bones) close, there is an overgrowth of the long bones. This causes the individual to grow abnormally tall and have increased muscle and visceral development. Weight increases, but body proportions are usually normal. Despite their size, these patients are usually weak. Other kinds of gigantism may be caused by certain genetic disorders or by disturbances in sex hormone production. Once identified, these children should be referred for further medical evaluation and follow-up.

Assessment
Collection of subjective data includes assessment of the patient's understanding of the disease process and his or her ability to verbalize emotional responses.

Collection of objective data requires frequent measurement of height. Assess the patient's use of adaptive coping measures and family interactions.

Diagnostic Tests
A GH suppression test may be done to evaluate GH levels (Mayo Clinic, 2021). In the patient with gigantism, baseline levels of GH are high. Blood levels of GH also are evaluated for diagnosis of gigantism.

Medical Management
Medical management of children with gigantism may include surgical removal of tumor tissue or irradiation of the anterior pituitary gland, with subsequent replacement of pituitary hormones as indicated. The health care provider then observes the child for the development of related complications, such as hypertension, heart failure, osteoporosis, thickened bones, and delayed sexual development.

Nursing Interventions and Patient Teaching
Nursing interventions primarily include early identification of children who are experiencing increased growth rates compared with other children their age. The child's height is recorded at each visit to the primary health care provider, and a deviation of two or more percentile levels from the median should be reported. The condition causes potential problems with self-image, especially if the child is a preteen who is a great deal taller than peers. Girls usually experience more emotional trauma in this situation than boys do. Be understanding and compassionate regarding the emotional and physical aspects of being taller than their peers.

Early diagnosis of these patients is essential because proper medical management can hinder the height a child will reach. Stress to the parents the importance of regular visits to the pediatrician or pediatric endocrinologist (a health care provider who specializes in endocrinology).

Prognosis
With new medical and surgical advances, the expected life span of these patients is longer than it was previously. The increased risk of cardiovascular and neurological complications result in life expectancy that is still less than average.

DWARFISM
Etiology and Pathophysiology
There are differing types of dwarfism or short stature. The condition may be caused by genetic mutations; GH deficiency; and other, unknown causes. *Hypopituitary dwarfism* is a condition caused by deficiency in GH. Most cases are idiopathic, but a small number can be attributed to an autosomal recessive trait. In some cases, the patients also lack ACTH, TSH, and the gonadotropins.

Clinical Manifestations
Short stature is the most obvious clue to a potential deficiency in GH. These patients are usually well proportioned and well nourished but appear younger than their chronologic age. If a child's height is below the third percentile, there is cause for follow-up. They may have problems with dentition as the permanent teeth erupt, because the jaws are underdeveloped (Mayo Clinic, 2018). Sexual development is usually normal but delayed. Many people with hypopituitary dwarfism are able to reproduce offspring of average height unless there is an accompanying deficiency in gonadotropins. Because only a small number of children with short stature or delayed growth have dwarfism, a thorough diagnostic workup is crucial.

Assessment

Subjective data include the patient's understanding of the disease process and emotional responses to it. A family history of dwarfism may reveal previously successful coping strategies. Encourage the patient to verbalize feelings. Affected children typically have normal intelligence. The child's history usually reveals a normal birth weight. It is important to determine when the child's growth retardation first was noted.

Collection of objective data includes regular measurement of height and weight to determine responses to GH and other hormones that may be administered. Review birth weight and length. Compare current height and weight with standard growth charts, and compare the child's growth pattern with that of siblings and other relatives at a comparable age.

Diagnostic Tests

Diagnostic tests include radiographic evaluation of the skull and skeleton. There is a review of differences between the patient's bone age and chronological age. Significant differences may signal a growth problem. MRI or a CT scan will be used to rule out a pituitary tumor. Definitive diagnosis is based on decreased plasma levels of GH. Note: Restrict the patient's oral intake after midnight for this test. Additional genetic testing may be indicated to distinguish specific types of dwarfism and to help in future family-planning decisions (Mayo Clinic, 2018).

Medical Management

Medical treatment involves replacement of GH by injection and the addition of other hormones as needed to correct deficiencies. If a tumor is the cause of dwarfism, surgery usually is indicated. Nurses should be aware that replacement of GH by injection is expensive and may prevent uninsured or underinsured parents from pursuing this treatment option.

Nursing Interventions and Patient Teaching

Exercise particular care to identify children with growth problems. The health care provider correlates the onset of growth retardation with symptoms of headache, visual disturbances, or behavior changes that may indicate a tumor, so be alert for these symptoms. Avoid making the parents feel guilty about any delay in seeking medical attention for their child.

Encourage the child to wear age-appropriate clothing and engage in activities with peers, because significant problems with self-esteem can occur in dwarfism. Emphasize the child's abilities and strengths instead of his or her physical size. Ensuring that older children and young adults have clothing that is consistent with their peers, fashionable, and age appropriate contributes to their emotional well-being.

Prognosis

Most of these patients lead fairly average lives, and many become parents of average-height children. Complications experienced are often of the musculoskeletal and cardiovascular systems. The life span of a patient with dwarfism is typically normal, depending on the management of complications.

DIABETES INSIPIDUS

Etiology and Pathophysiology

Diabetes insipidus is a metabolic disorder of the pituitary gland. Diabetes insipidus develops when there is a decrease in production of ADH from the posterior pituitary or the action of ADH is diminished. The condition may be transient or permanent. A decrease in ADH causes increased urinary output, which in turn results in dehydration and increased plasma osmolality—that is, a state of imbalance between the electrolyte and fluid components of the plasma.

The condition may be either primary as a result of a deficiency of ADH or secondary due to intracranial tumor, aneurysm, head injury, or infectious process such as encephalitis or meningitis.

Clinical Manifestations

Diabetes insipidus is characterized by significant polyuria (excretion of an abnormally large quantity of urine) and intense polydipsia (excessive thirst). The urine is extremely dilute, looking pale and clear like water. Associated urine specific gravity (the density of urine compared with that of water) is 1.001 to 1.005 (the normal range is 1.003 to 1.030). Normal urinary output is approximately 1.5 L/24 hours. Patients with diabetes insipidus may have a urinary output exceeding the normal volume and be high as 5 to 20 L/24 hours. The patient craves fluids and may drink 4 to 20 L of fluid daily yet still becomes severely dehydrated and has increased levels of sodium in the blood (hypernatremia) because of excess urine output. These patients continue to produce copious quantities of urine when unconscious after surgery or head trauma; if not prevented, diabetes insipidus under these circumstances can lead to hypovolemic shock (failure to adequately perfuse vital organs as a result of insufficient blood volume). Abnormalities in serum electrolytes may lead to changes in level of consciousness, tachycardia, tachypnea, and hypotension. Hypovolemic shock usually follows trauma and consequent blood loss; in these cases, the body increases its release of ADH in an effort to maintain blood volume; in diabetes insipidus–related hypovolemic shock, urinary output remains high rather than decreases.

Assessment

Subjective data include the patient's understanding of the relationship of symptoms (such as thirst and polyuria) to the underlying cause. The patient should be able to state the importance of not restricting oral fluids. Assess the severity of thirst. The patient may be embarrassed about the constant need to drink and then empty the bladder and voluntarily may restrict social contacts and work activities. The patient is weak, tired, and lethargic. Assessment of the patient should include symptoms indicating an electrolyte imbalance.

Collection of objective data includes assessment of skin turgor (the normal resiliency of the skin) and color and specific gravity of the urine and vital signs. Carefully monitor intake and output (I&O). The skin is dry, turgor is poor, and body weight is lost. Constipation may occur from lack of fluid in the bowel. Weigh the patient daily in the early morning, before breakfast. Determine whether the patient has nocturia because this may interrupt sleep patterns.

Diagnostic Tests

Diagnosis is based on clinical manifestations, urine specific gravity, and urine ADH measurement. The urine specific gravity often drops below 1.003, and the serum sodium level increases to more than 145 mEq/L (normal serum sodium level is 135 to 145 mEq/L). Because of hemoconcentration the serum osmolality may be greater than 300 mOsm/kg (normal is 280 to 300 mOsm/kg). The fluid deprivation (water deprivation) test may be ordered to determine how well the pituitary is producing ADH and to help rule out other causes. This test involves withholding fluids for a period of up to 12 hours. During the testing period, urine specific gravity and serum osmolality frequently are measured, as well as orthostatic vital signs. Beginning and ending weights also are obtained for comparison. A CT scan and radiographic evaluation of the sella turcica (the "Turkish saddle"–shaped depression in the sphenoid bone that houses the pituitary gland) may be done to help evaluate the pituitary structures.

Medical Management

Medical treatment involves intravenous (IV), subcutaneous, intranasal, or oral administration of synthetic ADH preparations in the form of desmopressin acetate (1-deamino-8-D-arginine vasopressin, or DDAVP). Coffee, tea, and other beverages containing caffeine usually are eliminated from the diet because of their possible diuretic effect. If the patient cannot match the urinary losses through oral intake, he or she is at risk for dehydration and severe hypernatremia. IV fluids of hypotonic saline or dextrose 5% in water are needed. Serum electrolyte levels require monitoring and management.

Nursing Interventions and Patient Teaching

Specific nursing interventions are aimed at protecting the patient from injury. The patient likely is fatigued from frequent ambulation to the bathroom to void and impaired sleep pattern. The patient may be at risk for injury or falls secondary to fatigue, exhaustion, and electrolyte imbalances. Carefully monitor the patient's I&O and document. Assess skin turgor frequently,

along with the condition of oral mucous membranes. Weigh the patient and record I&O daily. Do not limit oral fluids in an effort to reduce urinary output. Foods and beverages that promote diuresis, such as caffeine, should be avoided.

A patient problem and interventions for the patient with diabetes insipidus include but are not limited to the following:

PATIENT PROBLEM	NURSING INTERVENTIONS
Potential for Inadequate Fluid Volume, related to excessive urine production	Assess for signs and symptoms of dehydration (dry oral mucous membranes, poor skin turgor, soft eyeballs, lowered blood pressure, rapid pulse) Monitor electrolyte status carefully Measure I&O

Instruct the patient to wear some form of medical alert identification, such as a necklace or bracelet, stating the potential for and diagnosis of diabetes insipidus. Stress that the patient must remain under medical supervision for monitoring of the metabolic state because the condition may worsen with time.

Prognosis

The prognosis depends on the cause. Patients who survive usually are dependent on medication for the rest of their lives. With proper treatment, most patients can expect to live a relatively normal life.

SYNDROME OF INAPPROPRIATE ANTIDIURETIC HORMONE

Syndrome of inappropriate ADH (SIADH) occurs when the pituitary gland releases too much ADH. In response to ADH, the kidneys reabsorb more water, decreasing urinary output and expanding the body's fluid volume. The patient experiences hyponatremia (low sodium), hemodilution, and fluid overload without peripheral edema.

Etiology and Pathophysiology

ADH regulates the body's water balance. Synthesized in the hypothalamus, ADH is stored in the posterior pituitary gland. When released into the circulation, it acts on the kidneys' distal tubules and collecting ducts, increasing their permeability to water. This decreases urine volume, because more water is reabsorbed and returned to the circulation, which increases blood volume.

When the body's system of checks and balances malfunctions—whether from a tumor, medication, unrelated disease process, or some other cause—ADH may be released continuously, causing SIADH, which occurs more commonly in older adults.

ADH is released in response to stress. Be alert to patients who have the following risk factors and who are also in pain or undergoing stressful procedures:

- Medications, including anesthetics, opiates, barbiturates, thiazide diuretics, and oral hypoglycemics

- Malignancies (the most common cause of SIADH; cancerous cells are capable of producing, storing, and releasing ADH)
- Nonmalignant pulmonary diseases, including chronic obstructive pulmonary disease, tuberculosis, lung abscesses, and pneumonia
- Nervous system disorders, including head trauma, cerebral vascular accident, encephalitis, meningitis, and Guillain-Barré syndrome
- Miscellaneous causes, including lupus erythematous, adrenal insufficiency, and thyroid and parathyroid deficiencies

Clinical Manifestations

Clinically, SIADH is characterized by hyponatremia and water retention that progresses to water intoxication. The severity of the patient's condition is linked primarily to the sodium levels and the location of fluid accumulation. Most signs and symptoms appear when serum sodium levels fall below 125 mEq/L. Signs and symptoms include nausea, vomiting, irritability, confusion, tremors, seizures, stupor, coma, and pathologic reflexes.

Assessment

Subjective data include vague complaints. Hyponatremia triggers the earliest symptoms, which are nonspecific and could indicate other disorders. Assess for complaints or reports of cramping, anorexia, nausea, and headaches.

Collection of objective data includes assessment for hyponatremia. Fluid intake exceeds urinary output. The patient does not develop peripheral edema, because excess fluid is accumulating in the vascular system, not in the interstitial spaces; therefore, weight gain is not always noted with SIADH.

As water intoxication progresses and the patient's serum becomes more hypotonic, brain cells expand (become edematous), and as a result the later signs of SIADH are neurologic. The patient becomes progressively lethargic, with marked personality changes. The patient has seizures, and the deep tendon reflexes diminish or disappear altogether.

All electrolyte levels should be monitored and the patient assessed often for signs and symptoms of increases and decreases in electrolytes, either from the disease process or the implementing of treatments for correction.

Diagnostic Tests

The diagnosis of SIADH is made by simultaneous measurements of urine and serum osmolality. Serum osmolality is less than 280 mmol/kg (normal is 285 to 295 mOsm/kg). Laboratory tests show hyponatremia (sodium less than 134 mEq/L). The serum is diluted and the urine is concentrated. Urine specific gravity is greater than 1.032, and urine sodium is elevated because of concentration.

Medical Management

Fluid restrictions are necessary. Initially this limitation is 800 to 1000 mL/day. If severe hyponatremia persists, fluid intake may be further restricted. The health care provider orders fluid restriction, initially 800 to 1000 mL/day. Daily fluid intake should equal fluid output. If fluid restriction is adequate, tests show a gradual increase in serum sodium along with a decrease in body weight.

An IV hypertonic saline solution (3% to 5%) may be administered. The infusion is used to both correct sodium imbalances and pull fluids from edematous brain cells. The infusion rate is limited to avoid rapid rises in sodium levels.

The health care provider may order medications such as demeclocycline, a tetracycline derivative, and lithium carbonate. Both drugs interfere with the antidiuretic action of ADH and cause polyuria. Diuretics such as furosemide (Lasix) may be administered orally or intravenously to eliminate excess fluid, but only if the serum sodium is at least 125 mEq/L, or the drug may promote more loss of sodium. Taking furosemide increases losses of potassium, magnesium, and calcium; supplements may be needed.

Treatment also must be directed at eliminating the underlying problem. Surgical resection, radiation, or chemotherapy may be indicated for malignant neoplasms. If the causative factor is a medication, it is discontinued.

Monitoring the patient for signs and symptoms of further electrolyte imbalances is a priority nursing assessment. I&O should be monitored to ensure there is no significant fluid overload or signs of dehydration.

Nursing Interventions and Patient Teaching

The goals of nursing care are focused on assessment of the condition with documentation and reporting of changes. Timing of the assessment frequency is based on the patient's condition. Perform a neurologic examination and assess the patient's hydration status frequently. Auscultate lung sounds; crackles indicate fluid overload. Monitor the patient's oxygen saturation frequently. Carefully observe serum electrolytes, urine sodium, and urine specific gravity because overcorrection can cause hypernatremia. Weigh the patient daily and closely monitor I&O; output is the primary guide to regulating fluid intake.

Restriction of fluid intake prevents fluid overload. Provide and frequently reinforce education. Solicit patient input in scheduling fluid allotments and types of fluids. Patients on diuretic therapy may require supplementation of sodium and potassium. Instruct patients to avoid foods high in sodium content, which may promote thirstiness.

Use simple explanations when detailing the plan of care because anxiety can aggravate SIADH. If the patient reports nausea, obtain an order for an antiemetic before administration.

Patient problems and interventions for the patient with SIADH include but are not limited to the following:

PATIENT PROBLEM	NURSING INTERVENTIONS
Fluid Volume Overload, related to decreased urinary output	Obtain daily weight, same scales, same time Assess and record I&O Monitor laboratory results Administer medications as ordered Maintain dietary and fluid restrictions (fluids should be high in sodium; avoid salty foods) Monitor IV infusions (such as 3%–5% sodium chloride over several hours)
Potential for Compromised Oral Mucous Membranes, related to fluid restrictions of 500 mL/day	Provide frequent oral care; avoid alcohol-based mouthwashes Allow patient to choose fluids and to divide the allotted amount (such as half in morning, one-third in evening, and the remainder at night)

Patient teaching should be an ongoing part of nursing care. Be certain the patient understands the treatment plan, the rationale behind it, and the expected outcome. Provide information about signs and symptoms of SIADH, and tell the patient to alert the health care provider if any changes are noted. SIADH can recur after discharge.

Prognosis
SIADH resulting from an adverse reaction to medication, or secondary to a head trauma, is self-limiting. The ability to manage metabolic conditions determines the chronicity of the disease. SIADH is potentially dangerous but treatable. Early diagnosis and medical management improve the prognosis.

DISORDERS OF THE THYROID AND PARATHYROID GLANDS

HYPERTHYROIDISM
Etiology and Pathophysiology
Hyperthyroidism—also called *Graves disease,* exophthalmic goiter, and thyrotoxicosis—is a condition in which there is increased activity of the thyroid gland, with overproduction of the thyroid hormones T_3 and T_4, resulting in an exaggeration of metabolic processes. Graves disease (the most common cause of hyperthyroidism) occurs most frequently in women in the 20- to 40-year-old age group. Two percent of the female population is affected by Graves disease, compared with 0.2% of the male population. Graves disease is an autoimmune disorder of unknown cause.

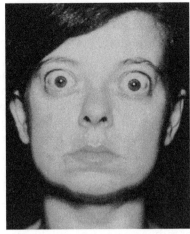

Fig. 11.6 Exophthalmos of Graves disease. (From Seidel HM, Ball JW, Dains JE, et al: *Mosby's guide to physical examination,* ed 5, St. Louis, 2003, Mosby.)

Clinical Manifestations
Clinical manifestations will range from mild to severe. The neck will display visible edema in the anterior region as a result of the enlarged thyroid. In severe cases, periorbital edema will cause exophthalmos (bulging of the eyeballs) (Fig. 11.6). The classic finding of exophthalmos occurs in 20% to 40% of patients with Graves disease. Exophthalmos is when the eyeballs are forced outward, resulting in incomplete closure of the eyelids; the exposed corneas become dry, with subsequent development of corneal ulcers and loss of vision.

Assessment
Subjective complaints of the patient include difficulty with mental focus and concentration and short-term memory loss. The patient may complain of dysphagia or may be hoarse. Unplanned weight loss is noted despite reports of a strong appetite. The patient reports feeling nervous, jittery, and excitable and may experience insomnia. Assess the patient for complaints of "heart palpitations" or other cardiac concerns, such as shortness of breath. These patients are emotionally labile and may overreact to stressful situations.

Objective data include changes in vital signs. The pulse is usually rapid, blood pressure is elevated, with cardiac arrhythmias noted. A bruit may be auscultated over the thyroid. The skin is warm and flushed, and the hair becomes fine and brittle. Female patients may cease to menstruate. Elevated body temperature may be accompanied by intolerance to heat, with profuse diaphoresis. The patient may have an increase in bowel movements. Note tremors of the hands. Behavior changes may include hyperactivity and clumsiness. Daily weighing usually shows weight loss.

Diagnostic Tests
The thyroid is controlled by the hypothalamus. Under normal conditions the thyroid secretes T_3 and T_4 in

response to TSH released by the pituitary. As the T_3 and T_4 levels in the blood increase, the pituitary stops secreting TSH—an example of the negative feedback loop described earlier in this chapter.

If the thyroid becomes impaired, its hormone secretion may not respond normally to TSH. It may secrete too much (hyperthyroidism) or too little (hypothyroidism) T_3 and T_4. Hyperthyroidism is confirmed by a decrease in TSH level (because the overactive thyroid is releasing high amounts of T_3 and T_4, which exert negative feedback on the pituitary gland, causing it to stop secreting TSH) and an elevation of the level of free T_4 (FT_4). Total T_3 and T_4 levels may be evaluated but are not as helpful in the diagnosis. Additional diagnostic tests include radioactive iodine uptake scans and thyroid scans, typically performed in an outpatient setting (Box 11.1).

Medical Management

Ablation therapy using radioactive iodine is the gold standard for treating hyperthyroidism. The goal is to destroy enough of the hypertrophied thyroid tissue to produce a normally functioning thyroid gland. Dosing is patient specific and often results in the development of hypothyroidism. The therapeutic dose of radioactive iodine is low, so no radiation safety precautions are necessary, with the exception of danger to pregnant women providing care.

Medical management for hyperthyroidism may include daily administration of drugs that block the production of thyroid hormones, such as propylthiouracil (PTU) or methimazole (Tapazole) (Table 11.2). The patient usually begins to notice a decrease in symptoms within 6 to 8 weeks after starting drug therapy. This may be followed after the acute stage by ablation therapy using a therapeutic dose of radioactive iodine ($Na^{131}I$ or $Na^{125}I$), based on the patient's age, clinical manifestations, and estimated weight of the thyroid.

Because of the possible development of hypothyroidism after this treatment, the patient must have adequate follow-up medical supervision. If a patient develops hypothyroidism after treatment, levothyroxine therapy will be needed. NOTE: ^{131}I is not a radiation hazard to the non-pregnant patient but absolutely is contraindicated during pregnancy. Pregnant health care professionals should not care for this patient for several days after treatment.

Surgery has fallen out of favor because of possible serious complications, such as hemorrhage, hypoparathyroidism, and vocal cord paralysis. Surgery still may be indicated for patients who cannot tolerate antithyroid drugs, are not good candidates for radioactive iodine therapy, have a possible malignancy, or have large goiters causing tracheal compression.

Surgical treatment for hyperthyroidism is subtotal thyroidectomy, a procedure in which approximately five-sixths of the thyroid is removed. If too much

---

Box 11.1   Diagnostic Tests for Hyperthyroidism

- T_3 (serum triiodothyronine): Measures the T_3 level in the blood. The normal level is 65–195 ng/dL. As with serum thyroxine (T_4), the serum T_3 level provides an accurate measurement of thyroid function. T_3 is less stable than T_4; an elevated T_3 determination is clinically important in the patient who has a normal T_4 level but has all the signs and symptoms of hyperthyroidism. In this patient the test may identify T_3 thyrotoxicosis.

- T_4 (serum thyroxine): Measures the T_4 level in the blood. The normal level is 5–12 mcg/dL. Some medications such as oral contraceptives, steroids, estrogens, and sulfonamides may be withheld for several hours before the T_3 and T_4 tests, but food and fluids are not withheld. Elevated levels of these tests usually indicate hyperthyroidism.

- Free T_4 (FT_4): Measures the active component of total T_4. Normal values are 1–3.5 ng/dL. Because this level remains constant, this is considered a better indication of function than T_4 and is useful in diagnosing hyperthyroidism and hypothyroidism. High FT_4 suggests hyperthyroidism; low FT_4 suggests hypothyroidism.

- Thyroid-stimulating hormone (TSH): Measures the level of TSH. Normal values are 0.3–5.4 mcg/mL. This is considered the most sensitive method for evaluating thyroid disease. It is generally recommended as the first diagnostic test for thyroid dysfunction. TSH is suppressed in hyperthyroidism and elevated in hypothyroidism.

- Radioactive iodine uptake (RAIU) test: Radioactive iodine, ^{131}I, is given by mouth to the fasting patient. After 2, 6, and 24 h, a scintillation camera is held over the thyroid to measure how much of the isotope has been removed from the bloodstream. A hyperactive thyroid may remove 35%–95% of the drug. This test may be affected by prior ingestion of iodine-containing substances or foods. A signed consent form is required for this test. Also note any allergy to iodine on the request form, along with medications currently being taken. No radiation precautions are necessary, except to ensure that pregnant health care professionals do not come in close contact with the patient.

- Thyroid scan: ^{131}I is given to the patient either orally or intravenously. If an intravenous dose is given, the scan may be done in 30–60 min. A scintillation camera positioned over the patient's thyroid sends images that are received on an oscilloscope and may be printed out on special paper. A signed consent form is required for this test. No radiation precautions are necessary.

---

tissue is taken, the gland will not regenerate after surgery, and hypothyroidism will result. Surgery usually is delayed, if possible, until the patient is in a normal thyroid (euthyroid) state because of the risk of excessive bleeding during thyroidectomy and postoperative thyroid crisis.

Patients with mild hyperthyroidism are admitted rarely to the acute care hospital. They are treated by

Table 11.2 Medications Commonly Used to Treat Hyperthyroidism and Hypothyroidism

MEDICATIONS	COMMON SIDE EFFECTS
Hyperthyroidism	
Iodine or iodine products (potassium or sodium iodide with strong iodine solution, potassium iodide, Lugol solution)	Nausea, vomiting, diarrhea, abdominal pain
Radioactive iodine (^{131}I or ^{125}I)	Sore throat, edema or pain in neck, temporary loss of taste, nausea, vomiting, painful salivary glands
Methimazole (Tapazole), propylthiouracil (PTU)	Rash or pruritus, vertigo, nausea, vomiting, loss of taste, paresthesias, abdominal pain
Hypothyroidism	
Levothyroxine (Synthroid, Eltroxin, Levo-T, Unithroid) Liothyronine (Cytomel) Liotrix (Thyrolar) Thyroid (Armour Thyroid, Thyrar)	Nervousness, irritability, tremors, insomnia, tachycardia, hypertension, palpitations, cardiac dysrhythmias, vomiting, diarrhea, nausea, appetite changes, weight loss, menstrual irregularities, leg cramps, fever

the health care provider in an office or clinic setting. However, the hospital nurse may come in contact with the hyperthyroid patient admitted for a different condition and also may care for these patients before and after thyroidectomy.

Nursing Interventions and Patient Teaching

The hyperthyroid patient needs more nutrients because of increased metabolism. Diet therapy usually consists of food high in protein. Increased vitamins (especially the B vitamins), minerals, and carbohydrates also are indicated. Losses in bone density may be attributed to hyperthyroidism. Supplementation with calcium and vitamin D is indicated to avoid the development of osteoporosis. Offer between-meal snacks. Food should be soft and easily swallowed if the patient has dysphagia (difficulty swallowing). Coffee, tea, and colas should be avoided because of their stimulant effect.

Preoperative teaching is extremely important for the patient who is scheduled for a thyroidectomy. Keep the environment as stable as possible to prevent increased stimulation. Include instructions on how to properly support the head while turning in bed or rising to a sitting or standing position. The nurse (or patient) places both hands behind the head and maintains anatomic position while the rest of the body is being moved. Also teach the patient to deep breathe. The health care provider determines whether postoperative coughing

is allowed because it strains the suture line. Inform the patient that a period of "voice rest" may be enforced for 48 hours postoperatively and that pencil and paper will be provided for writing notes instead of talking. Do voice checks every 2 to 4 hours, as ordered by the health care provider, to rule out damage to the laryngeal nerve resulting in inability to speak. Ask the patient to say "ah" and check for excessive hoarseness or voice change. Slight hoarseness is expected and should not cause alarm. Damage to the laryngeal nerve during surgery occurs in approximately 12.4% of cases, but the damage is not always permanent.

Postoperative management includes keeping the patient in a semi-Fowler's position, to decrease edema at the operative site and to enhance respiratory status, with pillows supporting the head and shoulders. Caution the patient to avoid hyperextending the head to prevent excess tension on the incision, which usually is made in a horizontal crease in the anterior neck. Have a suction apparatus and tracheotomy tray available for emergency use. A cool-mist humidifier at the bedside may help soothe the throat and prevent coughing. Check vital signs frequently, with special attention paid to the rate and depth of respirations and observations for any dyspnea (shortness of breath or difficulty breathing) related to edema in the operative site. Before giving any liquid orally, be sure the swallowing and cough reflexes have returned. Be alert for signs of internal or external bleeding; early signs of internal bleeding include restlessness, apprehension, increased pulse rate, decreased blood pressure, and a feeling of fullness in the neck. Later, cyanosis may develop, signaling an obstructed airway; provide for adequate airway management and notify the surgeon immediately. Inspect the dressing on the neck frequently for obvious external bleeding. Also check for bleeding at the sides and back of the neck and on top of the patient's shoulders because oozing blood may pool there as a result of gravity. Most surgeons allow a dressing to be reinforced as needed and loosened slightly if the patient complains that it is too tight.

Postoperatively, the diet initially consists of clear, cool liquids, progressing to soft food as tolerated. This is followed by a regular diet as soon as possible to help the patient regain lost weight and correct any nutritional deficiencies.

Another significant postoperative complication after thyroidectomy is tetany. One possible cause of tetany is the inadvertent removal of one or more of the parathyroid glands during surgery. Another is edema in the operative area, which occludes release of PTH into the bloodstream, resulting in a low serum calcium level (normal serum calcium is 9.0 to 10.5 mg/dL). The symptoms include numbness and tingling in the fingertips and toes and around the mouth. The patient also may have *carpopedal spasms* (muscle spasms in the wrists and feet) and increased pulse, respirations, and blood pressure, accompanied by anxiety and agitation.

Laryngeal spasm and stridor may occur. **Chvostek sign** is a clinical sign of abnormal spasm of the facial muscles when elicited by light taps on the facial nerve, which is located at the angle of the jaw. This is seen in patients who are experiencing hypocalcemia. **Trousseau sign** assesses for latent tetany, which is a carpal spasm that is induced by inflating a sphygmomanometer cuff on the upper arm to a pressure exceeding systolic blood pressure for 3 minutes; a positive result may be seen in hypocalcemia and hypomagnesemia. If untreated, the condition may progress to convulsions or lethal cardiac dysrhythmias. Emergency treatment of tetany is the IV administration of calcium gluconate, which always should be available postoperatively.

The other serious complication after thyroidectomy is thyroid crisis, or thyroid storm. Fortunately, it occurs rarely and usually can be attributed to manipulation of the thyroid during surgery, which causes the release of large amounts of thyroid hormones into the bloodstream. If thyroid crisis occurs, it usually does so within the first 12 hours postoperatively. In thyroid crisis, all the signs and symptoms of hyperthyroidism are exaggerated. In addition, the patient may develop nausea, vomiting, severe tachycardia, severe hypertension, and occasionally hyperthermia up to 106°F (41°C). Extreme restlessness, cardiac dysrhythmia, and delirium also may occur. The patient may develop heart failure as evidenced by decreased cardiac output secondary to cardiac strain and tachycardia. Diagnostic tests indicate increased FT_4 and decreased TSH.

The three goals of thyroid storm management are (1) to induce a normal thyroid state, (2) prevent cardiovascular collapse, and (3) prevent excessive hyperthermia. Emergency treatment of thyroid crisis includes administration of IV fluids, sodium iodide, corticosteroids, antipyretics, an antithyroid drug (such as PTU or methimazole), and oxygen as needed. Prompt, adequate treatment usually results in dramatic improvement within 12 to 24 hours.

Patient problems and interventions for the patient having a thyroidectomy include but are not limited to the following:

PATIENT PROBLEM	NURSING INTERVENTIONS
PREOPERATIVE	
Potential for Elevated Body Temperature, related to increased metabolism	Assess body temperature at regular intervals
	Regulate environment (room temperature, linens, clothing) to help keep patient comfortable
	Administer acetaminophen as prescribed
Insufficient Nutrition, related to increased metabolism	Encourage patient to eat prescribed diet and avoid caffeine
	Assess daily weight and food intake

PATIENT PROBLEM	NURSING INTERVENTIONS
POSTOPERATIVE	
Compromised Swallowing Ability, related to postoperative edema	Ensure swallowing and cough reflexes are present before oral intake
	Encourage patient to drink slowly and chew food thoroughly
Potential for Inability to Maintain Adequate Breathing Pattern, related to:	Monitor rate and depth of respirations
• Postoperative edema	Assess breath sounds and skin color
• Pain	Encourage slow, deep breaths at least hourly
	Position patient to maximize respiratory effort

Patient education after thyroidectomy includes stressing the importance of follow-up medical supervision. Thyroid function tests are done periodically to assess thyroid hormone levels. Before discharge, teach the patient proper care of the incision site and symptoms that may indicate development of an infection, in which case he or she should notify the surgeon immediately. Discuss with the patient the need for a high-calorie, high-protein, high-carbohydrate diet until weight is stable.

Prognosis

With adequate, appropriate medical or surgical treatment, these patients usually have a normal life expectancy. If exophthalmos is present, it may not completely resolve.

HYPOTHYROIDISM

Etiology and Pathophysiology

Hypothyroidism is one of the most common medical disorders in the United States. It occurs most often in women 30 to 60 years of age and is more common in older adults than previously thought. Hypothyroidism occurs when the thyroid fails to secrete sufficient hormones, slowing all of the body's metabolic processes. Causes include an autoimmune response, radiation therapy, pituitary disorders, or iodine deficiency. It sometimes results from medical or surgical treatment of hyperthyroidism (Mayo Clinic, 2020c). *Myxedema* denotes severe hypothyroidism in adults. It is characterized by edema of the hands, face, feet, and periorbital tissues. Congenital hypothyroidism is called *cretinism* and is estimated to occur in 1 of every 200 to 4000 births. The majority of these occurrences results when the thyroid does not develop in utero (NLM, 2020b). All infants in the United States are screened for decreased thyroid function at birth.

Clinical Manifestations

Clinical manifestations will depend upon the degree of the thyroid hormone deficiency. The absence of an adequate amount of thyroid hormone causes the body's metabolic processes to slow, resulting in decreased production of body heat, intolerance to cold, and weight gain. Atherosclerotic changes may result in coronary artery disease. Hypothyroidism may have adverse effects on the heart, with decreased cardiac output and contractility; the patient experiences decreased exercise tolerance and dyspnea on exertion. Early signs are weight gain, difficulty concentrating, constipation, and fluid/weight gain. Late signs include mood swings, infertility (in women), acute fatigue syndrome, and depression.

Assessment

Subjective data include a discussion of the patient's mental and emotional status. Reports of feelings of depression, paranoia, memory impairment, and as if their thought processes are sluggish are associated with hypothyriodism. Speech and hearing may be deficient. The patient is lethargic, forgetful, and irritable. Because of the body's slowed metabolism, cold intolerance, anorexia, and constipation may develop. Both men and women may experience decreased libido and reproductive difficulty.

Collection of objective data includes assessment of the skin and hair. Thinning hair and potential alopecia may be noted. The integument is dry and thickened. Facial features may enlarge to give the patient an edematous appearance with a masklike facial expression. The voice is characteristically low and hoarse. Decreased metabolism usually causes bradycardia, decreased blood pressure and respirations, and exercise intolerance. The patient has decreased ability to perform activities because of weakness, clumsiness, and ataxia. Assess the respiratory rate after administration of any central nervous system depressant. Evaluate the abdomen for distention because *myxedema ileus* (intestinal obstruction) may occur. Menorrhagia (excessive menstrual flow) is a frequent complaint of women with hypothyroidism. Infertility may result from the inhibition of ovulation.

Diagnostic Tests

Diagnosis of hypothyroidism is based on the physical examination and history and on appropriate laboratory tests, such as TSH, T_3, T_4, and FT_4 levels. Low levels of T_3, T_4, and FT_4 provide the underlying stimuli for TSH secretion. A compensatory elevation of TSH occurs in patients with primary hypothyroid states, and low levels of T_3, T_4, and FT_4 are present. Subclinical cases may go undiagnosed for years, so be aware of subtle clues while interviewing and caring for the patient.

Medical Management

Hypothyroidism is treated with hormone replacement therapy using desiccated animal thyroid (Armour Thyroid), T_4, or synthetic products such as levothyroxine (Levothroid, Synthroid, Levo-T) (see Table 11.2). Synthetic products typically are preferred over biological agents to treat hypothyroidism. The drugs usually are given in the morning to enhance nutrient

metabolism of ingested food during the daily meals. Teach the patient to take levothyroxine on an empty stomach. The patient initially is given a small dose, with increases as necessary until the desired effect is achieved. A maintenance dosage then is established. Early in treatment, the hormone level should be monitored about every 6 to 8 weeks until the patient's TSH level is normal and then tested at least annually. Monitor for adverse effects of drug therapy, which mimic the signs and symptoms of hyperthyroidism. The changes in the patient after the onset of therapy may be dramatic. Lifelong thyroid replacement therapy usually is required, as well as laboratory monitoring of T_3, T_4, and TSH levels to adjust the dosage and minimize the effects of hypothyroidism or hyperthyroidism as a result of a too-high dosage.

Nursing Interventions and Patient Teaching

Nursing interventions for the hospitalized patient with severe hypothyroidism focus on symptom management. Keep the room at least 70°F to 74°F (21°C to 23°C). Ensure the patient does not become chilled during bathing or other procedures. Allow extra time for physical care so that the patient does not feel rushed. Keep accurate records of bowel elimination because constipation may be severe. Stool softeners and bulk laxatives may be ordered. Provide a high-protein, high-fiber, low-calorie diet, and encourage increased fluid intake. The patient should avoid concentrated carbohydrates, such as sweets, to help prevent excessive weight gain. Monitor vital signs. Changes to heart rate and rhythm may signa cardiac involvement. Instruct patient to report chest pain or dyspnea. Caution the patient to not stop taking the thyroid hormone without consulting a health care provider. This medication must be taken for the rest of the patient's life. Because most patients with hypothyroidism are more susceptible to the effects of sedatives, hypnotics, and anesthetics, be alert for possible adverse effects if these agents are given.

Teach the patient to take the thyroid hormone on a consistent schedule, typically in the morning on an empty stomach. Taking the medication with food, vitamins, and minerals can impair absorption. In addition, the patient should inform the health care provider if the diet typically contains soybean flour, cottonseed oil, or walnuts, which can impair absorption.

Patient problems and interventions for the patient with hypothyroidism include but are not limited to the following:

PATIENT PROBLEM	NURSING INTERVENTIONS
Insufficient Cardiac Output, related to decreased metabolism	Assess pulse, blood pressure, skin color, and temperature
	Schedule nursing activities around patient's activity cycle, with rest periods as needed to conserve energy

PATIENT PROBLEM	NURSING INTERVENTIONS
Infrequent or Difficult Bowel Elimination, related to decreased peristaltic action	Assess frequency and character of stools Encourage increased intake of oral fluids and high-fiber foods

Regular checkups are essential to monitor labs and modify drug dosage as needed. Patient education topics include medication therapy. Discuss desired effects and potential side effects warranting reporting to the healthcare provider. Instruct the patient to eat well-balanced meals of high-fiber foods, such as fruits, vegetables, and whole-grain cereals and breads. The patient also needs an adequate intake of iodine, found in foods such as saltwater fish, milk, and eggs. Increased fluid intake helps prevent constipation. Tell the patient and the family that mental and physical slowness may still be present but should improve with thyroid replacement therapy.

Prognosis

Most patients with hypothyroidism do well with proper medical supervision, although they probably will have to take medication for the rest of their lives. In children, when T_4 replacement begins before epiphyseal fusion, the chance for normal growth is improved greatly.

SIMPLE (COLLOID) GOITER

Etiology and Pathophysiology

A simple, or colloid, goiter develops when the thyroid gland enlarges in response to low iodine levels in the bloodstream or when it is unable to use iodine properly. When the blood level of T_3 is too low to signal the pituitary to decrease TSH secretion, the thyroid gland responds by increasing the formation of thyroglobulin (colloid), which accumulates in the thyroid follicles and causes the gland to enlarge (Fig. 11.7). Most cases of simple goiter can be attributed to insufficient dietary intake of iodine, leading to this overgrowth of thyroid tissue.

Clinical Manifestations

The patient usually has no manifestations of overt thyroid dysfunction, and the diagnosis is based on the patient's physical appearance.

Assessment

Subjective data include the patient's emotional response to the unsightly enlargement of the thyroid. Encourage the patient to talk about his or her feelings. The patient may complain only of symptoms of dysphagia, hoarseness, or dyspnea related to the pressure of the enlarged gland against the esophagus and trachea. Dysphagia may make it difficult to eat and drink adequate amounts. Assess the patient for increasing dyspnea. Determine the patient's understanding of

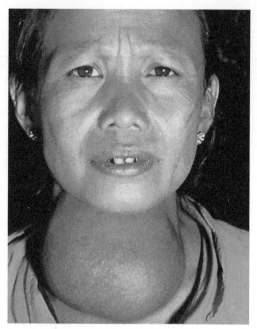

Fig. 11.7 Simple goiter. (Courtesy L.V. Bergman & Associates, Inc., Cold Spring, New York.)

the need for medication, diet therapy, and medical follow-up.

Collection of objective data includes assessment of increased goiter size, voice changes, and adequacy of food and fluid intake.

Diagnostic Testing

Diagnostic testing includes a thyroid scan or an ultrasound of the thyroid gland to determine function and structure. Serum tests to evaluate T_3, T_4, and TSH levels also are completed.

Medical Management

The thyroid may be only slightly enlarged, or it may be so enlarged that surgery is necessary to improve respiration or swallowing. Surgery also is performed sometimes for cosmetic effect, because this type of goiter can be unsightly and damage the patient's self-image and self-esteem. Lugol solution is one antihyperthyroid agent used in conjunction with other antihyperthyroid medications, to decrease or shrink the thyroid gland, typically before surgery. It also is used in cases in which surgical removal of the thyroid gland is not feasible or must be delayed (NLM, 2021).

If thyroidectomy is completed, most of the gland is removed. Medical treatment consists of oral administration of potassium iodide and foods high in iodine (such as seafood, seaweed, dairy, grains, iodized salt, and eggs) (Office of Dietary Supplements, 2021b).

Nursing Interventions and Patient Teaching

Nursing interventions after thyroidectomy (previously discussed) are aimed at prevention of complications such as bleeding, tetany, and thyroid crisis.

Patient problems and interventions for the patient with simple (colloid) goiter include but are not limited to the following:

PATIENT PROBLEM	NURSING INTERVENTIONS
Potential for Noncooperation or Nonconformity	Provide opportunities for patient to express feelings about treatment plan Correct misconceptions and reinforce previous medical instruction Stress importance of taking prescribed medications, having regular checkups, and avoiding any identified goitrogenic foods
Potential for Distorted Body Image, related to altered physical appearance	Develop open and trusting relationship so that the patient will express his or her feelings Discuss ways to disguise thyroid enlargement (scarves, high collars) Encourage and offer support groups for patients with similar situations

Stress the importance of adequate dietary intake of iodine by the patient. Medical supervision is recommended at regular intervals.

Prognosis

Most patients can expect to live a normal life after adequate treatment of goiter. If the thyroid becomes inactive, a diagnosis of hypothyroidism is made, and the patient is treated with conventional replacement therapy medications.

CANCER OF THE THYROID

Etiology and Pathophysiology

Cancer of the thyroid is a relatively rare malignancy. In 2020, nearly 53,000 new cases and more than 2100 deaths were reported. Risk factors include diets low in iodine (not common in the United States), radiation exposure, obesity, and gender. Whites are affected more often than other races. Women are impacted more than three times more often than men. For women, the diagnosis is more often made between the ages of 40 and 50 years. Cases in men are normally diagnosed between 60 and 70 years of age.

Clinical Manifestations

The principal clinical manifestation of thyroid cancer is a firm, fixed, small, rounded, painless mass or *nodule* that is felt during palpation of the gland. Only in rare instances are the symptoms of hyperthyroidism seen.

Assessment

Subjective data include the patient's use of adaptive coping methods to deal with the diagnosis. Also observe the support system provided by the patient's significant others. Assess the patient's understanding of the importance of medical follow-up, and for reports of trouble breathing, hoarseness, or difficulty in swallowing.

Objective data include progressive enlargement of the tumor area preoperatively, response to ^{131}I therapy, and skin involvement in the neck and torso after radiation therapy. Assess for trachea and vocal cord involvement as well.

Diagnostic Tests

Papillary thyroid cancer is suspected when a thyroid scan shows a "cold" nodule, indicating decreased uptake of ^{131}I. Benign adenomas and follicular cancers usually are visualized as "hot" nodules because of their increased uptake of the isotope. Thyroid function tests usually yield normal results. The health care provider uses ultrasound and CT scans of the thyroid to further investigate the thyroid and surrounding tissue. If the parathyroid gland is involved, the serum calcium level may be elevated as well. To confirm the diagnosis, a thyroid needle biopsy may be completed, but only by a skilled health care provider to avoid seeding of adjacent tissues. Metastasis could result, with the prognosis becoming much more grave.

Medical Management

Treatment of thyroid cancer is a total thyroidectomy, with subsequent lifelong thyroid hormone replacement therapy. If metastasis is present at the time of the initial surgery, a radical neck dissection may be performed. In addition, radiation therapy, chemotherapy, and administration of radioactive ^{131}I may be done.

Nursing Interventions and Patient Teaching

Nursing interventions are like those for the patient who has undergone thyroidectomy (see the previous section, "Hyperthyroidism"). As with a thyroidectomy for noncancerous lesions, the major postoperative complications are respiratory distress, recurrent laryngeal damage, hemorrhage, and hypoparathyroidism. Assess the patient's oxygen saturation, voice tone and presence, and surgical site and monitor for signs and symptoms of hypothyroidism and hypoparathyroidism, including serum calcium levels. Assess the posterior neck area as well. The drainage from the incision may pool at the posterior neck and not be obvious from the anterior view.

Patient problems and interventions for the patient with cancer of the thyroid include but are not limited to the following:

PATIENT PROBLEM	NURSING INTERVENTIONS
Anxiousness, related to situational crisis	Encourage patient to discuss feelings about upcoming surgery Monitor level of anxiety Maintain a calm environment; try to decrease stressors
Potential for Injury, related to increased metabolic action of thyroid hormone and decreased calcium serum levels	Monitor for signs and symptoms of decreased calcium (muscle spasms, irritability, tetany, and cardiac dysrhythmias) Monitor for signs and symptoms of hyperthyroidism and hypothyroidism (changes in vital signs, temperature intolerance, tremors or changes in sleep pattern)
Inadequate Fluid Volume, related to postoperative hemorrhage	Monitor incision and posterior neck for increased drainage Maintain accurate record of intake and output Monitor vital signs for changes such as increased pulse

Stress the importance of proper medical follow-up to monitor thyroid hormone replacement therapy and to help ensure prompt diagnosis of any metastatic lesions. Before discharge from the hospital, teach the patient proper care of the surgical incision. Include teaching on the possibility of surgically induced hypothyroidism (depending on the amount of thyroid gland removed), including the need to take thyroid replacement therapy correctly, and signs and symptoms of hyperthyroidism (if the dosage is too high).

Prognosis

The prognosis after treatment for thyroid cancer depends on the type of tumor. For papillary carcinoma the prognosis is excellent, and the 5-year survival rate for stages I and II is nearly 100%. For stages III and IV the rate is 93% and 51%, respectively; for follicular and anaplastic carcinomas, the prognosis is much less favorable (American Cancer Society [ACS], 2021).

HYPERPARATHYROIDISM

Etiology and Pathophysiology

Hyperparathyroidism involves overactivity of the parathyroid glands, with increased production of PTH. The cause of this condition may be a primary hypertrophy of one or more of the tiny parathyroid glands, usually in the form of an adenoma (benign growths that may evolve into adenocarcinomas). It also may result from chronic renal failure, pyelonephritis, or glomerulonephritis. Parathyroid carcinoma may in rare cases result in hyperparathyroidism with rapid progress and a grave prognosis. Hyperparathyroidism usually occurs in adults between 30 and 70 years of age, and it occurs twice as often in women. Risk factors include postmenopausal status, prolonged or severe calcium or vitamin D deficiency, lithium use, and radiation to the neck (Johns Hopkins Medicine, n.d.).

Clinical Manifestations

Assessment findings are often initially mild. The first symptoms noted may be the result of the elevated serum calcium levels. The patient may report nausea, vomiting, weakness, and fatigue. The hypercalcemia results as calcium leaves the bones and accumulates in the bloodstream. As a result, the bones become demineralized, causing skeletal pain, pain on weight-bearing, and pathologic fractures (fractures that result from slight or no trauma to diseased bone). The first presentation of the illness may be a patient seen for a fractured bone that is unrelated to trauma. The high level of calcium in the blood may lead to the formation of kidney stones.

Assessment

Collection of subjective data includes assessment of the severity of skeletal pain, the degree of muscle weakness, and the effectiveness of analgesics. It is important to determine nursing measures that contribute to the patient's comfort and mobility. As neuromuscular function decreases, the patient has generalized fatigue, drowsiness, apathy, nausea, and anorexia. Review for changes in bowel elimination patterns. Psychosocial changes include personality changes, disorientation, and even paranoia. Flank pain may indicate calculus (kidney stone) formation.

Collection of objective data includes careful observation for any skeletal deformity or abnormal movement of bone that may indicate a pathologic fracture. Observe the urine for quantity and the presence of hematuria and stones. There may be vomiting and weight loss. Hypertension and cardiac dysrhythmias may present significant problems. Changes in the serum calcium level may cause bradycardia and other cardiac irregularities. The level of consciousness may decrease to the level of stupor or coma.

Diagnostic Tests

Radiographic examination may reveal skeletal decalcification. Blood PTH levels are increased, as are alkaline phosphate levels. The patient should receive nothing by mouth for 8 to 12 hours before these tests. The serum calcium level is elevated, whereas the serum phosphorus level is decreased. Bone density measurements and x-rays also may be used to detect bone loss. Imaging, such as MRI, CT, and ultrasound, may be used to localize the adenoma. A sestamibi parathyroid scan is useful in determining the location of a parathyroid tumor. In this diagnostic test, a radioactive dye is injected into the patient's vein and the parathyroid gland absorbs the agent, which is then detectable on imaging (Buicko, 2017). The primary health care provider also may request 24-hour urine collection to determine calcium levels. An elevated urine calcium level is indicative of increased PTH levels. A differential diagnosis should be made to rule out multiple myeloma, Cushing syndrome, vitamin D excess, and other causes of hypercalcemia.

Medical Management

Treatment for hyperparathyroidism will be based upon the level of hormone elevation. If the levels are only mildly elevated and renal function is normal, the medical management may be conservative and consist of close monitoring of PTH levels.

Surgical removal of the abnormal tissue is the most common plan for condition management.

Nursing Interventions and Patient Teaching

Preoperative nursing interventions include helping restore fluid and electrolyte balance by encouraging increased oral fluid intake and by carefully monitoring IV fluid therapy. Monitor the patient's I&O. Furosemide may be used to promote a reduction of serum calcium levels. Thiazide diuretics are not used because they decrease renal excretion of calcium and thus increase the hypercalcemic state. Urine may be strained if the patient exhibits signs of kidney calculi. Monitor serum calcium levels. The diet should be low in calcium, eliminating milk and other dairy products. Antacids are high in calcium and should not be used. Accurately assess the patient's pain and administer prescribed analgesics as needed. Postoperatively, care for the patient in the same manner as after a thyroidectomy, with careful monitoring of I&O. These patients commonly retain fluid in the tissues after surgery and often have decreased urinary output. It is important to avoid overhydration at this point. Assess the patient frequently for signs of hypocalcemia, such as tetany, cardiac dysrhythmias, and carpopedal spasms (i.e., spasms of the hands or feet). If tetany does occur, it is treated with calcium gluconate intravenously.

Patient problems and interventions for the patient with hyperparathyroidism include but are not limited to the following:

PATIENT PROBLEM	NURSING INTERVENTIONS
Inability to Tolerate Activity, related to neuromuscular dysfunction	Help patient identify factors that increase or decrease activity tolerance and to eliminate or reduce painful, fatiguing activities Encourage patient to follow prescribed individualized activity or exercise program
Recent onset of pain, related to hormonal imbalances and physiologic variables	Assess factors that cause or worsen pain, and help patient adjust body mechanics or activity

PATIENT PROBLEM	NURSING INTERVENTIONS
Renal colic, related to physiologic variables	Encourage adequate fluid intake while assessing cardiac and urinary output

Teach the patient the principles of good body mechanics to prevent pathologic fractures during ambulation. Reassure the patient that bone pain should decrease gradually as electrolyte balance is restored and the condition is alleviated. Encourage the patient to participate in mild exercise as prescribed by the health care provider to regain muscle strength and promote bone health. Encourage the patient to consume plenty of water, monitor the amount of dietary calcium and vitamin D, and avoid smoking. Teach the patient that certain medications such as some diuretics and lithium can elevate the serum calcium level. Evaluate the home environment and develop a plan of changes necessary to prevent accidents, such as eliminating tripping hazards.

Prognosis

With proper medical or surgical treatment, the patient can maintain an average life expectancy. In patients with parathyroid carcinoma, the prognosis is grave.

HYPOPARATHYROIDISM
Etiology and Pathophysiology

Hypoparathyroidism occurs when there is decreased PTH, resulting in decreased levels of serum calcium. Idiopathic hypoparathyroidism is a rare condition, thought to be either autoimmune or familial in origin. The most common cause is the inadvertent removal or destruction of one or more of the tiny parathyroid glands during thyroidectomy. Other causes include previous radiation treatments to the neck area, an overdose of vitamin D or calcium, cancer (lymphoma or multiple myeloma), and a low magnesium level.

Clinical Manifestations

Decreased PTH levels in the bloodstream cause an increased serum phosphorus level and a decreased serum calcium level, resulting in neuromuscular hyperexcitability, involuntary and uncontrollable muscle spasms, and hypocalcemic tetany. Severe hypocalcemia may result in laryngeal spasm, stridor, cyanosis, and an increased possibility of asphyxia. Some patients have calcification of the basal ganglia in the brain, causing a parkinsonian syndrome with bizarre posturing and spastic movements.

Assessment

Collection of subjective data includes assessment of neuromuscular activity for symptoms such as dysphagia and numbness or tingling of the lips, fingertips, and occasionally feet and increased muscle tension leading to paresthesia (burning or prickling sensations) and stiffness. The patient may feel anxious, irritable, or depressed. The patient may experience headaches and nausea. Abdominal or flank pain may occur if a renal calculus attempts to pass down the ureter into the bladder. Assess the effectiveness of narcotics used to relieve renal colic.

Objective data include a positive Chvostek sign or Trousseau sign. If laryngeal spasm and stridor occur, cyanosis may appear. Cardiac output may decrease as a result of hypocalcemia, and the patient may develop dysrhythmias. Tetanic spasms of the extremities may be observed. The magnesium level should be monitored closely.

Diagnostic Tests
Diagnostic laboratory studies confirm the decreased serum calcium and PTH with increased urinary calcium, and increased serum phosphorus with decreased urinary phosphorus. Magnesium levels will also be diminished. Rule out other possible causes of hypocalcemia, such as vitamin D deficiency, kidney failure, and acute pancreatitis. Additional diagnostic testing includes electrocardiography, x-rays, and bone density scans.

Medical Management
The immediate treatment of hypoparathyroid tetany is IV administration of calcium gluconate or calcium chloride (10%). This drug irritates the vessel wall and always should be given slowly, at a rate not to exceed 1 mL/min. The patient may complain of a hot feeling of the skin or tongue. If given too rapidly, IV calcium can precipitate hypotension, serious cardiac dysrhythmias, or cardiac arrest. Electrocardiographic monitoring is indicated when administering calcium. After the initial IV dose, calcium may be continued in a slower IV infusion until tetany is controlled. Patients who continue to experience tetany may be sedated during the acute phases of treatment. Long-range therapies will include oral calcium supplements. Vitamin D promotes calcium absorption and aids in the reduction of serum phosphorus levels and will be prescribed. Magnesium supplementation may also be included. Thiazide diuretics aid in increasing serum calcium levels and may be utilized. In the event serum calcium levels cannot be maintained with oral therapies daily PTH injections can be prescribed.

Nursing Interventions and Patient Teaching
Once therapies begin, monitor for signs of hypercalcemia. The most common clinical manifestations of this are vomiting, disorientation, anorexia, abdominal pain, and weakness. Assess the patient for respiratory distress; renal involvement; and adverse reactions to calcium therapy, such as bradycardia, syncope, and hypotension. Use calcium cautiously in digitalized patients because it may cause digitalis toxicity. Cimetidine (Tagamet) interferes with normal parathyroid functioning and should be used carefully in these patients. The diet should contain foods high in calcium, such as low-fat dairy products, dark green vegetables, soybeans, tofu, and canned fish with the bones included.

Offer high-calcium snacks. Adults should consume 1000 mg of calcium each day. Women over age 50 need an additional 200 mg/day. This is in response to the increased mineral loss as a result of menopause (Office of Dietary Supplements, 2021a). If resistance to calcium intake is noted, supplements should be considered. A diet low in phosphorus is also important. Foods low in phosphorus include soy milk, white rice, jam, honey, lemon-lime soda, cucumbers, lettuce, peppers, tomatoes, and non-organ meats. Foods that contain elevated levels of phosphorus include deli meats, hot dogs, processed cheeses, and cornbread.

A patient problem and interventions for the patient with hypoparathyroidism include but are not limited to the following:

PATIENT PROBLEM	NURSING INTERVENTIONS
Potential for Injury, related to postoperative hypocalcemia	Assess for signs and symptoms of hypocalcemia (muscle spasms, laryngeal stridor, convulsion) Calcium therapy if needed

Teach the patient the early symptoms of hypocalcemia, with instructions to notify the nurse or health care provider if they occur. Draw blood levels of calcium and phosphorus periodically while the patient is hospitalized. Teach the patient to monitor the pulse for changes, maintain fluid balance, and use calcium supplements at home. Stress the need for lifelong treatment and follow-up care, including monitoring calcium levels three or four times a year.

Prognosis
For most patients, treatment keeps the symptoms under control, and those affected have a normal life expectancy.

DISORDERS OF THE ADRENAL GLANDS

ADRENAL HYPERFUNCTION (CUSHING SYNDROME)
Etiology and Pathophysiology
Cushing syndrome is a spectrum of clinical abnormalities caused by excess corticosteroids, particularly glucocorticoids. This syndrome may be caused by hyperplasia of adrenal tissue resulting from overstimulation by the pituitary hormone ACTH, by a tumor of the adrenal cortex, by ACTH-secreting neoplasms outside the pituitary (such as small-cell carcinoma of the lung), and by prolonged administration of high doses of corticosteroids. The body's protective feedback mechanism fails, resulting in excess secretion of the adrenal hormones: glucocorticoids, mineralocorticoids, and sex hormones.

Clinical Manifestations
This overabundance of corticosteroids produces the signs and symptoms commonly associated with

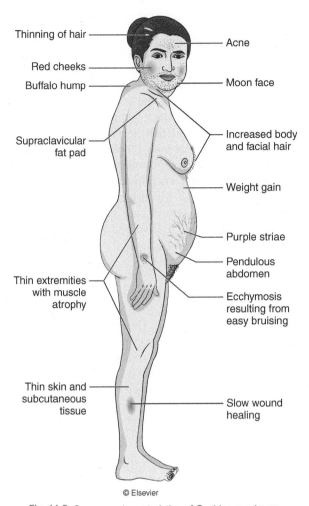

Thinning of hair

Acne

Red cheeks

Buffalo hump

Moon face

Supraclavicular
fat pad

Increased body
and facial hair

Weight gain

Purple striae

Pendulous
abdomen

Thin extremities
with muscle
atrophy

Ecchymosis
resulting from
easy bruising

Thin skin and
subcutaneous
tissue

Slow wound
healing

© Elsevier

Fig. 11.8 Common characteristics of Cushing syndrome.

Cushing syndrome, including moon face and buffalo hump. Weight gain, the most common feature, results from accumulation of adipose tissue in the trunk, face, and cervical spine area (Fig. 11.8). The arms and legs become thin as a result of muscle wasting. Hypokalemia (low potassium) is usually present. Hyperglycemia occurs because of glucose intolerance (associated with cortisol-induced insulin resistance) and increased glucose release by the liver. The patient usually has protein in the urine and increased urinary calcium excretion, which may lead to the development of renal calculi. Osteoporosis results from abnormal calcium absorption, and kyphosis (excessive curvature of the thoracic vertebra, or hunchback) may develop. The patient is susceptible to infections, but the symptoms may be masked and the infection not detected until it is life threatening.

Assessment

Collection of subjective data includes assessment of the patient's ability to concentrate. The patient may have mood disturbances such as irritability, anxiety, euphoria, insomnia, irrationality, and occasionally psychosis. Depression is common, and the possibility of suicide is an ever-present concern. Depression is also apparent

in patients with other endocrine disorders such as diabetes and hypothyroidism. When assessing the endocrine system, include an assessment of psychological demeanor. Be alert to subtle changes in the patient's affect, and take precautions to prevent the patient from inflicting self-harm. Patients of both sexes may experience loss of libido and alterations in self-esteem with concerns about sexual dysfunction. Encourage the patient to verbalize concerns about altered body image. Severe backache is often present and may signal a compression fracture of a vertebral body. Assess the severity of back pain and nursing measures that contribute to the patient's comfort. Appetite usually increases. Ensure that the patient understands the dietary restrictions (low sodium, controlled calories and carbohydrates with increased potassium) and the importance of medical follow-up.

Collection of objective data includes observation of the skin for ecchymoses and petechiae. The skin becomes thin and fragile, and wound healing is delayed. The patient may have weight gain and abdominal enlargement, with development of *striae* (a streak or linear scar that often results from stretching of the skin); this increased girth may contribute to difficulty with mobility. Monitor the patient's weight because peripheral edema and associated hypertension are common. Impaired carbohydrate metabolism results in hyperglycemia. Women may experience hirsutism (excessive body hair in a masculine distribution), menstrual irregularities, and deepening of the voice. Elevated body temperature may indicate an undetected infection.

Diagnostic Tests

Diagnosis usually is based on the patient's clinical appearance and laboratory test results. Plasma cortisol levels usually are elevated. Plasma ACTH levels may be increased or decreased, depending on the location of the tumor. Skull radiographic evaluation may detect erosion of the sella turcica in the presence of a pituitary tumor. Adrenal angiography aids in diagnosing an adrenal tumor. A 24-hour urine test for 17-ketosteroids and 17-hydroxysteroids shows increased levels. Blood glucose determination for hyperglycemia and urinalysis for glycosuria are other diagnostic tests associated with but not diagnostic of Cushing syndrome. An abdominal CT scan, MRI, and ultrasound may help localize an abdominal tumor.

Medical Management

Treatment is directed toward the causative factor. If an adrenal tumor is present, adrenalectomy usually is indicated for its removal. Pituitary tumors may be irradiated or removed surgically by transsphenoidal microsurgery. If the patient is unable to undergo surgery because of inoperable cancer elsewhere in the body or another preexisting condition, mitotane (Lysodren) therapy may be used. Mitotane alters the metabolism of cortisol in the periphery (in this case "peripheral metabolism" means elsewhere than in the adrenal gland), decreases the plasma corticosteroid level, and suppresses cortisol production—essentially providing a "medical adrenalectomy." This cytotoxic agent damages the adrenal glands and is given for at least 3 months, during which time the patient must be monitored for symptoms of hepatotoxicity, such as jaundice, gastrointestinal upset, and pruritus. The diet should be low in sodium to help decrease edema. Reduced calories and carbohydrates help control hyperglycemia, and foods high in potassium help correct hypokalemia. If Cushing syndrome has developed during the course of prolonged administration of corticosteroids (e.g., prednisone), one or more of the following alternatives may be tried: (1) gradually discontinuing corticosteroid therapy, (2) reducing the corticosteroid dosage, or (3) converting to an alternate-day regimen. Gradually tapering the corticosteroid is necessary to avoid potentially life-threatening adrenal insufficiency.

Nursing Interventions and Patient Teaching

Important nursing interventions include gentle handling to prevent skin impairment or excessive ecchymosis and frequent assessment for erythema, edema, or early signs of infection. Encourage the patient to turn frequently and ambulate as tolerated to eliminate undue pressure on bony prominences. Elbow and heel protectors and a pressure-reducing mattress or pad may help prevent decubitus ulcers in the bedridden patient. Encourage the patient to participate as fully as possible in typical ADLs, interspersing personal hygiene tasks with rest periods to prevent overtiring.

Patient problems and interventions for the patient with Cushing syndrome include but are not limited to the following:

PATIENT PROBLEM	NURSING INTERVENTIONS
Insufficient Knowledge, related to therapeutic regimen	Assess patient's understanding of prescribed medication and diet Encourage patient to wear a medical alert bracelet or necklace, and to carry a wallet identification card
Inability to Tolerate Activity, related to weakness and immobility	Assess patient's current activity tolerance, and identify priorities for energy expenditures Plan activity and rest periods with patient
Potential for Infection, related to: • Suppression of immune system • Lowered resistance to stress	Monitor patient for complaints of pain, purulent exudates, or decrease in function because the usual signs and symptoms of inflammation, such as fever and erythema, may not be present (Lewis et al., 2011) Practice meticulous handwashing before caring for patient

The patient's mental attitude is extremely important. Encourage verbalization of concerns and watch for the development of depression and suicidal thoughts. Help the patient understand the purpose of prescribed medications, such as mitotane, as well as possible side effects. It is important for the patient to wear a medical-alert bracelet or necklace and to carry a wallet card stating the diagnosis of Cushing syndrome. The patient may need to adjust to a major lifestyle change, and the aid of a community support liaison may be enlisted. Before adrenalectomy, teach the patient the importance of avoiding stress and infections. Postoperative teaching includes proper wound care and the symptoms of Addison's disease, which is sometimes an unavoidable sequela after this type of surgery.

Prognosis

Depending on whether the cause of the disease was benign or malignant and whether the treatment was successful or unsuccessful, the patient with Cushing syndrome can expect to have major lifestyle changes, possibly with many complications (osteoporosis, hypertension, frequent infections, loss of muscle mass and strength, and interference with other hormone levels). Life expectancy for a patient with Cushing syndrome is shortened, in part because of the multiple complications noted with the disease.

ADRENAL HYPOFUNCTION (ADDISON'S DISEASE)

Etiology and Pathophysiology

Adrenocortical insufficiency occurs when the adrenal glands do not secrete adequate amounts of glucocorticoids, mineralocorticoids, and androgens. It initially may be seen as Addison's disease, a rare primary condition; or it may result from adrenalectomy, pituitary hypofunction, or long-standing steroid therapy. The most common cause of Addison's disease is an autoimmune response: adrenal tissue is destroyed by antibodies against the patient's own adrenal cortex. Addison's disease can result from idiopathic adrenal atrophy or cancer of the adrenal cortex. Tuberculosis causes Addison's disease worldwide, and tuberculosis is on the rise. Other causes include infarction, fungal infections (e.g., histoplasmosis), acquired immunodeficiency syndrome, and metastatic cancer. Deficiencies in aldosterone and cortisol produce disturbances of the metabolism of carbohydrates, fats, and proteins, as well as sodium, potassium, and water. This results in electrolyte and fluid imbalance, dehydration, water loss, and hypovolemia (decreased plasma volume). Adrenal insufficiency most often occurs in adults younger than 60 years of age and affects both genders equally.

Clinical Manifestations

Because manifestations are usually not evident until 90% of the adrenal cortex is destroyed, the disease often is advanced before it is diagnosed. Clinical manifestations are related directly to imbalances in adrenal hormones, nutrients, and electrolytes.

Assessment

Subjective data include progressive weakness, fatigue, nausea, anorexia, and craving for salt. Orthostatic hypotension (or postural hypotension; a sudden drop in blood pressure provoked by standing up) may be associated with vertigo, weakness, and syncope, resulting in reluctance to attempt normal activities. The patient may complain of severe headache, disorientation, abdominal pain, or general joint and muscle pain, which could represent early symptoms of Addisonian crisis (see below). This patient tolerates stress poorly and feels anxious and apprehensive. It is important to assess emotional status and allow the patient to share feelings about his or her altered self-image. Also assess the patient's overall understanding of the disease process and the importance of medical treatment and follow-up.

Collection of objective data includes observation of changes in the color of the mucous membranes and the skin. Skin hyperpigmentation, a common feature, is seen primarily in sun-exposed areas of the body; at pressure points; over joints; and in creases, especially in palmar creases. The patient usually loses weight, often with vomiting and diarrhea. Hypoglycemia may contribute to fatigue; assess the patient's ability to perform ADLs. An abnormally low or abnormally high body temperature, orthostatic hypotension, hyponatremia, and hyperkalemia are signs of impending *Addisonian crisis*, a life-threatening emergency caused by insufficient adrenocortical hormones or a sudden sharp decrease in these hormones. Precipitating factors that can trigger an Addisonian crisis are stress-producing situations such as infections, surgery, trauma, hemorrhage, psychological stress, sudden withdrawal of corticosteroid hormone replacement therapy, after

adrenal surgery, or sudden pituitary gland destruction (Mayo Clinic, 2020a). See Table 11.3 for a comparison of Cushing syndrome and Addison's disease.

Diagnostic Tests

Laboratory studies show decreased serum sodium, increased serum potassium, and decreased serum glucose (Mayo Clinic, 2020a). Serum levels of cortisol, ACTH, and antibodies also are monitored. Fasting plasma cortisol levels and aldosterone levels are low with an ACTH stimulation test. The ACTH simulation test involves obtaining cortisol levels before and after injections of synthetic ACTH. A glucose tolerance test may yield abnormal results. Insulin and cortisol levels also are measured before and after the injection of insulin to monitor for increases and decreases. A CT and MRI of the abdomen may be indicated to assess the status of the adrenal glands. A CT scan and MRI of the pituitary gland also indicate the cause of the disease.

Medical Management

Medical treatment involves the prompt restoration of fluid and electrolyte balance and replacement of the deficient adrenal hormones. The most common form of replacement therapy is hydrocortisone, which has mineralocorticoid and glucocorticoid properties. Glucocorticoid dosage must be increased during times of physiologic stress to prevent Addisonian crisis. Fludrocortisone (Florinef) (a mineralocorticoid) also is administered. The diet should be high in sodium and low in potassium.

Treatment for the life-threatening emergency of an Addisonian crisis includes management of shock, high-dose hydrocortisone replacement therapy, and large volumes of 0.9% saline and 5% dextrose solutions to improve electrolyte imbalances and reverse hypotension.

Table 11.3 Nursing Assessment of Patients With Cushing Syndrome or Addison's Disease

AREA OF ASSESSMENT	CLINICAL MANIFESTATIONS IN CUSHING SYNDROME	CLINICAL MANIFESTATIONS IN ADDISON'S DISEASE
Cardiovascular	Mild to moderate hypertension	Postural hypotension, vertigo, syncope
Neurologic	Impaired memory and concentration, insomnia, irritability	Lethargy, headache
Musculoskeletal	Muscle weakness, muscle wasting in extremities, back and rib pain, kyphosis	Muscle weakness, fatigue, muscle aches, muscle wasting
Integumentary	Thin skin, red cheeks, acne, frequent petechiae and ecchymoses, increased body and facial hair, poor wound healing	Hyperpigmentation, decreased body hair
Self-care and self-concept	Tires easily; insomnia, malaise, negative feelings regarding changes in body	Tires easily; profound weakness, lack of interest in usual activities and relationships
Nutrition and fluid balance	Increased appetite, moderate weight gain, edema, buffalo hump, moon face, obesity of trunk, hyperglycemia; need for decreased salt intake, reduced calories and carbohydrate intake, increased potassium intake	Nausea and vomiting, fluid and electrolyte imbalance, dehydration, weight loss, hypoglycemia; need for increased salt and decreased potassium intake

Nursing Interventions and Patient Teaching

Carefully assess the patient's circulatory status, keep accurate I&O records, and record daily weight. Check skin turgor and offer fluids frequently. Monitor vital signs at regular intervals, paying attention to temperature and blood pressure. Also monitor the patient for response to prescribed steroid drugs, and promptly report any adverse effects to the health care provider. Keep the environment as free from stress as possible. Visitors and hospital personnel should be screened for infectious disease and excluded from the patient's room. Protect the patient from injury and advise the patient to rise slowly from a sitting or lying position if orthostatic hypotension is a concern. Continually assess the patient for signs of developing adrenal (Addisonian) crisis, manifested by a sudden, severe drop in blood pressure; nausea and vomiting; an extremely high temperature; and cyanosis, progressing to vasomotor collapse and possibly death. The patient should carry an emergency kit at all times with IM hydrocortisone, syringes, and instructions for use. Teach the patient and significant others to give an IM injection in case replacement therapy cannot be taken orally. Also advise the patient to consult with the health care provider to adjust (increase) medication doses during periods of physical or emotional stress. Patient education is imperative for long-term compliance in the management of Addison's disease.

Patient problems and interventions for the patient with Addison's disease include but are not limited to the following:

PATIENT PROBLEM	NURSING INTERVENTIONS
Potential for Infection, related to altered metabolic processes	Assess environment for stressors Screen visitors and personnel for contagious disease Monitor temperature routinely Stress the importance of taking prescribed medications
Potential for Injury, related to decrease in blood pressure on rising	Monitor vital signs (blood pressure and pulse) and for dizziness when rising Assist patient when rising, using a gait belt to prevent falls

Before discharge from the hospital, teach the patient the importance of adhering to the prescribed drug therapy; having regular medical checkups; and immediately reporting all illnesses, even a cold, to the health care provider. Emphasize that stress is one of the major precipitating factors in Addisonian crisis, and encourage the patient to minimize stress through cognitive behavior therapy, relaxation therapy, biofeedback, and mental imagery. Other conditions to avoid include overexertion, diarrhea, infection, decreased intake of salt, exposure to cold, and surgery. The patient must wear a medical alert bracelet and carry a wallet card stating that the patient has Addison's disease so that appropriate therapy can be initiated in case of trauma, accident, or crisis.

Prognosis

With long-term steroid therapy, adequate medical care, and follow-up, this patient has a fair prognosis.

PHEOCHROMOCYTOMA

Etiology and Pathophysiology

A *pheochromocytoma* is a rare tumor of the adrenal medulla that causes excessive secretion of a catecholamine (epinephrine and/or norepinephrine). These tumors occur most often in adults between 20 and 60 years of age and are usually benign; only about 10% are malignant. The secretion of excessive catecholamine results in severe hypertension.

Clinical Manifestations

Pheochromocytoma results in severe hypertension because of sympathetic nervous system stimulation. Other classic clinical signs and symptoms include anxiety, severe headache, diaphoresis, tachycardia, shortness of breath, feelings of extreme fright, and unexplained abdominal pain (NIH, 2020). Hypertensive crisis may occur, during which the blood pressure may fluctuate widely, sometimes as high as 300/175 mm Hg. Signs and symptoms may be triggered by an identifiable factor, such as overexertion or emotional trauma, or they may occur for no apparent reason. Extreme hypertension may result in stroke, kidney damage, and retinopathy. Cardiac damage may occur, resulting in heart failure.

Assessment

Subjective data during a hypertensive crisis include severe headache and palpitations. The patient may feel nervous, dizzy, and dyspneic and may experience paresthesia, nausea, and intolerance to heat. Anxiety is common, and the patient may have trouble sleeping. Question the patient about the occurrence of symptoms in relation to identifiable factors, such as excess stress or overexertion, and identify the coping methods used.

Collection of objective data includes frequent measurement of blood pressure and respiratory rate for increases and of pulse for tachycardia. The patient may have tremors, diaphoresis, dilated pupils, glycosuria, and hyperglycemia. Assess responses to prescribed medications.

Diagnostic Tests

The measurement of urinary metanephrines (catecholamine metabolites), usually performed as a 24-hour urine collection, is the simplest and most reliable test. Values are elevated in at least 90% of those with pheochromocytoma. Vanillylmandelic acid (VMA) also may be measured in a 24-hour urine sample. It should be noted that this test has more false negatives than that for urine metanephrines. Plasma catecholamines also are elevated. It is preferable to measure serum catecholamines during an "attack." A CT scan and MRI of the adrenal glands may help in locating the tumor.

Medical Management

Treatment is usually the surgical removal of the tumor. Surgery is more common via laparoscopic adrenalectomy than open abdominal incision. Preoperatively, the patient may be given alpha blockers including doxazosin, parazosin, and phenoxybenzamine to reduce blood pressure. Beta blockers (e.g., propranolol) to decrease tachycardia and other dysrhythmias also are used (NIH, 2020). Metyrosine may be given to help inhibit catecholamine production, and the drug must be continued on a long-term basis if the tumor is inoperable.

Nursing Interventions and Patient Teaching

Postoperative care is carried out in the same manner as for any major abdominal surgery, with the following special concerns. If the patient has undergone adrenalectomy, large amounts of hydrocortisone will be given. Watch carefully for fluctuations in blood pressure caused by adrenal manipulation during surgery, with subsequent release of epinephrine and norepinephrine. These fluctuations may be severe and life threatening if cardiovascular collapse occurs. The patient should avoid excess stress and must be allowed adequate time to rest; give sedatives to ensure this. Keep a careful I&O record and monitor IV infusions carefully. Vasopressors and corticosteroids may be given. The diet should be free from stimulants, such as coffee, tea, and soft drinks containing caffeine.

Patient problems and interventions for the patient with pheochromocytoma include but are not limited to the following:

PATIENT PROBLEM	NURSING INTERVENTIONS
Compromised Blood Flow to Tissue (Cardiopulmonary, Renal), related to hypertension	Monitor blood pressure and pulse and record intake and output Eliminate smoking and caffeine-containing beverages
Inability to Tolerate Activity, related to hypertension	Assist with gradual position changes from lying to sitting or standing Limit activity, as needed, to prevent increased hypertension

Follow-up 24-hour urine tests (for catecholamine metabolites or VMA) may determine when the levels have returned to normal. The patient then is considered cured and may resume normal activities. If the tumor is inoperable, the patient remains under lifelong medical supervision. Stress the importance of compliance with prescribed treatment. The patient should wear medical-alert identification and carry a wallet card. Teach the patient self-monitoring of blood pressure and when to call the health care provider if elevation occurs.

Prognosis

If undiagnosed and untreated, pheochromocytoma may lead to diabetes mellitus (DM), cardiomyopathy, and death. The prognosis after successful removal of the causative tumor is good; for an inoperable tumor, the prognosis depends on adequate medical management of hypertension.

DISORDERS OF THE PANCREAS

DIABETES MELLITUS

DM is a systemic metabolic disorder that involves improper metabolism of carbohydrates, fats, and proteins. It is centered on the body's use of insulin, a protein that allows the body's cells to absorb glucose from the bloodstream. DM is a chronic multisystem disease related to a decrease or absolute lack of insulin production by the beta cells of the islets of Langerhans in the pancreas or by impaired insulin use, or both. In patients who do not have DM, the beta cells are stimulated by increased blood glucose levels. Insulin secretion reaches peak levels about 30 minutes after meals and returns to normal in 2 to 3 hours. Between meals or during a period of fasting, insulin levels remain low, and the body uses its supply of stored glucose and amino acids to provide energy for the tissues. The beta cells of the pancreas continuously release insulin into the bloodstream in small amounts. A larger quantity (i.e., a *bolus*) of insulin is released after the intake of food. The average amount of insulin secreted by the beta cells of the pancreas in an adult is 40 to 50 units every 24 hours. The release of insulin in this systematic manner results in the body maintaining a normal blood glucose level between 70 and 100 mg/dL. In patients with DM, the body's insulin supply is either absent or deficient, or target cells resist the action of insulin. There are several types of DM, but in each type, hyperglycemia is the principal clinical manifestation.

There are two main types of DM: *type 1* and *type 2*. Type 1 formerly was called juvenile diabetes, juvenile-onset diabetes, or insulin-dependent DM. Type 2 formerly was called adult-onset diabetes, maturity-onset diabetes, or non–insulin-dependent DM. Because type 2 DM is becoming more common in children, and because some people with type 2 DM use insulin, these terms are no longer appropriate. Type 1 and type 2 DM have some distinct differences (Table 11.4). In type 1 an autoimmune disease (probably stimulated by a virus) eventually results in destruction of beta cells in the pancreatic islets and deficient insulin *production*; the patient retains normal sensitivity to insulin action. Within 5 years of diagnosis, all of the patient's beta cells have been destroyed and no insulin is produced. In type 2 DM the main problem is an abnormal resistance to insulin *action*. During pregnancy some women may experience gestational diabetes that results from hormonal changes causing insulin resistance in maternal cells (see FON Chapter 29).

Table 11.4	Comparison of Type 1 and Type 2 Diabetes Mellitus	
FACTOR	**TYPE 1**	**TYPE 2**
Age at onset	Usually 30 years or younger but can occur at any age	Usually age 35 years or older but can occur at any age Incidence is increasing in children
Body weight	Normal or underweight	80% are overweight
Symptoms at onset	Sudden; polyphagia, polydipsia, polyuria, weight loss, weakness, fatigue; glycosuria, hyperglycemia; acidosis, progressing to DKA	Gradual; may be asymptomatic at onset; later, may develop signs and symptoms of type 1 DM; others include slow wound healing, blurred vision, pruritus, boils or other skin infections; vaginal infections in women
Treatment	Diet, exercise, and insulin; may add subcutaneous insulin-enhancing drug (pramlintide [Symlin])	Diet and exercise; or diet, exercise, and oral hypoglycemic agents; or diet, exercise, oral hypoglycemic agents, and insulin during times of illness or stress; may add a subcutaneous insulin-enhancing agent such as exenatide (Byetta) or pramlintide
Incidence of complications	Frequent	Frequent
Psychosocial and sexual concerns	Irritability; disturbed body image; mood swings, depression; menstrual irregularities; decreased libido	Disturbed body image; amenorrhea; decreased libido; poor tolerance to stress

DKA, Diabetic ketoacidosis; *DM,* diabetes mellitus.

Regardless of the type of DM, all of these patients have impaired glucose tolerance. More than 32.4 million people in the United States have been diagnosed with DM. This reflects more than 10% of the US population. Of this number more than 7 million are undiagnosed and living without the benefit of treatment and care. Non-Hispanic whites reflect the population with the lowest incidence of DM. The highest levels of diabetes are found in African Americans (American Diabetes Association [ADA], 2018).

CAUSES AND COMPLICATIONS OF DIABETES MELLITUS

The exact cause of both types of DM is unknown. A number of factors contribute to its development: genetic predisposition, viruses (such as coxsackievirus B, rubella, and mumps), the aging process, diet and lifestyle, and ethnicity. Obesity is believed to be a major factor. The T lymphocytes may play a role in the autoimmune destruction of pancreatic insulin-producing cells.

Complications of DM impact all body systems. The elevated levels of serum glucose damages blood vessels, resulting in circulatory impairment. Cardiovascular complications include heart disease, hypertension, and stroke. Neurovascular complications include renal failure and erectile dysfunction. Neuropathy is a common complication that results in painful feet and fingers and the loss of sensation. This promotes safety risks such as falls and burns. Retinopathy may result in blindness. The skin has a greater risk for infection and impaired healing. Compliance with the diet and prescribed

medications and getting regular exercise are needed to prevent permanent damage. The complications from DM can be decreased significantly by properly maintaining the blood glucose level (60 to 99 mg/dL) and the hemoglobin A_{1c} (HbA_{1c}) level (less than 5% to 6%).

TYPE 1 DIABETES MELLITUS

Etiology

Type 1 DM results from progressive destruction of beta cell function in the pancreas as a result of an autoimmune process in a susceptible individual. The pancreatic islets of Langerhans cell antibodies and insulin autoantibodies cause an 80% to 90% reduction in beta cells before hyperglycemia and symptoms occur. Type 1 DM is characterized by autoimmune beta cell destruction, which is attributed to a genetic predisposition. Genetics plus infection with one or more viral agents and possibly chemical agents are believed to cause type 1 DM. It is not known whether these are the only factors involved.

The onset and progression of hyperglycemic signs and symptoms are usually more rapid and acute in type 1 DM than in type 2. Type 1 DM may occur at any age, but signs and symptoms usually appear before 30 years of age. The patient is usually thin. The patient is often hyperglycemic, with urine that is strongly positive for ketones (signs that fat is being used for energy instead of glucose because of a shortage of insulin), and depends on insulin therapy to prevent ketoacidosis (an abnormal buildup of acidic ketones in the blood) and to sustain life. Because they do not produce adequate amounts of endogenous insulin (i.e., insulin produced by the body), patients with type 1 DM must take regular injections of exogenous insulin (i.e., synthetic insulin) for optimal survival.

In prediabetes, *insulin resistance*—the lessening response of the body to the production of insulin by the pancreas—occurs. In the patient with insulin resistance, the serum glucose level may initially be normal, but the pancreas is working overtime to maintain that normal level. Excessive amounts of insulin are secreted by the pancreas to get a limited level of glucose control. The patient with insulin resistance should have the insulin level monitored in addition to the serum glucose level. The patient is treated with oral hyperglycemic agents if needed. If overweight, monitoring of caloric intake and regular exercise will aid in weight loss. The weight loss may also reduce levels of hyperglycemia and needed medications.

In type 1 DM there is no insulin resistance; there is a total absence of insulin production. It is diagnosed when the patient's pancreas does not produce insulin. Insulin then must be obtained through exogenous sources and administered mainly via the subcutaneous route (via insulin pump or injections). In serious situations, short-acting regular insulin can be administered via the IV route. People with type 1 DM are often healthy with the exception of the lack of insulin production. Although patients with type 1 DM are at risk for the typical complications of poor glucose control, they often do not have the history of high cholesterol, obesity, and high blood pressure that is noted with type 2 DM. Goals for treatment are to maintain a normal blood glucose level (60 to 99 mg/dL) via insulin administration, diet, and exercise. Clinical manifestations include the three *polys:* polydipsia (abnormal thirst partially because of the high glucose content of the blood and the kidney's attempt to dilute it), polyuria (frequent urination in response to the kidney's need to dilute and increase fluid intake), and polyphagia (increased food intake). Despite the increased consumption of food, the patient with type 1 DM often experiences weight loss because the body burns fat and protein instead of glucose for energy. Although there is plenty of glucose in the bloodstream, the body is unable to use it because there is no insulin available to move it into the cells. When the patient exercises, however, the muscles use glucose even if insulin is not available, which is why exercise is so important for maintaining the glucose level.

Pathophysiology

In normal metabolism the end products of digestion (glucose, fatty acids and glycerol, and amino acids) are absorbed into the venous circulation and carried to the liver, where they may be used immediately or stored for later use. The liver can change glycerol and fatty acids into glucose, and glucose into triglycerides, as needed. When glucose is not available as fuel or cannot be used, the liver changes fatty acids into ketone bodies. There are three types of ketones: beta-hydroxybutyric acid, acetoacetic acid, and acetone. The ketones serve as fuel for the muscles and as an energy source for the brain. Free glucose in the bloodstream always can be used by the brain and kidney because these tissues do not need insulin to move glucose molecules into brain cells or glomeruli.

Glucose also is stored in the form of glycogen in the liver. Glycogen can be changed back into glucose as needed by the body for energy. In the patient with DM, lack of proper amounts of insulin or its poor utilization impairs the use of glucose by the body. The excess glucose accumulates in the bloodstream, and hyperglycemia (greater than normal amounts of glucose in the blood) results.

To rid the body of this abnormal amount of glucose, the kidneys excrete it in the urine. This is called glycosuria (abnormal presence of a sugar, especially glucose, in the urine), a condition that necessitates an extra amount of water for proper dilution of the urine. The patient thus develops polyuria and also polydipsia. Often the patient is unable to drink enough fluid to compensate for polyuria and may become dehydrated.

Even though abundant glucose is available in the bloodstream, the body tissues cannot use it without the help of insulin, causing *polyphagia* (increased hunger and consumption of food) to develop. Despite increased intake, the body is unable to metabolize the food, and the patient loses weight. Because carbohydrates cannot be used properly, proteins and fats are broken down and ketone bodies are used excessively for heat and energy. Ketone bodies are acid substances, and acidosis may result. *Diabetic* ketoacidosis (DKA) (acidosis accompanied by an accumulation of ketones in the blood), formerly called *diabetic coma*, may develop and the patient could die. DKA is a severe metabolic disturbance caused by an acute insulin deficiency, decreased peripheral glucose use, increased fat mobilization, and ketogenesis.

Clinical Manifestations

The hallmark symptoms of type 1 DM include the three classic *polys*: polyuria, polydipsia, and polyphagia. As ketone bodies accumulate in the bloodstream, imbalances of sodium, potassium, and bicarbonate result.

Assessment

Subjective data include hunger, thirst, and nausea. In addition to frequent, copious urination, the patient may complain of nocturia, weakness, headaches, and fatigue. Visual complaints including blurring and halos around lights may be reported. Symptoms such as cold extremities, cramping pain in the calves and feet during exercise or walking, decreased sensation to pain and temperature in the feet, and numbness and tingling of the lower extremities may occur. Symptoms of delayed stomach emptying such as nausea, vomiting, and early satiety (feeling of being full after eating) may develop. Male patients may become impotent. A diagnosis of DM is a condition that will require life-long attention and care. Lifestyle changes may be challenging to the patient. Assess coping methods and knowledge about the disease process. Understanding of the care needs including diet planning, medication regimen, and exercise are needed to ensure the patient achieves optimal health and prevents complications Assess the patient's understanding of the importance of adhering to prescribed medical treatment and obtaining adequate follow-up.

Collection of objective data includes assessment of the skin because slow wound healing, furuncles, carbuncles, and ulcerations are common. Women with DM may have frequent urinary tract and vaginal infections, and vaginal discharge is often bothersome. In patients with type 1 DM, weight loss and muscle wasting may be seen. The skin on the lower extremities may appear shiny and thin, with less hair present. The legs and feet may feel cold to the touch, and there may be ulcerated areas. Gangrene of the toes is a dreaded sign. Assess the patient's ability to perform blood glucose testing and proper injection of insulin.

Diagnostic Tests

Diagnosis of DM is made based on clinical manifestations plus the patient's history and laboratory findings. The patient with a random blood glucose level greater than 200 mg/dL, a fasting plasma glucose level greater than 126 mg/dL, or a glucose 2-hour post-load level greater than 200 mg/dL should be evaluated further. Blood tests commonly performed include those listed in Box 11.2. Measurement of the patient's glycosylated hemoglobin (HbA$_{1c}$) permits the health care provider to see an average of glucose levels over the past 120 days. The average life span of a red blood cell is approximately 120 days. When the amount of glucose attached to the red blood cells is measured, the results indicate an average glucose level for the past 120 days (3 months). HbA$_{1c}$ is ideal for monitoring long-term compliance and regulating the blood glucose level. This benefits patient education and management because a one-time measurement of the blood glucose level shows only that day's management and may not reflect past glucose production.

The ADA recommends self-monitoring of blood glucose (SMBG) instead of urine testing in any patient with DM. Blood from a finger-stick is placed on a reagent strip, and a result is available for the patient in less than a minute. SMBG is the monitoring tool of choice because it provides an accurate picture of current blood glucose levels (Fig. 11.9).

The frequency of monitoring depends on the glycemic goals the patient and health care provider set and the intensity of the treatment regimen. The patient receiving two or more injections of insulin per day may want to test before meals and at bedtime every day. If glycemic control is relatively stable, the patient may

---

Box 11.2 Diagnostic Test for Diabetes Mellitus

- *Fasting blood glucose (FBG):* After an 8-h fast, blood is drawn. Normal is 60–100 mg/dL of venous blood; 126 mg/dL or greater is considered abnormal.
- *Oral glucose tolerance test (OGTT):* A blood sample is taken, and then, after the patient drinks fluid containing a known amount of glucose, the blood is sampled periodically for the next 3 h. An OGTT is usually not necessary for patients showing overt signs and symptoms of hyperglycemia, polyuria, polydipsia, and polyphagia, together with FBG levels of 126 mg/dL or greater.
- *Serum insulin:* Insulin is absent in type 1 diabetes mellitus (DM); normal to high in type 2 DM.
- *Postprandial (after a meal) blood glucose (PPBG):* Give a fasting patient a measured amount of carbohydrate solution orally, or have the patient eat a measured amount of foods containing carbohydrates, fats, and proteins. Draw a blood sample 2 h after completion of the meal. Elevated plasma glucose (more than 160 mg/dL) may indicate the presence of DM.
- *Patient self-monitoring of blood glucose (SMBG):* A blood sample is obtained by the finger-stick method, by either the patient or the nurse, and tested with a blood glucose–monitoring device.
- *Glycosylated hemoglobin (HbA$_{1c}$):* This blood test measures the amount of glucose that has become incorporated into the hemoglobin within an erythrocyte; these levels are reported as a percentage of the total hemoglobin. Because glycosylation occurs constantly during the 120-day life span of the erythrocyte, this test reveals the effectiveness of diabetes therapy for the preceding 8–12 weeks. Glycosylated hemoglobin levels remain more stable than plasma glucose levels and are evaluated by venipuncture every 6–8 weeks. Normal HbA$_{1c}$ is approximately 4%–6% of the total. There is an urgent need to reduce HbA$_{1c}$ values to below 7% to reduce complications. A result greater than 8% represents an average blood glucose level of approximately 200 mg/dL and signals a need for changes in treatment.
- *C-peptide test:* The production of insulin by beta cells of the pancreas begins with proinsulin, which consists of an A chain and a B chain connected by an amino acid chain called the C-peptide. The C-peptide is removed, allowing the A and B chains to fold and cleave together, creating the structure of insulin. The C-peptide remnant then is secreted into the bloodstream by the pancreas along with insulin. A patient's C-peptide level indicates whether any insulin is being produced. A newly diagnosed patient with DM often uses this test to determine whether he or she has type 1 or type 2 DM. Normal values are 0.5–2 ng/mL. The patient with type 1 diabetes is unable to produce insulin and therefore has decreased levels of C-peptide; C-peptide levels in patients with type 2 DM are normal or higher than normal.

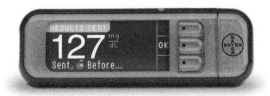

Fig. 11.9 Glucose sensor for self-monitoring of blood glucose. CONTOUR NEXT LINK blood glucose meter from Bayer sends results wirelessly to the insulin pump. (Copyright Bayer HealthCare Medical Care, Whippany, New Jersey.)

elect to test two or more times a day on certain days of the week. Testing usually takes place before meals, but it can occur any time the patient needs to know the way a factor, such as stress, is affecting the blood glucose level. How often SMBG results are recorded to guide therapy decisions should be determined jointly by the health care provider and the patient.

The technology used for SMBG changes rapidly, with newer and more convenient systems being introduced every year. Blood glucose monitoring based on noninvasive spectroscopy—in which a laser light is shone on the skin of the forearm or between finger and thumb—is being researched. Implantable sensors for continuous glucose monitoring also are being tested.

Urine testing for ketonuria is a valuable aid in determining the advent of DKA and is recommended for every patient with type 1 DM when the patient is experiencing hyperglycemia or acute illness.

Medical Management

Medical treatment for DM, regardless of type, consists of education, monitoring, meal planning, and exercise. Pharmacologic therapies also may be required to maintain a healthy serum glucose level. The overall goal is to assist people with DM to make changes in nutrition and exercise habits that lead to improved metabolic control. Additional goals include the following:

- Maintaining as near-normal blood glucose levels as possible by balancing food intake with insulin or oral glucose-lowering medications and activity levels. By maintaining near-normal glucose levels (60 to 99 mg/dL), the patient greatly reduces the risk of complications.
- Losing weight, especially in the case of a patient with type 2 DM who is overweight.
- Achieving optimal serum lipid levels.
- Consuming adequate calories for maintaining or attaining reasonable weight. Reasonable weight is defined as the weight the patient and health care provider decide is achievable and maintainable in the short term and the long term. This may not be the same as the usually defined desirable or ideal body weight. Adequate nutrition also means maintaining normal growth and development rates for children and adolescents and meeting increased metabolic needs during pregnancy, lactation, and recovery from illnesses.

- Preventing and treating acute complications such as hypoglycemia and long-term complications such as renal disease, neuropathy, hypertension, and cardiovascular disease.
- Improving overall health through optimal nutrition. The US Department of Agriculture's MyPlate food planning tool summarizes nutritional guidelines and nutrient needs for all healthy Americans and can be used by the patient with DM.

Diet. Nutritional therapy for the patient with DM is aimed at helping to achieve a normal blood glucose level of less than 126 mg/dL, an HbA_{1c} of 4% to 6%, and attaining or maintaining a reasonable body weight while ensuring proper growth and body maintenance. Nutritional therapy is the cornerstone of care for the person with DM. Dietary treatment, also called *medical nutrition therapy for diabetes,* involves individualized meal plans. Diets are based on ADA recommendations, and patients may obtain additional information and menus from that organization at no cost. A nutritionally adequate meal plan ideally should have a reduction in the total amount of fat, especially saturated fat, to lessen the risk of stroke and heart attack. Enlist the services of a dietitian for each newly diagnosed patient with DM. The menu must be individualized, taking into consideration the patient's age, weight, activity level, lifestyle, ethnic background, and food preferences. Assess the patient's ability to select and pay for groceries, prepare food, and properly store leftovers to ensure that he or she can follow dietary instructions after discharge. If the patient is living with family, teach the person who plans and prepares the meals how to accommodate the patient's dietary needs in the family menus.

Several years ago, the diabetic diet was regimented with "exchanges" allowed for the various food types. Today, the focus is on balance and healthy choice. The total number of calories needed per day is determined by a series of interrelated factors including age, gender, height, weight, level of activity, and overall weight goals. Adult women need between 1600 and 2400 calories daily. Adult men need more at 2000 to 3000 per day (U.S. Department of Health and Human Services [DHHS] and U.S. Department of Agriculture [USDA], 2015). Common approaches to diet planning are the "MyPlate" and carbohydrate counting. Using MyPlate, the patient engages in a process that encourages self-accountability and dietary variety. Exact measurements are not used and selections are more unrestricted, stressing moderation when selecting foods from the MyPlate food planning tool and reducing the use of simple carbohydrates, saturated fats, and alcohol. This diet may be used for the patient whose blood glucose levels are not extremely high, for the pediatric patient, or for the patient who does not adhere to the ADA diet. A normal 9-inch plate is used. The plate is then divided into three sections. The largest section occupies half of the plate. This portion of the plate is to be utilized for non-starch vegetables for the meal. A quarter of the plate is reserved for lean proteins. This may include lean meats or plant-based protein options. Sources of plant proteins are beans, nuts, tofu, lentils, and hummus. The remaining 25% of the plate is dedicated to carbohydrates. Foods in this section of the plate will have the most significant influence on the serum glucose levels. Examples include beans, fruits, starchy vegetables including potatoes, plantains, and pumpkin. Dairy products are included in this section (ADA, 2020).

Traditional *quantitative* diabetic diets involved following a recommended diet of 45% to 50% of total kilocalories from carbohydrates, 10% to 20% of total kilocalories from proteins, and no more than 30% of total kilocalories from fats. In recent years the rigid rules on carbohydrates have softened. Now the emphasis is on the total amount of carbohydrates consumed, rather than on the type. Once it was believed that a simple carbohydrate (sugar) would drive up blood glucose levels, so patients were advised to consume only complex carbohydrates. This has proven inaccurate. Some complex carbohydrates (rice, potatoes, and bread) produce a glycemic response similar to that caused by sucrose (table sugar), and others such as milk and fruit have less effect on blood glucose than most starches. As a result, sugars and complex carbohydrates are counted together as total carbohydrates.

Different carbohydrate foods affect the blood glucose level in different ways; this varying effect is termed the *glycemic index*. Foods having a lower glycemic index take longer to be digested, absorbed, and metabolized. This means the body takes longer to break down the food and there are smaller impacts of serum glucose levels. Examples include peanuts, lentils, raw apples, celery, and lettuce. Higher glycemic index foods provide a quick increase to glucose levels. These foods include white bread, breakfast cereals, and potatoes. Controlling serum glucose levels requires that an emphasis be placed not only on the amount of carbohydrate eaten but also on the glycemic index of those foods.

Insulin-dependent patients usually have mid-afternoon and bedtime snacks in addition to their regular three meals a day. It is important to distribute food intake evenly throughout the day, taking insulin dosage and exercise into consideration. The patient who plans to engage in strenuous exercise should be advised by the health care provider on dietary changes needed before, during, and after exercise, because exercise increases the absorption rate of insulin, thereby enabling muscles to use glucose more effectively.

Alcohol use by diabetics should be approached with restraint. The ingestion of alcoholic products should be discussed with the physician. Alcohol results in calories that provide no nutritional benefit. In addition, after alcohol ingestion the individual may experience hypoglycemia. Medication effectiveness can be impacted by alcohol ingestion. Diabetics choosing to drink should only do so when their glucose levels are under control. Alcohol use can promote complications (American Addiction Centers, 2021).

Exercise. The patient with DM should exercise regularly under the direction of the primary health care provider. The health care provider helps determine the best type of exercise for each patient. Exercise is beneficial not only because it aids in promoting proper use of glucose but also because it is important to the overall functioning of the cardiovascular system, leads to weight loss, and increases the patient's feeling of well-being. Of all the therapies available for treating type 2 DM, exercise is probably the least expensive and most cost effective. Exercise can reduce insulin resistance and increase glucose uptake for as long as 72 hours; it also reduces blood pressure and lipid levels. However, it can carry some risks, including hypoglycemia. Patients should have a complete physical examination before beginning a rigorous exercise program. Like medication, exercise can be adjusted to improve blood glucose control. With exercise, motivation is more important than facts and information. General guidelines are available, and the patient should be encouraged to discuss specific plans with the health care provider. If the patient's glucose is less than 100 mg/dL, a carbohydrate snack is necessary before beginning to exercise. If the glucose measures above 250 mg/dL, the patient may experience excess ketones (and ketoacidosis) during exercise and should consult the health care provider before exercising. Educate the patient to maintain a consistent, health care provider–approved level of exercise and to avoid sudden increases or decreases in exercise pattern.

Stress of acute illness and surgery. Emotional and physical stress can increase the blood glucose level and result in hyperglycemia. Total avoidance of stressful life situations in daily life is not possible. Such situations may necessitate extra insulin to avoid hyperglycemia.

Common stress-evoking situations include acute illness, pregnancy, and the controlled stress of surgery. The patient with DM who has a minor illness such as a cold or the flu should continue drug therapy and food intake. A carbohydrate liquid substitution such as regular soft drinks, gelatin dessert, or beverages such as Gatorade may be necessary. The patient should understand that food intake is important during this time because the body requires extra energy to deal with the stress of the illness.

Blood glucose monitoring should be done every 1 to 2 awake hours by either the patient or a person who can assume responsibility for care during the illness. Urinary output and the presence and degree of ketonuria should be monitored, particularly when fever is present. Increase fluid intake to prevent dehydration, with a minimum of 4 ounces per hour for an adult.

Instruct the patient to contact the health care provider when the blood glucose level exceeds 250 mg/dL; in such cases, fever, ketonuria, and nausea and vomiting may occur. The health care provider should supervise the necessary adjustments in the treatment regimen during times of stress. Eventually the well-informed patient will be able to make most adjustments independently based on experience.

Surgery is a controlled stress, and adjustments in the DM regimen can be planned to ensure glycemic control. The patient is given IV fluids and insulin immediately before, during, and after surgery when there is no oral intake. For the patient with type 2 DM who takes oral antidiabetic medications, usually the drugs are discontinued 48 hours before surgery, and the patient is treated with insulin during the surgical period. Explain to the patient that this is a temporary measure, not a worsening of DM. Treatment with short-acting or rapid-acting insulin allows more accurate control and adjustment in patient treatment.

Medications. Insulin and oral hypoglycemic drugs are the drugs of choice for patients with DM. Insulin administration is necessary for all patients with type 1 DM.

Insulin. In the past, insulin was obtained from the pancreas of cows and pigs. Currently only biosynthetic insulin is used. Biosynthetic insulin is produced by genetically altered common bacteria or yeast, using deoxyribonucleic acid (DNA) technology. This insulin exhibits chemical and biological properties identical to those of human insulin produced by human beta cells in the pancreas (Fig. 11.10). Insulin is a peptide hormone and is absorbed most commonly into the patient's bloodstream. Insulin is given subcutaneously, although IV administration of regular insulin can be done when immediate onset of action is desired. IV regular insulin is mixed in normal saline solution (0.9% sodium chloride). The amount of solution depends on the institution's protocol.

Insulins differ regarding onset, peak, action, and duration (Table 11.5). The specific preparation of each type of insulin is matched with the patient's diet and activity. By adding zinc, acetate buffers, and protamine to insulin in various ways, the onset of activity, peak, and duration times can be manipulated. Different combinations of these insulins can be used to tailor treatment to the patient's specific pattern of blood glucose levels.

Formulas are classified as follows:

Rapid-acting: Lispro (Humalog); aspart (NovoLog); glulisine (Apidra)

Short-acting: Regular insulin (Humulin R, Novolin R, ReliOn R)

Intermediate-acting: NPH insulin (Humulin N, Novolin N, and ReliOn N)

Long-acting: Glargine (Lantus), detemir (Levemir)

*Ultra-*long acting: Degludec (Tresiba)

Glargine is used once a day at bedtime and works around the clock for 24 hours. It is a "peakless" insulin that provides a continuous insulin level similar to the slow, steady (basal) secretions of insulin from a normal

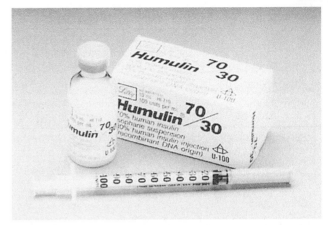

Fig. 11.10 Humulin 70/30 (70% human insulin isophane suspension and 30% human insulin injection [recombinant DNA origin]), containing 100 units of insulin per milliliter (U-100). Humulin is NPH (neutral protamine Hagedorn) insulin. Also shown is a disposable U-100 insulin syringe.

pancreas. Glargine must not be mixed in the same syringe with other insulins because it will interfere with their action (Fig. 11.11). Ultra-long-acting insulin may last up to 42 hours in the body. This allows for flexible injection times, as there are no peaks and the action is consistent.

If hyperglycemia occurs, elevated blood glucose is covered with sliding-scale regular insulin. Premixed combinations are 70/30 (70% NPH insulin and 30% regular insulin; trade names Humulin 70/30 [see Fig. 11.10] and Novolin 70/30) and 50/50 (50% NPH insulin and 50% regular insulin; trade name Humulin 50/50). Recently, two more combinations have become available: 75/25 insulin lispro (75% lispro protamine [intermediate-acting] and 25% lispro [rapid-acting]; trade name Humalog mix 75/25) and 70/30 insulin aspart (70% aspart protamine [intermediate-acting] and 30% aspart [rapid-acting]; trade name NovoLog mix 70/30). The premixed insulins are most helpful for those with stable insulin needs. Timing of insulin action to match food intake can be a challenge, and it tends to be more difficult for people with type 1 DM because their only source of insulin is by injection. Regular insulin is prescribed when a rapid onset of glucose-lowering action is needed, such as before meals and during periods of acute illness, surgery, or stress. Only regular insulin can be administered intravenously; thus it is used in emergencies.

A human insulin formula, called insulin lispro, begins to take effect in less than half the time of regular, short-acting insulin. Older insulin products must be taken subcutaneously 30 to 60 minutes before a meal; the newer lispro formula can be injected 15 minutes before a meal. This timing more closely mimics the body's own hormone activity. Lispro brings the most benefit to people with type 1 DM who take short-acting insulin before meals combined with a longer-acting insulin once or twice a day. Two additional rapid-acting insulins, aspart (NovoLog) and glulisine (Apidra),

Table 11.5   Types of Insulin and Their Use

TYPE OF INSULIN	SOURCE AND COLOR	INJECTION TIME (BEFORE MEAL)	RISK TIME FOR HYPOGLYCEMIC REACTION	ACTION	ONSET OF ACTION	PEAK ACTION	DURATION
Rapid Acting							
lispro (Humalog)	Human Clear	5–15 min	No meal within 30 min	Rapid	15–30 min	1–2 h	3–4 h
aspart (NovoLog)	Human Clear	5–15 min	No meal within 30 min	Rapid	15–30 min	1–3 h	3–5 h
glulisine (Apidra)	Human Clear	5–15 min	No meal within 30 min	Rapid	15–30 min	1–3 h	3–5 h
Short Acting							
Regular Humulin R Novolin R ReliOn R	Human Clear	30 min	Delayed meal or 3–4 h after injection	Short	30–60 min	2–4 h	6–8 h
Mixed							
NovoLog Mix 70/30 (neutral protamine aspart and aspart)	Human Cloudy	15 min	No meal within 30 min	Rapid and intermediate	15–30 min	2–10 h	12–16 h
Humalog mix 75/25 (neutral protamine lispro and lispro)	Human Cloudy	15 min	No meal within 30 min	Rapid and intermediate	15–30 min	2–10 h	12–16 h
NPH/regular mix 70/30 Humulin mix 70/30	Human Cloudy	30–60 min	Delayed meal or 3–4 h after injection	Short and intermediate	30–60 min	6–12 h	18–24 h
Novolin mix 70/30	Human Cloudy	30–60 min	Delayed meal or 3–4 h after injection	Short and intermediate	30–60 min	6–12 h	18–24 h
ReliOn N mix 70/30	Human Cloudy		Delayed meal or 3–4 h after injection	Short and intermediate	30–60 min	6–12 h	18–24 h
NPH/Regular Mix 50/50	Human Cloudy	30–60 min	Delayed meal or 3–4 h after injection	Short and intermediate	30–60 min	6–12 h	18–24 h
Humulin mi50/50	Human Cloudy	30–60 min	Delayed meal or 3–4 h after injection	Short and intermediate	30–60 min	6–12 h	18–24 h
Intermediate Acting							
NPH Humulin N, Novolin N, ReliOn N	Human Milky when mixed	30 min	4–6 h after injection	Intermediate acting	2–4 h	6–10 h	12–16 h
Long Acting							
glargine (Lantus) detemir (Levemir)	Synthetic Clear; do not mix with others	Usually take at 9 PM, once daily[a]	Starting dose should be 20% less than total daily dose of NPH	Long lasting	1–2 h	No pronounced peak	24 h[b]
Ultra-Long Acting							
Degludec	Synthetic Clear	flexible	None	Ultralong acting	1 hour	None	42 hours or longer

[a]May take at other times.
[b]For patients with type 1 diabetes, once or twice daily; for patients with type 2 diabetes, once daily.
From Lewis SM, Heitkemper MM, Dirksen SR, et al: *Medical-surgical nursing: assessment and management of clinical problems*, ed 7, St. Louis, 2007, Mosby.

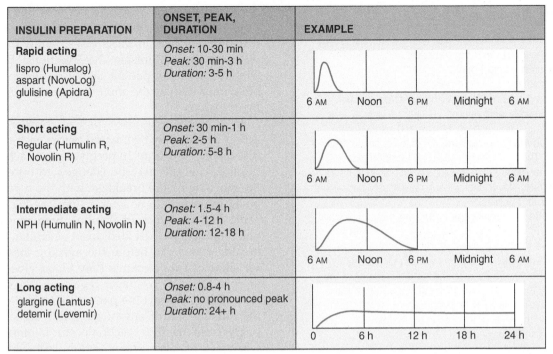

INSULIN PREPARATION	ONSET, PEAK, DURATION	EXAMPLE
Rapid acting lispro (Humalog) aspart (NovoLog) glulisine (Apidra)	*Onset:* 10-30 min *Peak:* 30 min-3 h *Duration:* 3-5 h	6 AM Noon 6 PM Midnight 6 AM
Short acting Regular (Humulin R, Novolin R)	*Onset:* 30 min-1 h *Peak:* 2-5 h *Duration:* 5-8 h	6 AM Noon 6 PM Midnight 6 AM
Intermediate acting NPH (Humulin N, Novolin N)	*Onset:* 1.5-4 h *Peak:* 4-12 h *Duration:* 12-18 h	6 AM Noon 6 PM Midnight 6 AM
Long acting glargine (Lantus) detemir (Levemir)	*Onset:* 0.8-4 h *Peak:* no pronounced peak *Duration:* 24+ h	0 6 h 12 h 18 h 24 h

Fig. 11.11 Commercially available insulin preparations, including onset, peak, and duration of action. (From Lewis SL, Heitkemper MM, Dirksen SR, et al: *Medical-surgical nursing: assessment and management of clinical problems*, ed 9, St. Louis, 2014, Mosby.)

with similar onset of action as lispro (Humalog), also are used. Insulins are used commonly in combination to mimic normal pancreatic insulin secretion.

When giving insulin, be careful to inject only into the *subcutaneous tissue* (between the fat and muscle layers), avoiding depositing the medication directly into the fat or muscle. Insulin administration requires the appropriate syringe. Most commercial insulin is available as U-100, indicating that each milliliter contains 100 units of insulin. U-100 insulin must be used with a U-100–marked syringe. For a user taking smaller doses of insulin, insulin syringes marked for 25, 30, or 50 units are available for use with U-100 insulins. One important distinction is that the 100-unit syringe is marked in 2-unit increments, whereas the 50- and 30-unit syringes are marked in 1-unit increments. Be certain that the patient gets the correct size of syringe and does not switch syringes, thus avoiding serious dosing errors. The Joint Commission now recommends using *units* instead of the abbreviation *U* on medication orders and medication administration records to decrease errors in dosing.

Insulin pens are another popular method of administering insulin. The pen serves the same function as a needle and syringe but is compact and portable, thus making it more convenient. Insulin pens are handy in that they contain all the necessary parts in one piece, but the user must also attach a needle and discard it after each use (Fig. 11.12). The units to be delivered are magnified on the pen, allowing more accurate dosing for the patient with visual impairment.

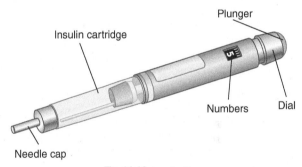

Fig. 11.12 Insulin Pen.

Needles are very fine, usually 25 to 32 gauge, so that they are as atraumatic to the tissue as possible. An open bottle of insulin currently being used does not have to be refrigerated. In fact, it is now believed that insulin should be administered at room temperature, not straight from the refrigerator, to help prevent insulin **lipohypertrophy** (a subcutaneous skin disorder in which a firm lump under the skin develops after long-term subcutaneous insulin injections). Lipohypertrophy can impede insulin absorption. Extra bottles are stored in the refrigerator. Box 11.3 offers guidelines for preparation of a dose of insulin, one or two types at a time.

Patients who self-inject insulin at home may want to have a family member oversee the procedure. Nurses administering insulin injections always must have another licensed person check and document the dose drawn up in the syringe to prevent medication errors. The patient with DM ideally should be taught self-injection technique before discharge from the hospital.

Box 11.3   Preparation of Insulin

1. Thoroughly wash hands with warm water and soap. Bring the insulin to room temperature; an injection of cold insulin can be painful.
2. Assemble all equipment needed, such as a properly calibrated insulin syringe with a prefitted needle, alcohol swab, and insulin.
3. Turn the insulin vial onto its side and gently rotate between the hands several times to be certain it is mixed. The precipitate should be blended evenly. This is not necessary with regular insulin because it has no precipitate. Never shake insulin vigorously because this creates air bubbles.
4. Clean the rubber stopper on the vial with an alcohol swab.
5. Remove the needle cover and draw in the same amount of air as units of insulin to be injected.
6. Insert the needle through the rubber stopper of the vial and then inject the air. Invert the bottle with the syringe unit attached, making sure the tip of the needle is below the level of the insulin so that air will not be drawn into the syringe.
7. Pull back slowly on the plunger, a few units past the desired dose of insulin.
8. Inspect for air bubbles in the syringe; if any are seen, gently tap the barrel until they rise to the top, then push back into the vial with the plunger to the level of the desired dose of insulin.
9. Holding on to the barrel and plunger, remove the syringe unit and put the needle cover back on. Always check an insulin dose with a second licensed nurse. Proceed with the injection procedure.

TWO INSULINS

1. Follow Steps 1 through 5 above.
2. Insert the desired amount of air into the vial of the longer-acting insulin first. Do not mix insulin glargine (Lantus) or detemir (Levemir) with any other insulin or solution.
3. Inject the desired amount of air into the shorter-acting insulin vial; leave the syringe unit in this vial; invert, and proceed through Steps 6 through 9, but do not inject yet. Set the vial of shorter-acting insulin out of reach to prevent accidental reuse.
4. Insert the needle into the vial of longer-acting insulin, being careful to hold on to the plunger so that none of the insulin in the syringe enters that vial.
5. Slowly pull the plunger to the level of the combined total of both types of insulin desired (such as regular 10 units, NPH 30 units, totaling 40 units). Do not pull extra units into the syringe. Take special care not to get any air bubbles into the syringe because they will displace some of the insulin and make the dose incorrect. If this happens, discard the whole syringe and start all over again. Check the insulin dose with a second licensed nurse.
6. If the dose is correct, proceed with the injection procedure.

Some patients are unable to perform this because of physical problems, intellectual incapacity, visual disturbances, or age. In these cases, family members or others must administer the injections. Before discharge, either the patient or the significant other, or both, must display the ability to correctly draw up and inject insulin.

In a newly diagnosed patient, regular or rapid-acting insulin may be injected before each meal. After reasonable control of hyperglycemia is achieved, the dosage schedule may be changed to once a day, in the morning before breakfast, with the type of insulin being intermediate or long acting (see Fig. 11.11 and Table 11.5 for types of insulin). Sometimes patients with DM take two divided doses of insulin, one before breakfast and one before the evening meal. Be alert for signs of hypoglycemia (low blood glucose) at the peak of action of whatever type of insulin the patient is receiving. Instruct the patient to notify a member of the nursing staff if any of the following signs of hypoglycemic (insulin) reaction occur: faintness, sudden weakness, excessive perspiration, irritability, hunger, palpitations, trembling, or drowsiness. Sometimes hypoglycemia signs and symptoms mimic a stroke, and a blood glucose level must be obtained immediately (Walker, 2011).

After appropriate blood glucose testing, the patient chooses an injection site. The subcutaneous pocket is the desired layer into which insulin should be injected. Insulin should not be injected into the muscle, because it enters the bloodstream too quickly and could cause hypoglycemia. Site selection is crucial, as is site rotation. The patient may choose sites on the abdomen (except for 2 inches [5 cm] around the navel), the upper arms, the anterior or lateral aspects of the thighs, and the hips or buttocks. The abdomen provides the fastest, least variable absorption, followed by the arms, thighs, and buttocks (Fig. 11.13). Patients may find it easier to keep track of their injection sites by recording each injection on a numbered chart.

Because of differing anatomic absorption rates of insulin, it currently is recommended that injections be given in all the available areas in a site, such as the thigh, before moving to another site. In this way, the patient with DM may take eight or more injections, spaced 1 to 1½ inches (2.54 to 3.81 cm) apart, and allow the tissues in other sites to recover more fully before being used again. This technique helps prevent lipohypertrophy, a condition that can lead to unsightly lumps under the skin and a decrease in insulin absorption. The technique for insulin injection is described in Box 11.4.

Several new delivery systems are available for patients who find injections emotionally and physically uncomfortable. These include automatic injectors, the jet stream (needleless) injector, the Insuflon indwelling insulin delivery service, and the button infuser.

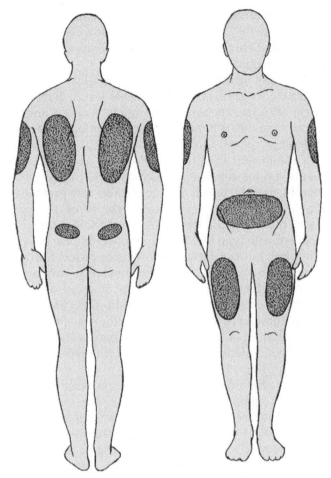

Fig. 11.13 Rotation of sites for insulin injections. (From Potter PA, Perry AG, Stockert PA, et al: *Fundamentals of nursing*, ed 8, St. Louis, 2013, Mosby.)

| Box 11.4 | Technique for Insulin Injection |

1. Follow the Steps in Box 11.3 to prepare the insulin dose.
2. Don disposable gloves.
3. Clean the injection site with an alcohol swab, using a circular motion. Allow the alcohol to dry. Place the swab between the last two fingers of the hand not used to inject the insulin.
4. Pick up the syringe and remove the needle cover and lay it aside. Hold the syringe like a dart.
5. Using the other hand, gently pinch up at least a 2-inch (5.1 cm) fold of tissue (not just the skin).
6. Quickly insert the needle into the top of the fold, entering the subcutaneous tissue. The needle should be inserted at a 90-degree angle unless the patient is very thin and has little subcutaneous tissue. In that case the angle may be reduced by up to 45 degrees to avoid intramuscular injection.
7. Release the skinfold and use that hand to steady the barrel of the syringe.
8. Inject the insulin slowly.
9. Place the alcohol swab against the needle hub, at the injection site, and pull the syringe unit straight out in one swift motion. Do not massage the site.
10. Carefully place the entire unit, uncapped, into the sharps container provided.
11. Record the injection site and insulin dose on a chart, computer, or other documentation sheet. Include the second licensed nurse who witnessed the insulin dose during preparation; ask this nurse to witness the dose given. Store insulin and other supplies properly.
12. When instructing a patient to self-inject insulin, use the following guidelines (if appropriate):
    - Aspiration is not necessary before injection.
    - The injection site does not have to be cleansed with alcohol.

Another method of insulin administration is continuous subcutaneous insulin infusion using an external infusion pump (Fig. 11.14). This small, battery-powered computerized device is worn on the user's body, usually in a pocket or on a belt. It is attached to a thin tube with a needle on the end, which is inserted into the subcutaneous tissue. A continuous, or basal, rate of rapid- or short-acting regular insulin delivery can be programmed, with bolus doses administered as needed. The insulin pump is as close a substitute as available to a healthy, working pancreas. It mimics the pancreas by releasing small amounts of rapid-acting insulin every few minutes. Buffered regular insulin may be substituted in patients unable to use rapid-acting insulin to improve postprandial blood glucose levels and long-term glucose control. The basal rate is designed to keep the blood glucose level steady between meals and during sleep. When food is eaten, the pump is programmed (at the touch of a button) to deliver a larger quantity (bolus) of insulin right away to cover the carbohydrate in the meal. The bolus can also be adjusted on the basis of blood glucose level and planned physical activity. For carefully selected and properly educated patients, the pump offers improved

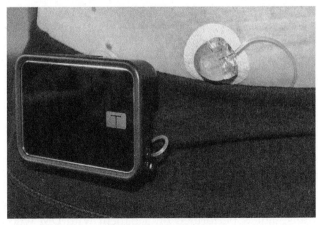

Fig. 11.14 Insulin pump.

flexibility in lifestyle, improved control of blood glucose and glycosylated hemoglobin (HbA_{1c}) levels (see Box 11.2), and freedom from multiple daily injections. Some disassembled insulin pump models can even be worn during bathing or while swimming. The insertion site is usually the abdomen, but the buttocks, thighs, arms, and sections of the back may be used, with the insertion site covered by a clear occlusive dressing, which usually is changed every other day.

Other treatments. Pramlintide (Symlin) is a subcutaneous agent that acts as an adjunct to insulin therapy, not a replacement for it. It decreases gastric emptying, glucagon secretion, and glucose output from the liver and increases satiety.

Another drug that may be used to treat hypoglycemic reactions in DM is glucagon, a hormone normally secreted by the alpha cells of the pancreas. It stimulates the liver to change stored glycogen into glucose, which then is released into the bloodstream. Glucagon is available in a purified, crystallized form for reconstruction and subcutaneous, IM, or IV administration in the event of loss of consciousness as a result of hypoglycemic reaction. The usual dose is 0.5 to 1 mg for adults, with smaller doses for children. Some form of oral protein and carbohydrate, such as milk and crackers, should be given after the patient regains consciousness. Many people with DM carry a commercially prepared kit containing glucagon and concentrated carbohydrate such as candy or glucose gel (see the Complementary and Alternative Therapies box).

Complementary and Alternative Therapies

Endocrine Disorders

- Herbal medicines used in the treatment of type 2 diabetes mellitus (DM) include aloe vera juice, beans (*Phaseolus* species), bitter gourd, karela (*Momordica charantia*), black tea (*Camellia sinensis*), fenugreek (*Trigonella foenum-graecum*), gurmar (*Gymnema sylvestre*), macadamia nut, and Madagascar periwinkle (*Catharanthus roseus*). Effects of these herbs include lowering of blood pressure (fenugreek), boosting of insulin production (gurmar), and increased use of available insulin (black tea).
- Kelp (*Fucus vesiculosus*) may help with weight loss in hypothyroid disorders. Milk thistle (*Silybum marianum*) is used for treatment and prophylaxis of chronic hepatotoxicity, inflammatory liver disorders, and certain types of cirrhosis.
- Yoga may help the patient with DM with diet control and may improve pancreatic function.

Selected patients with type 1 DM now have the option of a pancreas transplant. Usually a pancreas transplant is performed on a patient with DM who has end-stage renal disease and has already had a kidney transplant or will have one in the near future. Kidney and pancreas transplants usually are done at the same time. Patients who undergo kidney and pancreas transplantation must have lifelong immunosuppression therapy to prevent rejection of the transplants.

Nursing Interventions and Patient Teaching

People with DM may be hospitalized as a direct result of their disease process, or they may have a different primary diagnosis.

The daily routine for the patient with DM includes accurate monitoring of blood glucose levels, either by finger-stick specimens or by laboratory testing. Careful attention to diet is important; note the amount of food eaten at each meal and record it accurately.

If the patient with type 1 DM is ill, nauseated, or cannot eat for any reason (such as NPO [nothing by mouth] status), consult with the health care provider. Physiologic and psychological stress raises the patient's blood glucose level. Do not withhold insulin in a patient with type 1 DM without consulting the health care provider or reviewing the written orders for hypoglycemic episodes. Without insulin to promote glucose to enter the cells, the body must seek an alternative source for energy. Fats and protein are used. When these cells break down, ketones are formed. Accumulation of ketones results in ketosis and acidosis. If this situation is not corrected, the patient may develop DKA.

Often the primary health care provider recommends providing Popsicles or apple juice, which can compensate for a decrease in calories when a regular diet cannot be consumed. If the patient does not like the types of food on the meal tray, arrange for a dietitian to consult.

Good skin care is essential for the person with DM, because poor circulation can lead to the development of skin problems. Compromised skin integrity makes a patient with DM more susceptible to infection. In DM, elevated glycosylated hemoglobin in the red blood cells impedes the release of oxygen to the tissues. Elevated blood glucose levels also make some pathogens thrive and proliferate. Vascular changes decrease blood, oxygen, and nutrient supply to the tissues and affect the supply of white blood cells in the area, because if white blood cells do not function properly, phagocytosis is defective.

Report to the health care provider any abnormalities such as cuts, scratches, or lesions anywhere on the body, and treat them before infection develops. Special foot care is crucial for the patient with DM, because poor circulation and decreased nerve sensation or **neuropathy** (any abnormal condition characterized by inflammation and degeneration of the peripheral nerves) increase the danger of ulcers or other abnormal lesions developing into gangrene. The patient should be instructed to use a mirror for inspection of the feet if mobility is impeded, or to have a family member or friend inspect the feet on a daily basis. Many patients seek the services of a podiatrist for their foot care. The patient should wash the feet thoroughly with soap and water every day; dry them thoroughly; and inspect them carefully for cracks, blisters, or foreign objects, paying special attention to the area between the toes. Foot soaks or powders are not recommended. The patient should wear clean socks daily and avoid tight garters. The toenails should be clipped straight across so that the edges do not become ingrown. Never trim the toenails of a patient with DM without a health care provider's written order. Do not put hot water bottles or heating pads on the feet, because burns may occur and may not be felt. The patient should wear sturdy, properly fitting shoes, preferably with wide toe boxes, or molded shoes that are less constrictive. Medicare now reimburses patients with DM who have certain conditions for the cost of specially molded shoes. The patient should not go barefoot at any time. Notify the health care provider immediately of any injury to the toes or feet (see the Health Promotion box).

The patient with DM is encouraged to have eye examinations every 6 to 12 months to allow for early diagnosis and intervention of diabetes-related vision concerns such as retinopathy.

 Health Promotion

Foot Care for the Patient With Diabetes Mellitus

- Wash feet daily with a mild soap and *warm* water. Test water temperature with hands first.
- Pat feet dry gently, especially between toes.
- Examine feet daily for cuts, blisters, edema, erythema, and tender areas. If patient's eyesight is poor, have others inspect feet.
- Use lanolin on feet to prevent skin from drying and cracking. Do not apply between toes.
- Use mild foot powder on feet if perspiring.
- Do not use commercial remedies to remove calluses or corns.
- Cleanse cuts with *warm* water and mild soap, covering with clean dressing. Do not use iodine, rubbing alcohol, or strong adhesives.
- Report skin infections or nonhealing lesions to health care provider immediately.
- Cut toenails even with rounded contour of toes. Do not cut down corners. The best time to trim nails is after a shower or bath.
- Separate overlapping toes with cotton or lamb's wool.
- Avoid open-toe, open-heel, and high-heel shoes. Leather shoes are preferred to plastic ones. Wear slippers with soles. Do not go barefoot. Shake out shoes before putting on.
- Wear clean, absorbent cotton socks. Colored socks must be colorfast.
- Do not wear clothing that constricts circulation.
- Do not use hot water bottles or heating pads to warm feet. Wear socks for warmth.
- Guard against frostbite.
- Exercise feet daily either by walking or by flexing and extending feet in suspended position. Avoid prolonged sitting, standing, and crossing of legs.

Carefully watch the patient who is receiving insulin for development of hypoglycemia, especially when the particular kind of insulin being injected is at its peak

of action. Hypoglycemia is seen less frequently in patients receiving oral hypoglycemic medication, but it can occur.

The emotional aspects of DM are numerous, and many patients experience a period of denial after the initial diagnosis. Some patients become depressed. Because this disease affects all age groups, nursing interventions are tailored to fit the needs of each patient (see the Lifespan Considerations box). Patients with DM must have help in working through their feelings, so be a good listener and supportive. The patient who does not satisfactorily resolve any major problems in accepting the diagnosis of DM may be noncompliant with the treatment plan.

 Lifespan Considerations
Older Adults

Endocrine Disorders

- Diabetes mellitus (DM) is more prevalent in older adults. A major reason for this is that the process of aging involves insulin resistance and glucose intolerance, which are believed to be precursors to type 2 DM.
- The classic signs and symptoms of DM may not be obvious in older adults.
- Dietary management may be complicated by a variety of functional, social, economic, and financial factors.
- Hormone supplements must be administered with caution.
- Older adult patients with DM are at increased risk for infection and should be counseled to receive proper immunizations and seek regular medical attention for even minor symptoms. The older adult often has difficulty in managing DM.
- Some symptoms of hypothyroidism in the older adult are similar to those in a younger person but are more likely to be overlooked because the symptoms—fatigue, mental impairment, sluggishness, and constipation— often are attributed solely to aging. The older person with hypothyroidism has symptoms unique to the age set, including more disturbances of the central nervous system, such as syncope, convulsions, dementia, and coma. There is often pitting edema and deafness.
- The older patient with hyperthyroidism frequently has manifestations related only to the cardiovascular system, such as palpitations, angina, atrial fibrillation, and breathlessness. Signs and symptoms often attributed to "aging" actually may indicate an endocrine problem.

The nurse who supervises the patient in a home setting must encourage the patient to take the prescribed medication faithfully, eat the right kinds of food, test blood or urine correctly, and exercise regularly. If a family member is responsible for the patient's care, ensure that the caregiver is functioning adequately in this role. Some patients live alone and do well caring for themselves, with occasional visits from a home health or public health nurse. Others who have visual disturbances, circulatory problems, or other conditions may need daily visits and more actual nursing intervention, such as help with hygiene, meals, and insulin injections (see Nursing Care Plan 11.1).

Nursing Care Plan 11.1 | **The Patient With Diabetes Mellitus**

Ms. T. is an obese, 52-year-old, married patient with type 2 diabetes mellitus (DM) diagnosed 3 years ago. She was referred to a short-term ambulatory diabetes education program by her health care provider for instruction on insulin administration because she has not achieved blood glucose control with dietary measures.

Objective data included blood glucose 220 mg/dL, weight 200 pounds, and blood pressure 134/84 mm Hg. Collaborative nursing actions include teaching Ms. T. measures that will help her control blood glucose (insulin, diet, and exercise) and how to detect, prevent, and treat hypoglycemic reactions. The nurse reported Ms. T.'s work schedule to the health care provider and asked for insulin dosage alterations on weekends. The health care provider was unaware of her work schedule and stated that blood glucose control could not be optimum with this schedule.

PATIENT PROBLEM

Insufficient Knowledge: Self-injections, Self-monitoring of blood glucose (SMBG), related to lack of exposure

Patient Goals and Expected Outcomes	Nursing Interventions	Evaluation
Patient will independently self-administer insulin Patient will perform SMBG accurately Patient will use measurements obtained by SMBG to achieve blood glucose less than 126 mg/dL Patient will be able to detect and treat hypoglycemia	Support patient as necessary to self-inject insulin. Observe patient's skill in SMBG; correct as necessary. Review with patient the effect of activity, dietary intake, and insulin on blood glucose. Instruct patient on frequency and timing of SMBG. Review with patient signs and symptoms and treatment measures. Refer to dietitian for modification of diet necessary with insulin and for verification of diet knowledge.	Patient demonstrates safety in drawing up and self-administering insulin. Patient demonstrates accuracy in SMBG. Patient can verbalize the effect of activity, diet, and insulin on blood glucose. Patient can recite signs and symptoms of hypoglycemia and the correct immediate treatment to pursue.

PATIENT PROBLEM

Compromised maintenance of health, related to ineffective coping skills.

Patient Goals and Expected Outcomes	Nursing Interventions	Evaluation
Patient will state at least one change that will improve blood glucose control	Teach patient effects of stress, lack of exercise, and activity pattern on blood glucose level. Explore with patient willingness and ability to change behaviors: sleep activity, coping, and exercise. Engage patient in mutual problem solving; refrain from prescribing. Explore sources for long-term support in learning more effective coping skills; suggest support groups: • For patients with diabetes mellitus • For weight loss and maintaining weight loss • Available at work in health service program	Patient has enrolled in an exercise and weight reduction program to assist in achieving a reasonable weight and beneficial exercise.

CRITICAL THINKING QUESTIONS

1. Ms. T. received Humalog mix 75/25, 25 units subcutaneously at 7:30 AM. She followed the American Diabetes Association diet for her breakfast and lunch selections. At 3:00 PM she complains of being hungry, nervous, and tremulous. What are the immediate nursing interventions?
2. Ms. T. states, "I need to lose about 40 pounds, and I'm considering joining a weight reduction club." What would be some helpful suggestions by the nurse?
3. In discharge planning, the nurse notes that Ms. T. has poorly fitting shoes. What would be some important discharge patient teaching for foot care?

Acute complications. One of the acute complications of DM is coma, which may be attributed to three different causes. The first type of coma can occur during DKA, which results from inadequate amounts of insulin or from inadequate insulin use. The second type, hyperglycemic hyperosmolar nonketotic coma (HHNC), involves no acidosis or ketonemia (excessive levels of ketone bodies in the blood) but results from excess glucose, diuresis, and dehydration without adequate fluid replacement. The third type may occur during a hypoglycemic reaction, which results from an excess amount of insulin without an adequate amount of glucose present. These three complications are compared and contrasted in Table 11.6. (See also the Safety Alert boxes: Emergency Care for Hypoglycemic Reaction and Emergency Care for Hyperglycemic Reaction.)

Table 11.6   Comparison of Types of Diabetic Coma

ASSESSMENT	HYPERGLYCEMIC REACTION, DIABETIC KETOACIDOSIS	HYPOGLYCEMIC REACTION	HYPERGLYCEMIC HYPEROSMOLAR NONKETOTIC COMA
Type of diabetes	Type 1	Type 1 or type 2	Type 2
Cause	Inadequate insulin	Too much insulin or oral hypoglycemic agent	Inadequate insulin or oral hypoglycemic agent
Patient history	Omitted or insufficient dose of insulin, physical or emotional stress, gastrointestinal upsets, dietary noncompliance	Reduced food intake, delayed meal, too much exercise	Reduced fluid or food intake with increased urinary output, resulting in severe dehydration
Onset of symptoms	Hours to days	Minutes to hours	Days
Previous diagnosis of having diabetes	Almost always	Yes; on medication	Usually type 2 DM, on hypoglycemic agent
Age of patient	Usually younger patient	Usually younger patient	Usually older adult patient
Appearance of skin	Hot, dry, flushed	Cool, moist	Hot, dry; body temperature elevated
Breath	Fruity (from ketones)	Normal	Normal
Mucous membranes	Dry	Moist	Very dry
Respirations	Deep; may have Kussmaul respirations (air hunger) as a result of metabolic acidosis	Rapid, shallow	Normal
Neurosensory	Drowsiness to coma	Irritability, tremors, impaired consciousness, personality changes; may lose consciousness	Lethargy, decreased consciousness; may lose consciousness
Blood pressure	Low	Normal	Decreased
Glycosuria and ketonuria	Present	Absent	Glycosuria present; no ketonuria
Polyuria and polydipsia	Present	Absent	Present
Hunger	Absent; may have nausea and vomiting	Present; may be nauseated	Absent
Blood glucose level	Usually 300–800 mg/dL	Usually <50 mg/dL	600–2000 mg/dL; serum osmolality greatly increased
Emergency treatment	Insulin, usually regular	Glucose (oral or IV) or glucagon (subQ, IM, or IV)	Large amounts of intravenous fluids; regular insulin

GI, Gastrointestinal; *IM,* intramuscular; *IV,* intravenous; *subQ,* subcutaneous.

 Safety Alert

Emergency Care for Hypoglycemic Reaction

IMMEDIATE TREATMENT: IF CONSCIOUS

- Give patient 15–20 g of quick-acting carbohydrate in some form, such as 4–6 oz of orange juice or a regular soft drink (not a diet drink); half of a candy bar; commercially prepared concentrated glucose tablets or glucose paste; one tube of icing gel (small); 1 TBS of sugar or honey; six jellybeans or gumdrops; five or six pieces of hard candy or other roll candy; four animal crackers; or one granola bar. Offer another 5–20 g of quick-acting carbohydrate in 15 min if no relief is obtained.
- Give patient additional food, a longer-acting carbohydrate (e.g., slice of bread, crackers with peanut butter), after symptoms subside to maintain glucose level after the quick-acting (simple) carbohydrate has been metabolized.

IMMEDIATE TREATMENT: IF UNCONSCIOUS

- Administer glucose gel tube (follow package instructions) between the cheek and gums (in the buccal space).

- Give Glucagon injection (follow package and health care provider instructions for dosage and location).
- Administer IV bolus of 20–50 mL of dextrose 50% in water (ADA, n.d.)..

NURSING INTERVENTIONS DURING AND AFTER HYPOGLYCEMIC EPISODE

- Stay with the patient; check vital signs and do finger-stick blood glucose levels.
- Monitor for worsening of condition or relief of symptoms.
- If patient becomes unconscious, administer glucagon buccally, subcutaneously, intramuscularly, or intravenously.
- Be certain patient ingests food such as milk, six crackers with peanut butter, or one slice of cheese and six crackers after symptoms end (if able).
- Observe closely for 1–2 h after cessation of symptoms.
- Notify health care provider about the hypoglycemic reaction.
- Assess reason the reaction may have occurred.

Safety Alert

Emergency Care for Hyperglycemic Reaction (Diabetic Ketoacidosis)

USUAL TREATMENT DURING ACUTE STAGE
The nurse would expect the following orders from the health care provider:

- Start an intravenous (IV) line, using a large-gauge IV catheter, and begin fluid replacement, usually with normal saline (0.9% sodium chloride) at 1 L/h, until blood pressure is stabilized and urinary output is 30 to 60 mL/h. When blood glucose levels approach 250 mg/dL, add 5% dextrose to the fluid regimen to prevent hypoglycemia.
- Give regular insulin (the only kind that can be given intravenously) as a piggyback infusion, in 500 mL of normal saline. Administer the infusion with a pump controller. Adjust the infusion rate to obtain and maintain desired blood glucose levels.
- Determine blood glucose level hourly (self-monitoring of blood glucose [SMBG] method or venous sample).
- Provide IV replacement of potassium to help move insulin into cells; monitor serum potassium.
- Monitor arterial blood gas (ABG) values specifically for acidosis.
- Administer oxygen via nasal cannula or nonrebreather mask to maintain oxygen saturation at 95% or greater.
- Monitor cardiac status, with central venous pressure and Swan-Ganz monitoring if available.
- Insert Foley catheter and monitor intake and output (I&O) hourly.
- Assess vital signs and neurologic status.

NURSING INTERVENTIONS DURING AND AFTER DIABETIC KETOACIDOSIS

- Keep airway open (patent).
- Maintain patent IV infusion at prescribed rate.
- Keep accurate intake and output record.
- Do accurate blood testing for glucose and urine testing for acetone.
- Monitor vital signs frequently, and assess cardiac status on monitor.
- Assess breath sounds for fluid overload.
- Assess level of consciousness frequently, and perform neurologic checks as ordered.
- Assess the cause of diabetic ketoacidosis.

Another acute complication faced by the patient with DM is the increased risk for the development of infections of any kind. Hyperglycemia and ketonemia hinder the phagocytic action of leukocytes. Additionally, the potential for vascular injury associated with chronic diabetes further heightens risk. An infection may become more severe and last longer, with poor wound healing taking place. Infection increases the possibility of DKA and makes it harder to control the disease. Patients with DM often are hospitalized for treatment of infections that may be handled on an outpatient basis for the nondiabetic patient.

Chronic complications. Primary chronic complications associated with DM are those of end-organ disease, which results from damage to blood vessels (angiopathy) secondary to chronic hyperglycemia. Chronic complications of DM include blindness, cardiovascular problems, and renal failure (Fig. 11.15).

DM causes more cases of blindness in the United States than any other disease. Diabetic retinopathy involves progressive changes in the microcirculation of the retina, resulting in hemorrhages, scar tissue formation, and various degrees of retinal detachment. Surgical techniques such as laser beam coagulation of retinal vessels may improve vision for selected patients with early diagnosis. The risk for the development of glaucoma is greater in the patient with DM. Longevity of the disease, compliance with prescribed therapies, and aging are key factors in the development of the condition. Cataract development is 60% greater in the patient with DM.

Vascular changes in patients with DM, especially capillary changes, contribute to the development of renal sclerosis, often progressing to end-stage renal disease. Approximately 45% of patients with DM must undergo either peritoneal dialysis or hemodialysis as a result. DM contributes to accelerated atherosclerotic changes in the blood vessels, resulting in myocardial infarction, stroke, and gangrene in the lower extremities.

Nervous system manifestations (diabetic neuropathy) are seen commonly, which cause pain and decreased sensation in the extremities and contribute to the development of diabetic gangrene. Symptoms include pain and paresthesia. The pain—described as burning, cramping, itching, or crushing—is usually worse at night and may occur only at that time. Complete or partial loss of sensitivity to touch and temperature is common. Foot injury and ulcerations may occur without the patient ever feeling pain. At times the skin becomes so sensitive (hyperesthesia) that even light pressure from bed sheets cannot be tolerated.

Men with diabetes mellitus experience have an increased incidence of erectile dysfunction. As many as 75% of diabetic males may experience levels of impotence (Diabetes.co.uk, 2019). Impotence associated with DM is believed to result from damage to the sacral parasympathetic nerves. Patients of either gender may have orthostatic hypotension and bladder or bowel dysfunction.

Neuropathy affecting the autonomic nervous system also may result in gastropathy, a delayed gastric emptying that can produce anorexia, nausea, vomiting, early satiety, and a persistent feeling of fullness. These problems previously were referred to as *gastroparesis,* a term now reserved for the condition in which the stomach is severely affected and is very slow to empty solid foods. Metoclopramide (Reglan) stimulates gastric emptying and has been used in the treatment of gastroparesis.

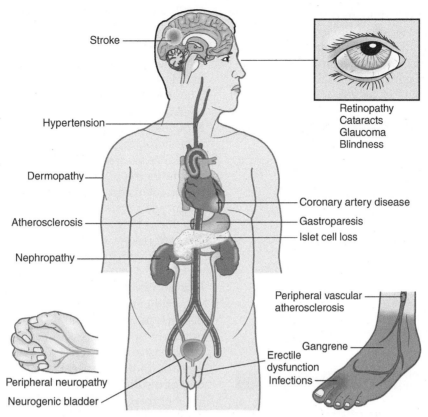

Fig. 11.15 Long-term complications of diabetes mellitus. (From Lewis SL, Heitkemper MM, Dirksen SR, et al: *Medical-surgical nursing: assessment and management of clinical problems*, ed 9, St. Louis, 2014, Mosby.)

Patient problems and interventions for the patient with DM include but are not limited to the following:

PATIENT PROBLEM	NURSING INTERVENTIONS
Impaired health maintenance, related to health beliefs	Instruct in proper self-injection of insulin; have patient perform return demonstration Reinforce instructions regarding availability of glucose and glycogen sources Remove potentially hazardous objects from environment
Potential for compromised maintenance of health	Establish therapeutic relationship so that patient can express negative feelings Correct misconceptions about treatment regimen Assist patient in setting long-term goals for lifetime optimal disease management Involve significant others when possible, and encourage communication between them and the patient Refer patient to appropriate agencies and services (local support groups, ADA)

Education for the person with DM has many important aspects, including the proper administration of insulin or oral hypoglycemic medications and their side effects; the signs and symptoms of hyperglycemia and hypoglycemia; methods of testing blood glucose levels and of urine testing for acetone; planning and preparing the prescribed diet; and personal hygiene, emphasizing skin and foot care. Stress the interrelationships of diet, medication, and exercise. Instruct the patient to visit the dentist regularly and an ophthalmologist annually. Because infections and illnesses of any kind could result in loss of diabetic control, instruct the patient to notify the health care provider at the first sign of any illness. Special plans for travel include taking extra insulin vials and syringes, carrying food and some form of concentrated carbohydrate, and arranging for SMBG or urine testing. Provisions for adequate rest time must be made because exhaustion can lead to changes in the overall condition.

Before discharge from the hospital, the patient should verbalize an understanding of how to prevent complications and display an interest in maintaining optimal wellness (see the Cultural Considerations box). Stress the importance of regular medical checkups. The social aspects of DM cannot be ignored. Patients need to learn about lifestyle adjustment and should wear a medical alert bracelet or necklace, and carry medical information wallet cards at all times. Decisions such as whether to attempt pregnancy should be considered thoroughly by women with DM. Above all, the patient must accept the responsibility for self-care and recognize that making the right choices can affect life expectancy and quality. A current trend is for hospitals to employ a diabetes nurse specialist to develop and implement patient and staff education (see the Home Care Considerations box).

Cultural Considerations

Chronic Conditions

- When caring for a patient with a chronic condition, the health care team should identify the patient's cultural background, values, and beliefs to identify appropriate regimens. This is particularly important in a condition such as diabetes mellitus, which may require major lifestyle changes for successful management.
- In assessing patients, it is important to consider the best way to communicate across cultures. For example, Asian and Mexican cultures consider asking a direct question and expecting a direct answer to be ill mannered and rude. Phrasing questions in a more indirect way fosters more effective communication.

Home Care Considerations

Diabetes Mellitus

- Most of the education for the patient with diabetes mellitus (DM) is provided outside of the hospital environment.
- Frequently, older adults have difficulty with mobility and changes in vision that may hamper the drawing up of insulin.
- Often there is missing information as to why control cannot be obtained; that missing link may be found during a home visit.
- DM caregivers and home care agencies often team up to provide specific care for the older adult.
- Home care personnel network with other community resources to improve the older adult's quality of life or help deal with economic issues.
- Diabetic management should include education in the following:
  - Motivation
  - Self-monitoring of blood glucose
  - Exercise
  - Nutrition therapy
  - Medications
  - Written treatment plan

Prognosis

Although the life expectancy for the person with DM usually is decreased, current research and recent advances have led to hope for a much better prognosis. Early diagnosis and prompt, accurate treatment are essential in promoting longevity. Quality of life has been enhanced by better ways to control hyperglycemia and by earlier recognition of developing complications. Life expectancy and quality of life are related directly to glycemic control.

TYPE 2 DIABETES MELLITUS

Etiology

Type 2 diabetes mellitus usually occurs in people who are older than 35 years of age, with about half of the people diagnosed being older than 55 at diagnosis. About 80% to 90% of patients with type 2 DM are overweight at the time of diagnosis. Type 2 DM often is diagnosed after the patient has suffered from high cholesterol, high blood pressure, obesity, and insulin resistance for some time. These disorders further complicate the type 2 patient's prognosis in terms of cardiovascular and neurologic risk factors. Most newly diagnosed patients with type 2 DM have had the disease for as long as 10 years without treatment, causing elevated risk for the development of serious complications before diagnosis.

Pathophysiology

The pathophysiologic factors that have been identified in type 2 DM include (1) decreased tissue (e.g., fat, muscle) responsiveness to insulin as a result of receptor or postreceptor defects; (2) overproduction of insulin early in the disease, but eventual decreased secretion of insulin (the result of beta cell exhaustion); and (3) abnormal hepatic glucose regulation. These factors result in what is often referred to as *peripheral insulin resistance*. This resistance stimulates increased insulin production as a compensatory response, which also may predispose the patient to weight gain.

Clinical Manifestations

Patients with type 2 DM have few classic symptoms. The patient is usually not prone to ketoacidosis except during periods of stress. The patient may be asymptomatic in the early stages of the disease but later may complain of symptoms associated with type 1, plus many others. These patients may not seek medical care until a severe complication such as kidney involvement, retinopathy, impotence, neuropathy, or gangrene occurs.

Assessment

The assessments for type 2 DM are similar to those of type 1. However, rather than weight loss and muscle wasting, most of these patients remain obese.

Diagnostic Tests

The diagnostic tests for type 2 DM are similar to those for type 1.

Medical Management

Patients with type 2 DM are encouraged to manage their disease with diet (control of carbohydrates and calories) as well as exercise. If cardiovascular disease is a concern, education to modify the diet is vital. The patient needs instruction in managing appropriate carbohydrates, calories, sodium (if hypertensive), fat, and cholesterol (if at risk for cardiovascular disease) and maintaining a healthy weight. Weight loss for the obese patient with type 2 DM tends to reverse this problem. Oral hypoglycemic agents are considered when the patient is unable to maintain normal glucose levels with the above-described lifestyle changes. In some cases, insulin is added to the treatment regimen to further control the disorder. These medications increase insulin production, improve cell receptor binding, regulate hepatic glucose production, and delay carbohydrate absorption from the small intestine.

When a patient with type 2 DM is hospitalized or otherwise experiences decreased mobility, medications (such as steroids), infection, and stress, the blood glucose levels often rise. The patient may require insulin to further manage blood glucose levels.

Oral hypoglycemics. Oral hypoglycemic medications are compounds used to treat type 2 DM, each having a different mechanism of action. Oral hypoglycemic agents are not oral insulin or a substitute for insulin. The patient must have some functioning insulin production for oral hypoglycemics to be effective.

Seven classes of oral drugs—sulfonylureas, meglitinides, alpha-glucosidase inhibitors, thiazolidinediones, and biguanide—are available for patients whose insulin production or use is inadequate because of type 2 DM (Table 11.7):

- *Sulfonylureas:* Sulfonylureas have blood glucose–lowering effects. They stimulate the pancreas to release insulin. A second generation of sulfonylureas, approved for use in the United States, includes glipizide (Glucotrol XL), glyburide (Diabeta, Glynase), and glimepiride (Amaryl). They are more potent than previous drugs and do not require renal excretion.
- *Meglitinides:* Meglitinides are a class of oral hypoglycemics that stimulate increased insulin release in the pancreas; they include repaglinide (Prandin) and nateglinide (Starlix).
- *Alpha-glucosidase inhibitors:* Alpha-glucosidase inhibitors are another class of oral hypoglycemics; they lower blood glucose by delaying carbohydrate absorption from the small intestine. This drug class includes acarbose (Precose) and miglitol (Glyset). The best way to gauge the effectiveness of therapy with acarbose and miglitol is to monitor the patient's 2-hour postprandial blood glucose level.
- *Thiazolidinediones:* Thiazolidinediones are a class of oral hypoglycemic medications that lower blood glucose by increasing insulin sensitivity at the insulin receptor sites on the cells. The two drugs currently available in this class are rosiglitazone (Avandia) (see Table 11.7) and pioglitazone (Actos). They are most appropriate for adults whose bodies produce insulin but cannot use it because of inadequate or ineffective insulin receptor sites.
- *Biguanides:* Metformin (Glucophage) is a *biguanide* glucose-lowering agent. It works primarily by reducing hepatic glucose production and lowers fasting blood glucose levels. It also enhances the tissue response to insulin and improves glucose transport into cells. Metformin usually does not promote weight gain and may help improve lipid levels. Metformin is used widely by itself and in combination with a sulfonylurea. Combined glyburide-metformin (Glucovance) is another oral hypoglycemic agent that may be prescribed.
  - SGT2 inhibitors assist the kidneys to remove excessive levels of glucose from the body.
  - DPP4 inhibitors provide assistance to the body after food ingestion. They encourage the pancreas to increase insulin release.

Once an oral drug becomes ineffective, simple substitution rarely works. But combination therapy can be highly effective. For example, oral drugs from two or more classes may be combined, or an oral drug may be combined with a bedtime dose of NPH or glargine insulin or detemir. Metformin and insulin are chosen commonly for combination therapy with sulfonylureas.

Other treatments. In addition to pramlintide (Symlin), exenatide (Byetta) can be used as an adjunct to insulin therapy for type 2 DM. It stimulates release of insulin from the pancreatic beta cells, decreases glucagon secretion, increases satiety, and decreases gastric emptying (Table 11.8). The heightened risk for renal complications makes it a contraindication to implement this treatment in patients already experiencing renal impairment.

GESTATIONAL DIABETES

Etiology
Risk factors for gestational diabetes include age over 25 years, family or personal history of diabetes or prediabetes, excess weight (body mass index >30), and nonwhite race. Complications include increased birth weight of baby (typically more than 9 lb [4.1 kg]), preterm delivery with respiratory distress syndrome, hypoglycemia in the infant after delivery, and risk for the mother to develop type 2 DM late in life.

Clinical Manifestations
Signs and symptoms of gestational diabetes are consistent with type 2 DM.

Assessment
The health care provider checks for gestational diabetes during the pregnant patient's prenatal visits, especially during the last half of the pregnancy.

Medical Management
The goal of therapy is to maintain a normal glucose level during pregnancy, using insulin, diet, and exercise as deemed appropriate by the health care provider. By maintaining normal glucose levels during pregnancy, the patient can decrease the risk of complications significantly.

Table 11.7 Classes of Oral Hypoglycemics

GENERIC NAME (TRADE NAME)	ACTION
Sulfonylureas	
glimepiride glipizide glyburide	Insulin secretagogues (i.e., chemicals triggering insulin release) stimulate the release of insulin from the pancreases.
Meglitinides	
nateglinide repaglinide	Insulin secretagogues, like the sulfonylureas, stimulate beta cells in the pancreas to increase insulin release. Their effects, which are glucose dependent, decrease when the patient's blood glucose level decreases. Requires functioning pancreatic beta cells.
Biguanides	
metformin	The biguanides work by reducing the action of the liver to reduce the liver's glucose production. The body's tissue responses to insulin is altered. Glucose transport into the cells is enhanced.
Alpha-Glucosidase Inhibitors	
acarbose miglitol	Alpha-glucosidase inhibitors compete with intestinal enzymes to digest carbohydrates. They delay carbohydrate absorption from the small intestine.
Thiazolidinediones	
pioglitazone rosiglitazone	Thiazolidinediones increase insulin sensitivity at insulin receptor sites on the cells. They are most appropriate for adults whose bodies produce insulin but cannot use it because of inadequate or ineffective insulin receptor sites.
SGT2 inhibitors	
Canagliflozin	Aid kidneys in the removal of glucose from the body
DPP-4 inhibitors	
Sitagliptin	Promote insulin release from the pancreas after dietary intake

Modified from Funnel MM, Barlage DL. Managing diabetes with "Agent Oral." *Nursing* 2004;34(3):36–40.

Table 11.8 Injectable Medications to Manage Type II Diabetes Mellitus

GENERIC NAME (TRADE NAME)	ACTION
Amylin mimetics; administered subQ	Used in combination with insulin therapy. It carries a black box warning because of its potential to cause severe hypoglycemia within 3 h of administration.
Incretin mimetics • liraglutide– • exenatide extended release	Incretin mimetics are prescribed for patients with type 2 diabetes meatus. The class promotes insulin secretion and suppresses glucagon release and appetite

❖ NURSING PROCESS FOR THE PATIENT WITH AN ENDOCRINE DISORDER

The role of the licensed practical nurse/licensed vocational nurse (LPN/LVN) in the nursing process as stated is that the LPN/LVN will do the following:

- Participate in planning care for patients based on patient needs
- Review patient's care plans and recommend revisions as needed
- Review and follow defined prioritization for patient care
- Use clinical pathways, care maps, or care plans to guide and review patient care

◆ ASSESSMENT

Hormones affect every body tissue and system, causing diverse signs and symptoms of endocrine dysfunction.

Endocrine disorders may have nonspecific or specific clinical manifestations. Some specific signs of endocrine dysfunction are the classic "*polys*" (polyuria, polydipsia, and polyphagia) in DM and exophthalmos in hyperthyroidism. Specific signs make the assessment easier, whereas nonspecific signs and symptoms, such as tachycardia, fatigue, and depression, are more problematic.

◆ PATIENT PROBLEM

Patient problems are determined from careful examination of patient data. Patient problem statements for the patient with an endocrine disorder may include but are not limited to the following:

- Compromised Maintenance of Health
- Distorted Body Image
- Impaired Coping
- Impaired Neurovascular Function

- Impaired Sexual Function
- Inability to Tolerate Activity
- Insufficient Knowledge
- Insufficient Nutrition
- Noncooperation or Nonconformity
- Potential for Impaired Self-Esteem due to Current Situation
- Potential for Inadequate Fluid Volume
- Potential for Infection
- Potential for Injury

◆ EXPECTED OUTCOMES AND PLANNING

The plan for management of patients with endocrine disorders must center on education to enable patients to understand their disorders, develop a healthy lifestyle, and prevent complications of their disease.

The care plan focuses on accomplishing individual goals and outcomes that relate to the identified patient problems. Examples of these include the following:

Goal 1: Patient will demonstrate safety in self-injections of insulin.

Evaluation: Patient independently administers insulin injection safely and accurately.

Goal 2: Patient will demonstrate SMBG.

Evaluation: Patient performs SMBG accurately.

◆ IMPLEMENTATION

A major nursing responsibility is to help patients gain self-management skills for their chronic endocrine disorder through teaching and counseling. Self-management skills are probably the major factor in controlling the health problem and maintaining an optimal quality of life. Self-management skills are implemented through education in the disease process, the management of medications, the management of nutrition, and the role of exercise; SMBG; hygiene; the prevention of complications; and assistance with psychological adjustment.

◆ EVALUATION

During and after patient educational teaching on self-management skills, assist in evaluating the success of the teaching by noting patient progress, based on stated goals and outcomes. For example, when the patient performs SMBG, observe the patient's skill, correct him or her as necessary, and evaluate the patient's technique to ensure accuracy. When patients are unable to meet expected outcomes, be ready to revise the care plan to promote success.

Get Ready for the NCLEX® Examination!

Key Points

- Endocrine glands are ductless glands that release chemicals (hormones) into the bloodstream to regulate body activities.
- The pituitary gland, located in the brain, is the master gland of the endocrine system.
- Hormones have a generalized effect on metabolism, growth and development, and reproduction.
- Endocrine glands regulate themselves by a series of negative feedback messages.
- Hormones secreted by the endocrine glands affect tissues of the entire body, and an imbalance in their levels may contribute to pathologic changes in many different systems.
- Acromegaly and gigantism, disorders of the pituitary gland, result in growth changes that may have a negative effect on the patient's self-image and self-esteem.
- Diabetes insipidus is a disorder of the posterior pituitary and must not be confused with diabetes mellitus, a disorder of the pancreas.
- Clinically, SIADH is characterized by hyponatremia and water retention that progresses to water intoxication.
- When caring for the patient with hyperthyroidism, provide for adequate rest periods and be sure that fluid and food intake meet the patient's nutritional needs.
- The emotions of the patient with hyperthyroidism are labile, so try to eliminate sources of stress from the environment, to help prevent emotional trauma.
- ^{131}I should not be administered to a pregnant patient because of risk to the fetus; nurses who are pregnant should not care for these patients.

- The thyroidectomy patient faces three life-threatening postoperative complications: hemorrhage, tetany, and thyroid crisis.
- The patient with hypothyroidism may experience sluggish mental and physical functioning, so be patient and allow adequate time for nursing routines.
- The prognosis for papillary adenocarcinoma of the thyroid is excellent because few of these tumors metastasize.
- When administering IV calcium chloride to any patient, be careful that none of the drug extravasates because tissue sloughing may result.
- The extreme hypertension often seen in patients with pheochromocytoma may result in cerebrovascular accident.
- Depression is common in patients who suffer from Cushing syndrome; be alert for suicidal thoughts and suicide attempts.
- The four main facets of medical treatment for the patient with DM are diet, SMBG, exercise, and medication.
- Type 1 DM usually is diagnosed first in people younger than 30 years of age; type 2 DM is found more commonly after age 35, and the incidence increases with age.
- As insulin resistance progresses, the pancreas secretes greater amounts of insulin to compensate. This in turn leads to progressive beta cell failure and a lessening of insulin production. Both beta cell dysfunction and insulin resistance are required for the development of hyperglycemia, the central metabolic characteristic of type 2 DM.
- The older person with diabetes may have a high blood glucose level before excreting any into the urine because of an increased renal threshold for glucose.

- The diabetic diet must be individualized, taking into consideration many factors, such as age, lifestyle, food preferences, and the ability to cook and store food.
- The person with type 1 DM must have access to a source of quick glucose at all times, in the event of a hypoglycemic reaction.
- Become familiar with the clinical manifestations of DKA, HHNC, and hypoglycemic reaction to properly assess diabetic patients, respond therapeutically, and educate them in self-care.
- Observe patients on insulin therapy and oral hypoglycemic medications during the time of peak action of the medication, and initiate treatment promptly if hypoglycemia develops.
- The nurse must be knowledgeable about various insulin types and characteristics.
- Two new insulin-enhancing drugs given subcutaneously are pramlintide and exenatide.
- There are five classes of oral hypoglycemic drugs: sulfonylureas, meglitinides, biguanides, alpha-glucosidase inhibitors, and thiazolidinediones.
- DKA can result in seizures, brain damage, or death for the patient with type 1 DM.

Additional Learning Resources

SG Go to your Study Guide for additional learning activities to help you master this chapter content.

Be sure to visit the Evolve site at http://evolve.elsevier.com/Cooper/adult/ for additional online resources.

Review Questions for the NCLEX® Examination

1. **Which hormones are responsible for "fight or flight"?**
   1. Estrogen and testosterone
   2. Follicle-stimulating hormone (FSH) and luteinizing hormone (LH)
   3. Epinephrine and norepinephrine
   4. Calcitonin and parathyroid hormone

2. **Which hormones are responsible for blood calcium levels?**
   1. Calcitonin and parathyroid hormone
   2. Estrogen and progesterone
   3. Melatonin and follicle-stimulating hormone (FSH)
   4. Thyroxine and parathyroid hormone

3. **What is the master gland of the body?**
   1. Thyroid gland
   2. Adrenal gland
   3. Pineal gland
   4. Pituitary gland

4. **Early in the day, a patient had a subtotal thyroidectomy. During evening rounds, you assess the patient, who now has nausea, a temperature of 105°F (40.5°C), tachycardia, and extreme restlessness. What is the most likely cause of these signs?**
   1. Diabetic ketoacidosis
   2. Thyroid crisis
   3. Hypoglycemia
   4. Tetany

5. **The nurse is caring for a patient recovering from a total thyroidectomy. The first night the patient experiences signs and symptoms of postoperative tetany. Which medication should the nurse anticipate will be ordered by the health care provider?**
   1. Sodium iodide PO
   2. Potassium chloride IV
   3. Magnesium sulfate IM
   4. Calcium gluconate IV

6. **The nurse is caring for a patient who had cranial surgery to remove a pituitary tumor 3 days ago, leaving the patient with partial left hemiparesis and diabetes insipidus. Which patient problem is of the greatest priority postoperatively?**
   1. Potential for Inadequate Fluid Volume, related to excessive loss via the urinary system
   2. Despair, related to development of chronic illness (hemiparesis and diabetes insipidus)
   3. Potential for Compromised Oral Mucous Membranes, related to dehydration
   4. Potential for Impaired Family Coping, related to chronic illness

7. **A male patient has hypoglycemia. To control hypoglycemic episodes, the nurse should recommend which of the following?**
   1. Increasing saturated fat intake and fasting in the afternoon
   2. Increasing intake of vitamins B and D and taking iron supplements
   3. Eating a candy bar if light-headedness occurs
   4. Consuming a low-carbohydrate, high-protein diet and avoiding fasting

8. **The nurse is assessing a postoperative thyroidectomy patient for damage to the laryngeal nerve. Which is most likely to suggest that damage may have occurred?**
   1. The patient complains of a slight sore throat.
   2. The patient's voice tone has changed slightly.
   3. The patient is unable to swallow fluids.
   4. The patient is becoming increasingly hoarse.

9. **The nurse is reviewing the plan of care for a patient newly diagnosed with type 1 diabetes mellitus. Which is the greatest priority in the care plan?**
   1. Teach the patient the effect of diet, exercise, and insulin on the blood glucose level.
   2. Refer the patient to the hospital dietitian for education about dietary needs.
   3. Instruct the patient on SMBG, observe return demonstrations, and correct the technique as needed.
   4. Review with the patient the desired effects of his medication, as well as possible side effects.

10. **The nurse is educating a patient who has had type 1 diabetes for the past year. Which statement demonstrates his need for additional teaching?**
    1. "If I want to lose weight, all I have to do is increase my dose of insulin."
    2. "I can have an occasional beer if it's calculated into my diet."
    3. "I will maintain better control of my blood sugar if I eat regular meals."
    4. "It is important that I eat properly, exercise regularly, and take my insulin injections."

11. The nurse is caring for a patient diagnosed with Addison's disease (adrenal hypofunction). The nurse's assessment reveals postural hypotension, fatigue, nausea, vomiting, and poor skin turgor. Which of these patient problems is of greatest priority at this time?

    1. Potential for Infection
    2. Potential for Inability to Regulate Body Temperature
    3. Pain
    4. Potential for Inadequate Fluid Volume

12. The nurse is caring for a patient who states the health care provider is prescribing an insulin that "takes effect in less than half the time of regular (short-acting) insulin." The nurse is aware that this patient has been prescribed which type of insulin?

    1. Humulin R, Novolin R
    2. Lispro (Humalog), aspart (NovoLog)
    3. Humulin N, Novolin N
    4. Humulin 70/30, Novolin 70/30

13. The nurse is aware that the polydipsia and polyuria experienced by a patient with poorly controlled diabetes are caused primarily by which of the following?

    1. The release of ketones from cells during fat metabolism
    2. Fluid shifts resulting from the osmotic effect of hyperglycemia
    3. Damage to the kidneys from exposure to high levels of glucose
    4. Changes in RBCs resulting from attachment of excessive glucose to hemoglobin

14. The nurse is planning care for an elderly patient with type 2 diabetes admitted to the hospital with pneumonia. What should the nurse understand about this patient?

    1. Must receive insulin therapy to prevent the development of ketoacidosis
    2. Has islet cell antibodies that have destroyed the ability of the pancreas to produce insulin
    3. Has minimal or absent endogenous insulin secretion and requires daily insulin injections
    4. May have sufficient endogenous insulin to prevent ketosis but is at risk for development of hyperosmolar coma

15. Which is an appropriate instruction for the patient with diabetes related to care of the feet?

    1. Use heat to increase blood supply.
    2. Avoid softening lotions and creams.
    3. Inspect all surfaces of the feet daily.
    4. Use iodine to disinfect cuts and abrasions.

16. The nurse is conducting a class for patients with diabetes in the community. What information should the nurse include in the educational plan? *(Select all that apply.)*

    1. Regular insulin (Humulin R) has an onset of action of 30 minutes to 1 hour.
    2. Lispro (Humalog) has an onset of action of 15 minutes.
    3. NPH (Humulin N) has an onset of action of 2 hours.
    4. Glargine (Lantus) has an onset of action of 6 to 10 hours.
    5. Lantus has a peak of 8 to 10 hours.

17. In the syndrome of inappropriate antidiuretic hormone (SIADH), what best describes the body's secretions?

    1. Too much antidiuretic hormone
    2. Too little antidiuretic hormone
    3. Too much diuretic hormone
    4. Too little diuretic hormone

18. The nurse is aware that SIADH is characterized by which clinical characteristics? *(Select all that apply.)*

    1. Peripheral edema
    2. Hyponatremia
    3. Water retention
    4. Brain cells becoming edematous
    5. Intake equal to output

19. The nurse is providing care to a patient with SIADH. What can most likely be anticipated to be included in the health care provider's orders?

    1. Increased fluid intake to 3000 mL/day
    2. Fluid restriction to 800 to 1000 mL/day
    3. Discontinue the ordered diuretics
    4. Antiemetics for complaints of nausea

20. The nurse is reviewing the plan of care for a patient with syndrome of inappropriate antidiuretic hormone (SIADH). What would nurse include in the interventions? *(Select all that apply.)*

    1. Daily weight
    2. Intake and output (I&O)
    3. Fluid restriction
    4. Foods high in sodium
    5. Assessment for abdominal sounds

21. The nurse is teaching a diabetic education class in the community. What information should the nurse include in the educational plan?

    1. Exercise leads to a decreased need for insulin.
    2. Insulin should be adjusted on the basis of the amount of protein ingested at each meal.
    3. During illness, the patient should avoid all insulin injections.
    4. Slow-healing wounds are expected and do not have to be reported to the health care provider.

22. What is an appropriate nursing intervention for a patient admitted into the hospital with signs and symptoms of diabetic ketoacidosis?

    1. Obtain blood glucose immediately.
    2. Administer NPH insulin intravenously.
    3. Give intravenous glucagon.
    4. Take vital signs every 4 hours.

23. Which is a principal clinical manifestation in the patient with pheochromocytoma?

    1. Darkly pigmented skin and mucous membranes
    2. Moon face and buffalo hump
    3. Severe hypertension
    4. Carpopedal spasms

24. A woman, 52, comes to the clinic after 2 years without an appointment. She explains that she has avoided going to her doctor for a couple of years because, she says, "…I've been afraid of bad news. I think I have cancer of the head—I mean, the whole head. First my eyes started bulging. And now look at this big tumor in my neck." The patient has visible edema in the anterior neck, consistent with hyperthyroidism, or Graves disease, rather than a tumor. She also exhibits exophthalmos, also consistent with Graves. Other symptoms include insomnia, weight loss, consistent hoarseness and episodes of feeling "jittery." Pulse is rapid, BP elevated, with bruit auscultated over the thyroid. Patient reports profuse diaphoresis and brittle hair. She is diagnosed with advanced hyperthyroidism and is referred to a surgeon. Hearing her options, the patient agrees that surgery is her best option. She is relieved to not have cancer and feels positive going into surgery for thyroidectomy. After surgery, she appears stable, but later in postop, she calls the nurse, sounding anxious. She reports numbness and tingling in the fingertips and toes and around the mouth. As the nurse enters her room, the patient also begins exhibiting muscle spasms in the wrists and feet as the monitor indicates a rise in pulse, BP, and respirations. The patient is now agitated, panicked, and thrashing.

Choose the *most likely* options to complete the statement below.

The **most likely** cause of these symptoms postoperatively is ____1____, which in turn is most likely caused by ____2____; emergency treatment involves ___3___.

Answers: The **most likely** cause of these symptoms postoperatively is **tetany**, which in turn is most likely caused by **low serum calcium due to edema that occludes release of PTH**; emergency treatment involves **IV calcium gluconate**.

OPTIONS FOR 1	OPTIONS FOR 2	OPTIONS FOR 3
Internal bleeding	Obstructed airway	IV calcium gluconate
Cyanosis	Hyperextension of the head	Emergency airway management
Head and neck edema	Low serum calcium due to edema that occludes release of parathyroid hormone	Use pillows to support head and shoulders
Dyspnea	Internal bleeding	Reduce tension on the anterior neck
Thyroid storm	Excess corticosteroids	Adjust to semi-Fowler's position
Tetany	Release of excess thyroid hormones into bloodstream	Mitotane therapy
Hypokalemia	Cushing syndrome	IV sodium iodide, corticosteroid, antipyretic, and methimazole

Objectives

Anatomy and Physiology

1. List and describe the functions of the organs of the male and female reproductive tracts.
2. Discuss menstruation and the hormones necessary for a complete menstrual cycle.

Medical-Surgical

3. Discuss the impact of illness on a patient's sexuality.
4. Discuss nursing interventions for the patient undergoing diagnostic studies related to the reproductive system.
5. Discuss the importance of the Papanicolaou test in early detection of cervical cancer and mammography as a screening procedure for breast cancer.
6. List nursing interventions for patients with menstrual disturbances.
7. Discuss the etiology and pathophysiology, clinical manifestations, assessment, diagnostic tests, medical management, nursing interventions, patient teaching, and prognosis for infections of the female reproductive tract.
8. Discuss four important points to be addressed in discharge planning for the patient with pelvic inflammatory disease.
9. List four problems pertinent to patients with endometriosis.
10. Identify the clinical manifestations of a vaginal fistula.
11. Describe the common problems with cystocele, and rectocele and the related medical management and nursing interventions.
12. Discuss the etiology and pathophysiology, clinical manifestations, assessment, diagnostic tests, medical management, nursing interventions, patient teaching, and prognosis for cancers of the female reproductive system.
13. Identify four patient problems pertinent to ovarian cancer.
14. Describe the preoperative and postoperative nursing interventions for the patient requiring major surgery of the female reproductive system.
15. Describe six important points to emphasize in teaching breast self-examination.
16. Compare four surgical approaches for cancer of the breast.
17. Discuss adjuvant therapies of breast cancer.
18. Discuss nursing interventions for the patient who has had a modified radical mastectomy.
19. List several discharge planning instructions for the patient who has undergone a modified radical mastectomy.
20. Discuss the etiology and pathophysiology, clinical manifestations, assessment, diagnostic tests, medical management, nursing interventions, patient teaching, and prognosis for inflammatory disorders of the male reproductive system.
21. Distinguish between hydrocele and varicocele.
22. Discuss the importance of monthly testicular self-examination beginning at 15 years of age.
23. Discuss patient education related to prevention of sexually transmitted infections.

Key Terms

amenorrhea (ă-měn-ŏ-RĒ-ă, p. 550)

candidiasis (kăn-dĭ-DĬ-ă-sĭs, p. 597)

carcinoma in situ (kăr-sĭ-NŌ-mă ĭn SĬ-tū, p. 571)

chancre (SHĂNG-kěr, p. 594)

Chlamydia trachomatis (klă-MĬD-ē-ă tră-KŌ-mă-tĭs, p. 597)

circumcision (sĭr-kŭm-SĬZH-ŭn, p. 539)

climacteric (klĭ-MĂK-těr-ĭk, p. 555)

colporrhaphy (kŏl-PŎR-ă-fē, p. 567)

colposcopy (kŏl-PŎS-kŏ-pē, p. 545)

cryptorchidism (krĭp-TŎR-kĭ-dĭz-ěm, p. 591)

culdoscopy (kŭl-DŎS-kŏ-pē, p. 546)

curettage (kū-rĕ-TĂHZH, p. 547)

dysmenorrhea (dĭs-měn-ō-RĒ-ă, p. 551)

endometriosis (ěn-dō-mē-trē-Ō-sĭs, p. 564)

epididymitis (ěp-ĭ-dĭd-ě-MĬ-tĭs, p. 589)

fistula (FĬS-tū-lă, p. 566)

introitus (ĭn-TRŌ-ĭ-tŭs, p. 541)

laparoscopy (lă-pă-RŎS-kŏ-pē, p. 546)

mammography (măm-MŎG-ră-fē, p. 548)

menorrhagia (měn-ō-RĂ-jă, p. 552)

metrorrhagia (mě-trō-RĂ-jă, p. 552)

panhysterosalpingo-oophorectomy (păn-HĬS-těr-ō-SĂL-pĭng-gō-ūf-ō-RĔK-tō-mē, p. 575)

Papanicolaou test (Pap test) (pă-pě-NĬ-kō-lō těst, smēr, p. 546)

perimenopause (p. 556)

phimosis (fĭ-MŌ-sĭs, p. 590)

procidentia (prō-sĭ-DĔN-shă, p. 567)

saline infusion ultrasound p. 573

sentinel lymph node mapping (SĔN-tĭ-něl lĭmf nŏd MĂP-ĭng, p. 580)

trichomoniasis (trĭk-ō-mō-NĬ-ă-sĭs, p. 596)

The period of life from conception through birth is made possible through the dynamics of the normally functioning male and female reproductive systems. Reproduction of like individuals is necessary for the continuation of the species. The male and female sex glands *(gonads)* produce the gametes *(sperm, ova)* that unite to form a fertilized egg *(zygote)*, the beginning of a new life.

ANATOMY AND PHYSIOLOGY OF THE REPRODUCTIVE SYSTEM

MALE REPRODUCTIVE SYSTEM

The organs of the male reproductive system include the testes, the ductal system, the accessory glands, and the penis (Fig. 12.1). These structures have various functions: (1) producing and storing sperm, (2) depositing sperm for fertilization, and (3) developing the male secondary sex characteristics.

Testes (Testicles)

The two oval testes (or testicles; the male gonads in animals) are enclosed in the *scrotum,* a saclike structure that lies suspended from the exterior abdominal wall. This position keeps the temperature in the testes below normal body temperature, which is necessary for viable sperm production and storage. Each testis contains one to three coiled *seminiferous tubules,* which produce the sperm cells. After puberty, millions of sperm cells are produced daily. The testes also produce the hormone *testosterone.* Testosterone is responsible for the development of male secondary sex characteristics.

Ductal System

Epididymis. Sperm produced in the seminiferous tubules immediately travel through a network of testicular ducts called the *rete testis.* These passageways contain cilia that sweep sperm out of the testes into the *epididymis,* a tightly coiled tube structure that lies superior to the testes and extends posteriorly. The smooth muscles within the walls of the epididymis contract in response to sexual stimulation. This forces the sperm to the ductus deferens.

Ductus deferens (vas deferens). The ductus deferens (also called the vas deferens) is approximately 18 inches (46 cm) long and rises along the posterior wall of the testes. As it moves upward, it passes through the inguinal canal into the pelvic cavity, loops over the urinary bladder, and joins with the ejaculatory duct. The ductus deferens and its accompanying nerves and blood vessels are enclosed in a connective tissue sheath called the *spermatic cord.* If a man chooses to be sterilized for birth control, it is a simple procedure to make small slits on either side of the scrotum and sever the ductus deferens. This procedure is called a *vasectomy.* It renders the man sterile because sperm can no longer be expelled.

Ejaculatory duct and urethra. Behind the urinary bladder, the ejaculatory duct connects the ductus deferens and seminal vesicle with the prostatic portion of the urethra. The ejaculatory duct is only 1 inch (2.5 cm) long. It unites with the urethra to pass through the prostate gland. Each of the two ejaculatory ducts empties into the prostatic urethra. The urethra passes through the prostate gland and extends the length of the penis, ending at the

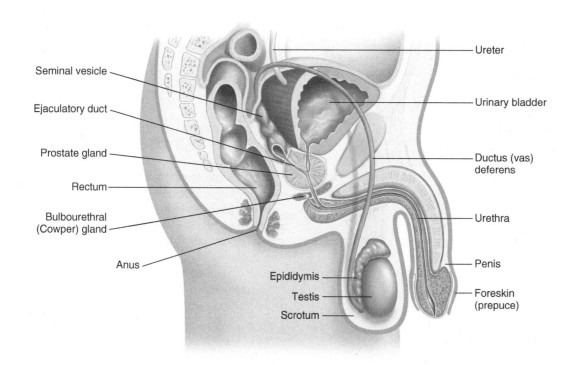

Fig. 12.1 Longitudinal section of the male pelvis, showing the location of the male reproductive organs. (From Patton KT, Thibodeau GA, Douglas MM: *Essentials of anatomy and physiology,* St. Louis, 2012, Mosby.)

urinary meatus (the opening through which urine passes). The urethra carries sperm and urine, but because of the urethral sphincter at the base of the bladder, it does not do so at the same time.

Accessory Glands

The ductal system transports and stores sperm. The accessory glands, which produce seminal fluid (semen), include the seminal vesicles, the prostate gland, and Cowper glands. With each ejaculation (2 to 5 mL of fluid), approximately 200 to 500 million sperm are released.

- *Seminal vesicles:* The seminal vesicles are paired structures that lie at the base of the bladder and produce 60% of the volume of semen. The fluid is released into the ejaculatory ducts to meet with the sperm.
- *Prostate gland:* The single, doughnut-shaped prostate gland surrounds the neck of the bladder and urethra. It is a firm structure, about the size of a chestnut, composed of muscular and glandular tissue. The prostate secretes alkaline fluid that contributes to the motility of sperm. Smooth muscle of the prostate contracts during ejaculation, expelling semen along the urethra. The ejaculatory duct passes obliquely through the posterior part of the gland. The prostate gland often hypertrophies with age, expanding to surround the urethra and making voiding difficult.
- *Cowper glands:* Cowper glands are two pea-sized glands under the male urethra. They correspond to Bartholin glands in women and provide lubrication during sexual intercourse.

Urethra and Penis

The male urethra has two purposes: conveying urine from the bladder and carrying sperm to the outside. The cylindrical penis is the organ of copulation. The shaft of the penis ends with an enlarged tip called the *glans penis.* The skin covering the penis, called the *prepuce,* or *foreskin,* lies in folds around the glans. This excess tissue sometimes is removed in a surgical procedure called circumcision to prevent phimosis (tightness of the prepuce of the penis that prevents retraction of the foreskin over the glans).

Three masses of erectile tissue, the *corpus spongiosum* and two *corpora cavernosa,* contain numerous sinuses that fill the shaft of the penis. With sexual stimulation the sinuses fill with blood, causing the penis to become erect. Sexual stimulation concludes with ejaculation, which is brought about by peristalsis of the reproductive ducts and contraction of the prostate gland. After ejaculation, the penis returns to a flaccid state.

Sperm

Spermatogenesis (the process of developing spermatozoa) begins at puberty and continues throughout life. Mature sperm consist of three distinct parts: (1) the head; (2) the midpiece; and (3) the tail, which propels the sperm. Once deposited in the female reproductive system, mature sperm live approximately 48 hours (or in some cases up to 5 days). If they come in contact with a mature egg, the enzyme on the head of each sperm bombards the egg in an attempt to break down its coating. It takes thousands of sperm to break the coating, but only one sperm enters and fertilizes the egg. The remaining sperm disintegrate. Once fertilization takes place, a chemical change occurs, making the ovum impenetrable for other sperm.

FEMALE REPRODUCTIVE SYSTEM

The organs of the female reproductive system include the ovaries, the uterus, the fallopian tubes, and the vagina (Fig. 12.2). These organs, along with a few accessory structures, produce the ovum, house the fertilized egg, maintain the embryo, and nurture the newborn infant. The ability to conceive and nurture this new human being requires the intricate balance of many hormones and the menstrual cycle.

Ovaries

The paired ovaries (the female gonads in animals) are the size and shape of almonds. They are located bilateral to the uterus and immediately inferior to the fallopian fimbriae. Each ovary contains 30,000 to 40,000 microscopic ovarian follicles. At puberty they release progesterone and the female sex hormone *estrogen,* and they release a mature egg during the menstrual cycle.

Fallopian Tubes (Oviducts)

The fallopian tubes are a pair of ducts opening at one end into the *fundus* (upper portion of the uterus) and at the other end into the peritoneal cavity, over the ovary. They are approximately 4 inches (10 cm) long with the fimbriae at the distal ends. The entire inner surface of the tubes is lined with cilia. When the mature (or graafian) follicle in the ovary ruptures and releases the mature ovum, the fimbriae sweep the ovum into the fallopian tube. Fertilization takes place in the outer third of this tube, and the fertilized ovum *(zygote)* is moved through the tube by a combination of muscular peristaltic movements and the sweeping action of the cilia. If the mature ovum is not fertilized, it disintegrates.

Uterus

The uterus is shaped like an inverted pear and measures 3 inches long by 2 inches wide (7.5 × 2.5 cm) in the nonpregnant state (Fig. 12.3). It is located between the urinary bladder and the rectum and consists of three layers of tissue: (1) the *endometrium,* or inner layer; (2) the *myometrium,* or middle layer; and (3) the *perimetrium,* or outer layer. The uterus is divided into three major portions (see Fig. 12.3). The *fundus* (upper, rounded portion) is the insertion site of the fallopian tubes. The larger midsection is the *corpus* (body). The smaller, narrower lower portion of the uterus is the *cervix,* part of which descends into the vaginal vault.

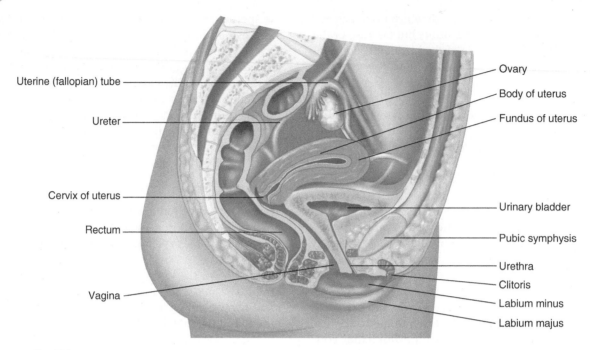

Fig. 12.2 Longitudinal section of the female pelvis, showing the location of the female reproductive organs. (From Thibodeau GA, Patton KT: *Structure and function of the body*, ed 14, St. Louis, 2012, Mosby.)

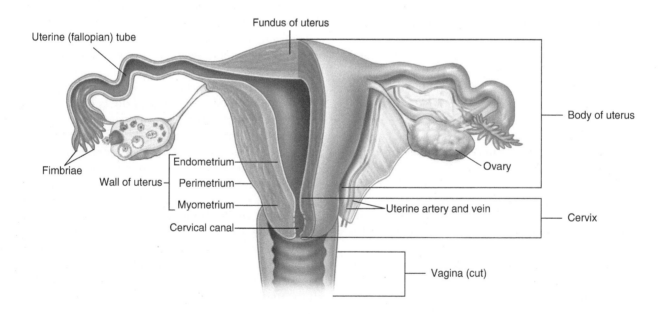

Fig. 12.3 Sectioned view of the uterus, showing its relationship to the ovaries and the vagina. (From Patton KT, Thibodeau GA: *The human body in health and disease*, ed 6, St. Louis, 2014, Mosby.)

Vagina

The vagina is a thin-walled, muscular, tubelike structure of the female genitalia, approximately 3 inches (7.5 cm) long. It is located between the urinary bladder and the rectum. The superior portion articulates with the cervix of the uterus; the inferior portion opens to the outside of the body. The vagina is lined with a mucous membrane, responsible for lubrication during sexual activity. The walls of the vagina normally lie in folds called *rugae*. This enables the vagina to stretch to receive the penis during intercourse and to allow passage of the infant during birth.

The external opening of the vagina is covered by a fold of mucous membrane, skin, and fibrous tissue called the *hymen*. For centuries, some cultures considered the hymen a symbol of virginity, but it is now known that rigorous exercise or the insertion of a

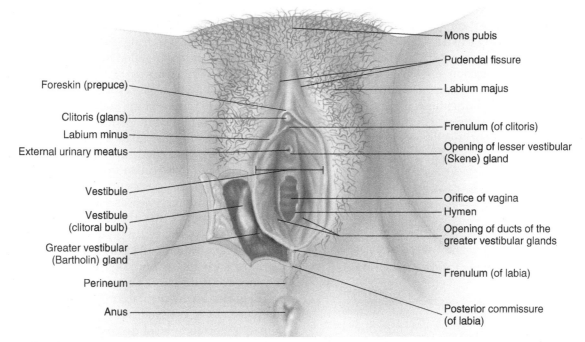

Fig. 12.4 External female genitalia (vulva). (From Patton KT, Thibodeau GA: *The human body in health and disease*, ed 6, St. Louis, 2014, Mosby.)

tampon may tear the hymen. If the hymen does remain intact, it is ruptured by *coitus* (intercourse).

External Genitalia

The reproductive structures located outside the body are the external genitalia, or *vulva*. These structures include the mons pubis, labia majora, labia minora, clitoris, and vestibule (Fig. 12.4).

Located superior to the symphysis pubis (where the iliac bones join at the front of the pelvis) is a mound of fatty tissue, covered with coarse hair. This structure is the *mons pubis*. Extending from the mons pubis to the perineal floor are two large folds called the *labia majora* (Latin, meaning "large lips"; singular, *labium majus*). These protect the inner structures and contain sensory nerve endings and an assortment of sebaceous (oil) glands and sudoriferous (sweat) glands. Directly under the labia majora lie the labia minora ("small lips"; singular, *labium minus*). These are smaller folds of tissue, devoid of hair, that merge anteriorly to form the prepuce of the clitoris. The *clitoris* is comparable to the male penis and is composed of erectile tissue that becomes engorged with blood during sexual stimulation.

The space enclosing the structures located beneath the labia minora is called the *vestibule*. It contains the clitoris, the urinary meatus, the hymen, and the vaginal opening (introitus).

Accessory Glands

Bilateral to the urinary meatus lie the paraurethral, or Skene, glands, the largest glands opening into the urethra. These glands secrete mucus and are similar to the male prostate gland. Bilateral to the vaginal opening are two small, mucus-secreting glands called the greater Bartholin glands (vestibular), which lubricate the vagina for sexual intercourse.

Perineum

The area enclosing the region containing the reproductive structures is referred to as the *perineum*. The perineum is diamond shaped and starts at the symphysis pubis and extends to the anus.

Mammary Glands (Breasts)

The breasts are attached to the pectoral (chest) muscles. Breast tissue is identifiable in both sexes. During puberty, the female breasts change their size, shape, and ability to function. Each breast contains 15 to 20 lobes, which are separated by adipose tissue. The amount of adipose tissue is responsible for the size of the breast. Within each lobe are many lobules that contain milk-producing cells; these lobules lead directly to the lactiferous ducts that empty into the nipple (Fig. 12.5).

The nipple is composed of smooth muscle that allows it to become erect. The dark pink or brown tissue surrounding the nipple is called the *areola*. Milk production does not start until a woman gives birth. At this time, under the influence of prolactin, the milk is formed. The hormone oxytocin allows milk to be released.

Menstrual Cycle

Menarche, the first menstrual cycle, usually begins at approximately 12 years of age. Each month, for the next 30 to 40 years, an ovum matures and is released about 14 days before the next menstrual flow, which occurs on average every 28 days. If fertilization occurs, menstrual cycling subsides and the body adapts to the developing fetus.

The menstrual cycle is divided into three phases: (1) menstrual, (2) preovulatory, and (3) postovulatory. This discussion uses the example of a 28-day cycle. On days 1 through 5 of the cycle (the menstrual phase), the endometrium sloughs off, accompanied by 1 to 2 ounces (30 to 60 mL) of blood loss. The anterior pituitary gland begins to release follicle-stimulating hormone (FSH); as the level of FSH increases, the egg matures within the graafian follicle (a pocket or envelope-shaped structure where the ovaries prepare the ovum; Fig. 12.6). From days 6 through 13 (pre-ovulatory phase), estrogen is released from the maturing graafian follicle. This estrogen causes vascularization of the uterine lining. On day 14, the anterior pituitary gland releases luteinizing hormone (LH), which causes the rupture of the graafian follicle and release of the mature ovum. The finger-like projections of the fallopian tubes (fimbriae) sweep the ovum into the fallopian tube. Once this mature ovum has been expelled, the follicle is transformed into a glandular mass called the *corpus luteum*. During days 15 through 28 (postovulatory phase), the developing corpus luteum releases estrogen and progesterone. If pregnancy occurs, the corpus luteum continues to release estrogen and progesterone to maintain the uterine lining until the placenta is formed, which then takes over the job of hormonal release. If pregnancy does not occur, the corpus luteum lasts 8 days and then disintegrates. Normally the corpus luteum shrinks and is replaced by scar tissue called *corpus albicans*. At this point the hormone level decreases over several days, and menstruation starts again.

EFFECTS OF NORMAL AGING ON THE REPRODUCTIVE SYSTEM

Menopause usually occurs in women between 42 and 58 years of age. The average age is 51. Whether it occurs earlier or later, menopause should not be considered abnormal. Cigarette smoking, family history, living at high altitudes, and surgical intervention or other disease management interventions are associated with early menopause. During menopause the menstrual flow ceases and hormone levels decrease. A woman may experience "hot flashes" (sudden warm feelings), which are caused by the decrease in estrogen production. Changes also occur in the reproductive organs. The vagina loses some of its elasticity, and the

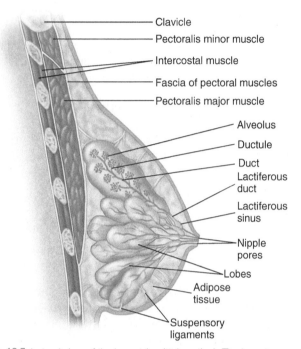

Fig. 12.5 Lateral view of the breast (sagittal section). The breast is fixed to the overlying skin and the pectoralis muscles by the suspensory ligaments of Cooper. Each lobule of secretory tissue is drained by a lactiferous duct that opens through the nipple. (From Patton KT, Thibodeau GA, Douglas MM: *Essentials of anatomy and physiology*, St. Louis, 2012, Mosby.)

Labels in Fig. 12.5: Clavicle; Pectoralis minor muscle; Intercostal muscle; Fascia of pectoral muscles; Pectoralis major muscle; Alveolus; Ductule; Duct; Lactiferous duct; Lactiferous sinus; Nipple pores; Lobes; Adipose tissue; Suspensory ligaments

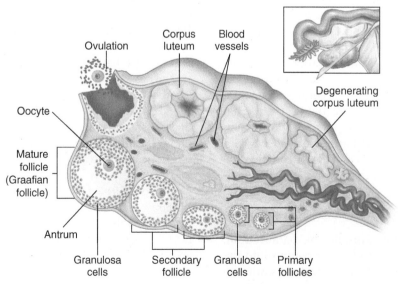

Fig. 12.6 Mammalian ovary showing successive stages of ovarian follicle and ovum development. (From Patton KT, Thibodeau GA: *Anthony's textbook of anatomy and physiology*, ed 20, St. Louis, 2013, Mosby.)

Labels in Fig. 12.6: Ovulation; Corpus luteum; Blood vessels; Degenerating corpus luteum; Oocyte; Mature follicle (Graafian follicle); Antrum; Granulosa cells; Secondary follicle; Granulosa cells; Primary follicles

breasts and vulva lose some adipose tissue, resulting in decreased tissue turgor. The bones also may become brittle and prone to osteoporosis.

Hormonal changes in men are more subtle. The impact of declining hormone levels are noted but not with the same emphasis as in women. Sperm production decreases but does not cease. In later years, testosterone production decreases but not dramatically.

Basically, as long as the older individual is healthy, nothing in the aging process prohibits normal sexual function (see the Lifespan Considerations box).

Lifespan Considerations
Older Adults

Reproductive Disorders

Women
- Many older women are reluctant to seek medical care for problems of the reproductive system. This may be related to cultural factors, embarrassment, or lack of knowledge. Routine gynecologic examination should continue as part of the overall physical examination, even after menopause.
- Certain forms of cancer of the reproductive tract are more common with aging. Any vaginal bleeding should be reported promptly to the health care provider, as should pelvic pain, pruritus, or skin lesions in the genital region.
- Decreased levels of estrogen and systemic diseases, such as diabetes, predispose older women to vaginitis.
- Breast cancer risk increases after 40 years of age. Breast examination should continue throughout the lifespan. The American Cancer Society (ACS) recommends an annual mammogram for women starting between ages 40 and 44 years. From age 55 women in consultation with their physician may opt to have mammograms annually or every other year (ACS, 2020a).

Men
- Decreased production of testosterone results in changes in the male reproductive system. Levels decline gradually with drops of 1% to 2% per year beginning in the third decade of life.
- Sexual interest often continues late in life. The ability to procreate can continue into the eighth decade.
- Chronic health problems, such as diabetes mellitus or hypertension, and many kinds of medication result in impotence in older men.
- Prostate enlargement is increasingly common with each decade after 40 years of age. Although this enlargement is usually benign, cancer of the prostate is a serious condition seen in older men. Ultrasonography of the prostate, when combined with rectal examination and prostate-specific antigen testing, is particularly useful in diagnosing prostate cancer.

HUMAN SEXUALITY

Sexuality and sex are two different things. *Sexuality* often is described as the sense of being a woman or a man. It has biological, psychological, social, and ethical dimensions. Sexuality influences life experiences, and

sexuality is influenced by life experiences. The term *sex* has a more limited meaning. It usually describes the biological aspects of sexuality such as genital sexual activity. Sex may be used for pleasure or reproduction. As a result of life's changes or by personal choice, sexual activity may be absent from a person's life for brief or prolonged periods. Some persons may choose to remain celibate.

The process by which people come to know themselves as women or men is not clearly understood. Being born with female or male genitalia and subsequently learning female or male social roles seem to be factors, although these do not explain differences in sexuality and sexual behavior. Such variations are more understandable if you remember that sexuality is intertwined with all aspects of self.

SEXUAL IDENTITY

Biological identity, or the differences between men and women, is established at conception and further influenced at puberty by hormones. *Gender identity* is the sense of being feminine or masculine. As soon as the infant is born (and sometimes before), the outside world labels the child as a girl or boy. Adults adjust their behavior to relate to a female or male infant. These varied patterns of interaction influence the infant's developing sense of gender identity.

Children explore and seek to understand their own bodies. By combining this information with the way in which they are treated, they begin to create an image of themselves as a boy or as a girl. By the age of 3, children are aware that they will remain boys or girls and that no outward change in their appearance will alter this. This understanding is part of the development of self-concept.

Gender role is the manner in which a person acts as a male or female in accordance with society's norms. Many believe that society influences female and male behavior and is thus the primary source of femaleness or maleness. Because society encourages certain behaviors according to one's gender, differences between individuals' sexual behaviors develop. Sexual behavior is a combined interaction of biological and environmental factors.

Cultural factors can be key ingredients in defining sex roles. Some cultures dictate roles as feminine or masculine (e.g., the man is the breadwinner, and the woman is the caregiver). Other groups have more flexible role definitions and encourage men and women to explore a variety of roles without labeling the behavior as feminine or masculine.

Sexual orientation is the clear and persistent erotic desire of a person for one sex or the other. There are heterosexual, homosexual, lesbian, and bisexual individuals, but the origins of sexual orientation are still not understood. Biological theorists describe orientation in genetic terms, meaning it is determined at conception. Psychological theorists attribute orientation to early learning experiences, believing that cognitive processes are the determining factor. Other theorists state that genetics and environment play roles in the development of sexual preference.

To some, the inward sense of sexual identity does not match their biological body. These people are known as *transgendered*. Researchers do not clearly understand how this occurs. (See *Foundations of Nursing*, Chapter 6). Transgendered people do not see their sexual identity as a choice; it is a clear and persistent orientation dating back to early childhood. In contrast, most homosexual men and women define themselves as satisfied with their gender and social roles; they simply have a persistent sexual attraction to members of the same sex.

A *transvestite* is most often a heterosexual man who periodically dresses like a woman; however, a transvestite may be a homosexual. Cross-dressing usually is done in private and kept secret even from those who are closest to him.

Because sexuality is linked to every aspect of living, any sexual choice involves personal, family, cultural, religious, and social standards of conduct. Ideas about ethical sexual conduct and emotions related to sexuality form the basis for sexual decision making. The range of attitudes about sexuality extends from a traditional view of sex only within marriage to a point of view that allows individuals to determine what is right. Sexual choices that overstep a person's ethical standard may result in internal conflicts.

Some people may judge sexual decisions as moral or immoral solely on the basis of religious standards; others view any private sexual act between consenting adults as moral. People will always have differing beliefs about sexual ethics. The debate over sexuality-related issues such as abortion, contraception, sex education, sexual variations, and premarital or extramarital intercourse will continue. Maintain a nonjudgmental attitude while caring for all patients.

TAKING A SEXUAL HISTORY

Because overall wellness includes sexual health, sexuality should be a part of the health care program. Yet health care services do not always include sexual assessment and interventions. The area of sexuality can be an emotional one for nurses and patients.

Giving patients information about sexuality does not imply agreement with specific beliefs. Patients need accurate, honest information about the effects of illness on sexuality and the ways that sexuality contributes to health and wellness. Provide this information without influencing patient choices. Professional behavior must guarantee that patients receive the best health care possible without diminishing their self-worth. Promotion of self-education and honest examination of sexual beliefs and values can help in reducing sexual bias.

Although there is no single approach to taking a sexual history, certain principles make it more comfortable for you and for the patient (Box 12.1):
- Obtain the sexual history early in the nurse-patient relationship, which indicates permission for patients to discuss sexual concerns. Traumatic situations such as those in which a rape or assault has taken place require a slower progression in data collection.
- Avoid overreacting or underreacting to a patient's comments; this aids in truthful data collection.
- Use language that the patient understands; you and the patient may need to define terms to ensure accurate data gathering.
- Move from the less sensitive to the more sensitive areas. This promotes a certain comfort level between you and the patient.
- At the end of the sexual history, ask if the patient has additional questions or concerns.

A brief sexual history assessment can be made and included in the nursing history through the use of three questions (Box 12.2). The questions may be adapted to address illness, hospitalization, life events, or any other relevant matter that influences or interferes with sexual health. The questions also may be adjusted to find out what the patient expects to happen as a result of procedures, medications, or surgery. Often

Box 12.1 Requirements for Taking a Sexual History

- Provision of privacy—a closed room
- An atmosphere of trust—ensure confidentiality
- Nurses' comfort with their own sexuality
- Nonjudgmental approach

HEALTH PROMOTION
Factors That Can Interfere With the Promotion of Sexual Health
- Lack of information
- Conflicting values system (attitudes and beliefs)
- Anxiety: Are specific attitudes, feelings, and actions "normal"?
- Guilt
- Lack of comfort with sexuality
- Invasion of privacy
- Lack of regard for hospitalized patient's need for time alone with significant other
- Manner in which the patient is touched
- Fear of being judged
- Lack of understanding of the effects of illness and treatment on sexual functioning

Box 12.2 Brief Sexual History

- Has your (illness, pregnancy, hospitalization) interfered with your being a (husband, wife, significant other, father, mother)?
- Has your (abortion, heart attack) changed the way you see yourself as a (woman, man)?
- Has your (colostomy, mastectomy, hysterectomy) changed your ability to function sexually (or altered your sex life)?

you do not need to ask the last two questions, because many patients voice their concerns about masculinity, femininity, and sexual functioning without further encouragement.

Nurses may intervene in sexual problems among patient populations through four strategies: (1) educating patient groups likely to have sexual concerns, (2) providing anticipatory guidance throughout the life cycle, (3) promoting a milieu conducive to sexual health, and (4) validating normalcy about sexual concerns.

ILLNESS AND SEXUALITY

Illness may change a patient's self-concept and result in an inability to function sexually. Medications, stress, fatigue, and depression also affect sexual functioning. Alcohol abuse can lead to a reduced sex drive and inadequate sexual functioning.

Changes in libido (sexual interest), desire, or ability fluctuate during an individual's life. A variety of factors can affect sexual libido. Health status has a strong influence on sexual interest and desire. Lack of interest or desire for sexual activity often occurs when patients are preoccupied with symptoms of illness. The sexual symptoms often disappear as patients recover from the acute phase of illness and resume sexual activity. Some illnesses—such as diabetes mellitus, end-stage renal disease, prostate cancer, certain types of prostate surgery, spinal cord injuries, and heart disease—may cause patients concern or may result in actual inability to function sexually.

Changes in the nervous system, circulatory system, or genital organs may lead to sexual health problems. Spinal cord injuries can interrupt the peripheral nerves and spinal cord reflexes that involve sexual responses. This can affect the ability to achieve orgasm. Some men and women who have spinal cord injuries have reported having satisfying orgasms in spite of denervation of pelvic structures.

An estimated 50% of men with diabetes mellitus are affected by sexual dysfunction at some point in the course of their disease. Chronic lack of glycemic control is associated with damage to vessels that serve the sex organs, resulting in an inability to achieve or maintain an erection. Sexual counseling is important to (1) provide accurate information about the sexual aspects of the disorder, (2) dispel the patient's incorrect assumptions and expectations, and (3) give advice to improve the patient's sexual self-esteem and dispel the guilt frequently found in both partners.

A mastectomy results in physical and emotional trauma. In addition to the resultant disfigurement, a patient must also grapple with the emotional implications of the cancer diagnosis and the impact of the physical changes on her relationship with her spouse or significant other. Problems that arise with pelvic irradiation for cancer of the cervix are much harder to treat than those of mastectomy; the entire physiology of the vagina is altered by the radiation, causing a true

loss of function. With a mastectomy the only function lost is the ability to nurse an infant. The goal for the patient and her partner is to face the issue in a straightforward manner, acknowledging the diagnosis and discussing their true feelings. If feelings are repressed rather than shared, the patient and her significant other may suffer. Therapeutic counseling before surgery can aid the patient's and partner's acceptance and recovery after surgery.

LABORATORY AND DIAGNOSTIC EXAMINATIONS

DIAGNOSTIC TESTS FOR WOMEN

A healthcare provider performs the pelvic examination, which involves visualization and palpation of the vulva, the perineum, the vagina, the cervix, the ovaries, and the uterine surfaces. During the pelvic examination, specimens frequently are obtained for diagnostic purposes. The bimanual pelvic examination progresses from the visualization and palpation of the external genital organs for edema and irritations to an inspection for abnormalities of the internal organs. To visualize the cervix and vaginal mucosa a vaginal speculum (an instrument used to enlarge the vaginal opening) is inserted. The health care provider may perform a rectovaginal examination to evaluate abnormalities or problems of the rectal area and the posterior internal organs (Box 12.3).

Colposcopy

Colposcopy (colpo, vagina or vaginal; and scopy, observation) provides direct visualization of the cervix and vagina. Douching or having intercourse within 24 hours of the examination is not recommended. These activities may mask abnormal cells and reduce the specimens available for collection. Women who are still experiencing menstrual periods are encouraged to schedule the procedure a few days after bleeding ceases for the month. Prepare the patient for a pelvic examination and explain the purpose of the procedure. Encourage the patient to void or have a bowel movement if needed. In the procedure, a speculum is inserted into the vagina. The vaginal walls may be swabbed with an iodine or vinegar solution to remove

Box 12.3	Endoscopic Procedures for Visualization of Pelvic Organs

- *Colposcopy:* Visualization of vagina and cervix under low-power magnification
- *Culdoscopy:* Insertion of a culdoscope through posterior vaginal vault into Douglas's cul-de-sac for visualization of fallopian tubes and ovaries
- *Laparoscopy:* Insertion of a laparoscope (with patient under general anesthesia) through small incision in abdominal wall (inferior margin of umbilicus), then insufflation of abdomen with carbon dioxide; permits visualization of all pelvic organs

surface mucus to improve visualization. A colposcope (a microscope adapted to visualize the vaginal walls and cervix) is inserted for inspection of the area. Tissue color, the presence of growths and lesions, and vascular condition are observed and specimens obtained as necessary. The procedure usually is not performed during menstruation (Mayo Clinic, 2020a).

Culdoscopy

Culdoscopy (*cul-de-sac*; and *scopy*, observation) is a diagnostic procedure that provides visualization of the uterus and uterine appendages (i.e., the ovaries and fallopian tubes). Before the procedure, prepare the patient for the vaginal operation with preoperative instructions. The patient is given a local, spinal, or general anesthetic. After the anesthetic is administered, the patient is assisted to a knee-chest position. The culdoscope (a thin, hollow endoscope with a camera at the end) is passed through the posterior vaginal wall. The area is examined for tumors, cysts, and endometriosis. During the procedure, *conization* (removal of eroded or infected tissue) may be done. A culdoscopy generally is performed on an outpatient basis. After the operation, assess for bleeding, assess vital signs, and monitor voiding.

Laparoscopy

Laparoscopy (examination of the abdominal cavity with a laparoscope, inserted through a small incision made beneath the umbilicus) provides direct visualization of the uterus and its appendages. Preparation of the patient includes insertion of a Foley catheter to maintain bladder decompression for an open view. The procedure is done with a general anesthetic. Carbon dioxide may be introduced to distend the abdomen for easier visualization. If a biopsy is to be done or organs are to be manipulated, a second incision may be made in the lower abdomen to allow for instrument insertion. The ovaries and fallopian tubes are observed for masses, ectopic pregnancy, adhesions, and pelvic inflammatory disease (PID). Tubal ligations may be done using this procedure. Instruct the patient of the probability of shoulder pain afterward because of carbon dioxide introduced into the abdomen.

Papanicolaou Test (Pap Test)

The Papanicolaou test (Pap test) is a simple way to detect cervical cancer in women. In this procedure, a speculum is used to widen the vagina, allowing access to the cervix. Exfoliative (i.e., peeling) and sloughed-off tissue or cells are collected from the cervix, stained, and examined.

In traditional Pap smears, the cells obtained on a brush and then placed in a cup of preservative of liquid solution. The specimens must be labeled with the date, time of the last menstrual period, and whether the woman is taking estrogen or birth control pills. Instruct patients not to douche, use tampons or vaginal

medications, or have sexual intercourse for at least 24 hours before the examination. Collect careful menstrual and gynecologic history.

The American Cancer Society highly recommends that every woman with a cervix begin annual Pap tests at 25 years of age. Between ages 25 and 65 years a "primary HPV test every 5 years. If primary HPV testing is not available, screening may be done with either a co-test that combines an HPV test with a Papanicolaou (Pap) test every 5 years or a Pap test alone every 3 years. a primary HPV test be completed every 5 years." Cervical screening may be stopped for women over the age of 65 years if they have been regularly screened for the previous decade and had normal results and experienced no cervical dysplasia for the previous 25 years. Women who have received the human papillomavirus (HPV) vaccine are encouraged to continue with their recommended age category screening (ACS, 2020a).

The health care provider may recommend more frequent testing for women with a history of multiple sexual partners or sexually transmitted infections (STIs), a family history of cervical cancer, or those whose mothers used diethylstilbestrol during pregnancy (NCI, 2019).

The pap test results may yield results that are negative, positive or inconclusive. Negative findings will indicate the woman will not need additional testing until the time defined by her age category. Abnormal findings of mild dysplasia will be monitored and follow-up testing completed. This provides a comparison of interpretation classifications of the cytologic findings and treatment recommendations. The Bethesda system is preferred because it allows better communication between the cytologist and the clinician. The Bethesda system evaluates the adequacy of the sample (i.e., whether or not it is satisfactory for interpretation) and provides a general classification of normal or abnormal findings and a descriptive diagnosis of the Pap test. Although the classification system used may vary, clinicians agree it is important to monitor Pap tests and ensure proper follow-up, including treatment of vaginal infections and colposcopy if necessary.

Pap tests have long been used to look for cervical cancer and precancerous cells. Nearly all cases of cervical cancer can be attributed to high-risk types of HPV. Twelve types of HPV have been identified as being high risk. There are several tests available that can identify the presence of HPV. Most tests identify the DNA of those HPV types deemed as high risk for causing cervical cancer.

Biopsy

Biopsies are procedures in which samples of tissue are taken for evaluation to confirm or locate a lesion. Tissue is aspirated by special needles or removed by forceps or through an incision.

A breast biopsy is performed to differentiate between benign or malignant conditions of the breast.

Breast biopsy is indicated for patients with palpable masses; suspicious areas appearing on mammography; and persistent, encrusted, purulent, inflamed, or sanguineous discharge from the nipples. The procedure may remove all or a portion of the suspicious growth. If the mass is palpable, the procedure is typically done on an outpatient basis.

Various techniques may be employed. The biopsy may be performed by fine-needle aspiration (FNA); stereotactic or ultrasound-guided core needle biopsy, under local anesthetic; or surgical biopsy, with general or local anesthetic:

- *Fine-needle aspiration:* In FNA, fluid is aspirated from a palpable breast mass and expelled into a specimen bottle. Pressure is placed on the site to stop the bleeding, and an adhesive bandage is applied. FNA may or may not require a local anesthetic, and typically is done in the health care provider's office.

- *Stereotactic or ultrasound-guided core needle biopsy:* Core needle biopsy is a reliable diagnostic technique to obtain a breast biopsy if an abnormal mass is seen on the mammogram. The skin is anesthetized, and a small incision is made. Under the guidance of ultrasound or stereotactic imaging, a biopsy gun is used to fire the core needle into the lesion to remove a sample of the mass. Compared with an open surgical biopsy, this procedure produces less scarring, requires only local anesthesia, is less expensive, and is done on an outpatient basis. Patients must be advised to stop aspirin or blood thinning products 3 to 5 days prior to the procedure and to avoid talcum powder and deodorant the day of the procedure (Cedars Sinai, 2021).

- *Open surgical biopsy:* In an open surgical biopsy, an excisional biopsy usually is performed in a portion of the breast to expose the lesion and then remove the entire mass. Specimens of selected tissue may be frozen and stained for rapid diagnosis. The wound is sutured and a bandage applied. The incision site is monitored for bleeding, tenderness, and erythema (Johns Hopkins, n.d.a.).

A cervical biopsy is done to evaluate cervical lesions and to diagnose cervical cancer. The biopsy generally is done without anesthesia. A colposcope is inserted through the vaginal speculum for direct visualization, the cervical site is selected and cleansed, and tissue is removed. The area then is packed with gauze or a tampon to check the blood flow.

An endometrial biopsy is performed to collect tissue for diagnosis of endometrial cancer and analysis for infertility studies. The procedure generally is performed at the time of menstruation, when the cervix is dilated and cells are obtained more easily. The cervix is anesthetized locally, a curette (a spoon-shaped instrument used to obtain samples from the wall of a cavity) is inserted, and tissue is obtained from selected sites of the endometrium.

Other Diagnostic Studies

Conization of the cervix is used to remove eroded or infected tissue or to confirm cervical cancer. A cone-shaped section is removed when the mass is confined to the epithelial tissue. After surgery the area is packed with gauze to control bleeding. The patient is observed for bleeding and generally discharged from the hospital the same day.

Dilation and curettage (D&C) (*curettage* is the scraping of material from the wall of a cavity or other surface; performed to remove tumors or other abnormal tissue for microscopic study) is a procedure used to obtain tissue for biopsy, to correct cervical stricture, and to treat dysmenorrhea. The patient is placed under general anesthesia, the cervix is dilated, and the uterine walls are scraped with a curette. Packing may be inserted for hemostasis, and a perineal pad is applied for absorption of drainage. After vaginal packing is removed, instruct the patient to monitor for excessive vaginal bleeding or malodorous drainage.

Cultures and smears are collected to examine and identify infectious processes, abnormal cells, and hormonal changes of the reproductive tissue. Specimens collected for smears are prepared by spreading ("smearing") the collected cells on a glass slide and covering the sample with a second slide or spraying it with a fixative. Specimens are handled aseptically, with care taken to avoid the transfer and spread of organisms. Cultures are taken from exudates of the breast, the vagina, rectum, and urethra. STIs and mastitis are diagnosed by isolation of the causative organisms. Treatment is prescribed according to the results of the culture.

Schiller's iodine test is used for the early detection of cancer cells and to guide the health care provider in doing a biopsy. An iodine preparation is applied to the cervix, and in its presence glycogen, which is present in normal cells, stains brown. Abnormal or immature cells do not absorb the stain. Unstained areas may be biopsied. This method of detection is valuable but not entirely reliable, because normal cells sometimes lack glycogen and malignant tissue sometimes contains glycogen. After the procedure the patient should wear a perineal pad to avoid stains on the clothing.

Radiographic examinations are performed to detect abnormal tissue, locate abnormal structures, and confirm the patency of ducts.

Hysterograms and hysterosalpingograms (images of the uterus and of the uterus and fallopian tubes, respectively) (Fig. 12.7) are taken to confirm (1) tubal abnormalities (adhesions and occlusions), (2) the presence of foreign bodies, (3) congenital malformations and leiomyomas (fibroids; noncancerous uterine growths), and (4) traumatic injuries. The patient is placed in the lithotomy position. A speculum is inserted into the vagina, a cannula is inserted through the speculum into the cervical cavity, and a contrast medium is injected through the cannula. As the contrast

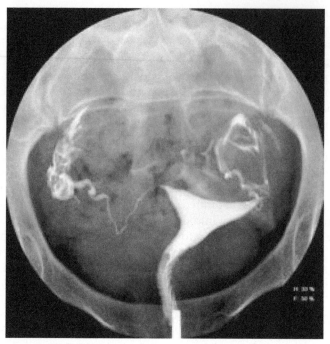

Fig. 12.7 Normal hysterosalpingogram in a young woman with primary infertility. The metal cannula within the external os is seen at the bottom of the figure. The uterine cavity and both fallopian tubes are normal in appearance. There is contrast spilling from both tubes into the pelvic peritoneal cavity, a normal finding.

medium progresses through the cavity, the uterus and fallopian tubes are viewed with a fluoroscope and films are taken.

Mammography is radiography of the soft tissue of the breast, done to allow identification of various benign and neoplastic processes, especially those not palpable on physical examination. Digital mammography is a newer technique that allows a clearer, more accurate image; it involves digitally coding x-ray images into a computer (traditional mammography images are captured on a film cassette). Digital images may be manipulated by the health care provider to enhance elements of concern found in the image. In addition, digital mammography is a more rapid assessment and reporting system. It is believed that the average breast tumor is present for 9 years before it is palpable. The ACS recommends that mammography be an annual option for women between the ages of 40 and 44 years. Annual mammography for women ages 45 to 54 is recommended. For women age 55 and older can transition to the screening every other year (ACS, 2020a).

When the mammography procedure is scheduled, advise the patient to refrain from using body powders, deodorants, and ointments on the breast areas, because this could cause false-positive results. Before the procedure the patient is given a gown and asked to remove jewelry and upper garments. The technician asks the patient to sit or stand in an upright position and rest one breast on the radiographic platform between to plastic imaging plates. During the imaging process, the patient will be asked to take a deep breath and hold it. The breast will be squeezed between the plates. The machine is rotated, the breast is again compressed, and a lateral view is taken. This procedure is repeated on the other breast. The patient may be asked to remain until the radiographic films are read.

Because of the greater density of breast tissue, mammography is less sensitive in younger women, which may result in more false-negative results. About 10% to 15% of all breast cancers can be detected only by palpation; they cannot be seen on mammography. Even if mammogram findings are unremarkable, all suspicious masses should be biopsied.

Women with a positive personal history of breast cancer or the presence of the BRACA gene should be evaluated by mammography accompanied by magnetic resonance imaging (MRI). This testing is recommended for women with a 20% or greater chance for the development of breast cancer in their lifetimes. An MRI is not recommended as a routine screening for all eligible women because of its high cost and greater risk of false positives as compared with mammograms.

Ultrasound is used for further exploration after an examination or mammography reveals a suspicious finding. It is a helpful diagnostic tool to differentiate a benign tumor from a malignant tumor. It is useful in women who have dense breasts with fibrocystic changes. Unlike a mammogram, ultrasound will not detect microcalcifications, which are often the precursors of breast cancer.

In pelvic ultrasonography, high-frequency sound waves are passed into the area to be examined, and images are viewed on a screen; this is similar to a radiographic film. Ultrasound is useful in detecting foreign bodies (such as intrauterine contraceptive devices [IUDs]), distinguishing between cystic and solid tumor bodies, evaluating fetal growth and viability, detecting fetal abnormalities, and detecting ectopic pregnancy. In general, it is noninvasive, safe, and painless. Encourage the patient to drink fluids beforehand. Explain that a full bladder is essential for the accuracy of the test.

Tubal insufflation (Rubin's test) involves transuterine insufflation of the fallopian tubes with carbon dioxide (*insufflation* is the blowing of gas, in this case carbon dioxide, into a body cavity). The procedure enables evaluation of the patency of the fallopian tubes and may be part of a fertility study. Tubal insufflation takes approximately 30 minutes and usually is performed on an outpatient basis. If the tubes are open, the gas enters the abdominal cavity. A high-pitched bubbling is heard through the abdominal wall with a stethoscope as the gas escapes from the tubes. The patient may complain of shoulder pain from diaphragmatic irritation. In this case a radiographic film shows free gas under the diaphragm. If the tubes are occluded, gas cannot pass from the tubes, and the patient will not report pain.

All pregnancy tests, regardless of method, are based on detection of human chorionic gonadotropin (hCG), which is secreted into the urine after fertilization of the ovum. Regardless of method, it is important to know that the tests do not indicate whether the pregnancy is normal. In addition, false-positive results may occur.

Serum CA-125 is a tumor antigen associated with ovarian cancer; it is positive in 80% of such cases. CA-125 antigen levels in the blood decrease as cancer cells decrease. CA-125 has been touted as a way to detect primary ovarian cancer, but unfortunately it does not do so. CA-125 is useful mainly to signal a recurrence of ovarian cancer and to monitor the response to chemotherapy treatment. If chemotherapy causes a progressive decline in CA-125, it is an accurate indicator of a good response and is a good prognostic sign. Other conditions—such as endometriosis, PID, pregnancy, gynecologic cancers, and cancer of the pancreas—may result in an elevation of serum CA-125.

DIAGNOSTIC TESTS FOR MEN

Testicular Biopsy

Testicular biopsy is a means to detect abnormal cells and the presence of sperm. The testing can be done by aspiration or through an incision. The anesthetic used depends on the technique. Post-biopsy care measures consist of scrotal support, ice pack, and analgesic medications. Warm sitz baths for edema also may be helpful. Instruct the patient to call the health care provider if bleeding or elevated temperature occurs.

Semen Analysis

Semen analysis is often one of the first tests performed on the male when evaluating fertility. Other indications include substantiating the effectiveness of a vasectomy, detecting a specimen on a suspected rape victim, and ruling out or determining paternity. Semen

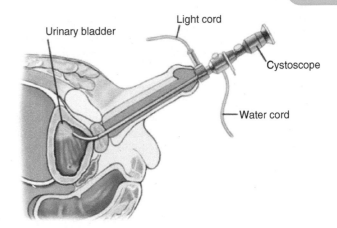

Fig. 12.8 Cystoscopy.

can be collected for testing by manual stimulation, coitus interruptus, or the use of a condom.

Prostatic Smears

Prostatic smears are obtained to detect and identify microorganisms, tumor cells, and even tuberculosis in the prostate. The health care provider massages the prostate by way of the rectum, and the patient voids into a sterile container that has been prepared with additive preservative. The specimen is collected and a smear is prepared in the laboratory.

Cystoscopy

In cystoscopy, a man's prostate and bladder can be examined by passing a lighted cystoscope (a specially adapted endoscope) through the urethra to the bladder (Fig. 12.8). Before the procedure, obtain a signed consent form and educate the patient about the procedure. The procedure may be performed with sedation or anesthesia. A numbing gel may be applied to the urethra to aid in the passage of the scope. After the cystoscopy the patient may have pink-tinged urine, and greater frequency and burning on urination. Baths may be restricted by some physicians. Warm compresses can be used to promote comfort when held at the urinary opening. Cystoscopy can be done for men and women to detect bladder infections and tumors.

Other Diagnostic Studies

Other diagnostic studies for men include the rectal digital examination and the test for prostate-specific antigen (PSA), a highly sensitive blood test. PSA, which normally is secreted and disposed of by the prostate, shows up in the bloodstream in cancer of the prostate and in a harmless condition called benign prostatic hyperplasia or prostate enlargement. The normal PSA level is less than 4 ng/mL. Elevated PSA levels in the bloodstream mean something must be checked. Even a slight increase in PSA level must be monitored closely; referral to a urologist for a biopsy is recommended. Still another study is the alkaline phosphatase (ALP) test. The normal ALP level is 35 to 142 units/L for men and 25 to 125 units/L for women. These specific tests are useful in diagnosing benign prostatic hyperplasia, prostatic cancer, bone metastasis in prostatic cancer, and other disease conditions.

The Reproductive Cycle

Menarche, the beginning of menses, designates the first menstrual cycle. Menarche occurs in late puberty and indicates that the body is capable of supporting pregnancy. Menarche traditionally occurs approximately 24 to 30 months after breast development. The age ranges from as young as 8 years to as old as 15 years. The average age of onset is 12 years. If a girl has not started menstruation by age 15 years, or if it has been longer than 3 years since breast development, a health care provider should be consulted. The length of the menstrual cycle varies from 24 to 32 days; the average cycle lasts 28 days. Day 1 of the menstrual cycle is the day that blood flow (called the *menstrual period*) begins. The flow lasts from 1 to 8 days; the average is 3 to 5 days. The amount of flow ranges from 10 to 75 mL; the average is 35 mL per cycle.

Help patients maintain their reproductive and sexual health by instructing or counseling women about personal hygiene. Personal cleanliness is a health habit that should be promoted for all patients and implemented in each care plan. Cleanliness is especially important during menstruation (see the Health Promotion box).

DISTURBANCES OF MENSTRUATION

Because of the relationship between the menstrual cycle and the body's mechanisms of hormonal secretion, a decrease or increase in activity of the hormonal glands can disturb menstruation. The most common disturbances include the following:

- *Amenorrhea:* Absence of menstrual flow
- *Dysmenorrhea:* Painful menstruation
- *Dysfunctional uterine bleeding (DUB):* Abnormal uterine bleeding
- *Menorrhagia:* Bleeding that is excessive in amount and duration
- *Metrorrhagia:* Bleeding between menstrual periods
  Another disturbance of the menstrual cycle is premenstrual syndrome (PMS), which is discussed later.

Suggested nursing diagnoses are anxiety, ineffective coping, fear, pain, deficient knowledge, and low self-esteem. Nursing interventions are based on specific behaviors, symptoms, and treatments.

AMENORRHEA

Amenorrhea (absence of menstrual flow) is normal before puberty, after menopause, during pregnancy, and sometimes during lactation. Menstrual flow also may be absent or suppressed as a result of hormonal abnormalities or surgical interventions such as a hysterectomy (surgical removal of the uterus).

Health Promotion

Health Teaching for Menstruation

KNOWLEDGE OF THE PHYSIOLOGIC PROCESS
- Factors that may alter the menstrual cycle: stress, weight loss, fatigue, exercise, acute or chronic illness, changes in climate or working hours, and pregnancy

PERSONAL HYGIENE
- Change tampons frequently to decrease risk of toxic shock syndrome.
- Consult health care provider if tampon use frequently causes discomfort.
- Take a daily shower for comfort; warm baths may relieve slight pelvic discomfort.
- Keep perineal area clean and dry; cleanse from anterior to posterior.
- Wear cotton underwear; remember that nylon pantyhose and tight-fitting slacks retain moisture and should not be worn for extended periods.
- Douching is not recommended because it changes the protective bacterial flora of the vagina and predisposes the woman to infection.

EXERCISE
- Exercise is not contraindicated and may help prevent or reduce discomfort.
- Modify exercise if fatigue occurs.

DIET
- Limit salt intake if fluid retention is present.
- Consult a health care provider if fluid retention persists after menstruation.

DISCOMFORT
- Ibuprofen and NSAIDs block prostaglandin production reducing abdominal discomfort Apply heating pad to abdomen or back.
- For prolonged, severe discomfort, consult a health care provider.

Etiology and Pathophysiology

Amenorrhea is classified as *primary* when menarche has not occurred by the age of 17 to 18 years. The other changes associated with puberty may or may not have taken place. This may be the result of hormonal imbalances or genetic disorders. Potential structural causes include congenital defects such as an imperforate hymen, blockages or narrowing of the cervix, missing uterus or vagina, or a vaginal septum. *Secondary amenorrhea* means menarche has occurred, but flow has ceased for at least 6 months. This diagnosis excludes those women who are pregnant, breast-feeding, or menopausal. Secondary amenorrhea may be due to frequent, vigorous exercise, as in female athletes; low body fat; anxiety or an emotional disorder such as depression; pituitary tumors; hyperactive thyroid gland; polycystic ovarian syndrome (PCOS); and medications such as oral and injectable contraceptives. Hormone levels may be altered significantly by antihypertensives and anti-depressive medications resulting in amenorrhea. Estrogen producing cells and eggs within the ovaries can be killed by chemotherapy also resulting in amenorrhea.

Although the primary manifestation is the absence of menstruation, there may be other symptoms present. Weight gain or loss may be reported. Additional changes that may signal hormonal imbalances include breast discharge, vaginal dryness, increased hair growth, changes in breast size, and voice changes.

Assessment

Early diagnosis and prompt management are necessary to prevent more serious reproductive and genital problems. Discussions concerning the presence or absence of menstruation should be included in the health teaching provided to girls and their parents about the progression of puberty and the onset of menses. Urge the sexually active woman to see a health care provider as soon as a menstrual period is missed. Women who suspect their amenorrhea is caused by menopause can be examined by a health care provider to confirm this.

Assess emotional or behavioral factors that may influence the menstrual cycle. A menstrual history includes a discussion of the number of menstrual periods, characteristics of prior periods, and any experience with amenorrhea. A review of medication and drug use history also is needed.

Diagnostic Tests

Confirming the absence of pregnancy is the first step. Beyond the preliminary workup and when pregnancy is not a possibility, the diagnostic study for primary and secondary amenorrhea is the same. This includes a pelvic examination. The pelvic examination determines the presence of structural abnormalities or the presence of growths. Serum studies review hormone levels including estradiol, FSH, prolactin, testosterone, and thyroid-stimulating hormone (TSH). An examination of internal structure may include a computed tomography (CT) scan, MRI, ultrasound, or hysterosalpingogram. Genetic testing also may be indicated.

Medical Management

Treatment is based on the underlying cause and must be determined on an individual basis. Hormonal therapy may be needed.

Nursing Interventions and Patient Teaching

A patient problem and interventions for women with amenorrhea include but are not limited to the following:

PATIENT PROBLEM	NURSING INTERVENTIONS
Anxiousness, related to loss of menstrual cycles	Acknowledge patient's feelings and provide emotional support Refer for counseling as necessary Explain diagnostic procedures Provide information, privacy, and consultation as indicated for sexual concerns

Encourage patients to comply with treatment and emphasize the importance of follow-up visits with the health care provider for treatment, therapy, and evaluation of treatment efficacy.

DYSMENORRHEA

Dysmenorrhea is uterine pain with menstruation, commonly called "menstrual cramps." Primary dysmenorrhea that is not associated with pelvic disorders usually develops when ovulatory function is established (before 20 years of age) and there is no underlying organic disease. Often it disappears or declines after pregnancy or by the time a woman is in her late 20s. The discomfort usually begins at the time of menstruation or in the first 2 days preceding (Cleveland Clinic, 2020). Secondary dysmenorrhea is painful menstruation in women who have normal periods. The cause is linked to disorders of the reproductive tract. Potential causes include fibroid tumors, endometriosis, PID, STIs, and PMS. Stress and anxiety are also related causes.

Dysmenorrhea is the greatest single cause of absenteeism among girls in school and women in the workplace. It is one of the most common health problems for which women seek treatment.

Etiology and Pathophysiology

The leading risk factors for dysmenorrhea are age (<20 years) and nulliparity (the condition of never having given birth). Other risk factors may include heavy periods, anxiety/depression, smoking, and attempts to lose weight. The causes of dysmenorrhea can be related to endocrine imbalance; an increase in prostaglandin secretions; or chronic illnesses, fatigue, and anemia. A recent theory proposes that dysmenorrhea may be caused by hypercontractility of the uterus resulting from higher-than-normal levels of prostaglandins. Conditions that cause general debilitation, such as inadequate diet and exercise, anemia, and fatigue, often are related to dysmenorrhea.

Assessment

Many women have systemic symptoms of breast tenderness, abdominal distention, nausea and vomiting, headache, vertigo, palpitations, and excessive perspiration. Assess the woman for colicky and cyclic pain and, infrequently, dull pain in the lower pelvis that radiates toward the perineum and back. This pain may be experienced 24 to 48 hours before menses or at the onset of menses. The family history is important, because dysmenorrhea has been reported to be significantly more common among mothers and sisters of women with dysmenorrhea. Secondary dysmenorrhea is suspected if the symptoms begin after 20 years of age. It has been described as a steady or cramping pain and may be specific to the site of pelvic disorder.

Diagnostic Tests

Diagnostic studies include a complete blood count and cultures to check for the presence of STIs. A pelvic examination is performed to assess for structural abnormalities. Ultrasonography, CT scans or MRI can be completed to provide imaging of the abdominal or pelvic cavity. Surgical diagnostics may involve a laparoscopy to visualize the reproductive and abdominal organs or structures. Hysterosalpingography or a D&C may be employed as well.

Medical Management

Treatment of secondary dysmenorrhea is aimed at the cause. Surgical and medication intervention may be appropriate, depending on the severity and underlying causes of dysmenorrhea.

Interventions that are helpful in the management of dysmenorrhea not related to organic causes include a nutritious diet rich in complex carbohydrates. High fiber intake also is recommended. Intake of caffeine, sugar, and alcohol should be limited. During episodes of dysmenorrhea drinking warm beverages and eating small, frequent meals is helpful. Local applications of heat and warm showers are helpful. Mild analgesics are prescribed. Medications for dysmenorrhea include over-the-counter prostaglandin inhibitors, such as ibuprofen (Motrin, Advil), celecoxib (Celebrex), and naproxen sodium (Anaprox). Oral contraceptives may be used to suppress ovulation by inhibiting prostaglandin levels (Table 12.1). Supplementation with vitamin B_6, vitamin B_1, omega 3 fatty acids, and vitamin E have been used to manage dysmenorrhea with some success. Physical activity and sexual intercourse can provide relief of discomfort.

Nursing Interventions and Patient Teaching

A patient problem and interventions for women with dysmenorrhea include but are not limited to the following:

PATIENT PROBLEM	NURSING INTERVENTIONS
Insufficient Knowledge, related to disease process and treatment	Present information on disease process, procedures to be performed, medications, and treatments
	Prepare for informational question-and-answer sessions according to patient needs
	Teach procedures patient must know how to perform
	Obtain feedback
	Be certain learning has taken place; reinforce teaching as needed
	Develop a trusting relationship
	Involve patient in care

Encourage a positive attitude and instruct women to maintain good posture, exercise, and practice good nutrition.

ABNORMAL UTERINE BLEEDING (MENORRHAGIA AND METRORRHAGIA)

Abnormal uterine bleeding may take many forms, including menorrhagia and metrorrhagia.

Menorrhagia is excessive bleeding at the time of regular menstrual flow. The excessive bleeding can be characterized as increased in duration (more than 7 days), increased in amount (more than 80 mL), or both. Potential causes may involve uterine growths or tumors, cancer of the uterus, hormonal imbalance, PID, medications such as aspirin, and disorders of coagulation. In younger women it may be attributed to hormonal or endocrine disturbances, but in older women it usually indicates inflammatory disturbances or uterine tumors. Uterine fibroids (also called *leiomyomas*) and endometrial polyps are common causes of menorrhagia in women in their 30s and 40s. Emotional or psychological problems may also affect uterine bleeding. The severity of menorrhagia usually is estimated in terms of the number of pads or tampons used in excess of those used for regular menstrual flow.

Metrorrhagia is the appearance of uterine bleeding between regular menstrual periods or after menopause. It merits early diagnosis and treatment because it may indicate cancer or benign tumors of the uterus and ovaries. Endometrial cancer must be considered for postmenopausal women experiencing spotting.

The diagnostic process begins with a complete health history and review of the symptoms being reported. Focus should be on the past menstrual history. This should include length of periods and characteristics of the bleeding. The age at menarche should be recorded as well. Medication history should include the use of oral contraceptives and the ingestion of prescription and over-the-counter medications. Review the patient's obstetric history. The sexual history should include partners, onset of regular sexual activity, and any past or present STIs.

Diagnostic evaluation includes a Pap smear and routine speculum and pelvic examination. Laboratory testing includes blood tests and may include thyroid function assessments, hormone levels, pregnancy testing, and complete blood count studies. Endometrial biopsy and ultrasonography also are used to diagnose gynecologic causes of menorrhagia and metrorrhagia. Endometrial ablation done by laser or electrosurgical technique has been successful with many patients with menorrhagia. Ablation destroys layers of the endometrium. This will halt or sharply reduce uterine bleeding. It is not as invasive or permanent as a hysterectomy but provides rapid relief for many women. Recovery is within days.

Nursing interventions for the woman who is experiencing bleeding abnormalities include assessment of bleeding and pain and review of the patient's concerns and feelings. The woman should be asked to keep a log of her menstrual and bleeding history. Recording the dates, type, and characteristics of the bleeding, and the number of pads or tampons used, is important.

Table 12.1   Medications for Reproductive Disorders

GENERIC NAME	ACTION	SIDE EFFECTS	NURSING IMPLICATIONS
acyclovir ointment	Antiviral agent, interferes with DNA synthesis needed for viral replication	Mild pain with transient burning; stinging, pruritus, rash, vulvitis	Apply ointment q 3 h or six times daily around the clock; cover all lesions; use gloves for self-protection when applying
clotrimazole	Interferes with fungal DNA replication; binds sterols in fungal cell membrane	Rash, urticaria, stinging, burning, peeling, blistering skin fissures, abdominal cramps, bloating, urinary frequency	Watch for allergic reactions; note therapeutic response (decrease in size and number of lesions); use gloves for application; can be used through menstrual cycle; avoid use of other vaginal creams or suppositories during therapy
conjugated equine estrogen	Affects release of gonadotropins; inhibits ovulation; is involved in adequate calcium use in bone structure	Nausea, peripheral edema, enlargement of breasts, breast tenderness, anorexia, vomiting, diarrhea, headache, thrombophlebitis, dizziness, depression	Notify health care provider of weight gain of ≥5 lb/week (11 kg/week) (patient may need diuretic); monitor BP; check liver function test; check Homans' sign for possible clots; give IV product slowly to prevent flushing
danazol	Synthetic androgen, causes atrophy of endometrial tissue; decreases FSH and LH, which leads to amenorrhea and anovulation	Fluid retention, virilization, androgenic effects, weight gain, amenorrhea, dizziness, headache, rashes, hepatic impairment	Check weight; monitor I&O; check for edema; give with food or milk to decrease gastrointestinal upset
elagoix	Lowers blood levels of estradiol and progesterone which reduces stimulation of endometrial tissue and related discomforts of the condition	Anxiety, depression and suicidal thoughts Hot flashes and night sweats Headache Nausea Insomnia	Monitor for mood changes Provide teaching and resources to engage if mood disorders result
estradiol transdermal system	Same as conjugated equine estrogen	Same as conjugated equine estrogen	Same as conjugated equine estrogen
fluconazole	Used to treat or prevent fungal infections	Nausea, stomach pain, diarrhea, headache, dizziness	Take medication with a full glass of water
medroxyprogesterone acetate	Inhibits secretion of pituitary gonadotropins, which acts to prevent follicular maturation and ovulation; stimulates growth of mammary tissue	Irregular bleeding, breast tenderness, masculinization of fetus, edema, cholestatic jaundice, thrombophlebitis, anorexia, acne, mental depression, weight gain or loss	Notify health care provider of weight gain of ≥5 lb/week; monitor BP at beginning of treatment and periodically thereafter; check liver function test; discontinue if patient is pregnant
metronidazole	Direct-acting amebicide-trichomonacide; binds, degrades DNA in infecting organism	Rash, headache, dizziness, fatigue, convulsions, blurred vision, nausea, vomiting, diarrhea, pseudomembranous colitis, albuminuria, neurotoxicity, metallic taste, disulfiram-type reaction with alcohol	Watch for allergic reactions and superinfection; check stool for parasites; give oral form with food; watch for vision problems; tell patient not to drink alcohol during therapy
miconazole nitrate	Same as clotrimazole	Vulvovaginal burning, itching, pelvic cramps, rash, urticaria, stinging, burning, contact dermatitis	Same as clotrimazole
nystatin	Same as clotrimazole	Rash, urticaria, stinging, burning	Same as clotrimazole

Continued

Table 12.1   Medications for Reproductive Disorders—cont'd

GENERIC NAME	ACTION	SIDE EFFECTS	NURSING IMPLICATIONS
oral contraceptives: estrogen-progesterone combinations	Inhibits ovulation by suppressing gonadotropins, FSH, and LH; alters genital tract to inhibit sperm penetration and inhibit implantation	Nausea, cramps, diarrhea, appetite change, acne, rash, increased BP, thrombophlebitis, edema, dysmenorrhea, bleeding irregularities, depression, fatigue, breast changes, cholestatic jaundice, optic neuritis	Monitor glucose, thyroid function, and liver function tests; check Homans' sign for clot detection; monitor BP; discontinue if patient is pregnant
terconazole	Same as clotrimazole	Vulvovaginal burning, itching, pelvic cramps, rash, urticaria, stinging, burning	Same as clotrimazole
testosterone cypionate	Increases weight by building body tissue; increases potassium, phosphorus, chloride, and nitrogen levels; increases bone development	Acne, flushing, gynecomastia, edema, hypercalcemia, nausea, cholestatic hepatitis, aggressive behavior, headache, anxiety, mental depression, androgenic and anabolic activity	Check weight daily; monitor BP; monitor growth rate in children; check electrolyte (potassium-sodium, chloride, calcium) and cholesterol levels; monitor liver function test
tioconazole ointment	Same as miconazole but two to eight times more potent	Vulvovaginal burning, itching, soreness, swelling	Same as clotrimazole
topical amphotericin B	Binds to ergosterol, altering cell membrane permeability in susceptible fungi	Urticaria, stinging, burning, dry skin, pruritus, contact dermatitis, staining of nail lesions	Cover lesions completely after cleansing and drying well; use gloves to prevent further infection; watch for allergic reactions; tell patient that it may discolor skin and clothing
topical nystatin	Interferes with fungal DNA replication; causes fungal cell membrane permeability	Rash, stinging, burning, urticaria, nausea, vomiting, anorexia, diarrhea	Watch for allergic reaction; use gloves for topical application; for vaginal preparation, tell patient that she may need protective perineal pads

BP, Blood pressure; *DNA,* deoxyribonucleic acid; *FSH,* follicle-stimulating hormone; *I&O,* intake and output; *IV,* intravenous; *LH,* luteinizing hormone.

Women of all ages need to be educated about the importance of follow-up care when abnormal uterine bleeding is detected initially. Menopausal women may believe that the return of bleeding is normal or a re-occurrence of menstruation. Vaginal bleeding in post-menopausal women is never normal. Education and assessment of women in this age group should include this vital health teaching.

PREMENSTRUAL SYNDROME

PMS is a grouping of symptoms that affect an estimated 90% of women experience PMS at some point during their childbearing years. The condition is timed to coincide with the woman's menstrual cycle.

Etiology and Pathophysiology

An exact cause for the condition is not known. There are many theories about potential causes for the condition. There are factors that have been identified as increasing risk for PMS. They include a history of depression, cyclic hormone changes and fluctuations of serotonin in the brain. The changes during the menstrual cycle with estrogen and progesterone levels is

believed to trigger the onset of symptoms. Risk factors for PMS include the following:

- Age 25 to 40 years, with symptoms worsening as menopause nears
- Diet high in sugar
- Personal or family history of depression
- History of postpartum depression

Premenstrual dysphoric disorder (PMD-D) is the term applied to a type of PMS that includes a severe mood disorder. PMD-D has similar symptomology but demonstrates an excessive response in one or more of the following: sadness or hopelessness; anxiety or tension; extreme moodiness; marked irritability or anger (USDHHS, 2018).

PMS occurs 7 to 10 days before the menstrual period and usually subsides within 1 to 2 days after the onset of the menstrual flow.

Clinical Manifestations

Symptoms are multiple and vary among individuals. Both physical and emotional manifestations are included and occur in the days leading up to the onset of menstruation. Most symptoms decrease and then subside in the days following the onset of menstruation. Behavioral symptoms include anxiety, mood swings, irritability, lethargy (inactivity), fatigue, sleep disturbances, and depression. Women may report difficulty concentrating or forgetfulness. Physical symptoms—such as headache, vertigo, backache, breast tenderness, abdominal distention, acne, paresthesia (burning or tingling) of hands and feet, and allergies—appear or may become worse. Many symptoms appear alone or in combination with other symptoms. Some women accept the symptoms as being normal and seek medical help only after the symptoms become severe or begin to affect their family processes and interactions with others.

Assessment

Subjective data are specific symptoms experienced by each woman. Maintaining a log of outlining the timing and symptoms experienced is encouraged. The records should be kept for at least three consecutive menstrual cycles. The collected information can be analyzed and symptoms treated accordingly.

Objective data pertinent to the syndrome include the inability to perform activities of daily living (ADLs) in the multiple roles of wife, mother, and career person.

Diagnostic Tests

PMS is diagnosed only after eliminating other possible causes for the symptoms. A focused health history and a physical examination are done to identify any underlying conditions, such as thyroid dysfunction, uterine fibroids, or depression that may account for the symptoms. No definitive diagnostic test is available for PMS.

Patients may be asked to keep a journal of their symptoms for two or three menstrual cycles (USDHHS, 2018). Tests include evaluation of estrogen and progesterone levels to rule out hormonal imbalances and determination of glucose levels; low levels may lead to irritability.

Medical Management

The goal of treatment is to manage the individual symptoms being experienced and to return the patient to optimal functioning. Therapies will vary between patients. No medication has been approved to specifically treat PMS. Medications prescribed are based upon the individual symptoms being experienced. Analgesics including aspirin, ibuprofen, or other NSAIDs are utilized. Diuretics are prescribed to treat fluid retention.

Hormonal therapies such as estrogen containing oral contraceptives are prescribed for some women. Ovulation is suppressed and, in some studies, shown to reduce symptomology tied to ovulation. Serotonergic antidepressants (SSRIs) including sertraline (Zoloft), paroxetine (Paxil), and fluoxetine (Prozac) show promise in managing both behavioral and physical symptoms (Hofmeister, 2016).

Dietary management includes small, frequent meals with limitations on intake of sugar, sodium, and caffeine. Whole grain and fiber intake reduce bloating and constipation Supplements of vitamin B_6, calcium, and magnesium may be administered as prescribed. Alcohol and smoking should be discontinued. Encourage regular exercise three or four times a week for 30 minutes, especially during the premenstrual interval. Exercise results in release of endorphins, leading to mood elevation. Techniques for stress reduction include yoga, meditation, imagery, and biofeedback training. Because fatigue may exaggerate PMS symptoms, adequate rest, sleep, and relaxation are helpful.

Nursing Interventions and Patient Teaching

A patient problem and interventions for the woman with PMS include but are not limited to the following:

PATIENT PROBLEM	NURSING INTERVENTIONS
Anxiousness, related to PMS	Encourage verbalization of feelings
	Acknowledge existence of syndrome and its symptoms
	Encourage patient to keep a menstrual symptom diary to document the cycle and nature of the symptoms
	Encourage patient to plan activities during the symptom-free part of her cycle
	Administer supplements of vitamin B_6, calcium, and magnesium as prescribed
	Encourage attending self-help groups and reading self-help literature; group support tends to reduce stress
	Provide emotional support in a nonjudgmental and caring manner
	Assist in identifying possible sources of anxiety and coping mechanisms

PMS, Premenstrual syndrome.

MENOPAUSE

The **climacteric** is the phase of the aging process of women and men who are making a transition from a reproductive phase to a nonreproductive stage of life. The female climacteric is called *menopause*. This term refers to the normal cessation of menses. Menopause may be hormonal, surgical, or pharmacologic. Hormonal menopause occurs in middle adulthood and marks the onset of physical changes, a decrease in hormone secretion, and the cessation of ovulation and menses. Surgical menopause results from the loss of hormone production after surgical intervention involving removal of the ovaries (bilateral salpingo-oophorectomy). Medication therapies can result in the onset of menopausal signs and symptoms. Medications to manage fibroid tumors include gonadotropin-releasing hormone (GnRH) agonists (e.g., euproide [Lupron]). This class of medication causes levels of estrogen and progesterone to fall, resulting in a menopausal state.

Perimenopause is experienced by most women as they near the middle adulthood years. During this period the level of estrogen produced begins to fall. This may begin as early as the early to mid-30s. Perimenopause (state of transition to menopause) may last for several years, with an average of 4 years. This stage lasts until the ovaries no longer produce estrogen and the woman has had a full year without a menstrual period.

Etiology and Pathophysiology

Menopause is the normal decline of ovarian function resulting from the aging process. Menopause begins in most women between 42 and 58 years of age (the average age being 51) and is characterized by infrequent ovulation, decreased menstrual function, and eventual cessation of the menstrual flow. Factors that have been linked to an earlier age at menopause include higher body mass index; cigarette smoking; and racial, ethnic, and socioeconomic factors.

Menopause may be induced artificially by such procedures as irradiation of the ovaries or surgical removal of both ovaries. Both cause menopause with all its physiologic changes, whereas ovaries left intact after a hysterectomy continue to function provided the woman has not yet reached the age of the climacteric. Menopause also may occur earlier because of illness, side effects of chemotherapy, or drugs.

Decline in ovarian function produces a variety of symptoms, including a decrease in the frequency, amount, and duration of the menstrual flow; spotting; amenorrhea; and polymenorrhea (increased number of menstrual periods). Symptoms can last from a few months to several years before menstruation ceases permanently. Menopause is not considered complete until 1 year after the last menstrual period.

Clinical Manifestations

Physical changes that occur in the body generally do not develop until after permanent cessation of menstruation. Changes in the reproductive system include shrinkage of vulval structures, atrophic vulvitis, shortening of the vagina, and dryness of the vaginal wall. A relaxation of supporting pelvic structures results from the decrease in estrogen. Cystitis and urinary frequency and urgency may appear as a result of changes in the urinary system. There is loss of skin turgor and elasticity; increased subcutaneous fat; decreased breast tissue; and thinning of hair of the axilla, the head, and the pubis. About 25% of postmenopausal women develop osteoporosis.

Assessment

Subjective data include a family history. Determine whether family members and significant others are aware of the transition and whether they are supportive. Note emotional illness if present. Hot flashes caused by glandular imbalances may become prominent. Other symptoms may include fatigue, vertigo, headache, nausea, dyspareunia (painful intercourse), palpitations, and chest and neck pain. Some experience a feeling of being unwanted, and some may fear growing old; both feelings could cause depression.

Collection of objective data includes an awareness that some patients may display frequent crying spells or outbursts of anger. Explore the use of contraceptives. Assess frequency, amount, and duration of the menstrual flow. Diaphoresis, weight gain, vomiting, and tachycardia may occur.

Diagnostic Tests

Tests include analysis of hormonal levels. Other diagnostic testing may be indicated by specific symptoms. Some examinations are performed to rule out conditions such as cancer.

Medical Management

The status of hormone replacement therapy (HRT) for postmenopausal women has been a source of study and discussion. Hormone replacement is used in menopausal women to help with some of the troubling manifestations associated with the loss of estrogen. Symptoms improved by the use of HRT include hot flashes, night sweats, and vaginal dryness. Therapies are also beneficial to maintaining bone density. Despite these positive findings there are risk factors for some women for the development of heart disease, stroke, and blood clots. Side effects of HRT include breast tenderness, cramping, bloating, and vaginal spotting. A change in dosage or type of prescribed therapies may help in the management of side effects. At present, studies suggest that women with moderate to severe symptoms of menopause be prescribed the lowest effective dose possible for the shortest duration possible (Banks, 2021). Women who still have their uterus are prescribed replacement estrogen and progesterone. If the woman has her uterus and progesterone is not included in the replacement therapy, there is an increased risk of endometrial cancer. Estrogen therapy is also used for women who no longer have a uterus (i.e., who have undergone a hysterectomy).

Nurses are in a good position to apprise their patients of the benefits, risks, and appropriate uses of HRT. HRT is used for short-term treatment of moderate to severe symptoms of menopause, such as hot flashes, night sweats, and vaginal dryness. At present, no data indicate how long HRT can be taken without the risk of cardiovascular or other adverse effects, and it is not known whether lower dosages lessen the risk of complications. In women with moderate to severe menopausal symptoms, it is assumed that risk can be minimized by providing HRT only until the severe symptoms disappear and using the lowest effective dosage. HRTs may be administered in a number of ways, including orally or by transdermal patch, gels, subcutaneous implants, creams, injections, and suppositories. Low-dose alternatives in HRT include the low-dose conjugated estrogen, medroxyprogesterone, containing either 0.45 mg of conjugated estrogens and 1.5 mg of medroxyprogesterone, or 0.3 mg of conjugated estrogens and 1.5 mg of medroxyprogesterone; or low-dose intravaginal estrogen products, such as estrogen topical vaginal cream (Premarin vaginal cream or Estrace) and low-dose vaginal rings. Because of the later diagnosis of breast cancer and colon cancer in women receiving combination HRT, closely scrutinize any abnormal mammogram and screen for colon cancer as part of the follow-up.

Most health care providers recommend calcium and vitamin D supplements, which are available in many forms; the generic calcium carbonate products are the most cost effective.

Herbals and dietary modification are also useful in the management of menopause-related symptoms. Phytoestrogens are compounds that mimic estrogen in structure. They are found in yams, lentils, oats, barley, sesame seeds, and tofu (Webber, 2020).

SSRIs, including the antidepressants paroxetine (Paxil), fluoxetine, and venlafaxine (Effexor), are an effective alternative to HRT in reducing hot flashes, even if the user is not depressed. Also known to relieve hot flashes are clonidine (Catapres), an antihypertensive drug, and gabapentin (Neurontin), an antiseizure drug (Mayo Clinic, 2020b).

Nonhormonal therapy. To relieve menopausal symptoms without the risks of HRT, several methods to decrease heat produced by the body and promote heat loss have been recommended. Reducing intake of caffeine and alcohol lowers the production of body heat. Suggestions to promote heat loss at night when hot flashes interfere with sleep include increasing air circulation, using light covers and loose-fitting clothing, and placing cool cloths on flushed areas. Acupressure and acupuncture are utilized to relieve the discomforts of menopause.

Nursing Interventions and Patient Teaching
Education regarding menopause should occur before its onset. Many women appreciate opportunities to discuss menopause. Set up an exercise program that includes movement and weight bearing to slow bone loss and modify coronary artery disease risk factors. Walking is an excellent weight-bearing exercise. Other exercises include bicycling, stationary cycling, and aerobic dancing three or four times per week.

Patient problems and interventions for the menopausal patient include but are not limited to the following:

PATIENT PROBLEM	NURSING INTERVENTIONS
Impaired Self-Esteem due to current situation, related to concerns about femininity, sexuality, and aging	Encourage patient and significant others to verbalize concerns
	Assess knowledge of menopause
	Provide education related to menopause
	Refer patient to couple, family, and sex therapy as appropriate
	Provide understanding and support
Insufficient Knowledge Regarding patient's physiologic and psychological changes related to menopause	Explain the process of climacteric and menopause, at a level the patient can understand
	Explain importance of keeping fit, eating a well-balanced diet, getting adequate rest and sleep, avoiding stress and fatigue, and continuing contraception until contraindicated by health care provider
	If estrogen replacement therapy is ordered, inform patient about side effects
	Instruct patient to report any vaginal bleeding occurring 6 months or more after last menstrual period
	Inform patient of the availability of water-soluble lubricants if needed before coitus

For patient teaching, emphasize that the climacteric is normal and self-limiting and that menopause is not the end of the patient's sex life. A nutritious diet and weight control improve physical condition, and an exercise program promotes vitality. Interest and participation in various activities help decrease anxiety and tension. Skin creams and lotions can be used to prevent drying, pruritus, and cracking skin. Encourage the woman to perform breast self-examination (BSE) monthly and to monitor calcium intake. Contraceptives should be used for 1 year after the last menstrual period. The patient can obtain a prescription for the treatment of pruritus or burning of the vulva. Women can practice Kegel exercises regularly to strengthen pelvic muscles (see the Health Promotion box). A water-soluble lubricant, such as K-Y jelly, can be used to prevent dyspareunia. Explain the side effects of any medications or hormonal therapy. Emphasize that an annual physical examination is important for maintaining good health.

 Health Promotion

Kegel Exercises

Kegel exercises are performed to help strengthen and tighten muscles that support the pelvic organs. These muscles (pelvic floor) are used to stop the flow of urine. To perform Kegel exercises while standing or sitting, tighten the pelvic floor muscles as hard as you can. Hold for 5 s, then release. Repeat at least 10 times. This exercise can be done as many as 40 to 50 times each day.

MALE CLIMACTERIC

Etiology and Pathophysiology

The climacteric is less pronounced in men and often may not even be apparent. The appearance of the climacteric phase is gradual and occurs between 55 and 70 years of age. There is a gradual decrease of testosterone levels and seminal fluid production. The impact is largely psychological, possibly because of the recognition of some reduction of sexual activity and interests.

Clinical Manifestations

Manifestations are mostly physiologic changes. Erections require more time and are not as full or firm. The prostate gland enlarges, and secretions diminish; seminal fluid decreases. The physical changes occur as the man grows older, and the most noticeable signs are loss or thinning of hair from the head, chest, axillae, and pubis. There may be some flushing and chilling. Muscle tone is decreased.

Assessment

Collection of subjective data reveals that the man is generally at the peak of his career or possibly considering retirement. He interprets his decreased sexual needs as a loss of productivity and sexual power. Therefore the assessment should invite verbalization of emotions with coping mechanisms.

Collection of objective data includes assessment of behaviors that may be causing the man stress and concern. Ask him to explore changes he has noted regarding his lifestyle and feelings of loss of self-worth.

Diagnostic Tests

Diagnostic tests include a complete physical examination to rule out abnormalities of structure and function. Hormone level assessments provide information about potential imbalances.

Nursing Interventions and Patient Teaching

A patient problem and interventions for men experiencing male climacteric include but are not limited to the following:

PATIENT PROBLEM	NURSING INTERVENTIONS
Impaired Coping related to situational crisis (climacteric)	Show understanding and concern
	Assist patient in identifying how the problem affects his life and future, his family, and significant others
	Encourage patient to talk about factors that could be influencing the way he sees the problem
	Assist patient in identifying strengths and coping skills and the nature and strength of situational support
	Collect data about current and potential sources of support
	Assist patient in planning alternative solutions
	Give positive reinforcement

Inform the patient that the climacteric is normal. Encourage the patient to verbalize his fears and to seek counseling if stress increases.

ERECTILE DYSFUNCTION

Erectile dysfunction (ED) is a man's inability to attain or maintain an erect penis that allows satisfactory sexual performance. In the past the condition was referred to as *impotence*. ED has largely replaced this terminology. ED may arise from a variety of causes:

- *Psychological causes:* ED may have a psychological basis, including stress, depression, and other mental conditions.
- *Organic causes:*
  - Anatomic anomalies may result in a physical defect in the genital structures
  - Atonic ED: Conditions associated with atonic ED include advanced syphilis; congenital spinal cord anomalies, such as spina bifida; spinal cord tumors; amyotrophic lateral sclerosis (Lou Gehrig disease); multiple sclerosis; and cord compression caused by a herniated disk
  - Surgical interventions, such as radical prostatectomy, often lead to ED
  - Low testosterone levels
  - Hypertension
  - Substance use/abuse

ED potentially can interfere with a man's self-esteem, relationships, confidence, and sense of well-being. The prevalence alone makes ED a significant condition. An estimated 30 million men in the United States experience ED. The rate of incidence increases with aging, with approximately 4% of men in their 50s affected by ED. This rate increases to 17% during the seventh decade of life. Among men in their 70s, the rate of incidence of ED nears 50%. ED in younger men may result from substance abuse, including alcohol or recreational drugs. Medical conditions associated with ED are diabetes mellitus, hypertension, renal disorders, cancer, coronary artery bypass surgery, and organ transplants. Understand ED by developing a broad understanding of the factors that contribute to the condition.

ED can result when the physiology of the erection faces interference. Stimulation sends impulses to the brain and to the corpora cavernosa of the penis. This results in its relaxation and allows blood to enter and fill the spaces. Pressure in the corpora cavernosa causes the penis to expand and harden. Many disorders have the ability to interfere with this process, thus causing ED (NIDDK, 2017).

Medical Management

Review of the patient's history is the first step. The information collected should include a detailed sexual history, medication and drug use, and past and current medical conditions.

Medical treatment is based on careful assessment of the causative factors. It is known that medications such as antihypertensives, antidepressants, antihyperlipidemic, diuretics, drugs for Parkinson disease, marijuana, cocaine, antianxiety agents, and some cardiac agents may cause ED. Illicit or abused substances such as alcohol, cocaine, and nicotine also are known to cause ED. Disease conditions such as diabetes mellitus or end-stage renal, heart, and chronic obstructive pulmonary disease also may be causative factors.

A drug named sildenafil citrate is prescribed as an oral therapy for ED. The physiologic mechanism of erection of the penis involves release of nitric oxide in the corpus cavernosum during sexual stimulation. The drug enhances smooth muscle relaxation and the inflow of blood in the corpus cavernosum, thus allowing erection to occur. For most patients, the recommended dose is 50 mg taken as needed approximately 1 hour before engaging in sexual activity. However, sildenafil may be taken from 30 minutes to 4 hours before sexual activity. Sildenafil has been shown to potentiate the hypotensive effects of nitrates; therefore, its

administration to patients who are using nitrates (either regularly or intermittently) in any form is contraindicated. Tadalafil is another anti-impotence agent for ED contraindicated for concurrent use with nitrates, nitric oxide, or alpha-adrenergic blockers. It should not be used in patients who have unstable angina, a recent history of stroke, life-threatening heart failure, uncontrolled hypertension, or myocardial infarction within 90 days. For most patients, the recommended dose is 10 mg before sexual activity (range, 5 to 20 mg; not to exceed one dose in 24 hours). A third anti-impotence agent is vardenafil, 10 mg, taken 1 hour before sexual activity (range, 5 to 20 mg; no more than once daily). This drug is not to be used with nitrates because of the potential for an unsafe decrease in blood pressure, which could result in myocardial infarction or stroke. The side effects of all three medications are similar and include headache, hypotension, and dyspepsia. Medications alone will not result in an erection. Sexual stimulation is needed.

Management also may include penile injections. Alprostadil and phentolamine are used for this purpose. The patient can self-inject the medication into the side or the base of the penis. The medications typically provide an erection that can last 20 to 40 minutes.

Mechanical devices are available for the patient with ED. The least invasive means may be the use of a vacuum pump device. The vacuum is placed over the penis and suction is applied by a hand-generated or battery-operated means. Once the erection occurs, a ring is placed over the base of the penis to maintain it (Mayo Clinic, 2021). Surgical implantation of a penile prosthesis may be performed as a same-day procedure or may require hospitalization for 5 or more days, depending on the patient and the device used (Fig. 12.9).

Nursing Interventions and Patient Teaching

The nurse is responsible for teaching the patient to administer prescribed medications and to watch for side effects. For patients who have received penile implants, inform the patient about signs and symptoms

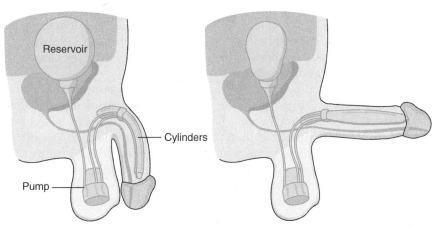

Fig. 12.9 The Scott inflatable prosthesis has erect and flaccid positions designed to mimic normal erectile function. (From Beare PG, Myers JL: *Adult health nursing*, ed 3, St. Louis, 1998, Mosby.)

of infection of the implant, including tenderness of the penis, fever, dysuria, and signs of urinary tract infection. Tell the patient to seek medical attention promptly if infection occurs.

INFERTILITY

Etiology and Pathophysiology

Infertility is defined as the inability to conceive after 1 year of sexual intercourse without birth control measures. If the woman is over the age of 35, the time period is reduced to 6 months. Primary infertility refers to couples who have never conceived. Secondary infertility refers to couples who have conceived but are now unable to do so. An estimated 10% to 15% of couples are infertile.

Men and women are able to conceive early in adolescence. Men retain the capability to father a child throughout their lives. Women do experiences changes in the levels of fertility as they age. As women reach their mid-30s there is a decline in ovulatory cycles. This decline is associated with drops in the ability to conceive a child. These declines continue until menopause.

The inability to conceive may be attributed to the woman or the man; in some cases both have factors resulting in infertility. Statistically, the causes are relatively evenly spread between the partners, with approximately one-third of the causes linked to the woman, the man, and to both combined (Mayo Clinic, 2019a)

Damage to sperm production, longevity, or sperm motility issues are the leading causes of male-related infertility. The sperm count may be diminished or absent. Structural abnormalities and low motility may account for infertility. Abnormally shaped sperm cannot penetrate and fertilize the ovum. Excessive heat exposure of the testicles associated with undescended testicles and hot tubs are implicated with male-based infertility. Inability to travel to the fallopian tubes as a result of poor motility will prevent conception as well. Additional male-related causes include hormonal imbalances, anatomic abnormalities, and genetic defects (NICHD, 2017). Lifestyle and other health-related behaviors also may affect male fertility. The use of alcohol and drugs, smoking, exposure to environmental toxins, and some medications may result in reduced or absent fertility. Illness such as cancer and the related treatments may render a man infertile.

Female-related causes of infertility include ovulatory issues, hormonal imbalances, and structural abnormalities. Ovulation-related disorders compromise the majority of female-related cases of infertility. Women who do not experience ovulatory menstrual cycles will not conceive. Hormonal imbalances can be linked to problematic levels of estrogen, progesterone, and FSH. These hormones are responsible for the maturation and release of the ovum from the ovaries as well as preparation of the uterus for implantation of the fertilized egg. Structural abnormalities may include scarring from STIs or endometriosis, abnormalities in the shape and size of the uterus, the presence of uterine fibroid tumors, and blockages in the fallopian tubes. Lifestyle factors that may play a part in a woman's fertility include increasing age, smoking, excessive alcohol use, athletic training, obesity, or being underweight.

Assessment

Collection of subjective and objective data includes physical examination and health histories for both partners to make the infertility assessment and prepare a treatment plan.

Diagnostic Tests

Specific testing is necessary to rule out systemic diseases such as diabetes mellitus, neoplasms, hepatic and renal diseases, and viral conditions. Genetic defects and disorders of the testes are explored. Diagnostic testing can produce a great deal of anxiety and stress. This testing may continue for fairly long periods with or without favorable results. Infertility testing can be expensive and may not be covered by some insurance carriers. Male testing is somewhat simpler and usually less expensive than female testing. If there is reason to suspect the man is infertile or sterile, it is appropriate to test him first. Male infertility testing includes semen analysis, which measures the quantity and quality of semen, volume of sperm cells, sperm motility, and sperm density; and endocrine imbalance testing, which explores possible disruption of the pituitary gonadotropins and testosterone production.

Female testing focuses on the ovulation process and function of the reproductive organs. Testing commonly includes (1) assessment of ovulatory functioning; (2) endometrial biopsy, which confirms ovulation and endometrial cyclic changes; and (3) hysterosalpingography and hysterography to assess the position and alignment of the reproductive organs.

Male and female interaction studies include (1) Huhner's test, which examines the cervical mucus for motile sperm cells after intercourse, at mid-menstrual cycle; (2) immunologic or immunoglobulin (antibody) testing for detection of spermicidal antibodies in the woman's serum; and (3) testing the man and woman for normalcy of their sex chromosomes.

Medical Management

The management of infertility problems depends on the cause. If infertility is secondary to an alteration in ovarian function, supplemental hormone therapy may be attempted to restore and maintain ovulation. Drugs used to induce ovulation include clomiphene citrate (Clomid) and bromocriptine (Parlodel). These drugs increase the risk for multiple births. Structural abnormalities may be investigated for surgical correction. Fibroid tumors and scar tissue may be candidates for surgery. Hormonal imbalances also may be treated pharmacologically. Progesterone may be administered by an injection or vaginal gel/jelly. If pregnancy results, it may also be continued until 10 to 12 weeks' gestation, when the placenta will be functioning and can take over the hormone production.

Poor cervical mucus may be a result of chronic cervicitis or inadequate estrogenic stimulation. Careful cauterization of the cervix may eradicate the chronic cervicitis, and the administration of estrogens can improve the quantity and quality of the cervical mucus.

Improving the patient's general health may help, especially when a debilitating or chronic illness is present. Eliminating or reducing psychological stress can improve the emotional climate, making it more conducive to achieving a pregnancy. Education of the couple regarding the probable time of ovulation and appropriate coital technique also may be indicated. Timing of sexual intercourse to the days preceding and at ovulation is best.

When a couple has not succeeded in conceiving even with infertility management, another option is intrauterine insemination with the partner's or a donor's sperm. If this technique does not succeed, in vitro fertilization (IVF) may be used. IVF is the removal of mature oocytes from the woman's ovarian follicles via laparoscopy, followed by fertilization of the ova with the partner's sperm in a Petri dish. When fertilization and cleavage have occurred, some of the resulting embryos are transferred into the woman's uterus. The procedure requires 2 or 3 days to complete and is used in cases of fallopian tube obstruction, decreased sperm count, and unexplained infertility. IVF is costly and emotionally stressful, but it has become an accepted therapy for infertile couples.

Assisted reproductive technologies (ARTs) have developed rapidly since the first IVF baby was born in 1978. ARTs include IVF, gamete intrafallopian transfer (GIFT), zygote intrafallopian transfer (ZIFT), cryopreserved embryo transfer (CPE), and donor oocyte programs. Current research could lead to a rapid expansion of these techniques. With the increased knowledge of freezing techniques for embryos (CPE), couples will have increased pregnancy potential. Researchers also are investigating the replication of normal tubal secretions. This tubal factor is important because the pregnancy rate is higher with GIFT and ZIFT than with IVF. Finally, the development of embryo biopsy and genetic engineering may allow for preconception techniques for those couples with identified genetic abnormalities. It also raises the possibility of gender selection. Thus noncoital reproduction poses many ethical, legal, and social concerns. All decisions related to infertility are influenced by the couple's age, their wishes, and the length of time they have been attempting to conceive.

Nursing Interventions and Patient Teaching

The nurse has a responsibility to teach and provide emotional support throughout the infertility testing and treatment period. Feelings of anger, frustration, sadness, and helplessness between partners and between the couple and health care providers may increase as more tests are performed. Infertility can generate great tension in a marriage as the couple exhausts their financial and emotional resources. Few insurance carriers cover the cost of infertility testing or the therapeutic measures associated with infertility. Shame and guilt may arise when other people become involved in such an intimate area of a relationship.

Recognizing and dealing with the psychological and emotional factors that surface can assist the couple in coping with the situation. Encourage couples to participate in a support group for infertile couples and in individual therapy. Continue providing information and emotional support as therapeutic measures are attempted. Give couples ample opportunity to plan what is financially realistic. IVF treatments can cost $10,000 to 15,000 per cycle in the United States (IHR, 2018).

Prognosis

The condition causing the infertility and the age of the woman are the primary deciding factors determining the outcome of infertility treatments. Women over age 40 have reduced chances of achieving pregnancy. An estimated 50% of couples who undergo diagnostic testing and treatments for fertility are able to conceive.

INFLAMMATORY AND INFECTIOUS DISORDERS OF THE FEMALE REPRODUCTIVE TRACT

Infections of the female reproductive tract are found most commonly in the vagina, the cervix, the fallopian tubes, and their adjacent areas. The vagina is lubricated and protected by normal flora, an acidic pH, and secretions from the vaginal and cervical cells.

A number of organisms can cause vaginal infections. Vaginal infections may be caused by bacteria, fungi, or viruses. Infections are more likely to occur when the flora and the acidity of the vagina are disturbed by medications (e.g., birth control pills, antibiotics), stress, malnutrition, douching, aging, and disease. Health-related concerns may include diabetes mellitus and pregnancy.

Organisms often are introduced from external sources by way of unclean douche nozzles, poor hygiene, inadequate handwashing, neglected nail care, soiled clothing, and intercourse. Vaginal infections can be transmitted sexually and will return unless both partners are treated.

VAGINITIS

Etiology and Pathophysiology

Vaginitis is a common vaginal infection. The cause of the condition may be bacterial or inflammatory. *Escherichia coli,* an organism found in feces and the rectum, is a common cause. Other potential pathogens include staphylococcal and streptococcal organisms; *Trichomonas vaginalis* (a flagellated protozoan); *Candida albicans* (a yeast-like fungus); and *Gardnerella vaginalis*, a coccobacillus.

If the patient changes perineal pads or tampons infrequently, the vaginal tract and inner groin become irritated. This creates a medium suitable for organism growth. Examination of the vaginal walls will show a profuse foamy (bubbly) exudate if the vaginitis is caused by *T. vaginalis*. If *C. albicans* is the causative agent, a thick, cheese like discharge results. Bacterial vaginitis produces a malodorous milky discharge.

Clinical Manifestations

The exudate in vaginitis is yellow, white, or grayish white; curdlike; and generally accompanied by pruritus, burning, and edema of the surrounding tissue. Voiding and defecation generally intensify the symptoms.

Assessment

Subjective data include menstrual history, age at menarche, length of cycles, duration and nature of flow, dysfunctions, birth control methods, medications taken, family history of diabetes mellitus, previous vaginal infections, and STIs. Ask about sexual practices and signs of infection in the sex partner. Dysuria may occur as a consequence of local irritation of the urinary meatus.

Collection of objective data includes observation for excoriations of the skin caused by scratching, in which case secondary infection may result. Observe the specific type of exudate.

Diagnostic Tests

Diagnostic tests include direct visual examination of the vagina, culture of the organism, and bimanual examination to assess for inflammation of the vagina and its surrounding tissues.

Medical Management

Vaginal infection can be treated by a variety of methods. The major goals of treatment are to (1) cure the infection, (2) prevent reinfection, (3) prevent complications, and (4) prevent infection of the sexual partner(s). Douching frequently is prescribed for treatment, as are local applications of vaginal suppositories, ointments, and creams. Advise the patient to use the medication at bedtime and to remain recumbent for more than 30 minutes after insertion to allow absorption and to prevent loss of any medication from the vagina. The patient may require oral medications appropriate to the infecting organism. During treatment the patient should refrain from intercourse or request that her partner use a condom (see Table 12.1).

Nursing Interventions and Patient Teaching

Advise the patient of the importance of hand washing before and after vaginal application of medications.

Douching too frequently can alter normal vaginal flora. Discourage douching unless specifically prescribed by the health care provider.

Most patients with vaginal infections are directed to abstain from sexual intercourse during treatment. The male partner's use of a condom until the symptoms of infection disappear may be advised. Treatment of the partner is based upon the underlying pathogen.

Prognosis

With proper treatment, the prognosis is good.

SENILE VAGINITIS OR ATROPHIC VAGINITIS

Low estrogen levels cause the vulva and vagina to thin and atrophy, becoming more susceptible to bacterial invasion. The subsequent exudate causes pruritus, edema, and skin irritations. Although the condition is seen most commonly after menopause, it may be experienced by any patient whose condition is associated with reductions in estrogen levels. Estrogen, vaginal suppositories, and ointments may be prescribed (Mayo Clinic, 2019b).

CERVICITIS

Cervicitis is the inflammation of the cervix. It may be caused by various causes but is linked to STIs such as chlamydia, gonorrhea, herpesvirus, HPV, and trichomoniasis. Bacteria including *Staphylococcus* and *Streptococcus* can cause cervicitis. Other potential causes may include cervical caps, diaphragms, or pessary devices. Allergic reactions to condoms, douches, or spermicides also may be implicated. Risk-increasing behaviors include multiple sexual partners, a history of STIs, and sexual intercourse at an early age. Therapy is specific to the causative organisms. Symptoms are dyspareunia (painful intercourse); vaginal pain; pelvic heaviness; abnormal vaginal bleeding; and a gray, white, or yellow vaginal discharge. If cervicitis remains untreated, the tissues are continually irritated and the infection may spread to other pelvic organs. Personal hygiene and frequent warm tub baths can minimize odor and discomfort. Avoid douching and limit tampon use. Local applications of vaginal suppositories, ointments, and creams usually are prescribed. Drug therapy also includes azithromycin, 1 g orally as a single dose, or doxycycline, 100 mg orally twice a day for 7 days; the partner is treated with the same drugs (Ollendorf, 2017). More advanced conditions may require more invasive therapies such as cryosurgery, electrocauterization, and laser therapy.

PELVIC INFLAMMATORY DISEASE

PID is any acute, subacute, recurrent, or chronic infection that may involve the cervix (cervicitis), uterus (endometritis), fallopian tubes (salpingitis), or ovaries (oophoritis) and may extend to the connective tissues lying between the layers of the broad ligaments (folds of peritoneum supporting the uterus).

Etiology and Pathophysiology

The most common causative organisms are *Neisseria gonorrhoeae*, streptococci, staphylococci, chlamydiae, and tubercle bacilli. PID can follow the insertion of a biopsy curette or an irrigation catheter, abortion, pelvic surgery, sexual intercourse, or pregnancy. The condition may occur with or without gonorrheal infection and may be mild or severe.

When conditions or procedures alter or destroy the cervical mucus, bacteria ascend into the uterine cavity. Pelvic examination and movement of the reproductive organs become painful. PID is serious because it may cause adhesions and sterility. Sexually active women with more than one partner are at increased risk for PID.

Clinical Manifestations

Signs and symptoms are temperature elevation, chills, severe abdominal pain, malaise, nausea and vomiting, and malodorous purulent vaginal exudate.

Assessment

Subjective data relate to the severity of the disorder, pain, time of onset, and frequency (primary infection or continuous reinfection). Sexual history, pelvic examinations, and pelvic procedures are important because they may reveal the origin of the pathogen. The patient may complain of lower abdominal and pelvic pain, dysmenorrhea, dysuria, and vulvar pruritus.

Objective data include the patient's knowledge, level of discomfort, and coping mechanisms. Assess the patient for fever and chills and the amount and characteristics of vaginal discharge. The vaginal discharge is purulent to thin and mucoid.

Diagnostic Tests

Diagnostic tests include Gram stains of secretions from the endocervix, urethra, and rectum. Culture and sensitivity testing identifies organisms and is helpful in selecting antibiotics for treatment. Ultrasound or MRI may be used to visualize the pelvic cavity. Vaginal ultrasonic examinations can aid in diagnosing abscesses and monitoring the treatment and healing process. Laparoscopic visualization of the pelvic inflammation may be necessary to confirm the extent of infection. Laboratory testing includes leukocyte count, C-reactive protein rates, and erythrocyte sedimentation rate, which are elevated.

Medical Management

The goal of treatment is to control and eradicate the infection by preventing it from spreading to other body systems. Treatment includes systemic antibiotics administered intravenously or intramuscularly. The antibiotics of choice are usually cefoxitin (Mefoxin) and doxycycline to provide thorough coverage against the responsible pathogens. Intercourse must be avoided for the entire time of treatment. The patient's partner(s) must be examined and treated as well. Pain control, rest, and adequate fluid intake are essential to the care. A corticosteroid often is added to the antibiotic treatment to aid in more rapid recovery and improvement in maintaining fertility.

Nursing Interventions and Patient Teaching

The patient usually is hospitalized to isolate the organism and plan treatment. Inform the patient and those assisting with the patient's care of all specific precautions and observe standard precautions. Use goggles if any splashing is likely. Nursing interventions include (1) assessing pain and administering prescribed analgesics as needed; (2) monitoring vital signs and progress of treatment; (3) providing fluids to avoid dehydration; (4) performing palliative measures for comfort such as bathing, changing of perineal pads, personal hygiene, and warm douches; (5) providing patient support with a positive, nonjudgmental attitude; and (6) positioning the patient in Fowler's position to facilitate drainage.

Patient problems and interventions for the patient with PID include but are not limited to the following:

PATIENT PROBLEM	NURSING INTERVENTIONS
Recent Onset of Pain	Manage pain with analgesics as ordered; assess effectiveness of pain-relief measures Provide comfort measures
Impaired Health Maintenance, related to insufficient knowledge of condition and complications	Teach patient about the significance of PID and the importance of complying with medication therapy

PID, Pelvic inflammatory disease.

Education of the patient should include the following:
- Discussion about the signs and symptoms to report to the health care provider
- Medication therapy
- Personal hygiene practices to reduce infection (hand washing and avoidance of tampons)

Prognosis

PID can lead to complications such as adhesions and strictures of the fallopian tubes as a result of scarring. Ectopic pregnancy risk is elevated. Infertility may result. Early diagnosis and treatment will reduce the potential for complications.

TOXIC SHOCK SYNDROME

Etiology and Pathophysiology

Toxic shock syndrome (TSS) is an acute bacterial infection commonly caused by *Staphylococcus aureus* or *streptococcus pyogenes*. It usually occurs in women who are menstruating and using tampons (particularly superabsorbent tampons), contraceptive sponge, or diaphragm. If the tampon is left in place too long, the bacteria may proliferate and release toxins into the bloodstream, causing TSS. Women at the greatest risk are those who insert tampons with their fingers instead of with inserters, women with chronic vaginal infections, and women with genital herpes. TSS can also occur in non-menstruating women. Additional risk factors include recent childbirth, miscarriage or abortion, surgery, and internal medical packing (Johns Hopkins Medicine, n.d.b.).

Clinical Manifestations: Often the patient has flu-like symptoms for the first 24 hours. Between days 2 and 4 of the menstrual period, the patient may have an elevated temperature (up to 102°F [39°C]), vomiting, dizziness, headache, diarrhea, myalgia, hypotension, and signs suggesting the onset of septic shock. Sore throat, headache, and a red macular palmar or diffuse rash followed by desquamation of the skin, hands, and feet may develop; urinary output is decreased, and the blood urea nitrogen (BUN) level is elevated. Disorientation may occur from dehydration and the release of toxins. Pulmonary edema and inflammation of mucous membranes may occur.

Assessment

Collection of subjective data includes determining whether the patient recently has used tampons and how long she used a single tampon before changing it. Obtain information about myalgia, sore throat, headache, and fatigue.

Collection of objective data includes assessing for edema. Assess the palms and soles for an erythematous rash. Desquamation and sloughing occur within 1 to 2 weeks after the rash. Note the patient's level of consciousness. Hypotension is a sign of TSS, as are nonpurulent inflammation of the conjunctiva and hyperemia of the oropharynx and vagina.

Diagnostic Tests

There is no definitive test for TSS. However, cervical-vaginal isolates of *S. aureus* are present 90% of the time. Blood tests demonstrate leukocytosis; thrombocytopenia; and elevated levels of bilirubin, BUN, creatinine, serum glutamic-pyruvic transaminase (alanine aminotransferase), serum glutamic-oxaloacetic transaminase (aspartate aminotransferase), and creatine phosphokinase. Blood and urine cultures should be taken along with throat cultures when appropriate.

Medical Management

Treatment of TSS varies because of the range in types and severity of symptoms. Antibiotic therapy is given according to the results of culture and sensitivity tests. Parenteral therapy is given to maintain proper fluid balance. Laboratory data are evaluated for electrolyte imbalance caused by vomiting and diarrhea, elevated BUN suggesting renal involvement, and elevated enzymes suggesting liver dysfunction. Dialysis may be indicated in the event of renal failure.

Nursing Interventions and Patient Teaching

When the patient is hospitalized, bed rest is prescribed and antibiotics are administered. Closely monitor vital signs and fluid status. If there is respiratory distress, oxygen therapy is instituted.

A patient problem and interventions for the patient with TSS include but are not limited to the following:

PATIENT PROBLEM	NURSING INTERVENTIONS
Inadequate Fluid Volume related to vomiting and diarrhea	Monitor amount, frequency, and characteristics of vomitus and diarrhea Assess tissue turgor for evidence of dehydration Assess patient for dry mucous membranes, and monitor parenteral fluids; give fluids and electrolytes as ordered Monitor intake and output (I&O)

As the use of tampons during menstruation has been linked to TSS, advise patients not to use superabsorbent tampons. If tampons are used, they should be alternated with the use of pads. Before it is used, a tampon should be inspected for flaws and discarded if any are noted. Tampons should be changed frequently (every 4 hours) and should be inserted carefully to avoid abrasions. Patients who have had TSS should not use tampons. Instruct the patient to wash her hands thoroughly before inserting a tampon. Advise women who are menstruating and develop a sudden high fever accompanied by vomiting and diarrhea to seek immediate medical attention. If the woman is wearing a tampon, she should remove it immediately.

Prognosis

TSS is a rare and sometimes fatal disease. The effect of the toxin on the liver, kidneys, and circulatory system makes this a potentially life-threatening condition. The prognosis depends on the severity of the disease and how quickly therapeutic measures are instituted to combat shock and renal failure, if present.

DISORDERS OF THE FEMALE REPRODUCTIVE SYSTEM

ENDOMETRIOSIS
Etiology and Pathophysiology

Endometriosis is a condition in tissue that lines the uterus (endometrial) appears outside of it. Endometrial tissue can be found on the ovaries, the fallopian tubes, and the uterus; within the abdominal cavity (the uterovesical peritoneum); and in the vagina (Fig. 12.10). Tissue is believed to spread through the lymphatic circulation, by menstrual backflow to the fallopian tubes and pelvic cavity, or through congenital displacement of the endometrial cells. The condition is common in

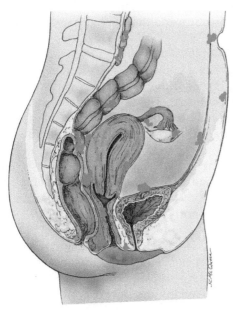

Fig. 12.10 Common sites of endometriosis. (From Lentz GM, Lobo RA, Gershenson DA, et al, editors: *Comprehensive gynecology*, ed 6, Philadelphia, 2013, Mosby.)

adolescents of childbearing age. An estimated 1 in 10 women are affected.

During the monthly cycle, hormones are secreted that cause changes in the uterine lining. As the endometrial prepares for a potential pregnancy it will become engorged and bleed. The displaced tissue will respond to the same hormones and then bleed despite its out of uterine location. The bleeding that results has no path of escape when not in the uterus. The repeated swelling and bleeding with each menstrual cycle results in inflammation and ultimately scar tissue. Adhesions can develop as areas with scaring form. Cyst development in the ovarian region may result. These are referred to as endometriomas. Rupture of these cysts may result in additional complications.

Risk factors for the development of endometriosis include a familial connection. Women having a mother or sister with the condition have an increased risk for developing it. Timing of menarche is also influential. Early onset of menses at age 11 years or younger is tied to endometriosis. Certain characteristics of the menstrual cycle are associated with endometriosis. Shorter cycles and heavier periods are seen in women having the condition. Delayed childbearing is also noted in endometriosis sufferers.

Clinical Manifestations

Dysmenorrhea is the most common complaint. Lower abdominal and pelvic pain with or without pain in the rectum, that may be unilateral or bilateral and may radiate to the lower back, legs, and groin, also is reported. Dyspareunia also is experienced frequently. Symptoms are more acute during menstruation and subside after menstruation.

Assessment

Subjective data include a history of the patient's symptoms, including pelvic pain with menstruation, aching, cramping, a bearing-down sensation in the pelvis, or lower back dyspareunia. The type of pain may indicate cysts that are about to rupture or infected tissue. The patient may reveal a history of menstrual irregularities such as amenorrhea.

Collection of objective data involves noting signs such as abnormal uterine bleeding, which appear 5 to 7 days before menses and last 2-3 days. Signs also may include infertility.

Diagnostic Tests

Diagnosing the condition will begin with a pelvic exam. Masses from cysts or thickening from scaring may be noted. Ultrasound will provide visualization of the pelvic organs. Cystic growths may be noted. The size of the structures can be ascertained with the ultrasound. MRI provides detailed visualization of the reproductive organs. Adhesions between structures and abnormal growths can be identified. Surgical visualization is completed with laparoscopy. The surgical procedure is done under general anesthesia. The organs are assessed for endometrial tissue growth and related scarring.

Medical Management

A chief complaint of the condition is the discomfort experienced. Due to the chronic nature of the diagnosis, narcotic medications are avoided unless the pain is severe. Nonsteroidal anti-inflammatory medications such as ibuprofen and naproxen are employed. Elagolix (Orilissa) is the only medication approved by the FDA specifically for the discomforts experienced in endometriosis. It is used for moderate to severe pain levels.

Hormonal therapies such as high-dose antiovulatory medications are used. These inhibit ovulation and induce a state physiologically similar to menopause, thus suppressing menstruation. Synthetic androgens such as danazol or a gonadotropin-releasing hormone agonist (GnRHa; e.g., leuprolide [Lupron]) may be prescribed to arrest proliferation of the endometrium and prevent ovulation, producing atrophy of the displaced endometrium. Hormonal contraceptives containing estrogen control and slow the growth of the endometrial tissue. Progestin only contraceptives will not impact endometrial tissue growth but will ease the menstrual blood flow or stop it completely. Unfortunately, the symptoms and progression of the disease return once the medications are discontinued. An interruption of the menstrual cycle slows the progress of the disorder. Some women who become pregnant are asymptomatic after pregnancy for extended periods of time.

Surgery may be indicated if the condition is severe. Laparoscopy in addition to being used to diagnose the condition allows for the removal of endometrial tissue outside of the uterus and adhesions. If the areas are too large to visualize with the laparoscopic procedures a laparotomy may be performed. Lasers can vaporize the small implants of endometrial tissue. Advanced cases of endometriosis may require a more drastic action, such as hysterectomy (removal of the uterus), oophorectomy (removal of the ovaries), and salpingectomy (removal of the fallopian tubes).

Nursing Interventions and Patient Teaching

Reinforce the health care provider's explanation of the expected results of treatment; instruct the patient regarding the dosage, frequency, and side effects of prescribed medications; and emphasize the importance of regular checkups and of reporting abnormal vaginal bleeding. Encourage verbalization of concerns and assist the patient with comfort measures. Endometriosis can impact fertility resulting in emotional anguish. Heating pads can provide relief of abdominal or back pain. Success has been reported with the use of acupuncture, TENS (transcutaneous electrical nerve stimulation), and yoga. Eating a balanced diet and regular physical activity are also helpful.

Patient problems and interventions for the patient with endometriosis include but are not limited to the following:

PATIENT PROBLEM	NURSING INTERVENTIONS
Pain related to displaced endometrial tissue	Institute comfort measures to cope with pain, such as medications and warm compresses to abdomen Maintain bed rest when pain is most severe
Impaired Sexual Function, related to painful intercourse or infertility	Emphasize importance of communicating fears and concerns that lead to anxiety

Prognosis

Approximately half of the women with endometriosis are infertile. Delaying childbearing by women with endometriosis is not recommended because worsening of the condition may result in a loss of fertility. Pregnancy and menopause stop the progression of the condition.

VAGINAL FISTULA

Etiology and Pathophysiology

A fistula is defined as an abnormal opening between two organs. Vaginal fistulas are caused by an ulcerating process resulting from cancer, radiation, weakening of tissue by pregnancies, and surgical interventions. Vaginal fistulas are named for the organs involved (Fig. 12.11). For example, a urethrovaginal fistula is an opening between the urethra and the vagina; a vesicovaginal fistula is an opening between the bladder and

the vagina; and a rectovaginal fistula is an opening between the rectum and the vagina.

Clinical Manifestations

Fistulas are recognized by their exudate, which has a distinct odor of urine or feces. In general, a bladder infection is present. The vesicovaginal fistula causes a constant trickling of urine into the vagina; a rectovaginal fistula allows feces and flatus to enter the vagina.

Assessment

Subjective data include the patient's understanding of the exudate that occurs and of any causative factors. The patient reports the presence of urine or feces from the vagina.

Collection of objective data includes noting any behaviors that indicate stress, anxiety, and pain. The patient may express feelings of decreased self-esteem because of the condition. Observe for urine or feces on the perineal pad.

Diagnostic Tests

Diagnostic testing includes a methylene blue instillation in the bladder, and an intravenous (IV) pyelogram or cystoscopy to assist in locating the fistula. Pelvic examination is performed.

Medical Management

Spontaneous healing is unlikely due to the continued exposure of the affected tissues to urine or stool. Smaller fistulas may be managed conservatively. The vesicovaginal fistula may be managed by transvesical or transvaginal application of a fibrin glue sealant or collagen plug, which is applied to close the fistula. To be successful the area will require drainage. Larger fistulas may require surgical intervention accompanied by urinary or bowel diversion. If the organ tissue is healthy, a surgical approach is recommended. The surgical approach may be similar to anteroposterior

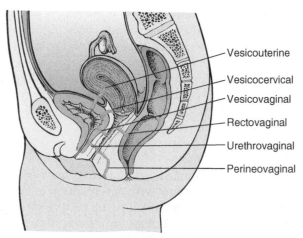

Fig. 12.11 Types of fistulas that may develop in the vagina and the uterus. (From Stenchever MA, Droegemueller W, Herbst AL, et al: *Comprehensive gynecology*, ed 3, St. Louis, 1998, Mosby.)

colporrhaphy, which is discussed later in this chapter. A diet high in protein, to promote healing, is recommended. Dietary fiber is beneficial to prevent constipation and straining. Antibiotics are included in the plan of treatment.

Nursing Interventions
Soiling from leakage of urine or stool into the vagina is disturbing for the patient. Sitz baths, deodorizing douches, perineal pads, and protective undergarments are necessary. If the fistula is repaired surgically, a Foley catheter is inserted postoperatively to prevent strain on the suture line by a full bladder.

Patient problems and interventions for the patient with vaginal fistula include but are not limited to the following:

PATIENT PROBLEM	NURSING INTERVENTIONS
Compromised Skin Integrity, related to exudates	Teach how to care for the skin with douches, creams, and sitz baths
Impaired Sexual Function, related to pain during sexual activity	Offer support and understanding of distress concerning sexual activities and self-esteem

Prognosis
Small vaginal fistulas may close spontaneously but more frequently will require surgery. If so, 4 to 6 months are required for the inflammation to subside before surgery can be attempted. After repair there are risks for infection, stool incontinence, bowel obstruction and recurrence.

RELAXED PELVIC MUSCLES
The most common problems resulting from relaxed pelvic muscles are as follows:
- *Displaced uterus:* A uterus that has moved away from its normal position
- *Prolapsed uterus:* A uterus that has protruded into the vaginal canal, or beyond the vaginal opening (*procidentia*)
- *Cystocele:* A bladder that has protruded into the vagina
- *Urethrocele:* A urethra that has protruded into the vagina
- *Rectocele:* A rectum that has protruded into the vagina
- *Enterocele:* A small bowel that has protruded into the vagina

Displaced Uterus
A displaced uterus can result from a traumatic childbirth experience. Scarring from PID or endometriosis can result in uterine displacement. The presence of fibroid tumors can result in the movement of the uterus from its normal anatomic position. Congenital abnormalities can cause displacement. Normally the uterus lies with the cervix at a right angle to the long axis of the vagina, and the body of the uterus is angled forward (see Fig. 12.2). The terms *retroversion* and *retroflexion* describe ways in which the uterus may be displaced: the retroverted uterus is aligned with the vagina and points toward the sacrum; the retroflexed uterus is flexed even farther backward. The patient with a displaced uterus has backache, muscle strain, leukorrhea (a whitish-colored discharge from the vagina), and heaviness in the pelvic area. The patient also tires easily. Treatment consists of a *pessary* (a rubber or plastic doughnut-shaped ring placed in the vagina, to help prop up the uterus) and possibly uterine suspension (a surgical procedure in which the uterus is repositioned).

Uterine Prolapse
Etiology and pathophysiology. Prolapse of the uterus is considered mild if the cervix drops to the lower vaginal segment. Moderate prolapses present with the cervix being visible at the vaginal opening. A severe prolapse, also termed a procidentia, results when the entire cervix protrudes through the vaginal opening (Fig. 12.12). Obstetric trauma, overstretching of the uterine muscle support system, multiple births, coughing, straining, the aging process, and lifting heavy objects contribute to uterine prolapse. Estrogen losses after menopause also are implicated in the condition.

Clinical manifestations. The patient complains of a feeling of "something coming down." She may have dyspareunia, a dragging or heavy feeling in the pelvis, backache, and bowel or bladder problems if cystocele or rectocele is also present. Stress incontinence is a common and troubling problem.

Medical management. Treatment is not undertaken unless the condition begins to result in increasing discomfort, impact daily life activities or the uterus drops into the opening of the vagina. The type of surgical procedure will be determined by the degree of prolapse, plans for future pregnancies, the woman's age and overall health, and the woman's desire to maintain vaginal function. Surgery generally involves a vaginal hysterectomy (i.e., removal of the uterus through the vagina) with anterior and posterior repair of the vagina and underlying fascia (Mayo Clinic, 2020c). It is also called an anteroposterior colporrhaphy (suture of the vagina) (also referred to as anterior posterior colporrhaphy or A&P repair).

When surgery is contraindicated, pessaries are used to provide uterine support. Before insertion of the vaginal pessary, the uterus is replaced manually in its normal position. Once inserted, the pessary holds the cervix in a posterior (anteflexed) position. When the pessary is properly placed, the woman is unaware of its presence and has no difficulty voiding or having intercourse. A variety of pessaries are available for the differing levels of prolapse. Every 3 to 4 months, the

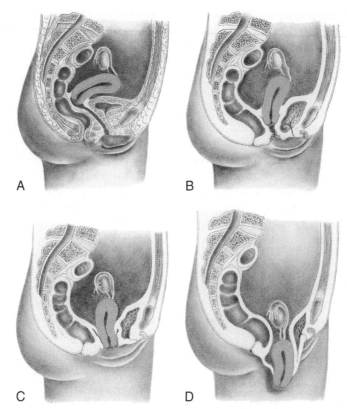

Fig. 12.12 Uterine prolapse. (A) Normal uterus. (B) First-degree prolapse of the uterus. (C) Second-degree prolapse of the uterus. (D), Third-degree prolapse of the uterus (procidentia). (From Seidel HM, Ball JW, Dains JE, et al: *Mosby's guide to physical examination*, ed 7, St. Louis, 2011, Mosby.)

pessary is cleaned and replaced by the woman, if possible, or by her health care provider. The vaginal walls should be assessed for signs of irritation. Pessaries that are unattended for long periods are associated with erosion, fistulas, and an increased incidence of vaginal carcinoma. Potential side effects of pessaries include foul-smelling discharge, vaginal ulcerations, and difficulty with normal sexual activity.

Cystocele and Rectocele

Etiology and pathophysiology. When the tissue, muscles, and ligaments that support the uterus and perineum have been stretched and weakened by childbearing, multiple births, or cervical tears, the organs gradually move into other positions. Relaxation of the tissues, muscles, and ligaments of the bladder may cause a displacement of the bladder into the vagina. This is referred to as a *cystocele* (Fig. 12.13A and B).

Clinical manifestations. Clinical symptoms are urinary urgency, frequency, and incontinence; fatigue; and pelvic pressure. A large cystocele prevents complete emptying of the bladder, which leads to bacterial growth and infection.

Relaxation of the supporting tissues to the rectum causes the rectum to move toward the posterior vaginal wall and form a rectocele (Fig. 12.13C and D). The rectocele causes constipation, rectal pressure, heaviness, and hemorrhoids.

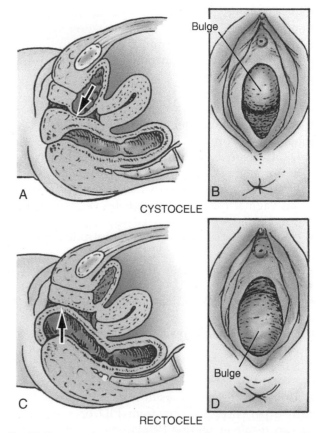

Fig. 12.13 A and B, Cystocele. C and D, Rectocele. (From Black JM, Hawks JH: *Medical-surgical nursing: Clinical management for positive outcomes*, ed 8, St. Louis, 2009, Mosby.)

Medical management. Cystocele and rectocele are corrected through anteroposterior colporrhaphy, a surgical repair involving shortening of the muscles that support the bladder and repair of the rectocele.

Nursing interventions and patient teaching. An important aspect of preoperative care for colporrhaphy is ensuring as clean an operative area as possible. Patients may be given a cathartic followed by enemas to be sure the bowel is completely empty. A liquid diet for 48 hours before surgery helps keep the bowel empty. A cleansing vaginal douche is given the evening before and the morning of surgery. Postoperative care includes checking vital signs and observing for hemorrhage. A Foley catheter usually is inserted into the bladder to keep it empty and to prevent pressure on sutures. Stool softeners often are prescribed. Small to scant amounts of vaginal bleeding will be noted.

Encourage early ambulation. Advise the patient against standing for long periods or lifting heavy objects. Coitus must be avoided until healing occurs, usually after about 6 weeks.

Prognosis. Surgical intervention to treat a cystocele and rectocele may result in complications such as infection, bladder injury causing urinary retention or urinary incontinence, or fistula development. An estimated 20% of women who undergo surgical correction experience reoccurrence of the prolapse.

LEIOMYOMAS OF THE UTERUS
Etiology and Pathophysiology
Leiomyomas (fibroids, myomas) are the most common benign tumors of the female genital tract. Fibroids are benign tumors arising from the muscle tissue of the uterus. The cause of leiomyomas is unknown. The number of women who have fibroid tumors is large. An estimated 20% to 80% of women have them. Fibroid tumor incidence increases with age, with their peak incidence during the 30s and 40s. During menopause the tumors shrink, as they are dependent on the body's ovarian hormones for their growth. Genetic factors are implicated in the development of fibroid tumors. A woman's risk for fibroids is increased threefold if her mother had them. African American women have a greater likelihood for their development than do white women. Obesity and dietary intake high in red meat and pork are linked to fibroid development. The size and number of leiomyomas vary. Most are found in the body of the uterus, but some occur in the cervix or involve the broad ligaments.

Clinical Manifestations
Small fibroid tumors are often asymptomatic. Increasing pressure of tumors on the uterus and pelvic organs may cause discomfort. These may include pain (including dysmenorrhea and dyspareunia), abnormal uterine bleeding, and menorrhagia. If the fibroid tumor becomes large enough to cause pressure on other structures, the patient may have backache, constipation, and urinary symptoms.

Assessment
Collection of subjective data includes asking the patient about pain with menstruation or abnormally heavy menstrual flow. Have the patient describe her symptoms, which may include pelvic fullness or heaviness, constipation, urinary frequency or urgency, and menorrhagia.

Collection of objective data includes assessing the patient for excessively heavy discharge of blood by observing the number and saturation of perineal pads.

Diagnostic Tests
Initially a pelvic examination will be performed. The health care provider may be able to palpate the tumors during the bimanual examination. Diagnostic tests to confirm the presence of fibroid tumors may include pelvic ultrasonography, MRI, x-rays, and a CT scan. More invasive studies include the hysterosalpingogram. Surgical intervention such as a laparoscopy or hysteroscopy may be used to visualize fibroid tumors.

Medical Management
The treatment of fibroid tumors depends on the patient's symptoms, her age and how close to menopause she is, and whether she wishes to become pregnant. Conservative nonsurgical management will be implemented if the tumors are not causing too-significant levels of discomfort. Pain management may include ibuprofen or acetaminophen. Women who experience heavy menstrual bleeding may require iron supplementation. Dysmenorrhea may be managed with low-dose oral contraceptives.

Myomectomy (removal of uterine myomas while leaving the uterus in place) is the procedure of choice for women hoping to maintain fertility. If during the surgery there is severe bleeding or an obstruction is found, a hysterectomy may still be necessary. Before surgical intervention medications may be prescribed to shrink the tumors. A GnRHa may be administered by injection or nasal spray or implanted. GnRHa medications place the woman in a medication-induced form of menopause. Side effects of the drug therapy include hot flashes, depression, reduced libido, and joint pain.

A hysterectomy is performed if the fibroids cause excessive vaginal bleeding, discomfort, or if the woman has no desire to maintain fertility. The hysterectomy is limited to removal of the uterus. The ovaries are preserved in the absence of other anomalies.

An increasingly used alternative treatment for uterine fibroids is uterine artery embolization. This procedure consists of injecting embolic material (small plastic or gelatin beads) into the uterine artery, which carries the material to the fibroid branches and thus occludes the arteries supplying blood to the tumor.

Deprived of oxygen and nutrients, the tumor shrinks over time and symptoms diminish.

Six months after uterine artery embolization, fibroids are typically about 50% smaller in most women, and in 80% to 90% of women the symptoms are considerably decreased or gone. About 5% of patients experience complications from the procedure, such as infection or permanent cessation of menstrual periods.

Nursing Interventions and Patient Teaching
Preoperative and postoperative nursing interventions are like those discussed for a patient who undergoes a hysterectomy. Reinforce the health care provider's explanation of the treatment plan—either a total hysterectomy or pelvic examination at regular intervals to monitor the status of the fibroid tumor. Instruct the patient about the dosage, frequency, and possible side effects of prescribed medications. Tell the patient with menorrhagia to include adequate iron in her diet to prevent iron deficiency anemia from the extra blood loss. Stress the importance of regular checkups to monitor the status of the fibroid tumor and encourage the patient to express her feelings and assist her with coping mechanisms.

A patient problem and interventions for the patient with fibroid tumors include but are not limited to the following:

PATIENT PROBLEM	NURSING INTERVENTIONS
Pain, related to fibroid tumors	Assess pain location, onset, and duration
	Administer analgesics as ordered.
	Provide comfort measures as needed

Prognosis
Fibroid tumors of the uterus tend to diminish and disappear spontaneously with menopause. They rarely become malignant. Infertility may result from a myoma that obstructs or distorts the uterus or fallopian tubes. Myomas in the body of the uterus may cause spontaneous abortions; those near the cervical opening may make the delivery of a fetus difficult and may contribute to postpartum hemorrhage.

OVARIAN CYSTS
Etiology and Pathophysiology
Ovarian cysts are benign tumors that arise from dermoid cells of the ovary or from a cystic corpus luteum or graafian follicle.

Clinical Manifestations
Ovarian cysts enlarge and are palpable on examination. They may cause no symptoms, or they may result in a disturbance of menstruation, a feeling of heaviness, and slight vaginal bleeding. Some individuals report sharp abdominal pain that may subside with rupture of the cyst.

Medical Management
The cysts may be removed by ovarian cystectomy. Often ovarian cysts are not removed if the patient is not experiencing debilitating symptoms.

Nursing Interventions
If surgery is performed, nursing interventions are similar to those for the patient undergoing an abdominal hysterectomy (i.e., removal of the uterus through an abdominal incision).

Prognosis
The prognosis is good; ovarian cysts do not become malignant.

CANCER OF THE FEMALE REPRODUCTIVE TRACT

Cancer is the second most common cause of death in women, and malignant tumors of the reproductive tract represent a significant portion of the total number of deaths from cancer (see the Cultural Considerations box).

Cultural Considerations
Cancer of Female Reproductive System
- Ovarian cancer is seen more frequently among white women than among African American women. Survival rates for African American women with ovarian cancer are less than those of white women.
- Japanese women have a low incidence of ovarian cancer. However, second- and third-generation Japanese women in the United States have much higher rates, similar to those of white women born in the United States. Dietary practices may explain this difference.
- Endometrial cancer occurs more frequently among white women than among African American women.
- The 5-year survival rate for endometrial cancer (all stages combined) is 80% for white women and 55% for African American women.
- Cervical cancer has a higher incidence among Hispanic, African American, and Native American women than among white women. The mortality rate for cervical cancer is more than twice as high among African American women as among white women.
- Jewish American women have a low incidence of cervical cancer.

Cervical cancer often affects women in their reproductive years. The cancer can be detected in its early stages with a diagnostic Pap test. Endometrial cancer is primarily a disease of women older than 50 years of age, but the incidence among younger women is increasing. Most cases of ovarian cancer occur in women older than 50, but malignant neoplasms of the ovaries may occur at any age. Ovarian cancer is largely "silent," that is, symptom free, until late in its progression, resulting in a relatively poor prognosis.

CANCER OF THE CERVIX
Cancer of the cervix is a neoplasm that can be detected in the early, curable stage by a Pap test. The rate of

cervical cancer has declined over the past few decades. This decline is attributed to Pap testing by women. Cancer of the cervix is usually a squamous cell carcinoma. An estimated 13,000 cases of cervical cancer were diagnosed in 2020. An estimated 4300 cervical cancer deaths occurred in 2020 (ACS, 2020b). The ease in availability of pap testing promote the high cure rate for those women who have an early diagnosis when the cancer is localized (92%). The survival rates decline consistent with spread of the disease by the time of diagnosis.

Etiology and Pathophysiology

Women who become sexually active in their teens are at an increased risk for cancer of the cervix, as are those who have had multiple sexual partners, had partners who had multiple sexual partners, and are of lower socioeconomic status. Cervical cancer risk is closely linked to sexual behavior, to STIs with several strains of HPV, and to smoking. Women who smoke have a 50% higher risk of developing cervical cancer than nonsmokers. Chronic infections and erosions of the cervix are most likely significant in the development of cancer.

Carcinoma in situ, including that of the cervix, is a term used to describe a preinvasive, asymptomatic carcinoma that can be diagnosed only by microscopic examination. Once diagnosed, it can be treated early without radical surgery. Carcinoma in situ of the cervix is 100% curable.

Clinical Manifestations

Cervical cancer is typically silent in the early stages and offers few symptoms. The two primary symptoms are leukorrhea and irregular vaginal bleeding or spotting between menses. Bleeding often occurs after coitus or after menopause. Bleeding is slight at first but increases as the disease progresses. The vaginal exudate becomes watery and then increases and becomes dark and bloody, with an offensive odor caused by necrosis (death of tissue) and infection of the tumor mass. As the cancer progresses, the bleeding may become constant and may increase in amount. With advanced stages the patient has severe pain in the back, upper thighs, and legs.

Assessment

Subjective data in the early stages of cancer of the cervix are not available, because the woman has no symptoms. If the tumor becomes more invasive, the patient experiences back and leg pain, weight loss, and malaise. Urge women to have regular health appraisals and pelvic examinations so that cancer of the cervix can be detected in its earliest stages.

Collection of objective data includes observing the sanitary pads for abnormal vaginal discharge. The vaginal exudate may be watery to dark red and malodorous. Note the number and saturation of the perineal pads. If the tumor becomes more invasive, assess the patient for anemia, fever, and lymphedema.

Diagnostic Tests

Cervical cancer is diagnosed with the following tests: (1) Pap test; (2) physical examination; (3) colposcopy and cervical biopsy; and (4) additional diagnostic studies, such as a CT scan, chest radiographic evaluation, IV pyelogram, cystoscopy, sigmoidoscopy, or liver function studies to determine the extent of invasion. The ACS recommends that cervical cancer screening begin at 25 years of age. Traditional Pap tests are less than 100% accurate in screening for cervical cell abnormalities, and false-positive and false-negative results do occur. A newer, liquid-based technique can reduce the number of inaccurate Pap tests results.

Medical Management

Gardasil is a vaccine that reduces the incidence of cervical cancer resulting from infection with HPV types 6, 11, 16, and 18. Vaccination is recommended to begin between ages 11 and 12 years in both male and female adolescents. It may be given as early as 9 years of age. To be effective, the vaccine should be given before a person becomes sexually active. The goal of these vaccines is to reduce the incidence of HPV-related genital disease, including precancerous cervical lesions and cervical cancer. In women the vaccine is provides protection from linked to HPV to the cervix, vaginal, anus, and vulva. Three injections are given over 6 months. The second dose is given 2 months after the first dose and the third dose 6 months after the first dose (Gardasil 9, n.d.).

Cervarix is a three-dose vaccine to prevent cervical cancer; cervical intraepithelial neoplasia (CIN) grades 1, 2, or worse; and adenocarcinoma in situ. It was approved by the FDA in 2009 for girls and young women 10 to 25 years old and is undergoing pediatric testing for use in 9-year-old girls. Cervarix is effective against HPV types 16 and 18, but it does not offer coverage against all the other types of HPV infection, nor is it effective after exposure to HPV (FDA, 2019).

Carcinoma in situ is treated by removal of the affected area. A variety of techniques can be used, including electrocautery, cryosurgery (use of subfreezing temperature to destroy tissue), laser, conization, and hysterectomy. Conization is the surgical removal of a cone-shaped section of the cervix and is particularly useful in preserving childbearing function.

Early cervical carcinoma can be treated with a hysterectomy or intracavitary radiation (see Chapter 17).

A radical hysterectomy with pelvic lymph node dissection may be required for more extensive lesions. Invasive cervical cancers generally are treated by surgery, radiation, or both, as well as chemotherapy (cisplatin-based) in some cases. Radiation may be external or internal (e.g., cesium, radium). Brachytherapy is a form of radiation therapy in which the source of radiation is implanted in the cervix. The patient is hospitalized for 48 hours for treatment. The treatment plan is tailored to each patient, based on the extent of the disease.

NURSING INTERVENTIONS AND PATIENT TEACHING

Nursing interventions should include verbal reassurance and support. In advanced cervical cancer, position the patient comfortably; change her position slowly; maintain her body alignment; provide pain relief measures; change the patient's dressings and sanitary pads often; and assess color, odor, and amount of drainage. Assess the skin for impairment. See the section "Abdominal Hysterectomy" for a description of nursing interventions for a patient undergoing a hysterectomy.

Patient problems and interventions for the patient with cancer of the cervix include but are not limited to the following:

PATIENT PROBLEM	NURSING INTERVENTIONS
Alteration in urinary elimination, related to postsurgical sensorimotor impairment	Connect indwelling catheter to closed gravity drainage. Give meticulous catheter care as indicated. Record color and amount of urinary output. Promote micturition at regular intervals when catheter is removed. Catheterize for residual urine as ordered
Potential for Impaired Self-Esteem due to Current Situation, related to body image change and value of reproductive organs	Encourage discussion with significant others. Relate importance of communicating anything that causes anxiety. Reinforce correct information to correct any misconceptions
Compromised Blood Flow to Peripheral Tissue, related to: • Pelvic surgery • Thrombophlebitis	Ensure that bed is not elevated in the knee gatch position. Assess proper placement of antiembolism stockings q 4 h as ordered. Assist in passive and active leg exercises every shift. Encourage ambulation. Assess legs for erythema, increased tenderness, and severe cramping every shift

The key to preventing cervical cancer and treating it in the early stages is education. Educate and encourage patients to be responsible for their health by having a yearly Pap test. Education about the HPV vaccine for females is very important. Encourage patients to seek prompt medical assistance for any abnormal vaginal exudate.

Prognosis

The prognosis is good if the cancer is treated in the early stages. It usually takes 2 to 10 years for squamous cell carcinoma to become invasive beyond the basement membrane and metastasize. Therefore early diagnosis and treatment are vital.

CANCER OF THE ENDOMETRIUM
Etiology and Pathophysiology

Cancer of the endometrium usually affects postmenopausal women. In 2020, an estimated 62,620 women will be diagnosed with endometrial cancer. Approximately 12,590 will succumb to the disease (ACS, 2020c). Endometrial cancer is usually an adenocarcinoma (a tumor originating from glandular epithelial cells). The tumor is more likely to be localized but may spread to the cervix, bladder, rectum, and surrounding lymph nodes. It is the most common malignancy of the female genital tract. Women at increased risk are those with a history of irregular menstruation, difficulties during menopause, obesity, hypertension, or diabetes mellitus; those who have not had children; and those with a family history of uterine cancer. Obesity is a risk factor because adipose cells store estrogen. Women who used estrogen replacement therapy to treat menopausal symptoms are more likely to develop endometrial cancer. Combined progesterone and estrogen replacement therapy (HRT) may largely offset the increased risk related to using only estrogen. Also at increased risk for developing endometrial cancer are women at high risk for developing breast cancer as well as those in an advanced stage of breast cancer who are taking tamoxifen, an antiestrogen drug that blocks estrogen receptors.

Carcinoma in situ is slow growing. Invasion and metastasis occur later, with expansion to the cervix and the myometrium and ultimately to the vagina, the pelvis, and the lungs.

Clinical Manifestations

Abnormal bleeding is seen in 90% of women diagnosed with endometrial cancer. This may include vaginal bleeding post menopause or bleeding between menstrual periods. As the disease progresses additional signs will include pelvic discomfort or pain, and weight loss without trying

Assessment

Collection of subjective data includes assisting the patient in identifying and reporting changes in reproductive or sexual health. The patient may report abdominal pressure, pain, and pelvic fullness. The patient will have a history of postmenopausal bleeding and leukorrhea. Pelvic and back pain and postcoital bleeding are late signs and symptoms.

Collection of objective data includes observing the color and amount of vaginal exudate on perineal pads. Assess the patient for enlarged lymph nodes.

Diagnostic Tests

The diagnostic process begins with a pelvic and rectal manual examination. An ultrasound will be included in the exam. This test may show abnormalities of the uterus. During the abdominal ultrasound the bladder will need to be filled to promote visualization. A transvaginal ultrasound provides more distinct imagine of the uterus. The saline infusion ultrasound (hysterosonogram) facilitates visualization of the uterus by infusing saline through a small catheter. The appearance of growths or thickening of the uterus will require further investigation. The endometrial biopsy is the definitive means to affix the diagnosis of endometrial cancer. The National Cancer Institute (NCI, 2021) reports that screening of asymptomatic or low-risk women by means of an endometrial biopsy is not encouraged. The Pap test is not a reliable diagnostic tool for endometrial cancer, but it can rule out cervical cancer.

Medical Management

Treatment of cancer of the endometrium depends on the stage of the tumor and the woman's health. Surgery, radiation, or chemotherapy may be used to remove the tumor and to treat metastasis. For early cancer of the endometrium, total abdominal hysterectomy with bilateral salpingo-oophorectomy (TAH-BSO) is done. The hysterectomy is performed abdominally as opposed to vaginally to allow the surgeon the ability to view the inside of the abdominal and pelvic cavities to assess for potential areas of concern and metastasis. Intracavitary radiation followed by a TAH-BSO may be done for the early stage of endometrial cancer (stage I). Patients with stage II disease may receive pelvic irradiation to shrink the tumor and to help prevent spread. Afterward the patient undergoes a hysterectomy. Patients with stages III and IV disease are uncommon, and treatment is based on the extent of the disease.

Nursing Interventions and Patient Teaching

See the section "Abdominal Hysterectomy," later in this chapter, for a description of nursing interventions for the patient undergoing a hysterectomy; also see Chapter 17 for care of the patient through intracavitary radiation.

Health teaching and follow-up after discharge should emphasize the need for regular physical examination by the health care provider and the importance of compliance with the prescribed treatment plan.

Prognosis

Cancer of the endometrium is primarily a slow-growing adenocarcinoma. Metastasis occurs late, and the sign of irregular vaginal bleeding often appears early enough to allow for cure of the disease. Approximately 66.7% of endometrial cancer patients are diagnosed when the disease is localized without spread to other parts of the body. The 5-year survival rate for this group of patients is 95%. The populations who are diagnosed once the disease has spread to nearby regions (21%) or metastasized (9%) experience a lessened rate of survival at the 5-year point of 69% and 16%, respectively (ACS Cancer Statistics Center, 2021). For those women whose cancer has spread, the rate is reduced significantly—only 25% at 5 years (NLM, 2020).

CANCER OF THE OVARY

Etiology and Pathophysiology

Ovarian cancer, the fifth most common cause of cancer death in women, is the leading cause of gynecologic death in the United States, following cancer of the uterine corpus. Risk for ovarian cancer increases with age. More than half are over the age of 63 years when diagnosed (ACS, 2021c).

It is estimated that over 21,400 women will be diagnosed with ovarian cancer in 2021 and nearly 14,000 will die from the disease (ACS, 2021c).

In the early stages the tumors are asymptomatic; when detected, they usually have spread to other pelvic organs. Nothing alters the magnitude of risk for ovarian cancer more than genetics. Hereditary ovarian cancer accounts for 5% to 10% of ovarian cancers. In general, the closer the relative with ovarian cancer and the younger the relative at diagnosis, the higher the risk is. Women at increased risk are those who are nulliparous or delay childbearing until age 35 years or after. Hormone therapies after menopause is tied to an increased risk for development of the cancer. Other risk factors include a high-fat diet and exposure to industrial chemicals such as asbestos and talc. Mitigating factors that reduce the risk of ovarian cancer include use of oral contraceptives, breastfeeding and carrying a fetus to term by the age of 26 years. Ovarian cancer commonly spreads by peritoneal seeding of the cancer cells. Common sites of metastasis are the peritoneum (the membrane that lines the abdominal cavity), the omentum (peritoneal folds that connect the organs to one another or to the abdominal wall), and bowel surfaces (ACS, 2021c).

Clinical Manifestations

In the early stages the symptoms may cause vague abdominal discomfort, flatulence, mild gastric disturbances, pressure, bloating, cramps, sense of pelvic heaviness, feeling of fullness, and change in bowel habits. Pain is not an early symptom. As the tumor progresses, abdominal girth enlarges from ascites (accumulation of fluid in the peritoneal cavity), and there is flatulence with distention. Other symptoms may include urinary frequency, nausea, vomiting, constipation, menstrual irregularities, and weight loss. A challenge of ovarian cancer management is the fact that it often is caught after the disease has spread. The symptoms usually include bloating, pelvic or abdominal pain, urinary disturbances, difficulty eating, or feelings of fullness. These symptoms are attributed easily to other benign disorders. Women who experience these symptoms are encouraged to seek prompt care with their health care provider.

Assessment

Collection of subjective data requires an awareness that cancer of the ovary is difficult to detect. The patient reports symptoms of abdominal discomfort, bloating, fullness, gastric disturbances (nausea, constipation), and urinary frequency.

Collection of objective data includes observing any increase in abdominal girth. The patient may void at frequent intervals because of pressure on the bladder. The patient may be dyspneic because of ascites and pressure on the diaphragm.

Diagnostic Tests

Although detecting ovarian cancer early is difficult, an annual bimanual pelvic examination may help to identify pelvic masses. Because the ovaries are movable and therefore harder to assess, screening for ovarian tumors requires a thorough examination, including bimanual and rectovaginal examination. Postmenopause palpable ovary syndrome (a palpable ovary in a woman 3 to 5 years past menopause) may indicate an early tumor. CT scan of the pelvis and abdomen is indicated if an ovarian mass is palpable. Definitive diagnosis of ovarian cancer usually is established by a tumor biopsy at the time of exploratory laparotomy, when staging and tumor debulking take place.

Ovarian cancer is diagnosed by palpation of a pelvic mass, aspiration of ascitic fluid, and detection of cancer cells in the fluid. A blood test to determine CA-125 is used to identify women with ovarian cancer. High levels of CA-125 are found in the blood of 80% of women with epithelial ovarian cancer. However, although the antigen test can help evaluate a woman's response to cancer treatment, it is controversial as an independent screening tool. Because of the test's lack of specificity and sensitivity, false-positive and false-negative results can occur. Many benign conditions, including endometriosis and fibroid tumors, can raise CA-125 levels above normal.

Vaginal ultrasonography, which also lacks specificity and sensitivity, may be used with pelvic examination and CA-125 antigen testing to monitor a woman at increased risk.

Medical Management

Treatment often involves surgery alone or in conjunction with radiation or chemotherapy. Treatment depends on the stage of ovarian cancer (see Chapter 17). Surgery may be a TAH-BSO and omentectomy (excision of portions of the peritoneal folds). In some very early tumors, only the involved ovary is removed, especially in young women who wish to have children. Injection therapy with luteinizing-hormone releasing

hormone (LHRH) antagonists (goserelin and leuprolide) may be indicated in premenopausal women. The therapy works by sharply cutting off the estrogen to the ovaries. The treatment is repeated every 1 to 3 months. Targeted therapy also may be employed. This type of therapy uses drugs or other substances such as antibodies to attack the cancer cells but not damage the normal cells.

Nursing Interventions

Nursing interventions for any patient with ovarian cancer include management similar to that for patients undergoing abdominal hysterectomy and receiving chemotherapy and external radiation (see Chapter 17). Because ovarian cancer is generally at an advanced stage when diagnosed, despite the woman's feeling well, support and encouragement to comply with the treatment regimen are important nursing interventions. As the disease progresses, become involved in activities to increase the patient's comfort.

Patient problems and interventions for the patient with cancer of the ovaries include but are not limited to the following:

PATIENT PROBLEM	NURSING INTERVENTIONS
Fearfulness related to diagnosis of cancer	Assist patient with recognizing and clarifying fears and with developing coping strategies for those fears Be an active listener
Impaired Self-Esteem due to Current Situation, related to body image change and value of reproductive organs	Encourage patient's comments and questions about condition Encourage discussion with significant others Provide factual information to correct any misconceptions

Prognosis

The overall 5-year survival rate for ovarian cancer ranges from 48% for invasive epithelial to 93% for germ cell tumors (ACS Cancer Statistics Center, 2021).

HYSTERECTOMY

A hysterectomy involves removal of the uterus; the cervix, fallopian tubes, ovaries, and other structures may also be removed. This procedure may be done for many conditions, including DUB, endometriosis, malignant and nonmalignant tumors of the uterus and cervix, and disorders of pelvic relaxation and uterine prolapse.

Various terms are used to describe removal of the uterus:

- *Subtotal hysterectomy:* A subtotal hysterectomy involves removal only of the uterus, either vaginally, abdominally, or laparoscopically. The cervix remains intact and the vagina retains its usual length. Intercourse is possible even though childbearing is not; leaving the cervical stump in place may play a role in a woman's sexual pleasure and orgasm. Estrogens are still released because the ovaries are still present. Menopause occurs naturally.
- *Total hysterectomy:* A total hysterectomy involves removal of the uterus and cervix, either vaginally, abdominally, or laparoscopically. The vagina remains intact, but somewhat shortened; intercourse is possible even though childbearing is not. Estrogens are still released because the ovaries are present. Menopause occurs naturally.
- *Total abdominal/laparoscopic hysterectomy with bilateral salpingo-oophorectomy (TAH-BSO/TLH-BSO):* Total abdominal/laparoscopic hysterectomy with bilateral salpingo-oophorectomy involves removal of the uterus, fallopian tubes, and ovaries; this is done abdominally (TAH-BSO) or laparoscopically (TLH-BSO). It is sometimes called a panhysterosalpingo-oophorectomy. Because the ovaries are removed, menopause is induced.
- *Radical hysterectomy:* A radical hysterectomy also includes removal of the pelvic lymph nodes; this is done abdominally. Because the ovaries are removed, menopause is induced.

VAGINAL HYSTERECTOMY

A vaginal hysterectomy is typically done for a prolapsed uterus. In this procedure the patient is placed in the lithotomy position, and the uterus is removed through the vagina. The vaginal route is not used as often as the abdominal approach; there are, however, clear advantages to the vaginal approach. Patients who are poor candidates for abdominal surgery or prolonged anesthesia may benefit from this option. The procedure is less expensive and requires a reduced period of hospitalization. A vaginal hysterectomy does not require an abdominal incision, which facilitates recovery. Postoperative discomfort is less than with the abdominal approach. There is a reduced risk for the development of complications. The most important disadvantage of the vaginal route is the necessarily limited view of the operative field for visualizing intrapelvic and intra-abdominal organs. Vaginal hysterectomy is not used in cases of large uterine fibroids, enlarged uterine size, or suspicions of malignancy.

ABDOMINAL HYSTERECTOMY

An abdominal hysterectomy is preferred when there is a need to explore the pelvic cavity and when the fallopian tubes and ovaries are to be removed. The laparoscopic hysterectomy may be performed when there is no need to have a more extensive visualization of the pelvic or abdominal cavities.

Nursing Interventions

Preoperative interventions. When the health care provider has explained the surgery to the patient, reinforce the explanation and answer any questions. Encourage verbalization of fears. Provide additional preoperative instructions to help the woman prepare for postoperative recovery. Instruct the patient how to turn, cough, and deep breathe.

Before a vaginal or abdominal hysterectomy, the colon is emptied to prevent postoperative distention. The patient may be on a low-residue diet for several days preoperatively. Enemas may be given the evening before surgery. An indwelling catheter is placed to decompress the bladder, to prevent trauma during surgery. The catheter normally is removed the day after surgery. An antiseptic vaginal douche may be ordered to decrease microbial invasion of the surgical site.

Surgical preparation of the skin on the abdomen, the pelvis, and the perineum often is performed in surgery. The patient signs a consent form, and oral intake after midnight is restricted. On occasion, ureteral stents are placed in the ureters for identification and to prevent possible trauma to the ureters during surgery.

Postoperative interventions. Nursing interventions after surgery focus on monitoring and recording patient status, preventing complications, and reporting concerns to the surgeon. The postoperative nursing assessment is performed at least every 4 hours during the first day after surgery. Lung fields are assessed. The patient is assisted to turn, cough, and deep breathe every 2 hours. Instruct the patient to splint the abdomen as needed. Incentive spirometry to encourage deep breathing is often prescribed during waking hours. Vital signs are assessed and compared with the preoperative baselines. Oxygen saturation levels are assessed. The urinary catheter is assessed to ensure patency (i.e., that it is unblocked). The amount of urine also must be recorded. Output less than 30 mL/h must be reported. The incidence of urinary retention after a hysterectomy is greater than after any other type of surgery, because some trauma to the bladder is unavoidable. The abdomen is assessed for distension and bowel sounds. As the postoperative period progresses assess for passage of flatus. The lower extremities are evaluated for redness or tenderness. Early ambulation is initiated to promote bowel activity and prevention of venous thrombus. When bowel sounds have returned and flatus is being expelled, the patient is allowed liquids by mouth and a gradual return to solid foods.

Patients undergoing pelvic surgery are susceptible to venous stasis and thrombophlebitis because of trauma to blood vessels. The patient usually is permitted out of bed on the first postoperative day. Encourage the patient to sit on the side of the bed and dangle her legs before standing and walking, to avoid postural hypotension. Encourage the patient to cough, deep breathe, and use an incentive spirometer to prevent postoperative pneumonia and atelectasis. Antiembolism stockings may be used to prevent thrombus or embolus formation, and the legs should be exercised frequently when the patient is in bed. Many health care providers prescribe intermittent pneumonic compression cuffs for the calves to prevent venous stasis, deep-vein thrombosis, and pulmonary embolism. The patient should avoid bending her knees. This could cause pooling of blood in the pelvic cavity, resulting in stasis in the lower extremities. The patient at risk for thromboembolic disease may receive low-dose heparin or low molecular weight enoxaparin (Lovenox) to prevent thrombus formation.

Analgesics such as morphine may be ordered for relief of pain. Slight vaginal drainage may occur for several days. Report any unusual bleeding to the health care provider. Observe the abdominal dressing on the patient with an abdominal hysterectomy for evidence of hemorrhage. Use surgical asepsis for the dressing change. The patient usually receives IV feedings for the first postoperative day. Carefully monitor the rate of flow and the condition of the IV site.

Patient problems and interventions for the patient who has had a hysterectomy include but are not limited to the following:

PATIENT PROBLEM	NURSING INTERVENTIONS
Prolonged Pain, related to metastatic process	Monitor and document pain characteristics
	Administer prescribed analgesics q 3–4 h to control pain
	Provide environment conducive to comfort and rest
Fluid Volume Overload, related to ascites	Monitor IV fluids
	Maintain accurate I&O
	Weigh patient daily
	Observe for signs of edema
	Measure abdominal girth daily
Impaired Family Coping, related to poor prognosis	Assess present coping abilities
	Encourage and allow time for verbalization of feelings
	Support patient's coping strengths, and discuss alternative coping measures
	Involve patient and significant others in nursing interventions and procedures

I&O, Intake and output; *IV,* intravenous.

Patient Teaching
Before discharge, the health care provider explains to the woman and her partner that they should not have sexual intercourse for 4 to 6 weeks after surgery. With an abdominal incision, there may be further restrictions on heavy lifting (nothing greater than 10 pounds), walking up and down stairs, and prolonged riding in the car. Riding in the car may cause pelvic pooling and development of a thrombus in the legs.

Inform the patient that vaginal drainage is normal for about 2 to 4 weeks after an abdominal hysterectomy. Advise her to avoid wearing any tight clothing such as a girdle or knee-high hose, which may constrict circulation to the surgical site and cause venous stasis.

Several signs and symptoms of infection should be reported to the health care provider if they occur: (1) erythema, edema, exudate, or increased tenderness along the surgical incision; (2) increased malodorous vaginal exudate; (3) a temperature of 101°F (38.3°C) or more; and (4) any problems with urinating, such as difficulty in starting to void, voiding too often, voiding small amounts, or a burning sensation while urinating (indicative of a bladder infection).

DISORDERS OF THE FEMALE BREAST

FIBROCYSTIC BREAST CONDITION
Etiology and Pathophysiology
Fibrocystic breast condition involves benign tumors of the breasts. The condition is common and impacts more than 50% of women at some point in their lives. It usually occurs in women 20 to 50 years of age and is rare in postmenopausal women. This suggests that the occurrence is related to ovarian activity.

The cysts are characterized by numerous cellular changes, with an abnormal amount of epithelial hyperplasia and cystic formation within the mammary ducts. The cysts rarely become malignant. Women experiencing fibrocystic breast condition are not at an increased risk for the development of breast cancer.

Clinical Manifestations
Cystic lesions are often bilateral and multiple. The cysts are soft, well differentiated, tender, and freely movable. The lumpiness and tenderness are more apparent mid cycle around ovulation and then subside just before menses. Some women may experience green to brown discharge that is non bloody.

Diagnostic Tests
The disorder is diagnosed by mammography or ultrasound and confirmed by biopsy. As a therapeutic measure, the cyst is aspirated by needle and syringe to empty the secretions, and the fluid is sent to the laboratory for cytologic examination to rule out a malignancy. Aspiration produces a turbid, nonhemorrhagic fluid that is yellow, greenish, or brownish.

Medical Management
When a cyst recurs in the same area and repeated aspirations are ineffective, surgical excision of the cyst may be done.

Conservative treatment is the usual approach to fibrocystic breast condition. The usefulness of eliminating methylxanthines (in coffee, tea, and cola) from the diet is still controversial, but it is the least expensive therapy. Many women have reported decreased symptoms after altering their diet, even though findings by palpation and mammogram were not significantly changed. Danazol may be prescribed to inhibit FSH and LH production, thereby decreasing ovarian production of estrogen. Danazol may cause weight gain, hot flashes, menstrual irregularities, hirsutism, and deepening of the voice. Vitamin E also may be prescribed, but its efficacy has not been proven.

Nursing Interventions and Patient Teaching
Instruct the patient to perform BSE 1 week after menses, to recognize the presence of cysts, and to note any changes. Breast tissue thickening, bloody nipple discharge or discomfort that lingers beyond the onset of menses warrant reporting.

ACUTE MASTITIS
Acute mastitis is an acute bacterial infection of the breast tissue, most commonly caused by *S. aureus* or streptococci. It is observed most often during lactation and late pregnancy. The infection may result from a clogged milk duct, inadequate cleanliness of the breasts, a nipple fissure, or infection in the infant. The breasts are tender, inflamed, and engorged, obstructing the milk flow.

Treatment involves application of warm packs, support of the area with a well-fitting brassiere (which also supplies comfort), and systemic treatment with antibiotics. Women who are breast-feeding are permitted to continue with nursing because this promotes emptying of the inflamed ducts and reduce the incidence of milk stasis.

CHRONIC MASTITIS
Chronic mastitis tends to develop in women between 30 and 50 years of age and is more common in those who have had children, have had difficulty with inverted and cracked nipples, and have had problems nursing their infants. A traumatic blow to the breasts causes the fat to necrose in the area and form abscesses. Increased fibrosis of the tissue causes cysts to form. The cysts are tender, painful, and palpable on examination. The disorder is generally unilateral and benign and most frequently occurs in obese women. Treatment is the same as for acute mastitis.

CANCER OF THE BREAST
Breast cancer is the second most common malignancy (after lung cancer) affecting women in the United States: approximately one of every eight American women will develop breast cancer during her lifetime. In contrast, the incidence of breast cancer in men is rare. Their likelihood for the development of breast cancer is 1 in 883. In 2020, an estimated 276,480 women will be diagnosed with breast cancer. Nearly 43,000 women will die during this same period. The deaths from breast cancer have declined since 2000. Improved diagnostic testing, increased availability of

mammography, promotion of self-breast exams and reduced usage of hormone replacement therapies are linked to this success.

Women over 60 years of age have twice the incidence of breast cancer as women ages 45 to 60. In women older than 55, 50% more patients have metastatic disease at presentation than do younger women. Vital to the process of detection are monthly BSEs, breast imaging with digital mammography and MRI or ultrasound to differentiate a cyst from a lesion and to detect small tumors before they can be palpated, and periodic breast examinations by a health care provider.

Etiology and Pathophysiology
The cause of breast cancer is unknown. The high incidence in women implies a hormonal cause (Box 12.4).

The primary risk factors are female gender, age greater than 50 years, North American or Northern European descent, a personal history of breast cancer, atypical hyperplasia or carcinoma in situ, two or more first-degree relatives with the disease, and a first-degree relative with bilateral premenopausal breast cancer. Other risk factors include early menarche, a first pregnancy after age 30, natural menopause after age 55, and one or more breast cancer genes. The inherited susceptibility genes, *BRCA1* and *BRCA2*, account for approximately 2% to 7% of all cases and confer an increased lifetime risk in these women (CDC,

---

Box 12.4 Predisposing Factors for Women at High Risk for Breast Cancer

- *Gender:* Being female introduces a high risk.
- *Age:* Higher incidence occurs among women over 40 years of age and in the postmenopausal phase of life. After age 60 the incidence increases dramatically.
- *Race:* White women, in the middle or upper socioeconomic class, are at higher risk.
- *Genetics:* The inherited susceptibility genes *BRCA1* and *BRCA2* account for approximately 5% of all cases and confer a lifetime risk in these women, ranging from 35% to 85%.
- *Family history:* This is especially important if a diagnosed family member had ovarian cancer, was premenopausal, had bilateral breast cancer, or is a first-degree relative (mother, sister, daughter).
- *Parity (total number of pregnancies):* Risk is decreased for women who gave birth before reaching 18 years of age; it is increased for women who are not sexually active, infertile women, and women who became pregnant for the first time after 30 years of age.
- *Menopause:* Menopause after 55 years of age increases the risk.
- *Obesity:* Weight gain and obesity after menopause increase the risk.
- *Other cancer:* Risk is increased for women diagnosed with some other form of cancer, such as endometrial, ovarian, or colon cancer; if cancer has appeared in one breast, it is more likely to occur in the other breast.

2020). Findings suggest that prophylactic removal of the breasts and/or ovaries in *BRCA1* and *BRCA2* carriers decreases the risk of breast cancer considerably, although not all women who choose this surgery would have developed cancer. Women who consider this option should have an opportunity for counseling before reaching a decision. Some research studies assessing the relationship between survival rates and obesity have found some evidence showing that obese women have a lessened survival rate for breast cancer. Current data indicate that tamoxifen and raloxifene decrease breast cancer risk in women who are at increased risk. With the exception of advancing age and being female, however, most women who develop breast cancer do not have any risk factors for the disease. That is why it is so important to encourage even healthy women to undergo screening examinations.

Breast cancer is usually an adenocarcinoma, arising from the epithelium and developing in the lactiferous ducts; it infiltrates the parenchyma (the functioning tissue of an organ other than the supporting or connective tissue). The cancer occurs most often in women who have not given birth or breast-fed a child. It occurs most often in the upper outer quadrant of the breast because this is the location of most of the glandular tissue. A slow-growing breast cancer may take up to 10 or more years to become palpable, or to reach the size of a small pea. Slow-growing lesions often are associated with a lower mortality rate. When referring to estimated growth rate of breast cancer, the term *doubling time* indicates the time it takes malignant cells to double in number. Assuming that the doubling is constant and that the neoplasm originates in one cell, a carcinoma with a doubling time of 100 days may not reach clinically detectable size (1 cm) for 8 years. Rapid-growing cancers have a much shorter preclinical course and a greater tendency to metastasize to regional nodes or more distant sites by the time a breast mass is discovered. In breast cancer, metastasis occurs via the lymphatic system and bloodstream (Fig. 12.14). The most common sites for metastasis are, in order, the bones, lungs, pleura, other breast sites, central nervous system, and liver.

Clinical Manifestations

Breast cancer is detected as a lump or mammographic abnormality in the breast. Breast tumors are usually small, solitary, irregularly shaped, firm, nontender, and nonmobile. There may be a change in skin color, feelings of tenderness, puckering or dimpling of tissue (peau d'orange—skin with the appearance and texture of an orange peel), nipple discharge, retraction of the nipple, and axillary tenderness.

Women should perform BSEs monthly, preferably 1 week after menses. Postmenopausal women should perform a BSE on the same day each month (Fig. 12.15). If there are questionable findings, the patient should immediately contact her health care provider (see the Patient Teaching box).

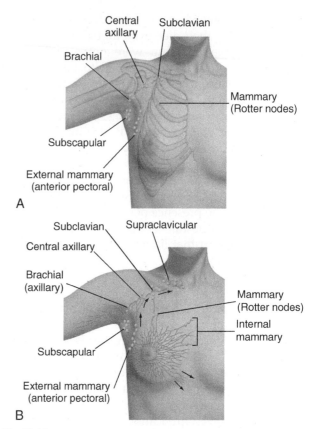

Fig. 12.14 (A) Lymph nodes of the axilla. (B) Lymphatic drainage of the breast. (From Seidel HM, Ball JW, Dains JE, et al: *Mosby's guide to physical examination*, ed 7, St. Louis, 2011, Mosby.)

Patient Teaching

Breast Self-Examination

- The majority of breast lumps are not cancer.
- Cancerous breast lesions are treatable.
- Breasts should be examined by premenopausal women each month, 7 or 8 days after conclusion of the menstrual period when they are least congested, and by postmenopausal women on the same day of each month.
- Visual inspection and palpation should be done.
- Visual inspection should be done when the woman is stripped to the waist and looking in a mirror, using the following arm positions: (1) arms at rest at sides, (2) hands on hips and pressed into hips, (3) contracting chest muscles, (4) hands over the head (torso in upright position), and (5) hands over the head (torso leaning forward).
- Palpation may be done in the shower, where the soap and water help the hands glide over the skin. However, examination of large breasts and axillae is better done in a supine position rather than while standing.
- The entire breast should be examined in a systematic way, moving clockwise, with a circular motion, or moving back and forth. Always include the axillae in the examination.
- Do not forget specific examination of the nipple, through compression for discharge, and the areola, through palpation.
- Report any changes to the health care provider.

Vertical strip	Circular	Wedge
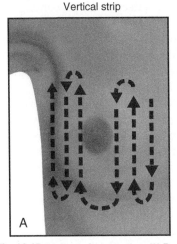	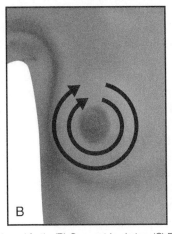	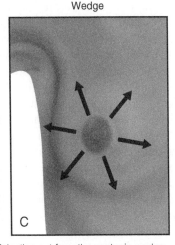
A	B	C

Fig. 12.15 Methods for palpation. (A) Back and forth. (B) Concentric circles. (C) Palpation out from the center in wedge sections. (From Seidel HM, Ball JW, Dains JE, et al: *Mosby's guide to physical examination*, ed 7, St. Louis, 2011, Mosby.))

Diagnostic Tests

The essential factors in the early detection of breast cancer are the regular performance of BSE, regular clinical breast examination (CBE), and routine mammography. The frequency of these examinations is determined by the woman's age, the presence of significant risk factors, and her medical history. Current guidelines accepted by the ACS regarding breast surveillance practices include the following:

- Monthly BSE starting at 20 years of age.
- Physical examinations of the breast by a trained health professional; CBE every 3 years between 20 and 40 years of age and every year for women 40 and older.
- Screening mammography annually beginning between 40 and 44 years of age. If a first-degree family member has a history of breast cancer, a screening mammogram is recommended at 35 years.
- MRI screening combined with mammograms for women with a significant family history or genetic tendencies.

Guidelines from the US Preventive Services Task Force established in 2009 recommend the following: (1) women age 40 to 49 should not receive routine screening mammography for breast cancer unless they are at an increased risk, but these women should decide for themselves when to begin mammography after weighing the risks and benefits; (2) women aged 50 to 74 years should receive screening mammography every 2 years (instead of annually); (3) routine BSE should no longer be taught. The Task Force states that this is not a recommendation against mammography for women in their 40s and BSE, but that there is not enough evidence to prove that women benefit from them (USPSTF, 2016).

Several techniques can be used to screen for breast disease or to diagnose a suspicious physical finding. Mammography is a radiographic technique used to visualize the internal structure of the breast. Mammography can detect tumors that cannot be felt by palpation. The minimum size detectable by physical examination is 1 cm. It takes 10 or more years to grow a tumor this size. Mammography can detect masses of 0.5 cm. Because tumors usually metastasize late in the preclinical course, earlier detection by mammography may prevent metastasis of smaller lesions.

Comparative mammography may show early cancer tissue changes. The diagnostic accuracy of mammography in combination with physical examination has significantly improved early and accurate detection of breast malignancies. In younger women, mammography is less sensitive because of the greater density of breast tissue, resulting in more false-negative results. Mammography will not reveal 10% to 25% of breast cancers. Masses should be biopsied, even if mammogram findings are unremarkable.

Definitive diagnosis of a mass can be made only by means of histologic examination of biopsied tissues. Biopsy techniques may include either FNA biopsy and cytologic examination or core-cutting needle biopsy, excisional biopsy, and incisional biopsy. Even if the lesion is nonpalpable, an FNA biopsy can be used. FNA and cytologic evaluation should be done only if an experienced cytologist is available, and all lesions read as negative are followed up by a more definitive biopsy procedure. If the aspirated specimen is positive for malignancy, the patient can be given this information at the same visit and begin learning about treatment issues.

Improved imaging techniques have reduced the radiation exposure that accompanies mammography to insignificant levels. Therefore the benefits of mammography outweigh the risks from radiation exposure. Ultrasound (echogram, sonogram) also can be used to differentiate a benign cyst (fluid filled) from a malignant mass (solid). An ultrasound will not detect microcalcifications, which are often the only indicators of very small tumors.

Other methods used to help diagnose and stage breast cancer include MRI and positron emission tomography (PET). MRI and PET scans are used to help differentiate between malignant and benign disease in select patients.

A diagnostic tool used before therapeutic surgery is the sentinel lymph node mapping, which identifies the initial lymph node(s) most likely to drain the cancerous cells. During this procedure a radioactive substance is injected around the breast biopsy site. The patient is then sent to the operating room, where a blue dye is injected as well. The area then is monitored to see which nodes take up the substances. The node that "lights up," containing the most radioactivity and blue dye, is considered the sentinel node and the one most likely to contain cancer cells. The identified node and at least two other nodes then are biopsied to see if they contain tumor cells. If they do not, it is likely that the more distant axillary nodes are cancer free. The nodes can be left intact, reducing the threat of complications such as edema, infection, pain, and loss of function of the arm. Sentinel lymph node dissection has been associated with lower morbidity rates and greater accuracy compared with complete axillary node dissection.

Spread to the axillary lymph nodes are one of the most important prognostic factors in early-stage breast cancer. Their close proximity to the breast makes them the first area to which they spread may be noted. Metastasis in axillary nodes can be determined by pathologic examination of as few as 6 to 10 nodes. The more nodes involved means the greater the risk of recurrence. Patients with four or more positive nodes have the greatest risk of recurrence. During examination, the lymph nodes can provide prognostic information that helps further determine treatment (chemotherapy, hormone therapy, or both).

Another diagnostic test useful for determining prognosis and treatment is estrogen and progesterone receptor status. Receptor-positive tumors commonly (1) show evidence of being well differentiated (see Chapter 17, Box 17.2), (2) have a more normal DNA content and low proliferation, (3) have a lower chance for recurrence, and (4) are hormone dependent and responsive to hormonal therapy. Receptor-negative tumors (1) are often poorly differentiated, (2) have a high incidence of abnormal DNA content and high proliferation, (3) frequently recur, and (4) are usually unresponsive to hormonal therapy (Komen.org, 2021a).

Medical Management

The intervention for treatment of breast cancer depends on the tumor stage, the patient's age and health, the hormonal status, and the presence of estrogen receptors in the tumor. Radiation, chemotherapy, and surgery alone or in combination are the most common modes of treatment for breast cancer (see Chapter 17).

Staging. After breast surgery and axillary dissection, the staging process is completed. Axillary lymph node dissection or sentinel lymph node mapping usually is performed regardless of the treatment option selected. Examination of nodes provides the most powerful prognostic data currently available. Also, removal of axillary

nodes is highly effective in preventing axillary recurrence, aids in decision making regarding adjuvant chemotherapy or hormonal therapy, and eliminates the need for axillary nodal radiation. Radiation of the axilla is equally effective in decreasing the incidence of axillary recurrence (see Fig. 12.14).

The most widely accepted staging method for breast cancer is the American Joint Committee on Cancer's TNM system. This system uses tumor size (T), nodal involvement and size (N), and presence of metastasis (M) to determine the stage of disease (Box 12.5).

Surgical intervention. Surgery plays a vital role in the management of breast cancer. Tissue biopsy, inspection and biopsy of lymph nodes in the axillary areas, radiologic examinations, and laboratory reports aid in making the decision to perform surgery.

Because estrogen can affect a tumor's invasive ability, it is suggested that premenopausal women be operated on during the menstrual phase, when estrogen levels are lower or opposed by progesterone.

Several surgical options are available for the removal of a breast carcinoma. In breast conservation surgery (termed *lumpectomy*), which conserves the breast, a circumscribed area is removed along with the tumor. This surgery is usually done when the tumor is small and located on the peripheral area of the breast. The breast contour and muscle support are preserved if possible. Axillary nodes often are removed in these breast-sparing procedures as well. Contraindications to lumpectomy or excisional biopsy include two or more separate tumors in separate quadrants of the breast, diffuse microcalcifications, a history of previous radiation to the region, a large tumor-to-breast ratio, a history of collagen vascular disease, large breasts, and a tumor located underneath the nipple.

One of the main advantages of breast conservation surgery and radiation is that it preserves the breast, including the nipple. The goal of the combined surgery and radiation is to maximize the benefits of cancer treatment and cosmetic outcome while minimizing risks. Disadvantages of this surgery plus radiation include the increased cost over surgery alone and the possible side effects of radiation. Lumpectomy is followed by 6 weeks of radiation.

A simple mastectomy involves removal of the entire breast. The skin flap is retained to cover the incised area. Pectoralis major and pectoralis minor muscles are left intact. The patient has the option of breast reconstruction.

A modified radical mastectomy may be performed if the tumor is 4 cm or larger, if it is invasive, or if the patient and health care provider decide this procedure is in the patient's best interest. In this operation all breast tissue, overlying skin, nipple, and pectoralis minor muscles are removed, as are samples of axillary lymph nodes and fascia under the breast. The pectoralis major muscle remains intact. The patient has the option of

Box 12.5   TNM System for Staging Breast Cancer

Breast cancer is staged using the TNM (tumor, node, metastasis) system, which categorizes the disease by tumor size and spread, lymph node involvement, and metastasis. The TNM system, which was developed by the American Joint Committee on Cancer and revised in 2003, works this way:

- *Tumor:* A number from 0 to 4 indicates the tumor's size and whether it has spread to nearby tissue (if it has not, this indicates a carcinoma in situ). Higher numbers indicate a larger tumor or wider spread. For example, a tumor labeled T1 is 2 cm or smaller; T4 indicates a tumor of any size that has spread to the chest wall or the skin.
- *Nodes:* A number from 0 to 3 indicates whether the cancer has spread to surrounding lymph nodes and, if so, the number of nodes that are affected. For example, N1 indicates a spread to one, two, or three lymph nodes under the arm on the same side as the breast cancer.
- *Metastasis:* M0 means the cancer has not spread to distant organs; M1 means the cancer has metastasized to other organs.
  All of this information is combined to determine an overall stage of 0 to IV.
- *Stage 0:* Refers to carcinoma in situ, in which the tumor is confined to the milk duct or the lobule, no lymph nodes have been affected, and no metastasis has occurred.
- *Stage I:* The tumor is 2 cm or smaller. Lymph nodes are negative. There is no distant cancer spread.
- *Stage IIA:* The tumor is 5 cm or smaller. It may have spread to one, two, or three axillary nodes. There is no distant cancer spread.
- *Stage IIB:* The tumor can be larger than 5 cm. Up to three lymph nodes may be involved, but there is no metastasis to other organs.
- *Stage IIIA:* The tumor may be more than 5 cm and has spread to more than 3 but fewer than 10 lymph nodes. No distant organs are involved.
- *Stage IIIB:* The tumor, regardless of size, has spread to the chest wall or the skin. There is lymph node involvement but no distant metastasis.
- *Stage IIIC:* Refers to any size tumor, including one that has spread to the chest wall or the skin. There is involvement of 10 or more lymph nodes, but no distant metastasis.
- *Stage IV:* The tumor can be any size. There is nodal involvement and metastasis to distant organs.

Data from American Cancer Society: Breast cancer stages, 2017.
Available at https://www.cancer.org/cancer/breast-cancer/understanding-a-breast-cancer-diagnosis/stages-of-breast-cancer.html and from Lewis SL, Dirksen SR, Heitkemper MM, et al: *Medical-surgical nursing: assessment and management of clinical problems*, ed 9, St. Louis, 2014, Mosby.

breast reconstruction, which can be performed immediately after the mastectomy or can be delayed until postoperative recovery is complete (about 6 months).

Most women diagnosed with early-stage breast cancer (tumors less than 5 cm) are candidates for either lumpectomy plus radiation or modified radical mastectomy. Overall 10-year survival with lumpectomy and radiation is about the same as with modified radical mastectomy (Komen.org, 2021).

Adjuvant therapies

Radiation therapy. Depending on the tumor's size, regional spread, and aggressiveness, radiation therapy often is prescribed. Radiation therapy may be used for breast cancer (1) as the primary therapy to destroy the tumor or as a companion to surgery to prevent local recurrence, (2) to shrink a large tumor to operable size, and (3) as palliative treatment for the pain caused by local recurrence and metastasis. Lumpectomy is almost always followed by radiation. Radiation therapy is usually started 2 to 3 weeks after surgery, when the wound is completely healed and the patient can comfortably raise her arm over her head. Contraindications include a diagnosis of breast cancer during the first or second trimester of pregnancy, delayed wound healing, collagen vascular disease, and previous radiation to the same breast.

In external beam radiation, the radiation procedure uses an external beam of high-energy protons. The treatments are usually done 5 days a week for 5 to 6 weeks. Adverse effects include fatigue and skin reactions such as erythema, pruritus, dryness, infection, and pain. The skin literally has a burned appearance.

Internal radiation, also known as implant radiation or brachytherapy, is a new procedure that is an alternative to traditional radiation treatment for early-stage breast cancer. The technique uses a balloon catheter to insert radioactive seeds into the breast after the tumor is removed (at the time of the lumpectomy or shortly thereafter into the tumor resection cavity). The seeds deliver a high dose of concentrated radiation directly to the site where the cancer is most likely to recur.

Chemotherapy. Patients who require postsurgical chemotherapy—typically those with lymph node involvement or metastasis to distant organs—receive antineoplastic medications, hormones, a monoclonal antibody, or a combination of these medications. Regimens for node-negative disease (i.e., cancer that has not spread to the lymph nodes) include cyclophosphamide, methotrexate, and 5-fluorouracil (Efudex), referred to as CMF; cyclophosphamide, doxorubicin, and 5-fluorouracil, or CAF; or doxorubicin and cyclophosphamide, commonly called AC. For those with node-positive disease, the regimens include CAF, AC followed by paclitaxel, doxorubicin followed by CMF, and CMF.

The most common adverse effects of traditional antineoplastic drugs are bone marrow suppression (which causes anemia, thrombocytopenia, and leukopenia), nausea and vomiting, alopecia, weight gain, mucositis, and fatigue. Agents such as filgrastim (Neupogen), which raise leukocyte counts, can combat the threat of infection that accompanies bone marrow suppression. Epoetin alfa (Procrit) is helpful in raising erythrocyte counts to help correct anemia. Other drugs typically ordered for chemotherapy patients are phenothiazines, such as prochlorperazine, and serotonin antagonists such as granisetron and ondansetron (Zofran). These drugs prevent or lessen nausea and vomiting.

Hormonal therapy. Estrogen can promote the growth of breast cancer cells if the cells are estrogen receptor positive. Hormonal therapy removes or blocks the source of estrogen, thus promoting tumor regression.

Two advances have increased the use of hormonal therapy in breast cancer. First, hormone receptor assays, which are reliable diagnostic tests, have been developed to identify women who are likely to respond to hormonal therapy. The tumor's estrogen and progesterone receptor status can be determined. These assays can predict whether hormonal therapy is a treatment option for women with breast cancer, either at the time of initial therapy or if the cancer recurs. Second, drugs have been developed that can inactivate the hormone-secreting glands as effectively as surgery or radiation. Premenopausal and perimenopausal women are more likely to have tumors that are not hormone dependent, whereas women who are postmenopausal are more likely to have hormone-dependent tumors. Chances of tumor regression are significantly greater in women whose tumors contain estrogen and progesterone receptors.

Estrogen deprivation can occur by destroying the ovaries by surgery, radiation, or drug therapy. Hormonal therapy can block or destroy the estrogen receptors. Hormonal therapy is used to treat recurrent or metastatic cancer but also may be used as an adjuvant to primary treatment.

Tamoxifen is the hormonal agent of choice in postmenopausal, estrogen receptor–positive women with or without lymph node involvement. Tamoxifen, an antiestrogen drug, blocks the estrogen receptor sites of malignant cells and thus inhibits the growth-stimulating effects of estrogen. It is commonly used in advanced and early-stage breast cancer to prevent or treat recurrent disease. Tamoxifen also may be used to prevent breast cancer in high-risk individuals. Side effects of tamoxifen are minimal but include hot flashes, nausea, vomiting, vaginal discharge, and other effects commonly associated with decreased estrogen. It also increases the risk of blood clots, cataracts, and endometrial cancer in postmenopausal women. Tamoxifen is not used in women desiring continued fertility.

Toremifene (Fareston), an antiestrogen agent similar to tamoxifen, is indicated as first-line treatment for metastatic breast cancer in postmenopausal women with estrogen receptor–positive or estrogen receptor–unknown tumors. Fulvestrant (Faslodex) may be given to women with advanced breast cancer who no longer respond to tamoxifen. This drug slows cancer progression by destroying estrogen receptors in the breast cancer cells. Fulvestrant is given intramuscularly on a monthly basis.

Aromatase inhibitor drugs, which interfere with the enzyme that synthesizes endogenous estrogen, are used to treat advanced breast cancer in postmenopausal women with disease progression. These drugs include anastrozole (Arimidex), letrozole (Femara), exemestane (Aromasin), and aminoglutethimide (Cytadren).

Research has shown that letrozole reduced the risk of recurrence of breast cancer and lengthens the period before reoccurrence in those who ultimately experienced a return of the disease (Breastcancer.org, 2017). Letrozole, previously approved by the FDA for advanced breast cancer, offers an option for extending treatment of early-stage disease. Letrozole, like tamoxifen, works by interfering with the hormone estrogen, which feeds breast cancer cells. Tamoxifen blocks estrogen receptors on the cells, whereas letrozole inhibits the creation of estrogen.

Bisphosphonates, such as pamidronate sodium (Aredia), are being used to delay bone metastases and reduce the occurrence of skeletal problems in patients with advanced breast cancer. This is done by reducing calcium loss to the bones and reducing the risk of fractures. The loss of bone also may be reduced with the use of bisphosphonates (clodronate, risedronate, ibandronate, zoledronate). Raloxifene (Evista), used to prevent bone loss, may also reduce the risk of breast cancer without stimulating endometrial growth. Raloxifene acts as an estrogen antagonist at the hormone-sensitive tissues of breast cancer and bone. Additional drugs that may be used to suppress hormone-dependent tumors include megestrol, diethylstilbestrol, and fluoxymesterone (Breastcancer.org, 2016).

Monoclonal antibody therapy. Another drug treatment for breast cancer is the monoclonal antibody trastuzumab (Herceptin). It is used to treat metastatic breast cancer in women who overexpress (i.e., have an excess amount of) a breast cancer cell antigen called HER2. Up to 30% of patients fall into this category.

Ovarian ablation. Another promising treatment option is ovarian ablation by means of a bilateral oophorectomy, which is used in combination with tamoxifen for metastatic disease.

Bone marrow and stem cell transplantation. Autologous (i.e., originating within self) bone marrow or stem cell transplantation combined with high-dose chemotherapy has been used to treat patients with advanced metastatic breast cancer. In this technique, patients donate their own bone marrow or peripheral blood, from which stem cells are harvested. They then receive high doses of chemotherapy, which causes bone marrow suppression. The patient subsequently undergoes autologous bone marrow or stem cell transplantation to reconstitute or "rescue" their hematopoietic (i.e., blood-forming) system to start producing blood cells.

Nursing Interventions

The health care provider discusses with the patient and the family the rationale for the specific surgical approach and the manner of coping with the cosmetic effects of and psychological response to the surgery. Patients will have questions about possible alternatives to standard or modified mastectomy.

The patient may be confused with so many options for therapy and surgical interventions. During this time, play an active role as listener, reinforce information provided by the health care provider, and encourage the patient to verbalize her concerns and recognize her feelings about the surgery. The emotional preparation of the patient may be more important than the physical preparation. Often she undergoes anticipatory grieving for the loss of a body part.

Preoperative preparation involves the patient, support group, and nursing staff so that progressive care can run continuously from admission through surgery, recovery, and the postoperative period. The initial admission assessment provides data that are helpful for the nurse and patient in planning care. Nursing diagnoses can be developed and a care plan individualized according to the patient's needs (Nursing Care Plan 12.1).

Assess and identify members of the patient's support system to know their strengths and concerns about the pending treatment and interventions. Support does not always need to come from the immediate family and close friends. Outside support and resources can come from co-workers, religious groups, oncology clinicians, psychologists, and Reach to Recovery support groups. It is important to openly discuss the patient's fears; establishing a therapeutic relationship with the patient and family enables this to happen.

Reach to Recovery volunteers are a source of information, encouragement, and support for women with breast cancer. The organization is based on the premise that rehabilitation for the cancer patient should include communication with and support from another who was in a similar situation and learned to cope and resume her normal activities.

Nursing interventions for patients who undergo modified radical mastectomy include monitoring vital signs and observing for symptoms of shock or hemorrhage, because many large blood vessels are involved in the procedure. Drains such as a Jackson-Pratt, Davol, or Hemovac drain may be placed in the axilla to facilitate drainage and to prevent formation of

---

🤝 Nursing Care Plan 12.1 | The Patient Undergoing Modified Radical Mastectomy

Ms. C., age 52, was diagnosed with ductal cell carcinoma of the left breast. She has undergone a left modified radical mastectomy.

PATIENT PROBLEM
Fearfulness, related to the cancer diagnosis and surgical intervention

Patient Goals and Expected Outcomes	Nursing Interventions	Evaluation
Patient will be able to state fears Patient will state she has made improvement in coping	Encourage patient to talk about specific fears and feelings about each fear. Provide a calm, supportive environment. Provide information on coping mechanisms. Encourage consultation with resource persons (psychologist, clergy, nurse specialist, Reach to Recovery). Use support of family and significant others. Encourage use of comfort measures, such as music. Encourage patient's comments and questions about surgery and postoperative care.	Patient verbalizes fear, has support of significant others, and expresses confidence in ability to cope.

PATIENT PROBLEM
Potential for Infection, related to surgical incision and presence of drain

Patient Goals and Expected Outcomes	Nursing Interventions	Evaluation
Skin will remain free of signs and symptoms of infection Vital signs and white blood cell (WBC) value will be maintained within normal limits	Assess skin integrity. Instruct patient on signs and symptoms of infection. Assess and report abnormal vital signs and elevated WBC count; skin changes; and comfort level. Observe and record amount of exudate. Check drainage tubing for patency. Instruct patient to examine remaining breast every month. Caution patient to avoid injections, vaccinations, taking of blood pressure, taking of blood samples, or insertion of intravenous line in affected area.	Incision has no erythema or purulent drainage. Temperature remains within normal range. WBC count remains normal.

Continued

Nursing Care Plan 12.1 The Patient Undergoing Modified Radical Mastectomy—cont'd

PATIENT PROBLEM

Distorted Body Image, related to loss of breast through modified radical mastectomy

Patient Goals and Expected Outcomes	Nursing Interventions	Evaluation
Patient will verbalize acceptance of altered body image as evidenced by absence of weeping, irritability, or verbalization of discomfort with present body; and by the attempting of difficult physical or mental tasks despite limitations Patient will demonstrate interest in her personal appearance Patient will verbalize plans to resume former activities	Encourage patient's comments and questions about surgery, progress, and prognosis. Encourage patient to discuss change in her body with husband or significant other. Reinforce correct information, and provide factual information to correct any misconceptions. Relate importance of communicating anything that causes anxiety. Encourage patient to verbalize and explore feelings regarding impact missing body part might have on patient's functioning as a sexual partner and in activities of daily living. Encourage patient to continue activities associated with femininity, such as fixing hair, using makeup, and wearing own apparel. Encourage patient to look at and touch the changed body part when she is ready. Encourage use of rehabilitation services (Reach to Recovery, Wellness Community).	Patient verbalizes feelings about surgery and change in body image; indicates beginning resolution of negative feelings toward self; and begins to accept altered body image.

CRITICAL THINKING QUESTIONS

1. Ms. C. confides in her nurse that she feels ugly and unattractive and she refuses to look at her incision. What would be a helpful approach by the nurse?
2. In assessing Ms. C., the nurse notes her holding her left arm guardedly in an adducted position. She does not use it for activities of daily living. What should effective patient teaching include?
3. What should be included in discharge teaching for Ms. C. to prevent trauma and infection of her left arm?

a hematoma. Postoperative dressings are usually constrictive and bulky and may tend to impede respiratory effort and cause pain and discomfort. Assess for excessive exudates on the dressing and in the axillary region. Place a smaller, less bulky dressing over the incisional site for the first postoperative day. When the vital signs are stable, place the patient in a 45-degree Fowler's position to promote drainage. Change the position frequently and encourage deep breathing and coughing.

Some patients may experience incisional pain for several days after surgery and when doing arm exercises. They may complain of numbness and referred pain in the arm of the operative area. The pain radiates to the shoulder and back because of the severance of the peripheral nerves. Most of the nerves regenerate, but there are cases of residual numbness.

No matter what type of surgery the patient has, pain management and wound care are priorities. The patient-controlled analgesia pump with morphine for 12 to 24 hours can provide pain management and allowing patient control over the dosing. Once the pump and the higher dosages of morphine are not needed, oral analgesics are employed.

Patient Teaching

Postoperative atelectasis must be avoided. Coughing, deep breathing, and positional changes are key.

Respiratory exercises including incentive spirometry are implemented shortly after surgery.

Health care providers differ in opinion about the best position for the affected arm. Some health care providers place the arm in the dressing and place it in a sling for a couple of days postoperatively. Some health care providers prefer to avoid slings. If the arm is not restricted by dressings, it may be elevated on a pillow with the hand and wrist higher than the elbow and the elbow higher than the shoulder joint. This facilitates the flow of fluids through the lymph and venous routes and prevent lymphedema (accumulation of lymph in soft tissues).

Early ambulation promotes respiratory health, reduces the risk of thrombophlebitis, and reduces constipation. Unless there are additional complications, ambulation will begin the day after the procedure. Assistance will be needed to get out of bed and ambulate. Woman may report feeling "unbalanced" due to the loss of breast tissue.

Protection of the arm on the operative side is important. Instruct the patient not to have any procedures involving the arm on the affected side. This includes blood pressure readings, injections, IV infusion of fluids, or the drawing of blood. Procedures on the operative side may cause edema or infection. Due to the removal of lymph nodes there is a heightened risk for infections. Infections can be caused from burns or breaks in the

Box 12.6   Hand and Arm Care After Breast Surgery

PREVENTION OF INFECTION
- Wear gloves when cleaning with harsh detergent.
- Wear gloves when gardening.
- Avoid injections, vaccinations, and venipuncture in involved arm.
- Use cuticle remover rather than cutting cuticles.
- Sew with a thimble.
- Avoid chapped hands; use lanolin cream daily.
- Take care when using equipment that might cut, scrape, or abrade.
- Shave underarms with an electric razor.
- Avoid insect bites; use insect repellent.

PREVENTION OF CONSTRICTING CIRCULATION
- Do not take blood pressure in involved arm.
- Wear loose clothing; avoid tight bra straps or tight sleeves.
- Wear watch or jewelry on uninvolved arm.
- Carry purse on uninvolved arm or shoulder.
- Prevent drag or pull:
  - Carry heavy packages on uninvolved arm.
  - Avoid motions that increase centrifugal force.

PREVENTION OF BURNS
- Wear padded mitts to reach into oven; use potholders.
- Prevent sunburn; use sunscreens with SPF of 15; cover arms during prolonged exposure.
- Immediately report any signs of erythema, edema, warmth, or pain.

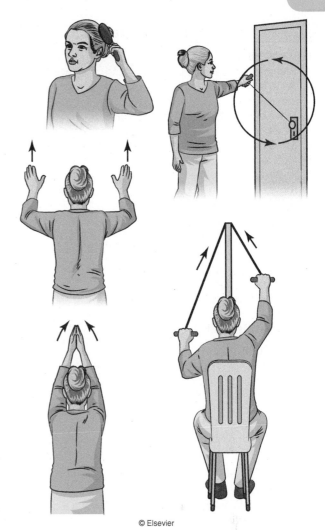

© Elsevier

Fig. 12.16 Exercises after mastectomy.

skin. Removing lymph nodes and channels increases the risk of developing lymphedema, even years after surgery. Once the incision has completely healed, a gradual exercise program should be initiated. This has the ability to control lymphedema if it develops. Lifting heavy objects with the affected arm for 6 to 8 weeks is necessary. Instruct the patient to avoid sleeping on the involved arm. Clothing on the affected arm should be nonconstricting. Bracelets and watches should be worn on the unaffected arm (Box 12.6).

Persistent edema is a challenge to manage. Diuretics and low-sodium diets often are prescribed. If the edema persists, an elastic stockinette is measured for precise fit to avoid venous flow constriction. The sleeve is applied from the wrist to the shoulder and worn when the patient is out of bed. When the patient is sleeping, position the arm to aid venous flow. If the lymphedema is severe, the health care provider may order a knit compression sleeve (Jobst extremity therapy) to manage the condition. A pneumomassage sleeve with automatic inflation and deflation can be placed on the arm. The compression pump is strictly contraindicated when there is evidence of acute phlebitis, perivascular lymphangitis, or cellulitis.

Isometric exercises are helpful for increasing the circulation and developing the collateral lymph system. The patient can open and clench fingers and squeeze a rubber ball in the first few postoperative days. This activity provides extension and flexion of the wrist and elbow; it is equivalent to sewing, knitting, typing, and playing piano when at home.

Preventing muscle contractures. Specific exercises may be ordered to restore the muscle strength and full range of motion of the affected area. Gentle exercises started early in the postoperative course help to decrease muscle tension and to regain muscle function more quickly. The nurse or the therapist should instruct the patient and encourage the continuation of the exercises on discharge. Many of the exercises may be incorporated into ADLs as they are resumed (Fig. 12.16 and Box 12.7). Exercising can be painful, but the patient can meet the challenge with the encouragement of a support group.

Body image acceptance. After losing a breast, many patients experience grief over the loss of the body part. This acute grief is like a crisis and may persist 4 to 6 weeks or longer. Adaptation and acceptance of the loss is needed to successfully cope. Counseling our participation in support groups is beneficial.

Initial coping mechanisms often begin to lose effectiveness at about 3 months, and a period of depression

| Box 12.7 | Postmastectomy Arm Exercises |

CLIMBING THE WALL
1. Stand facing wall with toes 6-12 inches from wall.
2. Bend elbows and place palms of hands against wall at shoulder level.
3. Move both hands parallel to each other up the wall as far as possible until incisional pull or pain occurs.
4. Move both hands down to starting position.
5. Goal is complete extension with elbows straight.
6. Activities that use the same action include reaching top shelves, hanging out clothes, washing windows, hanging curtains, and setting hair.

ELBOW PULL-IN
1. Extend arms sideways to shoulder level.
2. Clasp hands behind neck.
3. Pull elbows forward until they touch.
4. Return to position 2.
5. Unclasp hands and extend arms sideways at shoulder level.
6. Lower arms to side.

BACK SCRATCH
1. Place hand of unoperated side on hip for balance.
2. Bend elbow of affected arm, placing back of hand on small of back.
3. Work hand up the back slowly until fingers reach opposite shoulder blade.
4. Lower arm and straighten both arms.

ROPE PULL
1. Attach a rope over a shower rod, a hook, or the top of an open door.
2. Sit on a chair (with door between legs if using a door) and grasp each end of rope.
3. Alternately pull on each end, raising affected arm to a point of incisional pull or pain. (The goal is to raise the affected arm almost directly overhead.)

ensues. Provide anticipatory guidance for this eventuality. Special nursing interventions, in terms of psychological support and self-care education, are necessary if the cancer recurs. Participation in a cancer support group is important and has been found to have a clinically significant impact on survival.

When deep-breathing exercises are started immediately after surgery and the patient splints the area and exercises her arm, she will recognize the absence of the breast through touch. Dressing changes and incision cleansing with patient involvement make the absence real. Being involved and responsible for the dressing and incision allows a more personal approach to the patient. At this time, the nurse's support is important. Provide a mirror or seat the patient in front of a mirror so that she can see the operative site being cleansed and dressed. Be sensitive to the patient and be alert for signs of readiness to become involved in care and accept the loss of the body part. The incisional area may be erythematous and edematous, but the discoloration gradually lessens and the site becomes more comfortable. Encourage her to massage in cocoa butter or a cream to make the incisional line softer. Advise the patient that it takes time to accept the loss and to heal emotionally and physically.

Prosthesis. A breast prosthesis should not be worn unless authorized by the health care provider. Many breast forms are available. Forms are made of gels, molded silicone, and saline solution. Most forms are covered with soft fabric, are lightweight, and feel like breast tissue. There is a shape for each type of breast, because each body is different and each surgery is different. Forms have been developed that can be fitted for a right or left breast, slanted for the breast that was slanted, or formed with an outer curve that simulates the extension of a full breast under the axilla and upward on the chest. It is advisable to have a skilled fitter from a reliable company fit the prosthesis.

A well-fitted brassiere is essential before choosing the shape form. If the woman is active, she may desire a pocket or restraining cup. Some forms can be worn against the skin with no underpadding or bra cups. Most forms can be washed with water and mild detergent to keep them clean and supple. Many prostheses are waterproof and can be worn swimming; when wet, they do not "weigh down" the wearer.

When the patient is being fitted with a prosthesis, the best assurance that the fit is right is when each of the following is observed:
- The brassiere fits snugly around the rib cage.
- The prosthesis fills the bottom of the bra cup.
- The prosthesis projects the same as the remaining breast, with form bulk and nipples in position.
- The breasts are separated when the bra is centered.
- The top of the bra cup is filled and appears like the other breast.

Breast Reconstruction
The patient whose disease is limited to the breast may benefit from reconstructive surgery. The benefits of breast reconstruction include avoidance of an external prosthesis that has potential for slipping, greater choice of clothing (including lower necklines), and loss of self-consciousness about appearance. For many women, breast reconstruction is beneficial in improving self-esteem. Breast reconstruction can provide many women with a renewed sense of wholeness and a return to a normal state. The most important indicators for reconstruction are the patient's motivation and desire for the procedure. The primary determinant for the procedure is the patient's clinical status. Goals for reconstruction are to select the simplest type that meets the patient's needs and expectations and to match the opposite breast in size, shape, and contour.

Breast reconstruction can be performed immediately after surgery or at a later time. An increasing number of women are electing immediate reconstruction; this may prolong the initial hospitalization but eliminates the need for a second hospitalization and contributes to self-esteem. Others wait until they have completed adjuvant chemotherapy or radiation to be certain the area is disease free.

Breast implant. After the removal of the breast, the patient may desire reconstruction. The timing of onset varies. It may be initiated at the time of the mastectomy or be at a later date. It will take a few procedures to adequately prepare the breast area to receive the implant. Implants may be silicone or saline. The communication with the plastic surgeon will ideally begin prior to the mastectomy. This consultation will allow full discussion of the procedures that will be needed to complete the reconstruction. The patient benefits from a realistic discussion of the procedures, literature to review and photographs illustrating the process, healing stages and potential final results.

Pre-mastectomy health and wellness will impact the reconstruction process. Complications of breast reconstruction include infection, poor healing, pain, breast asymmetry, bleeding, changes in breast sensation and the development of scar tissue. Silicone implants carry the risk of leakage into the body.

Some researchers have suggested that the silicone filling or the implant covering can lead to autoimmune or connective tissue disease. Today most implants are saline filled instead of silicone.

Musculocutaneous flap procedure. Musculocutaneous flap surgery has made reconstruction possible for most patients who have undergone mastectomy, even when the pectoralis muscles have been removed or when nerve damage has resulted in muscle atrophy. The flap receives its blood supply from muscle, and also from the overlying layer of skin. At the same time that this procedure is performed, a silicone or saline breast implant may be inserted; if enough tissue is available, no implant is needed.

Musculocutaneous flaps most often are taken from the back (latissimus dorsi muscle) or the abdomen (transverse rectus abdominis muscle). When the latissimus dorsi musculocutaneous flap is used for reconstruction, a block of skin and muscle from the patient's back is used to replace tissue removed during mastectomy (Fig. 12.17E). The transverse rectus abdominis musculocutaneous (TRAM) flap is the most frequently used flap operation for breast reconstruction. The rectus abdominis muscles are paired, flat muscles running from the rib cage down to the pubic bone. Arteries inside the muscle branch at many levels, and these branches supply blood to the fat and skin across a large expanse of the abdomen. In the TRAM technique, the surgeon elevates a large block of tissue from the lower abdominal area, but leaves it attached to the rectus muscle (see Fig. 12.17A–D). This tissue then is tunneled under the skin or detached and placed as a "free flap" at the site of the breast reconstruction. The tissue is trimmed and shaped to form a breast mound similar to that of the opposite breast. An implant may be used in addition to the flap to achieve symmetry. The abdominal incision is closed in a fashion similar

to that of an abdominal hysterectomy or a "tummy tuck." This surgical procedure can last 2 to 8 hours, with recovery taking 4 to 6 weeks. Complications are consistent with other operative procedures and include bleeding and infection. Additional TRAM adverse effects include hernia in the abdominal area where the tissue was obtained, tissue necrosis resulting for an inability of the body to provide adequate perfusion to the transplanted tissue and scar tissue in the breasts.

Nipple reconstruction usually is performed as a separate procedure after the completion of breast reconstruction. Nipple construction is generally from available tissue at the site or harvested tissue from the opposite breast. New techniques allow the nipple to be created from tissue and subcutaneous tissue of the breast mound. Areola reconstruction is provided by obtaining pigmented skin from the upper thigh or by using skin from the lateral chest area. Newer procedures may employ a sutured tuck to create a nipple and using a tattoo for the areola.

 Home Care Considerations

Cancer of the Breast

- Explain the follow-up routine to the patient and emphasize the importance of beginning and continuing breast self-examination and annual mammography.
- Symptoms that should be reported to the health care provider include new back pain, weakness, constipation, shortness of breath, and confusion.
- If adjuvant therapy is to be used, give the woman specific instructions about appointment times and treatment locations.
- If applicable, stress the importance of wearing a well-fitting prosthesis. The return of a normal external appearance is important to most women.
- Often the husband, sexual partner, or family member may need assistance in dealing with his or her emotional reactions to the diagnosis and surgery for him or her to effectively support the patient.
- If difficulty in adjustment or other problems develop, counseling may be necessary for women with breast cancer to deal with the emotional component of a modified radical mastectomy and the diagnosis of cancer.

Prognosis

The 5-year relative survival rate for localized breast cancer is close to 100%. Survival rate for stage II at 5 years is about 93% and 72% for stage III. Once the cancer is metastatic the rate of survival drops to a 5-year rate of survival at 22% (ACS, 2021a). Breast cancer ranks second among cancer deaths in women. The most important prognostic factor is the stage of the disease and nodal involvement. Even having one to three nodes involved carries a 50% to 60% risk for metastatic recurrence (see Box 12.6 and the Home Care Considerations box: Cancer of the Breast).

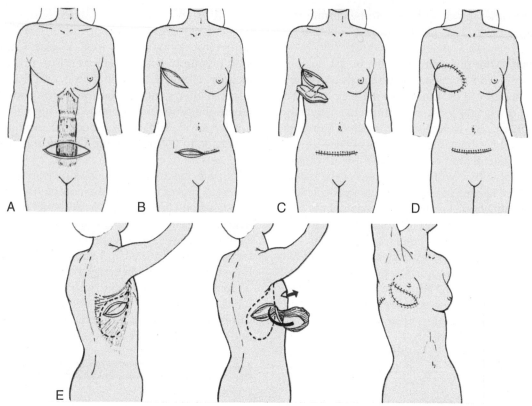

Fig. 12.17 Transverse rectus abdominis musculocutaneous (TRAM) flap. (A) Pedicle TRAM flap procedure is planned. (B) The abdominal tissue, still attached to the rectus muscle, nerve, and blood supply, is moved through a tunnel beneath the skin, from the abdomen to the chest. (C) The flap is trimmed to shape the breast. The lower abdominal incision is closed. (D) Nipple and areola are reconstructed after the breast has healed. € In the latissimus dorsi musculocutaneous flap, a block of skin and muscle from the patient's back is used to replace tissue removed during mastectomy. (From Belcher AE: *Cancer nursing*, St. Louis, 1992, Mosby.)

INFLAMMATORY AND INFECTIOUS DISORDERS OF THE MALE REPRODUCTIVE SYSTEM

PROSTATITIS

Etiology and Pathophysiology
Prostatitis refers to inflammation or infection of the prostate gland. The condition may be acute or chronic. The cause is most commonly bacterial. However, there are cases of nonbacterial prostatitis. Causative organisms in bacterial prostatitis include *E. coli, Klebsiella, Proteus, Pseudomonas, Streptococcus, N. gonorrhoeae,* and *Chlamydia trachomatis.*

Clinical Manifestations
The clinical manifestations of acute prostatitis include chills, fever, prostate pain and tenderness, and arthralgias. Specific urinary symptoms may include dysuria, frequency, nocturia, weak stream, and hesitancy. An exacerbation of chronic prostatitis often has a slower onset of symptoms. Symptoms of the chronic condition are not typically systemic and often include dysuria and recurrent urinary tract infections. The patient also may have acute urinary retention caused by prostatic edema. On palpation, the gland is tender, edematous, and firm. In chronic prostatitis, many patients may appear asymptomatic, but generally the symptoms are the same as in the acute phase but less intense.

Diagnostic Tests
Diagnosis is based on culture and sensitivity tests of the urethra, prostatic fluid, and urine for organism identification and appropriate antibiotic therapy. Prostatic fluid is collected by prostate massage and expression of fluid. The pH of the fluid generally is elevated. A rectal examination done by the health care provider reveals gland tenderness and edema.

Medical Management
Medical management includes antibiotic therapy such as the fluoroquinolones, doxycycline, minocycline, trimethoprim-sulfamethoxazole (TMP-SMZ). These compounds penetrate into the prostate and produce favorable treatment results (Brusch, 2020). For patients who have multiple sex partners, doxycycline may be ordered. Oral antibiotics are given for up to 4 weeks for patients with acute prostatitis and for 4 to 16 weeks for chronic prostatitis. The most common medications used for pain control are anti-inflammatory agents. Opioids should be used carefully because of the chronic nature of the pain. Periodic digital massage of

the prostate by the health care provider to increase the flow of infected prostatic secretions may be performed. Heat may be applied using sitz baths.

Nursing Interventions

Nursing interventions primarily focus on symptoms and include (1) a full explanation of antibiotic therapy and the need for compliance with treatment, which may be lengthy in chronic prostatitis; (2) supportive care such as bed rest to relieve strain and pain of the perineum and suprapubic area, sitz baths to promote muscle relaxation, and stool softeners to prevent straining on defecation; (3) monitoring of I&O; (4) bladder drainage with suprapubic catheterization if acute urinary retention develops into acute prostatitis (in acute prostatitis, passage of a catheter through an inflamed urethra is contraindicated); and (5) encouragement of follow-up for evaluation of the inflammation.

Patient problems and interventions for the patient with prostatitis include but are not limited to the following:

PATIENT PROBLEM	NURSING INTERVENTIONS
Recent Onset of Pain related to disease process	Assess type and location of pain; provide analgesics as ordered
	Encourage bed rest to promote comfort
	Provide nonpharmacologic comfort measures:
	• Assist patient with assuming comfortable position
	• Provide diversional activity
	• Provide a restful environmentInstruct patient on necessity of taking prescribed antibiotics and following orders for activity level
Potential for Impaired Self-Esteem due to Current Situation, related to: • Fear of impotence • Embarrassment	Encourage patient to express feelings Actively listen Encourage adaptive coping behaviors

Prognosis

Recurrent episodes of acute prostatitis may cause fibrotic tissue to form; such fibrosis causes a hardening of the prostate gland that initially may be confused with carcinoma. With treatment, the prognosis for bacterial prostatitis is favorable.

EPIDIDYMITIS

Etiology and Pathophysiology

Epididymitis is an infection of the cordlike excretory duct of the testicle, usually secondary to an infectious process (sexually or nonsexually transmitted). It is one of the common infections of the male reproductive tract. The infection often travels to the epididymis from the urethra. The causative organisms include *S. aureus*, *E. coli*, streptococci, chlamydia, and *N. gonorrhoeae*. The inflammation is associated with urethral strictures, cystitis, and prostatitis.

Symptoms can occur after trauma to the genital area, after instrumentation of the urethra and cystoscopy, and after physical exertion or prolonged sexual activity. Risk factors include being uncircumcised, recent surgery involving the urinary tract, structural issues, regular use of a urethral catheter, and unprotected sexual intercourse with multiple partners.

Clinical Manifestations

Severe pain appears suddenly in the scrotum and radiates along the spermatic tube. Additional sites for pain can include the groin, pelvic region, and lower abdomen. Testicular pain worsens with bowel movements. Edema appears and the patient develops a "duck walk" or "waddling gait" because of the sensitivity and pain that walking stimulates. The scrotal area becomes tender. Pyuria (pus in urine) or blood in the semen may be noted. Chills and fever are noted. The physical examination reveals swelling and tenderness at the affected testicle. Lymph nodes may be enlarged.

Diagnostic Tests

Diagnostic testing includes urinalysis and a complete blood cell count. The epididymis is massaged by the health care provider, and a fluid expression specimen is sent to the laboratory. The patient also may be tested for gonorrhea and chlamydia.

Medical Management

Medical management includes a regimen of bed rest and support of the scrotum. The use of antibiotics is important for both partners if the transmission is through sexual contact. Apply cold for relief of edema and discomfort. Administer antibiotic therapy as prescribed. If abscess formation occurs, incision and drainage of the scrotum may be required. Anti-inflammatory medications may be included in the treatment plan.

Nursing Interventions

Nursing interventions for patients with epididymitis include (1) bed rest during the acute phase of illness; (2) support of the testicular area, with scrotal support by elevation of the scrotum on a folded towel during bed rest and athletic support when ambulatory; (3) ice compresses to the area in the initial phase to hasten recovery; (4) explanation of the need for compliance with antibiotic therapy until all signs of inflammation have disappeared; and (5) advice to refrain from sexual intercourse during the acute phase.

Prognosis

Promptly treated, epididymitis can be resolved. The infection can be bilateral and may recur. Bilateral epididymitis can cause sterility. Untreated epididymitis leads to necrosis of testicular tissue. Abscesses and fistulas can form, and septicemia can develop, which can be fatal.

DISORDERS OF MALE GENITAL ORGANS

PHIMOSIS AND PARAPHIMOSIS

Etiology and Pathophysiology

Phimosis is a condition in which the prepuce (foreskin) is too small to allow it to be retracted over the glans penis. Phimosis is often congenital but may be a result of adhesions caused by local inflammation or disease and poor hygiene. The condition is rarely severe enough to obstruct the flow of urine but may contribute to local infection because it does not permit adequate cleansing.

Paraphimosis is an inability to return the retracted foreskin over the glans of the penis as a result of edema. If the foreskin is not placed back in the forward position, an ulcer can develop. Paraphimosis can occur when the foreskin remains contracted during perineal cleansing, use of a urinary catheter, or intercourse.

Medical Management

Circumcision may be performed to manage either condition. Paraphimosis is a urologic emergency requiring prompt intervention. Manual reduction is the first line of treatment attempted. It requires that the glans be pushed back and the foreskin returned to its original location. Chilling the penis with ice for a few minutes before this procedure may aid in reduction of the inflammation. A puncture method also may be used. This procedure engages the use of needles to puncture the foreskin to allow trapped fluid to escape. A tourniquet can be applied to the penis and needles used to aspirate blood from the glans in an attempt to reduce volume and allow for subsequent manual reduction. If none of the manual retraction methods are successful, the swollen foreskin may be incised surgically to allow for the glans to be freed and circulation restored.

Nursing Interventions

Assessment of the degree of swelling and management of discomfort are priorities for the nurse. Care of the patient experiencing either phimosis or paraphimosis also includes education and emotional support. After a circumcision a sterile petrolatum gauze dressing is applied and changed after each voiding. Regardless of the management of the condition, aftercare includes assessment of bleeding and urinary output.

HYDROCELE

Etiology and Pathophysiology

A *hydrocele* is an accumulation of fluid between the two layers of the *tunica vaginalis,* a membrane covering the testicle. The scrotum slowly enlarges as the fluid accumulates. Distinguishing a hydrocele from a cancerous testicular mass is fairly simple: when a strong light is directed from a point behind the scrotum (transillumination), the light passes through if the swelling is a hydrocele; if the swelling is a solid mass the light does not pass through. Pain occurs if the hydrocele develops suddenly. Most hydroceles occur in men older than 21 years of age, but they can occur in infants and children. A hydrocele also may develop as a result of trauma in the area, orchitis (inflammation of the testes), or epididymitis.

Medical Management

No treatment is indicated unless the swelling becomes large and uncomfortable, in which case treatment includes aspiration of fluid from the sac or surgical removal of the sac to avoid constriction of the circulation of the testicles. After aspiration the pain is relieved and the scrotum can be examined more easily.

Nursing Interventions

Nursing interventions consist of maintaining bed rest, scrotal support with elevation, ice to edematous areas, and frequent changes of dressings to avoid skin impairment.

Prognosis

With treatment, the prognosis is good.

VARICOCELE

Varicocele occurs when veins within the scrotum become dilated, usually after internal spermatic vein reflux. Obstruction and malfunctioning of the veins cause engorgement and elongation, preventing adequate drainage of blood from the testis. Symptoms include a "pulling" sensation that causes a dull aching and pain accompanied by edema of the scrotal area. Treatment involves sealing off the problem vein, either by ligation (tying it off) or by embolization (essentially plugging the vein, using a chemical agent or device); blood flow then is redirected into other, normal veins. Complications that may result from the condition include infertility (probably the result of increased testicular temperature) and shrinkage of the testicles. Nursing interventions after treatment include bed rest with scrotal support, ice on the incisional site, and medication for discomfort as ordered.

Ligation of the internal spermatic vein in the treatment of varicocele has been shown to improve semen quality.

CANCER OF THE MALE REPRODUCTIVE TRACT

The more common tumors of the male reproductive tract involve the testis, the prostate gland, and the penis. Most tumors of the male reproductive system are malignant.

CANCER OF THE TESTIS (TESTICULAR CANCER)

Etiology and Pathophysiology

Testicular cancer is the most common cancer in men ages 15 to 35 years of age. It is estimated that in 2020 about 9600 cases will be diagnosed and nearly 450 men will die from the condition. The risk for developing testicular cancer is only about 1 in 250 (ACS, 2021d). Risk factors for the development of this form of cancer include abnormal testicular development and cryptorchidism (failure of testes to descend into the scrotum). The condition is seen more in white men than in African American or Asian American men. A father or brother having had testicular cancer increases the risk for development. Men having human immunodeficiency virus (HIV) are at an increased risk. Most testicular cancers develop from embryonic germ cells. The two types of germ cell cancers are seminomas and nonseminomas. Seminomas are the most common and the least aggressive; nonseminoma testicular germ cell tumors are rare and very aggressive.

Clinical Manifestations

Testicular cancer may have a slow or rapid onset, depending on the type of tumor. The signs and symptoms of early disease include an enlarged scrotum and a firm, nontender, painless, smooth mass in the testicular area. Some patients complain of a dull ache or heavy sensation in the lower abdomen, perianal area, or scrotum. Acute pain is the presenting symptom in about 10% of patients. Some men may display gynecomastia (excessive breast tissue development).

Diagnostic Tests

Palpation of the scrotal contents is the first step in diagnosing testicular cancer. A cancerous mass is firm and does not transilluminate. Ultrasound of the testes is indicated when testicular cancer is suspected (e.g., a palpable mass) or persistent or painful testicular edema is present. If a testicular neoplasm is suspected, obtain blood to determine the serum levels of alpha-fetoprotein, lactate dehydrogenase, and hCG. A chest radiograph and CT scan of the abdomen and pelvis are obtained to detect metastasis.

Medical Management

Radical inguinal orchiectomy is usually the treatment of choice. This is the removal of the testis, epididymis, a portion of the gonadal lymphatics, and their blood supply. The remaining testis provides enough testosterone to maintain the man's sexual characteristics. However, he may have a lower sperm count and decreased sperm mobility. Surgery generally is followed by radiation or chemotherapy. Often a retroperitoneal lymph node dissection is performed to remove affected nodes and assist in determining the tumor stage. Staging a testicular tumor helps determine treatment.

Nursing Interventions and Patient Teaching

The most important aspect of care of patients who have or are at risk for a tumor of the testis is early detection by testicular self-examination (TSE). Young men should be taught to perform TSE monthly, beginning at puberty. Video media and illustrations are available as teaching aids and ideally should be introduced during high school or college physical education classes. Information about TSE is available on the ACS website and other websites. The examination takes 3 minutes and should be done monthly. The best time to perform a TSE is after a warm shower, when the scrotal skin is relaxed. The scrotum is checked for color, contour, and skin breaks. The left side is usually longer because the left testicle is suspended from a longer spermatic cord. Each testicle is palpated gently by grasping the scrotum in the center with the thumb and index finger (see the Patient Teaching box and Fig. 12.18). Normal testicles are firm but somewhat resilient, smooth, and mobile. If a testicle is indurated (hardened), carcinoma is suspected.

Prognosis

With the advent of tumor markers (which indicate the presence of disease and enable the health care provider to monitor its response to treatment), early detection, refined surgery, and effective chemotherapy are heralded as keys to the increases in survival rates. The survival rate is higher than 95% for those patients with cancer diagnosed and treated in the early stages. Testicular cancer metastasis occurs most commonly to the abdomen, lungs, the retroperitoneal region, and spine (ACS, 2021e).

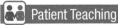 **Patient Teaching**

Testicular Self-Examination

- Examine the scrotum once a month.
- Perform testicular self-examination after a bath or shower, when the scrotum is warm and most relaxed.
- Grasp the testis with both hands and palpate gently between the thumb and index finger. The testis should feel smooth and egg shaped and be firm to the touch.
- The epididymis, found behind the testis, should feel like a soft tube (see Figs. 12.1 and 12.18).

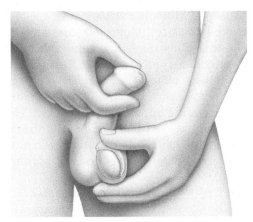

Fig. 12.18 Testicular self-examination. (From Harkreader H, Hogan MA: Fundamentals of nursing: caring and clinical judgment, ed 3, St. Louis, 2007, Saunders.)

CANCER OF THE PENIS
Etiology and Pathophysiology
Cancer of the penis is rare. The frequency is only 1 in 100,000 men and represents less than 1% of cancers in men. It generally appears in men older than 50 years of age. Men who have not been circumcised, have phimosis or smegma are at an increased risk. Infections such as HPV or HIV are associated with an increased risk for penile cancer. Social practices such as smoking and tobacco use are also implicated.

Clinical Manifestations
The tumor is painless, and a wartlike growth or ulceration on the glans under the prepuce is present. It is common for metastasis to occur to the inguinal nodes and adjacent organs.

Diagnostic Tests
Biopsy confirms the diagnosis.

Medical Management
Surgical intervention requires removal of as little tissue as possible, but it may be necessary to do a partial or total amputation of the penis and to remove the adjacent tissue and inguinal lymph nodes. When metastasis involves the bladder and rectum, more radical surgery may be needed, and outlets for urinary or fecal elimination are provided by creating an ileal conduit and a colostomy. The surgeon may place a suprapubic catheter into the bladder to drain the urine.

Nursing Interventions
Nursing interventions include providing emotional support. If amputation of the penis is required, the patient faces the psychological trauma associated with the loss of sexuality and the ability to urinate naturally. Monitor urinary output by suprapubic catheter or, if an ileal conduit was constructed, monitor urine in the urostomy bag. Elevation of the scrotum controls edema. Provide comfort measures to control pain.

SEXUALLY TRANSMITTED INFECTIONS

Today, despite sweeping advances in the diagnosis and treatment of communicable diseases, the incidence of infections transmitted through intimate or sexual activities continues to increase worldwide. STIs previously were called *sexually transmitted diseases* or *venereal diseases*. These infections usually are transmitted during intimate sexual contact. They may have other routes of transmission (e.g., from an infected mother to her newborn), occur with or without symptoms, and have long periods of asymptomatic infectivity.

Any sexually active person may be at risk for an STI. People who have frequent sexual contact with multiple partners and who engage in unprotected sexual activity are at increased risk. Commonly, those most

Table 12.2	Assessment of Risk Factors for Sexually Transmitted Infections Using the 5 Ps
5 Ps	**QUESTIONS TO ASK**
Past STIs	Have you ever had an STI in the past?
Partners	Have you had sex with men, women, or both? In the past 2 months how many people have you had sex with? In the past 12 months, how many partners have you had sex with? Is it possible that any of your partners in the past 12 months had sex with other partners while they were in a relationship with you?
Practices	To identify your personal risks for STIs we need to discuss your recent sexual activity. • Have you had vagina sex? Oral sex? • Anal sex?
Protection	What do you do to prevent STIs and HIV? How frequently do you protect yourself during sexual activity?
Pregnancy	What are you doing to prevent pregnancy? Are you using protection consistently?

HIV, Human immunodeficiency virus; *STIs*, sexually transmitted infection. Modified from https://www.cdc.gov/std/tg2015/clinical.htm#risk.

at risk are young, single, urban, poor, male, and homosexual. Some STIs can be managed but cannot be cured. Other STIs such as herpes simplex and HPV may persist without obvious outward symptoms and place unsuspecting individuals at risk. Collection of data to assess risk for STIs is an important role of the nurse (Table 12.2).

Despite the physical and emotional discomfort, the possibility of long-term disability (infertility, chronic infectivity), and advances in diagnosis and treatment that sharply decrease the period of infectivity, STIs continue to be among the world's most common communicable diseases. Four main factors are responsible: (1) unprotected sex, (2) antibiotic resistance, (3) treatment delay, and (4) sexual behavior patterns and permissiveness. The following is a discussion of some of the more commonly diagnosed STIs (see the Safety Alert box).

HERPES SIMPLEX
Etiology and Pathophysiology
Herpes simplex virus (HSV) is an infectious viral disease characterized by recurrent episodes of acute, painful, erythematous, vesicular eruptions (blisters) on or in the genitalia or rectum. The two closely related forms are designated types 1 and 2. Traditionally type 1 was designated as oral lesions and type 2 were genital lesions. The viral types can affect either body location. Among individuals 14 to 49 years of age, an estimated one in six has genital herpes.

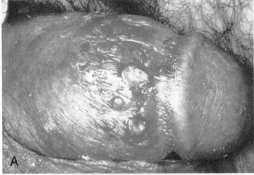
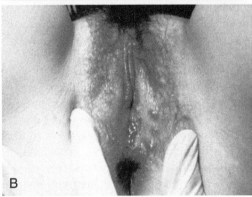

Fig. 12.19 Herpes simplex virus type 2 in male and female patients. Vesicular lesions on A, penis and B, perineum. (From Beare PG, Myers JL: *Adult health nursing*, ed 3, St. Louis, 1998, Mosby.)

! Safety Alert

Sexually Transmitted Infections

- Teach "safe" sex practices including abstinence, monogamy with an uninfected partner, avoidance of certain high-risk sexual practices, and use of condoms and other barriers to limit contact with potentially infectious body fluids or lesions.
- All sexually active women should be screened for cervical cancer. Women with a history of STIs are at greater risk for cervical cancer than women without this history.
- Inform patients of the new HPV vaccine for girls and boys beginning at ages 11–12 years to prevent HPV infection and the precancerous changes that lead to cervical cancer.
- Instruct patients in hygiene measures, such as washing and urinating after intercourse to rid the body of causative organisms.
- Explain the importance of taking all antibiotics as prescribed. Symptoms often improve after 1 or 2 days of therapy, but organisms may still be present.
- Teach patients about the need for treatment of sexual partners with antibiotics to prevent transmission of disease.
- Instruct patients to abstain from sexual intercourse during treatment and to use condoms when sexual activity is resumed, to prevent spread of infection and reinfection.
- Explain the importance of follow-up examination and reculture at least once after treatment (if appropriate) to confirm complete cure and to prevent relapse.
- Allow patients and partners to verbalize concerns to clarify areas that need explanation.
- Instruct patients about symptoms of complications and the need to report problems to ensure proper follow-up and early treatment of reinfection.
- Explain precautions to take, such as being monogamous; asking potential partners about sexual history; avoiding sex with partners who use IV drugs or who have visible oral, inguinal, genital, perineal, or anal lesions; using condoms; and voiding and washing genitalia after coitus to reduce the occurrence of reinfection.
- Inform patients regarding their state of infectivity to prevent a false sense of security, which may result in careless sexual practices and poor personal hygiene.

Clinical Manifestations

Signs include the appearance of fluid-filled vesicles 2 days to 2 weeks after exposure. In women the vesicles usually occur on the cervix, which is considered the primary site but also may be seen on the labia, rectum, vulva, vagina, and skin. In men vesicles are found on the glans penis, foreskin, and penile shaft (Fig. 12.19). Other lesions may appear on the mouth and anus. Vesicles may rupture and develop into shallow, painful ulcers; they are erythematous with marked edema and tenderness. Lymph nodes may become involved. Initial lesions last from 3 to 10 days, and recurrent lesions have a duration of 7 to 10 days. The primary infection may be accompanied by fever; malaise; myalgia; dysuria; and, in women, leukorrhea. Urination may be painful, the result of urine contacting active lesions.

After the initial outbreak has subsided, the virus lies dormant in the body. It may be triggered by illness, fatigue, injury, or stress in the individual. Recurrent outbreaks are typically less painful and shorter in duration. The frequency of subsequent outbreaks is individualized, with some people never having an outbreak and others experiencing them frequently.

Diagnostic Tests

Diagnosis is based on the physical examination and the patient history. The diagnosis is confirmed by the appearance of the virus on tissue cultures. Cultures are more frequently positive when the lesions are from a primary infection versus recurrent infections. Asymptomatic disease may be identified by serologic testing.

Medical Management

The skin lesions of genital herpes heal spontaneously unless secondary infection occurs. Encourage symptomatic treatment such as practicing good genital hygiene and wearing loose-fitting cotton undergarments. The lesions should be kept clean and dry. Frequent sitz baths may soothe the area and reduce inflammation. Pain may require a local anesthetic such as lidocaine (Xylocaine) or systemic analgesics such as codeine and aspirin. Advise patients to abstain from sexual contact while lesions are present. Transmission of the virus has been documented in the absence of symptoms, making the practice of safe sex necessary at all times.

Antiviral medications can be prescribed to manage the initial outbreak, subsequent outbreaks, or as a suppressive therapy to prevent outbreaks in the future. Treatment regimens of antiviral medications may include acyclovir (Zovirax), valacyclovir (Valtrex), and famciclovir. These medications do not cure the disease but reduce the severity of symptoms and shorten the duration of the outbreak. Therapy for the initial outbreak often is prescribed for 7 to 10 days. Subsequent outbreaks are managed with a 5-day course of therapy. Suppressive therapy requires that the individual take the daily medications to lessen outbreaks over time. Continued use of oral acyclovir for up to 5 years is safe and effective, but it should be interrupted after 1 year to assess the patient's episode recurrence rate. Adverse reactions to acyclovir are mild and include headache, occasional nausea and vomiting, and diarrhea. The safety of systemic acyclovir for the treatment of pregnant women has not been established. Acyclovir ointment appears to be of no clinical benefit in the treatment of recurrent lesions, either in speed of healing or in resolution of pain. IV acyclovir is reserved for severe or life-threatening infections in which hospitalization is required for the treatment of central nervous system infections (meningitis) or pneumonitis. Nephrotoxicity has been observed with high-dose IV use.

Nursing Interventions and Patient Teaching

Advise the patient to keep genital lesions clean and dry. Hands should be washed thoroughly after touching a lesion. Loose, absorbent underclothing is usually more comfortable than close-fitting clothing. Sitz baths decrease lesion discomfort and enhance urinary and bowel elimination. Teach the patient that sexual intercourse during the active lesion phase increases the risk of transmission and also may be painful. Patients should inform future sexual partners and health care providers of recurring or latent infections. Sexual transmission of HSV has been documented during asymptomatic periods; encourage the use of barrier methods, especially condoms. Inform the patient about the role of stress, poor nutrition, and insufficient rest in recurrences of signs and symptoms. Female patients need a yearly Pap test and should inform their health care provider in the event of pregnancy so that the disease can be monitored closely; there is a possibility of spontaneous abortion. Provide the patient with nonjudgmental support and with the contact number of the local herpes support group if one exists.

Prognosis

Genital herpes is a recurrent disease with no cure.

SYPHILIS

Etiology and Pathophysiology

The coiled spirochete *Treponema pallidum* causes syphilis. In 2018, there were more than 38,000 new cases of syphilis reported. An increase in syphilis rates since the early 2000s has been noted each year. In the 10 years between 2008 and 2018, the number of new cases reported has more than tripled. The population experiencing the highest number of cases are men who have sex with other men.

Syphilis is the third most frequently reported communicable disease in the United States, exceeded only by varicella (chickenpox) and gonorrhea. Transmission occurs primarily through sexual contact during the primary, secondary, and latent stages of the disease. In addition to sexual contact, syphilis may be spread through contact with infectious lesions and sharing of needles among drug addicts. Prenatal infection from the mother to the fetus is possible. The organism thrives in the warm parts of the body and can be destroyed by soap and water. The spirochete penetrates intact skin and openings in the mucous membranes of the genital organs, rectum, and mouth.

Clinical Manifestations

Syphilis has four stages—primary, secondary, latent, and tertiary—each with its peculiar signs and symptoms. The signs and symptoms of syphilis include the clean-based chancre (painless erosion or papule that ulcerates superficially with a scooped-out appearance) of primary syphilis to the skin rashes of secondary syphilis. Moist, raised, gray to pink lesions of the genital or perirectal skin; enlarged lymph nodes; fever; fatigue; or infections of the eyes, bones, liver, or meninges may occur. In the late stages of syphilis, dementia, pain or loss of sensation in the legs, and destruction of the aorta occur. Destructive inflammatory masses can appear in any organ. In tertiary or late-stage syphilis the heart and blood vessels (cardiovascular syphilis) and the central nervous system (neurosyphilis) frequently are involved. Spinal cord degeneration, partial paralysis, and various psychoses may result.

Diagnostic Tests

Diagnostic tests include the Venereal Disease Research Laboratory (VDRL) slide test and rapid plasma reagin (RPR) test. Both assesses the presence of serum antibodies for syphilis. The antibodies will be present if the body has been exposed to the infection. Gonorrhea and syphilis often appear together. Patients suspected of syphilis should also be screened for gonorrhea as well (CDC, n.d.).

Medical Management

Therapeutic management of syphilis is aimed at eradication of all syphilitic organisms. However, treatment cannot reverse damage that is already present in the late stage of the disease. Parenteral benzylpenicillin (penicillin G) remains the treatment of choice for all stages of syphilis. In patients who have an allergy to penicillin, tetracycline, erythromycin, and ceftriaxone are prescribed. All stages of syphilis should be treated.

Appropriate antibiotic treatment of maternal syphilis before the 18th week of pregnancy prevents infection of the fetus. Appropriate treatment after 18 weeks of pregnancy cures mother and fetus, because the antibiotics can cross the placental barrier. Treatment administered in the second half of pregnancy may pose a risk of premature labor. Some authorities recommend hospitalization and fetal monitoring of women at 20 weeks of gestation or later.

Carefully monitor all patients with neurosyphilis by periodic serologic testing, clinical evaluation at 6-month intervals, and repeated cerebrospinal fluid examinations for at least 3 years. Specific therapeutic management is based on the specific symptoms (CDC, n.d.).

Nursing Interventions
In addition to routine interventions for patients with STIs, monitor for drug reaction to penicillin, stress good handwashing technique, encourage follow-up visits with the health care provider, and inform the patient that he or she should absolutely not engage in sexual intercourse until cured.

Prognosis
Syphilis infection must be treated at the earliest stage possible. Patients treated in the primary and secondary stages have the highest potential positive outcome. Although syphilis can be cured in late stages, damage to the body is more difficult to manage. As the disease progresses physiologic damage may result. Advanced stages of syphilis may result in the formation of gummas (bumps on the skin, bones, or body organs), neurologic damage, and cardiovascular illness. About 20% of patients with tertiary syphilis who are not treated die of the condition. Untreated syphilis advances from the primary stage to the secondary stage, latent stage, and eventually the tertiary stage.

GONORRHEA

Etiology and Pathophysiology
Gonorrhea is caused by *N. gonorrhoeae,* a gram-negative diplococcoid bacterium, and almost exclusively follows sexual contact. It may be referred to as "the clap" or "the drip." It is the second most commonly reported STI in the United States (chlamydial infections are the most commonly reported). Gonorrhea rates remained stable from 1997 to 2000 after a 74% decline from 1975 to 1997. Since that time the rate of gonorrhea infections has sharply risen. The Centers

for Disease Control and Prevention estimate that 820,000 people are infected annually, but only half are diagnosed and reported. In 2019, a total of 616,392 cases were reported (CDC, 2021a). The highest incidence of gonorrhea occurs in adolescents and young adults of all racial and ethnic groups. African Americans are also a high-risk population. Gonorrhea is primarily an infection of the genital or rectal mucosa but is not limited to the genital organs; it can infect the mouth and throat through oral sex with an infected partner. It may also infect the eyes.

Clinical Manifestations
Some infected men may be asymptomatic after the incubation period. Typically within 2 to 5 days of exposure, symptoms develop. Signs and symptoms of urethritis, dysuria, infection with a profuse purulent discharge, and edema of the affected area are most common. A common sensation experienced by infected symptomatic individuals is that of "peeing razor blades." Most women remain asymptomatic but may show a greenish yellow discharge from the cervix. Other female signs and symptoms, depending on the infection site, are urinary frequency, purulent discharge from the urethra, pruritus, burning and pain of the vulva, vaginal engorgement and erythema, abdominal pain and distention, muscular rigidity, and tenderness. As the infection spreads, nausea, vomiting, fever, and tachycardia may develop. Other signs and symptoms are pharyngitis, tonsillitis, rectal burning, and purulent rectal discharge.

Diagnostic Tests
Diagnosis is determined by cultures from the site of infection to isolate and identify the organism. Cultures of the discharge or secretion can provide a definitive diagnosis after incubation for 24 to 48 hours. An important concern in the treatment for gonorrhea is coexisting chlamydial infection (see the section "Chlamydia" for more information). Chlamydia has been documented in up to 45% of gonorrhea cases. It is important to test for syphilis as well.

Medical Management
A history of sexual contact with a partner known to have gonorrhea is considered good evidence for the infection. Because of the short incubation period and high infectivity, treatment is instituted without awaiting culture results, even in the absence of signs or symptoms. Treatment of gonorrhea in the early stage is curative. Traditionally, the drug of choice for gonorrheal therapy was penicillin, but changes have been made because of (1) a rapid increase in the number of cases of gonorrhea caused by resistant strains of *N. gonorrhoeae* and (2) coexisting chlamydial infection.

There is no clinical distinction between infections caused by resistant or sensitive strains of *N. gonorrhoeae*. As a result, ceftriaxone, a penicillinase-resistant cephalosporin, has become part of the treatment plan. The most common treatment for gonorrhea is a single IM dose of ceftriaxone. Cefixime (Suprax) given orally one time is also effective. Other medications that may be used in the treatment of gonorrhea are ciprofloxacin, ofloxacin, and levofloxacin. The high frequency of coexisting chlamydial and gonococcal infections has led to the addition of doxycycline or tetracycline to the treatment plan. The expense of diagnosing chlamydial infection and the sequelae make this strategy cost effective. Patients with co-incubating syphilis are likely to be cured by the same drugs.

All sexual contacts of patients with gonorrhea must be treated to prevent reinfection after resumption of sexual relations. The "ping-pong" effect of re-exposure, treatment, and reinfection will cease only when infected partners are treated simultaneously. In addition, advise the patient to abstain from sexual intercourse and alcohol for 2 to 4 weeks. Sexual intercourse allows the infection to spread and can retard complete healing as a result of vascular congestion. Alcohol irritates the healing urethral walls. Caution men against squeezing the penis to look for further discharge. Follow-up examination and reculture should be done at least once after treatment, usually in 4 to 7 days. Treat relapse, reinfection, and complications appropriately.

Be alert to changes in CDC recommendations. Report the disease to infection control authorities as required by the local health agency.

Nursing Interventions and Patient Teaching

Advise patients that loose, absorbent underclothes, changed frequently after perineal or penile cleansing, enhance comfort. Sitz baths decrease lower abdominal discomfort and dysuria. Obtain laboratory specimens as ordered. Discuss alternative methods of birth control as appropriate. Encourage notification of present and past sexual partners of the diagnosis and stress the need for them to promptly seek medical care. Inform the patients that sterility may occur as a result of gonorrhea.

Prognosis

With treatment, gonorrhea is curable. The inflammation may clear up without serious results, or it may become chronic and produce urethral stricture. Complications include prostatitis, epididymitis, orchitis, arthritis, and endocarditis. It can result in sterility and PID in the female. No case of acute gonorrhea in the female should be considered cured until three consecutive negative smears of the cervix and Bartholin and Skene glands are obtained. The main cause of infections identified after completed treatment is reinfection, not treatment failure.

TRICHOMONIASIS

Etiology and Pathophysiology

Trichomoniasis is an STI caused by the protozoan *T. vaginalis*. In the United States, an estimated 3.7 million people are infected (CDC, 2021b). The incubation period is 4 to 28 days. Trichomoniasis usually is transmitted by sexual intercourse. On occasion, a newborn develops an infection from an infected mother. *T. vaginalis* thrives when the vaginal mucosa is more alkaline than normal. Frequent douching and use of oral contraceptives and antibiotics raise the normal pH of the vagina, making women more vulnerable to trichomoniasis.

Clinical Manifestations

Most men and approximately 70% of women are asymptomatic. The male signs and symptoms are mild to severe transient urethritis, dysuria, frequent urination, pruritus, and purulent exudate. In women, signs and symptoms include profuse, frothy, gray, green, or yellow malodorous discharge; pruritus; edema; tenderness of vagina; dysuria; frequency of urination; spotting; menorrhagia; and dysmenorrhea. Signs and symptoms may persist for a week to several months and may be more pronounced after menstruation or during pregnancy.

Diagnostic Tests

Diagnosis is based on microscopic examination of a vaginal discharge sample that identifies *T. vaginalis*.

Medical Management

Treatment for men and women is oral metronidazole (Flagyl) in small doses for 7 days or a single large dose. The patient should avoid alcoholic beverages, because alcohol can cause reactions such as disorientation, headache, cramps, vomiting, and possibly convulsions. Metronidazole can cause the urine to turn dark brown (see Table 12.1).

Nursing Interventions and Patient Teaching

Advise the patient to avoid alcohol during treatment; inform patients that their urine may turn dark orange or brown; and counsel patients to avoid douches, sprays, and powders during treatment. Teach the patient how to disinfect douche nozzles, applicators, diaphragms, and the toilet area. Encourage the patient to wear loose-fitting clothing and cotton underwear, to schedule follow-up visits with the health care provider, and to contact sexual partners so that they can get treatment.

Prognosis

With treatment, trichomoniasis is curable. Reinfection is common if sexual partners are not treated simultaneously. Chronic infection may develop in untreated cases.

CANDIDIASIS

Etiology and Pathophysiology

Candidiasis (thrush) is a mild fungal infection that appears in men and women. Candidal infections usually are caused by *C. albicans* and *Candida tropicalis*. The fungi are a part of the normal flora of the gastrointestinal tract, mouth, vagina, and skin. The infection often occurs when the glucose level rises from diabetes mellitus or when resistance is lowered from diseases such as carcinoma. Radiation, immunosuppressant drugs, hyperalimentation (IV feeding), antibiotic therapy, and oral contraceptives may predispose individuals to candidiasis. Infected men and women display signs of scaly skin; erythematous rash; and occasional exudates that appear under the breasts, between the fingers, and in the axillae, groin, and umbilicus.

Clinical Manifestations

If the mother is infected, a newborn can contract thrush during delivery. The infant may display a diaper rash. The infant's nails become edematous and have a darkened, erythematous nail base with purulent exudate. Thrush may appear on the mucous membranes of the infant's mouth as pearly, bluish white "milk-curd" lesions and cause edema and engorgement. The infant may have an edematous tongue that can cause respiratory distress. Poor feeding may be noted. The adult female patient may have a cheesy, tenacious white vaginal discharge accompanied by pruritus and an inflamed vulva and vagina. The adult male patient has signs of an infected penis with purulent exudate. Systemic infections are indicated by chills, fevers, and general malaise.

Diagnostic Tests

Diagnosis is based on evidence of a *Candida* species on a Gram stain of specimens collected from scraping of the vagina and penis, from pus, and from exudate from the mouth.

Medical Management

Treatment consists of managing any underlying condition, such as controlling diabetes mellitus, and discontinuing antibiotics and oral contraceptives. Nystatin is effective for superficial candidiasis; topical amphotericin B is effective for skin and nail infections.

Nursing Interventions and Patient Teaching

Emphasize the use of prescribed ointments, sprays, and creams as indicated for each part of the body affected. Teaching includes the method for inserting vaginal suppositories (to be inserted high into the vagina when in a dorsal recumbent position) and remaining on the back for 30 minutes to allow suppository absorption. Patients should encourage sexual partners to have an examination and treatment. Teach good handwashing techniques to avoid reinfection or the transfer of the fungi. Encourage pregnant women to accept treatment to prevent infection of the newborn at the time of delivery.

Prognosis

Candidiasis is curable with the use of the prescribed treatment.

CHLAMYDIA

Etiology and Pathophysiology

Chlamydia trachomatis, a gram-negative, intracellular bacterium, causes several common STIs. Cervicitis and urethritis are most common, but like gonococci, chlamydial organisms also cause epididymitis in men and salpingitis in women. Chlamydial infections are the most commonly occurring STI in the United States. They are responsible for about 20% to 30% of diagnosed PID cases. In 2019, there were more than 1,808,703 cases of chlamydial infections reported in the United States (CDC, 2021a). Almost two-thirds (61.0%) of all reported chlamydia cases were among persons aged 15–24 years. Increases in chlamydia rates are more likely a result of better screening and use of more sensitive tests, rather than an increase in the total burden of the disease in the United States (CDC, 2021a). Chlamydia can be transmitted during vaginal, anal, or oral sex.

Although men and women may have asymptomatic infection, women are more likely to be asymptomatic carriers even with deep pelvic infections, such as infection of the fallopian tubes and PID.

Clinical Manifestations

In men, signs and symptoms may include a scanty white or clear exudate, burning or pruritus around the urethral meatus, urinary frequency, and mild dysuria. Signs and symptoms of cervicitis in women may include one or more of the following: (1) vaginal pruritus or burning, (2) dull pelvic pain, (3) low-grade fever, (4) vaginal discharge, and (5) irregular bleeding. Symptoms of chlamydia may be absent or cause minor discomfort; therefore it has been called a silent disease. Females may develop a PID, which can result in infertility. For this reason the CDC (2014) recommends that all females younger than 25 years of age be screened routinely for chlamydia at their annual gynecologic examination. The CDC further advises annual screening of all women older than 25 years of age with one or more risk factors for the disease (CDC, 2014).

Diagnostic Tests

The direct fluorescent antibody test provides a ready basis for diagnosis. However, this test is less specific than a culture and may produce false-positive results. Culturing for chlamydial organisms should be done if the laboratory facilities are available. New techniques using nucleic acid amplification promise to surpass culture as the gold standard of chlamydial testing. Treatment can be initiated promptly, based on a confirmed diagnosis.

Medical Management

Chlamydial infections respond to treatment with tetracycline, doxycycline, azithromycin, or ofloxacin. For tetracycline, the dosage is 500 mg orally four times a day for at least 7 days. For doxycycline, the dosage is 100 mg two times a day. For ofloxacin, the dosage is 300 mg twice a day. Azithromycin (1 g in a single dose) offers the advantage of ease of administration, but safety for patients younger than 15 years of age has not been established. Alternative regimens include erythromycin, ofloxacin, and levofloxacin. Erythromycin is the drug of choice for use in pregnant patients. If this treatment is not tolerated, amoxicillin is an alternative. Follow-up care includes advising the patient to return if symptoms persist or recur, treating sexual partners, and encouraging the use of condoms during all sexual contact.

Because chlamydial infections are closely associated with gonococcal infections, both infections usually are treated concurrently, even without diagnostic evidence.

Nursing Interventions and Patient Teaching

Patients' physical symptoms often are complicated by their emotional responses to STIs. Depression, anger, fear, and guilt must be addressed if education and treatment are to be effective. Outcome also is influenced by educational and income levels, primary language, health insurance coverage, and support network. Patient education focuses on prevention (Box 12.8).

Prognosis

With treatment, chlamydial infection is curable. Reinfection occurs if sexual partners are not treated simultaneously. Chlamydial infections can be transmitted to infants during delivery, causing conjunctivitis and pneumonia. Poorly treated or untreated chlamydial infection can result in ectopic pregnancy or infertility.

ACQUIRED IMMUNODEFICIENCY SYNDROME

Acquired immunodeficiency syndrome (AIDS) is the ultimately fatal, advanced stage of infection with the retroviral HIV, which gradually destroys the cell-mediated immune system. For a more detailed discussion on this infection, see Chapter 16.

Box 12.8	Prevention of Sexually Transmitted Infections

- Reduce the number of sexual partners, preferably to one person.
- Avoid contact with individuals known to be infected or who are at risk of infection.
- Avoid contact with the genital area if signs and symptoms develop.
- Wash the hands and the genital-rectal area before and immediately after having intercourse.
- Pay special attention to washing the foreskin.
- An antiseptic mouthwash or gargle with hydrogen peroxide (1 part peroxide to 3 parts of water) may slightly reduce the risk of oropharyngeal sexually transmitted infection (STI).
- Use barrier (condom) contraceptives with new partners.
- Use a water-based lubricant as opposed to an oil-based lubricant.
- Void after intercourse.
- Avoid excess douching.
- If an STI infection is suspected, seek medical help immediately.
- Individuals with multiple sexual partners should have an STI examination twice a year or more if needed.

FAMILY PLANNING

Advances in drug therapy and family planning technology have made a range of options available for individuals wishing to prevent or plan conception. Birth control planning involves moral, religious, cultural, and personal values; be sensitive to these factors when discussing birth control with patients.

Numerous types of birth control procedures or devices can be employed. The selection of a method should be based on the patient's health, effectiveness of the method, cost, lifestyle, ease of use, and age and parity (total number of pregnancies) of the patient. The patient's willingness to comply with use and the couple's preference are two additional factors taken into consideration when selecting a method of contraception. Reinforce the information given by the health care provider and encourage patients to seek more information, directing them to the source.

Contraceptive methods and products can be categorized as surgical (Figs. 12.20 and 12.21), hormonal, barrier, and behavioral (Table 12.3).

❖ NURSING PROCESS FOR THE PATIENT WITH A REPRODUCTIVE DISORDER

The role of the licensed practical nurse/licensed vocational nurse (LPN/LVN) in the nursing process as stated is that the LPN/LVN will do the following:

- Participate in planning care for patients, based on patient needs
- Review patient's care plan and recommend revisions as needed

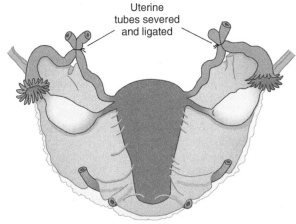

Fig. 12.20 Tubal ligation. Oviduct is severed and ligated. (From Lowdermilk DL, Perry SE, Cashion K, Alden KR: *Maternity and women's health care*, ed 10, St. Louis, 2012, Mosby.)

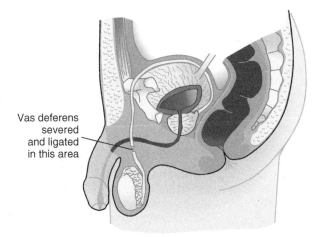

Fig. 12.21 Vasectomy. Sperm duct is severed and ligated. (From Lowdermilk DL, Perry SE, Cashion K, Alden KR: *Maternity and women's health care*, ed 10, St. Louis, 2012, Mosby.)

- Review and follow defined prioritization for patient care
- Use clinical pathways, care maps, or care plans to guide and review patient care

ASSESSMENT

People with reproductive disorders require skilled assessment by the nurse and the health care provider. Assessment occurs through observation of the patient during the patient health history and while doing baseline and continuing assessment of the patient's objective and subjective data.

Health history data should be relevant to the patient's developmental age. Information about reproductive health and sexuality can form a large portion of the collected data. This history is as important as the physical and emotional data in determining appropriate patient problems and interventions. Data collected about sexual health, sexual relations, birth control methods, STIs, and the use of chemical substances provide an opportunity to clarify any misconceptions or myths revealed during history taking.

Data Collection for Women

Data collection for adolescent and adult women focuses on the reproductive tract and the menstrual, gynecologic, and obstetric history.

The menstrual history encompasses menarche (onset of menstrual flow) through the climacteric (cessation of menstrual cycle), including (1) age of onset; (2) date of last menstrual flow; (3) usual amount and volume of flow (number of pads used per day); (4) presence of dysmenorrhea (painful menstruation), menorrhagia (excessive flow), amenorrhea (absence of flow), or metrorrhagia (excessive spotting between cycles); and (5) other difficulties during menses.

The gynecologic assessment includes data on (1) vaginal discharge (odor, color, frequency, and duration), (2) vaginal pruritus (itching), (3) vaginal irritation with coital activity, (4) date and results of the last Pap test, (5) birth control methods or kinds of contraceptives used, and (6) any family history of cancer of the reproductive system.

If the patient has conceived, information should be collected as to gravidity (number of pregnancies), parity (number of births), abortions, miscarriages, and stillbirths.

Assessment of the breast includes (1) tenderness of the breast areas; (2) pain; (3) masses in any specific areas; (4) presence of nipple discharge; (5) knowledge and frequency of BSE; and (6) date and results of last mammogram, if applicable.

Data Collection for Men

The data collected from the male adolescent and the adult man include (1) urologic history of voiding difficulties and any discharge from the penis; (2) characteristics of the urine (odor, color, amount, and frequency); (3) information on prostate and testicular problems; (4) frequency of PSA testing, if applicable; (5) masses or lesions on genitalia; (6) frequency of TSE; (7) frequency of professional testicular examination; (8) measures to prevent infections; and (9) birth control method. In addition, note concerns about sexual health voiced by the patient.

PATIENT PROBLEM

Possible patient problems for the patient with a reproductive disorder include but are not limited to the following:
- *Alteration in Urinary Elimination*
- *Anxiousness*
- *Compromised Blood Flow to Tissue*
- *Compromised Skin Integrity*
- *Distorted Body Image*
- *Fearfulness*
- *Impaired Coping*

Table 12.3   Methods of Birth Control

DESCRIPTION	SIDE EFFECTS AND COMPLICATIONS	PATIENT EDUCATION
TEMPORARY METHODS		
Combined		
Combination pill contains estrogen and progesterone (standard and low dose). Usually taken on 5th through 25th day of each cycle. Prevents ovulation; causes changes in endometrium; causes alterations in cervical mucus and tubal transport. Simple and unobtrusive in use. 99% effective. Failure from irregular or incorrect use.	*Side effects:* Weight gain, nausea and vomiting, spotting and breakthrough bleeding, postpill amenorrhea, breast tenderness, headache, melasma, irritability, nervousness, depression, and decreased libido. *Complications:* Benign liver tumors, gallstones, myocardial infarction, thromboembolism, stroke (smokers over age 35 years at higher risk). *Contraindications:* History of cardiovascular or liver disease, hypertension, breast or pelvic cancer; use caution with diabetes mellitus, sickle cell anemia. Provides no protection against HIV transmission.	Instruct patient in correct use of pills. Tell patient to take pill at the same time each day; if forgotten one day, take two the next day. Review side effects and contraindications. Explain that the patient should report cramps, edema of legs, chest pain. Discuss need for periodic (q 6–12 months) checkup of weight, BP, Pap test, hematocrit. Review danger signs of drug. Take drug history; ask about use of phenytoin, phenobarbital, antibiotic (ampicillin), which decrease contraceptive action. Inform patient that method is usually not recommended for women over age 35. Discourage smoking.
Morning-after pill, also called Plan B (norgestrel and ethinyl estradiol), contains ethinyl estradiol 50 mcg and norgestrel 500 mg. Another use of combined hormonal contraception. 98.4% effective. Creates hostile uterine lining and alters tubal transport.	Nausea for 1–2 days. Does not prevent an ectopic pregnancy. Patient is at risk for usual hormonal complications of abdominal pain, chest pain, cough, shortness of breath, headache, dizziness, weakness, leg pain.	Take two Ovral within 72 h of coitus. Repeat if vomiting occurs. Take second dose 12 h later. Menses should begin within 2–3 weeks. Start an ongoing method of contraception immediately after menses.
Progestin Only		
Progestin-only pills are taken daily, with no pill-free days. Preferred for women who are breast-feeding. Does not suppress lactation. Inhibits ovulation. Thickens cervical mucus. Alters uterine lining. Lower cardiovascular risk than combined pills.	Menstrual changes, breakthrough bleeding, prolonged cycles, or amenorrhea. Increase incidence of functional cysts of the ovary, ectopic pregnancy.	Use alternative contraception when starting POPs or if pill is missed. Take pill at same time every day. Keep record of menses and undergo pregnancy testing if 2 weeks late.
Medroxyprogesterone is a progestin-only drug given by injection q 3 mo. A private, convenient, and highly effective method. Efficacy similar to that of surgical sterilization.	May cause amenorrhea, headaches, bloating, and weight gain. Return of fertility may be delayed for several months after discontinuation.	Return q 3 mo for injection. Discontinue method for several months before planning to conceive.
Implanon is a thin, flexible rod containing 68 mg of etonogestrel that is inserted subdermally. The device provides contraceptive protection for up to 3 years.	Changes in menstruation patterns, breast tenderness, and weight gain.	Removal must be completed by a trained health care provider. Review patient history, as contraindications include a history of thrombolytic disease, liver disease, and undiagnosed vaginal bleeding.

Table 12.3   Methods of Birth Control—cont'd

DESCRIPTION	SIDE EFFECTS AND COMPLICATIONS	PATIENT EDUCATION
BARRIER METHODS		
Diaphragms are dome-shaped latex caps with a flexible metal ring (varies in size) covering the cervix. Inner surface is coated with spermicide before insertion. Provides mechanical barrier to sperm. Available by prescription, fitted by a professional. Continuing motivation to use is necessary. 87% effective. Failure from improper fitting or placement of device.	Allergy to latex or spermicide.	Demonstrate how to hold, insert, and remove device, using model. Allow for insertion and removal practice sessions. Advise patient that insertion may be done just prior to coitus, but removal should be 6–8 h after coitus. Tell patient to empty bowel and bladder before insertion. Give instructions for cleansing and storing, checking for holes or deterioration. Advise patient that diaphragm must be refitted after pregnancy, weight loss, or weight gain of 15 pounds or more. Advise patient that its use is not suitable if severe pelvic relaxation is present.
Cervical caps are rubber thimble-shaped shields covering cervix, held in place by suction. Spermicide in inner surface provides mechanical barrier to sperm. Fitted by professional. Effectiveness similar to that of diaphragm. Failure from dislodgment and improper fit.	Allergy to rubber; or spermicide, possible cervical irritation or erosion from suction.	Provide sufficient time for practice with insertion and removal (more time than for diaphragm). Give instructions for cleaning, storing, and inspecting for damage. Inform patient that it can be used with abnormalities of vaginal canal but not with cervical inconsistencies or PID.
Condoms		
Male: Thin rubber sheath fitting over erect penis, providing mechanical barrier to sperm. Simple method to use. No prescription necessary. 85% effective. Failure from tearing or slipping during coitus. Used with spermicide. Affords some protection against STIs and HIV transmission.	Possible allergy to rubber or latex; possible decrease in sensation and interference with foreplay.	Advise patient to roll sheath along entire penis, leaving slack at end to receive semen. Inform patient that sharp objects (fingernails) may tear the condom. Tell patient to hold sheath in place when penis is withdrawn to prevent emptying of sperm in or near vagina.
Female: Double-ring system fitted into the vagina up to 8 h before intercourse. No prescription necessary. Affords protection against HIV, cytomegalovirus, and hepatitis B.	No significant side effects; generally acceptable to couple.	Discuss insertion, lubrication, and method of removal. More expensive than male condoms.

Continued

Table 12.3 Methods of Birth Control—cont'd		
DESCRIPTION	SIDE EFFECTS AND COMPLICATIONS	PATIENT EDUCATION
OTHER METHODS		
Intrauterine devices (IUDs) are inserted into uterus; they are flexible objects made of plastic or copper wire (nonmedicated or medicated with substance to alter uterine environment), usually with attached string that protrudes into vagina. Contraception probably provided by inflammatory response in endometrium, preventing implantation. After insertion, no additional equipment necessary. 97% to 99% effective. Failure mainly from undetected expulsion. Most common type used today is Progestasert (contains progestins).	Increased menstrual flow, intramenstrual bleeding, and cramping, especially during early months of use. Possible complications include ectopic pregnancy, pelvic infection, perforation of uterus, infertility. Undetected expulsion of IUD may result in pregnancy.	Discuss techniques and experience of insertion and removal. Inform patient that insertion may be more difficult and expulsion and complications greater in nulliparous patients. Instruct patient to check for string in vagina after each period; report to health care provider if unable to locate. Discuss need for annual pelvic examination and Pap test.
Rhythm method requires periodic abstinence during fertile portion of menstrual cycle. Requires strong motivation, self-control. Complies with all religious doctrines. 60% to 65% effective. Failure from difficulty in determining precise day of ovulation, irregularity of menses.	Inaccurate or incomplete knowledge of menstrual cycle.	Discuss methods to establish baseline menstrual patterns and identify ovulation. Give instructions in use of calendar or basal body temperature method to determine ovulation and fertile period.
Permanent		
Tubal sterilization includes a variety of abdominal and vaginal surgical procedures (laparotomy, laparoscopy, culdoscopy) that permanently prevent sperm and ovum from meeting. Crushing, ligating, clipping, or plugging of fallopian tubes (potentially reversible procedure). Nearly 100% (99.96%) effective. Failure due to recanalization of fallopian tubes, erroneous ligation (see Fig. 12.20).	Bowel injury, hemorrhage, or infection.	Determine whether temporary contraceptives were used and reason for patient's dissatisfaction. Counsel regarding effects of procedure on physiology and sexual performance. Assist in obtaining written informed consent for procedure. Inform patient that procedure may require short-term hospitalization or can be done on outpatient basis.
Hysterectomy is surgical removal of uterus. 100% effective.	Bladder infection, vascular disorders, infection, hemorrhage, pain, psychological adjustment.	Assess or counsel regarding understanding of extent of surgery, altered physiology, complications, and sexual performance. Hysterectomy only performed for reasons other than contraception; sterility is secondary benefit when desired.
Vasectomy is bilateral surgical ligation and resection of ductus deferens.	Hematoma, edema, psychological adjustment (see Fig. 12.21).	Inform patient that procedure is usually done as outpatient procedure and takes 15 to 30 min. Tell patient that alternative form of contraception is needed until no sperm are seen on examination. Explain that procedure does not affect masculinity.

BP, Blood pressure; *HIV,* human immunodeficiency virus; *PID,* pelvic inflammatory disease; *STI,* sexually transmitted infection.

Modified from Lewis SL, Heitkemper MM, Dirksen SR, et al: *Medical-surgical nursing: assessment and management of clinical problems,* ed 7, St. Louis, 2007, Mosby.

Table 12.4	Planning and Setting Goals for the Patient With a Reproductive Disorder	
PATIENT PROBLEM	**GOAL**	**OUTCOME**
Impaired Coping, related to fear of positive diagnosis of breast cancer	Patient will attend cancer support group weekly.	Patient expresses fears of unfavorable outcome.
Insufficient Knowledge, regarding postoperative care at home after modified radical mastectomy	Patient will state four postoperative risks before discharge.	Patient verbalizes signs and symptoms of infection. Patient demonstrates exercises for affected arm. Patient verbalizes need to avoid injections and taking of blood or blood pressure in affected arm. Patient verbalizes need to examine remaining breast once a month.

- *Impaired Health Maintenance*
- *Impaired Self-Esteem due to Current Situation*
- *Impaired Sexual Function*
- *Insufficient Fluid Volume*
- *Insufficient Knowledge*
- *Potential for Infection*
- *Prolonged Low Self-Esteem*
- *Prolonged Pain*
- *Recent Onset of Pain*

◆ EXPECTED OUTCOMES AND PLANNING

Planning is a category of nursing behaviors in which patient-centered goals are established and strategies designed to achieve the goals and outcomes that relate to the identified patient problem (Table 12.4).

◆ IMPLEMENTATION

The implementation step for the patient with a reproductive disorder is the action-oriented phase of the nursing process, in which the nurse initiates and carries out the objectives of the nursing care plan. See the Complementary and Alternative Therapies box for additional treatment methods.

 Complementary and Alternative Therapies

Male and Female Reproductive Disorders

MALE REPRODUCTIVE SYSTEM
- Yohimbine *(Pausinystalia yohimbe)* for erectile dysfunction and impotence

FEMALE REPRODUCTIVE SYSTEM
- Biofeedback, therapeutic touch, and acupuncture for primary dysmenorrhea
- Black cohosh *(Cimicifuga racemosa)* for menstrual irregularity, premenstrual syndrome (PMS), and menopausal problems
- Chamomile *(Matricaria recutita, Chamaemelum nobile)* for menstrual cramps
- Chaste tree *(Vitex agnus-castus)* for PMS
- Evening primrose *(Oenothera biennis)* for PMS
- Feverfew *(Tanacetum parthenium)* for menstrual problems
- Sage *(Salvia officinalis)* for menstrual irregularity
- Soybeans and other legumes for their phytoestrogens that may help prevent breast cancer

Modified from Black JM, Hawks HJ: Medical-surgical nursing: Clinical management for positive outcomes, ed 8, Philadelphia, 2009, Saunders.

◆ EVALUATION

Examples of goals and their corresponding evaluative measures include the following:

Goal 1: Patient will be able to cope effectively.

Evaluative measure: Patient verbalizes fears and identifies two strategies for dealing with fear, such as questioning for clarification and relaxation breathing technique.

Goal 2: Patient will have adequate knowledge regarding postoperative care at home after modified radical mastectomy.

Evaluative measures: Patient states signs and symptoms of wound infection; lists proper arm exercises; verbalizes the need for BSE once per month; and states the need to avoid blood pressure checks, injections, and blood draws in affected arm.

Get Ready for the NCLEX® Examination!

Key Points

- Sperm are produced in the seminiferous tubules and stored in the epididymis.
- Testosterone, the male sex hormone, is responsible for male secondary sex characteristics.
- Seminal fluid is produced in the seminal vesicles, prostate gland, and Cowper glands.
- The male urethra serves the twofold purpose of conveying urine from the bladder and carrying the reproductive cells and secretions to the outside.
- The uterus consists of three layers of tissue: (1) endometrium, the inner layer; (2) myometrium, the middle layer; and (3) perimetrium, the outer layer.
- In the ovulating female, an egg matures each month in the graafian follicle, which is located in the ovary.
- The menstrual cycle prepares the body for the potential of pregnancy each month.
- Hormone levels systematically rise and fall in response to defined points in the menstrual cycle. Alterations in hormone levels will impact ovulation and menstruation.
- Early diagnosis and prompt management are necessary to prevent serious reproductive and genital problems.
- Health teaching for patients with menstrual disturbances includes a knowledge of the physiologic process, factors that alter menstruation, personal hygiene, exercise, diet, and pain management.
- Discharge planning is vital to prevent reinfection after PID.
- Pregnancy is encouraged in the patient with endometriosis, because it will slow the progress of the disorder; infertility is a complication as the condition continues.
- Menarche, the first menstrual cycle, usually begins around the age of 12 years.
- Serum CA-125 assessment is useful mainly to signal a recurrence of ovarian cancer and in monitoring the response to treatment.
- PSA is a highly sensitive blood test that is elevated in cancer of the prostate and in benign prostatic hyperplasia.
- There is no definitive test for TSS. However, cervical-vaginal isolates of *Staphylococcus aureus* are present 90% of the time with TSS.
- Vaginal fistulas are caused by an ulcerating process resulting from cancer, radiation, weakening of tissue from pregnancies, or surgical interventions.
- Correction of cystocele and rectocele is a surgical repair involving shortening of the muscles that support the bladder and repair of the rectocele. This is known as anteroposterior colporrhaphy.

- Screening tests for cervical abnormalities include routine Pap tests (a newer, liquid-based Pap test is recommended) and testing for HPV.
- Vaccines are now available that reduce the incidence of cervical cancer resulting from infection with HPV (types 6, 11, 16, 18).
- A panhysterosalpingo-oophorectomy involves removal of the uterus, fallopian tubes, and ovaries.
- In patients with breast cancer an axillary lymph node dissection usually is performed regardless of treatment options available. Examination of nodes provides the most powerful prognostic data currently available.
- A relatively new diagnostic tool used before therapeutic surgery for breast cancer is sentinel lymph node mapping, which identifies the first lymph node most likely to drain the cancerous cells.
- Overall, 10-year survival with lumpectomy and radiation is about the same as with modified radical mastectomy.
- After losing a breast, many patients experience acute grief that may last 4 to 6 weeks or longer. Grief makes the fact of loss real.
- Caution patients who have undergone a modified radical mastectomy to avoid injections, vaccinations, taking of blood pressure or blood samples, or insertion of IV line in the affected arm.
- Phimosis is a condition in which the prepuce is too small to retract over the glans penis.
- Young men should be taught to perform TSE monthly beginning at 15 years of age for detection of testicular carcinoma.
- Oral acyclovir is prescribed for primary genital herpes to shorten the duration of healing and to suppress 75% of recurrence with daily use.
- Parenteral penicillin remains the treatment of choice for all stages of syphilis. All stages of syphilis should be treated.
- Because of penicillin-resistant strains of *N. gonorrhoeae*, penicillin, the former drug of choice for treatment of gonorrhea, has been changed to ceftriaxone.
- Chlamydial infections respond to treatment with tetracycline, doxycycline, azithromycin, or ofloxacin. Erythromycin is the drug of choice for use in pregnant patients.

Additional Learning Resources

SG Go to your Study Guide for additional learning activities to help you master this chapter content.

Be sure to visit the Evolve site at http://evolve.elsevier.com/Cooper/adult for additional online resources.

Review Questions for the NCLEX® Examination

1. A patient visits her health care provider because of an increase in her abdominal girth and dyspnea during the past month. She is diagnosed as having ovarian cancer. The cause for these manifestations can be explained by what physiologic occurrence?

   1. Development of ascites
   2. Metastasis to the bowel
   3. Dilation of the alveoli
   4. Bladder distention

2. The nurse is discussing breast self-examination with a 30-year-old premenopausal patient. When should the nurse advise is the best time for the patient to perform her monthly self-examination of the breasts?

   1. During her menstruation
   2. 7 to 8 days after conclusion of the menstrual period
   3. The same day each month
   4. The 26th day of the menstrual cycle

3. A 52-year-old patient has ductal cell carcinoma of the left breast. After a modified radical mastectomy, a Davol drain is placed in the left axillary region. What is the primary purpose of this drain?

   1. To control numbness of her left incisional site
   2. To improve her ability to perform range-of-motion exercises on her affected side
   3. To facilitate drainage and to prevent formation of a hematoma
   4. To prevent postoperative phlebitis in her affected arm

4. A 35-year-old patient has undergone a vasectomy. Teaching for this patient should include what information? *(Select all that apply.)*

   1. The procedure is reversible if he later changes his mind.
   2. He should abstain from sexual intercourse until the incision is completely healed.
   3. He should apply warm compresses to the scrotum four times a day.
   4. He should return to the health care provider at regular intervals for sperm counts.
   5. Contraceptive use is indicated in the initial weeks after the procedure.

5. A 44-year-old patient is admitted for an abdominal hysterectomy. She is instructed that she will have a Foley catheter in place postoperatively. She asks the nurse how many days she will have the catheter in place. What is the best response by the nurse?

   1. "The indwelling catheter will probably remain in place for 1 week."
   2. "The indwelling catheter will be removed after you are fully awake from the anesthesia."
   3. "The indwelling catheter will generally be removed on the first postoperative day."
   4. "The indwelling catheter will remain in place for a few days after discharge."

6. A 60-year-old patient underwent a vaginal hysterectomy for a prolapsed uterus. The nurse is aware that patients undergoing pelvic surgery are more susceptible to what postoperative complications? *(Select all that apply.)*

   1. Wound dehiscence
   2. Postoperative loss of libido
   3. Urinary retention
   4. Venous stasis
   5. Thrombophlebitis
   6. Sexually transmitted infections (STIs)
   7. Pneumonia
   8. Pelvic inflammatory disease
   9. Sepsis

7. A 49-year-old obese patient has had a total abdominal hysterectomy. On the second postoperative day, the patient complains of increased pain in the operative site. She states, "It feels like something suddenly popped." With the symptoms presented, it would be likely that when the nurse removes the abdominal dressing she may note what occurrence?

   1. The wound has a purulent exudate.
   2. Dehiscence has occurred.
   3. The wound is indurated and tender.
   4. The wound is well approximated.

8. A 20-year-old patient goes to the health care provider's office with vaginal pruritus, burning, dull pelvic pain, and purulent vaginal discharge. A diagnostic test reveals she has chlamydia. What nursing interventions would best promote a successful patient outcome? *(Select all that apply.)*

   1. Encourage her to have her sexual partner(s) seek medical care as soon as possible to avoid reinfection of the patient.
   2. Recommend she abstain from sexual contact while lesions are present.
   3. Provide social and emotional support because the edematous, draining lymph nodes may be disturbing to the patient's self-image.
   4. Educate the patient that the causative organism is a spirochete that gains entrance into the body during intercourse.
   5. Discuss means to prevent future exposures to this infection.

9. A 23-year-old man is diagnosed with gonorrhea. Because of statements made in his patient interview, the nurse has established a patient problem of *Nonconformity*. Which is the most effective way to overcome *Nonconformity* for this patient?

   1. Telephone follow-up
   2. Case finding
   3. Single-dose treatment of ceftriaxone (Rocephin) IM
   4. Extensive patient education program

10. The nurse is teaching a group of teenagers about contraception and sexually transmitted infections (STIs). The nurse asks the students if they know which is the most prevalent STI. Which response by the participants is correct?

   1. Syphilis
   2. Chlamydial infection
   3. Gonorrhea
   4. Genital herpes

11. A 73-year-old patient comes to the health care provider's office with a complaint of constant seepage of feces from her vagina. These manifestations are most consistent with what condition?

   1. Rectovaginal fistula
   2. Vesicovaginal fistula
   3. Urethrovaginal fistula
   4. Rectocele

12. The American Cancer Society recommends that women have an annual screening mammography beginning at what age?

   1. 21 years
   2. 35 years
   3. 40 years
   4. 52 years

13. The first lymph node most likely to drain the cancerous site in a patient with breast cancer is known as the:

   1. axillary node.
   2. contaminated node.
   3. primary node.
   4. sentinel node.

14. While discussing breast cancer with a group of women, what should the nurse stress as the greatest risk factor for breast cancer?

   1. Being a woman over the age of 50 years
   2. Experiencing menstruation for 40 years or more
   3. Using estrogen replacement therapy during menopause
   4. Having a paternal grandmother with postmenopausal breast cancer

15. A patient diagnosed with breast cancer has been offered the treatment choice of breast conservation surgery with radiation or a modified radical mastectomy. Which statement by the patient concerning the lumpectomy with radiation indicates understanding of the procedure?

   1. "It preserves the normal appearance and sensitivity of the breast."
   2. "It provides a shorter treatment period with fewer long-term complications."
   3. "It has about the same 10-year survival rate as the modified radical mastectomy."
   4. "It has a much higher survival rate than the modified radical mastectomy."

16. The nurse is educating a patient who has undergone a modified radical mastectomy in ways to prevent lymphedema. What should the nurse include in the information provided? *(Select all that apply.)*

   1. Use a sling for the first 2 weeks after the procedure.
   2. Expose the arm to sunlight to increase circulation.
   3. Wrap the arm with elastic bandages during the night.
   4. Avoid unnecessary trauma (e.g., venipuncture, blood pressure) to the arm on the operative side.
   5. Elevate the hand and arm above the level of the chest.

17. The nurse plans early and frequent ambulation for a patient who has undergone an abdominal hysterectomy to: *(Select all that apply.)*

   1. prevent urinary retention.
   2. prevent deep-vein thrombosis.
   3. relieve abdominal distention.
   4. maintain a sense of normalcy.
   5. reduce postoperative nausea.

18. On the second postoperative day, a 63-year-old patient who underwent an abdominal hysterectomy complains of gas pains and abdominal distention. The patient has not had a bowel movement since surgery. Which nursing intervention will best stimulate peristalsis and relieve distention?

   1. Offering carbonated beverages
   2. Encouraging ambulation at least four times daily
   3. Administering a 1000-mL soapsuds enema
   4. Applying an abdominal binder

19. A 40-year-old patient has a history of multiple births in the past 15 years. Her health care provider is concerned she has a cystocele. What manifestations provide support to the diagnosis?

   1. Rectal pressure
   2. Dysmenorrhea
   3. Hemorrhoids
   4. Urinary frequency

20. The nurse is assisting the health care provider with a Pap test. What condition will be diagnosed by this diagnostic study?

   1. Cervical cancer
   2. Breast cancer
   3. Pelvic inflammatory disease
   4. Ovarian cancer

21. A patient has reported to the emergency department. The health care provider suspects toxic shock syndrome. What manifestations confirm this suspicion? *(Select all that apply.)*

   1. Sudden high fever
   2. Vaginal hemorrhage
   3. Diarrhea
   4. Sudden hypertension
   5. Headache

22. Lower abdominal and lower back pain that increases in severity during menstruation may signal which condition?

   1. Cervical polyp
   2. Ovarian tumor
   3. Endometriosis
   4. Uterine cancer

23. The nurse is reviewing the health history of an assigned patient. The patient was treated for pelvic inflammatory disease. What conditions may be noted in the patient's history as a result of the condition? *(Select all that apply.)*

   1. Vaginal discharge
   2. Infertility
   3. Hemorrhage
   4. Dyspareunia
   5. Dysmenorrhea

24. Which woman is most likely to develop toxic shock syndrome?

    1. The woman with multiple sexual contacts
    2. The woman who inserts tampons with her fingers
    3. The woman with untreated chronic PID
    4. The woman who has undergone multiple abortions

25. A patient is scheduled to have a Pap test. The nurse can provide correct information about preparing for the examination by including what information?

    1. Use a mild vinegar douche the night before the test.
    2. Abstain from intercourse 24 hours before the test.
    3. Take a warm tub bath the night before the test.
    4. Save a first-voided morning urine specimen.

26. A patient's husband tells the nurse that his wife, who has been diagnosed with inoperable ovarian cancer, is talking about dying and her fear of death. He asks the nurse for suggestions to help his wife. Which response by the nurse would be most helpful?

    1. "Your wife will probably die of another disease before she dies of ovarian cancer."
    2. "Talk of death is normal at this time, but will diminish in the future."
    3. "Your wife is expressing acceptance of the need for hospice care."
    4. "It is perfectly normal to want to talk about death. It is most helpful to support her by listening."

Care of the Patient With a Sensory Disorder

Objectives

Anatomy and Physiology

1. Describe structures and functions of the visual and auditory systems.
2. Explain normal vision and hearing physiologic processes.
3. Differentiate between abnormal and normal physical assessments of the visual and auditory systems.

Medical-Surgical

4. Describe two age-related changes and assessment findings in the visual and auditory systems.
5. Discuss the refractory errors of astigmatism, strabismus, myopia, and hyperopia, including etiology, pathophysiology, clinical manifestations, assessment, diagnostic tests, medical management, nursing interventions, and patient teaching.
6. Describe inflammatory conditions of the eye, including etiology, pathophysiology, clinical manifestations, assessment, diagnostic tests, medical management, nursing interventions, patient teaching, and prognoses.
7. Discuss Sjögren syndrome, ectropion, and entropion, including etiology, pathophysiology, clinical manifestations, diagnostic tests, medical management, nursing interventions, and prognosis.
8. Compare and contrast the nature of cataracts, diabetic retinopathy, macular degeneration, retinal detachment, and glaucoma, including the etiology, pathophysiology, clinical manifestations, assessment, diagnostic tests, medical management, nursing interventions, patient teaching, and prognoses.
9. Comprehend corneal injuries, including etiology, pathophysiology, clinical manifestations, assessment, diagnostic tests, medical management, nursing interventions, patient teaching, and prognoses.
10. Describe the various surgeries of the eye, including the nursing interventions and prognoses.
11. Differentiate between conductive and sensorineural hearing loss.
12. Describe the appropriate care of the hearing aid.
13. List tips for communicating with people with visual and hearing impairments.
14. Identify communication resources for people with visual and/or hearing impairment.
15. Describe inflammatory and infectious and noninfectious disorders of the ear, including etiology, pathophysiology, clinical manifestations, assessment, diagnostic tests, medical management, nursing interventions, patient teaching, and prognoses.
16. Explain the various surgeries of the ear, including the nursing interventions, patient teaching, and prognoses.

Key Terms

astigmatism (ă-STĬG-mă-tĭsm, p. 615)
audiometry (ăw-dē-ŎM-ĕ-trē, p. 638)
automated perimetry test (ĂW-tō-māt-ĕd pĕr-Ĭ-mĕt-rē, p. 608)
cataract (KĂT-ă-răkt, p. 621)
conjunctivitis (kŏn-jŭnk-tĭ-VĪ-tĭs, p. 617)
cryotherapy (krī-ō-THĔR-ă-pē, p. 625)
diabetic retinopathy (dī-ă-BĔT-ĭk rĕ-tĭn-NŎP-ă-thē, p. 624)
enucleation (ē-nū-klē-Ā-shŭn, p. 634)
glaucoma (glăw-KŌ-mă, p. 628)
Goldmann tonometry (GŌLD-măn tōn-Ŏ-mĕt-rē, p. 612)
hyperopia (hī-pĕr-Ō-pē-ă, p. 615)
keratitis (kĕr-ă-TĪ-tĭs, p. 619)
keratoplasty (kĕr-ă-tō-PLĂS-tē, p. 634)
keratotomy (kĕ-ră-TŎT-ŏ-mē, p. 616)
labyrinthitis (lăb-ĭ-rĭnth-Ī-tĭs, p. 645)
mastoiditis (măs-tŏy-DĪ-tĭs, p. 643)

miotics (mī-ŎT-ĭks, p. 630)
mydriatics (mĭd-rē-ĂT-ĭks, p. 612)
myopia (mī-Ō-pē-ă, p. 615)
myringotomy (mĭr-ĭn-GŎT-ŏ-mē, p. 643)
photocoagulation (fō-tō-kō-ăg-yū-LĀ-shŭn, p. 625)
refraction (rē-FRĂK-shŭn, p. 612)
retinal detachment (RĔ-tĭ-năl dē-TĂCH-mĕnt, p. 627)
Sjögren syndrome (SHĔR-grĕn SĪN-drōm, p. 620)
Snellen test (SNĔL-ĕn tĕst, p. 611)
stapedectomy (stā-pĕ-DĔK-tŏ-mē, p. 650)
strabismus (stră-BĬZ-mŭs, p. 615)
tinnitus (TĬ-nĭ-tĭs, p. 643)
tympanoplasty (tĭm-pă-nō-PLĂS-tē, p. 650)
umami (p. 651)
vertigo (VĔR-tĭ-gō, p. 639)
vitrectomy (vĭ-TRĔK-tŏ-mē, p. 635)

ANATOMIC STRUCTURES AND PHYSIOLOGIC FUNCTIONS OF THE VISUAL SYSTEM

ANATOMY OF THE EYE

The primary sensory system of the human body is the visual system. The visual system consists of highly sensitive tissues and structures that surround the eye and the many layered tunics of the globe (eyeball) that protect and control the refractory media and visual pathways. The eyes are 1-inch (2.5 cm) spherical structures that contain 70% of the sensory receptors of the body. The optic tracts contain more than 1 million nerve fibers that carry messages from the eyes to the brain, where they are interpreted. Only a small portion of each eye is visible externally; the remainder is enclosed in the *orbit*. The orbits consist of orbital bones of the face and cushioned in layers of fat. The orbital bones include the frontal, zygomatic, ethmoid, sphenoid, and lacrimal.

STRUCTURE OF THE EYE

External Structures of the Eye

The external structures of the eye include the eyebrows, eyelashes, lids, and the lacrimal apparatus. The primary function of the external structures is of a protective capacity. In addition to protection, three pairs of extraocular muscles control each eye. The extraocular paired muscles consist of (1) superior and inferior rectus muscles, (2) medial and lateral rectus muscles, and (3) superior and inferior oblique muscles. The extraocular muscles control eye movement via cranial nerves III (ocular nerve), IV (trochlear nerve), and VI (abducens nerve).

The *lacrimal apparatus* (Fig. 13.1) manufactures and drains tears to keep the eye moist and to sweep away debris that may enter the eye. Tears are composed of a watery secretion that contains salt, mucus, and a bactericidal enzyme, *lysozyme*. The lacrimal glands are located superior and lateral to each eye. Blinking causes tears to flow medially to the lacrimal ducts, which empty into the nasolacrimal ducts and drain into the nasal cavity.

The *conjunctiva* is a thin, transparent mucous membrane that lines the inner aspect of the eyelids and the anterior surface of the eye to the edge of the cornea. The lower conjunctival sac is where eyedrops and eye ointment medication usually are administered.

Internal Structures of the Eye

The eye is composed of three layers, or tunics (Fig. 13.2). The outermost layer of the eye is the fibrous tunic; it is composed of the sclera and the cornea. The *sclera* is a thick, white, opaque structure composed of collagen fibers meshed together and is known as the white of the eye. The sclera gives shape to the eye and, because of its toughness, protects the intraocular structures.

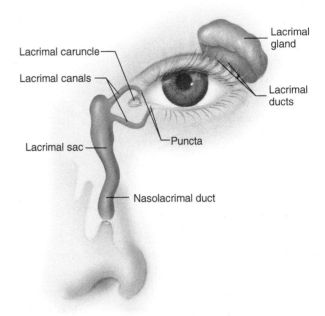

Fig. 13.1 Lacrimal apparatus. (From Patton KT, Thibodeau GA: *Anatomy and physiology*, ed 10, St. Louis, 2019, Elsevier.)

The *cornea* is the central anterior portion of the sclera. It is a transparent clear layer that covers the iris, which is the colored portion of the eye. The cornea allows light rays to enter the inner portion of the eye and is the first part of the eye that refracts (bends) light rays. The cornea is a dense layer that is uniform in thickness, nonvascular, and projects like a dome beyond the sclera. The cornea is one of the most highly developed, sensitive tissues in the body and is innervated by cranial nerve V (trigeminal nerve). The avascular cornea obtains oxygen primarily through absorption from the tear film layer that bathes the epithelium. A small amount of oxygen is obtained from the *aqueous humor* (watery fluid in front of the lens in the anterior chamber of the eye) through the endothelial layers. The degree of corneal curvature varies in each individual and progressively changes as the patient ages. The curvature is more pronounced in youth and changes to a more flattened curve in advancing age.

The junction of the sclera and cornea is called the *canal of Schlemm*. This tiny venous sinus, at the angle of the anterior chamber of the eye, drains the aqueous humor and funnels it into the bloodstream. This helps control intraocular pressure (IOP, the pressure within the eye).

The middle layer of the eye is the *vascular tunic*. It includes the choroid, the ciliary body, and the iris. The posterior portion of the vascular tunic is the *choroid*, which is a thin, dark brown membrane that lines most of the internal area of the sclera. It is extremely vascular and supplies nutrients to the retina. The anterior portion of the vascular tunic forms the ciliary body, which is an intrinsic muscular ring that holds the lens in place and changes its shape for near or distant vision. The

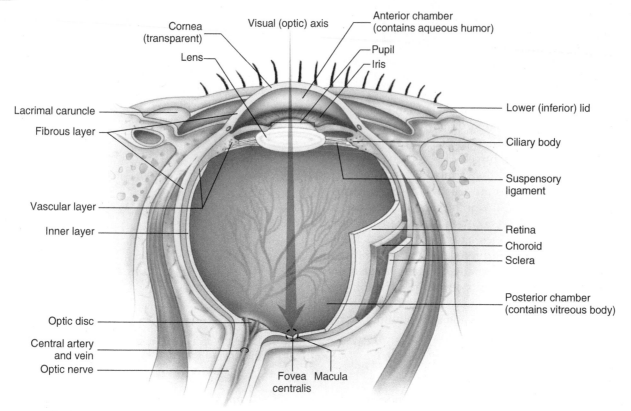

Fig. 13.2 Horizontal section through the eyeball. The eye is viewed from above. (From Patton KT, Thibodeau GA: *Anatomy and physiology*, ed 10, St. Louis, 2019, Elsevier.)

ciliary body also attaches to the *iris,* which is the pigmented part of the eye. The iris is a flat muscular ring located between the cornea and the lens and contains a round opening in the center, which is known as the *pupil.* The muscular ring of the iris surrounds the pupil to constrict and dilate according to light levels, much like a camera shutter. In darker light, the pupil dilates open to allow an increase of light to enter, and in brighter light the pupil constricts and becomes smaller to allow less light into the eye. Two sets of smooth muscles control the iris, which in turn controls the size of the pupil. In bright light, the circular muscle fibers of the iris contract and the pupil constricts; in dim light, the radial muscles contract and the pupil dilates. Pupillary constriction is a reflex that protects the retina from intense light and permits clearer, acute near vision.

The innermost tunic of the eye is the *retina.* The retina comprises nervous tissue membranes that receive images of external objects and transmits impulses through the optic nerve to the brain. The rods and cones are scattered throughout the retina except where the optic nerve exits the eye. The area where the retinal nerve fibers collect to form the optic nerve is known as the *optic disc;* this area is also called the *blind spot,* because of its lack of photoreceptors. Rods are receptors for vision in dim light and are unable to perceive color. The rods are located primarily in the periphery of the retina and are responsible for peripheral vision. Cones, which are located more centrally in the retina,

require bright light to perceive color. The cones are divided into three types, which are each sensitive to a different color: red, green, or blue. Rod and cone cells respond to light by way of photopsin, a photosensitive pigment, at their tips. The body requires vitamin A to synthesize photopsin.

Located in the center of the retina is the *fovea centralis,* a pinpoint depression composed only of densely packed cone cells. The fovea centralis contains the greatest concentration of cones of any area in the retina. This area of the retina provides the sharpest visual acuity and most acute color vision. Surrounding the fovea is the *macula,* an area of less than 1 mm^2 that has a high concentration of cones and is relatively free of blood vessels. The absence of the three types of cones causes color blindness, which is an inherited condition found primarily in males.

CHAMBERS OF THE EYE

The eye is divided into anterior and posterior chambers by the *crystalline lens,* a transparent, colorless structure that is biconvex, enclosed in a capsule, and held in place just behind the pupil by the suspensory ligament. The crystalline lens focuses light rays so that they form a perfect image on the retina. Anterior to the crystalline lens is the anterior chamber, which is filled with *aqueous humor,* a clear, watery fluid similar to blood plasma. The ciliary bodies of the choroid constantly secrete, drain, and replace aqueous humor to maintain normal IOP. Aqueous humor also helps maintain the eye's shape, keeps the retina attached to the choroid, and refracts light.

The posterior chamber is filled with *vitreous humor,* a transparent, jellylike substance that also gives shape to the eye, keeps the retina attached to the choroid, and refracts light. It differs from the aqueous humor in that it is not replaced continuously.

PHYSIOLOGY OF VISION

Light must travel through the cornea, the aqueous humor, the pupil, the crystalline lens, and the vitreous humor to reach the rods and cones of the retina. The image is transported via the optic nerve to the visual center of the cerebral cortex in the brain.

Four basic processes are necessary to form an image:
1. *Refraction:* The eye is able to bend light rays so that the rays fall onto the retina.
2. *Accommodation:* The eye can focus on objects at various distances. It focuses the image of an object on the retina by changing the curvature of the lens.
3. *Constriction:* The size of the pupil, which is controlled by the dilator and constrictor muscles of the iris, regulates the amount of light entering the eye.
4. *Convergence:* Medial movement of both eyes allows light rays from an object to hit the same point on both retinas.

NURSING CONSIDERATIONS FOR CARE OF THE PATIENT WITH COMMON EYE COMPLICATIONS

In caring for the patient with an eye disorder, review the following items:
- Eye pain, pruritus, photophobia, excessive tearing, dryness, floaters (dark to semitransparent spots in the visual field), light flashes, scotomas (diminished vision in a defined area of the visual field), halos around lights, diplopia (double vision), discharge, visual changes such as depth perception and peripheral vision changes, blind spots, or fading color vision
- Headaches
- Nystagmus (involuntary, rhythmic movements of the eyes)
- History of allergies
- Current medications, over the counter and prescription
- Side effects of any medications
- Use of visual assistive devices (glasses, contact lenses, or magnifying glasses)
- Adequacy of current eyewear prescription
- Personal habits related to care of eyewear
- Any previous eye injuries or surgeries

After gathering the information and reporting it to the health care provider, provide assistance with the eye examination. The results of the initial examination are compared with normal findings (Table 13.1).

Table 13.1   Normal Findings of the Adult Eye

AREA EXAMINED	FINDINGS
Eyelid	Blink reflex to light or touch intact. Lid margins just above the corneal borders
Eyeball	Eyeball does not protrude beyond the supraorbital ridge of the frontal bone. The eyeball is usually moist; moisture may be diminished in the older adult
Conjunctiva	Palpebral (eyelid): Pink, uniform blood vessels without discharge. Bulbar: Clear, tiny red vessels; in the older adult, the bulbar conjunctiva may lose luster
Sclera	Generally white; may have yellow-tan dots in a dark-skinned individual
Cornea	Transparent, smooth, convex. In the older adult, a gray ring around the cornea (arcus senilis) may be present as a result of lipid deposits
Iris	Round, intact, bilateral coloration. In the older adult, color may be paler and shape less regular
Pupil	Equal, round, reactive to light and accommodation. Response to light is equal bilaterally. In the older adult, constriction response may be slower
Internal eye (including retina, vessels, and optic disc)	Retina is intact. Vessel structure is intact and bilaterally similar in pattern. Optic disc has well-defined border
Visual Acuity	
Distant vision	20/20 (able to read line 11 of eye chart at a distance of 20 ft.)
Near vision	Able to read newspaper print at 14 inches
Peripheral vision	Side vision 90 degrees from central visual axis; upward 50 degrees; downward 70 degrees
Eye movement	Coordinated eye movement bilaterally
Color perception	Able to properly identify colors of major groups: red, blue, and green

LABORATORY AND DIAGNOSTIC EXAMINATIONS

After the review of the medical history and any complaints, an initial eye examination is performed. The goals of the examination are to evaluate visual acuity, visual fields, refraction, peripheral vision, and overall health of the eye and supportive structures. Additional diagnostic testing may be performed to assess for disorders or to determine progression of disease.

The most commonly performed examination is the Snellen test, which assesses visual acuity. The patient is placed 20 feet from the Snellen chart and asked to read lines (Fig. 13.3). The degree of vision is evaluated and

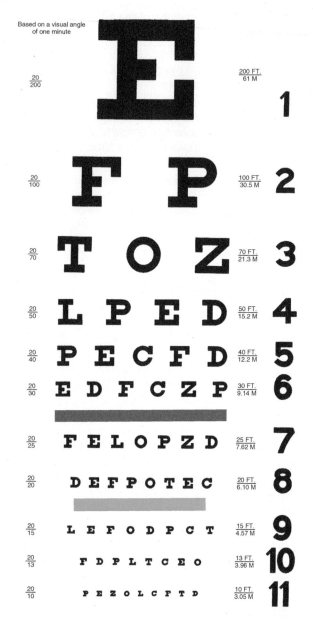

Fig. 13.3 Snellen chart. (From Patton KT, Thibodeau GA: *Laboratory manual for anatomy and physiology*, ed 10, St. Louis, 2019, Elsevier.)

the patient's acuity is assigned. Vision said to be 20/20 indicates that the individual has normal vision and can read at 20 feet the prescribed line. Vision identified as 20/40 indicates the patient can read at 40 feet what the normal eye can see at 20 feet. The chart is modified for children by using shapes or pictures.

Refraction refers to the bending of light rays as they enter the retina. An inability of the eye to accommodate the images seen is known as refractive errors. Refractive errors are diagnosed by asking the patient to sit with his or her chin resting on a supportive bar and looking into a device. The patient then is asked to read 20 feet away, using a variety of lenses. As the lenses are changed, the patient is asked to evaluate the clarity of the information viewed. The left and right eyes will be evaluated both individually and together. The result will determine the degree of visual acuity. Potential diagnoses of visual disorders include hyperopia, myopia, astigmatism, and presbyopia (Table 13.2).

Visual field assessment is key in the evaluation of vision. There are six visual fields. The examination identifies the loss or deterioration of any field. Sitting straight in front of the patient, the examiner reviews the patient's ability to see items as they are moved into the field of vision. The automated perimetry test places the patient in front of a computer-like device and asks him or her to stare at a screen and to press a button when flashes of light enter the field of vision (NLM, 2019).

The Amsler grid assesses for disturbances in central vision. It is used to evaluate the health of the macula, identifying conditions such as macular degeneration. Black grid markings are superimposed on a white background. A centralized black dot is used as the point of reference. The patient is asked to view the grid, concentrating on the dot, and report areas of distortion (Fig. 13.4).

The *slit lamp examination* uses magnification devices to view the eyelids, sclera, iris, conjunctiva, and cornea (Porter, 2018). A slit lamp also can help evaluate IOP by tonometry to detect glaucoma. Dilating drops (mydriatics) may be used to evaluate internal surfaces and will cause photosensitivity for a few hours after the examination. Conditions that may be diagnosed by this technique include cataracts, corneal injury, macular degeneration, and disorders of the retina, including detachment, vessel occlusion, and retinitis pigmentosa.

Retinal blood flow may be evaluated by *fluorescein angiography*. Dye is injected into vessels of the arm or hand. This is an invasive procedure requiring the patient's consent. The patient should be instructed that urine could be darkened or possibly orange for a few days after the test. Assess for allergies to seafood or iodine because this also may cause sensitivity to the dye used in the examination. Conditions that may be diagnosed by this test include retinal detachment, retinopathy, tumors, and macular degeneration (NLM, 2020a).

Today the measurement of IOP (*tonometry*) is done most commonly by puffing air onto the surface of the open eye (NLM, 2020b). The eye pressure is measured by evaluating how the light reflections change as the air hits the eye (Fig. 13.5). A more invasive study is Goldmann tonometry, in which the eye is numbed and a cone-shaped device is used to depress the eyeball gently to assess for internal pressure.

DISORDERS OF THE EYE

BLINDNESS AND NEAR BLINDNESS
Etiology and Pathophysiology
Blindness is a loss of visual acuity that ranges from partial to total loss of sight. Total blindness is defined as no light perception and no usable vision. Functional

Table 13.2   **Common Refractory Errors**

DESCRIPTION	ETIOLOGY AND PATHOPHYSIOLOGY	CLINICAL MANIFESTATIONS
Astigmatism: Defect in the curvature of the eyeball surface	May be hereditary or a muscular deficit Occurs when light rays cannot be focused clearly on a point on the retina because of an abnormal curvature of the cornea	Blurring of vision Difficulty focusing Complaints of eye discomfort
Esotropia: A form of strabismus in which one or both eyes turn in the direction of the nose	The eyes are unable to simultaneously fix on an object	Difficulty following objects visually
Exotropia: A form of strabismus in which one or both eyes turn outward, away from the nose		Only one eye focuses or is able to track a moving object
Hyperopia: Condition of farsightedness	May result from error of refraction in which rays of light entering the eye are brought into focus behind the retina	Inability to see objects at close range
Myopia: Condition of nearsightedness	Elongation of the eyeball or an error in refraction so that parallel rays are focused in front of the retina	Inability to see objects at a distance
Strabismus: Inability of the eyes to focus in the same direction; commonly referred to as being *cross-eyed*	May result from neurologic or muscular dysfunction, or may be inherited	The positions of the eyeballs are not symmetric

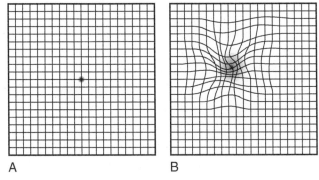

A   B

Fig. 13.4 Amsler grid. (From Miller RG, Ashar BH, Sisson SD: *The Johns Hopkins internal medicine board review: 2010–2011*, ed 3, Philadelphia, 2010, Mosby.)

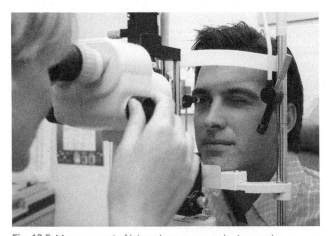

Fig. 13.5 Measurement of internal eye pressure by tonometry. (Copyright 1999–2012 Thinkstock. All rights reserved.)

blindness is present when the patient has some light perception but no usable vision. It may be congenital or acquired.

The Centers for Disease Control and Prevention estimates that in the United States approximately 1.02 million people are blind and more than another 3 million suffer a vision impairment that is uncorrectable. The number of blind individuals is expected to increase twofold by 2050 (CDC, 2020). The estimates for patients with visual problems and potentially blinding diseases range from 21 to 80 million people in the United States. *Legal blindness* refers to individuals with a maximum visual acuity of 20/200 with corrective eyewear and/or visual field sight capacity reduced to 20 degrees (the normal visual field range is 180 degrees).

Categories have been established to help determine the exact extent of vision loss and what assistive measures are appropriate for the individual. These categories range from low vision loss (20/70 to 20/200) to

three categories of blindness (20/400, 20/1200, and no light perception).

Congenital blindness results from various birth defects. Acquired blindness in adults occurs as a result of disorders such as diabetic retinopathy, glaucoma, cataracts, retinal degeneration, infections, tumors, and acute trauma.

Clinical Manifestations

The degree of vision loss depends on the extent of trauma or disease. Symptoms may include diplopia (double vision), blurred vision, pain, and presence of floaters or flashes of light in the visual field, light sensitivity, and burning of the eyes. Additional physical manifestations of the visually impaired patient may include loss of peripheral vision; halos (described as rainbow colors seen around lights); a sense of increased orbital pressure; bulging of the eye(s); and any difference in the appearance of an eye structure, such as the pupil.

The wide variety of emotions associated with blindness range from fear, anxiety, disorientation, depression, helplessness, and hopelessness to acceptance. The patient may experience poor interpersonal communication skills and coping mechanisms. Because self-care skills may be impaired, an individual who is blind may prefer isolation, causing additional physical and emotional difficulties.

Assessment

Subjective data may include patient reports of blurred vision, diplopia, loss of visual fields, halos, or increased pressure as early symptoms of eye disorders. It is important for the health care provider to determine the onset, severity, and duration of symptoms or pain, as well as any factors that relieve them.

Objective data may include a functional vision assessment (FVA). According to the American Foundation for the Blind (n.d.), an FVA investigates visual functionality for near task (closer than 16 inches [0.4 m]), intermediate task (16 inches to 3 feet [0.4 to 0.9 m]), and then a distance task (more than 3 feet). The assessment also includes visual acuity, visual field, contrast sensitivity, and color vision. It is also important to note the patient's compensation measures, such as use of a magnifying glass, as well as the effectiveness of the patient's current use of assistive eyewear.

Medical Management

Corrective eyewear is the first method of medical management for a partially sighted patient. If the visual defect results from an inflammatory disorder, medication appropriate to the causative agent is prescribed.

Additional assistive devices for a visually impaired patient include canes, guide dogs, magnifying systems, computers, and telescopic lenses. An eye specialist should evaluate the patient to determine which devices are best suited for the level of vision loss. Some of the more technologically complex devices are expensive and may not be covered by insurance.

Canes are the most frequently used devices for the partially or totally blind person. They are lightweight and portable and allow the patient simple maneuvering. The drawback is that canes usually do not help in detecting overhead objects. Guide dogs can be helpful in this respect; they allow the person who is visually impaired increased mobility that otherwise would be difficult to achieve independently. Trained guide dogs steer the patient away from obstacles and assist the patient to move through crowds. The guide dog is trained to detect curbs, stairs, and elevations that may cause the patient to fall or stumble.

The patient requires instruction on ambulatory safety before using ambulatory aids or assistants. Advise the patient to walk slowly; obtain verbal clues from the

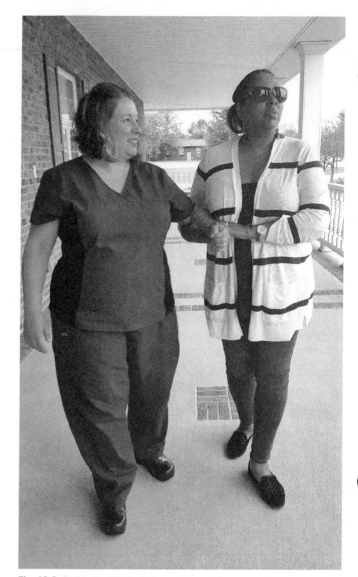

Fig. 13.6 Sighted-guide technique. The walking companion serves as the sighted guide, walking slightly ahead of the patient with the patient holding the back of the companion's arm.

walking companion, if present; and touch objects or borders with the tip of the cane to determine the boundaries of obstructions. The walking companion should precede the patient by about 1 foot, with the patient's hand on the companion's elbow for security (Fig. 13.6). Describe the surroundings when assisting the patient with visual impairment in new surroundings.

Surgical correction of the visual defect may provide improved eyesight. Laser surgeries provide excellent results in selected cases. Corneal transplants can restore vision in patients with corneal damage.

Nursing Interventions and Patient Teaching

Understand that the complications of loss of vision or blindness could result in physical and emotional manifestations by the patient. Assess the patient's ability to perform self-care and provide assistance with activities of daily living (ADLs) as needed. Allowing the patient adequate time to assist in self-care helps

Box 13.1	Guidelines for Communicating With People Who Are Visually Impaired

- Announce your presence when entering the room.
- Talk in a normal tone of voice.
- Do not try to avoid common phrases in speech, such as "See what I mean?"
- Introduce yourself with each contact (unless well known to the person).
- Explain any activity occurring in the room.
- Announce when you are leaving the room so that the blind person is not put in the position of talking to someone who is no longer there.

PATIENT PROBLEM	NURSING INTERVENTIONS
Fearfulness, related to visual loss or impairment	Determine the patient's level of fear Actively listen to the patient's concerns/fears and assist with addressing the issues with the appropriate resources
Potential for Injury, related to new/ unfamiliar environment	Orient the patient to the new environment Use therapeutic touch Avoid loud sounds that may startle the patient Use protective and assistive devices, such as side rails and canes Alter surroundings to create a safe environment (e.g., clear walkways, remove throw rugs)

foster independence and promotes the confidence of the patient to perform daily activities. Nursing interventions for patients with visual impairments must include consideration of emotional aspects, including appropriate communication (Box 13.1).

Vision loss affects not only the patient but also family, friends, and the community. Individuals have different coping mechanisms; consider this when caring for the visually impaired patient. Be aware of the services and devices available for the patient with a visual impairment and make appropriate referrals. Over time, with treatment and rehabilitation, the patient with visual impairment can develop the skills necessary to become independent in daily life. The primary resource for services for the patient who is legally blind is the local government; each state has a department for rehabilitation of the blind. The American Foundation for the Blind (www.afb.org) also lists agencies to assist and educate the patient with visual impairment.

Technological advances such as computers with voice recognition enable the patient to read, use the Internet, and communicate with others. Optical scanners can capture images and, by recognizing the written text, convert the images into identifiable characters and words. These then are recorded and played back, using a voice synthesizer. The information also can be saved as printed braille. Braille allows the patient to read, function effectively in the environment with signage, and enjoy an improved quality of living. Braille writers use advanced touch keyboards to record data for the production of written materials for the blind. Braille readers provide technology that allows for use of mobile phones and talking clocks (Hakobyan et al., 2013). Using a guide dog and a cane facilitates further independence. The nurse is responsible for patient education, providing assistance, counseling, and preventing complications for the patient with visual impairment. A comprehensive approach to care can help the patient with visual impairment successfully adjust to home, work, and society.

Patient problems and interventions for the patient with visual impairment include but are not limited to the following:

REFRACTORY ERRORS

An abnormally shaped eye and/or cornea may lead to refractive errors. These disorders result in blurred images because the eye is unable to bend the light from objects as they are viewed. Errors of refraction are treated with corrective lenses or by surgical intervention. Refractory errors can be progressive, requiring changes in the prescription for correction (see Table 13.2).

Common refractory errors (astigmatism, strabismus, myopia, and hyperopia) are described in Table 13.2.

MYOPIA

See Table 13.2.

Diagnostic Tests

Diagnosis of myopia commonly follows a visit to the health care practitioner because of the patient's inability to see distant objects clearly. After routine examinations by an optometrist the patient is assessed for corrective lenses or corrective refractory surgery.

Medical Management

The majority of patients are prescribed corrective eyeglasses or contact lenses. Patients who are unable or unwilling to wear corrective eyewear for occupational or cosmetic reasons may elect to seek surgical correction.

Surgical Management

Refractory surgery, such as reshaping the corneal curvature, is effective in treating the underlying complications causing visual problems. Myopia is the refractive error most commonly corrected by laser surgery. Patients are selected on the basis of the degree of myopia; the shape of the cornea; and the absence of medical conditions such as severe diabetes, glaucoma, or pregnancy. The usual age for correction is between 20 and 60 years. Radial keratotomy (RK), photorefractive keratectomy (PRK), laser-assisted in situ keratomileusis

(LASIK), laser thermal keratoplasty (LTK), and conductive keratoplasty (CK) surgeries are procedures used to correct myopia and markedly improve vision.

Radial keratotomy (RK) is a technique in which the surgeon makes partial-thickness radial incisions in the patient's cornea, leaving an uncut optical zone in the center. The patient must evaluate the risk of serious complications, such as operative infection and corneal scarring, when considering this procedure.

Photorefractive keratectomy involves the use of an excimer laser (a type of ultraviolet [UV] laser) to reshape the central corneal surface. It is used primarily to correct myopia but also is used for hyperopia and astigmatism. Evidence suggests that final visual acuity with this procedure is more predictable than with RK, at least in the short term.

Laser-assisted in situ keratomileusis is a procedure in which first a corneal flap is folded back and then an excimer laser removes some of the internal layers of the cornea. Afterward, the flap is returned to its normal position and allowed to heal in place. Evidence supports claims that LASIK creates earlier visual stability in patients with a high degree of myopia than with PRK (Mori, 2017).

Intracorneal implants, known as Intacs, are microthin rings implanted through incisions in the side of the cornea (Fig. 13.7). The corneal rings reshape the curvature of the cornea to improve visual acuity. Intacs are used for the patient who has keratoconus, a progressive disease in which the cornea thins. The Intac rings can be reshaped if necessary, and the effects on refractive error then are reversed completely (Nikolatus et al., 2016).

Nursing Interventions and Patient Teaching

The patient undergoing corrective surgery will leave the hospital or clinic shortly after surgery. An eye patch is placed on the operative site until the next morning. The patient can be up and around at home, but because of visual limitations, he or she may need some assistance. The patient may be photosensitive and complain of blurred vision initially, but his or her vision should improve quickly. The health care provider will schedule the patient for a follow-up examination the day after the surgery. Postoperative visual checkups are scheduled at 1 week and then monthly for 6 months. Patient problems and interventions for the patient with myopia are the same as for astigmatism and strabismus errors.

Instruct the patient preoperatively to stop wearing contact lenses 1 to 2 weeks before the surgical evaluation; contacts change the shape of the cornea and may alter the evaluation. Encourage rest the first day postoperatively. Inform the patient to notify the health care professional if pain persists after the first day of surgery. Educate the patient about the complications and symptoms that could occur postoperatively, including

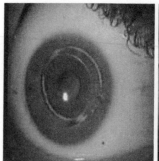
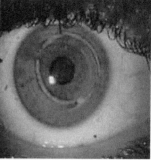

Fig. 13.7 Intacs. (From Kymionis GD, Siganos CS, Tsiklis NS, et al: Long-term follow-up of Intacs in keratoconus. *Am J Ophthalmol* 143:236–244, 2007.)

dry eyes, pain, photophobia, burning, itching, and infection. Inform the patient of the evaluation schedule for testing their functional vision in the postoperative period. Advise patients that postoperative visual acuity is not always 20/20 without glasses. The goals of operative interventions are to improve visual acuity. As a result of a slightly dilated pupil, the patient may experience a glare or halos from lights, which may require wearing glasses for night driving.

HYPEROPIA

Hyperopia is described in Table 13.2.

Diagnostic Tests

Common tests used in the diagnosis of hyperopia include ophthalmoscopy, retinoscopy, visual acuity tests, and refraction tests.

Medical Management

The primary treatment for farsightedness is corrective eyewear, either contact lenses or glasses. Some individuals may choose to self-treat these changes with over-the-counter eyewear until visual changes necessitate consultation with the eye care professional.

Nursing Interventions and Patient Teaching

Emphasize the importance of proper care of contact lenses (see the Health Promotion box). Eyeglasses should properly fit the bridge of the nose to eliminate slippage and an uneven level of each lens.

A patient problem and interventions for the patient with hyperopia include but are not limited to the following:

PATIENT PROBLEM	NURSING INTERVENTIONS
Insufficient Knowledge, related to lack of experience with corrective eyewear	Answer all questions the patient may have regarding eyewear maintenance
	Obtain literature on lens care
	Encourage follow up with the eye health care provider as directed

Health Promotion

Contact Lens Care

DO
- Wash and rinse hands thoroughly before handling contact lenses.
- Keep fingernails short and clean.
- Remove lenses from their storage case one at a time and place on the eye.
- Use the lens placement technique learned from eye care specialist.
- Use proper lens care products and clean the lenses as directed by the manufacturer. If using daily wear contacts, dispose of on a daily basis.
- Keep the lens storage kit clean.
- Wear lenses daily and follow the prescribed wearing schedule.
- Remove a lens if it becomes uncomfortable.
- Dispose of lenses if an eye infection occurs.
- Avoid potential corneal abrasions.
- Report any signs of photophobia, dryness, excessive burning, or tearing.
- Keep regular appointments with the eye care specialist.

DO NOT
- Use soaps that contain cream or perfume for cleansing lenses.
- Let fingernails touch lenses.
- Mix up lenses.
- Exceed prescribed wearing time.
- Use saliva to wet lenses.
- Use homemade saline solution or tap water to wet or clean lenses.
- Borrow lens cases or solution from others.

Nursing Interventions and Patient Teaching

The hospitalized patient wearing corrective eyewear requires daily assistance in cleaning and maintaining the eyewear. Eyeglass lenses should be cleaned daily with a clean, soft, dry cloth; check with the patient for special care instructions before cleaning. Check screw fittings to make sure they are secure. Contact lenses are cared for according to the manufacturer's directions. When not in use, place the lenses in a storage case. Take safety precautions when corrective eyewear is not worn.

A patient problem and interventions for the patient with astigmatism, strabismus, myopia, and hyperopia include but are not limited to the following:

PATIENT PROBLEM	NURSING INTERVENTIONS
Potential for Injury, related to visual changes	Provide adequate lighting in the environment
	Orient patient to the environment
	Remove small, movable objects from the path of the visually impaired patient

Encourage the patient to see an optometrist or ophthalmologist yearly to keep the eyewear prescription current. Instruct the patient on the use and care of eyewear; complications may result if the patient does not follow use and care instructions.

INFLAMMATORY AND INFECTIOUS DISORDERS OF THE EYE

HORDEOLUM, CHALAZION, AND BLEPHARITIS

The most common infections and inflammatory disorders of the eyelid are listed in Table 13.3 (Fig. 13.8).

Diagnostic Tests

Assess for the presence of visual disturbances. Diagnosis of the condition begins with assessment of the eyelid margin. Characteristics of the inflammation and the presence of drainage are noted. Culture and sensitivity tests of any drainage may be ordered.

Medical Management

The health care provider may prescribe anti-infective agents (cephalexin and erythromycin) and may perform localized incision and drainage of a cyst or stye with the patient under local anesthesia. Warm normal saline (0.9% NaCl) compresses are ordered for 10 to 20 minutes two to four times a day. Lid scrubs using no-tear baby shampoo may be ordered. Topical therapies are normally sufficient to manage the conditions. Recurrent or complicated infections may require oral or systemic antibiotic therapies.

Nursing Interventions and Patient Teaching

A primary objective of nursing care for the patient with an infectious or inflammatory process of the lids is prevention of the spread of infection. Hand hygiene is essential before contact with the eye. Discuss taking care with the application of warm compresses to ensure the skin is not injured. Gentle massage of the affected area may be prescribed. Provide accompanying teaching about this procedure.

Caution the patient to avoid irritating scents, fumes, or smokes, which may cause rubbing of the eyes, leading to further infection. Discourage the use of eye makeup until all inflammation subsides. Eye makeup should be replaced after an eye infection, and every 3 to 6 months thereafter, because of the potential for the makeup to harbor bacteria.

Prognosis

Some cases may resolve without treatment in 1 to 2 weeks. In the majority of patients, the inflammatory and infectious phases of these conditions respond favorably to topical antimicrobials. Surgical incision and drainage of cystlike formations result in minimal complications and are of low risk to the patient.

INFLAMMATION OF THE CONJUNCTIVA

Etiology and Pathophysiology

Conjunctivitis is a common disorder of the eye. It is responsible for 30% of all reported eye disorders. It involves an inflammation of the conjunctiva. Causes may be bacterial or viral infections, allergies, or environmental factors. It is commonly called *pinkeye*.

Table **13.3**   **Common Infections and Inflammatory Disorders of the Eyelid**

DESCRIPTION	ETIOLOGY AND PATHOPHYSIOLOGY	CLINICAL MANIFESTATIONS
Blepharitis: Inflammation of eyelid margins usually involving portion of the eyelid where the lashes grow	*Ulcerative:* Caused by bacterial infection, usually staphylococcal organisms *Nonulcerative:* Caused by psoriasis, seborrhea, or allergic response	Pruritus, erythema of eyelid, eyelid pain, photophobia Excessive tearing Matting during periods of extended closure such as sleep
Chalazion: Inflammatory cyst on the meibomian gland at the eyelid margin	Most often results from blockage of an oil gland in the eyelid May be the result of complications with a hordeolum (stye) Less frequently may be caused by infection	Discomfort, mass on eyelid, edema, visual disturbance Pressure may be felt as eyelid closes over cornea
Hordeolum: Acute infection of eyelid margin or sebaceous glands of the eyelashes; also called a *stye*	Frequently caused by staphylococcal organisms One or more pustules may form	Abscess localized to base of eyelashes, with edema of lid Warmth and redness Tenderness and pain that may diminish after pustule ruptures Tearing of eye Blurred vision Patient reports feelings of scratching sensation in the eye

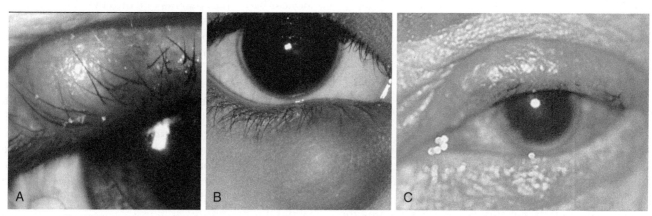

Fig. 13.8 (A) Hordeolum. (B) Chalazion. (C) Blepharitis. (A and B, from Kanski JJ: *Signs in ophthalmology: causes and differential diagnoses,* London, 2010, Mosby. C, from Kanski JJ: *Clinical ophthalmology: a test yourself atlas,* ed 2, New York, 2002, Butterworth-Heinemann.)

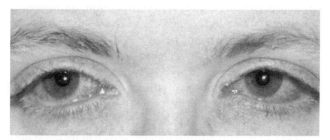

Fig. 13.9 Conjunctivitis. (From Palay DA, Krachmer JH: *Primary care ophthalmology,* ed 2, Philadelphia, 2005, Mosby.)

Although this typically occurs initially in one eye, it spreads rapidly to the unaffected eye (Fig. 13.9).

The hands usually transmit acute bacterial conjunctivitis after direct contact with a contaminated object. Pneumococcal, staphylococcal, streptococcal, gonococcal, and chlamydial organisms and *Haemophilus influenzae* are the major causative bacterial agents. The eye is an excellent medium for bacterial growth because of the moisture, warmth, and extensive vascularization of the eye. The disease is usually self-limiting, leaving no permanent impairment. Trachoma, a highly contagious form of conjunctivitis, is caused by a strain of *Chlamydia trachomatis.* Transmission is by direct contact with an ocular discharge. It is rare in the United States but is a major cause of blindness in Asian and Mediterranean countries.

Viruses of the respiratory tract may, in addition to causing a cold, lead to a secondary infection of the eye. The two most common viral agents are adenovirus and type 1 herpes simplex virus (HSV). Like bacterial conjunctivitis, viral conjunctivitis is highly contagious.

Clinical Manifestations

Contamination leads to an inflammatory process that produces erythema of the conjunctiva, edema of the lid, and a mucopurulent crusting discharge on the lids and cornea. If untreated, this infection leaves the eyelid scarred with granulations that invade the cornea, resulting in loss of vision.

Assessment

Subjective data include reports of pruritus, burning, and excessive tearing. During allergy seasons and exposures to environmental irritants these complaints may be increased.

Objective data include observing eyes that are erythematous with edema of the lid. Also look for dried exudate.

Diagnostic Tests

The conjunctiva is tested for bacteria and stained for microscopic examination.

Medical Management

Medical treatment is similar to that for blepharitis.

Nursing Interventions and Patient Teaching

The lid and lashes are cleansed of exudate with normal saline. Warm compresses are applied two to four times a day. When allergies are present, cold saline compresses may be ordered to control edema and pruritus. Eye irrigations with normal saline or lactated Ringer's solution may be prescribed to remove secretions. Administer topical antibiotics and adrenocortical steroid medications as ordered. Eye pads are contraindicated because they enhance bacterial growth.

A patient problem and interventions for the patient with conjunctivitis include but are not limited to the following:

PATIENT PROBLEM	NURSING INTERVENTIONS
Pain, related to inflammatory process	Apply warm or cold compresses Administer prescribed eye medications; ensure proper instillation of eyedrops and ointments; administer eye irrigation as prescribed Administer analgesics as ordered

Instruct patients and their family to avoid contact with infected eyes or soiled materials when an infection is present. Patients with infection should use individual washcloths and towels, separate from the rest of their family. Tell patients to wash their hands if contact is made with the eyes and before any treatments. Teach patients the steps to perform prescribed treatments such as irrigations, application of compresses, and medication administration; evaluate their ability to perform these steps before leaving the care of the nurse. Patients should avoid noxious fumes or smoke and should not wear contact lenses during the treatment period.

Prognosis

Conjunctivitis responds successfully to topical antimicrobials. Patient teaching reduces the risk of continued exposure and reinfection. Although highly contagious, the disease is self-limiting, leaving no chance of permanent visual impairment unless a chronic condition develops.

INFLAMMATION OF THE CORNEA

Etiology and Pathophysiology

Keratitis, an inflammation of the cornea, may result from injury; irritants; allergies; bacterial infections, including syphilis; viral infections such as HSV and varicella-zoster virus; fungal infections including Candida; and some nervous disorders. It may be superficial and involve the epithelial layer only or may invade the subepithelial layer and the endothelial membrane. The layers of the eye are innervated, and thus, inflammation causes acute pain. Ulcers may form in the membrane layers, resulting in scattered scarring of the corneal surface.

Pseudomonas, staphylococci, streptococci, and Haemophilus organisms are the most common bacterial causes of keratitis. The viral agent most often responsible for corneal inflammation is HSV. HSV keratitis is a growing problem, especially in immunocompromised patients. Keratitis can be triggered by stress, illness, and exposure to UV light. The condition may be associated with the use of ophthalmologic steroid medications. Overuse or abuse of topical steroids may injure epithelial cells. Contact lens wearing and having a history of eye injury also increase the risk for keratitis.

Another form of keratitis is acanthamoebic keratitis, which is caused by amebic parasites. The Acanthamoeba organism is found in the soil, airborne dust, fresh water, and the noses and throats of healthy humans. This organism is often resistant to antimicrobial agents. Contact lens wearers are more susceptible because traditional cleaning agents for lenses include rinsing with clean or distilled water. People who swim frequently are at greater risk because the organism is not killed by usual methods of disinfection, such as chlorine.

Clinical Manifestations

Severe eye pain is the most common symptom that differentiates this disease from other inflammatory eye diseases. If uncontrolled, keratitis may result in blepharospasms (involuntary blinking or spasms of the eyelid) and vision loss. Other symptoms include photophobia, tearing, edema, and visual disturbances.

Assessment

Subjective data include the duration and severity of the pain, the extent of light sensitivity (photophobia), and any vision loss.

Objective data include assessing the patient for facial grimacing, lacrimation, and photophobia.

Diagnostic Tests

An ophthalmoscopic exam including a slit lamp will be used. Assessment of the cornea's surface with stain may be employed to study ulcerations or other irregularities. Culture and sensitivity tests to determine the best agents to treat the condition will be completed.

Medical Management

Medical management includes topical antibiotic therapy. Systemic antibiotics may be prescribed for severe cases. Cycloplegic-mydriatic drugs paralyze the ocular muscles of accommodation and dilate the pupil. For viral keratitis, therapy includes corneal debridement followed by topical therapy with vidarabine or trifluridine (Viroptic) for 2 to 3 weeks. Corticosteroids are *contraindicated* because they contribute to a longer course, possible deeper ulceration of the cornea, and systemic complications. Drug therapy also may include antiviral therapy such as acyclovir (Zovirax). Analgesics are used to control pain associated with acute inflammation. Pressure dressings may be ordered to relax the eye muscle and decrease discomfort. These dressings often are applied to both eyes because the eyes move together. Warm or cold compresses two to four times daily are prescribed for symptomatic relief. Epithelial debridement of loose tissue may be performed. Surgical management involves a corneal transplant, known as *keratoplasty*.

Nursing Interventions and Patient Teaching

Nursing interventions for keratitis include control of pain, safety, and prevention of complications. Nursing diagnoses and interventions for the patient with keratitis are the same as for conjunctivitis. Provide information on self-care of a corneal abrasion. Also teach the patient to wash hands before instilling medication and to prevent infection by not rubbing the eyes. Instruct the patient to note any change in discharge or increase in pain and to notify the health care practitioner immediately.

Prognosis

Topical antibiotic, antiviral, or antifungal eye drops, when started promptly after diagnosis by culture, result in rapid healing and minimal visual impairment. Chronic keratitis may develop if treatment is delayed. Infection of the cornea can produce corneal ulcer and vision loss as a result of opaque scarring. Keratoplasty then may be indicated.

NONINFECTIOUS DISORDERS OF THE EYE

DRY EYE DISORDERS
Etiology and Pathology

Complaints of dry eye, caused by a variety of ocular disorders, are characterized by decreased tear secretion or increased tear film evaporation. Keratoconjunctivitis sicca (dry eye) is caused by lacrimal gland dysfunction, usually the result of an autoimmune reaction. If the patient with keratoconjunctivitis sicca has associated dry mouth, the patient may have primary Sjögren syndrome (an immunologic disorder characterized by deficient fluid production by the lacrimal, salivary, and other glands, resulting in abnormal dryness of the mouth, eyes, and other mucous membranes). Secondary Sjögren syndrome occurs in the presence of other systemic conditions such as rheumatoid arthritis, scleroderma, or systemic lupus erythematosus (Sjögren Foundation, n.d.).

Risk factors for the development of dry eyes include female gender and advancing age. Most cases occur in individuals older than age 50 years. Medications associated with the development of the condition include antihistamines, nasal decongestants, tranquilizers, oral contraceptives, and antidepressants. Dietary factors may be implicated. Diets that are low in Vitamin A and Omega 3 fatty acids are seen in individuals with dry eyes. The development of dry eye conditions may be noted after refractive eye treatment surgeries. In these patients, the condition may be time limited.

Clinical Manifestations

The eyes may appear reddened or contain stringy mucus. A variety of subjective complaints may be reported. Patients experience photosensitivity, eye fatigue, and blurred vision. These complaints may result in difficulty using computer aids and reading. The patient complains of a sandy or gritty sensation that typically worsens during the day and is better in the morning after eye closure with sleep.

Diagnostic Tests

The definitive test for dry eye, a noninfectious disorder of the lacrimal gland, is *Schirmer's test*. Schirmer's test involves the placement of filter paper in the lower lid of the eye. After 5 minutes the paper is removed and the moisture on the paper is evaluated. Normal results are 10 to 15 mm of wet paper. Fluorescein drops also are administered to assess the structural integrity of the cornea and the ability of tears to flow across the eye and through the lacrimal duct to the nose. Results of the fluorescein-staining test for excessive tear disorder are considered normal if the dye disappears from the lacrimal cul-de-sac within 1 minute.

Medical Management

Medical management for dry eye includes artificial tear replacement. Many nonprescription products are available. They should be used sparingly because preservatives in the drops or overuse can cause further irritation. Preservative-free drops are available and will not result in irritation after long-term use (AOA, n.d.). Cyclosporine, an immunosuppressant agent, is a prescription medication available to manage dry eye. It can increase tear production and reduce inflammation. It may take 3 to 6 months for the medication to provide noticeable improvement in the condition. Olopatadine is an antihistamine that eases the burning and itching associated with dry eye conditions. A slow dissolving insert that can thicken the tear film on the eye (hydroxypropyl cellulose) is a treatment for those experiencing severe dry eye conditions. Short-term corticosteroid drops may be prescribed to reduce inflammation in severe cases. Punctal plugs (temporary or permanent) may be inserted to close the tear ducts and keep the tears in the eyes longer.

Patients taking medications associated with the development of dry eye may have their prescriptions changed to medications that are less drying. If an infection accompanies the dry eye syndrome, antibiotic therapy may be prescribed. Eliminate as many environmental irritants as possible. High-efficiency particulate absorption (HEPA) filters are available to control pollen and dust levels in the home environment. If contact lenses cause local irritation and dry eye, a change in the prescription, type of lens, contact solution, or the addition of rewetting drops may be advised.

Surgical repair of an injured punctal sac by correctly aligning the eyelid margin or by probing an obstructed punctum (opening to the tear duct) is the recommended method of treatment to allow for tear absorption.

Nursing Interventions and Patient Teaching
The appropriate patient problem is *Pain, related to lack of natural eye moisture*. Interventions are similar to those for conjunctivitis. Instruct the patient on instilling eye medications, practicing appropriate hand and eye hygiene, and avoiding irritants.

Prognosis
Eyedrops alleviate the majority of symptoms caused by dry eye. Control of medical conditions minimizes discomfort and complications. Surgical repair of the punctual sac is a safe procedure and has a good prognosis.

ECTROPION AND ENTROPION
Etiology and Pathophysiology
Ectropion and entropion are two noninfectious disorders of the eyelid, causing an abnormal turning of the eyelid margins.

Ectropion is the outward turning of the eyelid margin. In the older patient, it is common for the orbicularis oculi muscle to be relaxed. Paralytic ectropion occurs when orbicularis muscle function is disturbed, as with Bell's palsy. Other causes of ectropion are birth defects, eyelid laceration, and burns of the conjunctival tissue.

Entropion is an inward turning of the eyelid. The lower eyelid margin is the most frequently involved. Entropion causes include atrophy of the eyelid tissue, spasms of the orbicularis oculi muscle, or scarring of the tarsal plate (dense connective tissue that stiffens the eyelid) caused by congenital conditions or eye trauma. Varying degrees of atonia commonly exist in the older adult orbicularis oculi.

Clinical Manifestations
Ectropion and entropion are characterized by abnormal positions of the eyelid, with tearing and corneal dryness. Redness of the sclera also may be present.

Assessment
Collection of subjective data includes noting the degree of vision loss and determining tear loss and dryness of the cornea.

Collection of objective data includes observing the extent to which the patient can perform ADLs and the presence of any eyelid margin inflammation.

Diagnostic Tests
The health care practitioner diagnoses these conditions after a visual and ophthalmologic examination.

Medical Management
Medical intervention consists of topical medications to reduce conjunctival and corneal inflammation or drying. Surgery is the preferred treatment. Resection of the tarsal plate, removal of the scarred tissue, or tightening of the orbicularis oculi muscle is the recommended treatment for permanent repair.

Nursing Interventions and Patient Teaching
Interventions for ectropion and entropion involve monitoring the medical treatment and reporting its progress. A patient problem statement for the patient with ectropion or entropion is *Impaired Sensory Awareness, related to edema and exudate*. Interventions include assistance in self-care activities, safety measures, observation for infection and inflammation, and medication and dressing treatments as prescribed.

Prognosis
Early diagnosis and treatment of eyelid disorders reduce the risk of conjunctival and corneal inflammation and scarring. Monitoring treatment reduces the need for surgical intervention and minimizes visual disturbances.

DISORDERS OF THE LENS

CATARACTS
Etiology and Pathophysiology
A cataract is a crystalline opacity or clouding of the lens (Fig. 13.10). The patient may have a cataract in one or both eyes. If they are present in both eyes, one cataract may affect vision more than the other. In the aging patient, opacification of the lens gradually occurs. About 50% of seniors between 65 and 74 years old have some degree of cataract formation. After 75 years of age, the percentage rises to about 70%. Cataract removal is the

most common surgical procedure for people greater than 65 years of age. When a cataract develops, the lens becomes foggy, decreasing visual acuity, and if a large enough portion of the lens becomes opaque, light cannot reach the retina.

Cataracts may be congenital (e.g., a result of exposure to maternal rubella) or acquired from systemic disease, trauma, toxins (e.g., radiation or UV light exposure, certain drugs such as systemic corticosteroids or long-term topical corticosteroids), and intraocular inflammation. Most cataracts are age related (senile cataracts). Systemic disorders associated with the development of cataracts include diabetes mellitus and hypertension. Smoking has been linked with the development of cataracts. Numerous factors contribute to cataract development. In senile cataract formation, it appears that altered metabolic processes within the lens cause an accumulation of water and alterations in the fiber structure. These changes affect lens transparency, causing vision changes.

Clinical Manifestations

Cataract symptoms are painless but include blurred vision, difficulty reading fine print, diplopia, photosensitivity, glare (the sense that normal light is too bright), abnormal color perception, and difficulty driving at night. Glare is due to light scatter caused by the lens opacities, and it may be significantly worse at night when the pupil dilates. The visual decline is gradual, and the rate of cataract development varies from patient to patient. The opacity can be seen in the center of the lens (see Fig. 13.10).

Assessment

Subjective data include blurred vision, often the first symptom expressed by the patient. Note any subjective complaints, such as "hazy" or "fuzzy" vision or abnormal color perception.

The gathering of objective data involves observing the patient for difficulty in reading, such as noting whether the patient brings a newspaper close to the eyes. Also note sensitivity to light.

Diagnostic Tests

Diagnosis is based on decreased visual acuity or other complaints of visual dysfunction. The opacity

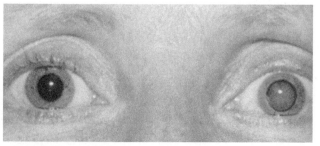

Fig. 13.10 Cataract in subject's left eye. (From Swartz MH: *Textbook of physical diagnosis*, ed 4, Philadelphia, 2002, Saunders.)

is directly observable by ophthalmoscope or slit-lamp microscopic examination. A totally opaque lens creates the appearance of a white pupil (see Fig. 13.10).

Medical Management

Monitor the patient for changes in vision associated with increasing cataract size. For many patients, the diagnosis is made long before they actually decide to have surgery. Often, changing the patient's eyewear prescription can improve the visual acuity, at least temporarily. If glare makes it difficult to drive at night, the patient may drive only during daylight hours and have a family member drive at night. When palliative measures no longer provide an acceptable level of visual function, the patient is an appropriate candidate for surgery. Surgery is the only definitive method of treatment and can be performed at any age. It can be done using a local or topical anesthetic, or under general anesthesia.

There are two surgical methods to improve vision: intracapsular and extracapsular extraction. Intracapsular extraction surgery involves removing the lens and its entire capsule. Although some surgeons still perform intracapsular extraction (and it may be necessary in instances of trauma), the intracapsular technique has been largely replaced by extracapsular extraction. In the extracapsular extraction method, the anterior capsule is opened and the lens nucleus and cortex are removed, leaving the remaining capsular bag intact. Healing is rapid with this method.

Phacoemulsification is the most common type of extracapsular cataract extraction. This technique uses ultrasound to break up and remove the cataract through a small incision, thereby reducing the healing time and decreasing the chance of complications.

During surgery the physician implants a synthetic intraocular lens in the posterior chamber behind the iris. At the end of the procedure, the patient receives injections of subconjunctival corticosteroid and antibiotics. Then an antibiotic and corticosteroid ointment are applied, and the patient's eye is covered with a patch and protective shield. The patch usually is worn overnight and removed during the first postoperative visit. Antibiotic and corticosteroid therapies continue for 1 to 2 weeks after surgery. The patient is encouraged to wear protective eyewear at night. During the day, the patient wears protected goggle-type sunglasses. Many refractive errors are corrected with the surgery. A patient who wore prescriptive eyewear before surgery may no longer need it. Even a patient needing prescription eyewear after surgery will likely have changes in the prescription.

Nursing Interventions and Patient Teaching

Preoperative and postoperative nursing care is a primary nursing responsibility (Nursing Care Plan 13.1). Cataract symptoms usually develop slowly and can be detected easily. Encourage patients to have

Nursing Care Plan 13.1   **The Patient With Cataracts**

Ms. J. is an 82-year-old who lives alone. She has developed bilateral cataracts and is admitted to same-day surgery for a right cataract extracapsular procedure with intraocular lens implantation.

PATIENT PROBLEM

Potential for Injury, related to altered visual acuity

Patient Goals and Expected Outcomes	Nursing Interventions	Evaluation
Patient will not have any evidence of injury Patient will have a safe environment in which she will avoid injury	**PREOPERATIVE** Instill eyedrops as prescribed, wearing clean latex or vinyl gloves. Administer preoperative medications or sedatives as ordered. Explain which postoperative procedures to expect, such as patches and eyedrops. **POSTOPERATIVE** Instill mydriatic-cycloplegic and corticosteroid eyedrops as prescribed while wearing clean latex or vinyl gloves. Instruct patient to avoid moving head suddenly, heavy lifting, bending over, coughing, sneezing, vomiting, and straining with elimination, which cause increased intraocular pressure. Keep eye patch or shield in position during specified hours. Instruct patient to avoid lying on the side of the affected eye on the night after surgery. Remove environmental barriers to ensure safety. Keep side rails up at all times. Plan all care with patient: Explain what will happen and when. Visit often and announce yourself on entering the room. Assist with deep-breathing exercises q 1–2 h. while awake. Check with health care practitioner for any special positioning or precautions. (If turned, position patient on the unaffected side.) Elevate head of bed 30 degrees as ordered. Assist with and teach active and passive range-of-motion exercises q 4 h. Provide increased activities and ambulation as ordered; assist as needed. Teach self-care activities, and assist as needed. Instruct family to remove unnecessary furniture and pick up objects that may be blocking pathways. Instruct patient that cataract surgery does not correct nearsightedness or farsightedness. Corrective lenses are still needed for these problems after surgery.	Patient experienced no injuries during the preoperative and immediate postoperative phase. Patient understands and demonstrates injury prevention measures in the home.

PATIENT PROBLEM

Anxiousness/Fearfulness, related to visual impairment

Patient Goals and Expected Outcomes	Nursing Intervention	Evaluation
Patient will voice decreased anxiety and fear	Observe level of patient and family anxiety. Note patient's coping mechanism related to vision loss. Encourage patient and family to vent feelings and concerns. Support patient and family's positive actions toward adapting to visual limitations.	Patient and family display trust and security after venting feelings.

CRITICAL THINKING QUESTIONS

1. Ms. J. puts her call light on and tells the nurse that she has severe pain and pressure in her right eye. What should be the initial response by the nurse?
2. What should be included in Ms. J.'s discharge planning to minimize the risk of injury to her operative eye?
3. In visiting with Ms. J., the nurse learns that Ms. J. enjoys embroidery and knitting. Ms. J. states that she is looking forward to resuming her handiwork. What should be included as appropriate patient teaching?

annual eye examinations. Surgery provides about a 90% success rate in achieving acceptable levels of vision. Unless complications occur, the patient is usually ready to go home within a few hours after the surgery, as soon as the effects of sedation have worn off. Postoperative medications usually include antibiotic and corticosteroid drops to prevent infection and decrease the postoperative inflammatory response. The ophthalmologist instructs the patient to avoid activities that increase IOP, such as bending, stooping, coughing, or lifting. Ophthalmologists also may recommend using an eye shield over the operative eye at night for protection. Discuss safety measures appropriate to vision alterations and instruct the patient to notify the health care practitioner of any complications, such as pain, erythema, drainage, or sudden visual changes. If sudden pain occurs, call the health care practitioner (see the Communication box and the Patient Teaching box).

Communication

Nursing-Patient Dialogue Regarding Postoperative Eye Surgery

Mrs. B., a 71-year-old patient, has been experiencing decreasing vision for the past 5 years. She seeks medical attention and is told that surgery is required to correct her condition. While talking to the patient, the nurse senses her reluctance to comply with postoperative treatment.

Patient: I'm too old to go through all the routines that the doctor wants me to. It involves too much.

Nurse: I know that surgery is a concern for you. You must have many emotions right now. It's understandable that you have concerns about your recovery.

Patient: There's so much to think about and remember.

Nurse: The doctor and our staff are here to help make your recovery as easy as possible for you. Can you tell me what bothers you the most?

Patient: What if I go home and fall? I could reinjure my eye or break something, like my hip.

Nurse: There are several things that you and your family can do to prevent any injury during your recovery. The nursing staff will provide education to you both before and after surgery to assist you with care after discharge.

Prognosis

Gradual loss of lens transparency increases the risk of injury because of vision loss. Carefully monitor patients for degeneration of the lens. The condition may be accompanied by secondary glaucoma, which further reduces visual acuity. Surgical intervention is advised to improve vision. Postoperative complications of cataract surgery are uncommon, but may include infection, hemorrhage, inflammation, glaucoma, and retinal detachment (Mayo Clinic, 2019). Complications may recur years after cataract surgery and should be reported to the ophthalmologist.

Patient Teaching

After Eye Surgery

- Discuss proper hand hygiene, which includes washing hands before and after caring for eyes, including the application of medications and dressing changes.
- Review signs and symptoms to report to the health care provider.
- Shaving, bathing, and washing of the face are permitted, but the patient must avoid excess water exposure and wetting of the area near the eyes.
- Shampoos and soaps must be used with caution near the eyes.
- Avoid the use of cosmetics for up to 4 weeks or as prescribed by the health care provider.
- Discuss personal hygiene.
- Normal symptoms include slight redness, mild watering, mild irritation, glare, and slight ptosis (drooping) of the upper eyelid. These symptoms may remain for 6–8 weeks after the operation.
- Abnormal symptoms include sudden onset of extreme pain, trauma or injury, decreased visual acuity, floaters, flashes of light, purulent drainage, or bleeding.
- Teach the patient postoperative restrictions on head positioning, bending, coughing, and the Valsalva maneuver to optimize visual outcomes and to prevent increased intraocular pressure (IOP).
- Postoperative restrictions include limitations on lifting, driving, and sexual relations for a period specified by the health care provider.
- Teach the prescribed medication therapies. Allow the patient to provide a return demonstration. Observe the use of aseptic technique.
- Instruct the patient to monitor pain and to take the prescribed medication for pain as directed and to report pain symptoms not relieved by medications.
- Make a follow-up appointment and provide a written appointment card for the patient.

DISORDERS OF THE RETINA

DIABETIC RETINOPATHY
Etiology and Pathophysiology

Diabetic retinopathy is a disorder of retinal blood vessels characterized by capillary microaneurysms, hemorrhage, exudates, and the formation of new vessels and connective tissue. Patients may present to their health care provider with visual alterations, which may lead to the initial diagnosis of diabetes mellitus. After 15 years with diabetes mellitus, nearly all patients with type 1 diabetes and 80% with type 2 diabetes have some degree of retinal disease accompanied by nephropathy. The incidence of diabetic retinopathy greatly increases in relation to how long the patient has diabetes mellitus and how well his or her blood glucose levels are controlled. The disorder occurs more frequently in patients with long-standing, poorly controlled diabetes mellitus (see the Cultural Considerations box).

The initial stage of diabetic retinopathy may last several years. The earliest and most treatable stages often produce no changes in vision. Because of this, the patient with diabetes must have regular dilated eye examinations by an ophthalmologist or optometrist for early detection and treatment. As the disease progresses, the blood vessels in the retina begin to widen and become tortuous. Microaneurysms then develop at the periphery, and small hemorrhages develop. These may disappear, but they leave in their place scars that can decrease vision. Increased capillary permeability causes protein exudate.

🌐 Cultural Considerations

Incidence of Hearing and Visual Problems

- Caucasians have a higher incidence of hearing impairment than African Americans or Asian Americans.
- The incidence and severity of glaucoma are greater among African Americans than among Caucasians.
- Hispanics have an increased incidence of diabetic retinopathy.
- Native Americans have an increased incidence of otitis media when compared with whites.
- Whites have a higher incidence of macular degeneration than Hispanics, African Americans, and Asian Americans.
- Inuits are susceptible to primary closed-angle glaucoma, resulting from a thicker lens and a shallow chamber angle.
- Native Americans and African Americans have a higher incidence of astigmatism than whites.

New blood vessels form on the retina and into the vitreous body as the disease progresses. These new vessels rupture, causing decreased vision. Some of the blood may be reabsorbed, which improves vision until another hemorrhage occurs. With progressive hemorrhages, the patient may have significant vision loss over time. Vitreous contraction and full retinal detachment can occur as the vessels and surrounding tissue become more fibrous and less flexible.

Clinical Manifestations
Symptoms include microaneurysms, which can be identified only by ophthalmoscopy in the initial stage. In the advanced stages, the patient has progressive vision loss and the presence of "floaters," which are minute products of the hemorrhage.

Assessment
Collection of subjective data includes assessment of the duration of the disease and how well the diabetes mellitus is controlled. Patients may have varying degrees of vision loss, from decreased vision to complete blindness. Assess each patient's knowledge of therapy and treatments.

Collection of objective data involves noting that in the early stages there are no symptoms; as the disease progresses, vision becomes diminished.

Diagnostic Tests
Indirect ophthalmoscopy shows dilated and tortuous vessels and narrowing or obliteration of the arteries. Opacities, hemorrhages, and microaneurysms can be visualized. Slit-lamp examination magnifies the lesions.

Medical Management
Surgical intervention includes early photocoagulation (see "Photocoagulation," below), cryotherapy (cryopexy), and/or vitrectomy (see "Vitrectomy" discussions). Photocoagulation uses a laser beam to destroy new blood vessels, seal leaking vessels, and help prevent retinal edema. A vitrectomy or cryotherapy may be performed when photocoagulation is not possible. A topical anesthetic is used in cryotherapy so that the probe can be placed directly on the surface of the eye to deliver therapy. When the probe is located properly on the eye, the tip of the probe creates a frozen area that extends through the external tissue and reaches a specific point on the retina. Vascular endothelial growth factor (VEGF) inhibitors may be injected into the retina. These medications work to stop the growth of the new blood vessels (Mayo Clinic, 2021).

Nursing Interventions and Patient Teaching
A patient problem and interventions for the patient with diabetic retinopathy include but are not limited to the following:

PATIENT PROBLEM	NURSING INTERVENTIONS
Insufficient Knowledge, related to unfamiliarity with therapeutic procedure	Determine patient's knowledge of purpose and procedures of photocoagulation, cryotherapy, or vitrectomy

Home care after surgery for the patient with diabetic retinopathy is the same as for any eye surgery.

Prognosis
The best treatment of diabetic retinopathy is early detection. Frequent eye examinations reduce the complication of vision loss, and modern laser technology is highly effective in reducing further damage to the retina and improving vision.

AGE-RELATED MACULAR DEGENERATION
Etiology and Pathophysiology
Age-related macular degeneration (ARMD) of the retina is characterized by slow, progressive loss of central and near vision. ARMD is the most common cause of vision loss in people older than 60 years. There is evidence of a genetic component of ARMD, and a positive family history for ARMD is a major risk factor. Additional risk factors include long-term exposure to UV light, hyperopia, cigarette smoking, gender (female), obesity, race, and light-colored eyes. Nutrition may play a role in the progression of ARMD. Dietary supplementation

with vitamin C, vitamin E, vitamin A (beta-carotene), copper, and zinc slows the development of advancing ARMD; however, it does not seem to have any effect on people with minimal ARMD.

There are two types of macular degeneration. The first is known as the *wet type* (also called *neovascular macular degeneration*). This is characterized by sudden new vessel growth in the macular region. The macula becomes displaced and scarring occurs. Because scarred cells no longer register light, vision loss is irreversible. Wet macular degeneration accounts for 10% of cases.

The second, known as the *dry type* (also called *non-exudative* or *non-neovascular macular degeneration*), occurs in 90% of cases. It is caused by degenerative changes, including lipid deposits. These are followed by slow atrophy of the macular region, including the retina. People with dry ARMD notice that reading and other close-vision tasks become more difficult. In this form, the macular cells have wasted or atrophied, resulting in decreased function. The patient may report, "Sometimes I see the image and sometimes it sort of blinks at me, like I have a short circuit."

Clinical Manifestations

The hallmark of ARMD is the appearance of drusen in the fundus (the interior surface of the eye), found on ophthalmoscopic evaluation. Drusen are yellowish exudates found beneath the retinal pigment epithelium and represent localized or diffuse deposits of extracellular debris. The main symptom of macular degeneration is gradual and variable bilateral loss of *central vision*. One eye may have a greater loss than the other and color perception also may be affected.

Assessment

The collection of subjective data includes asking the patient if he or she has noticed difficulty in distinguishing colors correctly. Assess for visual disturbances and coping mechanisms related to the loss of vision. Macular degeneration develops differently in each person, and therefore the symptoms may vary. However, some of the most common symptoms include (1) a gradual loss of ability to see objects clearly; (2) distorted vision, with objects appearing to be the wrong size or shape or straight lines appearing wavy or crooked; (3) gradual loss of clear color vision; (4) scotomas (blind spots in the visual field); and (5) a dark or empty area appearing in the center of vision.

The collection of objective data includes noting the degree to which the patient can centrally view objects.

Diagnostic Tests

Ophthalmoscopy is used to detect opacity, hemorrhage, and new blood vessel formation. The examiner looks for retinal detachment, drusen, and other fundus changes associated with ARMD, and any other abnormalities. Using an Amsler grid test may help define the involved areas. Fluorescein angiography is used to assess for the presence of leaking blood vessels and to confirm diagnosis.

Medical Management

Medications can be used to stop the growth of new blood vessels. Bevacizumab (Avastin) and pegaptanib (Macugen) are injected directly into the eye. Antibiotic drops may be prescribed to accompany the injections in an effort to prevent infection. Photodynamic therapy is a treatment for wet ARMD. This treatment uses intravenous verteporfin (Visudyne) and a "cold" laser. Verteporfin becomes active when exposed to the "cold" laser light wave. This procedure causes deconstruction of abnormal blood vessels but does not cause permanent damage to the retinal pigment epithelium and photoreceptor cells. The specific guidelines for use of this therapy in patients with wet ARMD are very strict, and only about 10% of patients are eligible for treatment. After delivery of this therapy the patient must understand that caution should be used to avoid direct exposure to sunlight and other intense forms of light for 5 days after treatment. Destruction of abnormal vessels may be performed with laser beam therapy. It has limited use. At present, there is no treatment for dry macular degeneration.

Unfortunately, central vision damaged by macular degeneration cannot be restored. However, because macular degeneration does not damage peripheral vision, low vision aids such as telescopic and microscopic special lenses, magnifying glasses, and electronic magnifiers for close work can be prescribed to help make the most of remaining vision. Often, with adaptation, people can cope well and continue to do most things they were accustomed to doing. High-dose nutritional supplements of zinc, beta-carotene, and vitamins C and E and a diet rich in fruits and dark green leafy vegetables is recommended (AMDF, n.d.).

Nursing Interventions and Patient Teaching

The patient needs patience and understanding to cope with the continuing loss of sight. Help the patient through the process of accepting loss of sight. Maintaining safety is important because only peripheral vision exists.

A patient problem and interventions for the patient with macular degeneration include but are not limited to the following:

PATIENT PROBLEM	NURSING INTERVENTIONS
Impaired Sensory Awareness, related to disease process	Note the extent of visual loss and the level of ability to perform ADLs; assist the patient in developing ways to perform these activities
	Determine the patient's support systems and solicit help if available

Instruct the patients about the disease process, stressing that peripheral vision will be maintained. Provide ways for the patient to maintain as much independence as possible, and help family and friends determine the areas in which to assist.

Prognosis

Early diagnosis of macular degeneration is critical to prevent blindness. Watchful waiting is the only approach to dry macular degeneration. Ophthalmic laser surgery is of limited benefit because of the gradual and progressive course of the disorder. Photocoagulation is preventive, not curative.

RETINAL DETACHMENT

Etiology and Pathophysiology

Retinal detachment is a separation of the retina from the choroid in the posterior area of the eye (Fig. 13.11). This usually results from a hole in the retina that allows vitreous humor to leak between the choroid and the retina. The immediate cause may be severe trauma to the eye, such as a contusion or a penetrating wound. In most cases, however, retinal detachment is the result of internal changes related to aging and sometimes inflammation of the eye. Retinal

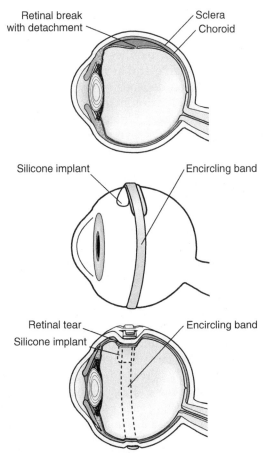

Fig. 13.11 Retinal break with detachment. Surgical repair by scleral buckling technique. (From Lewis SL, Bucher L, Heitkemper MM, et al: *Medical-surgical nursing: assessment and management of clinical problems*, ed 10, St. Louis, 2017, Mosby.)

detachment also may occur in debilitated patients when there is sudden, severe physical exertion. As the detachment progresses, it interrupts the transmission of visual images from the retina to the optic nerve. The result is a progressive loss of vision to complete blindness.

Clinical Manifestations

Symptoms include a sudden or gradual development of flashes of light, followed by floating spots, a "cobweb," a "hairnet," and loss of a specific field of vision. As the detachment progresses, patients may describe an enlarging dark spot in their visual field. Patients have described this as having a curtain or shade being drawn over their eye. This dark area may occur in any of the visual fields but typically begins in the peripheral visual field. The dark area may progress to include the entire visual field if the retinal detachment includes the entire retina.

Assessment

Subjective data include patient complaints of flashing lights unilaterally and floaters. Progressive vision restriction occurs in one area. If the tear is acute and extensive, the patient describes a sensation like a curtain being drawn across the eye. This is a painless condition, because the retina does not contain sensory nerves that relay sensations of pain.

Collection of objective data includes observing the patient for the ability to perform ADLs. Also assess the level of anxiety associated with coping.

Diagnostic Tests

Visual acuity measurements should be the first diagnostic procedure with any complaint of vision loss. Indirect and direct ophthalmoscopy are used to detect pallor of the retina and detachment. The gonioscopy is used to provide a view of the anterior chamber of the eye. It provides a magnified view of any retinal lesions. Slit-lamp examination magnifies the lesions. Ultrasound may be useful to identify a retinal detachment if the retina cannot be visualized directly (e.g., when the cornea, lens, or vitreous humor is hazy or opaque).

Medical Management

The treatment of choice is early corrective intervention. The typical time frame for retinal repair depends on the involvement of the macula. If the macula remains intact and the patient's central vision remains, then repair typically is done within 24 to 48 hours. If the macula is detached, the patient will have decreased central vision and the time frame for repair will be within 7 to 10 days. One of five procedures may be performed:

- *Laser photocoagulation* burns localized tears or breaks in the posterior portion of the eye, eventually sealing the tear or break.

- *Cryotherapy* freezes the borders of a retinal hole with a frozen-tipped probe. The probe is applied to the scleral surface directly over the retinal tear. The tear seals when the resultant inflammatory process produces scarring.
- *Electrodiathermy* burns a retinal break, using an ultrasonic probe. The probe is applied to the scleral surface directly over the retinal break. Sealing occurs from the resultant inflammatory and scarring process.
- *Scleral buckling* is an extraocular surgical procedure that involves indenting the globe of the eye so that the retinal pigment epithelium, choroid, and sclera move toward the detached retina. This not only helps seal retinal breaks but also helps relieve inward traction on the retina. The retinal surgeon sutures a silicone implant against the sclera, causing the sclera to buckle inward. The surgeon may place an encircling band over the implant if there are multiple retinal breaks, if the surgeon cannot locate suspected break(s), or if there is widespread inward traction on the retina (see Fig. 13.11). If present, subretinal fluid may be drained by inserting a small-gauge needle to facilitate contact between the retina and the buckled sclera. Scleral buckling usually is accomplished with the patient under local anesthesia. The patient may be discharged on the first postoperative day, or scleral buckling surgery may be performed as an outpatient procedure.
- *Pneumatic* (pertaining to air or gas) *retinopexy* is an intraocular procedure that involves the injection of a gas into the vitreous cavity to form a temporary bubble that closes retinal breaks and places pressure on the separated retinal layers. This bubble is temporary and is combined with laser photocoagulation or cryotherapy treatment. For several weeks after therapy, the patient must position his or her head in a forward position so that the bubble remains in contact with the retinal break.

Nursing Interventions and Patient Teaching

Postprocedure management includes cycloplegic, mydriatic, and anti-infective eyedrops. Eye patches are applied over only the operative eye or both eyes, allowing the eyes to rest for 1 or 2 days. Safety measures are essential because the eyes are patched. Depending on the procedure, how the patient's head may be positioned postoperatively may vary. If air is injected into the vitreous, the head is positioned with the unaffected eye upward and the patient lying on the abdomen or sitting forward for 4 to 5 days. Dark glasses are prescribed after removal of the eye patches to decrease the discomfort of *photophobia*. A patient problem and interventions for the patient with retinal detachment include but are not limited to the following:

PATIENT PROBLEM	NURSING INTERVENTIONS
Anxiousness, related to visual alterations	Allow the patient the opportunity to discuss feelings and fears about the possible loss of vision Answer questions honestly and educate the patient if misunderstandings still exist Provide a rationale for restrictions of activities and for procedures

Discuss with the patient temporary restrictions of physical activity after therapy (see the Patient Teaching box).

Patient Teaching

Retinal Detachment

- Refrain from strenuous physical activity, heavy lifting, or high-risk activities to reduce the risk of traumatic injury to the eye.
- Check with the health care provider about shampooing hair. Prevent getting shampoo or soap in the affected eye.
- Use correct techniques for administration of eye medications as discussed earlier in the chapter.
- Report to the ophthalmologist any signs of further detachment (flashes of light, increase in floaters, blurred vision).
- Report for medical follow-up visits as instructed.

Prognosis

Retinal detachment requires immediate treatment. Reattachment is successful in 90% of cases; the degree of sight restoration depends on the extent and duration of separation. Maximum vision is achieved within 3 months after surgery. Unless replaced, a detached retina slowly dies after several years. Blindness from retinal detachment is irreversible.

GLAUCOMA AND CORNEAL INJURIES

GLAUCOMA

Etiology and Pathophysiology

Glaucoma is not one disease but rather a group of disorders characterized by (1) increased IOP because of obstruction of the outflow of aqueous humor, (2) optic nerve atrophy, and (3) progressive loss of peripheral vision (Fig. 13.12). Glaucoma is found in people who are middle aged and older. Approximately 9% to 12% of all blindness in the United States results from glaucoma (Glaucoma Research Foundation, 2017). One in 50 whites is affected, whereas 1 in 10 African Americans will develop glaucoma. It is seldom seen in people younger than 35 years of age but may occur in infancy.

Open-angle glaucoma, also known as *primary open-angle glaucoma (POAG)*, represents 90% of the cases of primary glaucoma. In POAG the outflow of aqueous humor is decreased in the trabecular meshwork. In essence, the drainage channels become occluded, like a clogged kitchen sink. The course of the disease is slowly progressive and results from degenerative changes; often this occurs bilaterally.

Clinical Manifestations

In POAG the patient has no signs or symptoms during the early stages of the disease. As the symptoms become apparent, they include loss of peripheral vision (tunnel vision), eye pain, difficulty adjusting to darkness, halos around lights, and inability to detect colors. The IOP is elevated.

AACG produces excruciating pain in or around the eye, decreased vision, and nausea and vomiting. The sclera is erythematous, and the pupil is enlarged and fixed. The patient sees colored halos around lights and has an acute increase in IOP.

Optic disc cupping occurs as glaucoma progresses. This is visible by direct or indirect ophthalmoscopy. The optic disc becomes wider, deeper, and paler (light gray or white). Optic disc cupping may be one of the first signs of chronic open-angle glaucoma. Optic disc photographs are useful for comparison over time to demonstrate an increase in the cup-to-disc ratio and progressive blanching (Fig. 13.13).

Assessment

Collection of subjective data includes noting the time of day that eye pain occurs. Also assess frequency, intensity, and duration of the pain. Note complaints of peripheral vision loss, maladaptation to darkness, and halos seen around lights. Determine the severity of headaches and the presence of nausea and vomiting.

Collection of objective data includes noting a need for frequent eyeglass prescription changes. Elevated IOP is also present.

Diagnostic Tests

Tonometry is used to determine IOP (see Fig. 13.5). A patient with glaucoma tests above the normal range of 10 to 22 mm Hg. IOP is usually between 22 and 32 mm Hg in POAG. IOP may be 50 mm Hg or higher in AACG. Visual field studies show a decline in the patient's peripheral vision. Optic disc cupping occurs as glaucoma progresses and will lead to optic nerve damage over time.

Medical Management

Keeping the IOP low enough to prevent the patient from developing optic nerve damage is the primary focus of glaucoma therapy.

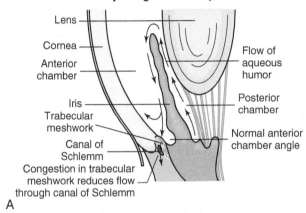

Slowly rising intraocular pressure

Lens
Cornea
Anterior chamber
Iris
Trabecular meshwork
Canal of Schlemm
Congestion in trabecular meshwork reduces flow through canal of Schlemm

Flow of aqueous humor
Posterior chamber
Normal anterior chamber angle

A

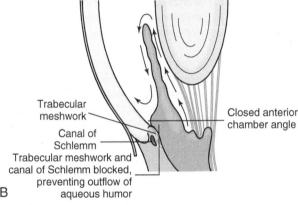

Rapidly rising intraocular pressure

Trabecular meshwork
Canal of Schlemm
Trabecular meshwork and canal of Schlemm blocked, preventing outflow of aqueous humor

Closed anterior chamber angle

B

Fig. 13.12 (A) Primary open-angle glaucoma (POAG). Congestion in the trabecular meshwork reduces the outflow of aqueous humor. (B) Acute angle-closure glaucoma (AACG). The angle between the iris and the anterior chamber narrows, obstructing the outflow of aqueous humor. (From Havener WH: *Synopsis of ophthalmology*, St. Louis, 1997, Mosby.)

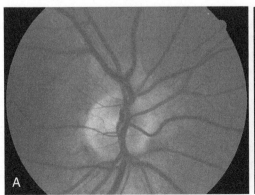
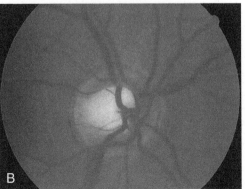

A   B

Fig. 13.13 (A) In the normal eye, the optic disc is pink with little cupping. (B) In the glaucomatous eye, the optic disc is bleached and optic cupping is present. (Note the appearance of the retinal vessels, which travel over the edge of the optic cup and appear to dip into it.) (From Lewis SL, Bucher L, Heitkemper MM, et al: *Medical-surgical nursing: assessment and management of clinical problems*, ed 10, St. Louis, 2017, Mosby.)

POAG is treated medically by the use of beta blockers, **miotics** (agents that cause the pupil to constrict), and carbonic anhydrase inhibitors (Table 13.4). A beta blocker, such as betaxolol hydrochloride (Betoptic), reduces IOP. Miotics, such as pilocarpine, constrict the pupil and draw the iris away from the cornea, allowing aqueous humor to drain out of the canal of Schlemm (see Fig. 13.12). Carbonic anhydrase inhibitors, such as acetazolamide (Diamox), decrease the production of aqueous humor, which results in lower IOPs. Surgery, which consists of a trabeculectomy or laser trabeculoplasty, is done when medications alone fail to control IOP. *Trabeculectomy* is the removal of corneoscleral tissue, usually the canal of Schlemm and trabecular meshwork. This produces an increase in the outflow of aqueous humor. Laser trabeculoplasty produces openings in the trabecular meshwork.

Table 13.4 Medications for Eye Disorders

GENERIC NAME	ACTION AND USE	SIDE EFFECTS	NURSING IMPLICATIONS
acetazolamide	Lowers intraocular pressure; used for open-angle glaucoma	Diarrhea, weakness, discomfort, urinary frequency, loss of appetite, nausea, vomiting, numbness in hands; contraindicated with severe renal, hepatic, or adrenocortical impairment	Know pregnancy and lactation cautions; give with food; in diabetes, it may increase blood and urine glucose levels; caution patient about drowsiness; monitor intake and output (I&O) and weight daily
betaxolol hydrochloride	Beta-adrenergic blocking agent that reduces formation of aqueous humor; used for open-angle glaucoma	Insomnia, irritation of eyelids, stinging on instillation, occasional tears, photophobia, systemic effects include possible disorientation, bradycardia, weakness, dyspnea	Know pregnancy cautions; do not touch dropper on eye; keep container tightly closed; determine intraocular pressure 4 weeks. after treatment; use cautiously in patients with history of heart failure or with diabetes mellitus
cyclopentolate hydrochloride	Anticholinergic drug that produces dilation of pupil and temporary paralysis of ciliary muscles; used in glaucoma; a diagnostic agent for angle-closure glaucomas	Ataxia, behavioral disturbances, tachycardia, disorientation, fever	Prevent contamination of dropper; warn patient of increased sensitivity to light and suggest sunglasses; contraindicated in angle closure glaucoma; use cautiously in older adults
dexamethasone	Decreases inflammation	Local irritation, retardation of corneal healing, blurred vision, eye pain, secondary eye infection	It may mask infection; use only for short term in children; tell patient not to wear contact lens during treatment; shake bottle before using; check with health care practitioner before using for future eye conditions; check with health care practitioner if condition does not improve in 5–7 days
gentamicin sulfate	Bactericidal antibiotic; used for treatment of blepharitis and conjunctivitis	Pruritus, erythema, edema, ocular discomfort, blurred vision (may occur for a few minutes after application)	Comply with full course of therapy; if no improvement occurs after a few days, check with health care practitioner
	Osmotic diuretic that reduces intraocular pressure; used for glaucoma	Fluid and electrolyte imbalance, chest pain, tachycardia, chills and fever, difficult urination	Administer by intravenous infusion; know pregnancy caution; duration of action is 1–3 h; monitor vital signs at least hourly and I&O, weight, and potassium levels daily
pilocarpine hydrochloride	Reduces intraocular pressure; used for open-angle glaucoma	Muscle tremors, nausea and vomiting, dyspnea, wheezing, bronchial spasms, local irritation	Encourage patient to have periodic intraocular pressure determinations; monitor for blurred vision or changes in vision; use cautiously in bronchial asthma and hypertension; apply light finger pressure on lacrimal sac 1 min after instillation of drops

Table 13.4 Medications for Eye Disorders—cont'd

GENERIC NAME	ACTION AND USE	SIDE EFFECTS	NURSING IMPLICATIONS
polyvinyl alcohol	Tearlike lubricant; used for dry eyes and eye irritations	Headache, burning, blurred vision, eye pain	Teach patient to instill; to avoid contamination of solution, warn patient not to touch tip of container to eye
sulfacetamide sodium	Broad-spectrum bacteriostatic anti-infective agent used in the treatment of ocular infections (conjunctivitis, corneal ulcers, trachoma, and chlamydial infections)	Pruritus, edema, erythema, other eye irritations	It is contraindicated in those with sulfonamide hypersensitivity; purulent exudate may inactivate drug; do not use silver preparations concurrently; encourage patient to comply with full course of treatment; store properly; discard solution if it discolors; warn patient to avoid sharing washcloths and towels with family members
timolol maleate	Beta-adrenergic blocking agent that reduces aqueous humor formation; used for open-angle glaucoma and hypertension; used with caution for patients who have heart conditions	Ocular sensitivity, severe irritation of eye or eyelid, systemic effects include cardiac failure, chest pain, disorientation, diarrhea, dizziness, exacerbation of asthma	It may mask hypoglycemia; measure intraocular pressure after 4 weeks. of treatment; avoid abrupt cessation; use cautiously in patients with bronchial asthma and heart conditions; know pregnancy and breastfeeding cautions; keep container tightly closed

Patient Teaching

Glaucoma

- Regular medical and ophthalmic care is required for the rest of the patient's life.
- Eye drops *must* be continued as long as prescribed even in the absence of symptoms; typically, treatment is lifelong.
- Blurred vision decreases with prolonged use.
- Avoid driving for 1 to 2 hours after administration of miotics.
- To prevent complications:
  - Press lacrimal duct for 1 min after eyedrop application to prevent rapid systemic absorption.
  - Keep reserve bottles of eyedrops at home.
  - Carry eyedrops when away from home.
  - Carry a card listing glaucoma as a diagnosis and the eyedrop solution prescribed.
  - There is no apparent relationship between vascular hypertension and ocular hypertension.
  - Report any reappearance of symptoms immediately to the health care provider.
  - If admitted to the hospital, alert the staff of the continued need for prescribed eyedrops.
  - Avoid the use of mydriatic or cycloplegic drugs (e.g., atropine) that dilate the pupils.

Medical marijuana use has become an increasingly popular option for reducing the IOPs associated with glaucoma. However, the effects of marijuana decrease IOP only for short time periods, typically 3 to 4 hours. For the patient to receive the benefits of consistently decreased IOPs with medical marijuana, the patient would have to consume the treatment six to eight times a day. Using medical marijuana at such a high frequency may leave the patient too impaired to lead an active lifestyle. The patient should be urged to consult with his or her health care provider concerning the use of both prescription and over-the-counter medications to avoid drug-related increases in IOP.

AACG is treated medically with osmotic diuretics, such as mannitol, carbonic anhydrase inhibitors, and miotics. Surgical treatments include peripheral iridectomy or iridotomy. Peripheral iridectomy is the surgical removal of part of the iris. The procedure is performed with the patient under local anesthesia. This procedure often restores drainage of the aqueous humor. Iridotomy is an incision into the iris of the eye to create an opening for aqueous flow; this is done under local or general anesthesia. Postoperatively, observe the patient for signs and symptoms of local hemorrhage, excessive or uncontrolled pain, and signs of excessive drainage from the eye.

Nursing Interventions and Patient Teaching

Nursing interventions involve protecting the patient's safety, monitoring compliance with therapy, and reinforcing discharge instructions. Depending on the practice setting, educate individual patients and families, groups of patients, or entire communities about the risks of glaucoma. In teaching, identify the increased incidence of glaucoma that occurs with age and the need for regular comprehensive ophthalmic examinations. Stress the importance of early detection and treatment in preventing long-term visual impairment. The current recommendation is for an ophthalmologic examination every 2 to 4 years for people between 40 and 64 years of age, and every 1 to 2 years for people 65 years of age or older. African Americans in every age group should have more frequent examinations because of the increased incidence and more aggressive nature of glaucoma in this patient population.

Glaucoma is a chronic condition requiring close observation for changes in condition. Follow-up care is needed to ensure that visual loss does not take place. The prescribed therapeutic regimen must be presented clearly to the patient and significant other(s). The implications of nonadherence must be addressed (see the Patient Teaching box for glaucoma). Information to be provided includes medication therapies, follow-up care, and signs and symptoms to report. Teach the patient about the purpose, frequency, and technique for administering prescribed medications. In addition to verbal instructions, give all patients written instructions that contain the information provided.

Prognosis

Today's method of medical and surgical management provides the patient with an excellent prognosis for a full recovery. Complications are few if care is obtained early in the course of the condition. When the patient ignores glaucoma or is noncompliant with therapy, blindness may occur. Regular eye examinations are required to detect and monitor for increased IOP. In general, once damage has occurred, the condition is irreversible. Surgery and medication can help lessen the complications from glaucoma.

CORNEAL INJURIES

Etiology and Pathophysiology

The cornea is composed of five layers of tissue and is uniform in nature. The cornea is nonvascular; therefore, no bleeding occurs from injury unless subcorneal structures are involved. The cornea is kept moist by tear production and is protected from daily insult by the eyelid. Any wound to the cornea can decrease the level of transparency, through scar formation.

Corneal injuries include the following:
- Foreign bodies
- Burns: chemical or thermal
- Abrasions and lacerations
- Penetrating wounds

Foreign bodies are the most common cause of corneal injury. Dust particles, propellants, and eyelashes may lodge in the conjunctiva or cornea. Blinking and tearing help to clear the irritant, but further irritation may occur from the upper lid, closing and moving the foreign body into deeper layers or over a wider area of the cornea.

Burns occur in the home and workplace. When burns affect the eye, it is a medical emergency. Burns are classified as chemical burns or thermal burns. Depending on what has caused a burn, the damage may be superficial or deep; regardless, it is essential to seek immediate emergency care after an exposure. Chemical irritants such as acids, alkalis, and metal flashes from acetylene blowtorches cause

significant pain, depending on the depth of chemical erosion.

Abrasions and lacerations are usually superficial scratches caused by fingernails or clothing. They may be painful, depending on the depth of the abrasion.

Penetrating wounds are the most serious corneal injuries. Eye structures may be injured permanently, resulting in total blindness. Infection may result from the introduction of microorganisms on the penetrating object.

Clinical Manifestations

Foreign bodies produce pain when the eye moves or the eyelid moves over the eye during blinking. Excessive tearing, erythema of the conjunctiva, and pruritus may occur. Acute pain and burning are the primary symptoms with any topical (surface) burn to the eye. Abrasions and lacerations produce mild to severe pain, depending on the depth of corneal involvement. The pain may be transitory and slight, or spasmodic and deep. Penetrating wounds result in varying degrees of pain. If underlying structures are involved, pain may be absent because the nerves have been severed.

Assessment

Foreign bodies. Subjective data include the time and type of exposure or injury. Assess the patient for the degree and severity of eye pain and vision loss. Ask about any first aid treatment provided. Objective data include observation of the foreign body and extent of damage. When the intracapsular area has been penetrated, fluids leak from the affected eye.

Burns. Subjective data include the degree of pain. It is important to assess the type of burn, thermal or chemical; the type of chemical exposure that caused the burn; and any first aid treatment that has been provided. Visual losses will be determined after examination by the health care professional.

Collection of objective data includes noting the extent of the burn in and around the eye, including eyelashes and eyebrows, and assessing the general condition of the eye and surrounding structures.

Abrasions and lacerations. Subjective data include the degree of pain after the incident and how the injury occurred. Note treatments used at the time of injury.

Collection of objective data includes assessing the degree of damage to the eye and surrounding structures and noting any vision loss.

Penetrating wounds. Subjective data include the duration of exposure and causative factors related to the injury. Assess the presence and severity of pain. Determine whether any first aid treatment was given.

Objective data include the type and size of the penetrating object. Note any fluid leakage from the eye and damage to surrounding structures.

Diagnostic Tests

Tests include visual and ophthalmoscopic examination, fluorescein staining, peripheral vision tests, and slit-lamp examination.

Medical Management

Foreign bodies are treated medically with a flush of normal saline when the object is near the sclera and conjunctiva; it then can be removed by a clean swab or tissue. Cotton is not used, because it may scratch the cornea. If the object is not flushed away easily, the individual must see an ophthalmologist to have the object removed. Antibiotic topical eye ointments are ordered.

Burns are treated medically with a 20-minute or longer normal saline flush immediately after burn exposure; this helps to prevent scar formation and subsequent loss of vision. Separate the eyelids while flushing the affected eye to ensure maximum irrigation. Thermal or chemical burns of the eye and surrounding eye structures are an emergency problem and require immediate medical treatment and examination by an ophthalmologist. After examination by an ophthalmologist, the patient with an eye burn may be prescribed topical antimicrobial medications.

Abrasions and lacerations of the eye are cleaned medically or flushed with a normal saline (0.9 NaCl) solution by the health care professional. Antibiotic therapy, usually topical, may be prescribed after injury (see the Safety Alert box).

Seek medical assistance immediately for eye injuries, burns, and foreign bodies that remain in the eye. Immediately after a penetrating wound injury, both eyes should be covered while the patient is transported to the hospital. Both eyes work in synchrony, so covering the unaffected eye prevents it from involuntarily moving with the other eye. A shield reduces further injury but must not touch the foreign object. A Styrofoam cup provides adequate coverage and is usually readily available. The foreign object should not be removed except by the ophthalmologist or surgeon after examination.

Nursing Interventions and Patient Teaching

Nursing interventions for foreign bodies include assisting with the required irrigation of the eye. For burns, assist with the flushing process and providing eye medications as ordered. For abrasions and lacerations, assist with cleaning the eye as ordered and providing general first aid.

When a patient has a penetrating wound, note whether the pupil on the affected side has become irregular in size. These results when the iris of the affected eye moves to occlude the wound area. Infection potential is high; therefore, topical and systemic antibiotics are ordered. If the wound is small, there may not be a need for surgical intervention. If the wound is large or deep, enucleation of the eye may be necessary.

Safety Alert

Eye Safety Measures

- Do not rinse eyes with unprescribed solutions.
- Discard any ophthalmic solution that is cloudy, discolored, contains particles, or that has been open for longer than 3 months.
- Do not self-treat an eye inflammation with a medication prescribed for a previous eye disorder.
- To avoid eye strain:
  - Use a good light for reading or doing work that requires careful visual focus.
  - When reading or focusing eyes for long periods, look at distant objects for a few minutes at repeated intervals to rest eyes.
- Avoid rubbing the eyes.
- Wash hands before and after touching the eyes.
- Wear safety glasses when engaging in activities that could injure the eyes. If injury occurs, seek immediate medical attention.
- Wear dark glasses for prolonged exposure to bright light (prolonged daylight exposure, activities in the snow, or on the water).
- Flush eyes immediately for 15–20 min or longer with cool water when any irritating substances are introduced. The Morgan lens traditionally is used to flush the eye in emergency cases (Fig. 13.14).
- Do not attempt to remove foreign bodies from the cornea; cover the eye with an eye shield (e.g., Styrofoam cup) to prevent excessive movement or touching of the eye. Seek medical attention immediately.
- If a speck of dust blows into the eye, pull the upper lid over the lower lid and let the tears wash the speck to the inner canthus (corner of the eye) or lower lid, where it may be removed safely. Irrigate the eye with cool tap water, if necessary.
- Eye makeup should be replaced every 3 months and with every eye infection to prevent the growth of bacteria or reinfection.
- Never share eye makeup, and when sampling makeup in stores use only fresh applicators and samples that have not been contaminated by multiple users. (The safest choice is to avoid store samples altogether.)

Effective and immediate therapy is crucial for any eye injury. If treatment is interrupted, ineffective, or not sustained, permanent eye damage will occur. The most frequent complications include infection, vision disturbances, and blindness. A patient problem for the patient with an eye injury will be *Recent Onset of Pain, related to inflammatory processes secondary to trauma or injury.* (See the preceding discussion on conjunctivitis.)

Ensure that the patient can apply ointments and dressings, if ordered. Instruct the patient in the use of other therapy devices, such as warm or cool compresses as needed. Teach proper handwashing techniques. The patient should wear dark sunglasses if cycloplegic or mydriatic eyedrops are used. Instruct the patient to avoid future exposures to chemical or environmental

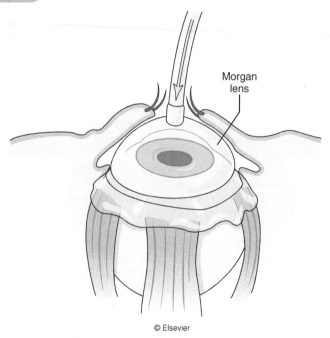

Fig. 13.14 The Morgan lens used to flush the eye in an emergency.

hazards. Ensure that the patient understands the discharge instructions, including the need for follow-up provider visits and symptoms to report. Determine the patient's knowledge about therapy, treatment, and the patient's ability to perform the necessary steps to care for his or her injury.

Prognosis

Immediate and appropriate treatment reduces the severity and complications of eye injuries. Superficial corneal abrasions usually heal without incident. Deeper abrasions or burns may result in permanent visual loss because of scarring.

SURGERIES OF THE EYE

ENUCLEATION

Enucleation of the eye is the surgical removal of the eyeball. It is often necessary after severe eye trauma but may be done because of other complications, such as malignant tumors. During the enucleation, an implant is inserted into the eye socket; this will allow the patient to have a prosthetic eye fitted and placed once the surgical wound has healed.

Nursing Interventions and Patient Teaching

The loss of an eye is extremely traumatic for the patient. Electing to have the procedure performed presents the patient with a difficult decision. The patient normally grieves the loss of the eye. The enucleation results in a life-altering change in appearance. There are concerns related to functionality, lost vision, and social implications (i.e., how others will perceive the patient). Priorities for care by the nurse include emotional support, open communication, and honest provision of information. Other nursing responsibilities include facilitating a therapeutic dialogue between the health care provider and the patient regarding the exact nature of the surgery and the expected course of therapy after the enucleation.

Postoperatively, apply a pressure dressing over the socket of the eye to control hemorrhage. Observe the dressing at least every hour for the first 24 hours. The recovery period includes a protective eye patch that will be worn for days to weeks after surgery. Ask the patient about any pain on the affected side of the head or any headache, which may indicate hemorrhage or infection. Report these findings to the health care provider immediately. Avoid routine postoperative procedures of coughing and turning onto the affected side to prevent sutures from dislodging or hemorrhage. The wound is healed adequately approximately 6 weeks after enucleation. An ocularist creates a prosthetic eye that fits the orbital socket and is designed to match the remaining eye. The patient must be educated in how to remove, cleanse, and insert the prosthesis carefully. Continued monitoring of the socket is necessary to ensure proper fit of the prosthesis, because changes, including atrophy of the socket, may occur.

KERATOPLASTY (CORNEAL TRANSPLANT)

Keratoplasty is the removal of the full thickness of the patient's cornea followed by surgical implantation of a cornea from a human donor. It is done to replace a damaged cornea resulting from trauma, ulceration, or congenital deformities. Keratoplasty is performed with the patient under local or general anesthesia. The transplanted tissue is sutured into place to maintain graft alignment and a watertight wound.

More than 40,000 corneal transplants are performed in the United States each year. Improved methods of tissue procurement and preservation, refined surgical techniques, postoperative topical corticosteroids, and careful follow up have decreased graft rejection. Immunosuppressants, medications that suppress the immune system and prevent rejection (e.g., cyclosporine), may be ordered postoperatively.

Corneal grafts usually are taken from the organ donor within 4 hours of death. An ideal donor is between 25 and 35 years of age who died from traumatic injury or an acute disease process. The corneas of people with chronic or communicable diseases—such as hepatitis, acquired immunodeficiency syndrome, or cancer—are not appropriate for transplantation. The eye bank will test donors for human immunodeficiency virus and hepatitis B and C. The donor's eye should have normal light perception and projection. The donor's tissue is best used within 5 days after removal.

Responsibilities of the nurse in a potential organ donation case are to notify the appropriate supervisory personnel and other agencies as directed by policy.

Nursing Interventions and Patient Teaching

Before surgery, encourage the patient to ask questions and express concerns related to the surgery. Teach the patient about the use of protective eyeglasses if a dilation-causing eye medication is to be used. Clean and prepare the surgical areas as ordered, usually with an antiseptic solution. Preoperative patient teaching includes deep breathing and turning to reduce any complications associated with surgery. Coughing is discouraged, because damage can occur to the surgical site. Maintain dietary restrictions, if ordered, and administer prescribed medications.

After surgery, ensure that correct postoperative positioning is maintained; the patient usually is positioned on the back or on the non-operative side. The health care provider should provide specific orders for activity limitations and care of the surgical site postoperatively. Use safety measures, including adequate lighting, clear paths, and orientation to unfamiliar environments, until the patient is able to ambulate safely. Prevent injuries by providing safety devices and orienting the patient to each new environment in the postoperative period. Anyone coming into the room should announce his or her presence. The patient should avoid bending, lifting, and straining for approximately 1 month to prevent increases in IOP or suture tension.

Reinforce the scheduled postoperative visits with the eye surgeon and other eye health care providers. Report any severe or progressive pain to the surgeon immediately, as well as any complaints of erythema, loss of vision, or photophobia that would occur with corneal rejection. Administer systemic and ophthalmic medications as prescribed. Maintain strict surgical asepsis during dressing changes. Staff, the patient, and the family must wash hands thoroughly before any contact with the eye area. Instruct the patient to avoid the use of irritants, including fragrant powders, perfumes, or eye makeup that may cause irritation, sneezing, or coughing and subsequent displacement of sutures. The patient should not rub the eye area to avoid contaminating the site or displacing sutures. Assess the patient's diversion activities; television usually is permitted, but reading is limited because the side-to-side movement of the eyes may loosen the sutures. If an eye patch or metal eyecup shield is ordered, demonstrate how to use and care for the device. The eye patch is applied snugly to inhibit the blink reflex and allow the eye to rest. The metal eye shield is used at night to protect the eye from trauma. Obtain discharge instructions from the health care provider regarding use of protective eyewear.

Prognosis

Because the cornea is avascular, healing is slow, and the incidence of infection is increased. Rejection of the donor tissue may occur. Teaching the patient and family to recognize the signs and symptoms of rejection is an essential part of the discharge planning.

PHOTOCOAGULATION

Photocoagulation is a nonsurgical procedure usually performed on an outpatient basis. A small, intense beam of light is directed into a small spot on the retina. The light converts to heat energy, and coagulation of tissue protein occurs. The structures of the eye remain undisturbed and only the sealing of leaks and destruction of offending tissue occur. The procedure is used to manage conditions such as ARMD and diabetic retinopathy.

Photocoagulation is useful in diabetic retinopathy to cauterize hemorrhaging vessels. It cannot increase visual acuity but can prevent further loss. Usually no hospitalization or postoperative medical management is required.

Nursing Interventions and Patient Teaching

Postoperative assessment for patients who have undergone photocoagulation therapy includes assessment of vision. They may have constriction of peripheral fields and a temporary decrease in central vision. A decrease in night vision and a headache from the laser's bright light also may occur.

Prognosis

Photocoagulation is used to prevent eye damage and is not curative. Minimal destruction of tissue occurs with photocoagulation. The procedure is nonsurgical; therefore, infection risk is minimal.

VITRECTOMY

A **vitrectomy** is the removal of excess vitreous fluid caused by hemorrhage and replacement with normal saline. The procedure allows for the removal of any existing scar tissue. The procedure is done to manage eye conditions such as retinal detachment, macular holes, and vitreous hemorrhage.

Postoperative management includes the application of topical eye medication for 4 to 6 weeks. Analgesics are prescribed for postoperative pain management. A pressure patch for the operative eye is placed immediately after surgery. Cold compresses may be used to reduce inflammation.

Nursing Interventions and Patient Teaching

The patient is required to lay on his or her abdomen or to sit forward, resting the non-operative side of the head on a table, to allow air that is in the eye to float against the retina. This position is maintained for 4 to 5 days.

Dark glasses are prescribed postoperatively to decrease the discomfort of photophobia. Postoperative care includes assessing the eye patch; applying cold packs; monitoring vital signs, especially for fever; and assessing the dressing for bleeding.

ANATOMY AND PHYSIOLOGY OF THE EAR

The external ear *(pinna,* or *auricle)* reveals only a portion of the complex organ of hearing. Within the ear are many structures that enable hearing and interpretation of sound and assist in maintaining equilibrium (balance). Anatomically, from the external structures to the internal structures, the ear has three distinct divisions: the external ear, the middle ear, and the inner ear (Fig. 13.15). The external ear and the middle ear deal exclusively with sound waves, whereas the inner ear deals with sound waves and equilibrium.

EXTERNAL EAR

The external ear is composed of the auricle (pinna) and the external auditory canal. The canal is shaped like a small, curved tube (about 1 inch [2.5 cm] in length). It extends into the temporal bone, ending at the *tympanic membrane*—a thin, semitransparent membrane. The tympanic membrane separates the external ear from the middle ear and transmits sound vibrations to the internal ear by means of the auditory ossicles. The external ear is designed to collect sound waves and channel them to the middle ear. The upper part of the pinna is composed of elastic cartilage, whereas the lower part, the lobe, is mainly fleshy tissue. The whole structure is attached to the skull by ligaments and muscles.

The walls of the external auditory canal are composed of cartilage-lined bone. The external auditory canal contains cilia (fine hairs) and specialized sebaceous glands called *ceruminous glands* that secrete cerumen (earwax). Together the cilia and cerumen protect the lining and inner ear from foreign bodies and potential sources of obstruction or infection.

MIDDLE EAR

The middle ear, or tympanic cavity, is a small, air-filled chamber located within the temporal bone. The *eustachian tube,* or auditory tube, is lined with a mucous membrane that joins the nasopharynx and the middle-ear cavity. During swallowing or yawning, the tube allows air to enter the middle ear, which equalizes the air pressure on either side of the tympanic membrane. Because the pharynx, the eustachian tube, and the middle ear are covered with a continuous mucous membrane, bacteria and viruses can travel easily from the throat to the middle ear. This often is seen in young children, in whom the eustachian tube is more level, making drainage difficult. The posterior wall of the middle ear opens into the mastoid process, an area filled with air spaces, which also aids in equalizing air pressure. Infection of the middle ear, if untreated, can spread to the mastoid process.

Extending along the middle-ear chamber are three small bones (ossicles) that carry sound waves from the external ear to the inner ear. These ossicles are named according to their shape: the *malleus* (hammer), the *incus* (anvil), and the *stapes* (stirrup). The internal surface of the tympanic membrane is connected to the first of these three bones, the malleus. The malleus transfers sound waves to the incus, which in turn transfers them to the stapes. The stapes pushes against the oval window, a small membrane that marks the beginning of the inner ear. When sound waves cause the tympanic

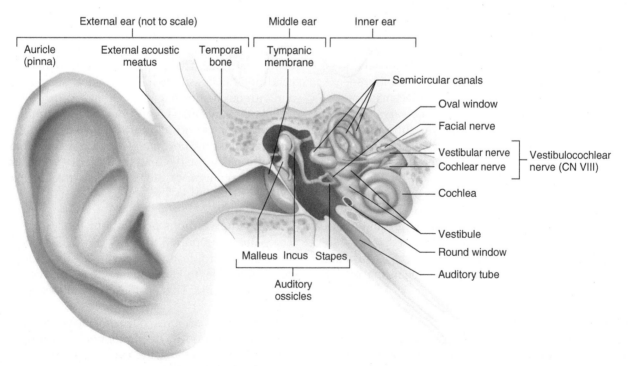

Fig. 13.15 External, middle, and inner ear (not to scale). (From Patton KT, Thibodeau GA: *The human body in health and disease*, ed 7, St. Louis, 2018, Elsevier.)

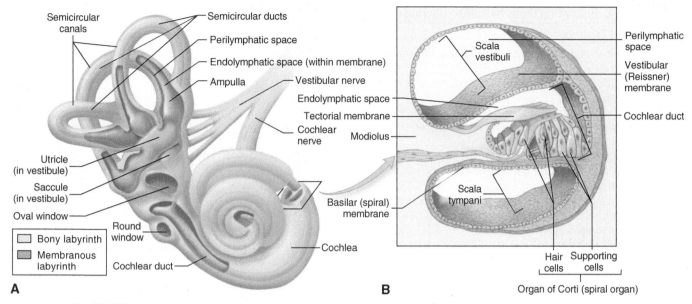

Fig. 13.16 The inner ear. (A) The bony labyrinth is the hard outer wall of the entire inner ear and includes semicircular canals, the vestibule, and the cochlea. Within the bony labyrinth is the membranous labyrinth *(purple)*, which is surrounded by perilymph and filled with endolymph. Each ampulla in the vestibule contains a crista ampullaris that detects changes in head position and sends sensory impulses through the vestibular nerve to the brain. (B) A section of the membranous cochlea. Hair cells in the organ of Corti detect sound and send the information through the cochlear nerve. Then vestibular and cochlear nerves join to form the eighth cranial nerve. (From Patton KT, Thibodeau GA: *The human body in health and disease*, ed 7, St. Louis, 2018, Elsevier.)

membrane to vibrate, that vibration is transmitted and amplified by the ear ossicles as it passes through the middle ear. Movement of the stapes against the oval window causes movement of fluid in the inner ear.

INNER EAR

The *labyrinth* is a series of canals making up the inner ear (Fig. 13.16). Structurally, it consists of the bony labyrinth, which is filled with a fluid called *perilymph*. The bony labyrinth has three subdivisions called the *semicircular canal* (associated with the sense of balance), the *vestibule*, and the *cochlea*. The membranous labyrinth is a series of sacs and tubes that contain a thicker fluid called *endolymph*. Endolymph and perilymph conduct sound waves through the inner-ear system.

The cochlea resembles a snail's shell and contains the *organ of Corti*, known as the organ of hearing. It contains many fine hair cell receptors, which respond to sound waves by stimulating the cochlear nerve (a branch of the eighth cranial nerve—the vestibulocochlear, or acoustic nerve), which transmits the message to the brain. These hair cells may become damaged over time from noise pollution (i.e., high-intensity sounds such as those produced by jet engines, factory equipment, and rock bands). Once these cells are damaged or destroyed, hearing becomes permanently impaired.

Deeper in the inner ear, past the cochlea, lies an oval central portion of the bony labyrinth known as the *vestibule*. The vestibule contains receptors that respond to gravity and provides information on which way is up and which way is down, enabling an individual to remain in an upright position. Extending upward from the vestibule are three semicircular canals responsible for maintaining balance and equilibrium. These canals contain sensory hair cells and endolymph. The motion of the endolymph stimulates the hair cells, which in turn stimulate the receptors to send the message to the brain for interpretation (see Fig. 13.16).

NURSING CONSIDERATIONS FOR CARE OF THE PATIENT WITH AN EAR DISORDER

Once the history and general assessment have been completed, focus on assessment of the ear. Additional information would include the following:

- Occurrence of ear drainage, tinnitus, vertigo, cerumen buildup, pressures, pain, and pruritus
- Other medical diagnoses that may affect hearing
- Family history
- Exposure to loud noises
- Behavioral clues indicating hearing loss (Box 13.2)
- History of medications use, specifically those known to be ototoxic
- Current medications for an ear disorder
- Side effects of medications, if any
- Associated speech pattern abnormalities
- Use of assistive hearing devices
- Use of home remedies that cause ear trauma

Communicate the gathered data to the appropriate personnel and document the findings in the patient record. The next step in the assessment process is to prepare the patient for the initial otoscopic diagnostic evaluation.

Box 13.2   Behavioral Clues Indicating Hearing Loss

Any adult who:
- Is irritable, hostile, and hypersensitive in interpersonal relations
- Has difficulty hearing upper-frequency consonants
- Complains about people mumbling
- Turns up volume on television and radio
- Asks for frequent repetition and answers questions inappropriately
- Loses sense of humor, becomes grim
- Leans forward to hear better; face becomes serious and strained
- Shuns large- and small-group audience situations
- May appear aloof and uninterested
- Complains of ringing in the ears
- Has an unusually soft or loud voice
- Repeatedly asks, "What did you say?"

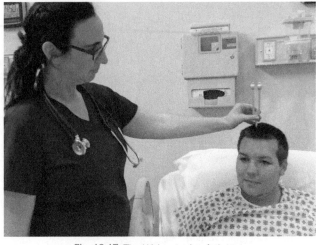

Fig. 13.17 The Weber tuning fork test.

LABORATORY AND DIAGNOSTIC EXAMINATIONS

OTOSCOPY

With an otoscope, the examiner can visualize the external auditory canal and the tympanic membrane. Normally the tympanic membrane is disk shaped and pearl pale pink. Otoscopy is the initial examination of the ear, performed before other testing. One of the nurse's responsibilities is to explain to the patient the purpose and procedure. Reassure the patient that otoscopy is a painless test requiring only about 1 to 2 minutes, with slight pulling of the ear upward and backward for an adult and down and back for a child.

WHISPERED VOICE TEST

General screening regarding the patient's ability to hear can occur with tests using the whispered and spoken voice. The examiner stands 12 to 24 inches (30 to 60 cm) to the side of the patient and speaks simple one- and two-syllable words in a low whisper. The patient is asked to repeat the words or information given. The examiner increases volume until the patient responds appropriately. Test each ear, with the patient covering the other ear. An accuracy of 50% is considered normal.

TUNING FORK TESTS

The two most common tests using tuning forks are the Weber test and the Rinne test. These tests are used to determine hearing loss and collect data related to the type of loss.

- *Weber test:* The *Weber test* is a method of assessing auditory acuity, especially useful in determining whether defective hearing in an ear is a conductive loss caused by a middle-ear problem or a sensorineural loss, resulting from a disorder in the inner ear or auditory nerve system. The test is performed by placing the stem of a vibrating tuning fork in the center of the patient's forehead or on the maxillary incisors. The sound is equally loud in both ears if hearing is normal. If the person has a sensorineural loss in one ear, the unaffected ear perceives the sound as louder. When conductive hearing loss is present, the sound is louder in the affected ear. The patient does not hear ordinary background noise conducted through the air and receives only vibrations by bone conduction (Fig. 13.17).

- *Rinne test:* The *Rinne test* is a method of distinguishing conductive from sensorineural hearing loss. The test is performed with tuning forks placed ½ inch (1.25 cm) from the external auditory meatus and the vibrating stem placed over the mastoid bone. While one ear is tested, the other is masked (Fig. 13.18). In sensorineural loss the sound is heard longer by air conduction, whereas in conductive hearing loss the sound is heard longer by bone conduction.

Nursing responsibility in the Weber test and the Rinne test includes explanation of the purpose and procedure of the tests. Stress that the patient needs to concentrate and use hand signals to indicate the ear in which the sound is heard in the Weber test and when it is no longer heard in the Rinne test. These tests can be performed in a few minutes and are painless and noninvasive measures.

AUDIOMETRIC TESTING

Audiometry is a test of hearing acuity. Audiometry is beneficial as a diagnostic test for determining the degree and type of hearing loss and as a screening test for hearing acuity. Various audiometric tests determine the lowest intensity of sound at which an individual can perceive auditory stimulus (hearing threshold), hear different frequencies, and distinguish different speech tones.

Nursing responsibilities include explaining the purpose and procedure of each test and reviewing any required responses by the patient.

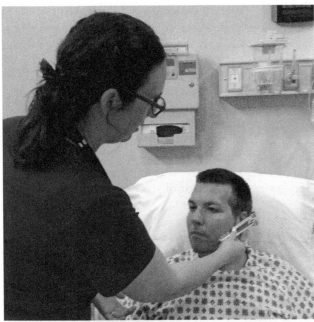

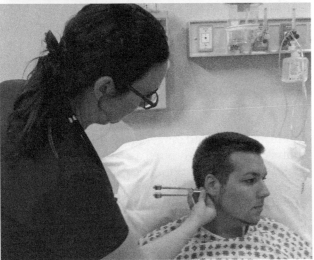

Fig. 13.18 The Rinne tuning fork test.

VESTIBULAR TESTING

The auditory and vestibular (balance and equilibrium) systems are closely related. Appropriate diagnosis depends on close observation of the patient's signs and symptoms to ascertain if they are related to balance or hearing loss. Ask the patient to describe the signs and symptoms that he or she is experiencing in accurate detail through the interview portion of the history.

Problems of the vestibular system may manifest as nystagmus or vertigo. *Nystagmus* is involuntary, rhythmic movements of the eye. The movements may be horizontal, vertical, rotary, or mixed. The sensation that the person or objects are moving or spinning is referred to as **vertigo**. Moving the head in any direction further heightens this feeling of vertigo. The Romberg and past-point tests are used for patients complaining of dizziness or disequilibrium.

- *Romberg test:* The *Romberg test* measures the patient's ability to perform specific tasks with eyes open and then with eyes closed. The normal response is to maintain balance throughout the entire test. An abnormal response (in which the patient loses balance when standing erect, feet together, eyes closed) indicates loss of the sense of position.
- *Past-point testing:* In past-point testing, the patient's ability to place a finger accurately on a selected point on the body is measured. Inability to correctly perform the test indicates a lack of coordination in voluntary movements.

Explain the purpose and procedure of each test. Institute safety measures to prevent patient injury during the Romberg test if the patient cannot maintain balance.

DISORDERS OF THE EAR

LOSS OF HEARING (DEAFNESS)

Hearing impairment is a state of decreased auditory acuity that ranges from partial to complete hearing loss. It is the most common disability in the United States affecting 28 million people. Among people older than 65 years of age, it is the third most common chronic condition. The quality of life for one-third of the adults in the United States between 65 and 75 years of age is decreased because of hearing impairments. Recognition, diagnosis, and early treatment may help prevent further impairment and damage.

The implications of hearing loss are great. Hearing is needed to develop speech and conceptual ability; thus hearing loss may affect personality development when the hearing impairment is severe and congenital. This may have implications for the person's education and socialization. As hearing loss increases, the person may withdraw socially because of the inability to understand and be understood; this could lead to isolation and depression (see the Health Promotion box).

Types of hearing loss

There are six types of hearing loss: conductive, sensorineural, mixed, congenital, functional (psychogenic), and central.

- In *conductive hearing loss,* sound is inadequately conducted through the external or middle ear to the sensorineural apparatus of the inner ear. Common causes are buildup of cerumen and otitis media with effusion. Other conditions that may result in conductive hearing loss are foreign bodies, otosclerosis, and stenosis of the external auditory canal. Sensitivity to sound is diminished, but clarity or interpretation of sound is not changed. Increased volume or amplification compensates for the conductive loss; therefore, a hearing aid may be helpful.
- In *sensorineural hearing loss,* sound is conducted through the external and middle ear in the normal way, but a defect in the inner ear results in its distortion, making discrimination difficult. Trauma,

Health Promotion

Facilitating Communication for People With Impaired Hearing

- If the patient wears a hearing aid, make certain it is in place, turned on, and functioning properly.
- Get the person's attention by raising an arm or hand.
- Ask permission to turn off the television or radio or turn down the volume.
- Ensure adequate lighting so that the patient will be able to understand or lip-read.
- Face the person when speaking.
- Lip-reading is a skill that not all hearing impaired are capable of achieving. Do not assume all people who are hearing impaired can lip-read.
- Speak clearly, but do not over accentuate words.
- Speak in a normal tone; do not shout or raise the pitch of voice. Shouting overuses normal speaking movements and may cause distortion in the sound that may be too loud for the person with sensorineural damage. If the person has conductive loss only, sometimes making the voice louder without shouting is helpful.
- If the person does not seem to understand what is said, express it differently. Some words are difficult to distinguish by lip-reading, such as *white* and *red*.
- Move closer to the person and toward the better ear if the person does not hear you.
- Write out proper names or any statement that you are not sure was understood.
- Do not eat, drink, chew gum, or cover your mouth when talking to a person with limited hearing.
- Observe for inattention that may indicate tiredness or lack of understanding.
- Use phrases rather than one-word answers to convey meaning. State the major topic of the discussion first and then give details.
- Do not show annoyance by careless facial expression. People who are hard of hearing depend more on visual clues for acceptance.
- Encourage the use of a hearing aid if the person has one; allow the person to adjust it before speaking.
- If in a group, repeat important statements and avoid asides to others in the group.
- Do not avoid conversation with a person who has hearing loss.

infectious processes, presbycusis, congenital conditions, and exposure to ototoxic drugs may cause this type of hearing loss. Destruction of the cochlear hair by intense noise also may cause sensorineural hearing loss. Amplifying sound with a hearing aid may help some people with this type of loss. However, many people have intolerance to loud noise and are not helped by a hearing aid.
- *Mixed hearing loss* is combined conductive and sensorineural hearing loss.
- *Congenital hearing loss* is present from birth or early infancy. It can be caused by anoxic injury (brain injury resulting from oxygen deprivation) or trauma during delivery, Rh factor incompatibility, or the mother's exposure during pregnancy to syphilis or rubella, or the use of ototoxic drugs.

- *Functional hearing loss* has no organic cause. It also is known as *psychogenic* or *nonorganic hearing loss*. Functional hearing loss may be caused by an emotional or psychological factor.
- *Central hearing loss* occurs when the brain's auditory pathways are damaged, as in a stroke or a tumor.

Clinical manifestations

Clinical manifestations vary, depending on the degree of hearing loss. Symptoms range from subtle clues, such as requests for repeating information, to more obvious signs of non-responsiveness.

Assessment

Collection of subjective data includes noting the onset and progression of the condition, deficit in one or both ears, family history, history of head trauma, mental status changes, exposure to noise, current medications, visual or speech disorders, and any other ear symptoms.

Objective data must include an assessment of behavioral clues that indicate a hearing difficulty (see Box 13.2).

Diagnostic tests

Conductive hearing loss produces lateralization of sound to the deaf ear in the Weber test. Results of the Rinne test show that sounds transmitted through bone conduction are heard longer than, or at least as long as, sounds transmitted through air conduction.

Sensorineural hearing loss produces lateralization of sound to the better ear in the Weber test. Results of the Rinne test show that air-conducted sounds are heard longer than bone-conducted sounds, but not twice as long.

Audiometric testing determines the type of hearing loss and the degree of impairment.

Medical management

Medical management depends on the type of impairment. Surgical procedures may be required. Hearing aids or cochlear implants may be used when appropriate. Cochlear implantation is performed in individuals with profound bilateral sensorineural hearing loss who receive no measurable assistance from hearing aids (see "Cochlear Implant," below, and Fig. 13.19).

Nursing interventions and patient teaching

Patients with partial hearing loss may benefit from a hearing aid. Help the patient care for the hearing aid as detailed in Box 13.3.

Emotional support of the patient as they become accustomed to wearing the hearing aid is needed. Some fear that the use of the device will be viewed as a sign of disability. Initially wearing the hearing aid for extended periods can cause discomfort. Common complaints include buzzing noises, loud background sounds and interference with cell phone or other electronic devices.

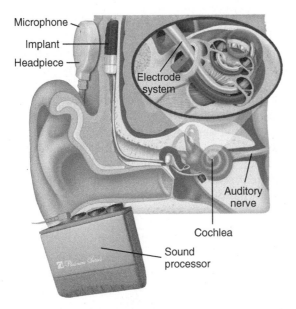

Fig. 13.19 Cochlear implant. (Lemmi FO, Lemmi CAE: *Physical assessment findings CD-ROM*, Philadelphia, 2000, Saunders.)

Box 13.3	Care of the Hearing Aid

DO
- Handle with care.
- Wash the ear mold or plug daily in mild soap and water.
- Dry the ear mold or plug thoroughly before reconnecting it to the receiver.
- Always keep extra batteries and cord available.
- When the hearing aid is not in use, turn the aid off and open the battery compartment.
- If the hearing aid whistles, reinsert the ear mold.
- If a hearing aid fails to work:
  - Check the on-off switch.
  - Inspect the ear mold for cleanliness.
  - Examine the battery for tightness of fit.
  - Examine the cord plug for tightness of insertion.
  - Examine the cord for breaks.
  - Replace the battery or cord.
  - Check for cracks in the tubing or ear mold.
  - Check to see that the ear mold and hearing aid are inserted in the correct ear.
  - Check that the ear mold or hearing aid is properly inserted.
  - Check that the volume control wheel is turned up to an appropriate setting.

DO NOT
- Put the hearing aid on a heated surface.
- Wash the hearing aid.
- Drop the hearing aid.
- Wear the hearing aid in the bath or shower.
- Wear the hearing aid overnight.
- Ignore a hearing aid that is "whistling."
- Use in contact with cream, oil, or hair spray when the hearing aid is on.

Most surprising to some is the discomfort that can be experienced by the sound magnification when wearing the aid. Follow up with the audiologist is indicated. Adjustments to the hearing aid may be indicated.

Patient problems and interventions for the patient with hearing loss include but are not limited to the following:

PATIENT PROBLEM	NURSING INTERVENTIONS
Impaired Sensory Awareness, related to disease process	Facilitate communication with the patient by following the interventions provided in the Health Promotion box for people with impaired hearing
Social Seclusion, related to loss of hearing	Assess factors that contribute to social isolation Identify support systems for patient Identify patient concerns Establish effective communication

Patient teaching

Assist the patient in learning to care for a hearing aid, if prescribed (see Box 13.3). Advise the patient to request that others speak slowly or more clearly and repeat if necessary.

Prognosis

Surgical repair of the injured structures increases the likelihood of restoring partial or complete hearing, especially when implants are used. Complications of surgery are rare. Technical advances also have improved the quality of hearing. Microtechnology has reduced the size of hearing aids so that they are almost undetectable.

INFLAMMATORY AND INFECTIOUS DISORDERS OF THE EAR

EXTERNAL OTITIS
Etiology and Pathophysiology

External otitis, or otitis externa, is an inflammation or infection of the external canal or the auricle of the external ear. It is sometimes called *swimmer's ear*. External otitis may be acute or chronic.

Allergies, bacteria, fungi, viruses, or trauma may cause external otitis. Common sources of allergic reactions can stem from nickel or chromium in earrings, chemicals in hair sprays, cosmetics, hearing aids, or medications (especially sulfonamides and neomycin). Common bacterial agents are *Staphylococcus aureus*, *Pseudomonas aeruginosa*, and *Streptococcus pyogenes*. Viruses including HSV and varicella-zoster virus, and fungi such as *Aspergillus* and *Candida*, can be a source of chronic infection and may be difficult to treat. The external ear also may be affected by skin disorders including eczema, psoriasis, and seborrheic dermatitis. External otitis is more prevalent during hot, humid weather. Excessive swimming in hot, humid weather may wash out the protective cerumen and lead to secondary infection.

Trauma from cleaning or scratching the ear canal with a foreign object (such as a cotton swab, bobby pin, or finger) may result in irritation and possible introduction of infectious organisms into the ear.

Cerumen in the older adult becomes dry and hard, making it difficult to remove adequately. As a result, the cerumen may become impacted, causing discomfort and decreased hearing. Certain activities allow moisture to become trapped in the ear, creating a medium for infection; these include using earphones, hearing aids, earplugs, earmuffs, and stethoscopes.

Malignant external otitis is a rare, lethal condition caused by *Pseudomonas* organisms, occurring mostly in patients with diabetes. It is a bone-destroying infection that quickly involves all surrounding ear structures.

Clinical Manifestations

The acute inflammatory or infectious process produces pain with movement of the auricle or chewing, and often the entire side of the headaches. Erythema, scaling, pruritus, edema, watery discharge, and crusting of the external ear may occur. Drainage may be purulent or serosanguineous. If the *Pseudomonas* organism is the cause of the infection, the drainage is green and has a distinct odor. Dizziness and decreased hearing also may be present if edema occludes the ear canal. With chronic external otitis there is usually pruritus and drainage but no pain with movement of the auricle.

Assessment

Collection of subjective data includes determining the onset, duration, and severity of pain, which is crucial to the assessment of inflammatory disease of the ear. An early indication of inflammation or infection of the ear is the complaint of ear pain accompanied by the patient gently pulling on the pinna. Ask the patient about any home remedies used to treat infections. Also assess knowledge of preventive measures.

Collection of objective data includes noting discharge amount, color, and odor, which may be watery or yellow with a pungent odor. Discharge from a fungal infection is black. The patient may have a partial loss of hearing or feel like the ear is occluded if the ear canal is edematous or is obstructed by adenoids (small clumps of lymphoid tissue in the back of the throat). Palpation of the external ear or pulling the pinna gently to examine the ear may produce pain.

Diagnostic Tests

Obtain a culture of exudates to identify bacterial, viral, or fungal organisms.

Medical Management

Oral analgesics may be used if the pain is severe. Corticosteroids (1% hydrocortisone) may be used to reduce edema to allow antibiotics to penetrate. Antimicrobial agents such as antibiotic or antifungal eardrops may be used to treat infections. The most commonly used contain neomycin (0.5%) or polymyxin B (10,000 units/mL). Systemic antibiotics are used only if the infection is severe. The specific antibiotic used depends on the results of the culture.

Nursing Interventions and Patient Teaching

Carefully clean the ear canal. Heat may be applied to the external ear for pain relief. Implement an adequate method of communication. Instill eardrops as prescribed.

A patient problem and interventions for the patient with external otitis include but are not limited to the following:

PATIENT PROBLEM	NURSING INTERVENTIONS
Pain, related to inflammatory process	Apply warm compresses as ordered Administer prescribed analgesics and instill ordered ear medications

Ensure that the patient has the information needed to prevent further infection and can adequately care for the infected ear at home.

Prognosis

External otitis responds favorably to topical antibiotic and corticosteroid eardrops. Systemic antibiotics rarely are required unless cellulitis is present. Acute external otitis may become a chronic problem. If the infection remains untreated and enters the brain, death can occur. The rare malignant external otitis media has a mortality rate of 50% to 75% unless the condition is treated.

ACUTE OTITIS MEDIA

Etiology and Pathophysiology

Acute otitis media, an inflammation or infection of the middle ear, is the most common disorder of the middle ear. Acute otitis media most often is caused by *H. influenzae* or *Streptococcus pneumoniae*. Gram-negative bacteria, such as *Proteus, Klebsiella,* and *Pseudomonas* organisms, usually cause chronic otitis media; however, additional sources of infection include allergies, exposure to cigarette smoke, mycoplasma, and several viruses.

Otitis media occurs more frequently in children, especially at 6 to 36 months of age, and in the winter and early spring. Children's shorter and straighter eustachian tubes provide easier access of the organisms from the nasopharynx to travel to the middle ear. The patient usually has had a recent upper respiratory tract infection that ascends via the eustachian tube and involves the lining of the entire middle ear. Typically, only one ear is affected.

Viral infections frequently cause a serous otitis media. Retraction of the tympanic membrane occurs with a buildup of sterile serous exudate. If there is a secondary bacterial infection, purulent exudate collects behind the tympanic membrane, causing it to bulge. This is called *purulent otitis media.*

Clinical Manifestations

The patient experiences a sense of fullness in the ear and also has severe, deep throbbing pain behind the tympanic membrane. This severe pain may disappear if the tympanic membrane ruptures. Hearing loss, tinnitus (a subjective noise sensation heard in one or both ears; ringing or tinkling sounds in the ear), and fever also may be present.

Assessment

Subjective data are the same as for external otitis. Objective data are the same as for external otitis, with the exception of noting pain on palpation of the external ear.

Diagnostic Tests

A culture of the purulent drainage is obtained to identify the causative organisms.

Medical Management

Antibiotic therapy is still the most common form of treating otitis media, and it may be based on results of the culture. Analgesics are prescribed for severe pain, as well as nasal decongestants. Sedatives may be prescribed for children to provide rest and pain relief in combination with local heat (Table 13.5).

Needle aspiration of secretions collected behind the tympanic membrane may be necessary. Myringotomy—a surgical incision of the tympanic membrane to relieve pressure and release purulent exudate from the middle ear—may be required to prevent spontaneous rupture. A tympanostomy tube may be placed for short- or long-term use. Prompt treatment of an episode of acute otitis media generally prevents spontaneous perforation of the tympanic membrane.

Nursing Interventions and Ppatient Teaching

Inner-ear pressure may cause discomfort, requiring an analgesic. Sedatives may be ordered for young children. Hearing loss also may occur, which means that clear, effective communication with the patient is essential. Alert parents of young patients to this fact and enlist their help in monitoring the level of loss.

Chronic otitis media caused by repeated attacks of acute otitis media may result in a permanent perforation of the tympanic membrane. The result is a slight to moderate conductive hearing loss.

A growth called *cholesteatoma* (a mass of epithelial cells and cholesterol in the middle ear) occurs when a tympanic membrane perforation allows keratinizing squamous epithelium of the external auditory canal to enter and grow in the middle ear. Enlargement is slow, but the mass can expand into the mastoid antrum and destroy adjacent structures. Unless removed surgically, a cholesteatoma can cause extensive damage to the structures of the middle ear; erode the bony protection of the facial nerve; create a labyrinthine fistula; or even invade the dura, threatening the brain.

Mastoiditis, an infection of one of the mastoid bones, may develop as an extension of a middle-ear infection that was left untreated or inadequately treated. Immediately report signs of mastoiditis, including earache, fever, headache, malaise, and large amounts of purulent exudate.

A patient problem and interventions for the patient with otitis media include but are not limited to the following:

PATIENT PROBLEM	NURSING INTERVENTIONS
Compromised Skin Integrity, related to edema and exudates	Note and report any purulent outer ear exudates
	Keep ear clean and dry; use sterile cotton to absorb drainage, if ordered
	Monitor temperature and report changes

Ensure that the patient and parents (if appropriate) are aware of the necessity to complete the entire course of antibiotic therapy. Children are fed upright to prevent nasopharyngeal flora from entering the eustachian tube. Instruct the patient to blow the nose gently, not forcefully. If a myringotomy has been performed, instruct the patient or the parents to change the cotton in the outer ear at least twice a day (see the Patient Teaching box).

Table 13.5 Medications for Ear Disorders

GENERIC NAME (TRADE NAME)	ACTION AND USE	SIDE EFFECTS	NURSING IMPLICATIONS
acetic acid	Antibacterial, antifungal, astringent; used for superficial infections of external auditory canal	Contact dermatitis, transient stinging	Clean ear first; use cotton plug for first 24 h; contact health care practitioner if condition worsens or no improvement occurs after 5–7 days; do not wash dropper—doing so may dilute medication
amoxicillin trihydrate	Systemic penicillin antibiotic used in acute otitis media	Anaphylaxis, skin rash, diarrhea	Use caution during pregnancy and lactation; take for full treatment period; consult with health care practitioner if no improvement occurs in a few days; take on full or empty stomach; check with health care practitioner about treating diarrhea; do not give if patient has penicillin or cephalosporin allergy

Continued

Table 13.3 **Medications for Ear Disorders—cont'd**

GENERIC NAME (TRADE NAME)	ACTION AND USE	SIDE EFFECTS	NURSING IMPLICATIONS
antipyrine and benzocaine	Analgesic; local anesthetic; used for otitis media; adjunct to cerumen removal	Contact dermatitis	Use caution during pregnancy and lactation; date bottle and discard after 6 months. from first use; do not use if eardrums are perforated; warm the bottle; position patient on side and fill ear canal; use cotton plug; wash dropper before replacing in bottle
carbamide peroxide	Cerumen removal	Contact dermatitis	Do not use if eardrum is perforated or if there is ear discharge; not recommended for children; avoid eyes; reevaluate if edema, erythema, or pain persists; use proper administration technique by allowing drops to enter ear canal; do not touch tip of dropper
cefaclor	Second-generation cephalosporin used to treat amoxicillin-resistant otitis media	Anaphylaxis, skin rash, joint pain; fever, diarrhea, abdominal cramping	Store suspension in refrigerator; give full course of therapy; tell patient not to use alcohol; give on full or empty stomach; do not give if patient has penicillin or cephalosporin allergies
colistin, neomycin, hydrocortisone, and thonzonium	Antibiotic-steroid-detergent used for susceptible disease of external auditory canal, mastoidectomy, and otitis media fenestration	Ototoxicity with prolonged use; contact dermatitis; hypersensitivity, including pruritus, skin rash, erythema, and edema	Do not heat bottle above body temperature; with herpes simplex, do not use if patient is infected; do not use if eardrum is perforated; use for 10 days only; keep dropper from touching skin; check with health care practitioner if signs and symptoms worsen or do not improve after 1 week.; shake well before using; use cotton plug to keep moist; change plug daily
dimenhydrinate	Anticholinergic antihistamine used in treatment of vertigo	Blurred vision, drowsiness, shortness of breath, painful urination, disorientation	Antihistamines may inhibit lactation; give no CNS depressants; give with food or milk; use caution during pregnancy in early months
meclizine hydrochloride	Anticholinergic antihistamine that acts as antiemetic, antivertigo agent; treatment and prophylaxis; possibly effective for diseases affecting vestibular system	Drowsiness, blurred vision, dry mouth	Use caution during pregnancy and breastfeeding; give with food, water, or milk; tell patient to avoid alcohol and central nervous system (CNS) depressants; not recommended for children under 12 years.
polymyxin B, neomycin, bacitracin, and hydrocortisone	Antibiotic and steroid used in the same way as Coly-Mycin S; used to treat swimmer's ear	Ototoxicity with prolonged use, contact dermatitis, pruritus, erythema, edema	Use caution during pregnancy and lactation; do not use if eardrum is perforated; keep dropper from touching skin; shake well before using; use cotton plug to keep moist; change plug daily
triethanolamine polypeptide oleate	Cerumen removal	Contact dermatitis	Fill ear canal; insert cotton plug after 15–30 min; irrigate ear canal with warm water
trimethoprim-sulfamethoxazole	Systemic antibacterial; used for acute otitis media; no sulfonamide allergy	Fever, itching, skin rash, photosensitivity, dizziness	Not recommended during lactation or pregnancy; emphasize importance of proper dental care; blood glucose levels may be affected in patients using oral antidiabetic agents; maintain adequate fluid intake; advise patient to avoid sun exposure; complete treatment; with pediatric suspension, shake well

Patient Teaching

Ear Infection

PREVENTION OF FURTHER INFECTION
- Protect the ear canals during showers (earplugs may be used to keep water out of the ears).
- Avoid swimming during active infection or after an eardrum has been perforated; avoid swimming in contaminated water.
- Continue antibiotic therapy for the prescribed number of days, even when symptoms disappear.
- Get adequate and early treatment of upper respiratory tract infections and allergic conditions.

CARE OF INFECTED EAR
- Use correct eardrop insertion or ear irrigations, as prescribed.
- Wash hands before and after medication administration to prevent secondary infection.
- Keep external ear clean and dry to protect skin from drainage.

SIGNS REQUIRING MEDICAL ATTENTION
- Fever
- Return of ear pain or purulent discharge

Prognosis

Middle-ear infections usually resolve completely with antibiotic therapy. Since the advent of treatment with antibiotics, the incidence of severe and prolonged infections of the middle ear has been reduced greatly. Chronic or untreated otitis media may lead to sound transmission hearing loss, which is successfully treated by tympanoplasty.

Mastoiditis is difficult to treat and may require intravenous antibiotic therapy for several days. Because children are affected most often, immediate treatment of the infection is crucial. Residual hearing loss may follow the infection. If early decalcification is present, intense antibiotic therapy and myringotomy usually can cure mastoiditis; if it has progressed to further destruction, simple mastoidectomy is necessary.

LABYRINTHITIS

Etiology and Pathophysiology

Labyrinthitis is an inflammation of the labyrinthine canals of the inner ear. Labyrinthitis is the most common cause of vertigo. A common cause is a viral upper respiratory tract infection that spreads into the inner ear; other causes include certain drugs and foods. The vestibular portion of the inner ear may be destroyed by streptomycin. Exposure to tobacco and alcohol also may be causative factors. A rarer form of labyrinthitis is caused by bacteria, which usually is associated with middle-ear and mastoid infections. Since the advent of antibiotics, bacterial labyrinthitis occurs infrequently.

Clinical Manifestations

Severe and sudden vertigo is the most common symptom of labyrinthitis. Other symptoms include nausea and vomiting, nystagmus, photophobia, headache, and ataxic gait.

Assessment

Subjective data include the frequency and duration of the vertigo and any safety measures taken by the patient during an attack. Assess other symptoms such as hearing ability, tinnitus, and nausea. Because fear is associated with the attacks, explore the patient's feelings.

Objective data include noting vomiting and any signs of nystagmus and laterality (favoring either the right or left side of the body). Assess the coloration and moistness of the skin to determine the extent of autonomic response (changes in heart rate, blood pressure, and respirations).

Diagnostic Tests

Electronystagmography, done to record involuntary movements of the eye, may show diminished or absent nystagmus with stimulation. Audiometric testing shows low-tone sensorineural hearing loss.

Medical Management

Labyrinthitis has no specific treatment. Usually antibiotics and dimenhydrinate (Dramamine) or meclizine (Antivert) for vertigo are prescribed. If nausea and vomiting persist, administer parenteral fluids.

Nursing Interventions and Patient Teaching

Note the frequency and degree of vertigo. Administer antibiotics and medications and assess fluid intake to ensure that dehydration does not occur.

Patient problems and interventions for the patient with labyrinthitis include but are not limited to the following:

PATIENT PROBLEM	NURSING INTERVENTIONS
Potential for Injury, related to altered sensory perception (vertigo)	Keep side rails up Note presence of vertigo before patient ambulates Supervise ambulation Caution the patient not to attempt ambulation alone and to call for assistance
Fearfulness, related to altered sensory perception (vertigo)	Explore patient's feelings about attack Teach patient concerning actions during an attack (see the Patient Teaching box) Reinforce health care practitioner's treatment orders

Instruct the patient about vertigo and how it is treated (see the Patient Teaching box).

Patient Teaching

Vertigo

- Nature of the disorder
- Physiologic basis for the vertigo
- Avoidance of any known precipitating factors
- Rationale for a low-salt diet
- Actions to take during an attack
  - Lie down immediately, and call for help if necessary at the first signs of an attack.
  - If driving when an attack occurs, pull over immediately to the curb.
  - Lie immobile and hold head in one position until vertigo lessens.
  - Ask for assistance when ambulating if dizzy.
- Take prescribed medications as instructed even if no recent attacks have occurred; check with the health care provider before discontinuing any medication.
- Seek medical attention for changes in symptoms or in the nature of attacks.

OBSTRUCTIONS OF THE EAR

Etiology and Pathophysiology

Ear canal obstruction usually is caused by impaction or excessive secretion of cerumen or by foreign bodies, including insects. Children often place beans, beads, pebbles, and small toys in their ears. Usually those objects are found on routine examination. Obstruction by cerumen can be caused when excessive amounts are produced by overactive glands or from impaction of cerumen in narrow or tortuous ear canals.

Clinical Manifestations

Obstruction may cause the ear to feel occluded. The patient may have tinnitus or buzzing, pain in the ear, and hearing loss.

Assessment

Collection of subjective data includes interviewing the patient about any possible foreign bodies being introduced into the ear and any home remedies used to remove the object. If the patient is a child, determine risk factors related to ear obstructions, such as beads or nuts.

Collection of objective data involves noting any presence of a foreign body in the external ear canal. Observe children for tugging of the pinna.

Diagnostic Tests

Otoscopic examination provides visualization of the possible causes of the obstruction.

Medical Management

Medical management includes removal of cerumen by irrigation or cerumen spoon. Remove foreign objects with forceps, if possible. Smother insects with drops of an oily substance and remove them with forceps. Medications, such as carbamide peroxide 6.5%, may be used to soften cerumen. Surgical removal of the foreign object may be necessary.

Nursing Interventions and Patient Teaching

Assist with the irrigation of the ear. Instill medications into the ear as ordered.

A patient problem and interventions for the patient with obstructions of the ear include but are not limited to the following:

PATIENT PROBLEM	NURSING INTERVENTIONS
Impaired Sensory Awareness, related to presence of foreign body causing obstruction	Note the presence and amount of hearing impairment and tinnitus Assure the patient (or parents) that once the obstruction is removed, any hearing loss or tinnitus should disappear

Inform the patient and parents about the danger of placing objects in the ears. Also reinforce the method for preventing cerumen obstruction by instilling prescribed drops at night. This is followed by hydrogen peroxide in the morning and cleaning with a soft cotton wick.

Prognosis

Ear canal obstructions caused by cerumen and foreign bodies resolve completely with treatment. Vertigo may be experienced temporarily until the ear canal dries. The older adult may become disoriented from the cerumen impaction and temporary loss of hearing.

NONINFECTIOUS DISORDERS OF THE EAR

OTOSCLEROSIS
Etiology and Pathophysiology

Otosclerosis is a condition characterized by chronic progressive deafness caused by the formation of spongy bone, especially around the oval window, with resulting ankylosis (stiffening, immobility) of the stapes. In otosclerosis, formation of new bone in adolescence or early adulthood progresses slowly. Gradually, normal bone in the otic capsule is replaced by highly vascular otosclerotic bone. This replacement bone is described as *spongy*. Calcification of the area follows, and fixation of the footplate of the stapes in the oval window causes tinnitus and then deafness.

Otosclerosis is an autosomal dominant genetic disease. Women are affected twice as often as men. Otosclerosis is bilateral in about 80% of patients. Frequently, pregnancy triggers a rapid onset of this condition. Previous ear infections are not believed to be related to otosclerosis.

Clinical Manifestations

The patient with otosclerosis experiences slowly progressive conductive hearing loss and low- to medium-pitched tinnitus. The deafness usually is noted first between the ages of 11 and 20 years.

Assessment

Subjective data include the degree and progression of hearing loss or tinnitus and mild dizziness to vertigo. Assess family history for the disease.

Objective data include assessment of behavioral clues related to hearing loss (see Box 13.2).

Diagnostic Tests

Otoscopy reveals a normal eardrum. A pink blush called *Schwartz sign* may be seen through the eardrum; this indicates a high degree of vascularity in active otosclerotic bone. The result of the Rinne test shows that sounds transmitted by bone conduction last longer than those transmitted by air conduction in the affected ear. Weber test results are the opposite of those for normal hearing. The Weber test and audiometric testing show a lateralization of sound, more to the affected ear. Audiometric testing may show minimal to total hearing loss. Tympanometry may reveal evidence of stiffness in the sound conduction system. Hearing loss ranges from mild in the early stages to total loss in the later stages.

Medical Management

Supplements such as fluoride, vitamin D, and calcium carbonate are sometimes used to attempt to stabilize the hearing loss that results from otosclerosis. It is believed that these supplements can slow hearing loss by preventing further bone resorption and promoting calcification of bony lesions. Hearing aids may be effective because there is normal inner ear function. Surgical treatment by stapedectomy restores this conductive hearing loss. The ear with greater hearing loss typically is repaired first.

Nursing Interventions and Patient Teaching

Patient problems and interventions of otosclerosis are specific to post-stapedectomy care. See the Patient Teaching box "After Ear Surgery" for relevant discussion.

Prognosis

Patients report varying degrees of success with hearing after stapedectomy surgery. For some patients, stapedectomy is successful in permanently restoring hearing. A hearing aid may further enhance sound conduction to more normal levels.

MÉNIÈRE DISEASE

Etiology and Pathophysiology

Ménière disease is a chronic disease of the inner ear characterized by recurrent episodes of vertigo, progressive unilateral nerve deafness, and tinnitus. Ménière disease is most common in women between 30 and 60 years of age. Risk factors include recent viral infection, stress, alcohol use, family history and allergies. There is no identified specific causation, but the condition is likely tied to a series of factors.

There is an increase in endolymph fluid, either from increased production or decreased absorption. This causes increased pressure in the inner-ear labyrinth. Attacks of severe vertigo, tinnitus, and progressive deafness result from this increased pressure. Usually one ear only is involved.

Clinical Manifestations

The patient experiences recurrent episodes of vertigo with associated nausea, vomiting, diaphoresis, tinnitus, and nystagmus. A sense of fullness in the ear and hearing loss may be present. These attacks last from a few minutes to several hours. Attacks may occur several times a year. Sudden movements often aggravate the symptoms.

Assessment

Collection of subjective data includes noting the frequency and severity of the vertigo attack. The patient may complain of tinnitus. Note the patient's history and knowledge of the disorder and circumstances that precipitate an attack. Assess actions taken by the patient during an attack and the degree of relief those actions provide.

Collection of objective data includes determining unilateral or bilateral hearing loss. Observe the patient for associated signs during an attack.

Diagnostic Tests

To confirm a diagnosis two or more episodes must be documented, accompanied by positive findings from other diagnostic tests. Diagnostic tests such as magnetic resonance imaging (MRI) or computed tomography (CT) often are ordered to rule out central nervous system disease. An audiogram demonstrates mild low-frequency sensorineural hearing loss. Tuning fork tests show a sensorineural deficit. Vestibular testing shows lack of balance.

Medical Management

There is no specific therapy for Ménière disease. Fluid restriction, diuretics, and a low-salt diet are prescribed in an attempt to decrease fluid pressure. Advise the patient to avoid caffeine and nicotine. Antiemetic medications to manage nausea and vomiting may be indicated.

Dimenhydrinate, meclizine, diazepam (Valium), diphenhydramine (Benadryl), and fentanyl with droperidol may be prescribed for use between attacks to reduce the vertigo. In acute attacks the medications may be given intravenously. Atropine also is given for its anticholinergic effect during these acute attacks.

Additional therapies are available for Meniere's disease. Rehabilitation to manage balance or unsteadiness that linger beyond the acute phase of the condition. A hearing aid can be beneficial for the impacted ear. Referral to an audiologist will be needed for this. A Meniett device is a small portable unit that is inserted into the ear and provides positive pressure pulses to the inner ear. A tympanostomy tube insertion is required (Li, 2020).

For preservation of hearing, surgical procedures may be performed. Approximately 5% to 10% of patients with Ménière disease require surgery. Surgical intervention may involve destruction of the labyrinth, insertion of drainage tubes into the subarachnoid space, or dissection of cranial nerve VIII (vestibular portion). These surgeries are relatively successful, with the preservation of hearing reported in 60% to 90% of patients. Postoperative care involves bed rest for the first 1 to 3 days, avoidance of sudden head movements for 1 to 2 weeks, and the implementation of safety precautions to avoid falls related to dizziness (Table 13.6).

Nursing Interventions and Patient Teaching

Maintain the prescribed low-salt diet and administer diuretics as ordered. Acute vertigo is treated symptomatically with bed rest, sedation, and antiemetics or with medications for motion sickness. Nursing interventions are planned to minimize vertigo and provide for patient safety. During an acute attack keep the patient in a quiet, darkened room in a comfortable position. The patient may have some auditory deficit, which requires alternative methods of communication. If the patient's tinnitus becomes distressing, an increase in background noise, such as music, may provide relief. Fluorescent or flickering lights or watching television may exacerbate symptoms and should be avoided. Have an emesis basin available because vomiting is common.

Patient problems and interventions for the patient with Ménière disease include but are not limited to the following:

PATIENT PROBLEM	NURSING INTERVENTIONS
Potential for Injury, related to sensory-perceptual alterations (vertigo)	Keep side rails up
	Assist with ambulation and instruct the patient to call for assistance before attempting to ambulate
	Have the patient sit or lie down when vertigo occurs
	Have the patient move slowly and avoid turning the head suddenly
	Administer medications as prescribed
	Position patient on unaffected side
	Stand in front of patient to prevent head turning
	Avoid bright or glaring lights around patient
	Place all needed supplies so that patient does not have to turn head
Social Seclusion, related to unpredictable vertigo attacks	Assess factors that contribute to social isolation
	Assess feelings of loneliness and abandonment
	Identify support systems for patient
	Identify patient concerns
	Establish effective communication

Provide information about a low-salt diet and the taking of diuretics. Warn the patient to avoid reading when vertigo or tinnitus is present. Instruct the patient to avoid smoking to prevent vasoconstriction. The patient should learn to identify precipitating

Table 13.6   Surgery for Ménière Disease

TYPE	DESCRIPTION	RESIDUAL	POSTOPERATIVE NURSING INTERVENTIONS
Surgical destruction of labyrinth	Extraction of membranous labyrinth by suction; access to inner ear through external canal (stapes and incus removed)	Destroys remaining hearing	Keep patient on bed rest and NPO until vertigo subsides in 1–3 days. Avoid sudden movement of head for 1–2 weeks. Take action to prevent falls from unsteadiness for 1–3 weeks.
Endolymphatic subarachnoid shunt	Insertion of drain tube from endolymphatic sac into subarachnoid space; access through mastoid	Preserves hearing in 60%–70% of patients	Monitor for vertigo (rare)
Cryosurgery	Application of intense cold to lateral semicircular canals to decrease sensitivity or to create an otic-periotic shunt; access through mastoid	Preserves hearing in 80% of patients	Monitor for dizziness for 2 days. Take action to prevent falls from unsteadiness for 2–3 weeks.
Vestibular nerve section	Dissection of cranial nerve VIII (vestibular portion); access through mastoid or by cranial drilling over roof of internal auditory canal	Preserves hearing in 90% of patients	Same as for surgical destruction of labyrinth

NPO, Nothing by mouth.

factors and the proper actions to take when an attack occurs: (1) sit or lie down immediately; (2) if driving, stop the car and pull over to the side of the road; and (3) keep medication available at all times (Nursing Care Plan 13.2).

Prognosis

Approximately 75% to 85% of patients experience improvement with medical management and supportive therapy. The remaining patients may, in time, require surgical intervention. Usually attacks occur

---

Nursing Care Plan 13.2   The Patient With Ménière Disease

Ms. L. is a 66-year-old patient admitted with Ménière disease. She complains of severe dizziness, nausea, vomiting, ringing in the ears, hearing loss, and an unsteady gait. She is accompanied by her husband of 35 years.

PATIENT PROBLEM
Anxiousness, related to effect of disorder

Patient Goals and Expected Outcomes	Nursing Interventions	Evaluation
Patient will voice and demonstrate decreased signs and symptoms of anxiety Patient will control her anxiety level	Encourage patient to explore concerns about decreased hearing and effects of vertigo attacks and to take action in relation to the concerns. Explore patient's knowledge of the disorder and correct misunderstandings. Educate patient on strategies that can give her back some control over her life. Suggest keeping an emesis basin, a pillow, a blanket, a cell phone, and a large sign with the words "HELP, POLICE" in the car in case of a sudden Ménière attack. Encourage realistic hope about expected hearing ability as described by health care practitioner. Refer patient to necessary support services, such as social worker or audiologist. Refer patient for more information to Vestibular Disorders Association (VEDA).	Patient states that level of anxiety has decreased.

PATIENT PROBLEM
Potential for Injury, related to vestibular auditory alterations

Patient Goals and Expected Outcomes	Nursing Interventions	Evaluation
Patient will describe actions to avoid vertigo Patient will remain free of injury Patient will remain safe from falls	Help patient identify avoidable actions that precipitate vertigo attacks. Encourage patient to move slowly and not turn head suddenly when vertigo is present. If tinnitus is distressing, increase background noises, such as music. If hearing is decreased: • Use measures to facilitate communication with hearing impaired. • Carry wax earplugs; even after losing some hearing, ears are often sensitive to loud noises, which can trigger vertigo. • Refer patient to audiologist, if appropriate. Keep side rails up when patient with vertigo is in bed. Assist with ambulation as needed. Encourage patient to sit or lie down and to remain immobile if signs of dizziness occur. Teach patient to stop car at side of road immediately at first signs of dizziness while driving.	Patient avoids physical environment that could cause injury. Patient does not manifest evidence of injury.

CRITICAL THINKING QUESTIONS

1. Ms. L. states that she would prefer going to the bathroom without the assistance of a nurse. What is an appropriate response by the nurse?
2. Ms. L. tells the nurse that she is depressed because of her unpleasant symptoms and wonders if she will ever feel well again. What would be a therapeutic reply?
3. The nurse notes an unpleasant odor from Ms. L.; her hair is unkempt, and she has poor oral hygiene. The nurse is preparing to give her a warm, therapeutic bed bath. Ms. L. states, "I feel too dizzy to take a bath." What nursing interventions would help promote personal hygiene and patient compliance?

several times yearly, until the disease either resolves itself or progresses to complete deafness in the affected ear.

SURGERIES OF THE EAR

STAPEDECTOMY

Stapedectomy is the removal of the stapes of the middle ear and insertion of a graft and prosthesis, performed to restore hearing in cases of otosclerosis. The stapes that has become fixed is replaced so that vibrations can again transmit sound waves through the oval window to the fluid of the inner ear.

Using a local anesthetic and an operating microscope for visualization, the surgeon removes the stapes and covers the opening into the inner ear with a graft of body tissue. One end of a small plastic tube or piece of stainless steel wire is attached to the graft, while the other end is attached to the two remaining bones of the middle ear, the malleus and the incus.

Nursing Interventions and Patient Teaching

Postoperative management consists of external ear packing to ensure healing; the packing is left in place for 5 or 6 days. Depending on the health care provider's preference, the patient remains in bed for approximately 24 hours and resumes activity gradually. Keep the patient flat with the operative side facing upward to maintain the position of the prosthesis and graft; make certain that the patient is not turned. Headache, nausea, vomiting, and dizziness are expected early in the postoperative period as a result of stimulation of the labyrinth intraoperatively. The patient's hearing does not improve until the edema subsides and the packing is removed by the health care provider (see the Patient Teaching box).

👥 Patient Teaching

After Ear Surgery

- Change cotton in ear daily as prescribed.
- Open mouth when sneezing or coughing and blow nose gently one side at a time for 1 week (to prevent increased ear pressure and infection).
- Keep ear dry for 6 weeks (to prevent infection).
- Do not wash hair for 1 week.
- Protect ear when outdoors, using two pieces of cotton.
- Protect ear with shower cap when bathing.
- Wear ear protection as necessary to prevent exposure to loud noises.
- Follow activity guidelines:
  - No physical activity for 1 week
  - No exercises or active sports for 3 weeks
  - Return to work in 1 week (3 weeks for strenuous work).
  - Avoid exposure to people with upper respiratory tract infections.
  - Avoid airplane flights for at least 1 week (to prevent effects of pressure changes).

Possible complications of the stapedectomy include infection of the external, middle, or inner ear. Displacement or rejection of the prosthesis or graft may occur, or perilymph fluid may leak around the prosthesis into the middle ear, causing tinnitus and vertigo.

Prognosis

During surgery the patient often reports an immediate improvement in hearing in the operative ear. Because of the accumulation of blood and fluid in the middle ear, the hearing level decreases postoperatively but does return to near-normal levels. After stapedectomy, 90% of patients experience an improvement in hearing, in many instances to near-normal levels.

TYMPANOPLASTY

Tympanoplasty is any of several operative procedures on the eardrum or ossicles of the middle ear to restore or improve hearing in patients with conductive hearing loss. These operations may be used to repair a perforated eardrum, for otosclerosis, or for dislocation or necrosis of a small bone of the middle ear.

Nursing Interventions

Postoperative management consists of bed rest until the next morning. Elevate the head of the bed 40 degrees, and keep the operative side facing upward. Medications include opioid analgesics, otic and oral antibiotics, and meclizine for vertigo.

After the operation, monitor and report the presence of bleeding; the amount, color, and consistency of drainage; and temperature. Note complaints of vertigo when the patient is getting out of bed; with sudden movements, nausea and vertigo may occur. Possible complications include infection and displacement of the graft.

Patient problems and interventions for the patient after a tympanoplasty include but are not limited to the following:

PATIENT PROBLEM	NURSING INTERVENTIONS
Compromised Physical Mobility, related to surgical procedure	Note patient's ability to comply with bed rest order Keep the patient's operative side up; do not allow the patient to be turned
Potential for Inability to Tolerate Activity, related to pain and vertigo	Keep side rails up When movement is allowed, begin gradually Administer prescribed medications for pain and vertigo as needed Assist with ambulation to prevent injury

Prognosis

Hearing will improve if there is no involvement of the ossicles.

MYRINGOTOMY

Myringotomy, also called *tympanotomy,* is a surgical incision of the eardrum. It is performed to relieve pressure and to release purulent exudate from the middle ear. The procedure is done with the patient under either local or general anesthesia. A myringotomy may be performed in one of two ways: (1) using a myringotomy knife, the surgeon makes a curved incision in the drumhead; or (2) a heated wire loop is touched for about 1 second to the drumhead, producing a 2-mm hole.

Nursing Interventions and Patient Teaching

Purulent exudate and fluid may drain immediately, requiring suctioning. Cotton placed in the ear absorbs drainage, which may continue for several days. Change the cotton frequently to avoid recontamination of the surgical area. The incision usually heals quickly with little scarring. Hearing usually is not disrupted.

Medications commonly used are tetracycline (Achromycin V) and polymyxin B (Neosporin) eardrops as anti-infective agents. Tylenol with codeine may be used for pain. Monitor for signs of bleeding and report any occurrence. Note incisional pain or hearing impairment.

Patient teaching involves providing the information in the Patient Teaching box "After Ear Surgery" and ensuring that the patient understands.

Prognosis

Once pressure is relieved, hearing is restored to more normal levels unless scarring is present.

COCHLEAR IMPLANT

The cochlear implant is a hearing device for the profoundly deaf. The system consists of a surgically implanted induction coil beneath the skin behind the ear and an electrode wire placed in the cochlea (see Fig. 13.19). The implanted parts interface with an externally worn speech processor. The system stimulates auditory nerve fibers by an electric current so that signals reach the brainstem's auditory nuclei and ultimately the auditory cortex. The implant is intended for the patient whose sensorineural hearing loss is either congenital or acquired. A small computer changes the spoken words into electrical impulses that are transmitted to the implanted cochlear coil. The ideal candidate is one who became deaf after acquiring speech and language. The adult who was born deaf or became deaf before learning to speak may be considered a candidate for a cochlear implant if she or he has followed an aural-oral educational approach.

The implant offers the profoundly deaf the ability to hear environmental sounds, including speech, at comfortable loudness levels. Multichannel cochlear implants also aid in speech production. Extensive training and rehabilitation are essential to receive maximum benefit from these implants. The positive aspects of a cochlear implant include providing sound to the person who heard none, improving the sense of security, and decreasing the feelings of isolation. With continued research, the cochlear implant may offer the possibility of hearing rehabilitation for a wider range of hearing-impaired individuals.

The deaf community is concerned with cultural pride. They believe that life without hearing is healthy and functional and that deafness is not a disease that must be cured. The National Association of the Deaf originally opposed the use of cochlear implants; it now endorses their use, stating, "cochlear implantation is a technology that represents a tool to be used in some forms of communication, and not a cure for deafness" (Munson, 2006).

OTHER SPECIAL SENSES

TASTE AND SMELL

The tongue of the average adult contains approximately 10,000 taste buds; some also are located on the inner aspect of the cheeks. It was once believed that there were specific receptors in specific locations on the tongue that were able to detect the individual taste sensations. This is no longer believed to be true. Traditionally there were four identified taste sensations. This has been expanded to include a fifth taste. Research is ongoing relating to the discovery of other potential tastes such as fat (InfomedHealth.org, 2011).

1. *Sweet:* Respond to sugar and other sweet substances
2. *Sour:* Respond to acid content of foods
3. *Salty:* Respond to metal ions within foods
4. *Bitter:* Respond to alkaline or basic ions within foods
5. *Umami (Savory):* Respond to flavors similar to meat broth. Amino acids glutamic acid or aspartic acid are responsible for this flavor profile.

The receptors for the sense of smell (olfactory receptors) are located in the roof, or the upper part, of the nasal cavity. On inhalation, an odor comes in contact with the olfactory receptors and the message is sent to the brain. Certain odors are remembered for a long time and stimulate certain memories. The body is not able to regenerate olfactory cells; once they are damaged, the sense of smell is impaired permanently.

TOUCH

The receptors for touch *(tactile receptors)* are located throughout the integumentary system. They respond to touch, pressure, and vibration.

POSITION AND MOVEMENT

Proprioception (sense of position) maintains the proper position of the body. *Proprioceptors* include any sensory nerve ending—such as those located in muscles, tendons, and joints—that responds to stimuli originating from within the body regarding movement and spatial position. The proprioceptors work in conjunction with the semicircular canals and the vestibule of the inner ear to maintain proper coordination. These systems work in conjunction to orchestrate the body's movements in running, walking, dancing, and many other activities. Once the proprioceptors receive information from the environment, they send it to the cerebellum for interpretation. Proprioceptors enable one to sense the position of the different parts of the body and to be aware of the movement of each.

EFFECTS OF NORMAL AGING ON THE SENSORY SYSTEM

As an individual ages, the crystalline lens of the eye hardens and becomes too large for the eye muscles, thus causing a loss of accommodation. This often results in a need for bifocals or trifocals. The crystalline lens loses some of its transparency and becomes more opaque, and glare begins to become a problem. The lens proteins are vulnerable to biochemical changes and exposure to UV light, resulting in cataract development. Hypertension and atherosclerosis lead to retinal vascular changes. ARMD also contributes to impaired vision. The pupils become smaller and decrease the amount of light that reaches the retina, resulting in a need for brighter lighting for reading.

Impaired hearing can result from age-related changes in the auditory system. A condition called *presbycusis,* a hearing deficit secondary to aging, can occur from numerous sources such as noise, vascular or systemic diseases, poor nutrition, ototoxic drugs, and pollution. These exposures occurring over the lifespan can damage the delicate hair cells of the organ of Corti, cause calcification of the ossicles of the middle ear, and interfere with sound conduction. Tinnitus (ringing in the ear) also may occur secondary to the aging process and prolonged exposure to loud noises.

Visual and hearing losses in the older adult can result in physical and psychosocial problems. Early detection of visual and hearing changes may enable the patient to maintain an active and productive lifestyle. The remaining senses undergo slight changes, including decreases in their reaction or threshold times, which results in slower responses or diminished sensation.

❖ NURSING PROCESS FOR THE PATIENT WITH A VISUAL OR AUDITORY DISORDER

The role of the licensed practical nurse/licensed vocational nurse (LPN/LVN) in the nursing process as stated is that the LPN/LVN will:

- Participate in planning care for patients based on patient needs
- Review patient's care plan and recommend revisions as needed
- Review and follow defined prioritization for patient care
- Use clinical pathways, care maps, or care plans to guide and review patient care

◆ ASSESSMENT

The complexity of the assessment for eye and ear disorders depends on the patient's disease or problem. Subjective data for eye and ear disorders include the following:

- Health history, including any acute or chronic disease
- History of current complaint
- Medications, including prescription, over-the-counter, and home remedies or folk medicines
- Surgery and other treatments

Collection of objective data includes external and internal assessment of the eye and ear. Use inspection and palpation to assess the external components of the eye and ear, noting any abnormalities. Review results of the internal examination of the eye and ear by the primary care provider. Note results of diagnostic tests. Because seeing and hearing are necessary for safety, communication, self-care, and psychosocial interaction, assess these areas as well.

◆ PATIENT PROBLEM

Nursing assessment identifies the patient's needs. Care is based on the patient problems that have been identified. Possible patient problems include the following:

- Anxiousness
- Compromised Maintenance of Health
- Compromised Social Interaction
- Fearfulness
- Impaired Health Maintenance
- Impaired Self-care (specify)
- Impaired Sensory Awareness
- Lonesomeness
- Potential for Injury
- Social Seclusion

◆ EXPECTED OUTCOMES AND PLANNING

Impairment of vision or hearing requires a major adjustment in the life of an individual. The patient must adjust to the loss and changes in lifestyle, whether the loss is permanent or temporary. The care plan focuses on achieving specific goals and outcomes that relate to the identified patient problems. Examples of these include the following:

Goal 1: Patient will remain free of injury.

Outcome: Patient and family inspect environment for potential hazards related to loss of vision or hearing.

Goal 2: Patient will remain socially active.

Outcome: Patient displays interest in social and recreational activities.

◆ IMPLEMENTATION

Measures used in the care of a patient with vision or hearing loss center around helping the patient remain physically and emotionally safe and secure and ensuring that the patient's needs are communicated and met while adjusting to the loss. Nursing interventions include promoting safety, assisting with ADLs, facilitating communication, and encouraging diversional activity. Also assess readiness to learn and teach health promotion practices (see the Patient Teaching boxes throughout this chapter). Consider the patient's culture, beliefs, values, and habits and the special needs of the older adult.

◆ EVALUATION

Systematic evaluation requires determining whether expected outcomes have been met. Refer to the goals and outcomes identified when assisting in planning care and evaluating the achievement of the goals. Examples of goals and their evaluative measures include the following:

Goal 1: Patient will remain free of injury.

Evaluative measure: Ask patient and family to describe what environmental changes must be made to ensure safety.

Goal 2: Patient will remain socially active.

Evaluative measure: Observe patient participating in social activities.

Get Ready for the NCLEX® Examination!

Key Points

- The five major senses are taste, touch, smell, sight, and hearing.
- The accessory structures of the eye are the eyebrows, eyelids, eyelashes, and the lacrimal apparatus.
- The three tunics of the eye are the fibrous tunic (sclera), the vascular tunic (choroid), and the retina.
- The two chambers of the eye are the anterior chamber, which contains aqueous humor, and the posterior chamber, which contains vitreous humor.
- Image formation at the retina requires four basic processes: refraction, accommodation, constriction, and convergence.
- The photoreceptors of the retina are the rods and cones. The rods control vision in dim light, and the cones control vision in bright light. The cones are also responsible for color vision.
- Light entering the eye must travel through the cornea, the aqueous humor, the pupil, the crystalline lens, the vitreous humor, and finally the retina.
- The ear is divided into external, middle, and inner ears.
- The external ear flap is called the pinna (auricle); it extends into the external ear canal.
- The middle ear contains the ossicles and the entrance of the eustachian tube and ends with the tympanic membrane.
- The inner ear contains the vestibule, the cochlea, and the semicircular canals.
- The organ of Corti is the organ of hearing; it is located within the cochlea.
- The semicircular canals are responsible for the sense of balance and equilibrium.
- The taste buds differentiate four basic tastes: sweet, sour, salty, bitter, and umami (savory).
- Normal aging causes decreased hearing and sight as a result of normal changes of the structures.
- Individuals who have chronic disease or are older than 40 should be examined yearly to detect eye abnormalities or to prescribe changes in therapy.
- Refractory errors include hyperopia, presbyopia, and astigmatism.
- Ranges of 20/20 to 20/40 vision are considered normal, whereas 20/200 with correction is defined as legal blindness.
- ARMD is divided into two classic forms: dry and wet. In dry ARMD, which accounts for 90% of patients with ARMD, the macular cells have wasted or atrophied. Wet ARMD is characterized by the development of abnormal blood vessels in or near the macula.

- Cataracts are opaque areas in the lens and may be removed by intracapsular or extracapsular extraction.
- Glaucoma is not one disease but rather a group of disorders characterized by (1) increased IOP and the consequences of elevated pressure, (2) optic nerve atrophy, and (3) peripheral visual field loss.
- Loss of hearing may result from cerumen buildup, infection, trauma, or use of ototoxic drugs, or it may be a congenital condition.
- Conductive hearing loss is a decrease in amplification, whereas sensorineural hearing loss is interference within the inner ear and nerve conduction.
- Prevention of serious complications of ear disorders, such as infections, mastoiditis, and brain abscess, requires early detection and treatment.
- *Potential for Injury* is the primary patient problem for the patient experiencing vertigo, which occurs in labyrinthitis and Ménière disease.
- An essential communication tip for speaking to the hearing impaired is to face the patient and to speak clearly without shouting.
- A cochlear implant is a hearing device for the profoundly deaf. The implanted device is intended for the patient with sensorineural hearing loss.

Additional Learning Resources

SG Go to your Study Guide for additional learning activities to help you master this chapter content.

Be sure to visit the Evolve site at http://evolve.elsevier.com/Cooper/adult for additional online resources.

Review Questions for the NCLEX® Examination

1. A patient is to have a laser treatment to cauterize hemorrhaging vessels caused by diabetic retinopathy. The patient asks the nurse what this procedure is called. Which response by the nurse is correct?

   1. Enucleation
   2. Scleral buckle
   3. Photocoagulation
   4. Trabeculoplasty

2. The parents want to know more about their child's conductive hearing loss. Which is the best explanation by the nurse?

   1. "Sound is delivered through the external and middle ear, but a defect in the inner ear results in distortion of sound."
   2. "Sound is inadequately delivered through the external or middle ear to the inner ear."
   3. "There is no organic cause, but a functional problem exists."
   4. "The brain's auditory pathways are damaged."

3. A patient has impaired hearing. Which action by the nurse would best facilitate communication?

   1. Face the patient when speaking.
   2. Overaccentuate words to make the communication more effective.
   3. Shout to allow the patient to hear.
   4. Use one-word phrases when speaking.

4. A patient tells the nurse he has dizziness. He states that the health care provider used another term. What term did the health care provider most likely use?

   1. Tinnitus
   2. Labyrinthitis
   3. Sensorineural
   4. Vertigo

5. A patient is diagnosed with an inner ear problem. For what symptom should the nurse monitor the patient closely?

   1. Echoing
   2. Intense pain
   3. Vertigo
   4. Loss of hearing

6. The nurse is evaluating a patient's eye as it adjusts to seeing objects at various distances. When documenting, how should the nurse identify this test?

   1. PERRLA
   2. Refraction
   3. Focusing
   4. Accommodation

7. A patient is suspected of having a retinal detachment. What signs/symptoms will provide support to this diagnosis? *(Select all that apply.)*

   1. "I have tunnel vision."
   2. "I am having a lot of pain in my eye."
   3. "It feels like I'm looking through cobwebs."
   4. "I see specks floating around the edges of my vision."
   5. "I feel like someone pulled a curtain over my eye."

8. Which of the following would be most hazardous in the home of a patient who is visually impaired?

   1. Area rugs
   2. Room carpeting
   3. Tile floor
   4. Concrete flooring

9. A patient arrives in the emergency room after an accident that resulted in a piece of metal penetrating the eye. What nursing action should be taken initially on the patient's arrival at the hospital?

   1. Apply a cool compress immediately.
   2. Lightly cover both eyes with an eye shield.
   3. Attempt to gently remove the object.
   4. Irrigate the eye with tap water.

10. A patient has just had cataract surgery. What information should the nurse include in the discharge instructions? *(Select all that apply.)*

    1. Wear an eye shield at night on the operative eye.
    2. Avoid bending, stooping, coughing, or lifting.
    3. Instill prescribed eyedrops into the conjunctival sac.
    4. Take an analgesic every 4 hours.
    5. Avoid lying on the affected eye for 2 weeks after surgery.

11. Which assessment finding would indicate a need for possible glaucoma testing? *(Select all that apply.)*

    1. Presence of "floaters"
    2. Halos around lights
    3. Progressive loss of peripheral vision
    4. Pruritus and erythema of the conjunctiva
    5. Lack of ability to adapt to darkness

12. While communicating with a patient, you notice a possible hearing deficit in one ear. Which nursing intervention would be appropriate?

    1. Shout in the affected ear.
    2. Speak clearly and in a slightly louder voice toward the patient's face.
    3. Plug the affected ear and shout in the unaffected ear.
    4. Speak more softly than usual in the affected ear.

13. The nurse is admitting an adult patient to a walk-in clinic. The patient complains of recent hearing loss. What does the nurse anticipate as the most probable cause of this patient's hearing loss?

    1. Cerumen buildup
    2. Ossification of the pinna
    3. Low batteries in the hearing aid
    4. Fluid in the ear

14. A 71-year-old patient complains of being severely dizzy. What instruction should the nurse give the patient?

    1. Avoid sudden movements.
    2. Avoid noises.
    3. Increase fluid intake.
    4. Lie on the affected side.

15. A patient who has been blind for the past 10 years is hospitalized with heart failure. What intervention should the nurse include in the plan of care?

    1. Keep all personal care items at a distance so that he won't bump into them.
    2. Schedule a consultation with an occupational therapist to teach activities of daily living.
    3. All personnel announce themselves when entering and leaving the room.
    4. Initiate a referral to the Department of Health and Human Services.

16. A patient has a family history of cataracts. He asks what early symptoms he should watch for that would alert him to the development of cataracts. What is the nurse's best response?

  1. Pain in the eyes
  2. Blurred vision
  3. Loss of peripheral vision
  4. Dry eyes

17. A patient is scheduled for a stapedectomy. What postoperative instructions should the nurse include in patient teaching? *(Select all that apply.)*

  1. Change cotton in external ear canal hourly.
  2. Gently blow through both nares simultaneously.
  3. Teach the patient to open the mouth when sneezing or coughing.
  4. Limit exercise or active sports for 3 weeks.
  5. Avoid exposure to people with upper respiratory tract infections.

18. A 15-year-old hearing-impaired patient is having problems communicating with the staff. Which behavior would improve communication? *(Select all that apply.)*

  1. Overaccentuating words
  2. Facing the patient when speaking
  3. Speaking in conversational tones
  4. Asking permission to turn off the television or radio
  5. Using written communication for most interactions

19. The nurse is caring for a patient with vertigo. What is the nurse's priority concern when caring for this patient?

  1. Safety
  2. Comfort
  3. Hygiene
  4. Quiet

20. While cleaning the garage, a patient splashed a chemical in his eyes. What is the initial action after the chemical burn?

  1. Transport to an emergency facility immediately.
  2. Cover the eyes with sterile gauze.
  3. Lubricate eye with petroleum-based jelly.
  4. Irrigate the eye with water for 20 minutes.

21. A patient visits the health care provider to have her vision tested using the Snellen eye chart. What instruction should the nurse provide to the patient?

  1. Use both eyes to read the chart.
  2. Read the chart from right to left.
  3. Cover one eye while testing the other.
  4. Use either eye because they will be the same.

22. A 78-year-old patient comes into the clinic complaining of progressive loss of vision in the center of the visual field. The nurse is aware that the patient is most likely experiencing symptoms of which disorder?

  1. Macular degeneration
  2. Primary open-angle glaucoma
  3. Color blindness
  4. Retinal degeneration

23. After cataract surgery a patient complains of sudden sharp pain in the operative eye. What is the most appropriate nursing action?

  1. Remove the metal eye shield to relieve pressure.
  2. Call the surgeon.
  3. Administer an analgesic.
  4. Document complaint of pain on chart.

24. A patient is asked to sign a surgical consent for treatment of otosclerosis. Which statement indicates correct understanding of the procedure?

  1. "It involves surgical repair of the external ear."
  2. "It means cutting the nerve in my ear."
  3. "It cleans the ear canal of wax."
  4. "It will help me hear sounds again."

25. The nurse receives medication orders for a patient with open-angle glaucoma. Which medication order does the nurse anticipate?

  1. Atropine, cyclopentolate hydrochloride
  2. Betoptic, pilocarpine hydrochloride
  3. Dexamethasone, Liquifilm
  4. Mannitol, Cyclogyl

26. A male junior in high school, age 17, is playing high school football when he is tackled particularly hard. He appears uninjured except for a slightly sore neck but develops a headache and earache later that night. Both are gone by morning, but he is left with some hearing loss, particularly with low-pitched sounds and whispers. He tells his parents and is taken to an otolaryngologist where, after hearing tests and a CT scan, he is diagnosed with otosclerosis, a usually genetic condition possibly triggered by a very tiny stress fracture to the bony tissue surrounding his inner ear. Fluoride, vitamin D, and calcium carbonate supplements are recommended to slow hearing loss, and he is given a trial use of a hearing aid. The hearing loss is slight and does not bother him. But in his senior year, the hearing loss gets worse and he cannot hear anything said when the team's in a huddle, so he returns to the otolaryngologist, where tests show that his hearing loss is even more profound than the patient has admitted to. He undergoes stapedectomy to insert a prosthetic device into the middle ear so that sound waves can reach the inner ear and restore hearing. Surgery and post-surgery go as expected, and the patient is released to home on Day 2 post-surgery. Within 24 hours, the nurse calls the patient and his mom at home for their scheduled telehealth follow-up. During the post-surgical evaluation, the patient says, "I have a question." He acknowledges that he cannot play football again just yet, but says, "Coach came to see me today, and it's official. We're going to State! So, I know I can't play or anything, but I don't see why I can't fly with the team so I can sit on the sidelines and watch my friends play. Coach says it's fine; he doesn't want me to miss out on our big moment. I'm pretty confident we're gonna take State."

Which statements or actions observed in the patient suggest a need for more follow-up, especially in terms of patient education?

___ Day 3 dizziness	___ Hearing has not improved
___ Day 3 packing has been removed	___ Coughs open-mouthed only
___ Day 3 nausea and headache	___ Day 3 of missing football practice
___ Patient has recently shampooed	___ Plans to fly with team in 2 days

Objectives

Anatomy and Physiology

1. Name the two structural divisions of the nervous system and give the functions of each.
2. List the parts of the neuron, and describe the function of each part.
3. Explain the anatomic location and functions of the cerebrum, the brainstem, the cerebellum, the spinal cord, the peripheral nerves, and cerebrospinal fluid.
4. Discuss the parts of the peripheral nervous system and how the system works with the central nervous system.
5. List the 12 cranial nerves and the areas they serve.

Medical-Surgical

6. List physiologic changes that occur with aging in the nervous system.
7. Explain the importance of prevention in problems of the nervous system, and give several examples of prevention.
8. Identify the significant subjective and objective data related to the nervous system that should be obtained from a patient during assessment.
9. Differentiate between normal and common abnormal findings of a physical assessment of the nervous system.
10. Discuss the Glasgow Coma Scale.
11. List common laboratory and diagnostic examinations for evaluation of neurologic disorders.
12. List five signs and symptoms of increased intracranial pressure and relate why they occur to physiology.
13. Identify nursing interventions that decrease intracranial pressure.
14. Discuss various neurologic disturbances in motor function and sensory-perceptual function.
15. Discuss the clinical manifestations of three types of headache.
16. Describe nursing interventions and teaching needs for the patient with headaches.
17. Describe nursing and medical measures to manage pain in the patient with neurological conditions.
18. List four classifications of seizures, their characteristics, clinical signs, aura, and postictal period.
19. Give examples of six degenerative neurologic diseases and explain the etiology, pathophysiology, clinical manifestations, assessment, diagnostic tests, medical management, nursing interventions, and prognosis for each.
20. Discuss the etiology, pathophysiology, clinical manifestations of stroke and the assessment, diagnostic tests, medical management, nursing interventions, and prognosis for a stroke patient.
21. Differentiate between trigeminal neuralgia and Bell palsy.
22. Discuss the etiology, pathophysiology, clinical manifestations, assessment, diagnostic tests, medical management, nursing interventions, and prognosis for Guillain-Barré syndrome, meningitis, encephalitis, and acquired immunodeficiency syndrome.
23. Explain the mechanism of injury to the brain that occurs with a stroke and traumatic brain injury.
24. Discuss the etiology, pathophysiology, clinical manifestations, assessment, diagnostic tests, medical management, nursing interventions, and prognosis for intracranial tumors, brain trauma, and spinal trauma.

Key Terms

agnosia (ăg-NŌ-zhă, p. 679)

aneurysm (ĂN-ūr-ĭ-zĭm, p. 699)

aphasia (ă-FĀ-zē-ă, p. 665)

apraxia (ă-PRĂK-sē-ă, p. 693)

ataxia (ă-TĂK-sē-ă, p. 685)

aura (ĂW-ră, p. 670)

bradykinesia (bră-dē-kĭ-NĒ-zē-ă, p. 687)

deep brain stimulation (DBS) (p. 689)

diplopia (dĭp-LŌ-pē-ă, p. 674)

dysarthria (dĭs-ĂHR-thrē-ă, p. 666)

dysphagia (dĭs-FĀ-jē-ă, p. 677)

flaccid (FLĂK-sĭd, p. 666)

Glasgow Coma Scale (GLĂS-gō KŌ-mă SKAL, p. 664)

global cognitive dysfunction (GLŌ-băl KŎG-nĭ-tĭv dĭs-FŬNK-shŭn, p. 710)

Guillain-Barré syndrome (GBS) (GĒ-yăn bă-RĀ, p. 706)

hemianopia (hĕm-ē-ă-NŌ-pē-ă, p. 666)

hemiplegia (hĕm-ē-PLĒ-jă, p. 677)

hyperreflexia (hī-pĕr-rĕ-FLĔK-sē-ă, p. 714)

neoplasm (p. 710)

nystagmus (nĭs-TĂG-mŭs, p. 685)

off times (p. 689)

paresis (pă-RĒ-sĭs, p. 666)

postictal period (pōst-ĬK-tăl PĒ-rē-ŏd, p. 680)

proprioception (prō-prē-ō-SĔP-shŭn, p. 666)

spastic (SPĂS-tĭk, p. 666)

stroke (strōk, p. 698)

unilateral neglect (ū-nĭ-LĂT-ĕr-ăl nĕ-GLĔCT, p. 666)

ANATOMY AND PHYSIOLOGY OF THE NEUROLOGIC SYSTEM

The nervous system is responsible for communication and control within the body. It interprets or processes the information received and sends it to the appropriate area of the brain or spinal cord, where the response is generated. The nervous system is the body's link with the environment. It works in conjunction with the endocrine system to maintain the body's homeostasis. The nervous system reacts in split seconds, whereas the hormones secreted by the endocrine glands work more slowly in initiating a response. The clinical picture for the patient with neurologic problems is often complex. Understanding these conditions requires knowledge of the anatomy and physiology of the nervous system.

STRUCTURAL DIVISIONS

The nervous system has two main structural divisions, the central nervous system (CNS) and the peripheral nervous system:

- *Central nervous system:* The CNS is made up of the brain and the spinal cord. It occupies a medial position in the body and is responsible for interpreting incoming sensory information and issuing instructions based on past experiences.
- *Peripheral nervous system:* The peripheral nervous system includes all the nerves that lie outside the CNS.

The peripheral nervous system contains two main divisions: the somatic nervous system and the autonomic nervous system:

- *Somatic nervous system:* The somatic nervous system sends messages to the CNS via sensory (or afferent) neurons and from the CNS to the skeletal muscles (voluntary muscles) via motor (or efferent) neurons.
- *Autonomic nervous system:* The autonomic system transmits messages from the CNS to the smooth muscle, the cardiac muscle, and certain glands. The autonomic system is sometimes called the *involuntary nervous system* because its action takes place without conscious control. It has two divisions: the sympathetic and parasympathetic.

CELLS OF THE NERVOUS SYSTEM

Two broad categories of cells exist within the nervous system. The neurons occupy the first category. Their role as transmitter is to carry messages to and from the brain and spinal cord (Fig. 14.1). The neuroglia or glial cells represent the second category; they support and protect the neurons while producing cerebrospinal fluid (CSF), which continuously bathes the structures of the CNS.

Neuron

A *neuron* (nerve cell) is the basic cell of the nervous system. It is a separate unit composed of three main

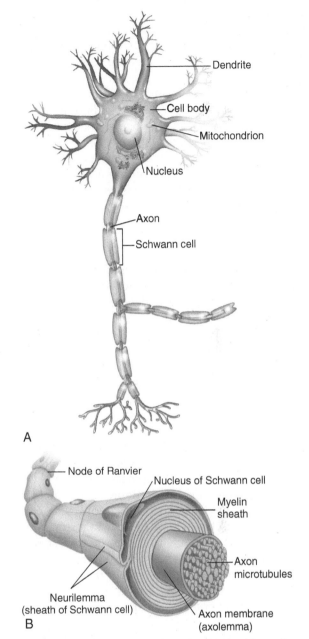

Fig. 14.1 (A) Diagram of a typical neuron showing dendrites, cell body, and axon. (B) Cross-section of a myelinated axon, showing the concentric, myelinated layers of the Schwann cell. (From Patton KT, Thibodeau GA: *The human body in health and disease*, ed 7, St. Louis, 2018, Elsevier.)

structures: the cell body, the axon, and the dendrites. The cell body contains a nucleus surrounded by cytoplasm. The axon is the cylindric extension of a nerve cell that conducts impulses away from the neuron cell body. The dendrites are branching structures that extend from the cell body and receive impulses. Between each neuron is a gap (space) called the *synapse*, defined as the region surrounding the point of contact between two neurons or between a neuron and an effector organ, and across which nerve impulses are transmitted through the action of a neurotransmitter.

All neurons are governed by the "all-or-none law," which means there is never a partial transmission of a message; the impulse is either strong enough to elicit a response or too weak to generate the message.

Neuromuscular Junction

The area of contact between the ends of a large, myelinated nerve fiber and a fiber of skeletal muscle is called the *neuromuscular junction*. The body's nervous system connects with the muscular system via these areas of contact. Neurotransmitters act to make certain that the neurologic impulse passes from the nerve to the muscle.

Neurotransmitters

Numerous chemicals called *neurotransmitters* modify or result in the transmission of impulses between synapses and at neuromuscular junctions. The best-known neurotransmitters are acetylcholine, norepinephrine, dopamine, and serotonin.

- *Acetylcholine* plays a role in nerve impulse transmission; it spills into the synapse area and speeds the transmission of the impulse. The enzyme cholinesterase then is released to deactivate the acetylcholine once the message or impulse has been sent. This happens rapidly and continuously as each impulse is relayed.
- *Norepinephrine* has an effect on maintaining arousal (awakening from a deep sleep), dreaming, and regulation of mood (e.g., happiness, sadness).
- *Dopamine* affects primarily motor function; it is involved in gross subconscious movements of the skeletal muscles. It also plays a role in emotional responses. A person with Parkinson disease has decreased dopamine levels and suffers involuntary, trembling muscle movements, or *tremors.*
- *Serotonin* induces sleep, affects sensory perception, controls temperature, and has a role in control of mood.

Neuron Coverings

Many neuron fibers (axons and dendrites) (see Fig. 14.1) are covered with a white, waxy, fatty material called *myelin*. Myelin increases the rate of transmission of impulses and protects and insulates the fibers. Axons leaving the CNS are wrapped in layers of myelin with indentations called the *nodes of Ranvier*. These nodes further increase the rate of transmission because the impulse can jump from node to node.

In the peripheral nervous system the myelin is produced by Schwann cells (see Fig. 14.1). The outer membrane of the Schwann cells gives rise to another layer called the neurilemma. The neurilemma is important because it helps regenerate injured axons. Thus regeneration of nerve cells occurs only in the peripheral nervous system. Cells damaged in the CNS result in permanent damage (paralysis) because they do not have a neurilemma and are not able to regenerate.

CENTRAL NERVOUS SYSTEM

The CNS is composed of the brain and the spinal cord and represents one of the two main divisions of the nervous system. It functions somewhat like a computer but is much more complex. The cranium protects the brain, and the vertebral column protects the spinal cord.

Brain

Specialized cells in the brain's mass of convoluted, soft, gray or white tissue coordinate and regulate the functions of the CNS. The brain is one of the largest organs in the body, weighing approximately 3 pounds (1.4 kg). It is divided into four principal parts: the cerebrum, the diencephalon, the cerebellum, and the brainstem.

Cerebrum. The cerebrum is the largest part of the brain (Fig. 14.2). It is divided into left and right hemispheres. The outer portion of the cerebrum is composed of gray matter and is called the *cerebral cortex*. It is arranged in folds, called *gyri* (convolutions); the grooves are called *sulci* (fissures). The connecting structure or bridge is called the *corpus callosum.* Two deep sulci subdivide the two hemispheres into four lobes that are named for the bones lying over them: the frontal lobe, the parietal lobe, the temporal lobe, and the occipital lobe. Each hemisphere of the cerebrum controls initiation of movement on the opposite side of the body. The functions of the cerebrum are multiple and complex. Specific areas of the cerebral cortex are associated with specific functions (Fig. 14.3 and Box 14.1).

Basal nuclei. The basal nuclei (formerly referred to as the basal ganglia) are additional islands of gray matter buried deep within the two cerebral hemispheres. They control automatic movement of the body as well as posture. This portion of the cerebrum regulates voluntary motor function, including the muscle contractions associated with walking and maintaining posture. The basal nuclei also are involved with thinking and learning (National Library of Medicine [NLM], 2020a).

Diencephalon. The diencephalon often is called the *interbrain.* It lies beneath the cerebrum and contains the thalamus and the hypothalamus. The thalamus serves as a relay station on the way to the cerebral cortex for some sensory impulses; it interprets other sensory messages, such as pain, light touch, and pressure. The hypothalamus, which lies beneath the thalamus, plays a vital role in the control of body temperature; fluid balance; appetite; sleep; and certain emotions, such as fear, pleasure, and pain. The sympathetic and parasympathetic divisions of the autonomic system are under the control of the hypothalamus, as is the pituitary gland. Thus the hypothalamus influences the heartbeat, the contraction and relaxation of the walls of the blood vessels, hormone secretion, and other vital body functions (see Fig. 14.2).

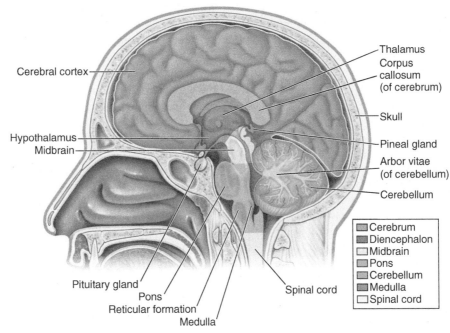

Fig. 14.2 Sagittal section of the brain. (From Patton KT, Thibodeau GA: *The human body in health and disease,* ed 7, St. Louis, 2018, Elsevier.)

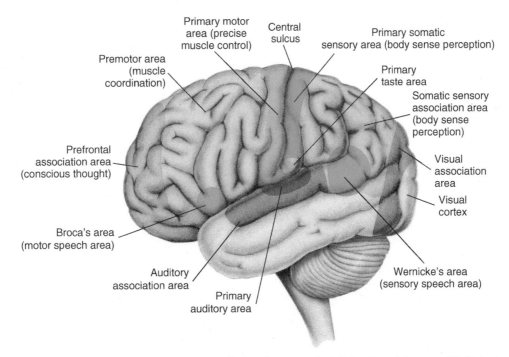

Fig. 14.3 Cerebral cortex. (From Patton KT, Thibodeau GA: *The human body in health and disease,* ed 7, St. Louis, 2018, Elsevier.)

Cerebellum. The cerebellum lies posterior and inferior to the cerebrum and is the second-largest portion of the brain. It contains two hemispheres with a convoluted surface much like the cerebrum. It is mainly responsible for coordination of voluntary movement and maintenance of balance, equilibrium, and muscle tone (a muscle's baseline degree of tension). It coordinates and smooths movement (e.g., the complex and quick coordination of many different muscles needed in playing the piano, swimming, or juggling). It is like the automatic pilot on an airplane in that it adjusts and corrects voluntary movement but operates entirely below the conscious level. Sensory messages from the semicircular canals in the inner ear send their messages to the cerebellum (see Fig. 14.2).

Brainstem. The brainstem is located at the base of the brain and contains the *midbrain,* the *pons,* and the *medulla oblongata* (see Fig. 14.2). These structures

Box 14.1   Functions of the Cerebrum

FRONTAL LOBE
- Written speech: Ability to write
- Motor speech, Broca's area: Ability to speak. Motor speech is mediated in Broca's area in the frontal lobe. When an injury to Broca's area (or the hemisphere in general) occurs, expressive aphasia can result and the patient will not be able to speak. The patient can produce only a garbled sound but can understand language and knows what he or she wants to say.
- Motor ability: Movements of body. The left side of the brain controls the right side of the body, and the right side of the brain controls the left side of the body.
- Intellectualization: The ability to form concepts, personality, emotion, behavior
- Judgment formation

PARIETAL LOBE
- Interpretation of sensory impulses from the skin, such as touch, pain, and temperature
- Recognition of body parts
- Determination of left from right
- Determination of shapes, sizes, and distances

TEMPORAL LOBE
- Wernicke's area: Language comprehension. When Wernicke's area is damaged in the person's dominant hemisphere, receptive aphasia results. The person hears sound, but it has no meaning, like hearing a foreign language.
- Integration of auditory stimuli

OCCIPITAL LOBE
- Interpretation of visual impulses from the retina

connect the spinal cord and the cerebrum. The brainstem carries all nerve fibers between the spinal cord and the cerebrum.

Midbrain. The midbrain forms the superior portion of the brainstem. It merges into the thalamus and the hypothalamus. It is responsible for motor movement, relay of impulses, and auditory and visual reflexes. It is the origin of cranial nerves III and IV.

Pons. The pons connects the midbrain to the medulla oblongata; the word *pons* means "bridge." It is the origin of cranial nerves V through VIII. The pons is composed of myelinated nerve fibers and is responsible for sending impulses to the structures that are inferior and superior to it. It also contains a respiratory center that complements respiratory centers located in the medulla.

Medulla oblongata. The medulla oblongata is the distal portion of the brainstem. It is the origin of cranial nerves IX and XII. The medulla controls heartbeat, rhythm of breathing, swallowing, coughing, sneezing, vomiting, and hiccups *(singultus).* A vasomotor center regulates the diameter of the blood vessels, which aids in the control of blood pressure.

Coverings of the brain and the spinal cord. The brain and the spinal cord are surrounded by three protective coverings called the *meninges:* (1) the dura mater, the outermost layer; (2) the arachnoid membrane, the second layer; and (3) the pia mater, the innermost layer, which

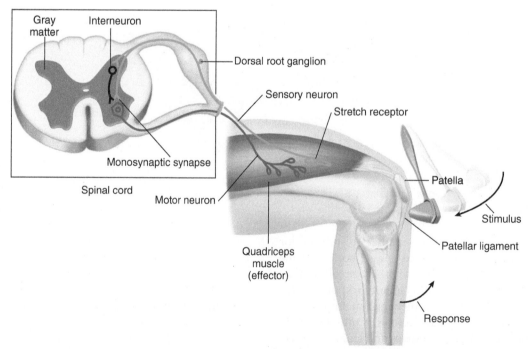

Fig. 14.4 Neural pathway involved in the patellar reflex. (From Patton KT, Thibodeau GA: *The human body in health and disease,* ed 7, St. Louis, 2018, Elsevier.)

provides oxygen and nourishment to the nervous tissue. These layers also bathe the spinal cord and the brain in CSF.

Ventricles. The four ventricles are spaces or cavities located in the brain. The CSF, which is clear and resembles plasma, flows into the subarachnoid spaces around the brain and the spinal cord and cushions them. It contains protein, glucose, urea, and salts; it also contains certain substances that form a protective barrier (the blood-brain barrier) that prevents harmful substances from entering the brain and the spinal cord.

Spinal Cord

The spinal cord is a 17- to 18-inch cord that extends from the brainstem to the second lumbar vertebra. It has two main functions: conducting impulses to and from the brain and serving as a center for reflex actions such as a knee jerk (Fig. 14.4). A sensory neuron sends the information to the spinal cord, a central neuron (located within the cord) interprets the impulse, and a motoneuron sends the message back to the muscle or organ involved. Thus a message is sent, interpreted, and acted on without traveling to the brain.

Peripheral Nervous System

The *peripheral nervous system* is made up of the motor nerves, the sensory nerves, and ganglia outside the brain and the spinal cord. It is composed of 31 pairs of spinal nerves, 12 pairs of cranial nerves, and the autonomic nervous system.

Spinal Nerves

The 31 pairs of spinal nerves are all mixed nerves. This means that they transmit sensory information to the spinal cord through afferent neurons and motor information from the CNS to the various areas of the body through efferent neurons. The spinal nerves are named according to the corresponding vertebra (e.g., *C1* for cervical spinal nerve 1, and *C2* for cervical spinal nerve 2).

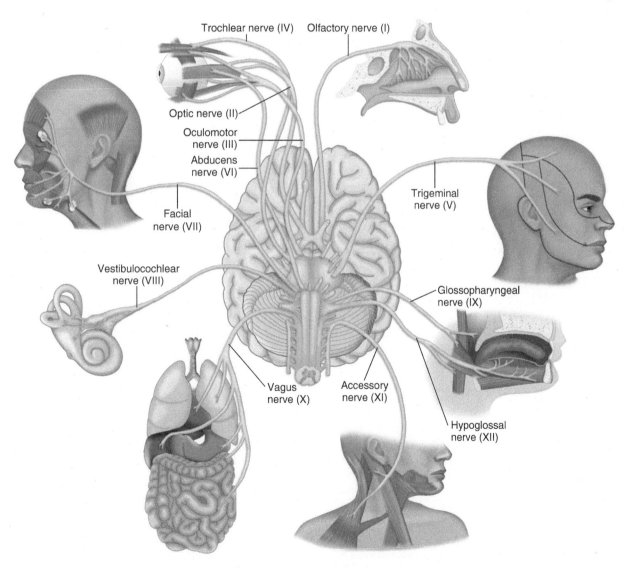

Fig. 14.5 Cranial nerves. (From Patton KT, Thibodeau GA: *The human body in health and disease*, ed 7, St. Louis, 2018, Elsevier.)

Cranial Nerves

There are 12 pairs of cranial nerves, which attach to the posterior surface of the brain, mainly the brainstem. Eleven of the pairs conduct impulses between the head, the neck, and the brain; the vagus nerve (cranial nerve X) also serves organs in the thoracic and abdominal cavities (Fig. 14.5). Table 14.1 lists the cranial nerves, their impulses, and functions.

Autonomic Nervous System

The autonomic nervous system controls the activities of the smooth muscle, the cardiac muscle, and all glands. The autonomic nervous system is not a separate nervous system but a subdivision of the peripheral nervous system.

It is misleading to think of this system as the automatic system, although most activity is performed on an unconscious level. Its primary function is to maintain internal homeostasis; for example, it strives to maintain a normal heartbeat, a constant body temperature, and a normal respiratory pattern.

To maintain this homeostasis, the autonomic system has two divisions: the *sympathetic nervous system* and the *parasympathetic nervous system*. These two divisions are antagonistic: one slows an action, and the other accelerates the action. These systems function simultaneously, but they are able to dominate each other as the need arises. In times of stress the sympathetic system takes over to prepare the body for "fight or flight." Heartbeat accelerates, blood pressure rises, and adrenal glands increase their secretions. To calm the body after a crisis, the parasympathetic system becomes dominant, slowing the heartbeat and decreasing the blood pressure and adrenal hormone output.

EFFECTS OF NORMAL AGING ON THE NERVOUS SYSTEM

The effects of aging on the nervous system are variable. The changes that occur include a loss of brain weight and a substantial loss of neurons (1% per year after age 50); the cortex loses cells faster than the brainstem. The remaining cells undergo structural changes. Aging also brings about a general decline in interconnections of dendrites, a reduction in cerebral blood flow, and a decrease in brain metabolism and oxygen use. The neurons may contain senile plaques, neurofibrillary tangles, and the age pigment lipofuscin. Older adults often have an altered sleep-to-wakefulness ratio, a decrease in the ability to regulate body temperature,

Table 14.1   Cranial Nerves

NERVE[a]	CONDUCTS IMPULSES	FUNCTIONS
I: Olfactory	From nose to brain	Sense of smell
II: Optic	From eye to brain	Vision
III: Oculomotor	From brain to eye muscles	Eye movements, extraocular muscles, pupillary control (pupillary constriction)
IV: Trochlear	From brain to external eye muscles	Down and inward movement of eye
V: Trigeminal Ophthalmic branch Maxillary branch Mandibular branch	From skin and mucous membranes of head to brain; from teeth to brain; from brain to chewing muscles	Sensations of face, scalp, and teeth; chewing movements
VI: Abducens	From brain to external eye muscles	Outward movement of eye
VII: Facial	From taste buds of tongue to brain; from brain to facial muscles	Sense of taste on anterior two-thirds of tongue; contraction of muscles of facial expression
VIII: Acoustic (vestibulocochlear)	From ear to brain	Hearing; sense of balance (equilibrium)
IX: Glossopharyngeal	From throat and taste buds of tongue to brain; from brain to throat muscles and salivary glands	Sensations of throat, taste, swallowing movements, gag reflex, sense of taste on posterior one third of tongue, secretion of saliva
X: Vagus	From throat, larynx, and organs in thoracic and abdominal cavities to brain; from brain to muscles of throat and to organs in thoracic and abdominal cavities	Sensations of throat, larynx, and thoracic and abdominal organs; swallowing, voice production, slowing of heartbeat, acceleration of peristalsis
XI: Spinal accessory	From brain to certain shoulder and neck muscles	Shoulder movements (trapezius muscle) and turning movements of head (sternocleidomastoid muscles)
XII: Hypoglossal	From brain to muscles of tongue	Tongue movements

[a]The first letter of the words in the following sentence are the first letters of the names of cranial nerves: "On Old Olympus's Towering Tops A Finn And German Viewed Some Hops." Many generations of students have used this or a similar mnemonic to help them remember the names of cranial nerves.

and a decrease in the velocity of nerve impulses. The blood supply to the spinal cord is decreased, resulting in slower reflexes.

Normal changes in the nervous system associated with aging are *not* the same as senility, organic brain disease, or Alzheimer disease (AD). Many older people reach old age with no functional deterioration of the nervous system. However, these normal changes may make care or rehabilitation of the older patient a challenge (see the Lifespan Considerations box).

Lifespan Considerations
Older Adults

Neurologic Disorder

- As neurons are lost with aging, neurologic function deteriorates, resulting in slowed reflex and reaction time.
- Tremors that increase with fatigue are common.
- The sense of touch and fine motor coordination diminish with aging.
- Most older people possess the ability to learn, but the speed of learning is slowed. Short-term memory is affected more by aging than is long-term memory.
- The incidence of physiologic dementia or organic brain syndrome—including Alzheimer disease, Pick disease, and multi-infarct dementia—increases with age.
- The incidence of stroke increases with age. Nerve irritation from arthritis, joint injuries, or spinal cord compression can cause chronic pain or weakness.
- Dementia is not a normal consequence of aging but may be a result of many reversible conditions, including anemia, fluid and electrolyte imbalance, malnutrition, hypothyroidism, metabolic disturbances, drug toxicity, hypotension, and a drug reaction or idiosyncrasy.

PREVENTION OF NEUROLOGIC PROBLEMS

Many conditions of the nervous system have no known cause. Other neurologic problems can be prevented or their effects reduced by modifying lifestyle factors. Neurovascular diseases are in part associated with defined risk factors. These risk factors are the same factors that increase the risk of cardiac disease, including high blood pressure, high blood cholesterol levels, cigarette smoking, obesity, stress, and lack of exercise.

Prevention of neurologic problems resulting from trauma is a major challenge. These injuries include spinal cord injury and head injury, which occur frequently in young people. Patient teaching on avoiding such injuries should include avoidance of drug and alcohol use, safe use of motor vehicles (e.g., using automobile seatbelts; wearing helmets with bicycles, motorcycles, and snowmobiles), safe swimming practices (e.g., not diving into shallow water), safe handling and storage of firearms, use of hardhats in dangerous construction areas, and use of protective gear as needed for sports (see the Safety Alert box).

Safety Alert
Preventing Neurologic Injuries

- One of the best ways to prevent head injuries is to prevent car and motorcycle accidents.
- Become active in campaigns that promote safe driving. Speak to driver's education classes regarding the danger of unsafe driving and driving after drinking alcohol or taking drugs.
- The use of seatbelts in cars and the use of helmets for riding on motorcycles are the most effective measures for increasing survival after accidents.
- Individual states have legislation requiring the use of automobile safety devices for children and adults.
- Recommend wearing protective helmets when engaging in potentially risky activities such as bike riding, horseback riding, and motorcycling.
- Encourage swimmers of all ages to refrain from diving into shallow water or areas in which water depth is unknown.

Neurologic diseases, such as meningitis or brain abscess, that occur as a result of infection sometimes can be prevented by prompt treatment of ear and sinus infections. Health teaching concerning immunizations to prevent diseases such as meningitis can reduce neurologic health concerns.

ASSESSMENT OF THE NEUROLOGIC SYSTEM

HISTORY

A comprehensive history is essential for diagnosing neurologic disease. This includes specifics about symptoms experienced and the patient's understanding and perception of what is happening. Obtaining information from family members or significant others also may be helpful. Follow the same format routinely to make certain information is complete.

For patients with suspected neurologic conditions, the presence of many symptoms or subjective data may be significant. These include the following:
- Headaches, especially those that first occur after middle age or those that change in character (e.g., headaches that are worse in the morning or awaken a person from sleep)
- Clumsiness or loss of function in an extremity
- Change in visual acuity
- Any new or worsened seizure activity
- Numbness or tingling in one or more extremities
- Pain in an extremity or other part of the body
- Personality changes or mood swings
- Extreme fatigue or tiredness

MENTAL STATUS

Assessment of the neurologic patient's mental status generally includes orientation (person, place, time, and purpose), mood and behavior, general knowledge (such as the names of US presidents), and short- and long-term memory. The patient's attention span and ability to concentrate also may be assessed.

Document the mental status in specific terms. Record as much information as possible to highlight the patient's status. For example, it is better to note "oriented to name, date, hospital, and purpose" than to note simply "oriented." Record actual statements made by the patient. Vary orientation questions to limit patients' ability to answer correctly simply because they have learned the right answers through repetition.

Level of Consciousness

Level of consciousness (LOC) is the earliest and most sensitive indicator of the patient's neurologic status. Changes in LOC are a result of impaired cerebral blood flow, which deprives the cells of the cerebral cortex and the reticular activating system (RAS) of oxygen. The RAS, located in the brainstem, is a functional system essential for wakefulness, attention, concentration, and introspection (*Mosby's Dictionary of Medicine, Nursing, & Health Professions*, 2017). A decreasing LOC is the earliest sign of increased intracranial pressure (ICP). LOC has two components: *arousal* (or wakefulness) and *awareness*. Wakefulness is the most fundamental part of LOC. If the patient can open his or her eyes spontaneously, in response to voice or to pain, the wakefulness center in the brainstem is still functioning. Awareness, a higher function controlled by the RAS, is the ability to interact with and interpret the environment. Awareness has four components, which are assessed as follows:

1. *Orientation:* Ask questions to determine the patient's orientation to person, place, time, and purpose.
2. *Memory:* Assess short-term memory; do not ask yes or no questions.

3. *Calculation:* Ask a simple math problem (e.g., "If you had four apples and you gave two away, how many apples would you have left?").
4. *Assessment of knowledge:* Ask the patient to name the president and something about current events.

Restlessness, disorientation, and lethargy may be seen first. Record observations in terms of behavior and signs—not labels such as "disoriented." Table 14.2 shows one method of classifying LOC.

Glasgow Coma Scale

The Glasgow Coma Scale (Table 14.3) is a quick, practical, and standardized system for assessing the degree of consciousness impairment in the critically ill and for predicting the duration and ultimate outcome of coma, particularly with head injuries. A patient's score on the Glasgow Coma Scale can change, along with the patient's health continuum. The Glasgow Coma Scale consists of a three-part neurologic assessment: eye opening, best motor response, and best verbal response.

The stronger the stimulus needed to obtain a response is, the lower the patient's score. The number values assigned to each part of the scale are added to yield an objective score. The score for a patient who is

---

Table 14.2   Levels of Consciousness

LEVEL	DESCRIPTION
Alert	Responds appropriately to auditory, tactile, and visual stimuli
Disorientation	Disoriented; unable to follow simple commands; thinking slowed; inattentive, flat affect
Stupor	Responds to verbal commands with moaning or groaning, if at all; seems unaware of the surroundings
Semicomatose	Is in an impaired state of consciousness, characterized by stupor, from which a patient can be aroused only by energetic stimulation
Comatose	Unable to respond to painful stimuli; corneal and pupillary reflexes are absent; cannot swallow or cough Is incontinent of urine and feces Electroencephalogram pattern demonstrates decreased or absent neuronal activity

---

Table 14.3   Glasgow Coma Scale: Measurement of Level of Consciousness[a]

CATEGORY OF RESPONSE	RESPONSE	SCORE
Eye-opening response	Spontaneous—open with blinking at baseline	4
	To verbal stimuli, command, speech	3
	To pressure (not applied to face)	2
	No response	1
Verbal response	Oriented	5
	Confused conversation, but able to answer questions	4
	words	3
	sounds	2
	No response	1
Motor response	Obeys commands for movement	6
	Purposeful movement to painful stimulus	5
	Withdraws in response to pain	4
	Flexion in response to pain (decorticate posturing)	3
	Extension response in response to pain (decerebrate posturing)	2
	No response	1

[a]The Glasgow Coma Scale provides a score ranging from 3 to 15; patients with scores of 3 to 8 are usually said to be in a coma. The total score is the sum of the scores in the three categories.
Modified from CDC n.d. Retrieved from https://www.cdc.gov/masstrauma/resources/gcs.pdf.

not neurologically impaired is 15; the lowest possible score is 3. In general, any score of 8 or less commonly is accepted as a definition of coma. The scale has a high degree of consistency even when used by staff of varied experience. There are some factors that may interfere with the outcomes of the scale. These are grouped into three categories: preexisting factors, effects of current treatments, and effects of other injuries or lesions. Language and cultural differences may act as barriers for the assessment. A hearing or intellectual deficit may result in impaired responses. Treatments such as pain medications or sedatives may influence the ability of the patient to appropriately respond. Coexisting conditions such as spinal trauma may result in altered findings (Glasgow Coma Scale, n.d.).

FOUR Score Coma Scale

The FOUR (Full Outline of UnResponsiveness) score coma scale is another method of assessment used by some facilities. This scale is used to assess patients with neurologic conditions that affect cognitive function such as stroke, craniotomy, and traumatic brain injury (TBI). Some feel it is a more user-friendly system to evaluate the neurologic status of patients. It also allows for improved evaluation of intubated patients, unlike the Glasgow Coma Scale. There are four categories: eye response, motor response, brainstem reflexes, and respiration pattern (Table 14.4). Each component is graded on a scale of 0 (worst response) to 4 (best response). The scores are not totaled, so there is not a *sum* score in this scale.

The FOUR score coma scale may be used as an alternative or complementary grading scale, along with the Glasgow Coma Scale (Foo, 2019). Facility policy and patient condition will determine if the Glasgow Coma Scale and/or the FOUR score coma scale will be used.

LANGUAGE AND SPEECH

It is important to assess the language and speech capability of the neurologic patient (see Box 14.1 and Fig. 14.3). Speech is a function of the dominant hemisphere, which is on the left side of the brain for all right-handed people and most left-handed people.

Aphasia

Aphasia is an abnormal neurologic condition in which the language function is defective or absent because of an injury to certain areas of the cerebral cortex. This most commonly involves Broca's area in the frontal lobe and Wernicke's area in the posterior part of the temporal lobe.

Aphasia can affect all areas of language, including speech, reading, writing, and understanding. Aphasia can manifest in various ways; some of its subdivisions are as follows:

- *Sensory aphasia,* or *receptive aphasia:* Inability to comprehend the spoken word or written word. Wernicke's area in the temporal lobe is associated

Table 14.4   FOUR Score Coma Scale

CATEGORY OF RESPONSE	RESPONSE	SCORE
Eye response (E)	Eyelids open or opened, tracking, or blinking to command	4
	Eyelids open but not tracking	3
	Eyelids closed, open to loud noise, not tracking	2
	Eyelids closed, open to pain, not tracking	1
	Eyelids remain closed with pain	0
Brainstem reflexes (B)	Pupil and corneal reflexes present	4
	One pupil wide and fixed	3
	Corneal or pupillary reflexes absent	2
	Corneal and pupillary reflexes absent	1
	Absent pupil, corneal, and cough reflexes	0
Motor response (M)	Thumbs up, fist or peace sign, to command	4
	Localizing to pain	3
	Flexion response to pain	2
	Extensor posturing	1
	No response to pain or generalized myoclonus status epilepticus	0
Respiration (R)	Not intubated, regular breathing pattern	4
	Not intubated, Cheyne-Stokes breathing pattern	3
	Not intubated, irregular breathing pattern	2
	Breathes above ventilator rate	1
	Breathes at ventilator rate or apnea	0

Updated source (also referenced in text):
Jabili R, Rezaei M: A comparison of the Glasgow Coma Scale Score with full outline of unresponsiveness scale to predict patients' outcomes in intensive care units. *Crit Care Res Pract*. Hindawi Publishing Corporation. 2014;2014:289803. https://doi.org/10.1155/2014/289803

with language comprehension. Pathologic conditions in this area result in receptive aphasia.
- *Motor aphasia:* Inability to speak or write, using symbols of speech (also called *expressive aphasia*). Broca's area in the frontal lobe mediates motor speech. Pathologic conditions in this area result in expressive aphasia.
- *Global aphasia:* Inability to understand the spoken word or to speak. Pathologic conditions in Broca's and Wernicke's areas result in global aphasia.
- *Anomic aphasia:* A form of aphasia characterized by the inability to name objects.

Dysarthria

Dysarthria is difficult, poorly articulated speech that usually results from interference in control over the muscles of speech. The general cause is damage to a central or peripheral nerve.

CRANIAL NERVES

Assessment of cranial nerve function is another important part of the neurologic assessment (see Fig. 14.5). The 12 pairs of nerves emerge from the cranial cavity through openings in the skull (see Table 14.1 for specifics of cranial nerve classification and assessment). The cranial nerves are tested in the following ways:

I (olfactory): Identification of common odors

II (optic): Testing of visual acuity and visual fields

III (oculomotor): Testing of ability of eyes to move together in all directions; testing pupillary response

IV (trochlear): Tested with oculomotor; testing eye movements

V (trigeminal): Jaw strength and sensation of face; corneal reflex

VI (abducens): Tested with oculomotor; testing eye movements

VII (facial): Ability of face to move in symmetry, identification of tastes

VIII (acoustic, or *vestibulocochlear):* Testing of hearing through whisper or other means and checking equilibrium and balance

IX (glossopharyngeal): Identification of tastes

X (vagus): Gag reflex, movement of uvula and soft palate

XI (spinal accessory): Shoulder and neck movement

XII (hypoglossal): Tongue motion

MOTOR FUNCTION

Evaluation of the neurologic patient's motor status detects abnormalities in the normal functioning of nerves and muscles. Motor function disturbances are the most commonly encountered neurologic symptom. In general, the motor status examination includes gait and stance, muscle tone, coordination, involuntary movements, and the muscle stretch reflexes.

Reflexes that usually are tested include biceps, triceps, brachioradialis, quadriceps, gastrocnemius, and soleus muscles. The examiner taps briskly over the muscle with a reflex hammer. The response is noted and graded on a scale, usually from 0 to 4+, with 4+ being hyperreflexic. The most important feature of any reflex pattern is not the absolute value on the scale but the comparison of one side of the body with the other. Stick figures are used commonly to record the bilateral values.

Damage to the nervous system often causes a serious problem in mobility. A complete loss of function is called *paralysis;* a partial loss of function is called paresis.

Injury or disease of motoneurons causes alterations in muscle strength, tone, and reflex activity. The specific signs and symptoms vary according to whether the lesion involves the upper motoneurons or lower motoneurons:

Lower motoneuron dysfunction: Muscles may be flaccid (weak, soft, and flabby and lacking normal muscle tone), with weak or absent deep tendon reflexes; muscle atrophy may occur; *fasciculations* (small, rapid muscle twitches) may occur and are localized, spontaneous, and involuntary.

Upper motoneuron dysfunction: Muscles may be spastic (prone to spasms, i.e., involuntary, sudden movements or muscular contractions), with increased reflexes (hyperreflexia). *Clonus* (alternating contractions and partial relaxation of a muscle, initiated by muscle stretching) may occur.

SENSORY AND PERCEPTUAL STATUS

The sensory examination is the most difficult part of the neurologic evaluation. Specific alterations in sensation that should be assessed include pain; touch; temperature; and proprioception, the body's sense, based on internal stimuli, of its own position and limb movements. This sensation enables one to know the position of the body without looking at it and to recognize objects by the sense of touch.

The sensory evaluation may reveal conditions of which the patient is unaware. An example is unilateral neglect, a condition in which an individual is perceptually unaware of and inattentive to one side of the body. Another perceptual problem is hemianopia, which is characterized by defective vision or blindness in half of the visual field.

In most clinical settings it is usually not feasible or necessary to complete the total neurologic examination during shift-to-shift assessments of the patient. However, in many settings, such as intensive care units, the neurologic checks may be done as frequently as every 15 minutes. The most important factors include orientation, LOC, bilateral muscle strength, speech, involuntary movements, ability to follow commands, and any abnormal posturing.

LABORATORY AND DIAGNOSTIC EXAMINATIONS

BLOOD AND URINE TESTS

Assessment of the neurologically impaired patient includes a variety of blood and urine tests. A culture of the urine may rule out infection involving the urinary tract. Other urine testing may indicate the presence of diabetes insipidus. Urine drug screens may be done to rule out drug use as a cause of lethargy or to identify specific drugs ingested.

Arterial blood gas (ABG) values are an important diagnostic tool for monitoring the oxygen and carbon dioxide content of the blood. These gas levels may be altered with neurologic diseases such as Guillain-Barré syndrome (GBS), which may affect breathing patterns.

Routine blood tests may help narrow the diagnosis of a neurologic disorder.

CEREBROSPINAL FLUID

Examination of the CSF can yield information about many neurologic conditions. CSF normally contains up to 10 lymphocytes per milliliter. An increase in the number of lymphocytes may indicate a bacterial, fungal, or viral infection. Low levels of CSF glucose may occur with bacterial and fungal infections such as meningitis. In the case of meningitis, a culture or smear examination is done to determine the causative organism. Spinal fluid protein is elevated when a degenerative disease or a brain tumor is present. Blood in the spinal fluid may indicate hemorrhage somewhere in the brain or spinal cord. A protein electrophoresis evaluation may give evidence of neurologic diseases such as multiple sclerosis (MS).

Lumbar Puncture

A lumbar puncture is often a part of the diagnostic workup for the patient who may have a neurologic problem. It is contraindicated in patients who may have increased ICP because the withdrawal of fluid may cause the medulla oblongata to protrude downward (herniate) into the opening at the base of the skull (the foramen magnum).

A lumbar puncture is done to obtain CSF for examination, to relieve pressure, or to introduce dye or medication. It is a common procedure, done in the patient's room or in the diagnostic imaging department. The procedure takes approximately 30 minutes.

The patient usually is positioned on the side with the knee and head flexed at an acute angle. This allows for maximal lumbar flexion and separation of the interspinous spaces. Some practitioners may choose to have the patient sit in a chair facing the back of the chair and lean forward over the back of the chair if they are removing a small amount of CSF. After anesthetizing the area with a local anesthetic, the health care provider inserts a hollow needle into the space between the lumbar vertebrae (often between L4 and L5, called the L4–L5 interspace), below where the spinal cord ends. The patient may feel slight pain and pressure as the dura is entered. The stylet within the hollow needle is removed to allow for collection and analysis of spinal fluid. A manometer attached to the needle is used to measure the CSF pressure. The first specimen of spinal fluid may contain blood from slight bleeding at the site of the puncture. This specimen should not be sent for cell count.

After the procedure, the patient may need to lie flat in bed for several hours. Assess the site of the puncture for any leakage, as evidenced by moisture on the bandage or around the puncture site. Assess for pain, numbness, and tingling in the extremities after the procedure. Back and leg pain may be experienced but should not be persistent. Acetaminophen may be given to manage minor discomfort. Approximately 30% of patients develop mild postprocedural headaches, believed to be caused by puncture of the dura during the procedure or with withdrawal of the needle, resulting in leakage of CSF. Headaches may begin within hours of the procedure, while some do not begin until more than 24 hours later. Nausea and vomiting may accompany the headaches. Options to manage the headache include bed rest, analgesics, rehydration, and ice applied to the head. Opioids are usually not helpful. Most postprocedural headaches are managed successfully with conservative interventions. A blood patch may be performed to provide relief for severe and lingering headaches (NLM, 2020b). This procedure involves the withdrawal of 20 to 30 mL of blood from a large vein, most commonly in the arm. The blood then is reinjected into the epidural space. The rationale behind the intervention is to provide a blood plug at the site of the dura's puncture to stop the leakage of spinal fluid.

OTHER TESTS

Routine radiographs of the head and vertebral column are useful for ruling out fractures of the skull and cervical vertebrae. Computed tomography (CT) scanning has reduced the use of skull radiography.

Computed Tomography Scan

The purpose of the CT scan is to detect pathologic conditions of the cerebrum and spinal cord, using a technique of scanning without radioisotopes. No special physical preparation is required for the test. A CT scan takes 20 to 30 minutes if done without contrast medium and about 60 minutes with contrast. If the use of contrast medium is anticipated, document and report to the health care provider any history of allergy to iodine and seafood, because iodine is present in the contrast medium. Kidney function should also be assessed since significant decreased kidney function can lead to acute or chronic renal failure when dye is used. If contrast medium is employed, the patient may be NPO for 4 to 6 hours before the testing begins. The procedure is painless, except for the slight discomfort when an intravenous (IV) line is started for injection of the contrast dye. There may be a brief metallic taste and flushing sensation as the medium is infused. The patient also may feel some discomfort from being required to lie still and may experience a sense of claustrophobia by being held in a small space.

During the procedure the patient lies face up (supine) with the head positioned within a rubber head holder to prevent air gaps between the machine and the scalp. The head is scanned in two planes simultaneously and at various angles. Each image that appears represents a specific layer of brain tissue. The computer displays a printout that indicates areas of increased density (e.g., tumors or thrombi).

Brain Scan

Like the CT scan, the purpose of a brain scan is to detect pathologic conditions of the cerebrum. It requires the use of radioactive isotopes and a scanner. No special physical preparation is required. The procedure takes approximately 45 minutes for the actual scan. The patient is injected with a radioisotope and then lies still while a scanner passes over the brain area. Concentrated areas of uptake are reflected. There are generally no adverse effects from the procedure and only minimal discomfort associated with the IV administration of the radioactive isotopes. Brain scans are being used less frequently than in the past because of the excellent results obtained from CT scans and magnetic resonance imaging (MRI).

Magnetic Resonance Imaging

MRI uses magnetic forces to image body structures. It is used to detect pathologic conditions of the cerebrum and the spinal cord and in the detection of stroke, MS, tumors, trauma, herniation, and seizure. Because MRI yields greater contrast in the images of soft tissue structures than does the CT scan, it is the diagnostic test of choice for many neurologic diseases. Advances in MRI techniques include diffusion-weighted imaging and magnetic resonance spectroscopy. Because MRI involves a magnetic force, watches, credit cards, and any metal from the clothing must be removed before entering the scanning room. Ask the patient about the presence of any metal in the body that would preclude the use of MRI, such as orthopedic appliances, older aneurysm clips and pacemakers, stents, and shrapnel.

During the procedure the patient lies supine with the head positioned in a head holder. The test may take as little as 20 minutes up to 60 minutes. The procedure is painless, except for the discomfort from lying still and possible feelings of claustrophobia when a "closed MRI" is performed. Warn the patient that the machine makes various loud noises during the scanning procedure.

Magnetic Resonance Angiography

Magnetic resonance angiography (MRA) uses differential radio waves and magnetic field signals to visualize flowing blood to evaluate extracranial and intracranial blood vessels. It is a noninvasive procedure for viewing possible occlusions in arteries. It provides anatomic and hemodynamic information. It can be used in conjunction with contrast media (contrast-enhanced MRA). MRA rapidly is replacing cerebral angiography in diagnosing cerebrovascular diseases. MRA has been useful to evaluate the cervical carotid artery and large-caliber intracranial arterial and venous structures.

Positron Emission Tomography Scan

Another evaluative measure that is similar to CT and MRI scans is the positron emission tomography (PET) scan. In this procedure the patient receives an injection of deoxyglucose combined with radioactive fluorine.

The area in question is scanned, and a color composite picture is obtained. Shades of color indicate the level of glucose metabolism, with abnormal levels suggestive of a pathologic state. PET scanning provides a noninvasive means of determining biochemical processes that occur in the brain. It is being used increasingly to monitor patients who have had a stroke or who have AD, Huntington disease, tumors, epilepsy, and Parkinson disease. As with the CT scan, discomfort is minimal. Inform the patient of the need to lie still for the duration of the scan, which is usually about 45 minutes.

Electroencephalogram

The electroencephalogram (EEG) provides evidence of focal or generalized disturbances of brain function by measuring the electrical activity of the brain. Among the cerebral disorders assessed by EEG are epilepsy, mass lesions (e.g., tumors, abscess, hematoma), cerebrovascular lesions, and brain injury. The test requires no special preparation, but encourage the patient to be quiet and rest before the procedure. An exception is a sleep-deprived EEG, during which the patient is kept awake the night before the test; the EEG usually is done first thing in the morning. An EEG usually takes about 1 hour to complete. The patient's hair and scalp should be clean. The electrodes are secured to the scalp with a gluelike substance called collodion, in a set pattern to cover all scalp areas. An EEG is painless.

The basic resting rhythm of the EEG is affected by opening the eyes or altering attention. Recordings sometimes are made while the patient is asleep or sleep deprived, when the seizure threshold may be lowered. Comparisons are made of different patterns of the recordings. After the test, allow the patient to rest. Assist the patient if necessary in washing the hair and removing the collodion from the scalp.

Myelogram

A myelogram is sometimes used to identify lesions in the intradural or extradural compartments of the spinal canal by observing the flow of radiopaque dye through the subarachnoid space. The most common lesion for which this test is used is a herniated or protruding intervertebral disk. Other lesions include spinal tumors, adhesions, bony deformations, and arteriovenous malformations. Before the procedure, assess and document the patient's baselines of lower extremity strength and sensation. Tell the patient that the procedure takes about 2 hours, it may involve slight discomfort as the dura is entered, and he or she may be asked to assume a variety of positions during the procedure.

Water-soluble iodine dyes such as iopamidol commonly are used because they are absorbed into the bloodstream and excreted by the kidneys. Preparation for this procedure is the same as for lumbar puncture. Before the dye is injected, ask the patient whether he or she has any allergies and specifically about any anaphylactic or hypotensive episodes related to other dyes.

The patient usually is positioned on the side with both knees and the head flexed at an acute angle to allow maximal flexion of the lumbar area for ease in performing the lumbar puncture. After the puncture is performed, the inner stylet is removed to allow drainage of CSF, measurement of pressure, and collection of specimens. The dye is instilled and the needle is removed. The patient then is turned to various positions so that the spinal cord can be visualized while fluoroscopic and radiopaque films are taken. The patient usually undergoes a CT scan 4 to 6 hours after a myelogram.

After the procedure, observe the puncture site for any leakage of CSF, and assess the strength and sensation of the lower extremities. Headache is fairly common. It may be accompanied by nausea and occasionally by vomiting. The patient should lie flat in bed for a few hours.

Angiogram

The angiogram (cerebral arteriography) is a procedure used to visualize the cerebral arterial system by injecting radiopaque material. It allows detection of arterial aneurysms, vessel anomalies, ruptured vessels, and displacement of vessels by tumors or masses.

Before the procedure the patient usually is given clear liquids, although in some institutions all oral intake is restricted. Assess the patient for any allergy to iodine because the dye contains iodine. If the femoral approach (through the leg) is to be used, mark the locations of the pedal pulse in both feet. If the carotid artery is used, measure the neck circumference as part of the baseline data. Immediately before the procedure, measure baseline vital signs and pulses and perform a neurologic check.

The test takes approximately 2 to 3 hours. The patient may become uncomfortable lying still for that length of time. When the dye is injected, most patients complain of feeling extremely hot, feeling flushed, and experiencing a metallic taste. The patient is positioned supine on the radiograph table. A local anesthetic agent is used to anesthetize the area of the puncture site. The catheter is introduced through the skin (percutaneously) and introduced into the relevant vessels. At times the catheter may be inserted directly into the carotid or vertebral arteries. After all injections are done, the catheter is withdrawn and pressure is applied to the puncture site for at least 15 minutes.

After the procedure, bed rest may be ordered, usually for 4 to 6 hours. Check vital signs and perform a neurologic check frequently (at times as often as every 15 minutes). Assess the puncture site frequently for the presence of a hematoma. With a femoral stick (i.e., when the puncture site is in the femoral artery), check the pulses distal to the site for evidence of arterial occlusion. With a carotid stick, assess whether the patient has any difficulty breathing or swallowing or an increase in the girth of the neck.

The patient undergoing this procedure is at risk for cerebrovascular accident and increased ICP. Promptly report any change in LOC or in other parts of the neurologic assessment.

MRA is replacing cerebral arteriography rapidly in many facilities.

Carotid Duplex

A carotid duplex study uses combined ultrasound and pulsed Doppler technology. A technician places a probe on the skin over the carotid artery and slowly moves the probe along the course of the common carotid to the bifurcation of the external and internal carotid arteries. The ultrasound signal emitted from the probe reflects off the moving blood cells within the vessel. The frequency of the reflected signal corresponds to the blood velocity. This response is amplified and is registered on a graphic record and also as sound. The graphic record registers blood velocity. Increased blood flow velocity can indicate stenosis of a vessel. Carotid duplex scanning is a noninvasive study that evaluates carotid occlusive disease. This study often is ordered when a patient has had a transient ischemic attack (TIA).

Electromyogram

An electromyogram (EMG) measures the contraction of a muscle in response to electrical stimulation. It provides evidence of lower motor neuron disease; primary muscle disease; and defects in the transmission of electrical impulses at the neuromuscular junction, such as in myasthenia gravis (MG). There is no special preparation for the test. The test takes approximately 45 minutes for one muscle study. Inform the patient that it is uncomfortable when the electrode is inserted into the muscle and when the electrical current is used. The muscle may ache for a short time after the procedure.

During the test an electrode is inserted into selected skeletal muscles. An electric current is passed through the electrode, and the machine graphs the variations of muscle potentials (voltage). After the procedure, assess the patient for signs of bleeding at the site of the electrode insertion. The patient may need an analgesic for discomfort and a rest period.

Echoencephalogram

An echoencephalogram uses ultrasound to depict intracranial structures of the brain. It is especially helpful in detecting ventricular dilation and a major shift of midline structures in the brain as a result of an expanding lesion. The preparation of the patient, the actual procedure, and aftercare are similar to those of the brain scan.

COMMON DISORDERS OF THE NEUROLOGIC SYSTEM

HEADACHES

Etiology and Pathophysiology

Headache is a common neurologic complaint; its significance and its causes vary. The source of recurring headache should be determined through careful physical examination with appropriate neurologic assessment.

The exact mechanism of head pain is not known. Although the skull and brain tissues are not able to feel sensory pain, pain arises from the scalp, its blood vessels and muscles, and the dura mater and its venous sinuses. Pain also arises from the blood vessels at the base of the brain and from cervical cranial nerves. Blood vessels may dilate and become congested with blood. Headaches are classified as primary or secondary. A primary headache is not one that is attributable to a physiological disorder. Vascular and tension types are classified as primary headaches. Secondary headaches are caused by underlying health disorders such as hypertension, dental problems, sinusitis, tumors, and head injuries,

- *Vascular headaches* include migraine, cluster, and hypertensive headaches.
- *Tension headaches* may arise from psychological problems related to tension or stress, or from medical problems such as cervical arthritis.

Migraine Headaches

The exact cause of migraine headaches is unknown. Genetics and environmental factors are often attributed to the cause of migraines. Abnormal metabolism of serotonin, a vasoactive neurotransmitter found in platelets and cells of the brain, plays a major role. Migraine headaches are three times more common in women than men. There is often a familial link. The age of onset is traditionally during the teen years and the peak is seen in the 30s. Hormonal changes and family history are also considered risk factors (Mayo Clinic, 2021b).

Patients with migraine often report experiencing prodrome symptoms in the days preceeding the onset of the headache. This may include symptoms such as constipation, fluid retention or mood changes. The aura is similar to the prodrome as it occurs prior to the onset of head pain. The aura are neurological symptoms. Auras most often are reported to occur in the half-hour preceding the attack but may occur up to 24 hours before the onset of pain. Each patient's aura is individualized but commonly includes visual field defects; unusual smells or sounds; disorientation; paresthesias; and, in rare cases, paralysis of a part of the body. Migraine headache pain is described classically as throbbing and pounding. It is often worse on one side of the head. Additional symptoms experienced during the headache include nausea, vomiting, sensitivity to light, chilliness, fatigue, irritability, diaphoresis, edema, and other signs of autonomic dysfunction. Migraine headaches may be triggered by a series of factors.

Assessment

Subjective data include the patient's understanding of the headache, possible causes, and any precipitating factors. It is important to determine migraine triggers. The list of common triggers is numerous, including too much wine or caffeine, sleep changes, certain foods and food additives, stress and certain medications (e.g., oral contraceptives). Determine what measures relieve the symptoms and the location, frequency, pattern, and character of the pain. This includes the site of return of the headache, time of day, and intervals between headaches. Also assess the initial onset of the headache, any symptoms that occur before the headache or associated symptoms, the presence of allergies, and any family history of similar headache patterns.

Diagnostic Tests

It is important to evaluate headaches that are not transient. Usual testing includes a neurologic examination, a CT scan (MRI or PET scan also may be done), a brain scan, and skull radiographs. Lumbar punctures are not commonly performed, but a lumbar puncture is not done if there is evidence of increased ICP or if a brain tumor is suspected, because quick reduction of pressure produced by removal of the spinal fluid may cause brain herniation. In these situations, a CT scan is done first.

Medical Management

Dietary counseling. Some foods may cause or worsen headaches. These include foods containing tyramine, nitrites, or glutamates (e.g., monosodium glutamate [MSG], often used in the preparation of Chinese foods and processed meats). Tyramine is an amino acid that helps to control blood pressure. It is found in foods including aged cheeses (cheddar and Swiss), cured meats, fermented cabbage (sauerkraut), and soy and fish sauces. Nitrites are present in curing substances used in the preparation of meats such as bologna, ham, hot dogs, and bacon. Other substances that may provoke headaches include vinegar, chocolate, yogurt, alcohol, fermented or marinated foods, and caffeine. Patients may not realize how often they are ingesting potential headache triggers; instructing them to keep a food diary is helpful.

Psychotherapy. Patients with headaches may respond to psychotherapy. This does not mean that the headache pain is not physiologic, but counseling can help the patient develop awareness of stress or triggering factors and deal with the pain. The patient may need help expressing feelings about intractable headache pain. Relaxation techniques can also be discussed to help with headache prevention and treatment.

Medications. Medications often are used to treat headaches. Mild migraine episodes may be managed with over-the-counter medications. Acetylsalicylic acid (aspirin), acetaminophen, or ibuprofen may be used. Using these medications more than 3 days per week can cause rebound headaches. For moderate to severe headaches, the triptans have become the first line of the therapy. Triptans are thought to act on receptors in the extracerebral, intracranial vessels that become dilated during a migraine attack. Stimulating these receptors constricts cranial vessels, inhibits neuropeptide release, and reduces nerve impulse transmission along trigeminal pain pathways. Triptans commonly prescribed include eletriptan, the seventh triptan to be marketed for treatment of migraine, joining almotriptan, frovatriptan, naratriptan, rizatriptan, sumatriptan, and zolmitriptan. Classified as selective serotonin receptor agonists, these drugs are indicated to treat acute migraine (with or without aura) in adults. In addition to relieving headache pain, the triptans also relieve the nausea, vomiting, and photophobia associated with an acute migraine attack.

Ergotamine preparations manage migraine headache pain by preventing the blood vessels in the brain from expanding and causing headaches. Ergotamine is combined with caffeine and the compounds are taken orally. They are most effective when taken at the first sign of migraine pain.

Another approach for managing migraine headaches is to prevent them by taking medications before the onset of pain. The decision to do this is based on the severity and frequency of headache pain. Topiramate taken daily has been an effective therapy for migraine prevention in adults. Other preventive drugs for migraine headaches include beta-adrenergic blockers (e.g., propranolol, atenolol), tricyclic antidepressants (e.g., amitriptyline), selective serotonin reuptake inhibitors (e.g., fluoxetine), calcium channel blockers (e.g., verapamil), divalproex, clonidine, and thiazide diuretics.

Some experiencing migraines also encounter nausea and vomiting during their headache experience. Their plan of care should include efforts to reduce these symptoms. Anti-emetic medications such as chlorpromazine, metochlopramide, or prochlorperazine may be administered.

Patients who experience frequent migraines may be evaluated for treatment to prevent their occurrence. These medication types are prescribed to reduce the incidence of migraines and reduce their duration. Medication classifications used in this manner include antihypertensive, antidepressant, and anti-seizure medications. Botox injections may be utilized to prevent or reduce migraine headaches.

Cluster headaches. Cluster headaches are named for the pattern with which they occur. These headaches occur almost daily for a period of time and then subside. They return and occur again, regularly. The period of attack may be a week to a year. The period of remission may be a month or longer. The exact cause is unknown, although theories support a sudden release of histamine or serotonin by the body. The pain of cluster headaches is usually one sided and is described as *burning, sharp,* and *steady.* It may be accompanied by watering of the eyes (tearing) and nasal stuffiness. Their onset is sudden and they often occur at the same time of day. Cluster headaches occur more commonly in men. They affect adolescents and middle-aged adults. Like migraine headaches, there are familial tendencies. The triggering factors for cluster headaches

are similar to those of migraine headaches but also include exertion, heat, and high altitudes (NLM, 2019a).

Diagnosis of cluster headaches usually is based on the presentation of symptoms. If the health care provider is present during an attack, Horner syndrome frequently is noted. This is the presentation of a small pupil or eyelid drooping on one side. These signs are not present in the absence of the headache. Other testing, such as MRI, may be performed to rule out other causes.

Because the pain associated with vascular cluster headaches is often severe, opioid analgesics, sometimes given intramuscularly, are used. Sumatriptan (Imitrex) may be prescribed to manage the headaches. Prednisone therapy may be initiated. During this type of intervention, the patient begins with a high dose of the steroid and then the doses gradually are reduced over time. Dihydroergotamine (DHE) may be injected and can stop pain within 5 minutes. It cannot be taken in conjunction with sumatriptan. Patients with cluster headaches usually feel fine between attacks, so no analgesic is needed during these times.

Tension headaches. Nonopioid analgesics often are used to treat tension headaches. These include acetaminophen, ibuprofen, and aspirin. Opioids are avoided because these drugs are often subject to abuse; it is much better to counsel patients to develop other ways to relieve tension headaches.

Nursing Interventions and Patient Teaching

Because stress and emotional upsets may precipitate some headaches and worsen others, the patient requires relaxation and rest. Help the patient with relaxation techniques, planned sleeping hours, and regular rest periods. Alcohol should not be used to relieve tension because it may become addicting and has been found to be a significant cause of cluster headaches. Regular physical exercise also may help prevent headaches, especially those caused by tension.

If a patient is suffering from a severe headache, plan nursing interventions so that only essential activities take place. Plan interventions so that the patient has adequate time to rest.

Comfort measures. Other treatments that may help a patient with a headache include cold packs applied to the forehead or base of the skull and pressure applied to the temporal arteries. People with migraine headaches are usually most comfortable lying in a dark, quiet room.

Identifying triggering factors. Triggering factors associated with severe and recurring headaches may include fatigue, alcohol, stress, seasonal climate changes, hunger, allergies, and menstruation. Help the patient identify these factors, if necessary, through ongoing observation or assessment of the patient's personality, habits, activities of daily living (ADLs), career plans, work habits, family relationships, coping mechanisms, and relaxation activities. The patient may keep a diary or journal to help collect this information.

Patient problems and interventions for the patient with headache include but are not limited to the following:

PATIENT PROBLEM	NURSING INTERVENTIONS
Anxiousness, related to pain	Provide quiet environment Encourage verbalization of concerns Provide diversional activities
Recent Onset of Pain or Prolonged Pain, related to disease process	Administer prescribed medications Provide comfort measures Maintain nonstressful environment Encourage pain reduction techniques as appropriate: rocking movements, external warmth, breathing patterns

Teaching is an important part of the nursing intervention for the patient with headaches. Topics include (1) avoidance of factors that trigger headaches; (2) relaxation techniques, including biofeedback; (3) maintenance of regular sleep patterns; (4) medications to be used (including dosage, actions, and side effects); and (5) the importance of follow-up care.

Prognosis

With proper treatment the person with headaches can expect to live a normal life. Changes in lifestyle may have to occur, especially during acute episodes of headache pain. The person may have to adjust to periodic headaches and rest until the headache resolves. Chronic headaches have a broad-reaching impact on the patient and family with regard to emotional well-being, physical impairment, and employment. Ninety percent of migraine patients are unable to function normally when a headache occurs. An estimated 25% of individuals who experience migraines have missed a day of work in the past 3 months. There are many types of headaches. For additional information, visit the National Headache Foundation website (https://headaches.org).

NEUROPATHIC PAIN

Etiology, Pathophysiology, and Clinical Manifestations

Neuropathic pain refers to pain originating from the peripheral or CNS caused by direct stimulation of the myelinated nervous tissue. It is characterized as a tingling or burning pain in areas of sensory loss. Neuropathic pain may result from postherpetic neuralgia, diabetic neuropathies, and trigeminal neuralgia; phantom limb pain is now considered a neuropathic pain. Patients may have disabling pain, caused by a disorder either within the nervous system or at a distant part of the body. Neuropathic pain may arise from lesions involving the peripheral cutaneous nerves, the sensory nerve roots, the thalamus, and the central pain tract (lateral spinothalamic tract) at some level. Each produces characteristic pain. Pain receptors are not adaptable—they are specific for pain only—and pain impulses continue

at the same rate as long as the stimulus is present. Pain receptors can be activated by cellular damage, certain chemicals such as histamine, heat, ischemia, muscle spasm, and sensations of cold and pruritus that go beyond a specific level of intensity.

Pain that is described as unbearable and does not respond to treatment is classified as *intractable*. It is chronic and often debilitating and may prevent the patient from functioning in everyday life.

Assessment

The perception of pain is highly subjective. Pain may vary from mild to excruciating. Subjective data include the patient's understanding of the pain; any precipitating factors; and measures that relieve stress, including medication. The site, frequency, and nature of the pain are important, as is the patient's usual coping patterns when under stress. Encourage the patient to use a pain scale to express the level of pain experienced. Associated symptoms and measures that make the pain worse are important subjective data.

Objective data may be limited when assessing neuropathic pain. Objective factors to assess are behavioral signs indicating pain or stress, a change in the ability to carry out ADLs, muscle weakness or wasting, vasomotor responses (such as flushing), abnormalities of spinal reflexes, and abnormalities noted during the sensory examination.

Diagnostic Tests

Diagnostic tests for the patient in pain may include electrical stimulation, used to define the pain to a greater degree. Psychological testing may be part of the workup. If back or neck pain is present, a myelogram usually is performed.

Medical Management

Nonsurgical methods of pain control. Neuropathic pain sometimes responds to other methods of pain control. These include transcutaneous electrical nerve stimulation and spinal cord stimulation. Both techniques use electrodes applied near the site of pain, or on or around the spine. The stimulator modifies the sensory input by blocking or changing the painful sensation with a stimulus that is perceived to be less or not at all painful. Acupuncture also is used to treat patients with neuropathic pain.

Nerve block. A nerve block is used to control intractable pain. It involves injecting a local anesthetic, alcohol, or phenol close enough to a nerve to block the conduction of impulses. Sources of pain often treated with a nerve block include trigeminal neuralgia, cancer, and peripheral vascular disease. The effect lasts from several months to several years. Pain and spasticity also may be controlled by means of an epidural catheter. Medication usually is administered continuously.

Medications. Medications often are used to treat patients with neuropathic pain. Anticonvulsant medications such as gabapentin (Neurontin) and carbamazepine (Tegretol) are often useful. Other medications include nonopioid analgesics such as acetaminophen, nonsteroidal anti-inflammatory drugs, and acetylsalicylic acid. Opioids do not appear as helpful for neuropathic pain, although they sometimes are used. Antidepressants—such as amitriptyline, doxepin, imipramine, and nortriptyline (Pamelor)—appear to be effective in treating neuropathic pain. The emphasis should be on helping the patient learn various other measures to control the pain.

Surgical methods of pain control. When intractable pain does not respond to more conservative measures, surgery may be necessary to reduce or eliminate the pain.

Nursing Interventions and Patient Teaching

Comfort measures. A patient with neuropathic pain may be uncomfortable and should be assisted to assume a position of comfort. For example, the patient with back pain should avoid movements that cause direct or indirect movement of the spinal cord. The patient may find lying in a supine position uncomfortable. Help the patient find a comfortable position and, if necessary, actively assist the patient in turning or moving. Straining when having a bowel movement can intensify pain, and a stool softener may be needed. Offer prune juice and a high-fiber diet and encourage the patient to drink up to 2000 mL/day or more of fluids.

Promotion of rest and relaxation. As with headache, stress and emotional upsets may precipitate or exacerbate neuropathic pain. Facilitate rest and relaxation, with planned sleeping hours and rest periods as needed.

Some patients with pain, especially intractable pain, may respond well to psychotherapy. This does not mean that the pain does not have a physiologic basis, but counseling can help the patient develop awareness of what makes the pain worse and how to cope with the discomfort.

Patient problems and interventions for the patient with neuropathic pain are the same as those listed previously for headache, with the addition of but not limited to the following:

PATIENT PROBLEM	NURSING INTERVENTIONS
Risk for Contractures or Muscle Atrophy, related to lack of use of a body part as a result of pain	Explain need for a regular exercise program to maintain joint mobility; provide range-of-motion (ROM) exercises to all body joints q 2–4 h Be positive and reassuring in approach
Inability to Feed, Bathe, Dress, or Toilet Self, related to pain	Assist with basic ADL needs as necessary, but encourage patient to participate as much as possible Provide sufficient time for ADLs Facilitate use of self-help devices as needed Provide for total hygiene as indicated

Teaching the patient with neuropathic pain is an important nursing intervention. Include the factors taught to the patient with headache, and help the patient become aware of physical methods such as positioning the body to increase comfort and structuring the home and work setting to minimize stress.

Prognosis
As with headache pain, neuropathic pain can in most cases be treated adequately. Lifestyle changes may be helpful in allowing the person to have a better quality of life.

INCREASED INTRACRANIAL PRESSURE

Etiology, Pathophysiology, and Clinical Manifestations
Increased ICP is a complex grouping of events that occurs because of multiple neurologic conditions. It often occurs suddenly, progresses rapidly, and requires surgical intervention. It is a potential complication in many neurologic conditions and rapidly can lead to death if not treated and reversed.

Increased ICP occurs in patients with acute neurologic conditions such as a brain tumor, hemorrhage, anoxic brain injury, and toxic or viral encephalopathies; it most commonly is associated with head injury. The Monro-Kellie doctrine states that the volume of the contents of the cranium (brain tissue, CSF, and blood) is constant. An increase in any constituent must be accompanied by a decrease in one of the others or else increased ICP will result. This is because the cranial vault is rigid and nonexpandable, that is, it does not allow for increases. Pressure may build up slowly over weeks or rapidly, depending on the cause. Usually one side of the brain is more involved, but both sides of the brain eventually become involved.

As the pressure increases within the cranial cavity, it is first compensated for by venous compression and CSF displacement. As the pressure continues to rise, the cerebral blood flow decreases and inadequate perfusion of the brain occurs. This inadequate perfusion starts a vicious cycle in which the carbon dioxide concentration in the blood ($PaCO_2$) increases, and the oxygen concentration (PaO_2) and pH decrease. These changes cause vasodilation and cerebral edema. The edema further increases the ICP, which causes increased compression of neural tissue and an even greater increase in ICP.

When the pressure buildup is greater than the brain's ability to compensate, pressure is exerted on surrounding structures where the pressure is lower. This movement of pressure is called *supratentorial shift* and can result in herniation. As a result of herniation of the brain, the brainstem is compressed at various levels, which in turn compresses the vasomotor center, the posterior cerebral artery, the oculomotor nerve, the corticospinal nerve pathway, and the fibers of the ascending RAS. The life-sustaining mechanisms of consciousness, blood pressure, pulse, respiration, and temperature regulation become impaired. A rise in systolic pressure and an unchanged diastolic pressure, resulting in a widening pulse pressure, bradycardia, and abnormal respiration, are late signs of increased ICP and indicate that the brain is about to herniate.

Assessment

Increased ICP must be detected early while it is still reversible. The ability to make accurate observations, interpret observations intelligently, and record observations carefully is most important for the nurse working with patients with increased ICP.

Subjective data for a diagnosis of increased ICP include the patient's understanding of the condition, any visual changes such as diplopia (double vision), a change in the patient's personality, and a change in the ability to think. The diplopia usually results from paralysis or weakness of one of the muscles that control eye movement. It often occurs fairly early in the process. Nausea or pain, especially headache, is also important. The headache is thought to result from venous congestion and tension in the intracranial blood vessels as the cerebral pressure rises. Headache that occurs with increased ICP usually increases in intensity with coughing, straining at stool, or stooping. It is usually present in the early morning and may awaken the patient from sleep.

Objective data include a change in LOC, which is the earliest sign of increased ICP. During assessment, it takes more stimulation to get the same response from the patient. Manifestations of a change in LOC include disorientation, restlessness, and lethargy. Record observations in terms of behaviors and signs and symptoms, not in terms of labels. Pupillary signs also may change with increased ICP. Pupillary responses are controlled by cranial nerve III (the oculomotor nerve). The pupils usually change on the same side as the lesion. The first and most subtle clue to trouble is that the pupil reacts, but sluggishly. As the brain herniates, the nerve is compressed—with the top part of the nerve being affected first. The *ipsilateral* pupil (when the lesion is in one hemisphere) remains dilated and is incapable of constricting. The pupil appears larger than that of the affected side and does not react to light. As the ICP increases and both halves of the brain become affected, bilateral pupil dilation and fixation occur. Dilating pupils that respond slowly to light are a sign of impending herniation. A pupil that is fixed and dilated, sometimes called a *blown pupil,* is an ominous sign that *must* be reported to the health care provider immediately (Fig. 14.6).

Changes in the blood pressure and pulse are seen with increasing ICP. Herniation causes ischemia of the vasomotor center, which excites the vasoconstrictor fibers, causing the systolic blood pressure to rise. If the ICP continues to increase, widening pulse pressure (i.e., increasing systolic pressure and decreasing diastolic pressure) occurs.

Pressure in the vasomotor center also increases the transmission of parasympathetic impulses through the vagus nerve to the heart, causing a slowing of the pulse. Widened pulse pressure, increased systolic blood pressure, deepening, irregular respirations, and bradycardia are together called *Cushing response.* It is considered an important diagnostic sign of late-stage brain herniation.

Brain herniation produces respiratory problems that are variable and related to the level of the brainstem compression or failure. The breathing pattern may be deep and stertorous (snorelike) or periodic (Cheyne-Stokes respiration). *Ataxic* breathing also may occur; this is an irregular and unpredictable breathing pattern with random, shallow, and deep breaths and occasional pauses. It is seen in patients with medulla oblongata damage. As ICP increases to fatal levels, respiratory paralysis occurs.

Failure of the thermoregulatory center because of compression occurs later with increased ICP. It results in high, uncontrolled temperatures. This hyperthermia increases the metabolism of brain tissue.

Compression of the upper motoneuron pathway (corticospinal tract) interrupts transmission of impulses to the lower motoneurons, and progressive muscle weakness occurs. Babinski's reflex, hyperreflexia, and rigidity are additional signs of decreased motor function. Seizures may occur. Herniation of the upper part of the brainstem may produce characteristic posturing when the patient is stimulated (Fig. 14.7). The worsening of motor problems is significant because it means that the ICP is continuing to increase.

Vomiting and singultus (hiccups) are two objective signs of increased ICP. The vomiting is often projectile and usually not preceded by nausea; this is called *unexpected vomiting.* Singultus is caused by compression of the vagus nerve (cranial nerve X) as brainstem herniation occurs.

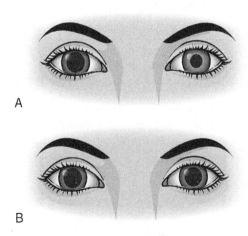

Fig. 14.6 (A) Unequal pupils, also called *anisocoria.* (B) Dilated and fixed pupils, indicative of severe neurologic deficit.

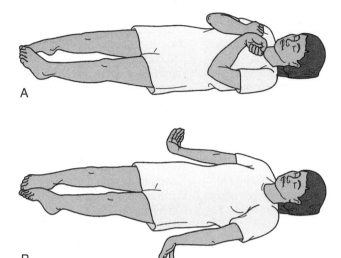

Fig. 14.7 Decorticate and decerebrate responses. (A) Decorticate response is characterized by flexion of the arms, wrists, and fingers with adduction of the upper extremities, and extension, internal rotation, and plantar flexion of the lower extremities. (B) Decerebrate response: All four extremities are in rigid extension, with hyperpronation of the forearms and plantar extension of the feet. (From Ignatavicius DD, Workman ML, Blair M, et al: *Medical-surgical nursing: Patient-centered collaborative care*, ed 8, St. Louis, 2016, Elsevier.)

One last objective sign is papilledema, which is detected with the use of an ophthalmoscope (usually by the health care provider). As ICP increases, the pressure is transmitted to the eyes through the CSF and to the optic disc at the back of the eye. As the optic disc becomes edematous, the retina also is compressed. The damaged retina cannot detect light rays. Visual acuity is lessened as the blind spot enlarges. *Papilledema* is also called a *choked disc*.

Diagnostic Tests

Diagnostic studies are aimed at identifying the presence and the underlying cause of increased ICP. The diagnosis of increased ICP is made by CT or MRI, which can show actual structural herniation and shifting of the brain. Because of CT and MRI, the diagnosis of increased ICP has been revolutionized completely and the therapeutic options greatly increased (Lewis et al, 2007).

Most of the time, acute increased ICP is a medical emergency, and diagnostic tests must be done quickly. Other tests include ICP measurement, EEG, cerebral angiography, transcranial Doppler studies, and PET. In general, lumbar puncture is not performed when increased ICP is suspected because of the possibility of cerebral herniation from the sudden release of the pressure in the skull from the area above the lumbar puncture. This can lead to pressure on cardiac and respiratory centers in the brainstem and potentially death (Pappu, 2016).

In postoperative or critically ill patients, internal measuring devices are used to diagnose increased ICP. One of the most common measuring devices requires the placement of a hollow screw through the skull into the subarachnoid space. The device is connected to a transducer and oscilloscope for continuous monitoring. Waveforms are produced that indicate the ICP.

Medical Management

The goals of treatment are to identify and treat the underlying cause of increased ICP. Preventing increased ICP may not be possible but preventing further increases in pressure with resulting damage to the brain is crucial. The medical treatment depends on the cause of the pressure. For example, surgery may be done to remove a tumor. If surgery is not possible, efforts are made to reduce the pressure through drug therapy or other measures.

Ensuring adequate oxygenation to support brain function is the first step in management of increased ICP. Endotracheal intubation may be necessary. ABG analysis guides the oxygen therapy. With controlled ventilation, the $PaCO_2$ can be lowered to below normal, which causes a slightly alkalotic pH. The decrease in $PaCO_2$ and the increase in pH will decrease vasodilation and decrease ICP. The goal is to maintain the PaO_2 at 100 mm Hg.

Mechanical decompression. Rapidly rising ICP can be relieved by mechanical decompression. This may include a craniotomy, in which a bone flap is removed and then replaced, or a craniectomy, in which a bone flap is removed and not replaced. Other means of decompression include drainage of the ventricles or of any subdural hematoma.

Internal monitoring devices are being used more frequently to diagnose and monitor increased ICP. Three basic monitoring systems are used: the ventricular catheter, the subarachnoid bolt or screw, and the epidural sensor. These monitoring devices detect pressure waves that can be used to indicate the status of ICP.

Medications. Three types of medications usually are administered to patients with increased ICP: osmotic diuretics, corticosteroids, and anticonvulsants. Osmotic diuretics also are called hyperosmolar drugs. They draw water from the edematous brain tissue. An example of this type of medication is mannitol. It begins to reduce increased ICP within 15 minutes, and its effects last for 5 to 6 hours. Loop diuretics such as furosemide, bumetanide, and ethacrynic acid also may be used in the management of increased ICP. Continuous midazolam and atracurium besylate infusions also are used.

Traditionally, health care providers have prescribed the corticosteroid dexamethasone. There are studies that demonstrate that corticosteroids may have limited value in managing head-injured patients. The use of corticosteroids in the care of head-injured patients was once standard. Studies have shown that patients managed with corticosteroid therapies reflect a higher mortality rate. Today, corticosteroids are not standard in the plan of care. However, those patients receiving this medication warrant close assessment of their blood glucose levels. Steroids can affect carbohydrate metabolism and glucose utilization and result in elevated blood glucose levels.

To prevent gastrointestinal ulcers and bleeding, patients receiving corticosteroids concurrently should be given antacids, histamine receptor blockers (e.g., cimetidine, famotidine), or proton pump inhibitors (e.g., omeprazole, pantoprazole).

Antiseizure medications are given to prevent seizures. Phenytoin is the most commonly given drug. It can be given intravenously but usually not intramuscularly because of poor absorption. Fosphenytoin is a short-term IV or intramuscular anticonvulsant in current use. Opioids and other drugs that cause respiratory depression are avoided.

Nursing Interventions and Patient Teaching

Therapeutic measures to reduce venous volume include the following:

- Elevate the head of the bed to 30 to 45 degrees to promote venous return.
- Place the neck in a neutral position (not flexed or extended) to promote venous drainage.
- Position the patient to avoid flexion of the hips, the waist, and the neck and rotation of the head, especially to the right. Avoid extreme hip flexion because this position causes an increase in intra-abdominal and intrathoracic pressures, which can produce a rise in ICP.
- Instruct the patient to avoid isometric or resistive exercises.
- Restrict fluid intake.
- Implement measures to help the patient avoid the Valsalva maneuver (any forced expiratory effort against a closed airway, such as straining during bowel movement). Avoid enemas and laxatives if possible.
- Have a Foley catheter in place if the patient is not alert because of the large amount of urine that is produced.
- Perform suctioning only as necessary and for no longer than 10 seconds, with administration of 100% oxygen before and after to prevent decreases in the PaO_2.
- Administer oxygen via mask or cannula to improve cerebral perfusion.
- Use a hypothermia blanket to control body temperature (increased body temperature increases brain damage).

Patient problems and interventions for the patient with increased ICP may include but are not limited to the following:

PATIENT PROBLEM	NURSING INTERVENTIONS
Inability to Maintain Adequate Breathing Pattern, related to neuromuscular impairment	Maintain patent airway; avoid flexion of neck Administer oxygen and humidification as ordered Provide oral nasopharyngeal airway as indicated for managing secretions; suction oropharynx as needed
Potential for Injury, related to physiologic effects of sustained ICP elevation	Elevate head of bed to 30 degrees Maintain body position; avoid semiprone or prone position Avoid compression of neck veins Check blood pressure, pulse, and respiration q 30 min Perform neurologic check q 30 min using Glasgow Coma Scale; report any findings below 8 to health care provider

The patient with increased ICP is often unresponsive. Share information about procedures that are being done with the patient and the family. This may help both to be as cooperative as possible.

Prognosis

The prognosis for the patient with increased ICP depends on the cause and the speed with which it is treated. The nurse assumes an important role in monitoring the patient for signs and symptoms of increased pressure. After herniation of the brain has begun as a result of pressure, there is little chance for complete reversal without significant brain damage.

DISTURBANCES IN MUSCLE TONE AND MOTOR FUNCTION

Etiology and Pathophysiology

Motor function disturbances are the most commonly encountered neurologic signs and symptoms. Damage to the nervous system often causes serious problems in mobility. An example of this is the patient with cerebral palsy.

Clinical Manifestations

Injury or disease of motoneurons results in alterations of muscle strength, tone, and reflex activity. Muscle tone may be described as *flaccid* (weak, soft, flabby, and lacking normal muscle tone) or *hyperreflexic* (excessive reflex responses). The specific clinical manifestations differ according to the location of the neurologic lesion.

Assessment

Subjective data for patients with motor problems include the patient's understanding of the problem and possible causes. Ask about the initial onset of the symptoms;

measures that improve symptoms; and the presence of clumsiness, incoordination, or abnormal sensation. If the lesion occurs suddenly, as in traumatic spinal cord injury, subjective symptoms may be minimal. If the motor deficit develops slowly, subjective symptoms may be so subtle that they are at first ignored.

Objective data include coordination, muscle strength, muscle tone, and muscle atrophy. Reflexes often are checked, as well as the presence of clonus or fasciculations and the ability to move muscles. Any abnormal gait is significant, as is a change in the ability to carry out ADLs.

Diagnostic Tests

One of the most common procedures for detecting pathologic conditions of muscle is the EMG. It detects the various types of electrical activity and abnormal patterns that may appear in resting muscle in the presence of disease.

Medical Management

Patients with motor problems may have spasticity. Muscle relaxants may be used to decrease tone and involuntary movements. Some commonly prescribed medications include baclofen, dantrolene, and diazepam. Baclofen has been used intrathecally to reduce spasticity. Common side effects of these drugs include drowsiness and vertigo. These side effects are increased by the use of alcohol or other depressants.

Some patients may have severe swallowing difficulty (dysphagia). This commonly results from obstructive or motor disorders of the esophagus and often is associated with neurologic problems. The patient with dysphagia often requires prefeeding and feeding exercises.

Some patients are at severe risk for aspiration. These patients may undergo videofluoroscopy with barium to determine which muscles are not working right and which types of food are safest. The procedure requires the patient to swallow a small amount of liquid or semisolid food, mixed with barium, while a fluoroscopic examination is being done.

For patients with paralysis, the eye on the affected side of the body may have to be protected if the lid remains open and there is no blink reflex. The patient is at high risk for corneal scratches or irritation. Irrigation with a physiologic solution of sodium chloride may be used, followed by eyedrops. An eye pad may be used to keep the eye closed, although an eye shield is preferable.

Nursing Interventions

Safety needs. Patients with paralysis have significant safety needs. This includes protection from falling, including the use of side rails when the patient is in bed and a chair restraint when the patient is in a chair, especially if balance cannot be maintained. If the patient also has a sensory problem, which often accompanies paralysis, he or she may not realize when part of the body is in danger. For example, a patient with a stroke may not be aware that a hemiplegic arm is hanging over the side of the wheelchair.

The eye on the affected side of the body should be cleaned and assessed for signs of infection on a regular basis, usually three times a day or more. Also inspect affected body parts for injury.

Regularly inspect the skin over bony prominences for signs of pressure. Paralyzed people are at risk for skin impairment, so teach them to turn themselves in bed and to reposition themselves in the bed or chair independently, if possible. If the patient is unable to turn independently, carry out this function. Usually the patient is turned from one side to another or from one side to the back to the other side. Repositioning also includes weight shifts, done by the patient or by staff. These weight shifts may include controlled leaning from one side to another or chair push-ups. If the patient is not able to do the activity, have him or her take responsibility for reminding staff when it is time to do weight shifting.

Inspect paralyzed or weakened areas at least daily for any signs of skin impairment. A mirror often is used to help the patient assess the skin so that he or she is not as dependent on staff or family.

Activity needs. The extremities of a person who has an acute motor problem may be flaccid at first. Spasticity of muscles develops gradually. The joints then become flexed and fixed in useless, deformed positions unless preventive measures are taken.

Carefully place the extremities in a normal anatomic position to prevent deformity. Counterpositioning may be helpful. In hemiplegia (paralysis of one side of the body), the affected upper extremity is pulled inward at the shoulder joint and the wrist drops; in the lower extremity, the knee flexes and the foot drops. In counterpositioning, the patient is placed so that the shoulder and upper arm are in abduction, the elbow is flexed, the wrist is dorsiflexed (i.e., the hand is bent upward, toward the top of the wrist), the knee is in neutral position, and the foot is dorsiflexed (i.e., pulled up toward the knee). If the person is supine, place a pillow between the upper arm and the body to hold the arm in abduction. Physical therapists and occupational therapists can provide splints and braces that can aid in positioning (Fig. 14.8).

Footboards may be used to prevent footdrop, although some believe that these contribute to increased spasticity and should not be used routinely for patients who have muscle spasms. High-top tennis shoes or other devices, such as splints or braces, can help prevent footdrop if therapy is initiated early. In some hospitals, casts are applied to patients' lower extremities to prevent footdrop or to reverse contractures. The presence of the cast impedes spasticity.

The prone position is excellent for patients who are able to tolerate it. Not only does this position decrease the chance of skin impairment but it also causes extension of the hip, the knee joints, and the ankles by means of gravity. A pillow placed under the chest may help patients comfortably assume this position.

Positioning of the paralyzed person is extremely important. Complications such as footdrop and flexion contractures of the knee seriously limit mobility. As a result, the level of self-care and independence is diminished. Most joint deformities in a paralyzed person are preventable with early and continuing nursing interventions.

In addition to positioning, interventions for the person with paralysis include ROM exercises to all joints. These may be passive (carried out by the nurse) or active (carried out by the patient). Passive ROM is indicated at least three times daily for all joints that the patient cannot voluntarily move.

Nutritional needs. Patience and persistence are often necessary in giving food and fluids to the patient with hemiplegia. Aspiration can occur and is related to loss of pharyngeal sensation, loss of oropharyngeal motor control, and decreased LOC. Consider consultation with a speech and language pathologist for a swallowing evaluation and recommendations for treatment (American Speech-Language-Hearing Association, n.d.). Important nursing measures include avoiding foods that cause choking, checking the affected side of the mouth for accumulation of food and resultant poor hygiene, not mixing liquids and solid foods, and encouraging the patient to take small bites. Adding a thickening agent (such as Thick-It) to liquids often helps prevent choking. If the patient has dentures, they should be worn. The patient should sit at a 90-degree angle with the head up and chin slightly tucked. The head should not be extended; encourage the patient to tip the head toward the unaffected side while swallowing. Avoid straws. Assistive devices for feeding include utensils with universal cuffs, covered plastic cups, scoop dishes, and plate guards. These enable the patient to be less dependent on the staff, and they are available through therapists in most hospitals.

Activities of daily living. During the acute rehabilitative phases of a motor problem, teach patients with paralysis how to carry out ADLs to the extent that they are able. A variety of devices are available to assist with dressing and grooming (Figs. 14.9 and 14.10). The occupational therapist becomes involved in many of these activities, including homemaking. Stress the concept of the rehabilitative team in managing these patients. Teach the patient to compensate for weakness or paralysis. Give the patient the time to do activities on his or her own if able. It is often easier and faster to do things for the patient, but this defeats the purpose of rehabilitation.

Psychological adjustments. The person with paralysis may need assistance in adjusting to body changes. The

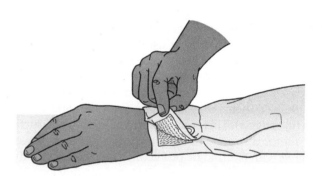

Fig. 14.9 Velcro shirtsleeve to facilitate closure. (From Hoemann SP: *Rehabilitation nursing: Process and application,* ed 2, St. Louis, 1996, Mosby.)

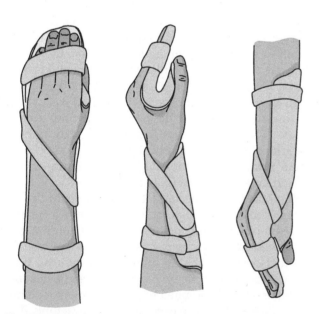

Fig. 14.8 Volar resting splint provides support to wrist, thumb, and fingers of patient after a cerebrovascular accident (stroke), maintaining them in a position of extension. (From Black JM, Hawks JH: *Medical-surgical nursing: Clinical management for positive outcomes,* ed 8, St. Louis, 2009, Saunders.)

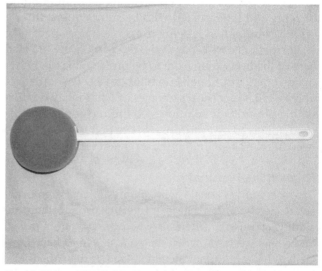

Fig. 14.10 Long-handled bath sponge. (From Sorrentino SA, Remmert LN: *Mosby's textbook for nursing assistants,* ed 8, St. Louis, 2012, Saunders.)

loss of the ability to function independently is traumatic, and the patient may have fears of rejection, loss of self-esteem, and concerns about the future. A grief reaction similar to that described for a death may occur. The patient may relate to the paralyzed part of the body as though it were not a part of him or her and may have nicknames for the body part. To help the patient cope with the loss of function and change in body image, praise the patient for achievements, encourage expression of fears and grief, and help him or her see that there is life after disability. It may be helpful to arrange a visit by someone with the same disability who has been rehabilitated successfully.

Patient problems and interventions for the patient with alterations in muscle tone and motor function include but are not limited to the following:

PATIENT PROBLEM	NURSING INTERVENTIONS
Compromised Physical Mobility, related to neuromuscular impairment	Perform active or passive range-of-motion (ROM) exercise q 4 h, to all extremities, neck, hands, fingers, wrists, elbows, and knees
	Provide physical therapy as ordered (massage and stretching exercises)
	Maintain planned rest periods
	Encourage ambulation to tolerance
	Arrange for necessary assistive devices for home care needs
Risk for Contractures or Muscle Atrophy, related to impaired functioning of body part	Perform hand, finger, and foot exercises; assist in active and passive ROM exercises q 2–4 h
	Assist patient with using supportive devices as indicated (overhead trapeze, braces, walker, cane)
	Encourage use of involved side when possible
	Instruct patient to use unaffected extremity to support weaker side (e.g., lift involved left leg with right leg or lift involved left arm with right arm)
	Turn q 2 h

Patient Teaching

Teaching is an extremely important part of caring for the person with motor problems. Appropriate teaching activities include safety needs, skin care, activity (ROM and positioning), medications (dosage, action, times, and side effects), good nutrition, ADLs, bowel and bladder care, and follow-up care. Written instructions reinforce teaching and give the patient something to refer to at home (see the Health Promotion box). Prepare family members to assume some of the care for the patient.

Health Promotion

The Patient With a Neurologic Disorder

- *Nutritional-metabolic pattern:* Neurologic problems can result in inadequate nutrition. Problems related to chewing, swallowing, facial nerve paralysis, and muscle coordination could make it difficult for the patient to ingest adequate nutrients.
- *Elimination pattern:* Bowel and bladder problems often are associated with neurologic problems, such as stroke, head injury, spinal cord injury, multiple sclerosis, and dementia. It is important to determine whether the bowel or bladder problem was present before the neurologic event to plan appropriate interventions.
- *Activity-exercise pattern:* Many neurologic disorders can cause problems in the patient's mobility, strength, and coordination. These problems can change the patient's usual activity and exercise patterns.
- *Sleep-rest pattern:* Sleep can be disrupted by many neurologically related factors. Discomfort from pain and inability to move and change to a position of comfort because of muscle weakness and paralysis could interfere with sound sleep.
- *Cognitive-perceptual pattern:* Because the nervous system controls cognition and sensory integration, many neurologic disorders affect these functions. Assess memory, language, calculation ability, problem-solving ability, insight, and judgment.
- *Self-perception–self-concept pattern:* Neurologic disease can alter drastically control over one's life and create dependency on others for daily needs.
- *Role-relationship pattern:* Ask the patient if neurologic problems have led to changes in roles, such as spouse, parent, or breadwinner. These changes can affect dramatically the patient and significant others.
- *Sexuality-reproductive pattern:* Assess the ability to participate in sexual activity, because many nervous system disorders can affect sexual response.
- *Coping–stress tolerance pattern:* The physical sequelae of a neurologic problem can seriously strain a patient's ability to cope. Often the pathology is chronic and stress from the life changes may require the patient to master and utilize multiple coping skills.
- *Value-belief pattern:* Many neurologic problems have serious, long-term, life-changing effects. These effects can strain the patient's belief system and should be assessed.

DISTURBED SENSORY AND PERCEPTUAL FUNCTION

Etiology and Pathophysiology

The presence of a lesion anywhere within the sensory system pathway, from the receptor to the sensory cortex, alters the transmission or perception of sensory information. The parietal cortex is of major importance in the interpretation of sensation. Loss of, decrease in, or increase in sensation of pain, temperature, touch, and proprioception results in difficulty in daily functioning. Any alteration lessens the patient's protection from inadvertent injury.

Sensory loss can affect proprioception, that is, the body's innate spatial sense. **Agnosia** is a total or partial loss, as a result of organic brain damage, of the ability to recognize familiar objects by sight, touch, or hearing or to recognize familiar people through sensory stimuli.

Assessment

Subjective data include the patient's understanding of the sensory disturbance, measures that relieve symptoms (including medications), and symptoms that occur with the sensory problem. An example is the person who experiences weakness of a hand and at the same time feels numbness and tingling. Collect information on the onset of the sensory problem and the specific site in the body.

Collection of objective data includes noting the patient's ability to perform purposeful movements or to recognize familiar objects.

Medical Management

Medical management will be determined by the underlying cause of the alteration in muscle tone and motor function.

Nursing Interventions and Patient Teaching

The most important nursing intervention for the patient with sensory dysfunction is to teach the patient protective measures. This includes helping the patient learn to inspect parts of the body that have no feeling, to protect sensitive body parts from the discomfort of linen rubbing over them, or exposure to dangerous temperatures such as dish and bathwater that is too hot. If a patient has a deficit in one sense, he or she should learn to compensate with another (e.g., the patient who learns to lip-read because of a hearing deficit; the patient with hemianopia who is taught to scan the printed page).

Patient problems and interventions for the patient with a sensory or perceptual problem are the same as those for the patient with a motor problem, with the addition of but not limited to the following:

PATIENT PROBLEM	NURSING INTERVENTIONS
Potential for Injury, related to sensory or perceptual disturbances	Maintain safe environment Teach patient to protect body parts that have decreased sensation Teach patient to inspect body parts for possible injury Protect patient from sustaining injury from hot liquid or heating pads

The teaching for a patient with a sensory deficit is essentially the same as that for the patient with a motor deficit.

OTHER DISORDERS OF THE NEUROLOGIC SYSTEM

Functioning of the neurologic system can be interrupted for a variety of reasons. These include conduction abnormalities, degenerative diseases, vascular problems, infection, tumors, trauma, and cranial and peripheral nerve disorders. Selected disorders in each area are discussed.

CONDUCTION ABNORMALITIES

EPILEPSY OR SEIZURES
Etiology and Pathophysiology

Seizure activity is the result of abnormal electrical activity within the brain. There are several conditions that may cause seizures. These include severe elevations in body temperature, drug use, electrolyte imbalance, brain tumors, brain infection, and epilepsy. Not all individuals experiencing seizure activity have epilepsy.

Epilepsy is a group of neurologic disorders characterized by recurrent episodes that may include convulsive seizure, sensory disturbances, abnormal behavior, and changes in LOC.

Cases of epilepsy have been recorded throughout history. Seizures occur in all races and affect men and women equally. There are no apparent geographic boundaries. In the United States approximately 3.4 million people suffer from active epilepsy, with 3 million being adults and 470,000 children affected (CDC, 2020b). The incidence rates are higher in the first year of life, decline through childhood and adolescence, plateau in middle age, and rise sharply again among older adults.

Clinical Manifestations

Seizures can be classified according to the features of the attack. The types include generalized tonic-clonic (grand mal), absence (petit mal), psychomotor (automatisms), jacksonian (focal), and miscellaneous (myoclonic and akinetic) seizures (Table 14.5).

Epilepsy is associated with paroxysmal, uncontrolled electrical discharges in the neurons of the brain that result in the sudden, violent, involuntary contraction of a group of muscles. The patterns or forms of seizures vary and depend on the area of the brain from which the seizure arises. The excessive neuronal discharges may result in a tonic convulsion, with alternate contraction and relaxation of opposing muscle groups. This gives the characteristic tonic-clonic jerking movements of the body. Seizures are followed by a rest period of variable length, called the postictal period (after a seizure). During this period the patient usually feels groggy and acts disoriented. Complaints of headache and muscle aches are common. Usually the patient sleeps after a seizure and may experience amnesia for the event.

When recurrent, generalized seizure activity occurs at such frequency that full consciousness is not regained between seizures; it is called status epilepticus. This is a medical emergency and requires medical and nursing interventions. Repeated seizures cause the brain to use more energy than can be supplied; the neurons become exhausted and cease to function, which may result in permanent brain damage or death. The most common

Table 14.5   Characteristics of Seizures

INCIDENCE	CHARACTERISTICS	CLINICAL SIGNS	AURA	POSTICTAL PERIOD
Generalized Tonic-Clonic (Formerly Called Grand Mal)				
Most common	Generalized; characterized by loss of consciousness and falling to the floor or ground if patient is upright, followed by stiffening of the body (tonic phase) for 10–20 s and subsequent jerking of the extremities (clonic phase) for another 30–40 s	Aura Cry Loss of consciousness Flashing lights or smells Partial loss of vision Fall Tonic-clonic movements Incontinence, cyanosis, excessive salivation, tongue or cheek biting	Yes	Yes Need for 1–2 h of sleep Headache, muscle soreness commonly felt May not feel normal for several hours or days after a seizure No memory of a seizure
Absence (Formerly Called Petit Mal)				
Occurs during childhood and adolescence Frequency decreases as child gets older Rarely continues beyond adolescence	Sudden impairment in or loss of consciousness with little or no tonic-clonic movement Occurs without warning Has tendency to appear a few hours after arising or when person is quiet	Sudden vacant facial expression with eyes focused straight ahead (staring spell) that lasts only a few seconds All motor activity ceases except perhaps for slight symmetric twitching about eyelids Possible loss of muscle tone May have an extremely brief loss of consciousness	No	No
Psychomotor (Automatisms; Also Called Partial Seizures)				
Occur at any age	Sudden change in awareness associated with complex distortion of feeling and thinking and partially coordinated motor activity Longer than absence seizures	Behaves as if partially conscious; may continue an activity that was initiated before the seizure, such as counting out change or picking items from a grocery shelf, but after the seizure does not remember the activity Often appears intoxicated Complex hallucinations or illusions May do antisocial things, such as exposing self or carrying out violent acts Autonomic complaints, such as shivering, lip smacking, repetitive movements that may not be appropriate Urinary incontinence	Yes	Yes Confusion Amnesia Need for sleep
Jacksonian-Focal (Local or Partial)				
Occur almost entirely in patients with structural brain disease	Depends on site of focus May or may not be progressive	Commonly begin in hand, foot, or face with numbness and tingling May end in tonic-clonic seizure	Yes	Yes
Myoclonic				
May antedate tonic-clonic by months or years	May be very mild or may have rapid, forceful movements	Sudden, excess jerk of the body or extremities; may be forceful enough to hurl the person to the floor or ground Brief seizures that may occur in clusters No loss of consciousness	No	No
Akinetic				
Not common	Peculiar generalized tonelessness	Falls in flaccid state Unconscious for a minute or two	Rarely	No

cause of status epilepticus is sudden withdrawal of anticonvulsant medications. The nursing interventions always involve ensuring that there is a patent airway and protecting the patient from injury. Medications to stop the seizure activity may be given in high doses that render the patient unconscious. The nurse must then assume total care of the patient's needs. Insert a Foley catheter and an IV line. Intubate the patient if necessary for ventilatory support. Protect the skin from injury. Take care with safety reminder devices such as bed check monitoring systems if the patient is awake and active so that they do not cause injury if the patient begins to have a seizure.

Assessment

Subjective data include the patient's awareness of the disorder and any precipitating factors. Assess whether an aura preceded the seizure. An aura occurs in many patients with generalized tonic-clonic seizures. *Aura* is a sensation (such as of light or warmth), emotion (such as fear), or a smell that may precede an attack of migraine or an epileptic seizure. An epileptic aura may be psychic, or it may be sensory with olfactory, visual, auditory, or taste hallucinations. The exact character of the aura varies from person to person. Awareness of an aura warns the person of the impending seizure and allows him or her to seek safety and privacy.

Objective data include the number of seizures occurring within a specific time, the character of the seizure, and any behaviors noted and injuries suffered. Describe the seizure as completely as possible, including duration, the patient's movements, whether the patient was incontinent, any cries or sounds that were made, and the level of alertness.

Diagnostic Testing

Diagnostic testing includes blood tests to assess for the presence of infection or chemical imbalances. A diagnosis of epilepsy cannot be made on the basis of a single seizure; epilepsy is a condition characterized by recurrent seizure activity. CT and MRI are performed to assess for the presence of lesions or to identify the location of seizure activity. PET scans may be used to pinpoint brain abnormalities. The most common test used to evaluate seizures is the EEG. It allows a specific diagnosis of the seizure.

Medical Management

Medications. In 60% of patients, seizure disorders are controlled by one or more antiseizure drugs, although the desire is to achieve monotherapy in order to decrease side effects of the medication (Ko, 2020). (Table 14.6). Therapy is aimed at preventing seizures because cure is not possible. Drugs generally act by stabilizing nerve cell membranes and preventing spread of the epileptic discharge. The choice of medication depends on the type of seizure. Failure to take the prescribed medication or an adequate

dose is often the cause of treatment failure. Blood levels may be checked to determine the therapeutic level of the medications taken. The primary goal of antiseizure drug therapy is to obtain maximum seizure control with minimum toxic side effects.

Surgical therapy. Pharmacologic therapies to control seizure activity are not possible for some patients with epilepsy. They may be considered candidates for surgical intervention. Surgery to manage seizure activity may include removal of the small area of the brain that is experiencing the misfiring and causing the seizures. This is called a *resection*. The connective tissue between the two hemispheres of the brain also may be severed in some cases (Mayo Clinic, 2021a).

Activities of daily living. Until seizures are controlled, patients should avoid activities such as driving a car, operating machinery, or swimming. Maintaining adequate rest and good nutrition is also important. Alcohol use should be avoided. If the patient is receiving long-term phenytoin therapy, good hygiene practices for the mouth and teeth are important because of the side effect of edematous and enlarged gums (gingival hyperplasia). The patient should wear a medical-alert bracelet or tag (see the Patient Teaching box).

 Patient Teaching

The Patient With Seizures

- Explain the need for the patient to continue taking medications even when seizure activity has stopped.
- Teach the patient about medications prescribed, including expected results, time and dosage, and side effects.
- Inform the patient that medical-alert bracelets, necklaces, and identification cards are available. The use of these medical identification tags is optional. Some patients have found them beneficial, but others prefer not to be identified as having a seizure disorder.
- Caution the patient to avoid the use of alcohol if taking antiseizure medications.
- Explain the need for good oral hygiene for people taking phenytoin (Dilantin) (a side effect is gingival hyperplasia).
- Stress the importance of adequate rest and a balanced diet.
- Educate about available community resources.
- Explain restrictions concerning driving.
- Explain the importance of follow-up care.
- A tonic-clonic seizure can be treated with monitoring the patient and keeping them safe; it is not necessary to send the patient to the hospital (or to call an ambulance) after a single seizure unless the seizure is prolonged, another seizure immediately follows, or extensive injury has occurred.
- In the event of an acute seizure, protect the patient from injury. This involves supporting and/or protecting the head, turning the patient to one side, loosening any constricting garments, and, if the patient is seated, easing him or her onto the floor.

Table 14.6   Medications for Preventing and Controlling Seizures

GENERIC NAME	USE RELATED TO SEIZURE TYPE	TOXIC EFFECTS
carbamazepine	Generalized tonic-clonic, psychomotor	Rash, drowsiness, ataxia
clonazepam	Absence seizures, akinetic, myoclonic, generalized tonic-clonic seizures	Drowsiness, ataxia, hypotension, respiratory depression
diazepam	Generalized tonic-clonic and status epilepticus, mixed	Drowsiness, ataxia
divalproex	Generalized tonic-clonic and myoclonic seizures	Sedation, drowsiness, behavior changes, visual disturbances, hepatic failure
ethosuximide	Absence seizures, psychomotor, myoclonic, akinetic	Drowsiness, nausea, agranulocytosis
felbamate	Seizures in children, generalized tonic-clonic seizures in adults; may be used to treat patients whose seizure disorders are refractory to other drugs	Irritability, insomnia, anorexia, nausea, headache; can cause aplastic anemia and hepatic failure
fosphenytoin sodium	Short-term parenteral (IV or IM) in acute generalized tonic-clonic seizures; used for status epilepticus and for preventing and treating seizures during neurosurgery	Dizziness, paresthesia, tinnitus, pruritus, headache, somnolence, ataxia, muscular incoordination, nystagmus, double vision, slurred speech, nausea, vomiting, and hypotension
gabapentin	Focal, generalized tonic-clonic in adults	Somnolence, fatigue, ataxia, dizziness, anorexia
lamotrigine	Focal, generalized tonic-clonic in adults	Rash, dizziness, tremor, ataxia, diplopia, headache, gastrointestinal upset, Stevens-Johnson syndrome (rare)
mephenytoin	Tonic-clonic, focal, psychomotor	Ataxia, nystagmus, pancytopenia, rash
oxcarbazepine	Generalized tonic-clonic and partial seizures	Feeling abnormal, headache, dizziness, vertigo, anxiety, blurred vision
phenobarbital	Generalized tonic-clonic, focal, psychomotor	Drowsiness, rash
phenytoin sodium	Generalized tonic-clonic, focal, psychomotor	Ataxia, vomiting, nystagmus, drowsiness, rash, fever, gum hypertrophy, lymphadenopathy
primidone	Generalized tonic-clonic, focal, psychomotor	Drowsiness, ataxia
topiramate, tiagabine, levetiracetam, zonisamide	Indicated for partial seizures and for secondary generalized seizures; currently used as adjunctive therapy	Topiramate: Somnolence, dizziness, ataxia, speech disorders and related speech problems, difficulty with memory, paresthesia, diplopia Tiagabine: Dizziness, lightheadedness, asthenia (lack of energy), somnolence, nausea, nervousness, irritability, tremor, thinking abnormally, difficulty with concentration or attention
trimethadione	Absence seizures	Rash, photophobia, agranulocytosis, nephrosis
valproic acid	Absence seizures	Nausea, vomiting, indigestion, sedation, emotional disturbance, weakness, altered blood coagulation

IM, Intramuscular; *IV,* intravenous.

Nursing Interventions and Patient Teaching

Care during a seizure. The primary goals of the nurse and the family caring for a patient having a seizure are protection from aspiration and injury and observation and recording of the seizure activity. Never leave the patient alone. If the patient is sitting or standing, lower him or her to the floor in an area away from furniture and equipment. Support and protect the head; if possible, turn the head to the side to maintain the airway. Loosen restrictive clothing around the neck if possible. Do not try to restrain the patient during the seizure. Do *not* try to pry open the jaw to insert a padded tongue blade. No objects should be placed in the mouth. After the seizure the patient may require suctioning and oxygen. Padded side rails may be used, especially if seizures often occur during sleep.

When a seizure occurs, carefully observe and record details of the event because the diagnosis and subsequent treatment often rest solely on the seizure description. Note all aspects of the seizure: What events preceded the seizure? When did the seizure occur? How long did each phase (aural [if any], ictal, postictal) last? What occurred during each phase?

Patient problems and interventions for the patient with seizures may include but are not limited to the following:

PATIENT PROBLEM	NURSING INTERVENTIONS
Inability to Clear Airway, related to mucus accumulation in oropharyngeal area during seizure	Place patient in side-lying position to prevent aspiration and ensure airway patency Suction secretions as needed
Potential for Injury, related to rapid onset of altered state of consciousness and seizure activity	If patient is out of bed during seizure activity, assist to the floor and remove objects that may harm him or her Provide privacy Maintain patent airway After the seizure, inform patient of seizure and reorient if necessary

Prognosis

Seizure disorders can affect a patient's emotional, economic, and social well-being. Society's attitude has improved, but epilepsy still carries a social stigma. Most states have legal sanctions against driving if one has epilepsy. The inability to maintain a driver's license can affect one's lifestyle negatively.

The majority of patients with seizures are able to control them with medications and can lead a fairly normal life. With most seizure disorders, the number and intensity of seizures stay constant. For patients who experience a first seizure as a result of a brain tumor or another brain pathologic condition, the prognosis is more uncertain.

DEGENERATIVE DISEASES

The term *degenerative diseases* refers to neurologic disorders in which there is a premature aging of nerve cells, which is caused by suspected metabolic disturbance or for which the cause is unknown. Six diseases are discussed: MS, Parkinson disease, AD, MG, amyotrophic lateral sclerosis (ALS), and Huntington disease.

MULTIPLE SCLEROSIS
Etiology and Pathophysiology

MS is a chronic, progressive, degenerative neurologic disease that affects many people. The cause is unknown, although genetics have been implicated, because there is a higher rate of the disease among relatives. Patients with the first signs and symptoms of MS have a proliferation of a certain type of immune

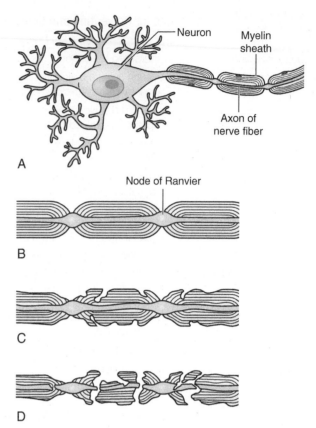

Fig. 14.11 Pathogenesis of multiple sclerosis. (A) Normal nerve cell with myelin sheath. (B) Normal axon. (C) Myelin breakdown. (D) Myelin totally disrupted; axon not functioning. (From Lewis SL, Heitkemper MM, Dirksen SR, et al: *Medical-surgical nursing: Assessment and management of clinical problems*, ed 9, St. Louis, 2014, Mosby.)

cell called *gamma delta T cells* in their spinal fluid. These cells are not found in patients who have had the disease for a long time. T cells, the "field commanders" of the immune system, usually defend the body from outside attackers. In MS, however, something goes wrong and induces the T cells to attack the body. Myelin damage occurs. The beginning mechanism may be a viral infection early in life that becomes apparent as an immune process later in life. A defective immune response also seems to have an important role in the pathology of MS.

The onset of signs and symptoms is usually between 15 and 50 years of age. Women are affected more often than men. The highest number of people with MS live in the Great Lakes area, the Pacific Northwest, and the North Atlantic states. MS is five times more prevalent in temperate climates between 45 and 66 degrees of latitude.

Multiple foci of *demyelination* are distributed randomly in the white matter of the brainstem, the spinal cord, optic nerves, and the cerebrum. During the demyelination process, the myelin sheath and the sheath cells are destroyed, causing an interruption or distortion of the nerve impulse so that it is slowed or blocked (Fig. 14.11). Areas of degeneration show evidence of partial healing, which explains the transitory nature of early signs and symptoms.

Clinical Manifestations

The onset is often insidious and gradual, with vague symptoms that occur intermittently over months or years, and thus the disease may not be diagnosed until long after the onset of the first symptom. Because of the wide distribution of areas of degeneration, the variety of signs and symptoms in MS is greater than in other neurologic diseases. These include visual problems, urinary incontinence, fatigue, weakness or incoordination of an extremity, sexual problems such as impotence in men, and swallowing difficulties. The majority of people have early remissions that may last for a year or more. The disease is characterized by chronic, progressive deterioration in some people and by remissions and exacerbations in others. Exacerbations may be related to fatigue, chilling, or emotional disturbances. With repeated exacerbations, progressive scarring of the myelin sheath occurs, and the overall trend is progressive deterioration in neurologic function.

Assessment

Subjective data include the patient's understanding of the disease. Eye problems such as diplopia, scotoma (partial loss of vision), and blindness may be present. The patient also may talk about weakness or numbness of a part of the body, fatigue, emotional instability, bowel and bladder problems, vertigo, or loss of joint sensation. Involvement of the cerebellum can result in ataxia (impaired ability to coordinate movement) and tremor. In men, impotence is significant. Pain is not a common symptom.

Objective data include documented abnormalities in neurologic testing; these may include nystagmus (involuntary, rhythmic movements of the eye; the oscillations may be horizontal, vertical, rotary, or mixed); muscle weakness and spasms; changes in coordination; or a spastic, ataxic gait. Cerebellar signs include ataxia, dysarthria, and dysphagia. There may be evidence of behavior changes such as euphoria, emotional lability, or mild depression. Urinary incontinence and intention tremors of the upper extremities may be present.

Diagnostic Tests

MS has no definitive diagnostic test; diagnosis is based primarily on history and clinical manifestations and the presence of multiple lesions over time as measured by MRI. Examination of the CSF in patients with MS may show elevated gamma globulin, a proliferation of gamma delta T cells in the initial phase, and an increased number of lymphocytes and monocytes. A CT scan may show enlargement of the cerebral ventricles. MRI scanning has been helpful in diagnosing

MS over time in the presence of multiple lesions; sclerotic plaques as small as 3 to 4 mm in diameter can be detected.

Medical Management

Medications. No specific treatment exists for MS, although immunosuppressants can help with symptom and disease progress. Medications known as *disease modifying therapies* (DMTs) are a key component in modifying the disease process (nationalMSsociety.org). Historically symptoms have been controlled with the use of adrenocorticotropic hormone (ACTH) and corticosteroids such as prednisone (Deltasone) or dexamethasone. These may be given orally, intramuscularly, or intravenously. The effects of ACTH and the steroids on the demyelinating process are unknown, although they probably help by reducing edema and acute inflammation at the site of demyelination. If steroids are used in high doses at the start of an exacerbation, the episode seems to resolve more rapidly. However, these drugs do not affect the ultimate outcome or degree of residual neurologic impairment from the exacerbation. If spasticity is a problem, drugs such as diazepam, dantrolene, and baclofen may help prevent or decrease the spasms. Immunomodulating drugs modify the disease process. Interferon beta-1b, given subcutaneously every other day, is indicated for use in ambulatory patients with relapsing-remitting MS to reduce the frequency of clinical exacerbations. Interferon beta-1a is similar to interferon beta-1b in efficacy and is used in similar patient groups with MS. It is given intramuscularly once a week. Another formulation of interferon beta-1a, Rebif, is administered subcutaneously three times weekly. Glatiramer acetate is used in relapsing-remitting MS. Glatiramer is not an interferon, but it is believed to help patients with MS by interrupting the inflammatory cycle and preventing the body's immune system from attacking the myelin coating that protects the nerve fibers. It is given subcutaneously daily. Mitoxantrone is a drug for the treatment of primary-progressive and progressive-relapsing MS. It is an immunosuppressant drug that reduces B and T lymphocytes. It is given intravenously monthly. Cardiac assessment and follow-up are needed because these medications may result in cardiac compromise. Many research studies are being conducted in the search for more effective medications to use in the treatment of MS.

Elimination. Urinary frequency and urgency may respond to propantheline. Cholinergic drugs such as bethanechol sometimes can help the patient with neurogenic bladder (loss of bladder control because of nervous system damage) by exerting a direct antispasmodic effect on smooth muscles. Because urinary tract infections are a major problem in MS, some patients are given prophylactic doses of medications such as trimethoprim-sulfamethoxazole or nitrofurantoin. Cystometric studies, done to evaluate bladder function, can help define the specific bladder problem. Some patients may need to be taught self-catheterization.

Encourage the patient to drink adequate fluids (at least 2000 mL/day). If the patient suffers from constipation, a stool softener such as docusate sodium may be used, as well as prune juice.

Nursing Interventions

Nutrition. A well-balanced diet with high-fiber foods and adequate fluids is important. Although there is no standard prescribed diet, a high-protein diet with supplemental vitamins often is recommended. Obesity makes it more difficult for the patient to meet daily needs and maintain mobility. The patient who is obese should be referred to a dietitian and be placed on a calorie-restricted diet that will help the patient lose weight slowly, while receiving adequate nutrition.

Skin care. Teach the patient with MS and/or the caregiver frequent turning to avoid skin impairment. Devices to relieve pressure, such as air mattresses, may be helpful. Because of sensory involvement, the patient may not feel discomfort that signals the need to change position.

Activity. Encourage patients with MS to exercise regularly but not to the point of fatigue. Physical therapy sometimes improves neurologic dysfunction. Exercise also helps daily functioning for patients with MS not experiencing an exacerbation. Exercise decreases spasticity, increases coordination, and retrains unaffected muscles to substitute for impaired ones. Water exercise is an especially beneficial type of physical therapy.

Daily rest periods may be helpful. During an acute exacerbation, patients often are kept as quiet as possible; this includes bed rest.

One side of the body often is more affected than the other. The patient must learn to stabilize the gait by leaning toward the less involved side. If the foot slaps forward while the patient is walking, teach him or her to put the foot down in a pronounced fashion and roll the weight forward on the side of the foot.

Control of environment. The patient should avoid hot baths because they often increase weakness. If summer travel is planned, the patient should travel in the coolest part of the day. If possible, the patient should be in air-conditioned surroundings during the summer.

People with MS do best in a peaceful and relaxed environment. They may have slow speech and be slow to respond. Sudden explosive emotional outbursts of crying or laughing also occur. The patient and family need support in dealing with this behavior.

Patient problems and interventions for the patient with MS may include but are not limited to the following:

PATIENT PROBLEM	NURSING INTERVENTIONS
Potential for Helplessness, related to physical limitations imposed by progressive physical deterioration, loss of body control, and threat to physical integrity	Provide emotional support, thorough explanations, and reassurance Be alert to emotional changes and mood swings Encourage the patient's participation and expression of needs and feelings Maintain planned rest periods Encourage self-care as indicated Provide physical care as indicated
Self-Care Impaired Inability to Bathe, Feed, Toilet Self, related to limitations in physical mobility imposed by disease process	Administer oral hygiene as needed Assist with or provide physical hygiene as indicated by physical ability Maintain appropriate bathing temperatures Administer oral hygiene q 4 h and as needed Catheterize intermittently as indicated; teach self-catheterization when possible Plan bladder dysfunction program as appropriate for spasticity or flaccidity Institute bowel control program (establish regular bowel routine, avoid constipation) Assist in dressing and grooming as indicated Provide nutritious, attractive meals

Patient Teaching

Teaching is important for the patient with MS and significant others. In late stages of the disease, the care functions usually are assumed by someone other than the patient. Important points include those for the patient with motor and sensory problems. In addition, stress the importance of spacing activities and avoiding temperature extremes and the potential for emotional lability. Make certain that the patient or the family has the address of the nearest MS society or support group.

Prognosis

The prognosis is variable. Some patients have MS for many years with few deficits, whereas other patients quickly become debilitated. The patient's ability to conserve energy and avoid stress may help prevent exacerbations. Exacerbations are treated and may resolve. The life expectancy for patients with MS has improved as treatments have improved. These individuals' life expectancy is approximately 5 to 10 years less than the average life expectancy.

PARKINSON DISEASE

Etiology and Pathophysiology

Parkinsonism is a syndrome that consists of a slowing down in the initiation and execution of movement (bradykinesia), increased muscle tone (rigidity), tremor, and impaired postural reflexes. Parkinson disease, a form of parkinsonism, is named after James Parkinson, who, in 1817, wrote a classic essay on "shaking palsy," a disease whose cause is still unknown today. Many other disorders resemble this disease, but their causes are known. These include drug-induced parkinsonism and vascular parkinsonism. Drug induced parkinsonism is typically related to drugs that alter brain dopamine levels, such as some antipsychotic and some antidepressant medications. The symptoms may stop after discontinuing the causative medication, but this can take anywhere from weeks to a year. Vascular parkinsonism is usually attributed to a series of small strokes. With both types of parkinsonism disorders, damage or loss of the dopamine-producing cells of the substantia nigra in the midbrain leads to depletion, in the basal ganglia, of dopamine that influences the initiation, modulation, and completion of movement and regulates unconscious autonomic movements. In cases of drug-induced parkinsonism, the dopamine receptors in the brain are blocked (Parkinson's Foundation, n.d.b.).

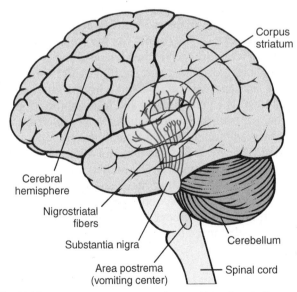

Fig. 14.12 Nigrostriatal disorders produce parkinsonism. Left-sided view of the human brain showing the substantia nigra and the corpus striatum *(shaded area)* lying deep within the cerebral hemisphere. Nerve fibers extend upward from the substantia nigra, divide into many branches, and carry dopamine to all regions of the corpus striatum. (From Lewis SL, Heitkemper MM, Dirksen SR, et al: *Medical-surgical nursing: Assessment and management of clinical problems*, ed 9, St. Louis, 2014, Mosby.)

According to the Parkinson's Foundation, Parkinson disease affects approximately 1 million people in the United States and more than 10 million people worldwide. Symptoms commonly occur after 50 years of age, with 4% being diagnosed before the age of 50. Peak onset of Parkinson disease is in the 60s. The average age of the patient with Parkinson disease is 65 years. There is an apparent genetic cause but no known cure. Men are 1.5 times more likely to develop Parkinson disease than women (Parkinson's Foundation, n.d.b.). Mayo Clinic (2020) suggests that additional risk factors include heredity, especially if more than one relative has the disease and prolonged exposures to toxins such as herbicides and pesticides.

Although patients with cerebrovascular disease may have parkinsonian-like symptoms, there is little evidence that parkinsonism is caused by arteriosclerosis. Distinguishing arteriosclerosis from true Parkinson disease is important for prognostic purposes. Patients with arteriosclerosis do not respond as well to treatment and are more likely to experience side effects of drug therapy. Most patients with parkinsonism have the degenerative or idiopathic form, for which the term *Parkinson disease* usually is reserved.

The pathology of Parkinson disease is associated with degeneration of the dopamine-producing neurons in the substantia nigra of the midbrain, which in turn disrupts the normal balance between dopamine and acetylcholine in the basal ganglia (Fig. 14.12). Major signs and symptoms, such as tremors, muscle rigidity, slowed movements, and impaired balance and coordination, occur when approximately 60% to 80% of dopamine-producing cells have been destroyed. It is believed that there is normally a balance between acetylcholine and dopamine in the basal ganglia. Any shift in the balance of activity (an increase in acetylcholine or a decrease in dopamine) seems to lead to parkinsonian-like symptoms. Dopamine is a neurotransmitter that is essential for normal functioning of the extrapyramidal motor system, including control of posture, support, and voluntary motion. In Parkinson disease the levels of dopamine-synthesizing enzymes and metabolites are reduced, and postmortem analysis of cross-sections of the midbrain shows loss of the normal melanin pigment in the substantia nigra and loss of neurons. In addition, deficient amounts of gamma-aminobutyric acid, serotonin, and norepinephrine have been found in basal ganglia and in the substantia nigra.

Clinical Manifestations

The onset of Parkinson disease is gradual and insidious, with a gradual progression and a prolonged course. In the beginning stages, only a mild tremor, handwriting changes, a slight limp, or a decreased arm swing may be evident. Later in the disease the patient may have a shuffling, propulsive gait with arms flexed and loss of postural reflexes (Fig. 14.13). Some patients may have a slight change in speech patterns. None of these alone is sufficient evidence for a diagnosis of the disease.

Because Parkinson disease has no specific diagnostic test, the diagnosis is based solely on the history, a thorough neurologic examination, and clinical features. A firm diagnosis can be made only when the patient has at least two signs of the classic triad: tremor, rigidity, and bradykinesia (slow or retarded movement). In the early stage of the disease there are subtle changes in cognitive function that can progress to dementia. The ultimate confirmation of Parkinson disease is a positive response to a low-dose trial of an antiparkinsonian medication, such as carbidopa-levodopa.

Tremor. Tremor, often the first sign, may be minimal initially, so the patient is the only one who notices it. This tremor can affect handwriting, causing it to trail off, particularly toward the ends of words. Parkinsonian tremor is more prominent at rest but disappears when the patient moves; it is aggravated by emotional stress or increased concentration. The hand tremor is described as "pill rolling" because the thumb and forefinger appear to move in a rotary fashion, as if rolling a pill, coin, or other small object. Tremor can involve the hands, diaphragm, tongue, lips, and jaw but rarely causes shaking of the head. Eventually tremors can become so pronounced

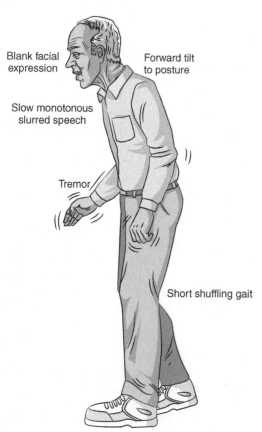

Blank facial expression

Forward tilt to posture

Slow monotonous slurred speech

Tremor

Short shuffling gait

Fig. 14.13 Characteristic appearance of a patient with Parkinson disease.

that the patient cannot hold a newspaper steady enough to read or make a call on a push-button telephone. Unfortunately, in many people a benign essential tremor has been diagnosed mistakenly as Parkinson disease. Essential tremor occurs during voluntary movement, has a more rapid frequency than parkinsonian tremor, and is often familial.

Rigidity. Rigidity, the second sign of the triad, is the increased resistance to passive motion when the limbs are moved through their range of motion. Parkinsonian rigidity is typified by a jerky quality when the joint is moved, like intermittent catches in the movement of a cogwheel. This is termed *cogwheel rigidity.* The rigidity is caused by sustained muscle contraction and consequently elicits a complaint of muscle soreness; fatigue and achiness; or pain in the head, the upper body, the spine, or the legs. Another consequence of rigidity is slowness of movement because it inhibits the alternating contraction and relaxation of opposing muscle groups (e.g., the biceps and triceps). Simple movements such as tying shoes and rising from a chair become a challenge.

Bradykinesia. Bradykinesia is particularly evident in the loss of automatic movements, which is secondary to physical and chemical alteration of the basal ganglia and related structures in the extrapyramidal portion of the CNS. In the unaffected patient, automatic movements are involuntary and occur subconsciously. They include blinking the eyelids, swinging the arms while walking, swallowing saliva, expressing oneself with facial and hand movements, and making minor postural adjustment. The patient with Parkinson disease does not execute these movements and lacks spontaneous activity. This accounts for the stooped posture, masked face (stiff facial muscles resulting in expressionless face), drooling, and shuffling gait (festination) that is characteristic of a person with this disease (see Fig. 14.13). The voice softens and loses modulation too, further contributing to communication problems. There may be evidence of bradykinesia in the patient's handwriting. The words become tiny and different from earlier handwriting samples. The patient often has a shuffling, propulsive gait that he or she is unable to stop until meeting an obstruction. In addition, there is difficulty initiating movement. Movements such as getting out of a chair cannot be executed unless they are willed consciously.

Assessment

Parkinson disease starts with subtle symptoms and progresses slowly. Subjective data include fatigue, incoordination, judgment defects, emotional instability, anxiety, depression, and heat intolerance. Assess the patient's understanding of the disease.

Objective data include tremor, which is the outstanding sign of the disease. This has been described as a pill-rolling motion of the fingers or a resting tremor. Bradykinesia is present with rigidity and loss of postural reflexes. Muscle rigidity leads to a masklike appearance of the face; slowed, monotonous speech; and drooling. Dysphagia, or difficulty swallowing, is a common late complication of neurologic degeneration, which poses the risk of choking and aspiration pneumonia. The patient may be constipated. There may be a scaly, erythematous rash (seborrheic dermatitis), particularly near the ears and eyebrows and in the scalp and nasolabial folds. Moist, oily skin is usually noted. Postural hypotension is prevalent and may be caused by failure of the arterial baroreceptors located in the aortic arch and the internal carotid arteries (Parkinson's Foundation, n.d.a.).

Diagnostic Tests

Parkinson disease has no definitive diagnostic tests. If there is a history of chronic dementia, the CT scan may show cerebral atrophy. The EEG may show minimal slowing, and the upper gastrointestinal evaluation may show decreased motility.

Medical Management

Medications. Treatment for Parkinson disease is based on easing the signs and symptoms of the disease. They often provide chemical substitution for dopamine or increase it in the body. They are referred to as dopaminergic. Levodopa is the most commonly prescribed medication for Parkinson disease. As levodopa passes through the brain, it is converted to dopamine. Carbidopa-levodopa (for 35 years, the gold standard of therapy) is effective, as the carbidopa protects levodopa from early conversion to dopamine outside the brain, thus enhancing the levels for the patient. Carbidopa also provides assistance with the nausea that may be experienced with levodopa. Recently an inhaled form of carbidopa-levodopa has been developed. It provides greater coverage in the prevention of symptoms between oral medication doses.

Dopamine agonists are also a common treatment for Parkinson disease. They do not enhance or replenish dopamine levels but cause the brain to believe dopamine levels are improving. These medications are not as strong carbidopa levodopa but cause fewer dyskinesia effects. Common side effects include sleepiness, confusion, visual hallucinations, and difficulty managing impulses (such as excessive shopping, gambling, and eating).

Amantadine hydrochloride is used to treat both tremors and Parkinson medication-induced extrapyramidal reactions.

Monoamine Oxidase Type B is an enzyme that breaks down dopamine in the body. MAO-B inhibitors are administered to reduce the body's breakdown of the enzyme, thus increasing dopamine levels. They may be prescribed singularly or in combination with other medication therapies to treat Parkinson disease.

Off times (also referred to as off episodes) result when there are periods of time in which there is a return to Parkinson symptomology or a failure to achieve improvement in symptoms of the disease. It may be caused by decreasing dopamine levels between medication doses as period of effectiveness comes to an end, medications dosages failing to achieve successful reduction of symptoms, and delays in the onset of symptom relief. Additional symptoms that may be experienced during the off times include difficulty with balance, feelings of exhaustion, and difficulty ambulating or speaking.

After prolonged treatment with some of the drugs, side effects such as dyskinesia (abnormal, involuntary muscle movements) may occur and the medication's effectiveness may decrease. Changes in the medication regimen may be indicated (Table 14.7). In the past medications were withdrawn and the patient given a drug holiday. This practice is not widely in use.

Surgery. Surgery that involves destroying portions of the brain that control the rigidity or tremor—so-called ablation surgery—has been used for Parkinson disease for more than 50 years. However, it has been replaced by deep brain stimulation (DBS). DBS involves placing an electrode in the thalamus, globus pallidus, or subthalamic nucleus and connecting it to a generator placed in the upper chest (like a pacemaker). The device is programmed to deliver a specific current to the targeted brain location. DBS can be adjusted to control symptoms and is reversible (the device can be removed). The procedure is nonablative and relatively safe and can improve dyskinesia (impaired ability to execute voluntary movements), gait, rigidity, and tremors. This procedure is often reserved for patients who have developed severe side effects to drug therapy or severe motor complications.

Medications are discontinued several days preoperatively so that signs and symptoms will be at their maximum at the time of surgery.

Another treatment approach for Parkinson disease involves human fetal dopamine cell transplants into the basal ganglia in an attempt to provide viable dopamine-producing cells to the brain.

Nursing Interventions

Activity needs. Physical and occupational therapies may be indicated to promote improved physical strength or to maintain physical capacity. Regular exercise needs to be incorporated in the daily routine. As the disease progresses, there will need to be revisions to the therapies and levels of exercise.

The disease will have impact on the activities of daily living. Rest and sleep are also affected. Pay special

Table 14.7   Medications for Disorders of the Neurologic System

GENERIC NAME	ACTION AND USE	SIDE EFFECTS	NURSING IMPLICATIONS
amantadine hydrochloride	Treats some cases of Parkinson disease and drug-induced extrapyramidal reactions, although its action in treatment of Parkinson disease is unknown	Nausea, vomiting, vision changes, dysrhythmias, disorientation, orthostatic hypotension, depression, fatigue	Tell patient to drink no alcohol; administer no CNS depressants; know pregnancy cautions; tell patient not to cease taking medication without conferring with health care provider and not to deviate from prescribed dosage; for best absorption, instruct patient to take after meals; if orthostatic hypotension occurs, instruct patient not to stand or change positions too quickly
baclofen	Reduces transmission of impulses from spinal cord to skeletal muscles; is antispasticity agent for treatment of spinal spasticity resulting from multiple sclerosis or spinal cord injury	Drowsiness, dizziness, disorientation, lightheadedness, hypotension, urinary frequency, possible increase in blood glucose level	Be aware of pregnancy cautions; give oral form with meals or milk to prevent gastrointestinal distress; watch for increased incidence of seizures in patients with epilepsy; tell patient to avoid activities that require alertness until CNS effects of drugs are known
benztropine mesylate	Blocks central cholinergic receptors, helping to balance cholinergic activity in basal ganglia; is indicated in treatment of mild cases of Parkinson disease and control of extrapyramidal reactions	Dizziness, drowsiness, depression, orthostatic hypotension, palpitation, tachycardia	Stress importance of following prescribed dosage; discontinue drug slowly; tell patient not to drink alcohol; advise patient of breast-feeding warnings; give with food; tell patient to rise slowly and notify health care provider of severe allergic reactions; do not give with antacids
carbidopa-levodopa	Increases levels of dopamine and levodopamine; is antiparkinsonian agent; improves modulation of voluntary nerve impulses transmitted to the motor cortex (lower dosage is needed than with single-dose therapy; efficiency may increase 75% when carbidopa and levodopa are used in combination)	Mental depression, mental changes, nausea and vomiting, orthostatic hypotension, dizziness, uncontrollable body movements	Give with food; give only as directed; effectiveness may take months; warn patient of breast-feeding and pregnancy cautions; caution patient about drowsiness and getting up too fast; lying down may affect control of blood glucose and darken urine
donepezil	Improves cholinergic function by inhibiting acetylcholinesterase; anti-Alzheimer agent; may temporarily lessen some of the dementia associated with Alzheimer disease, but does not alter the course	Diarrhea, nausea, vomiting, fatigue, headache, ecchymoses, atrial fibrillation, vasodilation	Monitor heart rate (may cause bradycardia); assess cognitive function periodically during therapy; administer in the evening just before bed; may be taken without regard for food
levodopa	Antiparkinsonian agent (mechanism of action is unknown); increases balance between cholinergic and dopaminergic activity to allow more normal body movements and alleviate signs and symptoms	Aggressive behavior, involuntary grimacing, head and body movements, depression, suicidal tendencies, orthostatic hypotension, nausea, vomiting, darkened urine, excessive and inappropriate sexual behavior	Do not give to patients with narrow-angle glaucoma; monitor patients receiving antihypertensive and hypoglycemic agents; advise patient to change positions slowly and dangle legs; protect drug from heat, light, moisture

Table 14.7   Medications for Disorders of the Neurologic System—cont'd

GENERIC NAME	ACTION AND USE	SIDE EFFECTS	NURSING IMPLICATIONS
memantine	Believed to act as an *N*-methyl-D-aspartate receptor antagonist to decrease glutamate, which is an excitatory neurotransmitter in the CNS; approved for the treatment of moderate to severe Alzheimer disease; does not prevent or slow neurodegeneration, but found in clinical studies to slow symptom progression	Dizziness, headache, constipation, hypertension, urinary frequency	Monitor I&O; do not give to patients with severe renal impairment; use cautiously in those with moderate renal impairment; be aware that conditions that increase urine pH, including severe urinary tract infections, lead to decreased excretion and increased serum levels
pyridostigmine bromide	Inhibits destruction of acetylcholine released from parasympathetic and somatic efferent nerves; causes acetylcholine to accumulate, promoting increased stimulation of receptor; is used in myasthenia gravis and by the oral route for senility associated with Alzheimer disease	Headache, seizures, bradycardia, hypotension, bronchospasm, increased bronchial secretions	Judging optimum dosage is difficult; monitor and document patient's response after each dose when using for myasthenia gravis; stress importance of taking drug exactly as ordered, on time, and in evenly spaced doses
selegiline hydrochloride	Monoamine oxidase (MAO) inhibitor used as treatment adjunct to levodopa and carbidopa-levodopa; may slow Parkinson disease and need for increased medication; may increase lifespan of people with Parkinson disease	Severe orthostatic hypotension, increased tremors, chorea, restlessness, grimacing, nausea and vomiting, slow urination, increased sweating, alopecia	Advise patient not to take more than 10 mg/day (there is no evidence that a greater amount improves effectiveness and it may increase adverse reactions); warn patient not to drink alcohol and drink only a little coffee; give with food; tell patient to rise slowly and notify health care provider of side effects; tell patient not to take over-the-counter cold remedies; monitor blood pressure and respirations
tacrine hydrochloride	Acts as reversible cholinesterase inhibitor, used for treatment of mild to moderate dementia of Alzheimer type	Bradycardia, nausea and vomiting, loose stools, ataxia, CNS disturbance, anorexia, agitation, increased serum transaminase levels, jaundice	Know risk of ulcers; monitor liver enzyme weekly for first 18 weeks; increase dosage at 6-week intervals; do not use NSAIDs concomitantly; be aware that it potentiates theophylline
trihexyphenidyl hydrochloride	Blocks central cholinergic receptors, helping to balance cholinergic activity of basal ganglia; is antidyskinetic and antiparkinsonian; controls some mild cases as an adjunct to more potent drugs; controls extrapyramidal reactions caused by drugs	Skin rash, eye pain, nervousness, headaches, tachycardia, urinary hesitancy, urine retention, dry mouth, disorientation	Do not give antacids or antidiarrheal agents within 1 h of giving medication; give with food; caution patient to rise slowly; use cautiously in patients with narrow-angle glaucoma and hypertension; warn patient to avoid activities that require alertness until CNS effects of drugs are known; tell patient to relieve dry mouth with cool drinks, ice chips, and hard candy

CNS, Central nervous system; *I&O,* intake and output; *NSAIDs,* nonsteroidal anti-inflammatory drugs.

attention to posture. Lying on a firm bed without a pillow may help prevent the spine from bending forward. Holding the hands folded behind the back when walking may help keep the spine erect and prevent the arms from falling stiffly at the sides. Problems secondary to bradykinesia can be alleviated by relatively simple measures. Advise patients who tend to "freeze" while walking to consciously think about stepping over imaginary or real lines on the floor, drop rice kernels and step over them, rock from side to side, lift the toes when stepping, and take one step backward and two steps forward. A patient who has difficulty rising from a sitting position can use a chair that gently propels him or her to an upright position. Do not hurry the patient because it will make the bradykinesia worse.

Nutrition. Diet is of major importance to the patient with Parkinson disease to avoid malnutrition, overnutrition, and constipation. When difficulty arises with eating patients may resist having an adequate diet. Patients with dysphagia and bradykinesia need appetizing foods that can be chewed and swallowed easily. Food should be cut into bite-sized pieces before it is served. Eating six small meals a day may be less exhausting than eating three large meals. Allow ample time for eating to avoid frustration and encourage independence. When the disease is advanced, aspiration is a real concern. Take care during feeding. Unless the disease is well controlled by medication, drooling can be a problem and increases with general excitement. When patients are dressed, garments with generous pockets for an ample supply of tissues help them to be less conspicuous. The types of exercise that may be engaged in may be limited as a result of progression of the disease. The reduction of exercise can lead to obesity. The diet needs to be balanced and include all food groups. The greatest intake should include proteins, fruits, and vegetables. Fruits and vegetables will provide fiber to aid in the reduction of constipation. Limit fat and sugar intake to avoid excessive empty calories.

Digestion and Elimination. The digestive changes that result from Parkinson disease cause nausea, constipation and difficulty voiding. The muscles involved in swallowing and digestion lead to nausea. The delay in movement of food through the body will result in constipation. Urinary challenges include feeling of urgency and hesitancy. Measures appropriate for the patient with MS also apply to these patients. Chronic constipation may be a real concern. The patient should be on a diet high in fiber and roughage for bulk. Encourage oral fluid intake, and use stool softeners, suppositories, and prune juice if necessary. Mild cathartics such as Milk of Magnesia are used if required. Daily exercise is also beneficial.

Patient problems and interventions for the patient with Parkinson disease are the same as those for the patient with MS, with the addition of but not limited to the following:

PATIENT PROBLEM	NURSING INTERVENTIONS
Compromised Physical Mobility, related to: • Rigidity • Bradykinesia • Akinesia	Assist with ambulation to assess degree of impairment and to prevent injury Perform active range-of-motion (ROM) exercises to all extremities to maintain joint ROM, prevent atrophy, and strengthen muscles Consult physical therapist or occupational therapist for aids to facilitate activities of daily living and safe ambulation Teach techniques to assist with mobility by instructing patient to step over imaginary line and rock from side to side to initiate leg movements; these techniques help deal with "freezing" (akinesia) while walking
Potential for Aspiration Into Airway, related to disease process	Ensure that, when eating, the patient sits at 90-degree angle with head up and chin slightly tucked, avoiding extending the head Provide soft-solid and thick-liquid diet because these consistencies are swallowed more easily Consult a speech therapist and a dietitian because they can provide specific plans to improve swallowing Encourage patient to take small bites Avoid use of straws

Patient Teaching

Education for the patient with Parkinson disease should include the importance of taking medications on the prescribed time schedule. Stress the need for good skin care and keeping active so that the patient remains as mobile as possible. Demonstrate proper ambulation and positioning to the patient and to the family if they will be taking care of the patient. Teach proper feeding techniques to reduce the risk of aspiration (see the Patient Problems box).

Prognosis

There is no cure for Parkinson disease. Parkinson disease is a chronic degenerative disorder with no acute exacerbations. If the patient takes medication as prescribed, signs and symptoms can be controlled for a long period. The care of the patient with Parkinson disease may eventually fall to family members and caregivers. The amount of care needed often increases as the disease progresses.

ALZHEIMER DISEASE

Etiology and Pathophysiology

AD is a chronic, progressive, degenerative disorder that affects the cells of the brain and causes impaired intellectual functioning. It is a common cause of dementia in the older person and affects men and women in equal numbers. Approximately 5.5 million Americans suffer from AD. It is estimated that 5 million of them are over age 65 years. Alzheimer may strike people in their 40s and 50s. AD is the sixth leading cause of death, with some estimates predicting it may move up to the third leading cause of death in the United States (National Institute on Aging, 2021). The cause is unknown, although research has shown a genetic link.

Changes in the brain of patients with AD include plaques in the cortex, neurofibrillary tangles (a tangled mass of nonfunctioning neurons), loss of connections between cells, and cell death (Fig. 14.14). This neuronal damage occurs primarily in the cerebral cortex and causes a decrease in brain size. These changes were first discovered in 1907 by the German neurologist Alois Alzheimer.

Studies have shown that individuals who engage in activities that require information processing (e.g., reading, learning a new language, doing crossword puzzles) have a lower risk of developing AD. Regular physical activity, leisure activities, and educational achievements throughout the life span may decrease AD risk (National Institute on Aging, 2017). Antioxidant-containing foods such citrus fruits, dark green vegetables, tomatoes, brown rice, and foods high in beta-carotene (sweet potatoes and carrots) are considered to lower the risk of the development of AD.

Clinical Manifestations

The Alzheimer's Association classifies the disease into three stages (Alzheimer's Association, n.d.). Some experts have developed increasingly advanced methods of staging patients with AD into more complex stages numbering up to seven. This textbook will highlight the three stages: early stage (mild), middle stage (moderate), and late stage (severe). In the early stage (mild) a person with Alzheimer has relatively mild memory lapses and may have difficulty using the correct word. Losing or misplacing objects is common. Planning and organizing becomes difficult. During this stage family and close friends may notice these subtle symptoms.

The middle stage (moderate) of AD may last for many years and is the longest stage of the disease. It is characterized by increased forgetfulness. The person with AD in this stage may forget their own address, phone number, or personal history. The person may be confused about where they are, experience changes in their sleep pattern, and demonstrate personality changes. Individuals may be able to perform ADLs with the assistance of others.

Late stage (severe) is the last stage of the disease. Trouble communicating, difficulty with walking, and lack of awareness of their surroundings are common characteristics. Difficulty swallowing eventually happens in this stage. The individual will need constant care in the late stage of AD. Hospice care is often initiated during this time.

The AD patient's behavior is neither intentional nor subject to self-control. Some patients develop psychotic manifestations (i.e., delusions, illusions, hallucinations). By the time a person reaches the third stage, he or she has total disorientation to person, place, and time. Motor problems such as apraxia (an inability to carry out learned sequential movements on command, perform purposeful acts, or use objects properly), *visual agnosia* (inability to recognize objects by sight), and *dysgraphia* (difficulty communicating via writing) interfere with the ability to carry out daily functions. Wandering is common. In the late stage, severe mental and physical deterioration is present. Total incontinence is common.

These stages may have some variations. All people with AD experience a steady deterioration in their physical and mental status, usually lasting 5 to 20 years until death occurs (Box 14.2).

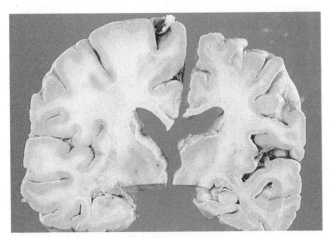

Fig. 14.14 Effects of Alzheimer disease on the brain. Note the normal brain on the left versus the Alzheimer brain on the right. (From National Institute on Aging: *Alzheimer's disease fact sheet.* (n.d.). Retrieved February 11, 2021, from https://www.nia.nih.gov/health/alzheimers-disease-fact-sheet)

Box **14.2**	**Ten Early Warning Signs of Alzheimer Disease**

1. Memory loss that disrupts daily life
2. Challenges in planning or solving problems
3. Difficulty completing familiar tasks at home
4. Confusion with time or place
5. Trouble understanding visual images and spatial relationships
6. New problems with words in speaking or writing
7. Misplacing things and losing the ability to retrace steps
8. Decreased or poor judgment
9. Withdrawal from work or social activities
10. Changes in mood and personality

Alzheimer's Association, 2020

Assessment

Memory loss is the first symptom usually noticed in AD, combined with the inability to carry out normal activities. Other evidence may be agitation or restlessness. It is important to rule out other conditions such as pernicious anemia, drug reactions, depression, or hormonal imbalances.

Diagnostic Tests

The diagnosis of AD is primarily one of exclusion. AD has no specific diagnostic test. A CT scan, EEG, MRI, and PET may be used to rule out other pathologic conditions. A family history of AD is significant. At times the diagnosis can be confirmed only at the time of autopsy.

Medical Management

The care of the patient with AD can be frustrating for the caregiver and the health care provider because the treatment options are so limited. Often medications make the condition worse. Lorazepam or haloperidol in small doses may be necessary to lessen agitation and unpredictable behavior. Treatment of depression in patients with AD may improve cognitive ability. Depression is treated most often with selective serotonin reuptake inhibitors such as fluoxetine, sertraline, fluvoxamine, and citalopram. Trazodone, an antidepressant, may help with problems related to sleep but also may cause hypotension. Three cholinesterase inhibitors, Donepezil, rivastigmine, and galantamine, may have short-term benefit for mild cognitive impairment. Memantine is the first drug approved for the treatment of moderate to severe AD. Memantine does not prevent or slow neurodegeneration, but it was found in clinical studies to slow symptom progression. Many clinical drug trials are trying to find drugs that manage the signs and symptoms of AD while limiting the rate of disease progression.

Nursing Interventions and Patient Teaching

Nursing interventions are directed toward maintaining adequate nutrition. This can be a challenge because often the patient will not sit still long enough to eat. Providing finger foods and letting the patient eat while walking may help. Frequent feedings with high nutritive value are important. Encourage fluids of at least 2000 mL/day (Nursing Care Plan 14.1).

Safety demands a special mention. Because of memory problems, patients with AD often do dangerous things, such as walking outside while undressed, turning on stoves, wandering away, and setting fires. Measures that the family can take include removing burner controls from the stove at night, double locking all doors and windows, and keeping the person under constant supervision. Disruptive behavior—including aggressive, agitated behavior—may occur. One frustrating part of the disease is that many patients sleep for only short periods and are awake most of the night.

Most of the time, education is directed at the family, because by the time the condition is diagnosed there is usually serious mental impairment. Help the family set a realistic schedule that also allows them time for rest and relaxation. The family may need to consider placing the patient in a long-term care facility. Put the family in touch with the local support group for AD.

Prognosis

Currently no effective treatment is available to stop the progression of AD, which occurs at a variable rate. The course of the disease can span 5 to 20 years, 4 to 8 years being the average (Cleveland Clinic, 2019). In 2010, between $159 and $215 billion was spent on AD care. By 2040, these costs are projected to jump to between $379 and more than $500 billion annually (CDC, 2020a). Ultimately, most patients die from complications such as pneumonia, malnutrition, and dehydration. Special Alzheimer units and family and nursing approaches may help the patient stay as productive and safe as possible. The burden on the individual, the family, caregivers, and society as a whole is staggering. Support groups for caregivers and family members have been formed throughout the United States to provide an atmosphere of understanding and to give current information about the disease and related topics such as safety and legal, ethical, and financial issues. Nurses often receive personal and professional satisfaction in participating in such support groups.

MYASTHENIA GRAVIS

Etiology and Pathophysiology

MG is an autoimmune disease of the neuromuscular junction, characterized by the fluctuating weakness of certain skeletal muscle groups. MG is an unpredictable neuromuscular disease with lower motoneuron characteristics. MG can occur at any age, even children, but most commonly occurs in women under 40 years of age and men over 60 (National Institute of Neurological Disorders and Stroke [NINDS], 2020d). According to the Myasthenia Gravis Foundation of America (n.d.), the incidence is about 20 in every 100,000 of the population (36,000 to 60,000 people).

With MG, no observable structural change occurs in the muscle or nerve. Nerve impulses fail to pass at the neuromuscular junction (the space between the nerve ending and muscle fiber), resulting in muscle weakness. MG is caused by an autoimmune process. It is thought to be triggered by antibodies that attack acetylcholine receptor sites at the neuromuscular junction. This attack damages and reduces the number of receptor sites, preventing conduction along the normal pathway at normal conduction speeds. Patients with MG have only about one-third as many acetylcholine receptors at the neuromuscular junction as is normal.

Some patients with MG have been found to thymus gland abnormalities. The thymus may be abnormally large or have a thymoma (a tumor of the thymus), and

Nursing Care Plan 14.1 | The Patient With Alzheimer Disease

Ms. A. is a 65-year-old who has been a seamstress. She has a history of progressive memory loss, paranoia, disorientation, and agitation. She was diagnosed as having Alzheimer disease 2 years ago. Her family kept her at home until 6 months ago, when she was admitted to a long-term care institution. The nursing history indicates that she is incontinent of urine about 50% of the time and expresses a great deal of anxiety, especially around new situations or people. She cries frequently and at times attempts to hit the staff.

PATIENT PROBLEM

Anxiousness, related to cognitive impairments

Patient Goals and Expected Outcomes	Nursing Interventions	Evaluation
Patient will demonstrate decreased anxiety as evidenced by decreased outbursts of agitation or crying, the ability to sleep through most of the night, and cooperation with care	Continue to assess presence of anxiety. Comfort patient when she is crying. Provide simple explanation for all procedures. Use calm, undemanding, unhurried approach. Keep nursing interventions consistent and simple. Assist patient in doing relaxation techniques. Maintain consistency of caregiver when able. Minimize patient's choices in care. Encourage patient to exercise. Offer snack at bedtime.	Patient sleeps 5–6 h per night. Patient remains calm with care. Patient experiences decreased episodes of crying or striking out at others.

PATIENT PROBLEM

Functional Inability to Control Urination, related to condition and cognitive impairment

Patient Goals and Expected Outcomes	Nursing Interventions	Evaluation
Patient will be continent Patient will be free of urinary tract infection	Take patient to bathroom on regular schedule. Encourage adequate fluid intake (at least 2000 mL/day). Determine patient's preference for fluid. Place sign on door indicating "Toilet" or "Bathroom," or with a picture. If patient has urgency, ensure closeness to bathroom. Simplify closures on clothing. Avoid fluids just before bed. Use disposable protective perineal garments (Attends) only as needed.	Patient is free of episodes of incontinence. Patient is free of infection. Patient will void when taken to the bathroom.

CRITICAL THINKING QUESTIONS

1. Ms. A. continually wanders about the long-term care facility. She is unable to sit at the table for an entire meal. She has lost approximately 20 lb in the past 3 months. What are some helpful measures to improve her nutritional status?
2. What are some helpful interventions to help Ms. A. obtain a better sleep pattern?
3. Ms. A. has difficulty in maintaining good personal hygiene. What are some methods for assisting Ms. A. in maintaining personal hygiene?

---

many have changes in the cellular structure of the thymus gland.

Clinical Manifestations

MG can occur in any muscle, but it is most commonly seen in muscle groups that control the eyes and eyelids, face, chewing, talking, and swallowing. In ocular MG the signs and symptoms include ptosis (eyelid drooping) and diplopia (double vision). MG may remain confined to the eye muscles. The generalized variety of MG may vary in presentation, from mild to severe signs and symptoms. The patient may complain initially of ptosis and diplopia. Skeletal weakness involving the muscles of the extremities, the neck, the shoulders, the hands, and the diaphragm; dysarthria; and dysphagia may follow. The vocal cords can become weak, and the voice can sound nasal. As the disease progresses, it affects the trunk and lower limbs, leading to difficulty with walking, sustained sitting, and raising the arms over the head. Usually the distal muscles (those of the lower arms, hands, lower legs, and feet) are not as affected as the proximal muscles (those closer to the center of the body). Muscle weakness may become so severe that the person cannot breathe without mechanical ventilation. Bowel and bladder sphincter weakness occurs with severe loss of muscle control. Extreme exacerbations of the disease, referred to as a myasthenia crisis, may be initiated by things such as infection, stress, or surgery. A myasthenia crisis is often a medical emergency since it often involves severe muscle weakness of the respiratory system, resulting in the need for mechanical ventilation until the crisis passes.

Assessment

Subjective data include the patient's understanding of the disease, complaints of weakness or double vision, difficulty chewing or swallowing, and any bowel or bladder incontinence.

Objective data include any documented muscle weakness on neurologic testing. Nasal-sounding speech may be noted; the voice often fades after a long conversation and breath sounds diminish. Note ptosis of the eyelids and weight loss if there are swallowing problems.

Diagnostic Tests

The diagnosis of MG starts with a history and physical examination, with emphasis on the neurological system. Examination with findings of weakness of various eye movements is often an indication that MG may be present. An EMG is very helpful in the diagnosis of MG, especially when the symptoms are mild. The IV anticholinesterase test is a reliable diagnostic test. Edrophonium, a short-acting cholinesterase inhibitor, which decreases the amount of cholinesterase at the neuromuscular junction while making acetylcholine available to muscles, is administered intravenously. The patient response is evaluated carefully. Shortly after the administration of IV edrophonium, muscle function improves dramatically in patients who have the illness. Another diagnostic test is serum testing for antibodies to acetylcholine receptors. While these antibodies are present in most patients with generalized myasthenia, there are some patients who will test negative but still have the disease based on other testing (NINDS, 2020d).

Medical Management

Medical management includes the use of anticholinesterase drugs such as neostigmine and pyridostigmine. These medications promote nerve impulse transmission and effectively alleviate symptoms. Corticosteroids may be used as an adjunct therapy. Immunosuppressive medications, including azathioprine, cyclosporine, and cyclophosphamide, are used because of MG's autoimmune component. Monoclonal antibody treatment is also currently used for those patients who test positive for the serum antibodies.

Plasmapheresis separates plasma from blood with a machine called a cell separator, which can be connected to the patient by means of a vascular cannula. This process removes the antibodies produced by the autoimmune response. Plasmapheresis can yield short-term improvement in symptoms and is indicated for patients in crisis or in preparation for surgery, when corticosteroids must be avoided.

Thymectomy is indicated for almost all patients with a thymoma. For some patients without thymoma, thymectomy may result in improvement in symptoms. Excision of the thymus reduces symptoms of MG in many patients. A thymectomy is a complex surgery, and patients with MG are at high risk for complications from anesthesia.

Another treatment option is the administration of IV immune globulin to reduce the production of acetylcholine antibodies. IV immune globulin is used for a severe relapse of MG.

During exacerbations of the disease, and when the respiratory status is compromised, the patient may require intubation and mechanical ventilation. A tracheostomy may be necessary.

Nursing Interventions and Patient Teaching

Respiratory problems typically occur in patients with MG. Upper respiratory tract infections occur because the patient may not have the energy to cough effectively, and pneumonia or airway obstruction may develop. Aspiration often occurs. During acute episodes of the disease, the patient may require hospitalization. Serial determination of vital capacity, minute volumes, and tidal volumes is done to assess the need for respiratory assistance. The patient also may be taught airway-protective techniques during swallowing (e.g., chin tuck, double swallow). Suctioning is done as needed, and if swallowing becomes impaired, a feeding tube may be necessary.

👥 Patient Teaching

Myasthenia Gravis

- Teach the importance of taking medication at the time prescribed and taking it early enough before eating or engaging in activities to obtain maximum relief.
- Explain how to adjust the medication dose to maintain muscle strength.
- Caution about medications to avoid.
- Teach the importance of seeking medical attention at the first sign of an upper respiratory tract infection.
- Explain the importance of eating only when sitting up, to prevent aspiration.
- Caution the patient to avoid crowds in flu and cold season.
- Explain how to adjust to daily activities to allow for leisure activities and rest periods.
- Explain planning to use minimal energy in activities that are essential so that energy may be conserved for activities that the patient enjoys.
- Advise patient to wear a medical-alert bracelet that identifies the patient as having myasthenia gravis.

People with MG may have to change daily patterns of activity. Help the patient and the family plan so that minimal energy is used in activities that are essential to remaining relatively self-sufficient, with energy left for leisure activities. Physical therapy such as ROM exercises may be beneficial for maintaining muscle function.

The patient with MG is usually able to adjust the medication depending on the symptoms. Also, the patient can have much control over preventing respiratory complications. Therefore teaching is important and should include those topics listed in the Patient Teaching box.

Prognosis

MG is a chronic disease. The course is variable with periods of exacerbation and remission. Some cases are mild, but others are severe, with death resulting from respiratory failure. Patients with a thymoma may experience improvement after a thymectomy.

AMYOTROPHIC LATERAL SCLEROSIS

Loss of upper and lower motor neurons is the major pathologic change in ALS, a rare, progressive neurologic disease that usually leads to death in 2 to 6 years. This disease became known as Lou Gehrig's disease when the famous baseball player was stricken with it in 1939. The onset is between 55 and 75 years of age, and men are slightly more likely to be affected than women. Being Caucasian or Hispanic also increases the risk. Studies also show that veterans are 1.5 to 2 times more likely to develop ALS, likely attributed to environmental toxins. The U.S. Department of Veteran Affairs recognizes ALS as a service-related disease (NIH, 2021).

For unknown reasons, motor neurons in the brainstem and spinal cord gradually degenerate in ALS. The dead motor neuron cannot produce or transport vital signals to muscle. Consequently, electrical and chemical messages originating in the brain do not reach the muscles to activate them.

Clinical Manifestations

The primary symptoms are weakness of the upper extremities (the hands are often affected first), dysarthria, and dysphagia. For some, weakness may begin in the legs. Muscle wasting and fasciculations (muscle twitching) result from the denervation of the muscles and lack of stimulation and use. Death usually results from respiratory tract infection secondary to compromised respiratory function.

Diagnostic Tests

An EMG is a common test performed when diagnosing ALS. A similar test called a nerve conduction study (NCS) is also frequently performed. This test measures electrical activity of the nerves and muscles by assessing the nerve's ability to send a signal along the nerve or to the muscle. Additional testing includes an MRI and lab testing to rule out other disorders.

Medical Management

Current medications used in the treatment of ALS include riluzole and edaravone. Riluzole is thought to add a few months to the life of a person diagnosed with ALS by reducing damage to motor neurons by decreasing levels of glutamate, which transports messages between nerve cells and motor neurons. Edaravone decreases the intensity of symptoms. Other medications are ordered to treat the symptoms of ALS such as muscle spasms and excessive respiratory secretions. Physical, speech, and respiratory therapy are essential for treatment and management of the symptoms of ALS. Consultation with a nutritionist is also important in order to maximize the diet in support of weakening muscles (NINDS, 2021).

Nursing Interventions and Patient Teaching

This illness is devastating because the patient remains cognitively intact while wasting away. The challenge of nursing interventions is to guide the patient in the use of moderate-intensity, endurance-type exercises for the trunk and limbs, because this may help reduce ALS spasticity (Mayo Clinic, 2019). Support the patient's cognitive and emotional functions by facilitating communication, providing diversional activities such as reading and companionship, and helping the patient and the family with advanced care planning and anticipatory grieving related to loss of motor function and ultimate death. Respiratory failure is the greatest cause of death for the patient with ALS.

Prognosis

Unfortunately, there is no cure for ALS. Most patients live 3 to 5 years after diagnosis of ALS. Supportive care and management of symptoms is of upmost importance. There is a great deal of ongoing research and support for the ALS Foundation.

HUNTINGTON DISEASE

Huntington disease is a genetically transmitted autosomal dominant disorder that affects men and women of all races. The offspring of a person with this disease have a 50% risk of inheriting it. The diagnosis often occurs after the affected individual has children. The onset of Huntington disease is usually between 30 and 50 years of age. In the United States, an estimated 3 to 7 per 100,000 people, usually of European ancestry, have Huntington disease (NLM, 2020c).

Diagnosis is based on family history, clinical symptoms, and the detection of the characteristic deoxyribonucleic acid (DNA) pattern from blood samples. People who are asymptomatic but who have a positive family history of Huntington disease face the dilemma of whether to get tested. If the test is positive, the person will develop Huntington disease, but at what age and to what extent cannot be determined.

Like Parkinson disease, the pathology of Huntington disease involves the basal ganglia and the extrapyramidal motor system. Huntington disease involves an overactivity of the dopamine pathway. The net effect is an excess of dopamine, which leads to symptoms that are the opposite of those of parkinsonism. The clinical manifestations are characterized by abnormal and excessive involuntary movements (chorea). These are writhing, twisting movements of the face, limbs, and body. The movements get worse as the disease progresses. Facial movements involving speech, chewing, and swallowing are affected and may cause aspiration and malnutrition. The gait deteriorates, and ambulation eventually becomes impossible. Perhaps the most devastating deterioration is in mental functions, which include intellectual decline, emotional lability, and psychotic behavior. Because there is no cure, therapeutic management is palliative. Antipsychotic (e.g., haloperidol), antidepressant (fluoxetine, sertraline), and antichorea (clonazepam) medications are prescribed and have some effect. These medications only treat the symptoms; they do not alter the course of the disease.

The goal of nursing management is to provide the most comfortable environment possible for the patient and the family by maintaining physical safety, treating the physical symptoms, and providing emotional and psychological support. Because of the choreic movements, caloric requirements are as high as 4000 to 5000 calories/day to maintain body weight. As the disease progresses, meeting caloric needs becomes a greater challenge when the patient has difficulty swallowing and holding the head still. Depression and mental deterioration also can compromise nutritional intake. Genetic counseling is important. DNA testing can be done on fetal cells obtained by amniocentesis or chorionic biopsy. Genetic testing can determine whether a person is a carrier. No test is available to predict when symptoms will develop.

This disease presents a great challenge to health care professionals. There is a large risk for depression and suicide in patients diagnosed with Huntington disease. Death usually occurs 10 to 30 years after the onset of symptoms (Cleveland Clinic, 2020).

STROKE

Etiology and Pathophysiology

Stroke (cerebrovascular accident or CVA) is an abnormal condition of the blood vessels of the brain, characterized by hemorrhage into the brain or the formation of an embolus or thrombus that occludes an artery, resulting in ischemia of the brain tissue normally perfused by the damaged vessels. A stroke should be treated as a medical emergency, just as one would with a myocardial infarction (heart attack).

Prompt medical attention at the first sign of symptoms is needed to reduce disability and death. Stroke is the most common disease of the nervous system. It is estimated that 795,000 people in the United States suffer a stroke annually, with 87% being ischemic strokes. It is ranked as the fifth leading cause of death in the United States. Every 40 seconds someone suffers a stroke and every 4 minutes there is a death due to a stroke. Strokes affect people in all age groups, but the risk increases with age. Approximately one in four strokes occur in people who have previously had a stroke. Strokes leave many people with serious, long-term disability. Of those who survive, more than half suffer mobility impairment. Common long-term disabilities include hemiparesis (weakness on one side of the body), inability to walk, complete or partial dependence in ADLs, aphasia, and depression (CDC, 2021a) (see the Cultural Considerations box).

🌐 Cultural Considerations

Stroke

A high mortality rate from strokes exists among African Americans, possibly as a result of the high frequency of hypertension, obesity, and diabetes, as well as less access to healthcare. Thrombotic strokes are twice as common among African Americans as among whites. Hemorrhagic strokes are almost twice as common among African Americans as among whites. Hispanics have a higher death rate from stroke than do other ethnicities (CDC, 2021a).

Strokes are classified as ischemic or hemorrhagic, based on the underlying pathophysiologic findings. Ischemic strokes are thrombotic and embolic. As previously mentioned, these account for 87% of strokes. The remaining 13% are hemorrhagic strokes,

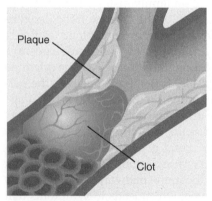

A **Thrombotic stroke.** Cerebral thrombosis is a narrowing of the artery by fatty deposits called *plaque*. Plaque can cause a clot to form, which blocks the passage of blood through the artery.

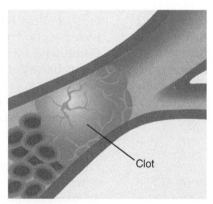

B **Embolic stroke.** An embolus is a blood clot or other debris circulating in the blood. When it reaches an artery in the brain that is too narrow to pass through, it lodges there and blocks the flow of blood.

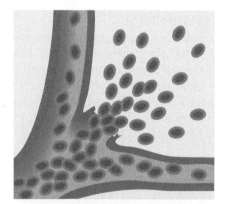

C **Hemorrhagic stroke.** A burst blood vessel may allow blood to seep into and damage brain tissues until clotting shuts off the leak.

Fig. 14.15 Three types of stroke. (From Lewis SL, Bucher L, Heitkemper MM, et al: *Medical-surgical nursing: Assessment and management of clinical problems*, ed 10, St. Louis, 2017, Elsevier.)

which result from bleeding into the brain tissue itself (Fig. 14.15). Many underlying factors also contribute atherosclerosis, atrial fibrillation, heart disease, hypertension, kidney disease, peripheral vascular disease, and diabetes mellitus. Other risk factors include family history of stroke, obesity, high serum cholesterol, cigarette smoking, stress, cocaine use, and a sedentary lifestyle. Newer low-dose oral contraceptives have lower risks for stroke than early forms of birth control pills, except in those individuals who are hypersensitive and smoke. Hypertension is the single most important modifiable risk factor. Stroke risk is two to four times more likely to occur due to hypertension. Atrial fibrillation is responsible for about 25% of strokes (NINDS, 2020b). Diabetes is another major risk factor for stroke. Diabetes affects vessels throughout the body, including the brain. Well-controlled diabetes can decrease the chance of stroke. Carotid artery stenosis, also called carotid artery disease, is defined as the narrowing of the carotid arteries that supply blood to the brain, usually from plaque buildup (atherosclerosis) in the inner lining of the artery. It is responsible for the vast majority of TIAs that affect patients annually. Recent studies have reviewed the risk for stroke in women taking hormone replacement therapies. Although the studies indicate that there may be a slight increase in risk, low-dose estrogen therapy in women without significant risk factors is considered safe (Medline Plus, 2021).

Clinical Manifestations

A stroke can affect many body functions, including motor activity, elimination, intellectual function, spatial perception, personality, affect, sensation, and communication. The functions affected are related directly to the artery involved and the area of brain it supplies. Permanent damage can result from a stroke because of anoxia of the brain. The vessel most commonly affected is the middle cerebral artery. The patient may be unconscious and may experience seizures as a result of generalized ischemia and the brain's response to abrupt hypoxia.

Ischemic stroke. Deficient blood flow to the brain from a partial or complete occlusion of an artery results in an ischemic stroke. Ischemic strokes are either *thrombotic* or *embolic* and account for nearly 90% of all strokes (American Stroke Association [ASA], n.d.).

Thrombotic stroke. Thrombosis is the most common cause of stroke, and the most common cause of cerebral thrombosis is atherosclerosis. Additional disease processes that cause thrombosis are hypertension or diabetes mellitus, both of which accelerate the arteriosclerotic process. Additional risk factors associated with thrombotic strokes include coagulation disorders, polycythemia vera, arteritis, chronic hypoxia, and dehydration. In 30% to 50% of individuals, thrombotic strokes have been preceded by a TIA. Stroke resulting from thrombosis is seen most often in the 60- to 90-year-old age group. Thrombosis occurs in relation to injury of a blood vessel wall and formation of a blood clot. The lumen of the blood vessel becomes narrowed, and if it becomes occluded, infarction occurs. Thrombosis develops readily where atherosclerotic plaques already have narrowed blood vessels. Thrombi usually occur in larger vessels, especially the internal carotid arteries.

Symptoms of this type of stroke tend to occur during sleep or soon after arising. This is thought to result partly because recumbency lowers blood pressure, which can lead to brain ischemia. Postural hypotension also may be a factor. Neurologic signs and symptoms frequently worsen for the first few hours after a stroke and peak in severity within 72 hours as edema increases in the infarcted areas of the brain.

Embolic stroke. Embolism is the second most common cause of stroke. People who have a stroke resulting from embolism are usually younger. The emboli most commonly originate from a thrombus in the endocardial (inside) layer of the heart, often caused by rheumatic heart disease, mitral stenosis and atrial fibrillation, myocardial infarction, infective endocarditis, valvular prostheses, and atrial septal defects. Less common causes of emboli include air, fat from long bone (femur) fractures, amniotic fluid after childbirth, and tumors. The embolus travels upward to the cerebral circulation and lodges where a vessel narrows or bifurcates. They most frequently occur in the mid-cerebral artery.

Hemorrhagic stroke. Hemorrhagic stroke accounts for approximately 13% of all strokes and results from bleeding into the brain tissue or subarachnoid space. The bleed causes damage by destroying and replacing brain tissue. The peak incidence of aneurysms occurs in people who are 35 to 60 years of age. Women are affected more frequently than men.

An aneurysm is often the cause of hemorrhage. An aneurysm is a localized dilation of the wall of a blood vessel usually caused by atherosclerosis and hypertension or, less frequently, by trauma, infection, or a congenital weakness in the vessel wall. It ruptures as a result of a small hole that occurs in a part of the aneurysm. The hemorrhage spreads rapidly, producing localized damage and irritation to the cerebral vessels. The bleeding usually stops when a plug of fibrin platelets is formed. The hemorrhage begins to absorb within 3 weeks. Recurrent rupture is a risk 7 to 10 days after the initial hemorrhage. The patient with intracerebral hemorrhage has no forewarning; has rapid, severe symptoms; and has a poor prognosis for recovery. Fifty percent of patients die soon after the aneurysm. Only about 20% are functionally independent after 6 months.

Transient ischemic attack. TIA refers to an episode of cerebrovascular insufficiency with temporary episodes of neurologic dysfunction lasting less than 24 hours and often less than 15 minutes. Most TIAs resolve within 3 hours. TIAs may be caused by micro-emboli that temporarily occlude the blood flow or by the narrowing of small vessels in the brain. TIAs also often occur in patients with carotid artery stenosis, which causes decreased blood flow to the brain. The most common deficits are contralateral weakness of the lower face, hands, arms, and legs; transient dysphasia; numbness or loss of sensation; temporary loss of vision of one eye; or a sudden inability to speak. Other symptoms may include tinnitus, vertigo, blurred vision, diplopia, eyelid ptosis, and ataxia. Between attacks the neurologic status is normal.

A TIA should be considered a forerunner of a stroke. Testing after a TIA includes a complete laboratory workup, x-rays, ultrasound of the carotid arteries and heart, MRI, CT, and thorough cardiac testing to determine the cause of the TIA. Evaluation must be done to confirm that the signs and symptoms of a TIA are not related to other brain lesions, such as a developing subdural hematoma or an increasing tumor mass. CT of the brain without contrast media is the most important initial diagnostic study.

The major importance of TIAs is that they warn the patient of an underlying pathologic condition. Approximately 40% of patients who experience TIAs will have a stroke in 2 to 5 years. The patient is given medications that prevent platelet aggregation, such as aspirin, ticlopidine, dipyridamole, and clopidogrel. Aspirin is the most frequently used antiplatelet agent. An anticoagulant medication (e.g., oral warfarin) is the treatment of choice for individuals with atrial fibrillation who have had a TIA.

Surgical interventions for the patient with TIAs from carotid artery disease include carotid endarterectomy (CEA) or percutaneous transluminal angioplasty and stenting.

- *Carotid endarterectomy:* In CEA the atheromatous lesion is removed from the carotid artery to improve blood flow. CEA surgery causes a reduction in stroke and vascular death. This surgery is reserved for patients with occlusions of 70% to 99% of blood flow. The long-term benefit of CEA is based on the severity of the preoperative stenosis. In patients with stenosis of 30% or less, surgery actually increases the risk for an ipsilateral stroke in the first 5 years postoperatively. There has been no proven effect within 5 years when the stenosis is 31% to 40% and only a marginal improvement in patients with 50% to 69% stenosis. However, the greatest benefit occurs when the stenosis is 70% or more (National Institute of Neurological Disorders and Stroke, 2016).
- *Percutaneous transluminal angioplasty:* In percutaneous transluminal angioplasty a balloon is inserted to open a stenosed artery to permit increased blood flow. This procedure is used to treat patients with clinical manifestations related to stenosis in the vertebrobasilar or carotid arteries and their branches. The risk of the angioplasty procedure is the possibility of dislodging emboli, which can travel to the brain or retina.

Assessment

Subjective data include the description of the onset of symptoms; the presence of headache; any sensory deficit, such as numbness or tingling; the inability to think clearly; and visual problems. In the case of a hemorrhage, the headache may be described as sudden and explosive. Assess the patient's ability to understand the condition.

Objective data include hemiparesis or hemiplegia, any change in the LOC, signs of increased ICP, respiratory status, and aphasia. The exact clinical picture varies, depending on the area of the brain affected (Fig. 14.16). A lesion on one side of the brain affects motor function on the opposite (contralateral) side of the body. When the middle cerebral artery is affected, as is most common, the signs and symptoms seen include contralateral paralysis or paresis, contralateral sensory loss, dysphasia or aphasia if the dominant hemisphere is involved, spatial-perceptual problems, changes in judgment and behavior if the nondominant hemisphere is involved, and *contralateral (homonymous) hemianopia* (Fig. 14.17).

In right-handed people and in most left-handed people, the left hemisphere is dominant for language

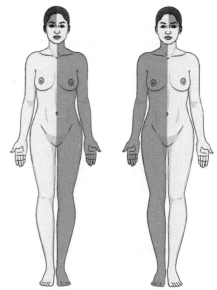

Right brain damage
(Stroke on right side of the brain)
- Paralyzed left side: hemiplegia
- Left-sided neglect
- Spatial-perceptual deficits
- Tends to deny or minimize problems
- Rapid performance, short attention span
- Impulsive, safety problems
- Impaired judgment
- Impaired time concepts

Left brain damage
(Stroke on left side of the brain)
- Paralyzed right side: hemiplegia
- Impaired speech/language aphasias
- Impaired right/left discrimination
- Slow performance, cautious
- Aware of deficits: depression, anxiety
- Impaired comprehension related to language, math

Fig. 14.16 Manifestations of right-sided and left-sided stroke.

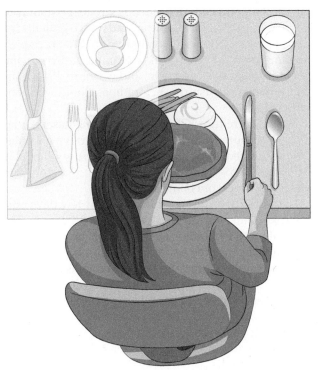

Fig. 14.17 Spatial and perceptual deficits in stroke. Perception of a patient with homonymous hemianopia shows that food on the left side is not seen and thus is ignored.

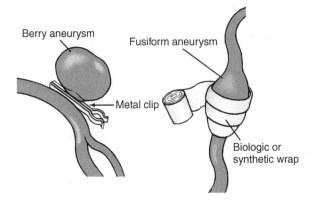

Fig. 14.18 Clipping and wrapping of aneurysms. (From Lewis SL, Heitkemper MM, Dirksen SR, et al: *Medical-surgical nursing: Assessment and management of clinical problems*, ed 9, St. Louis, 2014, Mosby.)

skills. Language disorders affect expression and comprehension of written and spoken words. When a stroke damages the dominant hemisphere of the brain, the patient may experience *aphasia* (total loss of comprehension and use of language). A stroke affecting Broca's areas of the brain (located in the frontal lobe of the brain) results in the person having difficulty with the ability to articulate words (*expressive aphasia*), but the ability to make vocal sounds and to understand written and spoken words remains intact (see Fig. 14.3 and Box 14.1). *Receptive aphasia* results when the stroke damages the area of the brain known as Wernicke's area (located in the temporal lobe). Patients with receptive aphasia have difficulty comprehending spoken and written communication.

A stroke patient may experience *dysarthria*, which is difficult or poorly articulated speech. Dysarthria is a result of deficits in the muscular control of speech related to damage that has occurred to the central or peripheral motor nerves (*Mosby's Dictionary of Medicine, Nursing & Health Professions*, 2017). Some stroke patients have a combination of aphasia and dysarthria.

Diagnostic Tests

CT and MRI are the tests most commonly used in the diagnosis of a stroke. The earlier the stroke is diagnosed, the better the chance for recovery from the potential effects. Cardiac testing as well as an EEG will likely be performed during the diagnostic stage. PET also may be useful in assessing the extent of tissue

damage by showing the brain's metabolic activity. After TIAs, a cerebral angiogram may be done as well as a Doppler study of the carotid arteries. A cerebral angiogram also allows for a detailed evaluation of the vasculature of the brain.

Medical Management

If the patient has had a hemorrhagic stroke as a result of an aneurysm, surgery may be necessary to prevent a rebleed. The surgery consists of performing a craniotomy; tying off or clipping the aneurysm; and removing the clot to prevent rebleeding into the brain (Fig. 14.18). An aneurysm often causes vasospasm in the brain as blood in the subarachnoid space becomes an irritant. Vasospasm narrows blood vessels in the brain, decreasing perfusion to the areas they supply with blood. It can occur whether or not the patient has surgery. The amount of blood in the subarachnoid space can directly affect the degree of vasospasm. Less invasive than surgery is an endovascular procedure in which a catheter is introduced through a major artery (usually the femoral artery) and guided toward the aneurysm to treat the bleed and prevent the aneurysm from rupturing (ASA, n.d.b.).

Vasospasm typically occurs in 30% to 60% of cases between postoperative days 4 and 12. The mortality rate is as high as 50%. If it is not treated rapidly, it can cause cerebral ischemia or cerebral anoxia, leading to severe mental and physical deficits or death. Any patient with subarachnoid hemorrhage should be started on the calcium channel blocker nimodipine within 96 hours of bleeding and receive it for 21 days to prevent vasospasm.

Research indicates that select patients with *acute ischemic stroke* can benefit from thrombolytics such as tissue plasminogen activator (tPA, alteplase), which digests fibrin and fibrinogen and thus lyses the clot. Because tPA is clot specific in its activation of the fibrinolytic system, it is less likely to cause hemorrhage than streptokinase or urokinase. Patients who are treated within 3 hours of the onset of symptoms are at least 30% more likely than patients who do not receive timely treatment to recover with little or no disability after 3 months (ASA, n.d.b.). Some patients may be eligible for treatment for up to 4.5 hours depending on condition related factors. Although thrombolysis improves the chances of recovery by up to 30%, only 2% to 3% of ischemic stroke patients receive it because they do not seek treatment soon enough.

Endovascular embolectomy may be performed to remove blood clots inside the brain (and can be done up to 8 hours after acute stroke onset). Using a catheter inserted into the femoral artery physicians may maneuver a device into the brain to manage the clot. Using x-ray assistance the catheter reaches the clot and it is entrapped (Fig. 14.19). Next the balloon catheter is inflated to prevent forward flow temporarily while the blood clot is withdrawn. The clot is enclosed in the balloon catheter and removed from the body. The balloon is deflated and blood flow is restored to the brain. This is an intervention that may be successful for larger clots that are not as responsive to pharmacological attempts to completely dissolve them. This procedure may be used in conjunction with tPA (Mayo Clinic, 2021c).

Patients with stroke symptoms need to be triaged, transported, and treated as rapidly as patients experiencing an acute myocardial infarction. In administration of thrombolytic drugs, the single most important factor is timing. Patients are screened carefully before treatment is initiated. This includes blood tests for coagulation disorders, recent history of gastrointestinal bleeding, and a CT or MRI scan to rule out hemorrhagic stroke. In patients with acute ischemic stroke, thrombolytic therapy increases short-term mortality, increases (but not by a statistically significant amount) symptomatic or fatal intracranial hemorrhage, decreases long-term death rate, and decreases dependence in terms of ADLs. The decision to use thrombolytic therapy should be based on a discussion of the risks and benefits with the patient and the family (Cruz-Flores, 2018). Some patients would accept a high risk of death from hemorrhage in an attempt to improve their chances of escaping permanent aphasia or dependency. Others prefer to avoid interventions that carry significant risk. Patients with stroke caused

by thrombi and emboli (ischemic strokes) also may be treated with platelet inhibitors and anticoagulants (after the first 24 hours if treated with tPA) to prevent the formation of more clots. Common anticoagulants include heparin, enoxaparin, and warfarin. Platelet inhibitors include aspirin, ticlopidine, clopidogrel, and dipyridamole.

Drugs to reduce ICP, such as dexamethasone, may be given. Suppositories such as bisacodyl generally are prescribed to be given daily or every other day. However, some health care providers order stool softeners, laxatives, or enemas.

Fluids may be restricted for the first few days after a stroke in an effort to prevent edema of the brain. The patient is fed IV fluids, or a nasogastric or gastrostomy tube may be inserted and tube feedings begun.

The length of time the patient remains in bed depends on the type of stroke suffered, deficits noted, and the health care provider's judgment regarding early mobilization. Some health care providers prescribe fairly long periods of rest after strokes, whereas others believe in early mobilization—1 or 2 days after the accident occurred.

Nursing Interventions

Carefully monitor the patient's neurologic status. The neurologic assessment includes the Glasgow Coma Scale (see Table 14.3) or the FOUR score coma scale (see Table 14.4), LOC, pupillary responses, assessment of any type of aphasia or dysarthria, vital signs, and extremity movement and strength. Interventions in the initial phase are directed toward preventing neurologic deficits and early detection of increased ICP.

Because nutrition is a concern and the patient may have difficulty swallowing at first, tube feedings and IV fluids may be necessary. See the patient problem statements and accompanying interventions to assist in feeding the patient with dysphagia.

If the patient is responsive after the onset of the stroke, help the patient assume as much self-care as possible. This includes teaching the patient one-handed dressing techniques and one-handed feeding techniques if motor deficits have occurred. It is important to reinforce teaching by other members of the patient's health team.

The patient with a stroke may be incontinent at first. Remove the urinary catheter (if there is one) as soon as possible to prevent urinary tract infection and delayed bladder retraining. Because of the lower incidence of urinary tract infections, an intermittent catheterization program may be used for patients with urinary retention. Place the patient on a bladder training program to assist in regaining continence. This usually includes taking the patient to the bathroom every few hours and encouraging fluids (at least 2000 mL/day), with the majority given between 8 a.m. and 7 p.m. Assess the patient's normal bowel pattern before the stroke and include this in the nursing care

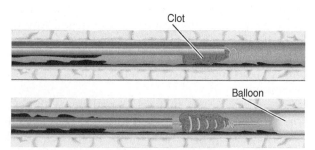

Fig. 14.19 The MERCI retriever is used to remove blood clots in patients who are experiencing ischemic stroke. (From Lewis SL, Heitkemper MM, Dirksen SR, et al: *Medical-surgical nursing: Assessment and management of clinical problems*, ed 9, St. Louis, 2014, Mosby.)

plan if possible. If the patient has difficulty with communication, a picture of a bathroom or toilet can be useful.

Return of motor impulses and movement in involved extremities occurs in stages, lasting from hours to months. Recovery also may halt at a specific stage and progress no further. Return of function is significant for functional use of extremities but also increases the possibility of contractures. Appropriate nursing interventions to prevent contractures include passive exercise, active exercise, strength building of the unaffected side, and early ambulation to promote the return of muscle function.

Patients may experience a loss of proprioception with a stroke. Neurologic deficits of apraxia and agnosia (a total or partial loss of the ability to recognize familiar objects or people) also may occur. Assist the patient with activities by repeating directions and demonstrating care. If the patient has hemianopia, which is common, approach the patient from the nonparalyzed side for care. Teach the patient to scan past midline to the side with the deficit. These patients also may fail to recognize that they have a paralyzed side. This is called *unilateral neglect* (described in the section "Sensory and Perceptual Status"). Teach the patient to inspect this side of the body for injury and to protect it from harm. These patients often show poor judgment and may move impulsively or unsafely. Observe for this and take safety precautions if needed until the patient can learn to compensate for this lack of judgment. Patients who have had a stroke may have difficulty controlling their emotions. Emotional responses may be exaggerated or unpredictable. Depression and feelings associated with changes in body image and loss of function can make this worse. Patients also may be frustrated by mobility and communication problems.

To foster the patient's self-esteem, always treat the patient as an adult, not as a child. Praise and reinforce the patient's successful efforts and gains in self-care.

Communication problems. Many stroke patients have speech problems, including dysarthria and aphasia. A speech pathologist evaluates and treats the patient with language disorders. The patient may be frustrated and should be approached in an unhurried manner. Often the patient does much better with communication when not feeling pressured to speak. Giving the patient a communication board may be helpful. The use of computers to assist with communication also may be beneficial. Wait for the patient to communicate, rather than prompting or finishing the sentence before the patient has a chance to find the appropriate word. Inability to articulate does not mean that the patient has decreased cognitive abilities.

Patient problems and interventions for the patient who has had a stroke include but are not limited to the following:

PATIENT PROBLEM	NURSING INTERVENTIONS
Compromised verbal communication, related to ischemic injury	Speak slowly and distinctly Ask questions that can be answered by yes or no (or by signals) Try to anticipate patient needs Provide a call signal within reach of the unaffected hand Begin speech therapy as soon as possible Use a communication board when necessary
Insufficient Nutrition, related to impaired ability to swallow	Provide IV fluids and tube feedings as prescribed during the initial period Request a consultation to speech therapist for assessment of swallowing problems Assess ability to swallow before initiating feedings Position patient with head elevated and turned to unaffected side during feedings Provide foods initially that are easier to swallow (soft foods, except for mashed potatoes) Thin liquids are often difficult to swallow and may promote coughing; thicken liquids with a commercially available thickening agent (e.g., Thick-It) Do not use milk products because they tend to increase the viscosity of mucus and increase salivation Use a training cup for fluids as necessary Do not use a straw Inspect mouth for food trapped in cheek pockets Be patient when feeding patient and provide directions for swallowing as needed. Ensure that meals are unrushed and nonstressful Encourage patient to feed self as soon as possible; provide self-help devices as necessary Provide scrupulous oral hygiene after meal because food may collect on the affected side of the mouth

Patient Teaching

Teaching for a patient with a stroke should include techniques to compensate for the deficits suffered as a result of the stroke. In this the nurse functions as part of the rehabilitation team. Begin rehabilitation at the time of admission to the acute care facility. The patient will probably attend occupational and physical therapy and perhaps speech therapy. Depending on the patient's status, the patient's rehabilitation potential, and available resources, the patient may be transferred to a rehabilitation facility or unit.

If the patient is receiving medications (e.g., for hypertension or anticoagulation), teach the patient and the family about side effects and the dosing schedule. Discuss plans for follow-up. Also teach the patient's family techniques to enhance safety and communication. If the patient has a problem with dysphagia, teach the family appropriate communication techniques. Because of the long-term nature of caring for the stroke patient, caregivers are at high risk for stress. Referral to an appropriate stroke support group is needed. Write instructions for the patient or the family to refer to after discharge. Most rehabilitation centers also include therapeutic leaves as a way to test the family's skills and knowledge. Each pass or leave has specific goals; obtain feedback from the family about additional teaching that may be needed. Also educate the family and the patient about perceptual problems associated with stroke and techniques to compensate for these deficits (e.g., writing down instructions for the patient who has trouble carrying out an activity alone).

Prognosis

The prognosis for patients with a stroke depends on the size of the lesion in the brain and the patient's premorbid status. More than 140,000 deaths occur in the United States each year as a result of strokes. Of those who survive, 50% to 70% are functionally independent; however, 15% to 30% have a permanent disability. The most frequent long-term disabilities include hemiparesis, inability to ambulate, aphasia, depression, and complete or partial dependence in ADLs. In the United States, the annual cost of stroke was estimated to be more than $46 billion per year (CDC, 2021). With therapy, significant functional gains can be made, even when paralysis or weakness continues. Many patients are able to return home and remain independent after a stroke. With new medical treatment for selected patients, using tPA for thrombolysis or mechanical clot removal, the prognosis is greatly improved.

CRANIAL AND PERIPHERAL NERVE DISORDERS

TRIGEMINAL NEURALGIA
Etiology and Pathophysiology

Trigeminal neuralgia is one specific kind of peripheral nerve problem. It is caused by pressure on or degeneration of the trigeminal nerve (cranial nerve V), and its cause is unknown. It is also called *tic douloureux*. It usually affects people in middle or late adulthood and is slightly more common in women. The pathophysiology is not fully understood.

Clinical Manifestations

Trigeminal neuralgia is characterized by excruciating, knife-like, or lightning-like shock in the lips, upper or lower gums, cheek, forehead, or side of the nose. The pain radiates along one or more of the three divisions of the fifth cranial nerve (Fig. 14.20). The fifth cranial nerve has motor and sensory branches. In trigeminal neuralgia the sensory (or afferent) branches, primarily the maxillary and mandibular branches, are involved. The pain typically extends only to the midline of the face and head because this is the extent of the tissue supplied by the offending nerve. The attacks are usually brief, lasting only seconds to 2 to 3 minutes, and are generally unilateral. Recurrences are unpredictable; they may occur several times a day or weeks or months apart. Areas along the course of the nerve are known as *trigger points,* and the slightest stimulation of these areas may initiate pain. People with trigeminal neuralgia try desperately to avoid triggering them. Precipitating stimuli include chewing, toothbrushing, a hot or cold blast of air on the face, washing the face, yawning, or even talking.

Medical Management

Antiseizure medications such as carbamazepine, phenytoin, valproate, gabapentin, oxcarbazepine, lamotrigine, and topiramate are the drugs used to treat trigeminal neuralgia pain. Antispasmodic, muscle-relaxing agents such as baclofen may be used alone or in combination with antiseizure medications. Absolute alcohol may be injected into the peripheral branches of the trigeminal nerve and provides relief for weeks to months by damaging the nerves, thus blocking pain signals. Biofeedback, acupuncture, and megavitamins are other therapies used.

Permanent relief of pain often is obtained by surgery, with several different options available. Options

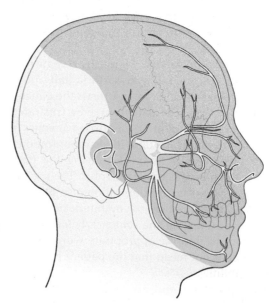

Fig. 14.20 Pathway of trigeminal nerve and facial areas innervated by each of the three main divisions of this nerve.

for surgical treatment include resecting the sensory root of the trigeminal nerve (traditional surgical method), microvascular decompression, and gamma knife radiosurgery. Discussion between the surgeon and patient, as well as patient risk factors and current condition, determines which surgical approach is the most appropriate.

Nursing Interventions
It is common for patients with trigeminal neuralgia not to have eaten properly for some time, because eating causes pain. They may be undernourished and dehydrated. They may not have washed, shaved, or combed the hair for some time. Oral hygiene often has been neglected. Measures to increase comfort for patients before surgery or for patients being treated nonsurgically are listed in Box 14.3.

Prognosis
The acute pain seldom lasts more than a few seconds or 2 or 3 minutes, but it is excruciating. The onset of pain can occur at any time during the day or night and may recur several times daily for weeks at a time. Some patients have continuous discomfort and sensitivity of the face. Although this condition is considered benign, the severity of the pain and the disruption of lifestyle can result in almost total physical and psychological dysfunction or even suicide. Permanent relief of pain frequently is obtained only by surgery.

BELL PALSY (PERIPHERAL FACIAL PARALYSIS)
Etiology and Pathophysiology
Bell palsy is thought to be caused by an inflammatory process involving the facial nerve (cranial nerve VII), anywhere from the nucleus in the brain to the

Box 14.3	**Comfort Measures for Patients With Trigeminal Neuralgia**

- Keep room free of drafts; moderate temperature.
- Avoid touching the patient's face.
- Do not urge patients to wash or shave the affected area or to comb the hair during acute attack.
- Stress the importance of hygiene, nutrition, and oral care and convey understanding if previous oral neglect is apparent.
- Provide lukewarm water and soft cloths and cotton saturated with solutions that do not require water for cleaning the face.
- A warm mouthwash or small, soft-bristled toothbrush assists in promoting oral care.
- When analgesia is at its peak, conditions are optimum for instructing in matters of hygiene. Many patients, however, prefer to execute their own care, as they fear inadvertent injury at the hands of someone else.
- Avoid hot or cold liquids, which trigger pain.
- Puree food and ensure that it is lukewarm. If necessary, suggest that food be taken through a straw.

periphery. Although the exact etiology is not known, there is evidence that viral infections such as herpes simplex, herpes zoster, Epstein-Barr, and adenovirus may be the cause. The reactivation of these viruses causes inflammation, edema, ischemia, and eventual demyelination of the facial nerve, creating pain and disturbances in motor and sensory function. Any of the three branches of the facial nerve may be affected. The disorder can be unilateral or bilateral. It can affect any age group but is more common in the 15- to 45-year-old age range and affects approximately 40,000 people each year (NINDS, 2020a).

Clinical Manifestations
With Bell palsy there is usually an abrupt onset of numbness, stiffness, or drawing sensation of the face. Unilateral weakness of the facial muscles usually occurs, resulting in a flaccidity of the affected side of the face with inability to wrinkle the forehead, close the eyelid, pucker the lips, smile, frown, whistle, or retract the mouth on that side. The face appears asymmetric, with drooping mouth and cheek. Other symptoms include loss of taste, altered chewing ability, reduction of saliva on the affected side, pain behind the ear on the affected side, and ringing in the ear or other hearing loss.

Medical Management
Bell palsy has no specific therapy. Electrical stimulation or warm moist heat along the course of the nerve may help. Stimulation may maintain muscle tone and prevent atrophy. Corticosteroids, especially prednisone, are started immediately, preferably before paralysis is complete. When the patient improves to the point that the corticosteroids are no longer necessary, they should be tapered off over a 2-week period. If HSV is implicated in a case of Bell palsy, treatment with acyclovir, alone or in conjunction with prednisone, is used. Additional antiviral agents to treat HSV, including valacyclovir and famciclovir, also have been used in the management of Bell palsy.

Nursing Interventions
Protection of the eye when the eyelid does not close is important. Eye shields used at night help prevent excessive drying and damage to the cornea. Artificial tears may be ordered and should be administered as directed. Massage of the affected areas sometimes is recommended. Active facial exercises may be prescribed for 5 minutes three times a day. These include wrinkling the brow and forehead, closing the eyes, and puffing out the cheeks.

Prognosis
Most patients recover fully within 3 to 6 months, although recovery may take as long as a year. The extent of the nerve damage generally is an indication of how long the recovery process will take. Recovery of taste

is the first sign of improvement; if it occurs within the first week, it signals a good chance for full recovery of motor function. Another favorable sign is if paralysis remains incomplete within the first 5 to 7 days. Permanent paralysis occurs only in a few cases, and rarely does the disorder recur.

INFECTION AND INFLAMMATION INDUCED PATHOLOGY

Etiology and Pathophysiology
Infection or inflammation commonly interferes with function. Some specific conditions include meningitis, encephalitis, brain abscess, Guillain-Barre syndrome (GBS), herpes zoster, neurosyphilis, poliomyelitis, and acquired immunodeficiency syndrome (AIDS). Only GBS, meningitis, encephalitis, brain abscess, and AIDS are discussed in this chapter.

The nervous system may be affected by a variety of organisms and may suffer from toxins of bacteria and viruses. These toxins reach the nervous system from a variety of sources, including adjacent bones, blood, or lymph. Meningitis can occur as a result of an invasive procedure such as surgery.

Assessment
Subjective data include a history of infection, such as an upper respiratory tract infection, and discomfort such as headache or stiff neck. The initial onset of symptoms, difficulty in thinking, and weakness may be important. Assess the patient's understanding of the condition.

Objective data include behavioral signs indicating discomfort or disorientation and an inability to carry out ADLs. Physical assessment may reveal abnormalities; fever, vomiting, abnormal CT results, seizures, altered respiratory patterns, tachycardia, or meningeal irritation. Also assess the patient's LOC and orientation.

Diagnostic Tests
Many infections of the nervous system can be diagnosed by examining the CSF. A CT scan or an EEG also may be done.

Nursing Interventions and Patient Teaching
Patient problems and interventions for the patient with an infection or inflammation are the same as those for the patient who has had a stroke, with the addition of but not limited to the following:

PATIENT PROBLEM	NURSING INTERVENTIONS
Elevated Body Temperature, related to inflammatory response to central nervous system infection	Assess temperature q 2 h and as needed Provide cooling measures as needed; avoid cooling to point of shivering
	Administer antipyretics and antibiotics as ordered
	Monitor parenteral fluids as ordered
	Control exposure to extremes in temperature
	Assess temperature, pulse, and respiration q 2 h as indicated
Recent Onset of Confusion, related to neurophysiologic response to infection	Introduce self to patient and establish rapport to prevent agitation
	Relate date, time of day, and recent activities
	Speak in kind tone, using short, simple sentences
	Maintain a therapeutic environment

Education for the patient with an infection includes teaching about the disease process, the treatments involved, and the expected outcomes. If the patient is seriously ill, the initial teaching involves the family. Other aspects of teaching for motor and sensory problems also may be relevant for the patient with an infection or inflammation, depending on the signs and symptoms demonstrated.

GUILLAIN-BARRÉ SYNDROME (POLYNEURITIS)
Etiology and Pathophysiology
Guillain-Barré syndrome (GBS) is also called *acute inflammatory polyradiculopathy* or *postinfectious polyneuritis*. It is an acute, rapidly progressing, and potentially fatal form of polyneuritis. It results in widespread inflammation and demyelination of the peripheral nervous system. The disease affects people of all ages and is seen equally in men and women and only affects 1 in 100,000 each year. The etiology is unknown, but it is thought to be an autoimmune reaction involving the peripheral nerves, most often after a respiratory or gastrointestinal viral infection. GBS rarely is seen as a result of surgery, viral immunizations, or Epstein-Barr virus (NLM, 2019b).

The peripheral nervous system is composed of 31 pairs of spinal nerves, 12 pairs of cranial nerves, and various plexuses and ganglia. Each nerve cell, or neuron, is composed of several parts, including the axon. Responsible for transmitting nerve impulses, axons are wrapped in segments of insulation called the myelin sheath, which is composed of Schwann cells (see Fig 14.1).

In GBS, the antibodies attack the Schwann cells, causing the sheath to break down (a process called *demyelination*) and the uninsulated portion of the nerve to become inflamed. Nerve conduction is interrupted, causing the classic signs of muscle weakness, tingling, and numbness. These signs begin in the legs or feet and work their way upward, perhaps because the signals to and from the legs are most vulnerable because they have to travel the longest distance. The demyelination is self-limiting. Once it stops, the Schwann cells rebuild the lost insulation. Remyelination, and therefore recovery, occurs in reverse; it starts at the top of the body and proceeds downward.

Clinical Manifestations

There is variation in the pattern of the onset of weakness and in the rate of progression of signs and symptoms. The progression may stop at any point. The patient may have difficulty swallowing, breathing, and speaking if cranial nerves VII, IX, and X are involved. Symmetric muscle weakness and lower motoneuron paralysis are present. The paralysis usually starts in the lower extremities and moves upward to include the thorax, the upper extremities, and the face. Respiratory failure may occur if the intercostal muscles are affected. Fluctuating blood pressure may occur as a result of effects on the autonomic nervous system.

Diagnostic Tests

GBS is diagnosed by elimination of other reasons for the signs and symptoms and by the characteristic muscle weakness. A CT scan may be ordered to rule out tumors or stroke. Changes in the respiratory status may aid in the diagnosis. A lumbar puncture is done. CSF in patients with GBS commonly has elevated protein levels. The health care provider may order a nerve conduction velocity study to test for slow impulse transmission. Electromyography and nerve conduction studies are markedly abnormal. A history of a recent infection is considered important.

Medical Management

Once GBS is suspected, hospitalization is essential. The patient's condition can deteriorate rapidly into paralysis that affects the respiratory muscles.

Adrenocortical steroids are used to treat the signs and symptoms of GBS. It also has been found that therapeutic plasmapheresis (the removal of unwanted or pathologic components from the patient's blood serum by means of a continuous-flow separator) in the first 2 weeks of GBS leads to decreased severity and length of symptoms. An alternative to plasmapheresis is IV immune globulin. Patients receiving high-dose immune globulin need to be well hydrated and have adequate renal function.

Patients who develop respiratory failure require mechanical ventilation and may require a tracheostomy. ABG monitoring and pulmonary function tests are used to assess the respiratory status. If the patient has severe paralysis and is expected to have a long recovery period, a gastrostomy tube may be placed to provide adequate nourishment.

Nursing Interventions

Closely monitor respiratory function. If the patient requires mechanical ventilation, be aware that cognition (the mental faculty or process by which knowledge is acquired) is not impaired and that the patient requires reassurance. The patient also may need to be fed intravenously or through a nasogastric tube. Attention to the prevention of complications, such as contractures, pressure ulcers, and loss of ROM, is important to allow complete recovery. Initiate physical therapy early in the course of the disease to prevent contractures. Administer medication, such as gabapentin or a tricyclic antidepressant such as amitriptyline, to help reduce neuropathic pain. Assess the patient's vital signs and motor strength frequently. Monitor the patient for signs of hypoxia.

Prognosis

Of the people suffering from GBS, 70% experience a full recovery. After 3 years approximately 30% report residual weakness. Long-term weakness is experienced by 15%. Post-disease reports of fatigue are common (NINDS, 2020c). The recovery period may vary from weeks to years. Those not recovering completely have some degree of permanent neurologic deficit. In general, recovery from the disease occurs in the reverse order of how the paralysis or weakness occurred. The level of supportive care received during the acute stage of the illness has a direct correlation to the recovery.

MENINGITIS

Etiology and Pathophysiology

Meningitis is an acute infection of the meninges. It often is caused by one of several bacteria, including pneumococci, meningococci, *Neisseria meningitidis*, staphylococci, streptococci, and *Haemophilus influenzae*; it also can be caused by viral agents. The bacteria cause an inflammatory reaction in the pia mater, with pus accumulation in the arachnoid space, high protein and white blood cell levels in the CSF, and possible injury to nervous tissue.

Meningitis can be classified as bacterial (septic) or viral (aseptic). The incidence of bacterial meningitis is higher in fall and winter, when upper respiratory tract infections are common. Pathologic changes that can occur include hyperemia (excess blood; engorgement) of the meningeal vessels, edema of brain tissue, increased ICP, a generalized inflammatory reaction with exudation of white blood cells into the subarachnoid spaces, and associated hydrocephalus (in infants) caused by exudate occluding the ventricles.

Clinical Manifestations

Two abnormal signs that occur with meningitis are *Kernig's sign* (the inability to extend the legs completely without extreme pain) and *Brudzinski's sign* (flexion of the hip and knee when the neck is flexed). The onset of meningitis is usually sudden and is characterized by severe headache, stiffness of the neck, irritability, malaise, and restlessness. The patient develops nausea and vomiting; delirium; and increased temperature, pulse rate, and respirations.

Diagnostic Tests

A CT of the head is ordered to rule out increased ICP. A lumbar puncture to obtain CSF is performed, unless ICP is increased. The CSF is sent to the laboratory to identify the pathogen responsible for causing the meningitis.

Medical Management

Rapid diagnosis and treatment are crucial in caring for the patient with bacterial meningitis. When meningitis is suspected, cultures are collected and diagnosis is confirmed. Treatment of meningitis includes multiple antibiotics given intravenously over a 2-week period. Medication options include ampicillin, penicillin, vancomycin, piperacillin, and third-generation cephalosporin (usually ceftriaxone [Rocephin] or cefotaxime for treating bacterial meningitis). Corticosteroids (dexamethasone) are given intravenously to decrease ICP. Anticonvulsants are given to prevent seizures. Aseptic (viral) meningitis is treated with supportive therapy, such as maintaining bed rest, ensuring fluid and electrolyte balance, and providing rest and comfort measures. Treatment with antiviral medication is debatable because the disease is usually self-limiting unless encephalitis has developed.

Nursing Interventions

Respiratory isolation is required until the pathogen can no longer be cultured from the nasopharynx. This usually is accomplished after 24 hours of effective antibiotic therapy. Other nursing interventions include the general care given a critically ill patient who may be irritable, disoriented, and unable to take fluids. Dehydration is common, generally requiring IV fluid replacement therapy. Keep the room darkened and noise to a minimum because any increase in sensory stimulation may cause a seizure. If the patient is disoriented, safety precautions should be implemented. Fever must be managed because it increases cerebral edema and the frequency of seizures. Neurologic damage may result from an extremely high temperature over a prolonged time. Acetaminophen may be used to reduce fever. On occasion, patients do not respond to acetaminophen; these patients may require the use of a cooling blanket to lower the body temperature.

Prophylactic antibiotic therapy for family and friends in close contact with a patient with bacterial meningitis may be recommended to destroy the causative bacteria that may have colonized in the nasopharynx.

Some forms of bacterial meningitis can be prevented by vaccination. The pneumococcal vaccine may be given to adults age 65 and older and other high-risk adults. The meningococcal vaccine is effective against *N. meningitidis* and is recommended for patients ages 11 to 12 and a booster given at age 16. If the primary dose was given at age 13 to 15 years the booster can be given at age 16 to 18. If the primary dose was given at age 16 or older, a booster is not necessary. The *H. influenzae* vaccine has significantly decreased meningitis caused by this organism in children (CDC, 2019).

Prognosis

With most cases of meningitis, the prognosis for complete recovery is good. The prognosis depends on the speed with which the infection is diagnosed and antibiotics are administered. With severe cases of meningitis, residual neurologic damage or death may occur.

ENCEPHALITIS

Encephalitis is an acute inflammation of the brain and usually is caused by a virus. Many different viruses have been implicated in encephalitis; some are associated with certain seasons of the year and endemic to certain geographic areas. Epidemic encephalitis is transmitted by ticks and mosquitoes. Nonepidemic encephalitis may occur as a complication of measles, chickenpox, or mumps.

Encephalitis is a serious, sometimes fatal disease. The infection affects 10,000 to 20,000 people in the United States each year. Overall mortality rate ranges from 5% to 20%, with the highest mortality rate in encephalitis caused by HSV and the eastern and Venezuelan equine viruses. Unfortunately, HSV encephalitis is the most common form of viral encephalitis. Cytomegalovirus encephalitis is a common complication in patients with AIDS.

Manifestations resemble those of meningitis, but they have a more gradual onset. They include headache, high fever, seizures, and a change in LOC. Early diagnosis and treatment of viral encephalitis are essential for favorable outcomes. Brain imaging techniques such as MRI and PET, along with viral studies of CSF, allow for earlier detection of viral encephalitis.

Medical management and nursing interventions are symptomatic and supportive. Cerebral edema is a major problem, and diuretics (mannitol) and corticosteroids (dexamethasone) are used to control it. The disease is characterized by diffuse damage to the nerve cells of the brain, perivascular cellular infiltration of glial cells, and increasing cerebral edema. The sequelae of encephalitis include mental deterioration, amnesia, personality changes, and hemiparesis.

Acyclovir and vidarabine are used to treat encephalitis caused by HSV infection. Acyclovir has fewer side effects than vidarabine and is often the preferred treatment. The mortality rate for well treated viral encephalitis is 8% (Howes, 2018). Long-term consequences include memory impairment, epilepsy, anosmia, personality changes, behavioral abnormalities, and dysphasia. For maximal benefit, antiviral agents should be started before the onset of coma.

West Nile Virus

West Nile virus (WNV) has been found commonly in humans and birds and other vertebrates in Africa, Eastern Europe, western Asia, and the Middle East, but it was not documented in the United States until 1999. The virus can infect humans, birds, mosquitoes, horses, and some other animals (CDC, 2021c).

The principal route of human infection with WNV is through the bite of an infected female mosquito. Mosquitoes become infected when they feed on infected birds. When the virus is injected into humans by a mosquito, it can multiply and possibly cause illness. The incubation period ranges from 2 to 14 days. The majority (70% to 80%) of people who become infected with the virus do not have any type of illness. Those who develop West Nile fever have flulike manifestations of fever, headache, back pain, myalgia, and anorexia, lasting only a few days and without any long-term health effects. Less than 1% of people infected with WNV develop encephalitis or meningitis. *WNV meningitis* usually is associated with a sudden onset of febrile illness, headache, chills, and neck pain. Patients with *WNV encephalitis* often have fever; headache; altered LOC; disorientation; behavioral and speech disturbances; and other neurologic signs such as hemiparesis, seizures, and coma. Even in areas where the virus is circulating, however, few mosquitoes are infected with the virus. The chances of becoming severely ill from any one mosquito bite are extremely small.

The current standard for diagnosing WNV is by testing blood or CSF with the immunoglobulin M (IgM) antibody capture enzyme-linked immunosorbent assay (ELISA) and immunoglobulin G indirect ELISA. The IgM test may not be positive when symptoms first occur; however, it becomes positive in most infected people within days of symptom onset. Someone recently vaccinated against yellow fever or Japanese encephalitis can also have a positive IgM antibody test result.

WNV cannot be transmitted through casual contact such as touching or kissing a person who has the disease. However, in a small number of cases, the virus has been transmitted through blood transfusion, organ transplantation, breast-feeding, and pregnancy (from mother to fetus).

The risk of becoming infected with WNV can be reduced by applying insect repellent to exposed skin. Choose an insect repellent that contains *N,N*-diethyl-3-methylbenzamide (DEET) and that provides protection for the amount of time to be spent outdoors. Also spray clothing because mosquitoes can bite through thin clothing. Wearing long-sleeved shirts, long pants, and socks while outdoors can reduce the risk. Take special precautions from April to October, the months when mosquitoes are most active.

DEET is the gold standard in currently available over-the-counter insect repellents. DEET was developed in 1946 by the US Army for use by military personnel in insect-infested areas. It has been used worldwide for more than 40 years and has a remarkable safety profile. Toxic reactions can occur, and they usually are linked to misuse of the product, such as massive exposure resulting from chronic use. Reports of greatest concern involve encephalopathy caused by DEET exposure. Most adverse reactions, though, are less serious, involving eye irritation and inhalation irritation (related to spraying repellent in the eyes or inhaling it).

DEET has been classified as a group D carcinogen (not classifiable as a human carcinogen). For casual use, a 10% to 35% concentration provides adequate protection. The American Academy of Pediatrics recommends limiting DEET repellents to a 30% maximum concentration when used on infants and children. The EPA states that normal use of DEET does not present a health hazard concern to the general population, including children. (U.S. Environmental Protection Agency [EPA], 2021)

Other means of decreasing the mosquito population and thus decreasing the possibility of transmission of the WNV include the following:

- Limit outdoor activities between dusk and dawn.
- Place mosquito netting over infant carriers or strollers when outdoors.
- Use mosquito repellents and wear long-sleeved shirts or pants when exposure is likely.
- Store any containers that may become filled with standing water, such as cans, flowerpots, or trash cans, indoors.
- Install or repair window and door screens so that mosquitoes cannot get indoors.

If WNV infection is confirmed, treatment is supportive, intended to manage symptoms, such as headache, fever, and nausea. In more severe cases, patients may need intensive therapy, often involving hospitalization for IV fluids, airway management, respiratory support, and prevention of secondary infections such as pneumonia. To manage WNV encephalitis, the patient may receive interferon alfa-2b, steroids, antiseizure medications, or osmotic diuretics.

Infected people have a transient viremia, making transmission of the virus via donated blood, organs, or tissue possible, but this is very rare. As with many viruses, contact with the blood of an infected person could lead to transmission of the virus; therefore use the same standard precautions as with all patients.

BRAIN ABSCESS

Brain abscess is an accumulation of pus within the brain tissue that can result from a local or a systemic infection. Direct extension from ear, tooth, mastoid, or sinus infection is the primary cause. Other causes of brain abscess formation include septic venous thrombosis from a pulmonary infection, infective endocarditis, skull fracture, and a nonsterile neurologic procedure. Streptococci and staphylococci are the primary infective organisms.

Clinical manifestations are similar to those of meningitis and encephalitis and include headache and fever. Signs of increased ICP may include drowsiness, confusion, and seizures. Focal symptoms may be present and reflect the local area of the abscess. For example, visual field deficits or psychomotor seizures are common with a temporal lobe abscess, whereas an occipital abscess may be accompanied by visual impairment and hallucinations.

Antimicrobial therapy is the primary treatment for brain abscess. Other manifestations are treated symptomatically. If drug therapy is not effective, the abscess may have to be removed if it is encapsulated. In untreated cases the mortality rate approaches 100%. Seizures occur in approximately 30% of the cases. Nursing interventions are similar to those for management of meningitis or increased ICP.

Other infections of the brain include subdural empyema, osteomyelitis of the cranial bones, epidural abscess, and venous sinus thrombosis after periorbital cellulitis.

HUMAN IMMUNODEFICIENCY VIRUS AND ACQUIRED IMMUNODEFICIENCY SYNDROME

Etiology and Pathophysiology

HIV and AIDS can have serious implications for the nervous system. Both the peripheral and CNS can be affected. More than 40% of patients with HIV infection develop some type of neurological symptoms (Krel, 2018). Patients develop neurologic signs and symptoms either from infection with HIV or as a result of associated infections. See Chapter 16 for a discussion of advanced HIV and AIDS.

Clinical Manifestations

Patients with AIDS may have AIDS dementia complex (ADC), which originally was known as subacute encephalitis (Kopstein, 2020). They may exhibit difficulty concentrating or a recent memory loss, which may progress to a **global cognitive dysfunction** (generalized impairment of intellect, awareness, and judgment). Patients also may experience opportunistic infections such as meningitis, HSV, cytomegalovirus, toxoplasmosis, and cryptococcal meningitis. Primary malignant lymphomas of the CNS also may develop.

Diagnostic Tests

The diagnostic tests used to determine whether a neurologic problem is related to AIDS include serologic studies, analysis of CSF through a lumbar puncture, CT scan, and MRI. At times, a cerebral biopsy may be necessary to make the differential diagnosis.

Medical Management

Treatment of the patient with neurologic problems related to AIDS depends on the infection. Methods of treatment include administration of antiviral, antifungal, and antibacterial agents. Antiretroviral therapy (ART) and highly active retroviral therapy (HART) have helped in decreasing neurologic problems. Seizures are sometimes noted when the brain is affected. Seizures are controlled with diazepam, phenytoin, or fosphenytoin.

Nursing Interventions

The patient is likely to be disoriented and may need to be reoriented frequently. Safety measures such as padded side rails may be necessary to prevent injury to the patient, who may have seizures. The patient may experience pain and have difficulty sleeping. Administer medications as needed and structure activities to avoid waking the patient. Visual problems also may be associated with the disease; be careful to orient the patient to nursing interventions.

Most patients with AIDS experience depression and a sense of powerlessness about the disease. They may isolate themselves from others. Encourage patients to talk about their fears and concerns, help them find emotional support, and refer them to a support group. Above all, maintain a nonjudgmental attitude, regardless of how the patient contracted the disease.

The patient may be incontinent of bowel and bladder. Encourage an active bowel and bladder program. If the patient has diarrhea, keep the rectal area as clean and dry as possible and administer antidiarrheals if ordered. The patient also may have nausea. Offer foods that the patient likes in small, frequent meals. Tube feedings or total parenteral nutrition may be needed if the patient agrees.

Prognosis

The prognosis for the patient with AIDS and consequential neurological complications has been much improved over the years due to treatment with ART and HART. Patients live many years with no complications because of these treatments. Mean survival in advanced neurological complications without the use of ART is 3 to 6 months. With the use of ART and HART the mean survival rate is that of the general HIV-affected population (Kopstein, 2020).

BRAIN TUMORS

Etiology and Pathophysiology

Brain tumors may be primary to the brain or be the result of metastases from another location. There are more than 150 different types of brain tumors. All areas and structures of the brain can be affected. Tumors may be benign or cancerous. The majority of tumors are benign and not primary to the brain. It is estimated that there are more than 700,000 people living with a brain tumor and another 80,000 will be diagnosed in 2018 (American Brain Tumor Association, n.d.). A primary brain tumor, or **neoplasm** (any abnormal benign or malignant mass), originates from the tissues of the brain and forms when changes occur in the genetic structure of normal brain cells (neurons and glial cells). Changes may be caused by a genetic predisposition, an environmental trigger, or both; the causes of most primary brain tumors are unknown. Most benign tumors affect the meninges, whereas most malignant tumors (78%) are gliomas. These tumors develop from the supporting cells of the brain, which are referred to as *glia*. Benign tumors include meningiomas and pituitary adenomas. Metastatic brain tumors occur in an estimated one in four patients with cancer. Brain tumors are named for the tissues from which they arise.

Assessment

Subjective data include the patient's understanding of the diagnosis, changes in personality or judgment, and abnormal sensations or visual problems. The patient may complain of unusual odors with tumors of the temporal lobe. The patient may report difficulty with the ability to think, speak, or articulate words. Patients with brain tumors usually experience headaches as a prominent early symptom. The headache is typically more severe in the morning. Loss of balance and dizziness are common complaints. The patient also may experience paresis (weakness) and vision changes.

Objective data include motor strength, gait, the level of alertness and consciousness, and orientation. Assess the pupils for response and equality. In some patients, the initial sign of a brain tumor is new-onset seizures. Seizure activity commonly occurs at some time among patients with brain tumors. Cognitive changes in memory, speech, concentration, and communication are also common. The patient's family may report a change in the patient's personality. Speech impairments, cranial nerve abnormalities, and signs and symptoms of increased ICP are also significant.

Diagnostic Tests

No one procedure is entirely diagnostic of brain tumors, but a CT scan is often the basis for the diagnosis. Other tests that may be performed include the brain scan, MRI, PET scans, and the EEG. Arteriography, as well as a biopsy, also may be done.

Medical Management

The general method of treatment for brain tumors includes surgical removal when feasible, radiation, and chemotherapy. The choice of therapy depends on the tumor type and where it is located. A combination of methods often is used. The blood-brain barrier may limit the effectiveness of chemotherapy when used as adjuvant therapy or to treat tumor recurrence.

Surgery. A surgical opening through the skull is called a *craniotomy*. After removing the bone, the surgeon makes an incision into the meninges and removes the tumor. The removed bone is preserved carefully and may be replaced at the end of surgery if there is no indication of infection or increased ICP. Sometimes the bone cannot be returned; the removal of part of the skull without replacement is called a *craniectomy*. Before the craniotomy/craniectomy

a less invasive procedure, a stereotactic biopsy, may be performed to obtain a sample of the tumor tissue. It involves drilling a small hole through the patient's skull, after which the tumor biopsy is obtained.

Brain tumor surgery has become increasingly successful because of computerized devices called *surgical navigation systems.* These systems help pinpoint tumors and guide the neurosurgeon during the surgery. Tumors that once were considered inoperable now can be removed because their location can be mapped accurately by a surgical navigation system.

Nursing Interventions

Preoperative preparation of the patient and the family is important. Specific fears may be related to a permanent change in appearance, dependency, and possible death. A baseline neurologic assessment is important. Explain treatments and procedures, including shaving the hair. Usually, hair is shaved in the operating room. Prepare the family for the patient's appearance after surgery.

Postoperative care depends on the patient's condition. Most patients spend one or two nights in an intensive care unit under close nursing observation with frequent neurologic checks. Assess the patient carefully for indications of increased ICP. The patient may have residual motor or sensory problems as a result of the tumor or surgery. A ventriculoperitoneal shunt (i.e., a catheter draining excess fluid from the brain to the abdomen) may be inserted if increased ICP is an issue.

Patient problems and interventions for the patient with a brain tumor are the same as those for the patient who has had a stroke, with the addition of but not limited to the following:

PATIENT PROBLEM	NURSING INTERVENTIONS
Impaired Neurovascular Function, Visual, auditory, kinesthetic, tactile, related to compression or displacement of brain tissue	Maintain method of communication Provide for social environment Provide orientation and appropriate level of stimuli
Recent Onset of Confusion, related to: • Altered circulation • Destruction of brain tissue	Protect patient from self-injury Provide soft safety reminder devices as indicated Assist patient in self-care activities Speak in kind tone, using short, simple sentences Give one direction at a time Relate date, time of day, and recent activities Maintain a therapeutic environment Keep equipment and personal possessions in same place Encourage socialization

Prognosis

The outlook for the patient with a brain tumor depends on whether the tumor is benign or malignant and on its size and location. In the past, the diagnosis of a brain tumor had a very high mortality rate within weeks of the diagnosis. Better diagnostic tools and new treatment modalities have increased the life span and quality of life for many patients with primary and metastatic brain tumors. The life span for many patients diagnosed with a brain tumor is now years rather than weeks.

TRAUMA

Interference with neurologic function can occur as a result of trauma. Parts of the nervous system commonly subjected to trauma include the brain, the spinal cord, and peripheral nerves. Only the first two are discussed in this chapter.

HEAD INJURY OR TRAUMATIC BRAIN INJURY

Etiology and Pathophysiology

The term *head trauma* is used primarily to signify craniocerebral trauma, or head injury, which includes an alteration in consciousness, no matter how brief. The current term used most often for a head injury is TBI. In the United States, an estimated 2.8 million head injuries occur annually, with 837,000 being children. These injuries account for more than 30% of all injury-related deaths in the United States. The most common causes of TBI in the United States are falls and motor vehicle collisions. Almost 50% of emergency department (ED) visits due to TBI is due to falls in the 0- to 17-year age group and 81% in the 65 years and older category. Falls and motor vehicle crashes were the first and second leading causes of all TBI-related hospitalizations (52% and 20%, respectively), while intentional self-harm accounts for 33% of TBIs. Head injury can result from recreational activities, sports-related trauma, and assaults (CDC, 2021b).

Craniocerebral trauma may result in injury to the scalp, skull, and brain tissues. Injuries vary from minor scalp wounds to concussions and open fractures of the skull with severe damage to the brain. The amount of obvious damage is not indicative of the seriousness of the trouble. Effects of severe head injury include cerebral edema, sensory and motor deficits, and increased ICP.

Injuries to the brain can result from direct or indirect trauma to the head. Indirect trauma is caused by tension strains and shearing forces transmitted to the head by stretching the neck. Direct trauma occurs when the head is directly injured. Indirect trauma results in an *acceleration-deceleration* injury, with rotation of the skull and its contents. Bruising or contusion of the occipital and frontal lobes, the brainstem, and the cerebellum may occur.

Clinical Manifestations

Head injuries may be open or closed. Open head injuries result from skull fractures or penetrating wounds. The amount of injury with this type of wound is determined by the velocity, mass, shape, and direction of the impact. A skull fracture (linear, comminuted, depressed, or compound) also may occur. Fractures of the base of the skull are more serious because they are near the medulla.

Closed head injuries include concussions (a violent jarring of the brain against the skull), contusions, and lacerations. Lacerations of the scalp bleed profusely because of the extensive vascularity in the region. Hemorrhage resulting from craniocerebral trauma may occur in the scalp or in the epidural, subdural, intracerebral, and intraventricular areas. Epidural and subdural hematomas require careful and continuous observation. Epidural hematomas resulting from arterial bleeding form as blood collects rapidly between the dura mater and skull. If lethargy or unconsciousness develops after the patient regains consciousness, an epidural hematoma may be suspected and needs immediate treatment.

A subdural hematoma forms as venous blood collects below the dura. Because the bleeding is under venous pressure, subdural hematoma formation is relatively slow. The clot causes pressure on the brain surface and displaces brain tissue. If a patient who has been conscious for several days after head injury loses consciousness or develops neurologic signs and symptoms, suspect a subdural hematoma. Subdural hematomas may be classified as acute, subacute, or chronic.

Assessment

Subjective data include the patient's understanding of the injury and the resulting pathologic processes. Determine how the injury happened and whether the patient has headache, nausea, or vomiting. Note abnormal sensations and a history of loss of consciousness and of bleeding from any orifice.

Objective data include the status of the respiratory system, level of alertness and consciousness, and size and reactivity of the pupils; check these frequently. Also assess the patient's orientation, motor status, vital signs, bleeding or vomiting, and abnormal speech patterns. The presence of *Battle's sign* (ecchymosis [a small hemorrhagic spot] behind the ear) usually indicates fracture of a bone of the lower skull (Fig. 14.21).

Diagnostic Tests

CT, MRI, and PET scans are the primary diagnostic imaging examinations in assessing soft tissue injuries.

Medical Management

Immediate care of the patient with a head injury is directed toward lifesaving measures and the maintenance of normal body function until recovery is ensured. It is extremely important to maintain a patent

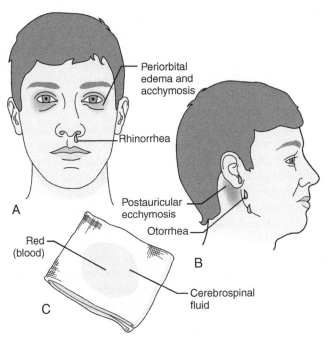

Fig. 14.21 (A) "Raccoon eyes" and rhinorrhea (nasal discharge). (B) Battle's sign (postauricular ecchymosis) with otorrhea (discharge from the ear). © Halo or ring sign.

airway and ensure adequate oxygenation. Suctioning may be necessary (but never through the nose because of the possibility of a skull fracture), along with the administration of oxygen. Check ABG levels. Stabilize the cervical spine; assume neck injury with head injury until diagnostic examination proves otherwise.

Medications are used to reduce cerebral edema and increased ICP, which are common problems in patients with head injuries. Medications include mannitol and dexamethasone. Codeine or other analgesics that do not depress the respiratory system are used for pain control. Anticonvulsants may be given to prevent seizures. Take measures to control elevated temperatures, because hyperthermia increases brain metabolism, resulting in brain damage.

Nursing Interventions
Check the patient's ears and nose carefully for signs of blood and serous drainage, which indicate that the meninges are torn and spinal fluid is escaping. *Do not attempt to clean out the orifice.* If there is evidence of drainage from the nose, the patient should not cough, sneeze, or blow the nose. If there is a question about whether the drainage is CSF, a glucose test strip (e.g., Tes-Tape) will show a positive reaction for glucose. Meningitis is a possible complication when communication with the meninges and the nose or ears occurs.

The patient with a head injury often shows a loss of memory and loss of initiative. Behavioral problems associated with a lack of judgment and restlessness also may occur. Restlessness may be caused by the need for a change of position, pain, or the need to empty the bladder. These patients require firm but gentle care, with specific guidelines for what behavior is allowed.

Medications to decrease agitation may be needed. It is not helpful to argue with patients but redirecting their attention may help. Memory aids such as a logbook or written schedule can assist with orientation.

The length of convalescence depends on the amount of brain damage and how rapid the recovery is. Many patients with head injury recover physically but have behavioral and psychological problems that make it difficult for them to function independently.

Patient problems and interventions for the patient with a head injury are the same as for the patient who has had a stroke, with the addition of but not limited to the following:

PATIENT PROBLEM	NURSING INTERVENTIONS
Compromised Social Interaction, related to cognitive and affective deficits from neurophysiologic trauma	Encourage and support verbalization about feelings, medical conditions, and current treatment; listen nonjudgmentally
	Build trust through consistency and kept promises
	Involve patient in care plan
	Give full attention to patient during verbal interactions and recognize qualities to promote self-esteem

Patient Teaching
A patient with a mild head injury may be seen in the ED but not be admitted to the hospital. Teach the patient about observations for complications such as increased drowsiness, nausea, vomiting, worsening headache or stiff neck, seizures, blurred vision, behavioral changes, motor problems, sensory disturbances, or decreased heart rate. Teaching for patients with a head injury who have residual deficits severe enough to require rehabilitation is similar to that needed for patients with motor or sensory problems.

Prognosis
The outcome for a patient with a head injury is often unpredictable. The extent of damage or recovery is not positively correlated with the amount of damage seen in surgery or on CT scan. Even minor head injuries can have residual effects. The person with a head injury is more prone to injuries and problems related to the brain damage (Newsome Melton, n.d.). Personality changes may result after a head injury. These changes may be short term or permanent. These changes may include depression, mood swings, confusion, anger, and social inappropriateness. Rehabilitation centers for TBIs are increasing in number and positive outcomes are greatly impacted

for patients receiving intense inpatient therapy in these facilities.

SPINAL CORD TRAUMA

Etiology and Pathophysiology

Spinal cord injury from accidents is a common and increasing cause of serious disability and death. There are currently 294,000 Americans living with SCI, and 17,810 new cases occur each year. Spinal cord injuries affect males significantly more than women: nearly 80% of injuries involve men, with the average age being 43 years of age. Automobile accidents are the most common cause, followed by falls, violence (mostly gunshot wounds), and sports or recreational activities respectively (United Spinal Association, 2020).

The soft tissue of the spinal cord is protected by the vertebral column. Injuries to this column include a simple fracture, compressed or wedge fracture, comminuted or burst fracture, or dislocation of the vertebrae (Fig. 14.22). As a result, the cord is often damaged. Severe traumatic lesions of the spinal cord may result in total transection of the spinal cord or tearing of the cord from side to side at a particular level, with a complete loss of spinal cord function. This total transection is also called a *complete cord injury.* With this type of injury, all voluntary movement below the level of the trauma is lost. A partial transection, or *incomplete injury,* of the cord also may occur. Tetraplegic patients (formerly referred to as quadriplegic) are those who sustain injuries to one of the cervical segments of the spinal cord. Paraplegic patients are those whose lesions are confined to the thoracic, lumbar, or sacral segments of the spinal cord. The signs and symptoms of an incomplete spinal injury vary (Table 14.8).

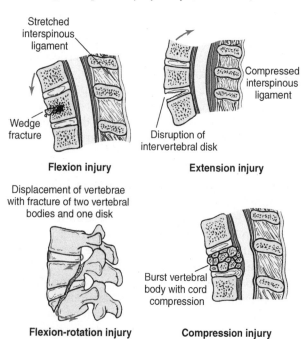

Fig. 14.22 Mechanisms of spinal injury. (From Lewis SL, Heitkemper MM, Dirksen SR, et al: *Medical-surgical nursing: Assessment and management of clinical problems,* ed 7, St. Louis, 2007, Mosby.)

Clinical Manifestations

Initially, in most spinal cord injuries, there is a period of flaccid paralysis and a complete loss of reflexes below the level of trauma. Sensory and autonomic functions are also lost. The loss of systemic sympathetic vasomotor tone may result in vasodilation, increased venous capacity, and hypotension. This is called *areflexia,* or spinal shock, and is temporary. During this time the patient may need temporary respiratory support.

One important complication of spinal cord injury is autonomic dysreflexia or hyperreflexia, a neurologic condition characterized by increased reflex actions. It occurs in patients with cord injuries at the sixth thoracic vertebra or higher and most commonly in patients with cervical injuries. Autonomic dysreflexia is an abnormal cardiovascular response to stimulation of the sympathetic division of the autonomic nervous system; the condition occurs as a result of stimulation of the bladder, large intestine, or other visceral organs (Fig. 14.23). The clinical signs include severe bradycardia, hypertension (systolic blood pressure up to 300 mm Hg), diaphoresis, "goose flesh," flushing (above the level of the lesion), dilated pupils, blurred vision, restlessness, nausea, severe headache, and nasal stuffiness. Patients tend to develop individual signs and symptoms of this condition and are soon able to recognize them. The most common causes of this condition include a distended bladder or a fecal impaction. It is a medical emergency that requires immediate treatment to prevent a stroke, blindness, or death (Box 14.4).

In most cases of spinal cord injury, men experience impotence, decreased sensation, and difficulties with ejaculation. Impaired fertility is common. The experience of orgasm is described as different than before the injury. Women with spinal cord injury are able to continue to perform sexually, although perception of sexual pleasure usually is altered.

Assessment

Subjective data include information about the nature of the injury, any dyspnea, and unusual sensations. The presence of pain, any loss of consciousness, and the absence of sensation on sensory examination are important to assess.

Objective data include the level of alertness and consciousness; orientation; pupil size and reactivity; motor strength; skin integrity; and bowel and bladder status, including distention. Assess for other injuries, such as fractured bones or head injury.

Diagnostic Tests

Radiographs often are taken first to detect any cervical vertebral fracture or displacement. A spinal tap or myelogram also may be done to detect occlusion. A CT scan and MRI may help rule out spinal cord injury.

Medical Management

Immediate care after spinal cord injury is directed toward realignment of the bony column in the presence

Table 14.8 Functional Level of Spinal Cord Injury and Rehabilitation Potential

LEVEL OF INJURY	MOVEMENT REMAINING	REHABILITATION POTENTIAL
Tetraplegia		
C1–C3 Often fatal injury, vagus nerve domination of heart, respiration, blood vessels, and all organs below injury	Movement in neck and above, loss of innervation to diaphragm, absence of independent respiratory function	Ability to drive electric wheelchair equipped with portable ventilator by using chin control or mouth stick, headrest to stabilize head; computer use with mouth stick, head wand, or noise control; 24-h attendant care, able to instruct others
C4 Vagus nerve domination of heart, respirations, and all vessels and organs below injury	Sensation and movement in neck and above; may be able to breathe without a ventilator	Same as C1–C3
C5 Vagus nerve domination of heart, respirations, and all vessels and organs below injury	Full neck, partial shoulder, back, biceps; gross elbow, inability to roll over or use hands; decreased respiratory reserve	Ability to drive electric wheelchair with mobile hand supports; indoor mobility in manual wheelchair; able to feed self with set-up and adaptive equipment; attendant care 10 h/day
C6 Vagus nerve domination of heart, respirations, and all vessels and organs below injury	Shoulder and upper back abduction and rotation at shoulder, full biceps to elbow flexion, wrist extension, weak grasp of thumb, decreased respiratory reserve	Ability to assist with transfer and perform some self-care; feed self with hand devices; push wheelchair on smooth, flat surface; drive adapted van from wheelchair; independent computer use with adaptive equipment; attendant care 6 h/day
C7–C8 Vagus nerve domination of heart, respirations, and all vessels and organs below injury	All triceps to elbow extension, finger extensors and flexors, good grasp with some decreased strength, decreased respiratory reserve	Ability to transfer self to wheelchair; roll over and sit up in bed; push self on most surfaces; perform most self-care; independent use of wheelchair; ability to drive car with powered hand controls (in some patients); attendant care 0–6 h/day
Paraplegia		
T1–T6 Sympathetic innervation to heart, vagus nerve domination of all vessels and organs below injury	Full innervation of upper extremities, back, essential intrinsic muscles of hand; full strength and dexterity of grasp; decreased trunk stability, decreased respiratory reserve	Full independence in self-care and in wheelchair; ability to drive car with hand controls (in most patients); independent standing in standing frame
T7–T12 Vagus nerve domination only of leg vessels, GI and genitourinary organs	Full, stable thoracic muscles and upper back; functional intercostals, resulting in increased respiratory reserve	Full independent use of wheelchair; ability to stand erect with full leg brace, ambulate on crutches with swing (although gait difficult); inability to climb stairs
L1–L2 Vagus nerve domination of leg vessels	Varying control of legs and pelvis, instability of lower back	Good sitting balance; full use of wheelchair; ambulation with long leg braces
L3–L4 Partial vagus nerve domination of leg vessels, GI and genitourinary organs	Quadriceps and hip flexors, absence of hamstring function, flail ankles	Completely independent ambulation with short leg braces and canes; inability to stand for long periods

GI, Gastrointestinal.
From Lewis SL, Dirksen SR, Heitkemper MM, et al: *Medical-surgical nursing: Assessment and management of clinical problems,* ed 8, St. Louis, 2011, Mosby.

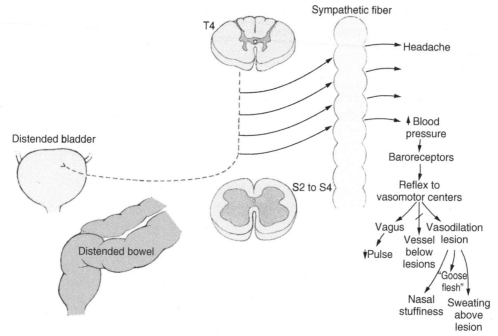

Fig. 14.23 Pictorial diagram of cause of autonomic hyperreflexia (dysreflexia) and results. (From Monahan FD, Sands JK, Neighbors M, et al: *Phipps' medical-surgical nursing: Health and illness perspectives*, ed 8, St. Louis, 2007, Mosby.)

of fractures or dislocations. This may involve simple immobilization, skeletal traction, or surgery for spinal decompression. Skeletal traction may include Crutchfield tongs (Fig. 14.24), halo traction, or a Stryker or Foster frame. Bracing may be used for thoracic or lumbar injuries. Often surgical decompression is not performed until after a period of skeletal traction if the injury involves the cervical region. In patients seen within 8 hours of injury, high-dose methylprednisolone is given.

Nursing Interventions and Patient Teaching

Throughout all stages of hospitalization of the patient with a spinal cord injury, nursing and medical interventions are directed toward restoring structural or body integrity. All efforts are taken to ensure that the skin is intact, that contractures do not develop, and that ROM is maintained. Early mobilization is important. When patients, especially those with tetraplegia, begin to sit up, it may be necessary to wrap the legs with thromboembolism stockings to encourage venous return. Slowly increasing the angle of sitting up is essential to prevent hypotension. A recliner wheelchair is usually necessary.

Usually, an indwelling catheter is inserted initially; later bladder training is started (see Chapter 10). Chronic indwelling catheterization increases the risk of infection. Intermittent catheterization should begin as early as possible. This helps maintain bladder tone and decreases the risk of infection. Encourage fluid intake of more than 2000 mL/day. Encourage cranberry juice to decrease renal calculus (kidney stone) formation.

Box 14.4	**Emergency Care for Autonomic Dysreflexia or Hyperreflexia**

- Unless contraindicated, place patient in sitting position to decrease blood pressure.
- Check patency of catheter for kinking. If catheter is occluded, insert new catheter immediately.
- Check rectum for impaction.
- If it is necessary to remove impaction, use an anesthetic ointment.
- Administer ganglionic blocking agent such as hexamethonium or a vasodilator such as nitroprusside (Nipride) as ordered if conservative measures are not effective.
- Continue monitoring blood pressure.
- Send urine for culture if no other cause is found; urinary tract infection can lead to symptoms of autonomic dysreflexia.

Patients usually are started on a bowel program early in their hospital stay. At first, bisacodyl suppositories are given at regular intervals (usually every other night). This is followed by digital stimulation to promote peristalsis. The goal is to eliminate the need for suppositories. Other aids to bowel programs are the use of adequate fluids (usually at least 3000 to 4000 mL/day, unless contraindicated), stool softeners, and prune juice.

Patient problems and interventions for the patient with a spinal cord injury are the same as those for the patient with a motor or sensory problem, with the addition of but not limited to the following:

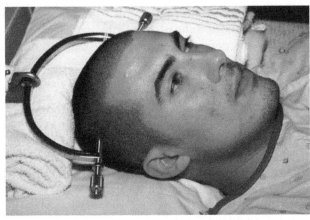

Fig. 14.24 Patient with Crutchfield tongs inserted into skull to hyperextend. (Courtesy Michael S. Clement, MD, Mesa, AZ.)

PATIENT PROBLEM	NURSING INTERVENTIONS
Impaired Neurovascular Function, related to neurophysiologic trauma to spinal cord above sixth thoracic vertebra	See Box 14.4 for emergency interventions
Alteration in Urinary Elimination, related to sensory-motor impairment	Check carefully for voiding and for distention of bladder
	Teach patient intermittent self-catheterization if indicated
	Teach patient Credé's maneuver as indicated
	Insert an indwelling catheter if ordered; administer meticulous aseptic technique in changing catheters
	Teach patient signs of infection
	Encourage patient to have a genitourinary checkup at least yearly
	Maintain fluid intake of 3000–4000 mL/day unless contraindicated
	Use adult perineal protector for incontinency, if necessary

Teaching of the patient with a spinal cord injury includes education about autonomic dysreflexia and about sexual functioning after spinal cord injury. Other teaching points are found in the sections of this chapter dealing with the patient with motor or sensory problems.

Prognosis

In cases of complete spinal cord injury, there is little chance for return of function. However, the paraplegic or tetraplegic patient can live a satisfying life with adaptations and assistance. Today, with improved treatment strategies, especially advancements in physical and occupational therapy, the outlook for many spinal cord injury patients is much improved. As with TBIs, the number of inpatient rehabilitation facilities has increased over the years and therapies have greatly improved. Care should be taken to prevent infections, such as urinary tract or respiratory tract infections, since infections are a leading cause of death in spinal cord injury patients. In patients with incomplete cord lesions, the amount of function regained is variable and often unpredictable. Recovery attained within the first 6 months is often a good indication of how complete recovery will be.

❖ NURSING PROCESS FOR THE PATIENT WITH A NEUROLOGIC DISORDER

The role of the licensed practical nurse/licensed vocational nurse (LPN/LVN) in the nursing process as stated is that the LPN/LVN will:
- Participate in planning care for patients based on patient needs
- Review patient's plan of care and recommend revisions as needed
- Review and follow defined prioritization for patient care
- Use clinical pathways, care maps, or care plans to guide and review patient care

◆ ASSESSMENT

People with neurologic deficits require skilled assessment by a nurse and a health care provider. Assessment includes observing the patient during the patient history. Nursing assessment is an ongoing process and should be tailored to meet the patient's needs. For example, hourly neurologic checks will not be as detailed as the initial assessment.

While interviewing the patient, obtain data about subjective complaints, such as pain, dizziness, or vision difficulties. Also assess the ability to speak and reason. Observations may also include vital signs, data about gait, symmetry of body parts, evidence of pain, or seizure activity. During ongoing assessments, data usually are obtained about pupil size, level of alertness, ability to perform motor tasks, changes in LOC, and ability to speak. Because subtle changes in neurologic status often can be the first sign of a complication, be alert for small changes in the neurologic assessment and report these to the proper person.

◆ PATIENT PROBLEM

Nursing assessment helps identify the patient's needs for care and observation. The actual care of the patient then is based on the patient problems that have been identified. Possible patient problems for a patient with a neurologic disorder include but are not limited to the following:
- *Compromised Blood Flow to Tissue*
- *Compromised Physical Mobility*
- *Compromised Swallowing Ability*

- *Compromised Verbal Communication*
- *Grief*
- *Impaired Family Coping*
- *Impaired Neurovascular Dysfunction*
- *Inability to Bathe Self*
- *Inability to Feed Self*
- *Inability to Toilet Self*
- *Insufficient Knowledge*
- *Insufficient Nutrition*
- *Potential for Contractures or Muscle Atrophy*
- *Potential for Falling*
- *Potential for Infection*
- *Prolonged Pain*
- *Recent Onset of Confusion*
- *Recent Onset of Pain*
- *Slow or Delayed Ability to Remember*

◆ EXPECTED OUTCOMES AND PLANNING

The plan for providing neurologic assessment and care should focus on the type of deficit the patient is experiencing and possible complications. Consider a patient's preferences and mental status. The type of care required determines the supplies and equipment needed. Schedule necessary care around tests and procedures and the patient's need for rest.

The care plan focuses on achieving specific goals and outcomes that relate to the identified patient problem. Examples of these include the following:

Goal 1: Patient's cerebral perfusion will be maintained.
Outcome: Patient remains awake, alert, and oriented; coma scale score remains the same or improves.
Goal 2: Patient will maintain optimal nutrition.
Outcome: Patient maintains or attains optimal weight, and laboratory values indicating nutritional health are within normal limits.

◆ IMPLEMENTATION

Nursing interventions for the patient with a neurologic disorder include those that maintain cerebral perfusion and other functioning, as well as those that prevent complications such as skin breakdown, falls, or contractures. Certain principles guide nurses in providing neurologic care:

- The neurologic system is a complex system that produces a wide variety of neurologic signs and symptoms.

- Identical disorders may result in different sets of signs and symptoms in different patients.
- The maintenance of cerebral perfusion is of utmost importance.
- The patient with a neurologic illness is prone to complications.
- Disorders of the nervous system produce physical problems and a wide variety of cognitive difficulties.

While providing care to meet the patient's specific challenges, also assess the patient's readiness to learn. At times the family must receive the primary teaching because the patient is unable to understand. Consider the patient's preferences and background in delivering care. Encourage the patient to be as independent as possible and give appropriate feedback. Preserve the patient's dignity and privacy whenever possible. Also consider the special needs of older patients (see the Lifespan Considerations box in the section "Effects of Normal Aging on the Nervous System").

◆ EVALUATION

Evaluate the success of planned interventions during and after care is given. The process is ongoing and dynamic because the patient's condition often changes. Always be ready to revise the care plan as needed. For example, if a patient has new episodes of confusion after surgery, notify the health care provider, increase safety measures, and assess more frequently.

Ongoing systematic evaluation requires determining whether specific outcomes have been met. The evaluation is specific to measure the goals identified. Examples of goals and their corresponding evaluative measures include the following:

Goal 1: Patient will be free of infection.
Evaluative measure: Assess patient for any signs of infection such as increased temperature, frequency of urination, erythematous incision, elevated white blood cell count, or confusion.
Goal 2: Patient will remain alert and oriented in thought processes.
Evaluative measure: Ask patient to respond to orientation questions. Observe ability to engage in conversation and to carry out care activities.

Get Ready for the NCLEX® Examination!

Key Points

- The nervous system is the body's link with the environment. It allows the interpretation of information and appropriate action.
- The two main structural divisions of the nervous system are the CNS and the peripheral nervous system.

- The CNS is composed of the brain and the spinal cord.
- The peripheral nervous system is composed of the nerve cells lying outside of the CNS. It is divided into the somatic nervous system and the autonomic nervous system.
- A nerve cell is composed of three parts: the dendrites, the cell body, and the axon.

- The brain and the spinal cord are protected by the bony coverings (skull and vertebral column), the CSF, and the three meninges (pia mater, arachnoid mater, and dura mater).
- The cerebrum is the largest part of the brain and contains five major areas: motor, sensory, visual, speech, and auditory. The cerebrum governs the ability to reason and make judgments.
- The diencephalon lies beneath the cerebrum and contains the thalamus and hypothalamus. The thalamus serves as a relay station. The hypothalamus has several roles, such as temperature control, water balance, and appetite.
- The cerebellum is the second largest portion of the brain and is responsible for coordination of skeletal muscles and maintenance of balance and equilibrium.
- The peripheral nervous system is composed of the cranial nerves, the spinal nerves, the somatic nervous system, and the autonomic nervous system.
- The autonomic nervous system contains two subdivisions: the sympathetic nervous system and the parasympathetic nervous system. The sympathetic nervous system speeds things up, and the parasympathetic nervous system slows things down.
- Normal changes of aging are not the same as senility, AD, or organic brain damage.
- The source of prolonged or unusual headaches should be determined through neurologic testing because it may be a symptom of a serious pathologic condition.
- A lumbar puncture should not be done if there is evidence of increased ICP because of the danger of brain herniation.
- Any increase in the volume of one of the contents of the cranium (brain, blood vessels, and CSF) results in increased ICP because the cranial vault is rigid and does not expand.
- Classic signs of increased ICP include restlessness, disorientation, headache, contralateral hemiparesis, an ipsilaterally dilated pupil, and visual changes that include blurring and diplopia.
- Nursing intervention measures can significantly influence ICP.
- Epilepsy is a transitory disturbance in consciousness or in motor, sensory, or autonomic functions with or without loss of consciousness, caused by sudden, excessive, and disorderly electrical discharges of the brain.
- Early signs and symptoms of MS are usually transitory.
- Stroke, or "brain attack," is the most common disease of the nervous system and can be caused by thrombus, embolus, or hemorrhage. The term *brain attack* is used to describe stroke and communicates the urgency of recognizing stroke signs and symptoms and treating their onset as a medical emergency, just as one would with a myocardial infarction.
- The MERCI device, a blood clot remover, can be used for up to 8 hours after acute stroke onset to remove blood clots from arteries deep inside the brain.
- Helpful nursing interventions for the patient with AD include using nonverbal cues or demonstrations as adjuncts to verbal cues, providing few choices, and not hurrying the patient.
- Trigeminal neuralgia (tic douloureux) is characterized by excruciating, burning pain that radiates along one or more of the three divisions of the fifth cranial nerve.

- With Bell palsy, there is usually an abrupt onset of numbness, a feeling of stiffness, or a drawing sensation of the face.
- Of the people suffering from GBS, 85% regain complete function.
- A majority of patients with advanced HIV disease and AIDS have neurologic symptoms that result from infection with HIV itself or from associated complications of the disease.
- Many patients with head injury may recover physically, but they will have behavioral and psychological problems that make it difficult for them to function independently.
- The signs and symptoms of intracranial tumors result from both local and general effects of the tumor.
- Autonomic dysreflexia in the patient with spinal cord injury is a medical emergency that demands quick nursing interventions.
- The first sign of increased ICP may be a declining state of consciousness.
- It is important to document patients' behaviors in terms of what is seen, not what is inferred.
- It is estimated that less than 1% of people infected with WNV will develop encephalitis or meningitis, a more severe form of the disease.

Additional Learning Resources

SG Go to your Study Guide for additional learning activities to help you master this chapter content.

Be sure to visit the Evolve site at http://evolve.elsevier.com/Cooper/adult/ for additional online resources.

Review Questions for the NCLEX® Examination

1. **A patient is admitted to the hospital with a diagnosis of transient ischemic attack (TIA). The patient asks the nurse to explain to him what a TIA is. Which statement by the nurse is most accurate?**

   1. "A TIA is the result of permanent cerebrovascular insufficiency."
   2. "An episode of a TIA may last up to 2 days."
   3. "A TIA is often a precursor to a stroke."
   4. "A TIA generally occurs once and never occurs again."

2. **A 35-year-old patient is being seen for complaints of headache, which she has experienced for the past month. Her health care provider wants to rule out a brain tumor. What diagnostic tests will be most helpful in formulating this diagnosis? *(Select all that apply.)***

   1. Brain scan
   2. Positron emission tomography (PET) scan
   3. Lumbar puncture
   4. Electroencephalography
   5. Magnetic resonance imaging (MRI)

3. A nurse in the emergency department of her community hospital is teaching a group of high school students how to prevent head and spine injuries. What should the nurse include in the presentation? *(Select all that apply.)*

   1. Use helmets for bicycles, motorcycles, and skateboarding.
   2. Use helmets when participating in contact sports.
   3. Never drive or ride with someone under the influence of alcohol or drugs.
   4. Wear seatbelts and shoulder harnesses when driving or riding in a car.
   5. Avoid diving in water less than 6 feet deep.

4. A 70-year-old with back pain is scheduled to have a myelogram in the morning to rule out a pathologic condition of the spine. In preparing him for the procedure, what statement by the nurse is accurate?

   1. "We will be assessing your mental status frequently after the procedure."
   2. "You will need to lie completely supine and still during the procedure."
   3. "You will be able to ambulate immediately after the test."
   4. "We will ask you if you have any numbness or tingling in your legs after the procedure."

5. The nurse assesses an 80-year-old who has had a stroke and determines that she has difficulty swallowing. A videofluoroscopy with barium was performed to rule out aspiration. The rehabilitation team in the skilled nursing facility determined that she can eat a soft diet with one-to-one supervision. Which action is important to prevent aspiration?

   1. Tipping the head toward the unaffected side while swallowing
   2. Extending the head during swallowing
   3. Mixing solids and liquids to facilitate swallowing
   4. Encouraging the patient to drink with a straw to make swallowing easier

6. A 12-year-old has a history of generalized tonic-clonic seizures. The nurse educates the patient and his family by including which teaching points?

   1. Most people feel normal immediately after the seizure.
   2. It is important to place a tongue blade in his mouth during the seizure.
   3. The tonic phase of the seizure usually lasts for 3 to 4 minutes.
   4. It is not uncommon to lose consciousness during this type of seizure.

7. A patient was involved in a snowmobile accident. On admission to the emergency department, he is receiving oxygen and is intubated. His Glasgow Coma Scale score is 6. About 10 minutes after arrival, he is noted to have a widened pulse pressure, increased systolic blood pressure, and bradycardia. Which finding indicates to the nurse that late-stage increased intracranial pressure (ICP) is present? *(Select all that apply.)*

   1. Deepening respirations
   2. Supratentorial shift
   3. Cushing's response
   4. Medullary reflex
   5. Shallow respirations

8. A 76-year-old who has had Parkinson disease for the past 6 years has now been admitted to a long-term care facility. The nurse doing the admission interview and assessment notices which characteristic sign of the disease? *(Select all that apply.)*

   1. Bradykinesia
   2. Increased postural reflexes
   3. Sensory loss
   4. Tremor
   5. Rigidity

9. A 13-year-old student is admitted to the pediatric unit with possible meningitis. The nurse finds that the patient cannot extend her legs completely without experiencing extreme pain. The nurse correctly documents this as which sign?

   1. Brudzinski's sign
   2. Battle's sign
   3. Kernig's sign
   4. Cosgrow's sign

10. A patient is diagnosed with Bell palsy after reporting a feeling of stiffness and a drawing sensation of the face. What is important to teach her about the disease?

    1. There is a heightened awareness of taste, so foods must be bland.
    2. There may be an increased sensitivity to sound.
    3. The eye is susceptible to injury if the eyelid does not close.
    4. Drooling from increased saliva on the affected side may occur.

11. The nurse is caring for a patient with a spinal cord injury who displays symptoms of autonomic dysreflexia. What intervention should the nurse implement first?

    1. Sit the patient upright, if permitted.
    2. Check for bladder distention.
    3. Give nitroprusside (Nipride) as ordered.
    4. Assess vital signs.

12. When teaching a patient with Parkinson disease, which response would indicate the need for further education?

    1. "If I miss an occasional dose of the medication, it doesn't matter much."
    2. "I need to exercise at least some every day."
    3. "I need to be sitting straight up with my chin slightly tucked so I won't choke when I eat or drink."
    4. "I should eat a diet high in fiber and roughage to decrease my constipation."

13. The nurse is caring for a patient who suffered a cervical spinal cord injury. What injury can most likely be anticipated?

    1. Tetraplegia
    2. Hemiplegia
    3. Paraplegia
    4. Paresthesia

14. The nursing care plan for a patient with increased intracranial pressure will include what as the most therapeutic position for the patient?

1. Keep the head of the bed flat.
2. Maintain the head of the bed at 30 degrees.
3. Increase the head of the bed's angle to 30 degrees with patient on left side.
4. Use a continuous-rotation bed to continuously change patient position.

15. During admission of a patient with a severe head injury to the emergency department, what is the highest priority assessment for the nurse?

1. Patency of airway
2. Presence of a neck injury
3. Neurologic status with the Glasgow Coma Scale
4. Cerebrospinal fluid leakage from the ears or nose

16. When caring for a patient who has undergone a craniotomy, what is the primary nursing intervention?

1. Preventing infection
2. Ensuring patient comfort
3. Avoiding need for secondary surgery
4. Preventing increased intracranial pressure

17. A right-handed patient has right-sided hemiplegia and aphasia from a stroke. What is the most likely location of the lesion?

1. Left frontal lobe
2. Right brainstem
3. Motor areas of the right cerebrum
4. Medial superior area of the temporal lobe

18. A patient experiencing transient ischemic attacks (TIAs) is scheduled for a carotid endarterectomy. The patient asks the nurse what this procedure is. The nurse correctly responds with which response?

1. "This procedure promotes cerebral flow to decrease cerebral edema."
2. "This procedure reduces the brain damage that occurs during a stroke."
3. "This procedure helps prevent a stroke by removing atherosclerotic plaques obstructing cerebral blood flow."
4. "This procedure provides a circulatory bypass around thrombotic plaques obstructing cranial circulation."

19. Which sign or symptom of late-stage increased intracranial pressure should the licensed practical nurse/licensed vocational nurse (LPN/LVN) be aware of? (Select all that apply.)

1. Increase in systolic blood pressure
2. Widening of pulse pressure
3. Bradycardia
4. Unequal pupils that react slowly to light
5. Tachycardia

20. What nursing interventions should the nurse include in the plan of care for a patient who has had a stroke with right-sided hemiplegia and expressive aphasia? (Select all that apply.)

1. Allow the patient ample time to verbalize his needs.
2. Encourage self-help behaviors as much as possible, such as feeding.
3. Monitor the patient's neurologic status once a day.
4. Perform range-of-motion (ROM) to affected extremities every shift.
5. Implement the use of a communication board for the patient to use as needed.

21. The nurse is caring for a patient with myasthenia gravis. The patient asks the nurse about the causes of the disease. Which response by the nurse is correct?

1. "Myelin sheath breakdown has caused your myasthenia gravis."
2. "Degeneration of the dopamine-producing neurons in the midbrain most commonly causes the disease."
3. "Antibodies attacking the acetylcholine receptors, damaging them, and reducing their number is the most likely cause of myasthenia gravis."
4. "Myasthenia gravis is usually caused by inflammation of cranial nerve VII."

22. A patient who has been experiencing recent seizure activity is preparing to have diagnostic testing performed. The health care provider has explained that the test will provide a graphic recording of the electrical conduction activities of the brain. The patient understands that which test will be performed?

1. Electrocardiogram (ECG)
2. Magnetic resonance imaging (MRI)
3. Positron emission tomography (PET)
4. Electroencephalogram (EEG)

23. A patient has been diagnosed with Bell palsy. This condition affects which cranial nerve?

1. Cranial nerve V
2. Cranial nerve VI
3. Cranial nerve VII
4. Cranial nerve VIII

24. When reviewing the medical plan of treatment for a patient with Guillain-Barré syndrome, which therapies are considered to be most therapeutic?

1. Avonex and Betaseron
2. Thymectomy and Zarontin
3. Depakote and Zarontin
4. Plasmapheresis and intravenous immune globulin

25. Which plan of care is considered beneficial for select patients who have experienced an ischemic stroke?

1. Intravenous (IV) edrophonium in the first 3 hours
2. Anticholinesterase in the first 3 hours
3. Thrombolytic such as tissue plasminogen activator (tPA) in the first 3 hours
4. Intravenous immune globulin in the first 3 hours

26. A woman, 43, begins having chest and back pain in a movie theatre. She tries to ignore the pain, but it quickly becomes worse, spreading to her neck and arms, and shooting down her back. She begins coughing and starts gasping for air, alarming her husband, who stands and calls for a doctor or an ambulance. EMTs quickly arrive and she is rushed to the emergency department (ED). Her husband rides along, holding her hand. The patient is obese and her husband says that she has a history of high blood pressure, high cholesterol, and atherosclerosis. Family history includes connective tissue disorder, although he is unsure what type. Auscultation reveals aortic insufficiency murmur; neurologic exam is normal; 12-lead electrocardiogram (ECG) shows sinus tachycardia. The ED physician suspects a vessel anomaly or mass that could be preliminary to an eminent arterial aneurysm.

The patient is sent immediately for an emergency presurgical angiogram via femoral stick. The nurse begins to prep the patient, keeping in mind risks associated with the procedure itself.

Place a check mark to indicate each potential issue in the left column is *most associated specifically* with this patient's procedure. Check all that apply.

POTENTIAL ISSUES WITH ANGIOGRAPHY	PROCEDURE-RELATED RISK
Allergy to iodine	
Risk for possible cerebrovascular accident	
Risk for increased intracranial pressure	
Difficulty swallowing	
Risk for hematoma or arterial occlusion	
Risk for sudden increase in girth of neck	

Objectives

1. Explain the concepts of immunocompetence, immunodeficiency, and autoimmunity.
2. Differentiate between natural and acquired immunity.
3. Compare and contrast humoral and cell-mediated immunity.
4. Review the mechanisms of immune response.
5. Discuss five factors that influence the development of hypersensitivity.
6. Identify the clinical manifestations of anaphylaxis.
7. Outline the immediate aggressive treatment of systemic anaphylactic reaction.
8. Discuss the two types of latex allergies and recommendations for preventing allergic reactions to latex in the workplace.
9. Discuss selection of blood donors, typing and cross-matching, storage, and administration in preventing transfusion reaction.
10. Explain an immunodeficiency disease.
11. Discuss the cause of autoimmune disorders.
12. Explain plasmapheresis in the treatment of autoimmune diseases.

Key Terms

adaptive immunity (ă-DĂP-tĭv ĭ-MŪ-nĭ-tē, p. 725)

allergen (ĂL-ěr-jěn, p. 725)

anaphylactic shock (ăn-ĕ-fĭ-lăk-tĭc, p. 731)

antigen (ĂN-tĭ-jěn, p. 725)

attenuated (ă-TĔN-ū-āt-ĕd, p. 728)

autoimmune (ăw-tō-ĭ-MŪN, p. 729)

autologous (ăw-TŎL-ŏ-gěs, p. 734)

cellular immunity (SĔL-ū-lěr ĭ-MŪ-nĭ-tē, p. 726)

humoral immunity (HŪ-mŏr-ĕl ĭ-MŪ-nĭ-tē, p. 726)

hypersensitivity (hī-pěr-sěn-sĭ-TĬV-ĭ-tē, p. 729)

immunity (ĭ-MŪ-nĭ-tē, p. 724)

immunization (ĭm-ū-nĭ-ZĀ-shŭn, p. 726)

immunocompetence (ĭm-ū-nō-KŎM-pě-těns, p. 723)

immunodeficiency (ĭm-ū-nō-dě-FĬSH-ĕn-sē, p. 729)

immunogen (ĭm-Ū-nō-jěn, p. 726)

immunology (ĭm-ū-NŎL-ŏ-jē, p. 724)

immunosuppressive (ĭm-ū-nō-sŭ-PRĔ-sĭv, p. 734)

immunotherapy (ĭm-ū-nō-THĔR-ă-pē, p. 726)

innate immunity (ĭ-NĂT ĭ-MŪ-nĭ-tē, p. 724)

lymphokines (LĬM-fō-kīnz, p. 725)

plasmapheresis (plăz-mă-fě-RĒ-sĭs, p. 735)

proliferate (prō-lĭf-ě-RĀT, p. 725)

NATURE OF IMMUNITY

The human body exists in an environment of antagonistic forces that constantly are attacking and threatening its integrity. In response to these onslaughts, the body exhibits a wide array of adaptations to protect against external and internal harmful agents. This chapter deals with those mechanisms.

The word *immune* is derived from the Latin word *immunis,* meaning "free from burden." Immunology is an evolving science that essentially deals with the body's ability to distinguish self from nonself. The body makes this distinction through a complex network of highly specialized cells and tissues that are collectively called the *immune system.* The immune system (also called the *host defense system*) is critical to our survival.

The immune system provides a function to the human body that allows for survival of the entire system.

The body has specialized organs, tissues, and cells working to protect it. The overriding function of the system is to protect the body from disease and compromise. To achieve this goal the body produces specialized cells that are designed to detect and destroy harmful pathogens from the body and remove damaged cells from the body. Additional functions of this system include the trigger of temperature elevation and mucus production.

When the immune system responds appropriately to a foreign stimulus, the body's integrity is maintained; this is called *immunocompetence.*

Immunocompetence is the immune system's ability to mobilize and use its antibodies and other responses to stimulation by an antigen. If the immune response is too weak or too vigorous, homeostasis is disrupted, causing a malfunction in the system. This is called *immunoincompetence.* With disruption of the homeostatic balance of the immune system, a number of diseases develop. Examples of inappropriate immune responses can be classified into four categories:

1. Allergies
2. Immunodeficiency
3. Autoimmune disorders
4. Attacks on beneficial foreign tissue

Allergies are caused by hyperactive responses against environmental antigens. These include medication allergies as well as allergies to allergens such as dust, mold, and pet dander. Immunodeficiency disorders include acquired immunodeficiency syndrome (AIDS) as well as therapy-induced immunodeficiency from treatments such as chemotherapeutic agents given for cancer and immunosuppressant medications given to prevent a reaction to organ transplantation. In addition, some individuals are born with immune deficiency disorders, in which the function or development of immune components is impaired (Fernandez, 2021). Autoimmune disorders include systemic lupus erythematosus, celiac disease, thyroid disease, inflammatory bowel disease, type 1 diabetes, multiple sclerosis, myasthenia gravis, psoriasis, rheumatoid arthritis, and many other common diseases. Attacks on beneficial foreign tissue include organ transplant rejection and transfusion reactions. These disorders have been discussed in content areas that are closest to their most common clinical manifestations.

Immunity is the quality of being insusceptible to or unaffected by a particular disease or condition. Immunity has two major subclassifications: innate (natural) and adaptive (acquired) (Fig. 15.1). Innate immunity is nonspecific, whereas adaptive immunity is specific. The study of the immune system is termed immunology.

INNATE (NATURAL) IMMUNITY

The body's first line of defense, innate immunity, provides physical, mechanical, and chemical barriers to invading pathogens and protects against the external environment. The innate system includes intact skin and mucous membranes, cilia, stomach acid, tears, saliva, sebaceous glands, and secretions and flora of the intestines and vagina. These organs, tissues, and secretions provide biochemical and physical barriers to disease. The first line of defense provides nonspecific immunity to the individual (Table 15.1).

The nonspecific response of phagocytes, such as neutrophils and macrophages, as well as the response of lymphocytes, are also part of innate or natural immunity to disease. Macrophages include any phagocytic cell involved in defense against infection. When organisms pass the epithelial barriers, phagocytes become activated. Phagocytes also migrate through the bloodstream to the tissues for the body's second line of defense against disease. Phagocytes engulf and destroy microorganisms that pass the skin and mucous membrane barriers. These cells also assist in the immune response by carrying antigens to the lymphocytes.

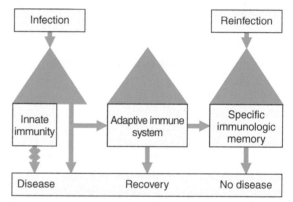

Fig. 15.1 When an infectious agent enters the body, it first encounters elements of the innate immune system. These may be sufficient to prevent disease; if not, a disease will result and the adaptive immune system is activated. The adaptive immune system helps the patient recover from the disease and establishes a specific immunologic memory. When the patient is exposed to the infectious agent a second time, his or her body is able to fight the disease, resulting in no illness developing with this exposure. The individual has acquired immunity to the infectious agent.

Table 15.1	Innate (Natural) and Adaptive (Acquired) Immunity	
CHARACTERISTICS	**INNATE (NATURAL)**	**ADAPTIVE (ACQUIRED)**
Physical barriers	Physical defense: skin and mucous membranes. Mucous membranes line body cavities such as the mouth and stomach. These cavities secrete chemicals (saliva and hydrochloric acid) that destroy bacteria. Cilia, tears, and flora of the intestine and vagina also provide natural protection	None
Response mechanisms	Nonspecific: Mononuclear phagocytic system; inflammatory response	Specific immune response: Humoral immunity, cellular immunity
Soluble factors	Chemical defense: Lysozyme, complement, acute-phase proteins, interferon	Antibodies, lymphokines
Cells	Phagocytes, natural killer (NK) cells	T cells, B cells
Specificity	None	Present
Memory	None	Present

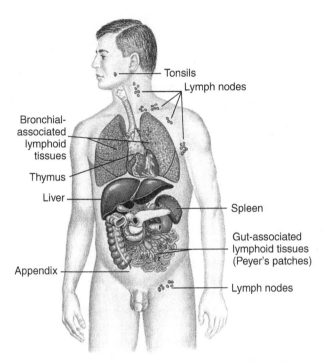

Fig. 15.2 Organization of the immune system. (From Grimes D: *Infectious diseases*, St. Louis, 1991, Mosby.)

ADAPTIVE (ACQUIRED) IMMUNITY

If the components of innate or natural immunity fail to prevent invasion or to destroy a foreign pathogen, the adaptive (acquired) immune response assists in the battle. This is the body's second line of defense against disease. Adaptive immunity provides a specific reaction to each invading antigen and has the unique ability to remember the antigen that caused the attack. The adaptive immune system is composed of highly specialized organs, cells, and tissues, including the thymus gland, the spleen, bone marrow, blood, and lymph (Fig. 15.2). Adaptive immunity includes humoral and cell-mediated immunity. The adaptive immune system's specificity results from the production of antibodies in the cells. Antibodies develop naturally after infection or artificially after vaccinations (Box 15.1).

Lymphocytes include the T and B cells (Fig. 15.3) and the large, granular lymphocytes also known as natural killer (or NK) cells. Approximately 70% to 80% of the lymphocytes are T cell lymphocytes. When activated, T cells release compounds called *lymphokines*. Lymphokines attract macrophages to the site of infection or inflammation and prepare them for attack. T cells cooperate with the B cells to produce antibodies but do not produce antibodies themselves. T cells are responsible for cell-mediated immunity and protect the body against viruses, bacteria, fungi, and parasites. T cells also provide protection in allografts (the transfer of tissue between two genetically dissimilar individuals of the same species) and against malignant cells.

B cells make up approximately 20% to 30% of the lymphocyte population. B cells trigger the production

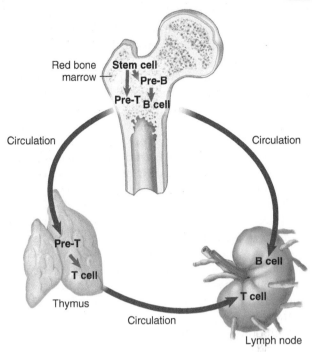

Fig. 15.3 Origin and processing of B and T cells. B and T cells originate in red bone marrow. B cells are processed in the red marrow, whereas T cells are processed in the thymus. Both cell types circulate to other lymph tissues. B cells produce antibodies to destroy specific foreign antigens (humoral immunity). T cells attack and destroy antigens (cell-mediated immunity). (From Patton KT, Thibodeau GA: *Anatomy and physiology*, ed 10, St. Louis, 2019, Elsevier.)

Box 15.1 Types of Acquired Immunity	
ACTIVE	**PASSIVE**
Natural immunity: Results from exposure to the infectious agent *Artificial immunity:* Results from immunization or vaccination with an antigen	*Natural immunity:* Results from the passage of maternal antibodies from mother to child *Artificial immunity:* Results from the injection of antibodies from other sources

of antibodies and proliferate (increase in number) in response to a particular antigen (a substance recognized by the body as foreign and that can trigger an immune response). An antigen is usually a protein that causes the formation of an antibody and reacts specifically with that antibody. B cells migrate to the peripheral circulation and tissues and eventually are filtered from the lymph and stored in the lymphoid tissue of the body. The initial formation of B cells does not require antigen stimulation or any other environmental stimulus; however, B cell proliferation depends on antigen stimulation. B cells are responsible for humoral immunity. B cells produce antibodies that protect against bacteria, viruses, and soluble antigens.

HUMORAL IMMUNITY

Humoral immunity (a form of immunity that responds to antigens) is mediated by the B cells. B cells produce antibodies in response to antigen challenge. On first exposure to a given antigen, a primary humoral response is initiated. This response is generally slow compared with subsequent antigen exposures. When a second exposure occurs, memory B cells cause a quick response, regardless of whether the first exposure was to an antigen or to immunization. Immunization is a process by which resistance to an infectious disease is induced or increased.

T lymphocytes can be categorized into T-helper (CD4) and T-suppressor (CD8) cells. T-helper cells coordinate the immune response by activating phagocytes and other T cells, and by stimulating B cells to produce antibodies (National Institute of Allergy and Infectious Diseases [NIAID], 2014). T-suppressor cells maintain the humoral response at a level appropriate for the stimulus.

Antibodies produced by one's own body are said to provide active immunity. Active immunity develops as the body defends itself from the presence of an active infection or results from immunizations against an antigen. In contrast, temporary, or passive, immunity is provided by antibodies that are formed by one person in response to a specific antigen and administered to another person. Passive immunity can occur as antibodies pass through the placenta or through breast milk. Other examples of passive immunity include antivenom given after a snake bite and immunoglobulin administered after exposure to prevent infection.

Even though humoral immunity is mediated by the B cell population, T-helper cells and T-suppressor cells are vital to the immunocompetent person. Immunocompetence is the ability of an immune system to mobilize and deploy its antibodies and other responses after stimulation by an antigen. The number and functions of the T-helper cells and T-suppressor cells help determine the strength and persistence of an immune response. The normal ratio of T-helper cells to T-suppressor cells in the body is 2:1 (Ignatavicius and Workman, 2016). When this ratio is disrupted, autoimmune and immunodeficiency diseases occur. Many factors can weaken the immune response, including the aging process, viruses, radiation, and chemotherapeutic drugs. Anxiety, stress, and loneliness also affect the immune response, as do lack of sleep and a lack of key nutrients.

Exposure to antigen and response with antibody may activate either the complement system or an antigen–antibody reaction:

Complement system: One of 25 complex enzyme serum proteins that together compose a system that breaks down bacteria and releases lysosomes to destroy bacteria.

Antigen-antibody reaction: The antigen-antibody reaction results in mast cells releasing histamine, which produces the symptoms of allergy. When symptoms of allergy occur, the antigen is referred to as an allergen (a substance that can produce a hypersensitivity reaction in the body but may not be inherently harmful). When immunity results, the antigen is referred to as an immunogen (any agent or substance capable of provoking an immune response or producing immunity).

CELLULAR IMMUNITY

Cellular immunity, also called *cell-mediated immunity*, is the mechanism of acquired immunity characterized by the dominant role of T cells. Cell-mediated immunity results when T cells are activated by an antigen. Whole cells become sensitized in a process similar to that which stimulates the B cells to form antibodies. Once these T cells have been sensitized, they are released into the blood and body tissues, where they remain indefinitely. On contact with the antigen to which they are sensitized, they attach to the organism and destroy it. Cellular immunity is involved in resistance to infectious diseases caused by viruses and some bacteria.

Cellular immunity is of primary importance in immunity against pathogens that survive inside cells, including viruses and some bacteria (e.g., *Mycobacterium* organisms), immunity against fungal infections, and tumor immunity. Cellular immunity also can have negative effects, including rejection of transplanted tissues, contact hypersensitivity reactions, and certain autoimmune diseases (Box 15.2). Hypersensitivity reactions are cell-mediated responses of the body (Box 15.3).

COMPLEMENT SYSTEM

Immunology dates back to the 19th century. Researchers recognized that blood plasma contained a substance necessary to complete the destruction of bacteria. The complement system includes approximately 25 serum enzymatic proteins that interact with one another and with other components of the innate (natural) and adaptive (acquired) arms of the immune system. Normally, complement enzymes are inactive in plasma and body fluids. When an antigen and antibody interact, the complement system is activated. The complement system functions in a "step-by-step" series, much like the clotting mechanism (see Chapter 7), but with a different purpose (Ignatavicius and Workman, 2016). The complement system can destroy the cell membrane of many bacterial species, and this action attracts phagocytes to the area.

GENETIC CONTROL OF IMMUNITY

The genetic role in immunity is currently a subject of intense research. A genetic link exists to well-developed

Box 15.2	The Four Rs of the Immune Response

- *Recognize self from nonself:* Normally the body recognizes its own cells and does not produce antibodies to fight those cells. An immune response generally is triggered only in response to agents that the body identifies as foreign. Autoimmune disorders disrupt the ability to differentiate self from nonself, and the immune system attacks the body's own cells as if they were foreign antigens.
- *Respond to nonself invaders:* The immune system responds by producing antibodies that target specific antigens for destruction. New antibodies are produced in response to new antigens. Deficits in the ability to respond may be the result of immunodeficiency disorders.
- *Remember the invader:* The ability to remember antigens that invaded the body in the past allows a quicker response if subsequent invasion by the same antigen occurs.
- *Regulate its action:* Self-regulation allows the immune system to monitor itself by "turning on" when an antigen invades and "turning off" when the invasion has been eradicated. Regulation prevents the destruction of healthy or host tissue. The inability to regulate could result in chronic inflammation and damage to the host tissue.

Box 15.3	Review of Mechanisms of the Immune Response

- The skin and mucous membranes are natural barriers to infectious agents. When these barriers are crossed, the immune response is triggered in the immunocompetent host.
- The first time an antigen enters the body, the antigen is processed by macrophages and presented to lymphocytes. Responses of B cells to the antigen in humoral immunity require interaction with T-helper cells, which assist B cells to respond to the antigen by proliferating, synthesizing, and secreting the appropriate antibody. Antigens then are neutralized by antibodies or can form immune complexes or be phagocytosed by macrophages or neutrophils.
- Humoral immunity responds to antigens such as bacteria and foreign tissue. Humoral immunity is the result of the development and continuing presence of circulating antibodies in the plasma. Humoral immunity consists of antibody-mediated immunity. *Humoral* means body fluid, and antibodies are proteins found in plasma. Therefore the term *humoral immunity* .
- Cellular immunity is the primary defense against intracellular organisms, including viruses and some bacteria (e.g., mycobacteria). In cellular immunity the antigen is processed by macrophages and recognized by T cells. T cells produce lymphokines, which further attract macrophages and neutrophils to the site for phagocytosis, or cytotoxic killer T cells can respond directly.
- Immunodeficiency is an abnormal condition of the immune system in which cellular or humoral immunity is inadequate and resistance to infection is decreased. The immunodeficiency diseases sometimes are classified as B cell (antibody) deficiencies, T cell (cellular) deficiencies, and combined T and B cell deficiencies.
- Hypersensitivity reaction is an inappropriate and excessive response of the immune system to a sensitizing antigen. In hypersensitivity reactions, the antigen is an allergen. Humoral reactions, such as anaphylactic hypersensitivity, are immediate. Cellular reactions are delayed reactions. Examples of delayed reactions include contact dermatitis, tissue transplant rejection, and sarcoidosis (Ignatavicius and Workman, 2016).

immune systems and poorly developed or compromised immune systems. In addition, researchers are finding that genes responsible for immune function are different in middle age from genes responsible for immune function in early adulthood.

EFFECTS OF NORMAL AGING ON THE IMMUNE SYSTEM

With advancing age, there is a decline in the immune system, As the body ages the response to infection slows. This delay allows for illness to more easily impair the body. Decreased immune function may be responsible for the increased incidence of cancer, infections, and autoimmune disorders seen in older adults (National Library of Medicine [NLM], 2020). Older adults are also more susceptible to infections (such as influenza and pneumonia) from pathogens that they were relatively immunocompetent against earlier in life.

Aging does not affect all aspects of the immune system. The bone marrow is relatively unaffected by increasing age. The thymus gland is largest between infancy and preadolescence. Then as the body ages it is gradually replaced by fat. This results in a sharp reduction in both size and activity (Haroun, 2018). T and B cells show deficiencies in activation, transit time through the cell cycle, and subsequent differentiation, but the most significant alterations seem to involve T cells . As thymic output of T cells diminishes, the differentiation of T cells in peripheral lymphoid structures increases. Consequently, there is an accumulation of memory cells rather than new precursor cells responsive to previously unencountered antigens.

Delayed hypersensitivity response, as determined by skin testing with injected antigens, is frequently decreased or absent in older adults. The clinical consequences of a decline in cell-mediated immunity are evident. Older adults have an increased risk of death from cancer (see the Lifespan Considerations box).

Lifespan Considerations

Older Adults

Immune Disorder

- Older adults are at increased risk for inflammation and infections resulting from changes in natural defense mechanisms.
- Pathogens are able to enter through breaks in fragile, dry skin, increasing the risk of skin infections.
- Decreased movement of respiratory secretions increases the risk of respiratory tract infections.
- Decreased production of saliva and gastric secretions increases the risk of gastrointestinal infections.
- Decreased tear production increases the risk of eye inflammation and infections.
- Structural changes in the urinary system that lead to urinary retention or stasis increase the risk of urinary tract infection.
- Signs and symptoms of infection tend to be more subtle than those in younger individuals. Because older adults have decreased body temperature, fever may be more difficult to detect. Changes in behavior such as lethargy, fatigue, disorientation, irritability, and loss of appetite may be early signs of infection.
- Immune system functioning declines with advanced age. Research is continuing.
- The older adult's immune system continues to produce antibodies, so immunization for diseases such as pneumonia and influenza is recommended.
- Older adults who have chronic illnesses are generally at increased risk for infection.
- Medications commonly taken by the elderly such as antidepressants, statin drugs for elevated cholesterol, proton pump inhibitors for heartburn, and steroids also can reduce the immune system response.

IMMUNE RESPONSE

There are two ways of helping the body to develop immunity: immunization and immunotherapy. The theory behind immunization is that controlled exposure to a disease-producing pathogen develops antibodies while preventing disease. The first immunization is credited to Edward Jenner, who observed that individuals who had had cowpox became immune to the disease. The idea of administering "attenuated [weakened] microbes" developed, and the scientific approach was applied by Louis Pasteur. Vaccines and toxoids are altered, or attenuated (the process of weakening the virulence of a disease organism), to reduce their power without affecting their ability to stimulate the production of antibodies. After immunization, the immune system mounts a greater response to a second encounter with an antigen. The vaccine, or toxoid, stimulates humoral immunity, which provides protection from disease for months to years.

The Centers for Disease Control and Prevention (2019) recommend the following immunizations for adults with no contraindications:

- Influenza vaccine every year.
- Tetanus, diphtheria (Td) vaccine every 10 years; Tetanus, diphtheria, and pertussis (Tdap) once after age 19.
- Varicella vaccine: two doses if there is no evidence of immunity to varicella.
- Human papilloma vaccination (HPV) for women 19 to 26 years of age: three doses if not previously vaccinated.
- Human papilloma vaccination (HPV) for men 19 to 21 years of age: three doses if not previously vaccinated. If having sex with men, vaccine should be given for men ages 19 to 26 years if not previously vaccinated.
- Herpes zoster: two doses for adults aged 50 and older.
- Measles, mumps, and rubella (MMR): two doses if there is no evidence of immunity.
- Pneumococcal 13 (PCV13): one dose.
- Pneumococcal 23 (PCV23): one to three doses depending on indication. One dose is required after the age of 65.
- Hepatitis A: two to three doses if at risk for hepatitis A for persons 1 year and older.
- Hepatitis B: three doses if at risk for hepatitis B available for all age groups.
- Meningococcal: one or more doses if at risk for meningitis, available beginning at age 11 to 12 years.
- *Haemophilus influenzae* type B: one to three doses if at risk for *Haemophilus influenzae* type B available for children under the age of 5 years and for older children and adults who have qualifying medical conditions.

Immunotherapy is a special treatment of allergic responses wherein the patient receives doses of the offending allergens over a period of 1 to 3 years to develop immunity gradually. Immunotherapy consists of injecting a person with a very diluted antigen (allergen) to which the patient has a type I hypersensitivity. The strength of the dilution is increased weekly until a maintenance dosage is reached. The theory is that immunotherapy assists the individual in building tolerance to the allergen without developing fever or increased signs and symptoms. *Desensitization* is another term used for immunotherapy. It is indicated for patients with clinically significant disease for whom avoidance of the allergen or treatment with medication is inadequate. It is considered safe in properly selected patients but is a lengthy, expensive process with a potential for severe anaphylaxis.

Immunotherapy may be administered during the allergy season, before allergy season, or year-round (perennial). Perennial therapy is most widely accepted because it allows for a higher cumulative dose, which produces a better effect. Perennial therapy usually begins with a very diluted dose of the allergen that is increased progressively each week over the course of up to 18 weeks or more. Immunotherapy is administered subcutaneously. The patient should be observed for at least 20 minutes after administration because a hypersensitivity reaction or anaphylaxis may occur. In the event of anaphylaxis during immunotherapy, the treatment protocol includes the administration of epinephrine chloride given subcutaneously.

Most patients begin immunotherapy at the health care provider's office on a weekly basis. Home administration by the patient or a family member is acceptable once the maintenance level is reached, which often takes 1 to 2 years. Some patients may require immunotherapy for up to 5 years. Interrupted regimens because of illness may place the patient at risk for reaction. Consult the health care provider before administering a dose of diluted allergen if the patient's maintenance immunotherapy was interrupted by illness or other factors.

DISORDERS OF THE IMMUNE SYSTEM

Immune system failure occurs in several ways and expresses itself in mild to severe form. The system can malfunction at many points while attempting to provide the body with protective defense. Failures may be the result of genetic factors, developmental defects, infection, malignancy, injury, drugs, or altered metabolic states.

The severity of altered immune response disorders ranges from mild to chronic to life-threatening. The disorders are categorized as follows:
1. Hypersensitivity disorder involves an allergic response and tissue rejection.
2. Immunodeficiency disease involves an altered and failed immune response.
3. Autoimmune disease involves extensive tissue damage resulting from an immune system that seemingly reverses its function to one of self-destruction. See Box 15.2 for the four Rs of the immune response.

HYPERSENSITIVITY DISORDERS
Etiology and Pathophysiology
Hypersensitivity is characterized by an excessive reaction to a particular stimulus. A hypersensitivity reaction is an inappropriate and excessive response of the immune system to a sensitizing antigen. Hypersensitivity disorders arise when harmless substances, such as pollens, danders, foods, and chemicals, are recognized as foreign. The body mounts an immune response in much the same way it does to any foreign protein. The host becomes sensitive after the first exposure and on subsequent exposure exhibits a hypersensitivity reaction. Chronic exposure leads to a chronic allergy response, which ranges from mild to incapacitating signs and symptoms.

Hypersensitivity disorders are believed to be caused by a genetic defect that allows increased production of immunoglobulin E (IgE) with release of histamine and other mediators from mast cells and basophils (Buelow and Routes, 2015). Humoral reactions, mediated by the circulating B lymphocytes, are immediate. Cellular reactions, mediated by the T lymphocytes, are delayed hypersensitivity reactions. Exposure to antigen may occur by inhalation, ingestion, injection, or touch (contact). Signs and symptoms caused by histamine release include vasodilation, edema, bronchoconstriction, mucus

Box 15.4 **Factors Influencing Hypersensitivity**

- *Host response to allergen:* The more sensitive the individual, the greater the allergic response.
- *Exposure amount:* In general, the more allergen the individual is exposed to, the greater the chance of a severe reaction.
- *Nature of the allergen:* Most allergic reactions are precipitated by complex, high-molecular-weight protein substances.
- *Route of allergen entry:* Most allergens enter the body via gastrointestinal and respiratory routes. Exposure to venoms through bites or stings and injectable medications presents a more severe threat of allergic response.
- *Repeated exposure:* In general, the more often the individual is exposed to the allergen, the greater the response.

secretion, and pruritus. Hypersensitivity reactions may be local (gastrointestinal, skin, respiratory, conjunctival) or systemic (anaphylaxis). The exact mechanism and pathway of these inflammatory responses are not clearly understood.

A combination of interrelated factors increases the severity of symptoms (Box 15.4). Disorders that result from hypersensitivity, which are discussed in other chapters, include urticaria, angioedema, allergic rhinitis, allergic conjunctivitis (hay fever), atopic dermatitis, and asthma. Many cases of asthma are attributed to an allergic response to a specific allergen.

Assessment
Assessment should involve predominantly the integumentary, gastrointestinal, respiratory, and cardiovascular systems. Be aware of the seasonal nature of the complaints.

Subjective data include pruritus, nausea, and uneasiness.

Objective data include sneezing, excessive nasal secretions, lacrimation, inflamed nasal membranes, skin rash or areas of raised inflammation, diarrhea, cough, wheezes, impaired breathing, and hypotension.

Hypersensitivity illnesses are diagnosed largely through patient history and physical examination. The most important diagnostic tool is a detailed history, including the following:
1. Onset, nature, and progression of signs and symptoms
2. Aggravating and alleviating factors
3. Frequency and duration of signs and symptoms

Assess environmental, household, and occupational factors. Common offenders include pollen, spores, dust, food, drugs, and insect venom. Many but not all offenders are seasonal. Signs and symptoms generally vary from mild upper respiratory tract manifestations, such as sneezing and excessive nasal secretions, to watery, itching eyes. Skin signs and symptoms are often eczema-like or urticarial (hives). Diarrhea may be a gastrointestinal complaint in some individuals. More severe signs and symptoms include those of the lower respiratory tract, such as coughing, wheezing, chest discomfort, breathing difficulties, and shock, which could be followed by cardiovascular collapse and respiratory arrest. The complete history assists in an accurate diagnosis (see the Health Promotion box).

Health Promotion

Assessing the Patient With Allergies

- Obtain a comprehensive history that covers family allergies, past and present allergies, and social and environmental factors, especially the physical environment.
- Identify the allergens that may have triggered a reaction.
- Determine the time of year that an allergic reaction occurs as a clue to a seasonal allergen.
- Obtain information about any over-the-counter or prescription medications used to treat allergies.
- In addition to identification of the allergen, find out about the clinical manifestations and course of allergic reaction.
- Ask about pets, trees, and plants on the property; air pollutants; and floor coverings, houseplants, and cooling and heating systems in the home and workplace.
- Have the patient keep a daily or weekly food diary with a description of any untoward reactions.
- Screen for any reaction to medication.
- Review questions about the patient's lifestyle and stress level in connection with allergic symptoms.

The physical examination should include a thorough assessment of the skin, the middle ear, the conjunctiva, the naso-oropharynx, and the lungs.

Diagnostic Tests

Laboratory studies are usually not necessary unless allergic signs and symptoms are severe or last an extended amount of time. A complete blood count with differential to identify the type of white blood cells that are elevated, skin testing, total serum IgE levels, and a specific IgE level for a particular allergen may be ordered. The latter test is called a *radioallergosorbent test* (RAST).

Medical Management

Treatment of hypersensitivity disorders includes the following:
- Symptom management with medications
- Environmental control
- Immunotherapy

The most effective treatment is environmental control, which includes avoidance of the offending allergen. Pollens are seasonal and can be avoided at season peaks with air conditioning and limited time spent outdoors. Mold spores can be reduced by maintaining dry conditions and using air filters. House dust can be controlled by damp dusting, use of air filters, and decreased use of carpet and overstuffed furniture. Most other offending allergens (e.g., food, drugs, chemicals, and stinging insects) should be avoided if possible.

Medications are used to treat and alleviate signs and symptoms. Antihistamines compete with histamine by attaching to the cell surface receptors and blocking histamine release. Antihistamines must be initiated soon after exposure or taken on a regular basis. Drowsiness, mucous membrane dryness, and occasionally central nervous system excitation are side effects of some antihistamines. Examples of antihistamines include pseudoephedrine (Actifed), diphenhydramine (Benadryl), chlorpheniramine (Chlor-Trimeton), and brompheniramine (Brovex). Nonsedating antihistamines include cetirizine (Zyrtec), loratadine (Claritin), and fexofenadine (Allegra). The nonsedating antihistamines are more desirable for those who experience drowsiness with antihistamine use (Table 15.2).

Leukotriene inhibitors are agents that significantly reduce symptoms of an allergic reaction caused by the release of leukotrienes from mast cells and basophils. Three are currently available in the United States. Montelukast (Singulair) and zafirlukast (Accolate) act as leukotriene receptor blockers, and zileuton (Zyflo) inhibits the production of leukotrienes.

Patient Problems

Patient problems for patients with hypersensitivity include the following:
1. Potential for Injury, related to exposure to allergen
2. Inability to Tolerate Activity, related to malaise
3. Potential for Infection, related to inflammation of protective mucous membranes

Patient Teaching

Patient teaching should revolve around the specific diagnosis. Advise the patient with seasonal allergies to avoid offending allergens and ensure that he or she understands the therapeutic medication plan. Focus on health promotion and health teaching for self-care management (see the Safety Alert box).

Safety Alert

Treating the Patient With a Hypersensitivity Reaction

- List all of the patient's allergies on the chart, the nursing care plan, and the medication record.
- After an allergic disorder is diagnosed, therapeutic treatment is aimed at reducing exposure to the offending allergen, treating the symptoms, and, if necessary, desensitizing the person through immunotherapy.
- All health care workers must be prepared for the rare but life-threatening anaphylactic reaction, which requires immediate medical and nursing interventions.
- Instruct the patient to wear a medical alert bracelet listing the particular drug allergy.
- For a patient allergic to insect stings, commercial bee sting kits containing epinephrine and a tourniquet are available. Teach the patient to apply the tourniquet and self-inject the subcutaneous epinephrine. The patient should wear a medical-alert bracelet and carry a bee sting kit whenever he or she goes outdoors.

Table 15.2   Medications for Hypersensitivity Reactions

GENERIC NAME (TRADE NAME)	ACTION	SIDE EFFECTS	NURSING IMPLICATIONS
dexamethasone	Corticosteroid	Anxiety, nausea, acne, easy bruising, increased appetite	Do not use for extended period; use cautiously with patients with diabetes or peptic ulcers
diphenhydramine (Benadryl)	Antihistamine	Drowsiness, confusion, nasal stuffiness, dry mouth, photosensitivity, urine retention	Use cautiously with central nervous system depressants, including alcohol; tell patient to avoid driving or hazardous activity because of drowsiness
epinephrine (Epinephrine chloride, EpiPen)	Alpha-adrenergic agonist and beta-adrenergic agonist	Nervousness, tremor, headache, hypertension, tachycardia, ventricular fibrillation, stroke	Do not use with monoamine oxidase inhibitor; use cautiously in patients with hyperthyroidism, hypertension, diabetes, and heart disease
fexofenadine (Allegra)	Nonsedating antihistamine	Headache, drowsiness, blurred vision, hypotension, bradycardia, tachycardia, dysrhythmias (rare), urinary retention	Same as for loratadine
flunisolide	Corticosteroid (inhaled)	Headache, transient nasal burning, epistaxis, nausea, vomiting	Not effective for acute episodes; use regularly; teach care and cleaning of inhaler; if symptoms do not improve in 3 wk, consult health care provider
loratadine (Claritin)	Nonsedating antihistamine	Dry mouth, headache, red and irritated eyes	Store in tight container at room temperature. Teach patient and family to avoid driving or other hazardous activities if drowsiness occurs

Anaphylaxis

Etiology and Pathophysiology. The most severe IgE-mediated allergic reaction is anaphylaxis, or systemic reaction to allergens. Anaphylaxis, or **anaphylactic shock**, is an acute and potentially fatal hypersensitivity (allergic) reaction to an allergen. Allergens that cause anaphylaxis include the following:

- Venoms
- Drugs, such as penicillin and aspirin
- Contrast media dyes
- Insect stings (such as bees and wasps)
- Foods such as eggs, shellfish, and peanuts
- Latex
- Vaccines

The hypersensitivity reaction results in a sudden severe vasodilation as a consequence of the release of certain chemical mediators from mast cells. Vasodilation causes an increase in capillary permeability, which causes fluid to seep into the interstitial space from the vascular space.

Clinical Manifestations. In anaphylaxis, the reaction occurs rapidly after exposure, from seconds to a few minutes. A massive release of mediators initiates events in target organs throughout the body. Skin and gastrointestinal signs and symptoms may occur, although respiratory and cardiovascular signs and symptoms predominate. Fatal reactions are associated with a fall in blood pressure, laryngeal edema, and bronchospasm, leading to cardiovascular collapse, myocardial infarction, and respiratory failure. Anaphylactic reactions are classified as mild, moderate, and severe.

Assessment. Early recognition of signs and symptoms and early treatment may prevent severe reactions and even death. In general, the more rapid the onset, the more severe the outcome is. The patient may have a feeling of uneasiness that increases to a sense of severe apprehension, and then a fear of impending death. The skin may or may not be involved. Urticaria, pruritus, and angioedema may be present in mild and moderate anaphylaxis, whereas cyanosis and pallor may be seen in severe reactions. Upper respiratory signs and symptoms range from congestion and sneezing to edema of the lips, the tongue, and the larynx with stridor and occlusion of the upper airways. Lower respiratory signs and symptoms occur soon thereafter and include bronchospasm, wheezing, and severe dyspnea. Gastrointestinal signs and symptoms increase from nausea, vomiting, and diarrhea to dysphagia and involuntary stools. The patient may have cardiovascular signs and symptoms such as tachycardia and hypotension. Signs and symptoms may worsen, and the patient may display coronary insufficiency, vascular collapse, dysrhythmias, shock, cardiac arrest, respiratory failure, and death.

Medical Management. Immediate aggressive treatment is the goal in anaphylaxis. At the first sign, the prescribed dose of epinephrine 1:1000 is given subcutaneously for mild symptoms. It may be repeated at 5- to 20-minute intervals as prescribed by the health care provider. Epinephrine produces bronchodilation and vasoconstriction and inhibits the further release of chemical mediators of hypersensitivity reactions from mast cells. The effects of epinephrine take only a few minutes. Epinephrine 1:10,000 at 5- to 10-minute intervals may be administered intramuscularly or intravenously for a severe reaction as prescribed by the health care provider. Diphenhydramine 50 mg to 100 mg may be given intramuscularly or intravenously as indicated for allergic signs and symptoms. If moderate to severe signs and symptoms occur, IV therapy with volume expanders and vasopressor agents such as dopamine (Intropin) may be initiated to prevent vascular collapse, and the patient may be intubated to prevent airway obstruction. Oxygen may be administered by a non-rebreather mask. Intubation or a tracheostomy may be required for oxygen delivery if progressive hypoxia exists. Place the patient in a recumbent position, elevate the legs, and keep the patient warm.

Nursing Interventions and Patient Teaching. Nursing interventions begin by assessing respiratory status, including dyspnea, wheezing, and decreased breath sounds. Also assess circulatory status, including dysrhythmias, tachycardia, and hypotension. Monitor vital signs continually. Other assessments include (1) intake and output (%49%26%4f); (2) mental status, including anxiety, malaise, confusion, and coma; (3) skin status, including erythema, urticaria, cyanosis, and pallor; and (4) gastrointestinal status, including nausea, vomiting, diarrhea, and incontinence.

The diagnosis most often is made by a history of signs and symptoms. Looking at and listening to the anxious patient should be leading factors in suspecting anaphylaxis. Question the patient about recent exposure to known antigens that cause anaphylaxis (Box 15.5). Most laboratory studies are not beneficial.

Box 15.5	Common Allergens Causing Anaphylaxis

DRUGS	VENOMS	FOODS
Vaccines	Honey bees	Cow's milk
Allergen extracts	Wasps	Peanuts
Enzymes	Hornets	Brazil nuts
Penicillins		Cashew nuts
Sulfonamides		Shellfish
Cephalosporins		Egg albumin
Dextrans		Strawberries
Hormones		Chocolate
Contrast media		Soy
Anesthetic agents		

A patient problem and interventions for the patient with anaphylaxis include but are not limited to the following:

PATIENT PROBLEM	NURSING INTERVENTIONS
Inability to Maintain Adequate Breathing Pattern, related to: • Edema • Bronchospasm • Increased secretions	Maintain airway Administer high-flow oxygen via nonrebreather mask Endotracheal intubation or a tracheostomy will be established for oxygen delivery if progressive hypoxia exists Administer prescribed medications Keep the patient warm Monitor vital signs Suction if necessary Anticipate intubation with severe respiratory distress

Reassure the patient during procedures. After the event, teach the patient about avoidance of the allergen, advise him or her to wear or carry medical alert identification, and teach the patient to prepare and administer epinephrine subcutaneously.

Prognosis. If the signs and symptoms are left untreated, anaphylaxis can lead to death in a relatively short time.

Latex Allergies

Allergy to latex products has become an increasing problem, affecting patients and health care professionals. The increase in allergic reactions coincided with the sharp increase in glove use after the introduction of universal precautions against infectious diseases in 1992 when the Occupational Safety and Health Administration (OSHA) mandated universal bloodborne pathogen precautions and the use of gloves by health care workers. It is estimated that 8% to 12% of health care workers regularly exposed to latex are sensitized (OSHA, n.d.). The more frequent and prolonged the exposure is, the greater the likelihood will be of developing a latex allergy. In addition to gloves, latex-containing products used in health care may include blood pressure cuffs, stethoscopes, tourniquets, IV tubing, syringes, electrode pads, oxygen masks, tracheal tubes, colostomy and ileostomy pouches, urinary catheters, anesthetic masks, and adhesive tape.

Latex proteins can become aerosolized through powder on gloves and can result in serious reactions when inhaled by sensitized individuals. Health care agencies are advised to use powder-free gloves. Certain food proteins are similar to some proteins in rubber. An allergic reaction to latex also may result in an allergic reaction to some foods. Bananas, avocados, kiwi fruit, tomatoes, apples, chestnuts, and melons are common foods to result in an allergy if one is allergic to latex.

Types of Latex Allergies. Two types of latex allergies that can occur are type IV allergic contact dermatitis and type I allergic reactions. Type IV contact dermatitis is caused by the chemicals used in the manufacturing of latex gloves. It is a delayed reaction that occurs within 6 to 48 hours. Typically the person first has dryness, pruritus, fissuring, and cracking of the skin, followed by erythema, edema, and crusting at 24 to 48 hours. Chronic exposure can lead to thickening and hardening of the skin, scaling, and hyperpigmentation. The dermatitis may extend beyond the area of physical contact with the allergen.

A type I allergic reaction is a response to the natural rubber latex proteins and occurs within minutes of contact with the proteins. These types of allergic reactions can range from skin erythema, urticaria, rhinitis, conjunctivitis, or asthma to full-blown anaphylactic shock. Systemic reactions to latex may result from exposure to protein via various routes, including the skin, mucous membranes, inhalation, or blood.

Nursing Interventions. Identification of patients and health care workers sensitive to latex is crucial in preventing adverse reactions. Collect a thorough health history and history of any allergies, especially for patients with any complaints of latex contact symptoms. Not all latex-sensitive individuals can be identified, even with a thorough history. Risk factors include long-term exposure to latex products (e.g., health care personnel, individuals who have had multiple surgeries, rubber industry workers) and a history of hay fever, asthma, and allergies to certain foods previously listed.

The National Institute for Occupational Safety and Health (NIOSH) has published recommendations for preventing allergic reactions to latex in the workplace (NIOSH, 2014):

- Non-latex gloves are recommended for tasks that are not likely to involve contact with infectious materials such as blood (e.g., food preparation, routine housekeeping, and maintenance).
- Workers at high risk of allergic reaction should be screened periodically to detect symptoms early and control or eliminate latex exposure.
- Appropriate work practices should be followed. For example, workers should wash their hands with a mild soap and dry thoroughly after removing latex gloves. Areas contaminated with latex-containing dust should be identified and cleaned, and ventilation filters and vacuum bags used in those areas should be changed frequently.
- Workers should be provided with education programs and training materials about latex allergy.
- Workers showing symptoms of latex allergy should consult a doctor experienced in treating the problem, and workers with a known allergy should avoid latex exposures, wear a medical alert bracelet, and follow their doctor's advice for dealing with allergic reactions.

Use latex precaution protocols for patients identified as having a positive latex allergy test or a history of signs and symptoms related to latex exposure. Many health care facilities have created latex-free product carts that can be used for patients with latex allergies.

Transfusion Reactions

Transfusion reactions are hypersensitivity disorders, best illustrated by reactions that occur with mismatched blood. Preventing transfusion reactions requires careful selection of blood donors, followed by careful typing and crossmatching of blood from donor to recipient. Proper storage of blood and adherence to the administration protocol are critical. Blood and blood components must be refrigerated at specific temperatures until a half hour before administration. Blood must be administered within 4 hours of removal from refrigeration, and blood components within 6 hours. Donor and recipient numbers are specific and must be checked thoroughly, and the patient must be identified with an armband. Administer all blood and blood products through microaggregate filters. Monitor for adverse effects.

Transfusion reactions are labeled mild, moderate, and severe. The most severe reactions occur within the first 15 minutes, moderate reactions occur within 30 to 90 minutes, and mild reactions may be delayed to late in the transfusion or hours to several days after transfusion.

Mild transfusion reaction signs and symptoms include dermatitis, diarrhea, fever, chills, urticaria, cough, and orthopnea. Treatment includes (1) stopping the transfusion; (2) notifying the health care provider; and (3) administering saline, steroids, and diuretics as ordered. The health care provider may give instructions to restart the transfusion at a slower rate and to continue to monitor the patient.

Moderate reactions, resulting in fever, chills, urticaria, and wheezing, occur after the first 30 minutes of administration. In the event of a moderate reaction, stop the transfusion, continue with saline, and notify the health care provider. Antihistamines and epinephrine may be ordered. The health care provider will decide whether to continue the transfusion.

Chills seen with mild or moderate transfusion reactions may be caused by the rapid infusion of cold blood, or may be due to a reaction against monocytes, granulocytes, lymphocytes, or leukocytes present in the donated blood.

A severe transfusion reaction often includes fever, chills, pain in the lower back, tightness in the chest, tachycardia, a drop in blood pressure, and blood in the urine. Patients may report a sense of "impending doom." Hemolytic reactions can result in kidney damage, requiring dialysis, or death if the transfusion is not stopped as soon as the first signs of a reaction appear.

If a severe reaction occurs, the transfusion is stopped immediately, saline is administered to maintain venous access, and the blood or blood product, along with the tubing, is returned to the laboratory for immediate testing. Further nursing responsibilities after a blood transfusion reaction include (1) following hospital protocol for collecting required blood and urine specimens to assess for hemolysis; (2) filling out a transfusion reaction record; and (3) documenting the transfusion reaction on required facility forms and in the patient's health record.

The best method for preventing transfusion reaction is an autologous transfusion (i.e., use of one's own blood) for replacement therapy. The blood can be frozen and stored for as long as 3 years. Usually the blood is stored without being frozen and is given to the person within a few weeks of donation.

Delayed Hypersensitivity

Delayed hypersensitivity reactions, occurring 24 to 72 hours after exposure, are mediated by T cells accompanied by release of lymphokines. Delayed reaction contact dermatitis, such as after contact with poison ivy, is one example. Another example is tissue transplant rejection.

Transplant Rejection. Transfer of healthy tissue or organs from a donor to a recipient has been done for many years. The immune process that protects the body from foreign protein is the same process at work in tissue transplant rejection. Knowledge of the function of the immune system has enabled medical experts to find a way to control the rejection process. Now the body is prepared before tissue transplantation to decrease the chances of rejection.

Autografting is the transplantation of tissue from one site to another on the same individual and is generally successful because there is a reduced likelihood of rejection. *Allografting* is the transplantation of tissue between members of the same species. Allografts commonly are used after trauma, especially on full-thickness burns, and in reconstructive surgery. *Isografting* is the transfer of tissue between genetically identical individuals (e.g., identical twins). Because few humans are born with an identical sibling, the allograft is the most common form of tissue transplant.

Antigenic determinants on the cells lead to graft rejection via the immune process. Therefore, antigenic determinants in recipient tissue and donor tissue are matched as closely as possible before transplantation. Tissue matching leads to a better chance of success.

Tissue rejection does not occur immediately after transplantation. It takes several days for vascularization to occur. Seven to 10 days after blood supply is adequately established, sensitized lymphocytes may appear in sufficient numbers for sloughing to occur at the site.

Graft rejection is slowed through the use of chemical agents that interfere with the immune response. These chemical agents include corticosteroids, cyclosporine (Neoral, Sandimmune), and azathioprine (Imuran). Administration of these chemical agents is referred to as immunosuppressive therapy—the administration of agents that significantly interfere with the immune system's ability to respond to antigenic stimulation.

Infection is a threat to the immunosuppressed patient. Meticulous aseptic technique is required when caring for these individuals. Prophylactic antibiotic therapy may be advisable, and good skin care is necessary. The frequency of bedside visits for staff and family should be limited. Do not allow people with infection near the patient.

Immunodeficiency Disorders

Immunodeficiency is an abnormal condition of the immune system in which cellular or humoral immunity is inadequate and resistance to infection is decreased. The first evidence of immunodeficiency is an increased susceptibility to infection. The problem can manifest as recurrent or chronic infection. Unusually severe infection with complications or incomplete clearing of an infection also may indicate an underlying immunodeficiency.

When the immune system does not protect the body adequately, an immunodeficient state exists. Immunodeficiency disorders involve an impairment of one or more of the following immune mechanisms:
- Phagocytosis
- Humoral response
- Cell-mediated response
- Complement response
- Combined humoral and cell-mediated deficiency

Immunodeficiency disorders are *primary* if the immune cells are improperly developed or absent, and *secondary* if the deficiency is caused by illnesses or treatment. Primary immunodeficiency disorders are rare and often serious, whereas secondary disorders are more common and may be less severe.

Primary Immunodeficiency Disorders

The basic categories of primary immunodeficiency disorders include the following:
- Phagocytic defects
- B cell deficiency
- T cell deficiency
- Combined B cell and T cell deficiency

Secondary Immunodeficiency Disorders

Drug-induced immunosuppression is the most common type of secondary immunodeficiency disorder. Immunosuppressive therapy is prescribed for patients to treat a wide variety of chronic diseases, including inflammatory, allergic, hematologic, neoplastic, and autoimmune disorders. Immunosuppressive therapy also is used to prevent rejection of a transplanted organ. Some of these immunosuppressive drugs are cyclosporine, mycophenolate mofetil (CellCept), and azathioprine. Immunosuppression is also a serious side effect of cytotoxic drugs used in cancer chemotherapy. Generalized leukopenia often results, leading to a decreased humoral and cell-mediated response. Secondary infections are common in immunosuppressed patients.

Stress may alter the immune response. This effect involves interrelationships between the nervous, endocrine, and immune systems.

A hypofunctional immune system exists in young children and older adults. Immunoglobulin levels decrease with age and lead to a suppressed humoral immune response in older adults. Thymic involution (i.e., shrinking of the thymus) occurs with aging, along with a decreased number of T cells. The incidence of malignancies and autoimmune diseases increases with aging and may be related to immunologic deterioration.

Malnutrition also alters cell-mediated immune responses. When protein is deficient over a prolonged period, the thymus gland atrophies and lymphoid tissue decreases. In addition, susceptibility to infections increases.

Radiation destroys lymphocytes either directly or through depletion of stem cells. As the radiation dose is increased, more bone marrow atrophies, leading to severe pancytopenia and severe suppression of immune function.

Surgical removal of lymph nodes, thymus, or spleen can suppress the immune response. Splenectomy in children is especially dangerous and may lead to septicemia from simple respiratory tract infections.

Hodgkin's lymphoma greatly impairs the cell-mediated immune response, and patients may die of severe viral or fungal infections. Viruses, especially rubella, may cause immunodeficiency by direct cytotoxic damage to lymphoid cells. Systemic infections can place such a demand on the immune system that resistance to a secondary or subsequent infection is impaired.

AUTOIMMUNE DISORDERS

Autoimmune disorders entail the development of an immune response (autoantibodies or a cellular immune response) to one's own tissues; in other words, these disorders are failures of the tolerance to "self." Autoimmune disorders may be described as an immune attack on the self and result from the failure to distinguish "self" protein (self-antigens) from "foreign" protein.

For some unknown reason, immune cells that are normally unresponsive (tolerant to self-antigens) are activated. T cells and B cells can have tolerance to self-antigens. An alteration in T cells alone or in both B cells and T cells can produce autoantibodies and

autosensitized T cells that cause pathophysiologic tissue damage. The particular autoimmune disease depends on which self-antigen is involved.

Autoimmune diseases tend to cluster, so a given person may have more than one autoimmune disease (e.g., rheumatoid arthritis and Addison's disease). The same or related autoimmune diseases may be found in other members of the family. This observation has led to the concept of genetic predisposition to autoimmune disease.

The pathophysiology of autoimmune responses is not clearly understood. Environmental factors, including smoking, viral infections, and low vitamin D levels, have been found to trigger autoimmune diseases in susceptible people (Wein, 2013). In addition, high salt intake may be associated with the autoimmune response (Wein, 2013). Many illnesses are now believed to be in this classification, including pernicious anemia, Guillain-Barré syndrome, scleroderma, Sjögren syndrome, rheumatic fever, rheumatoid arthritis, ulcerative colitis, male infertility, myasthenia gravis, multiple sclerosis, Addison disease, autoimmune hemolytic anemia, immune thrombocytopenic purpura, type 1 diabetes mellitus, glomerulonephritis, and systemic lupus erythematosus.

Plasmapheresis

Plasmapheresis is the removal of plasma that contains components causing, or thought to cause, disease. When plasma is removed, it is replaced by substitution fluids such as saline or albumin. Therefore the term *plasma exchange* more accurately describes this procedure (Fig. 15.4).

Plasmapheresis has been used to treat autoimmune diseases such as systemic lupus erythematosus, glomerulonephritis, myasthenia gravis, thrombocytopenic purpura, rheumatoid arthritis, and Guillain-Barré syndrome. The rationale is to remove pathologic substances present in plasma. Many disorders for which plasmapheresis is being used are characterized by circulating autoantibodies (usually of the immunoglobulin G [IgG] class) and antigen–antibody complexes. Immunosuppressive therapy prevents recovery of IgG production, and plasmapheresis prevents antibody rebound (in which posttreatment autoimmune antibody concentrations exceed their pretreatment level) that often occurs after immunosuppressive therapy.

In addition to removing antinuclear antibodies (an autoantibody that reacts to nuclear material) and antigen-antibody complexes, plasmapheresis also may remove inflammatory mediators (e.g., complement) that are responsible for tissue damage. In the treatment of systemic lupus erythematosus, plasmapheresis usually is reserved for the patient experiencing an acute attack and who is unresponsive to conventional therapy.

Plasmapheresis involves the removal of whole blood through a needle inserted in one arm and circulation of the blood through a cell separator.

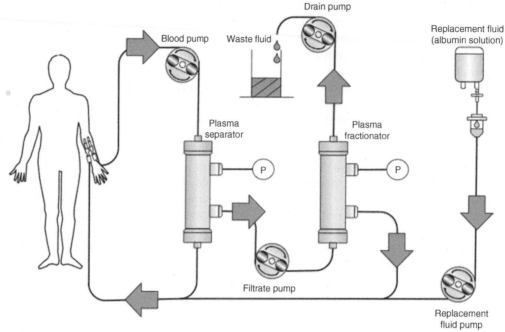

Fig 15.4 Plasmapheresis is the process of removing blood from the body and then separating the plasma. The blood cells are returned to the body and the plasma is replaced using an alternative fluid, such as normal saline or lactated Ringer's solution. (From Iwami, D., Miura, M., Chiba, Y., et al, 2018. Optimal settings for double filtration plasmapheresis with targeted removal rate of preexisting antibody in antibody-incompatible kidney transplant. Transplantation Proceedings, 50(10), 3478-3482).

The separator divides the blood into plasma and its cellular components by centrifugation or membrane filtration. Plasma, platelets, white blood cells, or red blood cells can be separated selectively. The undesirable component is removed, and the remainder is returned to the patient through a vein in the opposite arm. The plasma is generally replaced with normal saline, lactated Ringer's solution, fresh frozen plasma, plasma protein fractions, or albumin. When blood is removed manually, only 500 mL may be taken at one time. Apheresis procedures allow for greater than 4 L of plasma to be managed in a 2- to 3-hour period.

As with administration of other blood products, be aware of side effects associated with plasmapheresis. The most common complications are hypotension and citrate toxicity. Hypotension is usually the result of vasovagal reaction or transient volume changes. Citrate is used as an anticoagulant and may cause hypocalcemia, which may manifest as a headache, paresthesias, and dizziness.

Get Ready for the NCLEX® Examination!

Key Points

- The two major forms of immunity are innate (natural) and acquired (adaptive).
- T lymphocytes, B lymphocytes, and macrophages are the three major cell types active in acquired immunity.
- B lymphocytes produce antibodies. T lymphocytes do not produce antibodies but assist the B cells. T lymphocytes release lymphokines.
- Macrophages trap, process, and present antigen to T lymphocytes.
- Autoimmune disorders are failures of the body's tolerance to "self."
- Plasmapheresis is used to treat autoimmune diseases such as systemic lupus erythematosus, glomerulonephritis, myasthenia gravis, thrombocytopenic purpura, rheumatoid arthritis, and Guillain-Barré syndrome.

- Infection is a primary threat to the immunosuppressed patient. Aseptic technique is required when caring for these patients. Good skin care is necessary.
- Careful selection of blood donors and careful typing and crossmatching of blood are important to prevent transfusion reaction.
- Early recognition of signs followed by early treatment may decrease the severity of an allergic reaction.
- The five factors influencing the hypersensitivity response are: host response to allergen, exposure amount, nature of the allergen, route of allergen entry, and repeated exposure.
- Two types of latex allergies are type IV allergic contact dermatitis and type I allergic reactions. Type IV is caused by the chemicals used in the manufacturing of latex gloves, whereas the type I allergic reaction is a response to natural rubber latex proteins.

Additional Learning Resources

SG Go to your Study Guide for additional learning activities to help you master this chapter content.

Be sure to visit the Evolve site at http://evolve.elsevier.com/Cooper/adult/ for additional online resources.

Review Questions for the NCLEX® Examination

1. Which immune disorder results from a failure to tolerate "self"?
   1. immunodeficiency disorders
   2. hypersensitivity disorders
   3. desensitization disorders
   4. autoimmune disorders

2. The nurse is caring for a patient who has had a kidney transplant. What should be included in the care of a patient with a suppressed immune system?
   1. prophylactic antibiotic therapy
   2. meticulous aseptic technique
   3. restriction of all visitors
   4. antineoplastic medication administration

3. Which statements describe innate, or natural, immunity? *(Select all that apply.)*
   1. The body's first line of defense against disease, which protects locally against the external environment.
   2. The body's second line of defense against disease, which protects the internal environment.
   3. Includes stomach acid, saliva, and secretions/flora of the intestine and vagina.
   4. Mediated by B cells to produce antibodies in response to antigenic challenge.
   5. Provides an immunity that is specific.
   6. Responds with neutrophils, macrophages, and lymphocytes.

4. The activation of T cells by antigens indicates that which type of immunity is developing? *(Select all that apply.)*
   1. innate immunity
   2. adaptive immunity
   3. humoral immunity
   4. cellular immunity

5. The nurse is caring for a patient with a history of numerous allergies. What is the most important teaching concept?
   1. immunotherapy regimen
   2. avoidance of the allergen
   3. antihistamine administration
   4. adrenaline administration

6. Humoral immunity is mediated by which type of cells?
   1. T cells
   2. B cells
   3. macrophages
   4. myeloblasts

7. After a bee sting, the patient's face becomes edematous and she begins to wheeze. Based on this assessment, the nurse would be prepared to administer which medication?
   1. aminophylline
   2. diphenhydramine
   3. epinephrine
   4. diazepam

8. Which is another term for desensitization?
   1. autoimmune disorders
   2. adaptive immunity
   3. immunotherapy
   4. immunodeficiency disease

9. The nurse gave an intramuscular penicillin injection to a patient. What assessment finding would be most indicative of a systemic anaphylactic response?
   1. increased blood pressure
   2. bradycardia
   3. urticaria
   4. wheezing

10. A 38-year-old patient is receiving 2 units of packed red blood cells at 125 mL/h. Fifteen minutes after the start of the blood transfusion, the nurse notes the following vital signs: pulse 110 beats/min, respirations 28 breaths/min, blood pressure 98/58 mm Hg, and temperature 101°F. The patient is shivering. What is the nurse's initial action?
    1. Slow the infusion rate.
    2. Stop the infusion.
    3. Administer aspirin as ordered for elevated temperature.
    4. Report the findings to the nurse manager.

11. A 72-year-old patient is admitted to the hospital with a diagnosis of immunodeficiency disease. What is the primary nursing goal?
    1. Reduce the risk of the patient developing an infection.
    2. Encourage the patient to provide self-care.
    3. Plan nutritious meals to provide adequate intake.
    4. Encourage the patient to interact with other patients.

12. The patient tells the nurse he is overwhelmed. There is so much he must do to keep his new kidney functioning, and then rejection may still occur. Which patient problem statement is appropriate?
    1. Impaired Coping
    2. Distorted Body Image
    3. Potential for Unsafe Health Behaviors
    4. Impaired Self-Esteem due to Current Situation

13. A patient experienced an anaphylactic reaction to an antibiotic. What are the correct nursing interventions for anaphylaxis? *(Select all that apply.)*
    1. Assess vital signs every 4 hours
    2. Assess respiratory status frequently
    3. Maintain patent airway
    4. Administer epinephrine as ordered
    5. Monitor vital signs frequently

14. A patient comes to the clinic for his weekly allergy injection. He missed his appointment the week before because of a family emergency. Which action is appropriate in administering the patient's injection?

   1. Administer the usual dose of the allergen.
   2. Double the dose to account for the missed injection the previous week.
   3. Consult with the health care provider about decreasing the dose for this injection.
   4. Reevaluate the patient's sensitivity to the allergen with a skin test.

15. Type I allergic reaction to latex is a response to the _____ _____ _____.

16. The most common allergens that cause an anaphylactic reaction include: *(Select all that apply.)*

   1. Leafy, green vegetables
   2. Bees, wasps
   3. Shellfish
   4. Peanuts
   5. Oranges

17. Which illnesses are believed to be caused by an autoimmune disorder? *(Select all that apply.)*

   1. Rheumatoid arthritis
   2. Lung cancer
   3. Systemic lupus erythematosus
   4. Guillain-Barré syndrome
   5. Cardiovascular disease

18. The nurse advises a friend who asks the nurse to administer his allergy injections that:

   1. It is illegal for nurses to administer injections outside of a medical setting.
   2. He is qualified to do it if the friend has epinephrine in an injectable syringe provided with his extract.
   3. Avoiding the allergens is a more effective way of controlling allergies and allergy shots are not usually effective.
   4. Immunotherapy should be administered only in a setting where emergency equipment and drugs are available.

19. A patient is undergoing plasmapheresis for treatment of systemic lupus erythematosus. The nurse correctly recognizes which statement about the procedure? *(Select all that apply.)*

   1. Plasmapheresis will be used to remove the T lymphocytes from the blood that are responsible for producing antinuclear antibodies.
   2. Plasmapheresis will remove normal particles in her blood that are being damaged by autoantibodies.
   3. Plasmapheresis will replace the plasma that contains antinuclear antibodies with a substitute fluid.
   4. Plasma removed during the procedure will be replaced by normal saline.
   5. A side effect of the procedure is hypertension.

20. The nurse is collecting information from a patient during a hospital admission. Which allergen reports are concerning and may reveal an increased risk for latex allergies? *(Select all that apply.)*

   1. Strawberries
   2. Kiwi
   3. Celery
   4. Mangos
   5. Broccoli
   6. Chestnuts
   7. Walnuts
   8. Peanuts
   9. Almonds

21. The patient diagnosed with myasthenia gravis is undergoing plasmapheresis to treat the condition. During the procedure up to _____ mL of fluid is removed. Then, fluid replacement using lactated Ringer's solution, normal saline, frozen plasma, _____, or _____ is used.

Objectives

1. Describe the agent that causes HIV disease and the history of HIV.
2. Define AIDS by using the current terminology from the Centers for Disease Control and Prevention.
3. Explain the differences between HIV infection, HIV disease, and AIDS.
4. Describe the progression of HIV infection.
5. Discuss how HIV is and is not transmitted.
6. Describe patients who are at risk for HIV infection.
7. Discuss the pathophysiologic features of HIV disease.
8. List signs and symptoms that may be indicative of HIV disease.
9. Discuss the laboratory and diagnostic tests related to HIV disease.
10. Discuss the issues related to HIV antibody testing.
11. Describe the multidisciplinary approach in caring for a patient with HIV disease.
12. List opportunistic infections associated with advanced HIV disease (AIDS).
13. Discuss the nurse's role in assisting the HIV-infected patient with coping, grieving, reducing anxiety, and minimizing social isolation.
14. Discuss the importance of adherence to HIV treatment.
15. Discuss the use of effective prevention strategies in the counseling of patients.
16. Define the nurse's role in the prevention of HIV infection.

Key Terms

acquired immunodeficiency syndrome (AIDS) (ŭ-KWĪRD ĭm-yū-nō-dĕ-FĬSH-ĕn-sē SĬN-drŏm, p. 748)

adherence (ăd-HĔR-ĕns, p. 757)

CD4+ lymphocyte (SĒ DĒ FŌRPLŬS LĬM-fō-sīt, p. 745)

Centers for Disease Control and Prevention (CDC) (SĔN-tŭrz FŌR dĭz-ĒZ kŭn-TRŌL ĂND prĕ-VĔN-shŭn, p. 739)

HIV disease (ĀCH Ī VĒ dĭz-ĒZ, p. 748)

human immunodeficiency virus (HIV) (HYŪ-mĭn ĭm-yū-nō-dĕ-FĬSH-ĕn-sē VĪ-rŭs, p. 740)

Kaposi's sarcoma (kă-PŌS-sĕz sär-KŌ-mŭ, p. 739)

opportunistic (ŏp-pŏr-tū-NĬS-tĭk, p. 741)

phagocyte (făg-ō-SĪT, p. 748)

Pneumocystis jiroveci pneumonia (nū-mō-SĬS-tĭs yē-rō-VĔT-zē nū-MŌN-yŭ, p. 749)

retrovirus (rĕ-trō-VĪ-rŭs, p. 745)

seroconversion (sĕr-ō-kŏn-VĔR-zhŭn, p. 744)

seronegative (sĕr-ō-NĔG-ă-tĭv, p. 752)

seroprevalence (sĕr-ō-PRĔV-ŭ-lŭns, p. 742)

vertical transmission (VŬR-tĭk-ŭl trănz-MĬSH-ŭn, p. 743)

viral load (VĪ-rŭl LŌD, p. 743)

virulent (VĬR-ū-lĕnt, p. 741)

wasting (WĀST-ĭng, p. 764)

NURSING AND THE HISTORY OF HIV DISEASE

As early as 1979, physicians in New York and California were identifying cases of Pneumocystis jiroveci (formerly *Pneumocystis carinii*) pneumonia, an unusual pulmonary disease caused by a fungus that infects primarily people who have suppressed immune systems. The fungus is found commonly in the environment but does not normally have an adverse affect on people who are healthy. An estimated 20% of adults may carry the fungus at any time. During the time when the acquired immunodeficiency syndrome (AIDS) epidemic was at its peak, the majority of people with advanced AIDS developed this lung infection. The use of prophylactic antibiotics significantly has decreased the number of cases of this condition among patients with AIDS (CDC, 2021k). Also, during the height of the epidemic, physicians noted an increase in the number of people with Kaposi's sarcoma, a rare cancer of the skin and mucous membranes characterized by blue, red, or purple raised lesions (Fig. 16.1) that occurred mainly in men of Mediterranean descent. Of interest was that these two diseases were occurring at alarming rates in clusters of young homosexual men whose immune systems were failing. Researchers at the Centers for Disease Control and Prevention (CDC), a division of the US Public Health Service that investigates and reports on various diseases, soon learned that this immune disorder also was affecting people who used

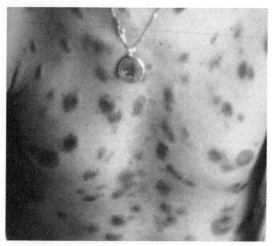

Fig. 16.1 Kaposi sarcoma. (Courtesy Paul A. Volberding, MD, University of California, San Francisco. US Department of Veterans Affairs.)

injection drugs and patients with hemophilia. Later, the immune disorder also was identified in heterosexual men and women.

The origins of **human immunodeficiency virus (HIV)** remain somewhat obscure, and why HIV gave rise to the AIDS epidemic (some resources refer to HIV/AIDS as a pandemic) only in the 20th century has not yet been determined. The earliest case of HIV infection has been dated to 1959. It was identified in the Democratic Republic of Congo through different methods of molecular clock analysis. It also has been estimated that HIV began to radiate from its source in approximately the 1930s (Buonaguro et al., 2007). The escalating epidemic probably resulted from the combination of significant cultural and sociobehavioral changes, the use of nonsterile needles for parenteral injections and vaccinations, and the unintended contamination of products used for medical treatments.

HIV has been recognized as a clinical syndrome since the early 1980s. Several researchers have, however, identified patients who may have fit the CDC's Case Surveillance definition before that time. The unusual and rapid deterioration and death in 1969 of a 15-year-old boy (Robert R.) in St. Louis from aggressive, disseminated Kaposi sarcoma suggests that his may have been the first confirmed death from HIV infection in the United States (Garry et al., 1988). This patient had no international travel experience, which suggests that other individuals were infected with HIV as well. This also implies that HIV may have existed in some form in the United States since at least the 1960s.

HIV is known as *zoonotic*, an organism that has been able to cross from an animal species to humans. A similar virus (called *simian immunodeficiency virus*) was noted in primates and probably crossed into humans by way of the hunting and consumption of these animals in Africa. Other examples of zoonotic transmission include severe acute respiratory distress syndrome, anthrax, rabies, hantavirus, and West Nile virus (World Health Organization [WHO], 2020). HIV began to spread in the middle to late 1970s, but because of the long incubation period, the viral epidemic progressed undetected in most countries. When the virus began causing widespread disease in the 1980s, it provoked fear among laypeople and health care providers. It was also a challenging time for health care workers because they knew they were observing a new pathogen whose route of transmission was not completely understood. In spite of the stigmas and fears that emerged (and still exist to some extent), nurses were at the forefront of providing care to affected patients. Nurses met the challenges of providing and coordinating services, organizing community-based organizations, teaching about prevention, and helping patients deal with a terminal disease. Interestingly, we find ourselves today in a similar situation with the current COVID-19 Coronavirus pandemic. Nurses are at the forefront caring for patients once again.

There are three stages of HIV. Stage 1 is the stage of acute HIV infection. This occurs within 2 to 4 weeks of transmission of the infection and manifests as if the patient had influenza. During this stage, patients are very infectious with elevated numbers of the virus in their blood and some bodily fluids. Stage 2 is known as chronic HIV infection. The patient is often asymptomatic during this stage with low levels of the virus present in their blood. The virus reproduces slowly and the patient may stay in this stage for 10 years or longer without medication. With medication the patient may never progress to stage 3. Towards the end of this stage the patient often becomes symptomatic. Stage 3 is when the patient develops AIDS, and this stage carries the same name. This is the most severe stage of the infection. Patients develop opportunistic infections because their immune systems have been damaged by the HIV infection. Their viral loads are elevated and they are very contagious. Their CD4 count drops to less than 200 cells/mm. They may experience fever, chills, sweating, swollen lymph nodes, weight loss, and weakness (CDC, 2021b).

The CDC (1981) published a notation about some patients with signs and symptoms that later would be attributed to AIDS. The signs and symptoms listed were related to the development of opportunistic infections. Such infections occur when the body's immune system has been weakened. Since that time, AIDS was known as one of the most challenging infectious diseases of the 20th and 21st centuries. Great advancements in treatment have made HIV and AIDS a much more manageable disease. In 1982, the CDC issued a statement that blood and other body fluids may be vehicles for transmitting the disease and that precautions must be used with all blood and body fluids.

The discovery of a second HIV strain was major and alarming at the time, because it was the first clue that HIV could mutate rapidly. This capability for rapid mutation has become the trademark of this virus. It represents an immense challenge for scientists as they search for vaccine strategies. HIV type 1 (HIV-1) is found worldwide and is the prevalent strain in most places, including the United States, Europe, and Central Africa. HIV-1 and HIV type 2 (HIV-2) are spread in the same ways and have similar signs and symptoms. Infection with either of these viral strains also results in opportunistic infections with progression to AIDS. HIV-1 infection is much more common in the United States, and worldwide, than HIV-2 infection. Despite HIV-1 being the predominant form of HIV infection in this country, it is important for testing to determine which infection an individual might have. Treatment varies based on the type of HIV infection (Peruski, 2020).

HIV-1 is much more **virulent** (toxic) than HIV-2. People with HIV-2 infection tend to be identified as long-term nonprogressors. Patients infected with HIV-2 develop problems with immunodeficiency more slowly. However, these patients can progress to AIDS with lower viral load levels than patients with HIV-1.

Since the first cases of AIDS were reported in 1981, the CDC has revised the HIV case definition several times in response to improved laboratory and diagnostic methods (CD4$^+$ and viral test results). Diagnostic criteria changes also allow for distinguishing between HIV-1 and HIV-2 infection and early HIV identification (Peruski, 2020). The current definition, used by all states and US territories, allows the disease to be monitored consistently for public health purposes. These revisions to the HIV surveillance case definition took into account the advances in diagnostic methods and treatment to provide more accurate information on the numbers of life-threatening illnesses and deaths that are **opportunistic** (caused by normally nonpathogenic organisms in a host whose resistance has been decreased by such disorders as HIV disease) among HIV-infected individuals (Peruski, 2020).

It was not until 1987, after the CDC reported three cases of occupationally acquired HIV infection in health care providers, that universal guidelines for blood and body fluid precautions, or *standard precautions,* were developed for the prevention of occupational exposure. These guidelines forever changed the way health care personnel protect themselves and other people from the spread of bloodborne pathogens. That same year, the Association of Nurses in AIDS Care was established to address the needs of individuals with HIV disease and to provide a professional forum for nurses, who often faced discrimination as a result of providing care to HIV-infected patients.

By that time, a broad spectrum of individuals, including children, adults, and people from all socioeconomic groups, were affected by this disorder (see the Lifespan Considerations box). Nurses became instrumental in establishing education and treatment standards, in collaboration with community-based organizations. Today nurses constitute the largest group of health care professionals who care for individuals with HIV disease, which stresses the importance of prevention and influencing policymakers. HIV nursing provides lessons that can be useful in other patient populations as well: the importance of patient education, adherence to medical regimens, prevention, and health-promoting behaviors.

Lifespan Considerations
Older Adults

HIV Disease

- In 2013, people who were 50 years old and older accounted for 42% of all residents of the United States who were living with diagnosed HIV infection (CDC, 2020b).
- Improved treatments and prophylactic medications are contributing to longer life spans in individuals with HIV disease, which has made the disease chronic.
- Because the immune system's ability to fight infection decreases with age, HIV disease progresses faster and complications increase among older adults with HIV infection.
- Divorced and widowed people are beginning to date again and may be having sex with multiple partners without recognizing their risk for becoming infected with HIV. Age-related changes to women's vaginal tissue may increase their risk for acquiring HIV.

SIGNIFICANCE OF THE PROBLEM
Disease Burden

Throughout the world, HIV is one of the leading causes of death and results in more deaths than does any other disease caused by infection. As of 2018 approximately 1.2 million people were living with HIV infections in the United States, and approximately 13% are unaware that they have the disease (HIV.gov, 2021b). In 201518, 15,820 deaths occurred in the United States due to people diagnosed with AIDS.

Sub-Saharan Africa has been hit especially hard. Since 2015, 3.5 million HIV infections have been reported in this region along with 820,000 deaths (UNAIDS, 2020). Death related to AIDS is associated largely with poor access to prevention and treatment services. Since 2005, the number of people infected with HIV has declined steadily (AVERT, 2021a). This decreasing infection rate is thought to be related to increased access to antiretroviral treatments. Managing and treating this disease will remain a challenge for years to come, especially in the sub-Saharan region of Africa.

In the United States, approximately 40,000 new cases of HIV are diagnosed each year. Since 2014, there has been a 7% decrease in diagnosed cases. The highest rate of infection is in people between the ages of 25 to 34 years (31.5% of cases) (HIV.gov, 2021b).

TRENDS AND MOST AFFECTED POPULATIONS

Beginning in 1996, the use of *highly active antiretroviral therapy* (ART) in people with HIV infection increased greatly in the United States. Since that time, fewer people with HIV infection have developed AIDS. New HIV and AIDS cases affect various racial groups, ethnic groups, geographic areas, and demographic populations; thus this epidemic has affected nonwhite people, women, heterosexuals, and people who use injection drugs. However, people with HIV are living longer (CDC, 2021e).

The CDC reported that the population of men who have sex with other men (MSM) constitutes the biggest proportion of HIV patients, accounting for 69% of the total number of HIV infections in male patients 13 years of age and older. Heterosexuals in general make up 24% of new HIV diagnoses (CDC, 2021e). The HIV infection rates among the MSM population decreased from 71% in 1983 to 44% in 1996. Holmberg (1996) predicted that this rate would continue to decrease to approximately 25%.

During the first 25 years of this epidemic, the distribution of new cases on the basis of ethnicity and race changed (see the Cultural Considerations box). Disproportionate numbers of Hispanic Americans and African Americans have been infected with HIV. In 2018, African American males (adolescents and adults) accounted for 42% of the total number of HIV cases that were diagnosed (CDC, 2021a). African American adults and adolescents are 10 times more likely to receive a diagnosis of AIDS than are white adults and adolescents. The primary risk factor for African American men who developed HIV was sexual contact. Young gay and bisexual men accounted for 83% of all new HIV diagnoses in people aged 13 to 24 in 2018 (includes young gay and bisexual men who inject drugs) (CDC, 2021c).

Some African American MSM identify themselves as heterosexuals because of the stigma and homophobia issues. Many African American MSM are secretive about their homosexuality or choose not to identify their sexual orientation. Prevention programs are challenged when people do not identify themselves as engaging in risky behaviors or having increased risk factors.

Initially the face of HIV was predominately homosexual men and people who used injection drugs. Rates of infection among heterosexual women from 2014 to 2018 have decreased 9%, but the rate for women who inject drugs has increased by 7%. Currently, an estimated 16% of HIV sufferers are women (CDC, 2021j).

Rates of new infections of Hispanic/Latino Americans has been stable (CDC, 2020f). Many socioeconomic and cultural factors have contributed to this epidemic and associated prevention challenges in the US Hispanic and Latino communities. For Hispanic men and women, the primary risk factor for developing HIV is sex with men. If current rates continue to trend, the CDC reports that 25% of Hispanic/Latino MSM may be infected with HIV during their life (CDC, 2021c). Rates of other sexually transmitted infections (STIs), including chlamydia, gonorrhea, and syphilis, are also higher among Hispanic Americans than among non-Hispanic white Americans (CDC, 2021c).

🌐 Cultural Considerations

HIV Disease

- Since 2000, Hispanic/Latino Americans have accounted for 56% of the United States' growth in population. The rate of **seroprevalence** (occurrence of disease within a defined population at one time) is higher among Hispanic/Latino Americans than among white Americans, and as a result, HIV prevention education is important. In 2018, Hispanic/Latino Americans represented 27% of new HIV infections (CDC, 2020c).
- Barriers to prevention include difficulty providing care in a nonthreatening environment where health care providers are viewed as authorities.
- Undocumented residents, including Hispanic Americans, are reluctant to seek HIV care because this condition disqualifies them for US legal residency and they fear deportation. In addition, nearly 75% of Hispanic Americans are members of the Catholic Church, which historically has been opposed to sex outside marriage, sex between men, and artificial birth control. These beliefs complicate prevention efforts that stress the use of condoms.
- Because of the deportation threat, Hispanic American patients may not share important health information with health care providers.
- In assessment and interventions, nurses should be sensitive to language and cultural differences.
- Nurses should provide a safe, supportive environment for assessment and treatment and should advocate for patients who need treatment, regardless of ability to pay for services or residency status.

Data from Centers for Disease Control and Prevention (CDC): HIV: Hispanics/Latinos. Available at: https://www.cdc.gov/hiv/group/racialethnic/hispaniclatinos/.

Transient Hispanic populations often have difficulty receiving access to health care because of social structure, language barriers, and migration patterns (CDC, 2021c). The predicaments caused by poverty limit access to appropriate health care, housing, and HIV prevention. All these factors may increase directly or indirectly risk factors for HIV infection in the Hispanic population.

As treatment for HIV has advanced, the progression from HIV to stage 3 (AIDS) has slowed, resulting in a decreased mortality rate among people infected with HIV. The data from the period of 2010 to 2017 shows an overall decline in HIV related deaths. This decline was noted in all groups including those with greater population percentages (CDC, 2020c). Advanced treatment options mean that people are living longer after their HIV diagnoses. Unfortunately, in countries where HIV-infected people are without adequate access to health care, HIV infection is still one of the leading causes of death.

TRANSMISSION OF HUMAN IMMUNODEFICIENCY VIRUS

Despite significant research into the modes of transmission of HIV, considerable fear and misinformation about HIV transmission, perhaps more than for any other disease, still exists. Health care providers and patients must be knowledgeable about modes of transmission and behaviors that put them at risk for HIV infection. Modes of transmission have remained constant throughout the course of the HIV epidemic. Health care providers also need to remember that transmission of HIV occurs through sexual *practices,* not sexual *preferences.*

The patterns in the spread of HIV changed considerably during the first two decades of the epidemic in the United States (Henry J. Kaiser Family Foundation, 2021). Most cases of HIV in the United States are diagnosed in MSM. In the United States, HIV diagnoses that are attributable to injection drug use have shown recent decline. The number of estimated pediatric HIV cases diagnosed each year has declined since 1992. This decline is associated with the increased compliance with universal counseling and testing of pregnant women and the use of ART by HIV-infected pregnant women and their newborns (Henry J. Kaiser Family Foundation, 2021).

HIV is an *obligate virus,* which means it must have a host organism to survive. The virus cannot live long outside the human body. HIV transmission depends on the presence of the virus, the infectiousness of the virus, the susceptibility of the uninfected recipient, and any conditions that may increase the recipient's risk for infection. HIV is transmitted from human to human through infected blood, semen, rectal secretions, cervicovaginal secretions, and breast milk. Deep mouth kissing favors transmission if both partners have open sores or bleeding gums and one partner is infected with HIV. Eating food that has been prechewed by a person infected with HIV can transmit the virus (only documented cases are with infants) (HIV.gov, 2019). If these infected fluids are introduced into an uninfected person, HIV can be transmitted to that person. In addition to the aforementioned body fluids, HIV also is found in pericardial, synovial, cerebrospinal, peritoneal, and amniotic fluids. Vertical transmission (transmission from a mother to a fetus) of HIV can occur during pregnancy, during delivery, or through postpartum breast-feeding (transmitted in the breast milk). Conditions that affect the likelihood of infection include the duration and frequency of exposure, the amount of virus inoculated into the recipient, the virulence of the organism, and the recipient's defense capability (immune system). Although HIV has been found in other body fluids such as saliva, urine, tears, and feces, there has been no evidence that these substances are vehicles of transmission, unless the fluids contain visible blood.

HIV generally is not transmitted by casual contacts, such as hugging, dry kissing, shaking hands, or sharing food and utensils. Contact with domestic animals or insects; coughing or sneezing; or through sharing objects such as pencils, computer keyboards, or telephones are behaviors that are not linked to transmission of the virus.

The two most common modes of HIV transmission are anal or vaginal intercourse and sharing contaminated injecting drug equipment and paraphernalia. Once infected, an individual is capable of transmitting HIV to other people at any time throughout the disease spectrum, even when the infected host appears healthy and has no obvious signs of the infection. In HIV infection, the viral load (amount of measurable HIV virions in the blood) peaks quickly after infection and during the later stages of the disease. During these periods, a recipient's unprotected exposure to an infected host increases the likelihood of transmission. However, it is important to remember that HIV can be transmitted during the entire disease spectrum.

SEXUAL TRANSMISSION

Sexual intercourse remains the most common mode of transmission of HIV in the world today and is responsible for the majority of the world's total HIV cases. Sexual activity provides the potential for the exchange of semen, cervicovaginal secretions, and blood. Important risk factors are the presence of HIV in one or both partners and the occurrence of behaviors that put one or both partners at risk for transmission. Some individuals become infected with HIV after a single unprotected sexual encounter, whereas others remain free from infection after hundreds of such encounters.

Although the majority of HIV transmissions in the United States occur among MSM via receptive anal intercourse, heterosexual transmission via anal intercourse is becoming increasingly prevalent. Heterosexual couples may prefer this method of sexual expression or use it because it eliminates the risk of pregnancy. Unfortunately, the most risky sexual activity is unprotected receptive anal intercourse. Because the rectum is generally tighter and the rectal mucosa is less lubricated than the vagina, the rectal mucosa may be torn, providing an excellent portal for the virus to enter the bloodstream.

During any form of sexual intercourse (anal, vaginal, oral), the risk of infection is considerably higher for the receptive partner, although infection can be transmitted to an insertive partner as well. The receptive partner generally has prolonged exposure to semen (HIV.gov, 2021a). Other factors that may increase the risk of sexual transmission include ulcerating genital diseases, such as herpes simplex virus (HSV) and syphilis; chancres secondary to STIs; intact (uncircumcised) foreskin; sex that is "forceful or vigorous"; immunosuppression resulting from drug use; and drug use that may lead to high-risk behavior. Infection risk for HIV also can be increased during intercourse when the infected partner has a high viral load (CDC, 2021i). The viral load often is increased in the primary and late stages of infection. Oral-genital transmissions have been reported, and the HIV transmission risk increases if the receiving partner already has an STI that has caused open sores, such as HSV infection.

PARENTERAL EXPOSURE

Injecting Drug Use

HIV may be transmitted by exposure to contaminated blood through the accidental or intentional sharing of injecting equipment and paraphernalia. Such equipment includes syringes, needles, cookers (spoons or bottle caps used for mixing the drug), and filtering equipment (such as cotton balls and rinse water) (CDC, 2021d). People who use injection drugs are the population with the second highest rates of HIV exposure, following MSM (CDC, 2021f). Although typically seen in large metropolitan areas, injection drug use occurs in smaller cities and rural areas as well. Such drugs are not limited to illicit drugs; HIV can be transmitted via contaminated equipment used to inject steroids, vitamins, and insulin.

People who use injection drugs confirm needle placement in a vein by drawing back blood into the syringe; the substance is then injected into the vein. Other factors that put people who use illicit injection drugs at risk for HIV include poor nutritional status, poor hygiene, and impaired judgment resulting from mood-altering substances. People who use illicit injection drugs are also less likely to use condoms during sexual intercourse and may engage in sexual activity in exchange for drugs. The long-term effects of illicit injection drug use include increased risk for other diseases, such as hepatitis B, hepatitis C, and other blood borne illnesses.

Blood and Blood Products

Since 1985, blood banks in the United States have screened all donated blood for HIV-1 antibodies and, since 1992, for HIV-2 antibodies. Blood banks also have implemented procedures to identify blood donors who may be at high risk for infection with HIV. Blood from donors who are deemed to be at high risk or that yields test results positive for HIV is discarded. In addition to HIV, blood currently is screened for human T-lymphotropic virus types 1 and 2 (HTLV-1 and HTLV-2), hepatitis B virus, treponema pallidum (syphilis), West Nile virus, *Trypanosoma cruzi* infection (Chagas disease), and hepatitis C virus (US Food and Drug Administration [FDA], 2021).

Every year, a small number of blood donations come from donors who are infected with HIV but in whom the HIV antibody was undetected. When a blood donor has not yet undergone seroconversion (a change in serologic test results from negative to positive as antibodies develop in reaction to an infection), the current HIV antibody test cannot detect the infection. In the past, there was a 22-day window during which the donor could donate infected blood in which HIV would not be detected by the HIV-1 and HIV-2 antibody test. Since 1995, however, blood also has been screened for HIV-1 p24 antigen. With this addition, this window has been reduced to 16 days. In 1999, the nucleic acid amplification test was introduced; this test detects HIV-1 RNA and has reduced the window to only 11 days. By 2008 only four people were infected with HIV after receiving a blood product transfusion (CDC, 2010). The blood came from three separate donors, and the blood tested negative for HIV with all currently available HIV tests (CDC, 2010). Currently, a person's risk for acquiring HIV through a blood transfusion is estimated to be about 1 per 1.5 million (CDC, 2010). Before 1985, people who received replacement clotting factors for blood coagulation difficulties (e.g., hemophilia) were at increased risk of contracting HIV. Since 1985, a recombinant technique is used to manufacture the clotting factors or the clotting factors are treated with chemicals or heated to kill the HIV.

Occupational Exposure

Almost 25,000 adults who developed AIDS before 2003 were health care workers. This number represents 5% of all AIDS cases among adults who had a known occupation.

The CDC distinguishes between two types of HIV seroconversion. When the infection is "documented," it means that the individual had a documented exposure related to occupation and developed HIV disease. A "possible" infection indicates that the individual worked in a high-risk setting with exposure to blood or other body fluids related to occupation; however, no exposure event was documented.

As of 2019 in the United States, only 58 health care workers were infected with HIV. Safe practices regarding blood borne pathogens in the health care workplace has proved successful. The use of proper PPE as well as safety needles and needless systems have attributed to the low percentage of health care worker HIV infection while at work. The risk of exposure to HIV from a needlestick injury is less than 1% and transmission by direct skin contact with fluids is less than 0.1% (Familydoctor.org, 2019).

Most of the health care workers who have been infected with HIV are nurses. The second largest group is laboratory clinicians, and the third largest group is physicians (nonsurgical). Other health care workers with possible exposures included emergency medical technicians, health care aides, housekeepers, and maintenance workers. Most of the infections occurred after a needlestick injury with resulting puncture wound. Exposures are thought to be underreported because such reporting is voluntary. If a health care worker does have a needlestick that results in exposure to a known source of HIV infection, the risk for contracting HIV is low, at approximately 0.3%.

Needlesticks that occur when a health care worker is exposed to patients with known HIV infection are known as *percutaneous exposures.* If the exposure involves a hollow-bore needle filled with blood that had previously been placed in the patient's vein or artery, then the transmission risk of HIV is increased.

The transmission risk also is increased if the health care worker suffers a deep injury at the time of the exposure. Scalpels, suture needles, and smaller gauge injection needles also pose a risk for transmission, but that risk is much lower. If only the mucous membranes are exposed during the incident, then the risk for seroconversion is only 0.09%. There is a low risk for seroconverting if the health care worker's skin is not intact and is exposed to blood or body fluids.

Unfortunately, antiretroviral medications used as post-exposure prophylaxis antiretroviral are hepatotoxic. When ART is given to a health care worker after a documented exposure, it may result in severe hepatitis that may necessitate liver transplantation.

Perinatal (Vertical) Transmission

HIV infection can be transmitted from a mother to her infant during pregnancy, at the time of delivery, or after birth through breast-feeding. It is the most common way for children to be infected with HIV. In the United States, it is estimated that approximately 25% of infected mothers transmit HIV to their infants and that approximately 50% to 70% of the transmissions occur late in utero or during birth. The rate of vertical transmission varies around the world. Factors such as the stage of maternal HIV disease (transmission is more likely to occur during the initial and later stages of infection, when more of the virus is circulating in the mother's blood and body fluids), a decreased CD4+ cell count or high viral load, the presence or absence of STIs, and the mother's nutritional status play a role in vertical transmission. Factors that increase the risk of transmission during delivery include extreme prematurity; lack of health care; gestational complications that lead to extended labor; the mixing of maternal and fetal blood; newborn ingestion of maternal blood, amniotic fluid, or vaginal secretions; skin excoriation in the newborn; and being the first child born in a multiple gestation. HIV-infected mothers are cautioned to use formula in place of breast-feeding because breastmilk is another way to transmit the infection to infants (HIVinfo.nih.gov, 2020c).

Clinical trials have demonstrated that the administration of a combination of antiretroviral medications to pregnant women who are infected with HIV can reduce transmission to approximately 1% of infants. These infants are given HIV medications for 6 weeks after birth to prevent the development of HIV infection in case of exposure.

In addition to drug therapy, substantial advances have been made in understanding the pathophysiology, treatment, and monitoring of HIV infection. These advances have resulted in changes in the standard of care for patients, including pregnant women, with HIV infection. More aggressive combination drug regimens that provide maximal viral suppression are now recommended. Although pregnancy alone is not a reason to defer treatment, the use of anti-HIV drugs during pregnancy requires special consideration. Unfortunately, no long-term data regarding the long-term effects on the fetus exist. Because of this, offering ART to HIV-infected women—whether primarily to treat HIV infection or to reduce the likelihood of perinatal transmission—should be accompanied by a discussion of the known and unknown short- and long-term benefits and potential risks. Women who are taking HIV medications during pregnancy are encouraged to enroll in the Antiretroviral Pregnancy Registry (Clinicalinfo.hiv.gov, n.d.).

Current recommendations call for routine HIV counseling and voluntary HIV testing of pregnant women and women considering pregnancy. An HIV-infected pregnant woman should be given information to make an informed decision about treatment options. The HIV transmission rates from mother to child have been reduced because of several recommended interventions, including ART, formula feeding, and cesarean section. In developed countries, this number is 1.1 out of 100,000 births (Irshad, 2021). In countries where ART is not available and mothers continue to breast-feed, the infection rate by age 2 for children born to HIV-infected mothers is much higher. Infants born to HIV-infected mothers have positive HIV antibody results as long as 15 to 18 months after birth. This finding is caused by maternal antibodies that cross the placenta during gestation and remain in the infant's circulatory system. HIV infection can be diagnosed earlier by means of an HIV viral culture or measuring the amount of HIV RNA or viral load through polymerase chain reaction (PCR) or branched-chain DNA (bDNA) testing.

PATHOPHYSIOLOGY

HIV is classified as a "slow" retrovirus or a lentivirus. After infection with these types of viruses, a long time passes before specific signs and symptoms appear. HIV requires cells for replication. The virus takes over the host cell and reproduces viral copies of it. Retroviruses are made of RNA. Most organisms' genetic material is made up of DNA. The retrovirus uses reverse transcriptase, an enzyme, to make its RNA change to DNA. This process allows the virus to be incorporated into the host's genetic material.

HIV can cross over into the host in the dendritic immune cells that are located in the mucosal layer of the vulva, the vagina, the rectum, and the penis. The exterior layer of the dendritic cell passes the virus into the interior portion of the cell. The virus is released into the lymphatic system via tissue or lymph nodes. Then the virus binds to a CD4+ lymphocyte (a type of white blood cell; a protein on the surface of cells that normally helps the body's immune system combat disease), by which it can travel farther into the lymphatic system and begin the cycle of infection (HIVinfo.nih.gov, 2020d).

The attachment of the viral particle to the host cell's CD4⁺ receptor and co-receptor (CCR5 or CXCR4) is the first step in replication of the virus (Fig. 16.2). The HIV virion enters the host cell when the virus binds to the cell. After binding to the cell, co-receptors are needed to continue the fusion process and to enable the viral particle to eject two copies of the virus's RNA. Inside the cell, HIV reverse transcriptase changes the viral RNA into DNA. A full copy of this DNA is created and broken down into smaller, more functional pieces that are moved to the nucleus of the cell. The HIV DNA moves into the nucleus of the cell, where viral integrase helps insert it into the DNA of the host. The inserted virus is called a *provirus*. After activation, the cell makes a new copy of HIV by using viral proteins. Afterward, there is an abnormal amount of immune activation. This perpetuates the progress of the HIV infection because it creates more CD4⁺ cells that will be under attack by HIV and eventually will exhaust the immune system. The number of CD8⁺ T cells that are activated at this time is related directly to an increased risk of developing advanced HIV infection, or AIDS. However, the HIV can remain dormant for years if the CD4⁺ cell remains inactivated. It has been difficult to control HIV completely because of its ability to remain undetected. Patients with HIV are advised to continue taking their antiretroviral medications (HIVinfo.nih.gov, 2020d).

New viral proteins are created when the infected CD4⁺ cell converts DNA into RNA. This process is called *transcription*. The process relies on the host cell and the viral genetic material. The new RNA is messenger RNA (mRNA), and it is returned from the nucleus back into the cytoplasm. In the cytoplasm, mRNA is used as a template to begin making HIV protein. This process is called *translation*. The protein sequence of the mRNA is changed back into RNA, and this makes up the outer envelope and inner core of HIV. After translation, the genetic materials become smaller and smaller pieces of viral material. The viral protease chunks the genetic products into smaller pieces so that they can infect more CD4⁺ host cells. This HIV protease is specific to this virus and is targeted by a class of medications called *protease inhibitors* (PIs) that are used to manage HIV. The envelope's viral proteins are joined together inside the host cell's membrane, with the core proteins, RNA, and enzymes just inside the membrane.

HIV then "buds" by pinching off this cell. One infected CD4⁺ cell has the ability to make thousands of cell copies quickly. The CD4⁺ cell dies as a result of this replication process. As time goes on, so many CD4⁺ cells are destroyed that the immune system becomes dysfunctional and opportunistic infections develop within the host.

INFLUENCES ON VIRAL LOAD AND DISEASE PROGRESSION

HIV replicates quickly after entering the host body. It can produce billions of copies rapidly, which infect CD4⁺ cells and the lymphatic system (Fig. 16.3). The viral load of the host during the early stage of the infection can be extremely high and increases risk of virus transmission to other people who are exposed. The severity and progression of the infection are related to the host's infection with other STIs, age, and immune response. Basic host immune defenses (cellular and humoral) help limit replication and slow progression of HIV. Unfortunately, these immune responses cannot completely eliminate HIV from the host. The host can continue to appear healthy even when infected with the virus (Table 16.1). Some patients live with the virus for at least 10 years without any treatment and appear healthy. They are referred to as *long-term nonprogressors*.

Many factors can increase HIV disease progression. People who use drugs and engage in high-risk sexual behavior are less likely to employ infection-preventive methods. Poverty, incarceration, immigration status, and co-infection with STIs also can contribute to a person's risk for HIV infection (CDC, 2016). This population of infected individuals are unlikely to seek testing or treatment when infection is identified. This leads to continued transmission among this population.

The virus can make amazing numbers of copies of itself daily (NIAID, 2018). HIV contained in blood plasma has a half-life of less than 2 days. While the virus continues to replicate, many millions of CD4⁺ cells are produced and destroyed each day. The viral load in the patient's blood determines how quickly the CD4⁺ cells are destroyed.

The HIV viral load in the blood can remain low or difficult to detect for weeks or even months after the initial exposure and infection (Fig. 16.4). When the immune system responds, the viral load decreases quickly as the body effectively contains the infection. Normally, antigens that are deemed foreign intermingle with B cells. At this stage, antibodies are produced. T cells start a cell-based immune response. In the early stages of the infection, the antibodies are able to reduce the viral load. T cells are beckoned to the lymph nodes, where the virus is trapped (see Table 16.1). The virus replicates in the lymph system (nodes, tissue, spleen, and tonsils).

The lymphatic system carries the infection from one site to another. During this time, the HIV-infected person does not have any signs or symptoms. Over time, the lymphatic system is damaged by the HIV. The virus enters the blood, which increases the rate of disease progression. The body is not able to mount an adequate response to new infections. The immune system damage is apparent on examination of B cell dysfunction, but more important CD4⁺ cells are destroyed and their levels depleted (see Fig. 16.2).

The HIV Life Cycle

HIV medicines in seven drug classes stop ⏹ HIV at different stages in the HIV life cycle.

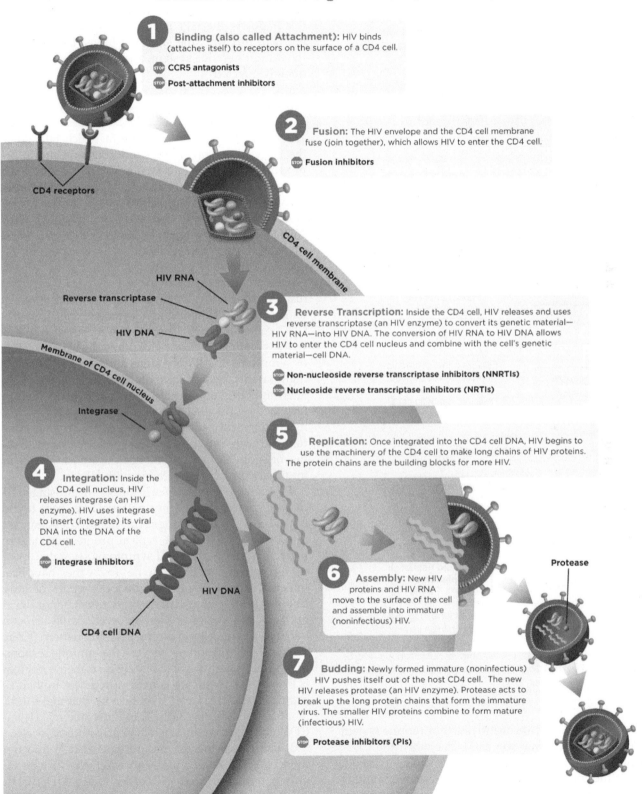

① **Binding (also called Attachment):** HIV binds (attaches itself) to receptors on the surface of a CD4 cell.

⏹ **CCR5 antagonists**

⏹ **Post-attachment inhibitors**

② **Fusion:** The HIV envelope and the CD4 cell membrane fuse (join together), which allows HIV to enter the CD4 cell.

⏹ **Fusion inhibitors**

CD4 receptors

CD4 cell membrane

HIV RNA

Reverse transcriptase

HIV DNA

③ **Reverse Transcription:** Inside the CD4 cell, HIV releases and uses reverse transcriptase (an HIV enzyme) to convert its genetic material— HIV RNA—into HIV DNA. The conversion of HIV RNA to HIV DNA allows HIV to enter the CD4 cell nucleus and combine with the cell's genetic material—cell DNA.

⏹ **Non-nucleoside reverse transcriptase inhibitors (NNRTIs)**

⏹ **Nucleoside reverse transcriptase inhibitors (NRTIs)**

Membrane of CD4 cell nucleus

Integrase

⑤ **Replication:** Once integrated into the CD4 cell DNA, HIV begins to use the machinery of the CD4 cell to make long chains of HIV proteins. The protein chains are the building blocks for more HIV.

④ **Integration:** Inside the CD4 cell nucleus, HIV releases integrase (an HIV enzyme). HIV uses integrase to insert (integrate) its viral DNA into the DNA of the CD4 cell.

⏹ **Integrase inhibitors**

HIV DNA

CD4 cell DNA

Protease

⑥ **Assembly:** New HIV proteins and HIV RNA move to the surface of the cell and assemble into immature (noninfectious) HIV.

⑦ **Budding:** Newly formed immature (noninfectious) HIV pushes itself out of the host CD4 cell. The new HIV releases protease (an HIV enzyme). Protease acts to break up the long protein chains that form the immature virus. The smaller HIV proteins combine to form mature (infectious) HIV.

⏹ **Protease inhibitors (PIs)**

Fig. 16.2 Life Cycle of HIV Cell.

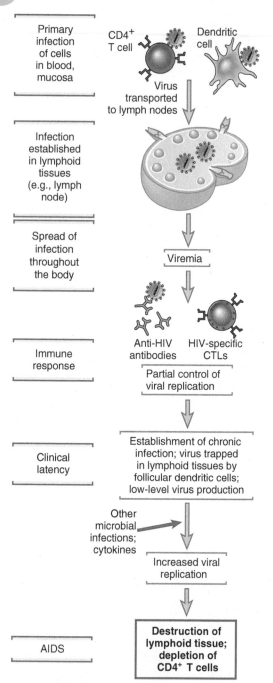

Fig. 16.3 Viral load in the blood and the relationship to CD4+ lymphocyte cell count over the spectrum of human immunodeficiency virus (HIV) disease. *AIDS*, Acquired immunodeficiency syndrome; *CTL*, cytotoxic T lymphocyte. (From Abbas AK, Lichtman AH, Pillai S: *Basic immunology: Functions and disorders of the immune system*, ed 4, St. Louis, 2013, Saunders.)

As the CD4+ cells are destroyed, the immune system fails. Immune dysfunction can occur when the CD4+ lymphocyte count falls below 500/mm³ of blood. When the count falls below 200/mm³, severe immune system dysfunction is apparent. This results in the development of possibly fatal opportunistic infections in the host.

Monocytes can be infected by HIV because some of them also have CD4+ receptors. When a monocyte is infected, it can change into a phagocyte (a cell that ingests and digests bacteria). When a phagocyte is infected with HIV, it merely works as a factory to create more HIV. An infected phagocyte can rupture as a result of a normal local inflammatory response. When this happens, the HIV is spread even deeper into the body. In this way, the skin, the lungs, bone marrow, the central nervous system, and lymph nodes become directly infected.

SPECTRUM OF HIV INFECTION

The term HIV disease (the state in which HIV enters the body under favorable conditions and multiplies, producing injurious effects) encompasses the immune system's progressive dysfunction that is produced by the viral activity within the host. HIV disease replaces the previous term *AIDS-related complex* (ARC) (Table 16.2). Acquired immunodeficiency syndrome (AIDS) (the end stage of HIV infection, in which the CD4+ cell count is 200/mm³ or lower) occurs as the disease progresses and the body is damaged severely by opportunistic infections. At this stage, the host's body can no longer protect itself and is injured (see Fig. 16.3). The CD4+ cell count is 200/mm³ or less. People can live for years with the infection before they develop any signs or symptoms of HIV. The signs and symptoms include night sweats, weight loss, diarrhea, unexplainable fevers, and fatigue. The viral course of HIV depends on host factors. The host has an increased risk for morbidity and mortality when he or she has inadequate access to health care services, is of lower socioeconomic status, or is under the care of a health care provider with minimal experience in dealing with HIV.

Progression from the early stages to end-stage HIV disease varies greatly. Three patterns have been found: typical progression, long-term nonprogression, and rapid progression. In the typical progression pattern, patients develop signs and symptoms several years after seroconversion. Many do not know they have been infected with HIV and can infect others. In the long-term nonprogression pattern, patients may not develop signs and symptoms even 30 years after seroconversion. The long-term nonprogression pattern is rare; it is thought to be longer because the immune response of affected patients is very intense, so their viral load is lower. Also, there are genetic differences in their receptors (CCR5) on CD4+ lymphocytes that make it difficult for the HIV to attach. This allows their CD4+ and CD8+ cells to be maintained at nearly normal levels.

When reviewing the progression of HIV infection there are factors that are seen when the disease begins to transition from HIV infection to AIDS (CDC, 2021b). Several common factors are found: their cytotoxic T cells (CD8+ cells) are dysfunctional and unable to contain HIV, the level of virus remains very high throughout the infection, and HIV antibodies are minimal.

Table 16.1   Types of White Blood Cells and Their Involvement in HIV Disease

WHITE BLOOD CELL (WBC) TYPE	DESCRIPTION	ROLE IN HIV DISEASE
Neutrophils	Normally constitute 50%–75% of all circulating leukocytes and are capable of phagocytosis Important in the inflammatory response and the first line of defense against infection Short life span	Neutropenia (WBC deficiency) commonly occurs in advanced HIV disease. Drug-induced neutropenia is common, especially with drugs used to treat *Pneumocystis jiroveci pneumonia*, toxoplasmosis, CMV retinitis, or colitis and with NRTIs.
Monocytes, macrophages	Constitute about 3%–7% of all WBCs Involved in the inflammatory response Capable of processing antigens for presentation to T cells Have CD4+ receptors Macrophages: distributed throughout tissue and capable of phagocytosis	Monocytes and macrophages serve as a reservoir for HIV. When activated by stimulation with interferon (inflammatory response), they produce neopterin. Neopterin levels are increased in HIV disease.
Basophils, mast cells	Both: involved in acute inflammation Mast cells: breakdown releases histamine and other factors	In HIV infection, these cells may inhibit leukocyte migration.
T helper cells (CD4+ or T4 cells)	Contain CD4+ receptors Considered the "conductor" of the immune system because of their secretion of cytokines, which control most aspects of the immune response	These cells are the major target of HIV. Progressive infection gradually destroys the available pool of T helper cells so that the overall CD4+ cell count drops. Lower CD4+ cell counts correspond to more immunodeficiency and the onset of opportunistic infections. Infection with HIV can impair T helper cell function without killing the cell.
Cytotoxic T cells or cytotoxic T lymphocytes (CTLs; CD8+ cells)	Contain CD8+ receptors and produce cytokines in a more limited manner than do CD4+ cells Combat viral and bacterial infections and are involved in direct killing of target cells by binding to them and releasing a substance that can perforate the cell membrane	Numbers of these cells increase in HIV infection. This increase represents the cellular response to infection. The strength of this initial cellular response has been shown to predict progression to AIDS (i.e., better cell response implies slower disease progression). Cytotoxic T cells kill T helper cells infected with HIV.
Natural killer (NK) cells	Large granular lymphocytes involved in cell-mediated immune response Able to kill target cells because target cells are coated with antibody that binds to receptors on the surface of NK cells, allowing the NK cell to attach Kill target cells by releasing a substance that triggers lysis (breakdown of cell wall) of cell	Counts and structure of these cells remain normal in patients with HIV infection, but they are functionally defective.
B cells	Produce antibodies specific to an antigen Capable of being stimulated by T helper cells	B cells are involved in the humoral response to HIV infection and produce a variety of antibodies against HIV. They are present throughout the course of HIV disease.

CMV, Cytomegalovirus; *HIV*, human immunodeficiency virus; *NRTI*, nucleoside reverse transcriptase inhibitor; *WBC*, white blood cell.

The term *acquired immunodeficiency syndrome* has been defined for surveillance and reporting purposes; it is not used alone to characterize serious disease caused by HIV infection (see Table 16.2).

ACUTE RETROVIRAL SYNDROME

Viral replication occurs during the acute infection period. The viral load peaks at millions of copies of virus per milliliter of plasma. The viral load declines right before the appearance of detectable antibodies that can be measured in the blood. The viral set point, or stabilizing of the viral load, is reached 4 to 6 months after exposure. This viral set point is important because some researchers believe it to be a prognostic indicator of long-term survival: that is, the lower the viral set point, the longer the individual will survive with HIV disease. Postexposure prophylaxis (PEP), begun as soon as possible after exposure, may help lower this viral set point. This theory is demonstrated in cases in which health care personnel initiate PEP medications after an exposure and do not undergo seroconversion.

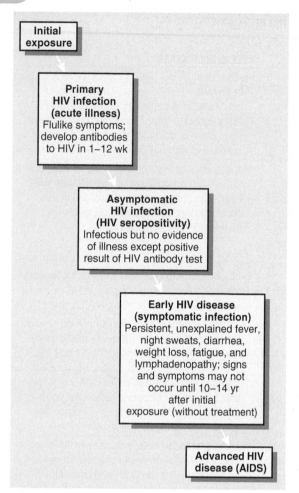

Fig. 16.4 Spectrum of human immunodeficiency virus (HIV) disease and associated signs and symptoms at various stages of the disease process. *AIDS*, Acquired immunodeficiency syndrome.

Table 16.2	Proper Terms Related to HIV and AIDS
MISLEADING PHRASES	**MORE ACCURATE PHRASES**
High-risk groups	High-risk behaviors
Infection with AIDS	HIV infection
AIDS test	HIV antibody test
AIDS positive	HIV positive
AIDS victim or patient	Person living with HIV or AIDS
AIDS carrier	HIV-infected person

AIDS, Acquired immunodeficiency syndrome; *HIV*, human immunodeficiency virus.

Table 16.3	Acute HIV Infection: Frequency of Associated Signs and Symptoms
SIGN OR SYMPTOM	**FREQUENCY (%)**
Fever	96
Headache	32
Lymphadenopathy	74
Nausea and vomiting	27
Pharyngitis	70
Hepatosplenomegaly	14
Rash	70
Weight loss	13
Myalgia or arthralgia	54
Thrush	12
Diarrhea	32
Neurologic symptoms	12
Oral or genital ulcers	5–20

HIV, Human immunodeficiency virus.
From the Department of Health and Human Services Panel on Antiretroviral Guidelines for Adults and Adolescents. Guidelines for the Use of Antiretroviral Agents in HIV-1 Infected Adults and Adolescents.

Seroconversion, as defined previously, is the development of antibodies from HIV, which takes place approximately 5 days to 3 months after exposure (generally within 2 to 4 weeks) (HIVinfo.nih.gov, 2020e). This process is accompanied by a flulike or mononucleosis-like syndrome consisting of fever, night sweats, pharyngitis, headache, malaise, arthralgias, myalgias, diarrhea, nausea, and a diffuse rash prominent on the trunk. These symptoms last approximately 1 to 2 weeks, although some symptoms may last for several months. Seroconversion illness occurs in approximately 89% of HIV-infected people. HIV antibodies appear in 95% of people within 3 months of infection, and seroconversion occurs in 99% within 6 months. The viral load during the period of seroconversion is extremely high, with a short-term drop in CD4$^+$ cells. The CD4$^+$ cell level quickly returns to normal as the immune system mounts an attack against the viral infection; as a result, viral loads exist at nearly undetectable levels in the blood. In most people with HIV infection, the acute retroviral illness is mild and may be mistaken for a cold or other minor viral infection (Table 16.3).

EARLY INFECTION

The median time between HIV infection and the development of end-stage HIV disease, or AIDS, in an untreated individual is between 8 and 14 years. This phase of HIV disease sometimes is called the *asymptomatic phase* because the HIV-infected individual looks and feels healthy. Some individuals have vague symptoms of a viral infection, including fatigue, headaches, low-grade fever, and night sweats. Because many of the symptoms of early infection are nonspecific, a diagnosis of HIV infection may not be made. Consequently, individuals may continue to engage in risky sexual and drug-using behaviors. Although seemingly healthy, the HIV-infected individual can transmit HIV to others. Lack of knowledge of one's HIV antibody status puts one at risk for earlier development of more advanced disease because changes in behaviors, such as those that promote health, are not instituted. Furthermore, if an individual is aware of being infected with the virus, early intervention with antiretroviral medications may prolong the asymptomatic phase and prevent progression to AIDS.

EARLY SYMPTOMATIC DISEASE

The early symptomatic phase of HIV infection occurs when the CD4$^+$ cell count drops below 500/mm^3. Early symptoms include constitutional problems such as persistent, unexplained fevers; recurrent drenching night sweats; chronic diarrhea; headaches; and fatigue. These signs and symptoms become severe enough to affect activities of daily living. A physical examination may reveal persistent generalized lymphadenopathy; recurrent or localized infections; and neurologic manifestations, such as numbness and tingling or weakness in the extremities (Box 16.1).

One of the most common infections in individuals with early symptomatic disease is oral candidiasis (thrush), a fungal infection that is rare in healthy adults (see Fig. 16.4). Other infections that signal immune dysfunction include varicella-zoster virus (shingles), persistent vaginal candidiasis (yeast infections), and increased frequency of oral or genital HSV outbreaks. Oral hairy leukoplakia, a condition related to the Epstein-Barr virus, and oral thrush are early indicators of HIV disease and prognostic markers for disease progression. Because of this, dental health professionals have a key role in identifying cases of early HIV disease.

Persistent generalized lymphadenopathy is defined as enlargement ($\geq$1 cm) of two or more lymph nodes, located in places other than the inguinal region that persists for at least 3 months. This condition may be present for many years before AIDS is diagnosed.

Neurologic manifestations of HIV disease occur in more than 90% of individuals who are infected. Neurologic symptoms include peripheral neuropathies, headaches, aseptic meningitis, cranial nerve palsies, and myopathies. These conditions may be caused by the HIV infection or may be side effects related to antiretroviral medications.

Several cofactors may influence a more rapid progression of HIV disease. In very young children and very old adults, the disease progresses more quickly. Concurrent infections such as HSV, cytomegalovirus, or Epstein-Barr virus affect progression. Drug and alcohol use, including smoking, may suppress the immune system. Malnutrition also is known to affect immune function, but further study relative to HIV is needed.

AIDS

AIDS is the term used to describe the end stage, or terminal phase, of the spectrum of HIV infection. The CDC has developed specific diagnostic criteria that must be present to make this diagnosis. These conditions are more likely to occur with severe immunosuppression. As HIV disease progresses, the CD4$^+$ lymphocyte count decreases, and the ratio of CD4$^+$ to CD8$^+$ cells (T helper cells to T suppressor cells), which is normally 2 to 1, gradually shifts, resulting in more CD8$^+$ than CD4$^+$. The amount of virus detectable in the blood increases rapidly and remains high despite pharmacologic interventions. The number of white blood cells also may decline, and the person's reactivity to skin tests, such as purified protein derivative (tuberculin), is decreased or absent. An individual is said to be anergic if no skin response is noted.

Without treatment, people with AIDS can expect to survive approximately 3 years, but this varies greatly. With the advent of more effective antiretroviral and opportunistic disease prophylaxis, the life span of an individual infected with HIV is difficult to predict (HIVinfo.nih.gov, 2020f). Morbidity in people with advanced HIV disease also varies widely. Some people are severely ill and die rather quickly, whereas others have only to make minor adjustments in their lifestyle to cope with medical regimens or physical symptoms, such as fatigue or pain. Significant advances in the management of HIV disease have made it resemble a chronic illness. The effects of therapy on mortality have been significant: The number of new AIDS cases reported to the CDC every year has leveled off. This can be attributed to effective prophylaxis for opportunistic infections and to the development of ART.

Box 16.1	Signs and Symptoms of HIV Infection

- Abdominal pain
- Chills and fever
- Cough (dry or productive)
- Diarrhea
- Disorientation
- Dyspnea
- Fatigue
- Headache
- Lymphadenopathy (any disorder of the lymph nodes or lymph vessels)
- Malaise
- Muscle or joint pain
- Night sweats
- Oral lesions
- Shortness of breath
- Skin rash
- Sore throat
- Weight loss

HIV, Human immunodeficiency virus.

LABORATORY AND DIAGNOSTIC EXAMINATIONS

Strong evidence shows that early intervention postpones the onset of severe immunosuppression. Encourage individuals at risk for HIV infection to seek HIV antibody testing, and educate them in how to decrease the risk of HIV transmission.

HIV ANTIBODY TESTING

Patients need to understand the implications of an HIV antibody test (Box 16.2):

- Nucleic acid tests (NAT) test the blood to determine if the HIV is present and the viral load (how much virus is present). This test is able to detect HIV sooner than other tests. This test is expensive, so it is not usually used for routine screening. It is mostly used if the patient has had a probable exposure to an HIV infected person. The results for this test typically take several days.
- Antigen-antibody testing detects HIV antibodies and antigens. The antigen called p24 is present if the patient has HIV. This test is done by venipuncture, but a rapid test is available by performing a finger-stick. The rapid test takes about 30 minutes or less for results.
- HIV antibody tests can detect antibodies in the blood or oral fluid. This test is available in a lab or at home testing. The oral fluid test can provide results in as little as 20 minutes or less.
- A result that is seronegative (the state of lacking HIV antibodies as confirmed by blood test) is not an assurance that the individual is free of HIV infection; seroconversion may not yet have occurred.
- Testing will provide an indication of exposure from 10 to 90 days following exposure, depending on the type of test.

Box 16.2   Tests Used to Detect HIV Infection

ANTIBODY DETECTION TESTS
Screening Tests
- Agglutination assays (blood or clean-catch urine specimen)
- Oral fluid test (swabbing of the cheek and gum)
- Urine screening test

Confirmatory Test
- Nucleic acid tests (NAT) antigen/antibody tests
- Indirect immunofluorescent antibody assay
- Radioimmunoprecipitation assay (RIPA)

ANTIGEN DETECTION TESTS (P24 ANTIGEN)
HIV Viral Load Tests/ Nucleic Acid Determination Assays
- Reverse transcriptase–polymerase chain reaction (RT-PCR)
- Branched-chain DNA (bDNA)
- Nucleic acid sequence–based amplification (NASBA)

Viral Culture Method
- HIV culture

Activated Immune Markers
- Neopterin
- β_2-microglobulin
- Absolute CD4$^+$ cell count
- Percentage of CD4$^+$ cells
- Percentage of CD8$^+$ cells
- CD4$^+$/CD8$^+$ cell ratio

HIV, Human immunodeficiency virus.

- A seronegative result does not mean that an individual is free from risk of infection. If an individual continues to engage in risky behaviors, such as unprotected sexual intercourse or use of contaminated needles or drug paraphernalia, transmission may occur (Box 16.3) (CDC, 2021h).

CD4$^+$ CELL MONITORING

Monitoring CD4$^+$ cells is one of the laboratory parameters used to track the progression of HIV disease. As the disease progresses, the number of CD4$^+$ cells decreases. The more significant the loss, the more severe the immunosuppression becomes. The CD4$^+$ cell count is the best marker of the immunodeficiency associated with HIV infection. As such, the CD4$^+$ cell count influences making decisions about antiretroviral and prophylactic drug therapy and is used to evaluate specific complaints related to the risk for contracting particular opportunistic infections. For example, *Mycobacterium avium* complex and cytomegalovirus infections are rare in patients with CD4$^+$ cell counts higher than 50/mm^3. *P. jiroveci* pneumonia and cryptococcosis are unusual in patients with CD4$^+$ cell counts higher than 200/mm^3. The CD4$^+$ cell count is not a perfect surrogate marker of immunodeficiency, and factors such as the patient's clinical status always must be taken into account.

The CD4$^+$ cell count reflects the number of CD4$^+$ cells per cubic millimeter (or per microliter) of blood. It does not indicate the total number of CD4$^+$ cells in the body. Millions of new CD4$^+$ cells are produced daily and cleared by normal body processes (unrelated to the virus). The absolute CD4$^+$ cell count can vary greatly in the same individual, depending on the time of day the blood is drawn; which laboratory is used; and the presence of acute illness or other factors, such as alcohol. The patient should be advised to continue to use the same laboratory, draw blood at the same time of day, and avoid testing on days when they are acutely ill or under abnormal stress. When using the CD4$^+$ cell count to make important treatment decisions, such as initiating prophylaxis for opportunistic infections, collect two separate samples a few weeks apart.

VIRAL LOAD MONITORING

The ability to detect HIV viral load measurements in plasma is a significant advancement in the monitoring of HIV disease. Viral load or burden is a quantitative measure of HIV viral RNA in the peripheral circulation, or the level of virus in the blood.

Three quantitative assay tests are available to measure viral load levels: nucleic acid sequence–based amplification (NASBA), reverse transcriptase–polymerase chain reaction (RT-PCR), and bDNA. Even very small numbers of infected cells can be detected by identifying virions. These tests can be used only to identify HIV.

| Box 16.3 | Counseling Before and After HIV Antibody Testing |

GENERAL GUIDELINES

- People who are being tested for HIV are commonly fearful of the test results; therefore carry out the following steps:
  - Establish rapport with the patient.
  - Assess the patient's ability to understand counseling.
  - Determine the patient's access to support systems.
- Explain the following benefits of testing:
  - Testing provides an opportunity for education that can decrease the risk of new infections.
  - Infected patients can be referred for early intervention and support programs.
- Discuss the following negative aspects of testing:
  - Breaches of confidentiality have led to discrimination.
  - A positive test result affects all aspects of the patient's life (personal, social, economic) and can raise difficult emotions (anger, anxiety, guilt, thoughts of suicide).

PRETEST COUNSELING

- Determine the patient's risk factors and when the last exposure risk occurred. Individualize counseling according to these parameters.
- Provide education to decrease future risk of exposure.
- Provide education that will help the patient protect sexual and drug-sharing partners.
- Discuss problems related to the delay between infection and an accurate test result:
  - Testing must be repeated at intervals for 6 months after each possible exposure.
  - The patient needs to abstain from further high-risk behaviors during that interval.
  - The patient needs to protect sexual and drug-sharing partners during that interval.
- Discuss the possibility of false-negative test results, which are most likely to occur during the period between infection and seroconversion.
- Provide information regarding the confidentiality of results.
- Explain that a positive test result shows HIV infection, not AIDS.
- Explain that the test result does not establish immunity.

- Assess the patient's support systems; provide telephone numbers and resources as needed.
- Discuss the patient's personally anticipated responses to test results (positive and negative).
- Outline assistance that will be offered if the test result is positive.

POSTTEST COUNSELING

- If the test result is negative, reinforce pretest counseling and prevention education. Remind the patient that test must be repeated at intervals for 6 months after the most recent exposure risk.
- Explain the need to report positive test results to the state health department and CDC.
- Discuss the importance of partner notification.
- If the test result is positive, understand that the patient may be in shock and not hear what is said after receiving that news.
- Provide resources for medical and emotional support, and help the patient get immediate assistance.
- Evaluate the patient's suicide risk, and follow up as needed.
- Determine need to test other people who have had high-risk contact with the patient.
- Discuss retesting to verify results. This tactic provides hope for the patient, but, of more importance, it keeps the patient in touch with health care professionals. While waiting for the second test result, the patient has time to think about and adjust to the possibility of being infected with HIV.
- Encourage optimism:
  - Remind the patient that treatments are available.
  - Review health habits that can improve the immune system.
  - Arrange for patients to speak to HIV-infected people who are willing to share and assist patients with new diagnoses during the transition period.
  - Reinforce that an HIV-positive test result means the patient is infected but does not necessarily mean that the patient has AIDS.

AIDS, Acquired immunodeficiency syndrome; *CDC,* Centers for Disease Control and Prevention, *HIV,* human immunodeficiency virus.
Modified from Bradley-Springer LA, Fendrick R: *HIV instant instructor cards,* El Paso, TX, 1994, Skidmore-Roth; and Consolidated Guidelines on HIV Testing Services: 5Cs: Consent, Confidentiality, Counselling, Correct Results and Connection 2015. Geneva: World Health Organization; 3, 2015. PRE-TEST AND POST-TEST SERVICES. Available from: https://www.ncbi.nlm.nih.gov/books/NBK316035.

Important characteristics of viral load monitoring include the following:

- In all clinical stages of the illness, HIV virus detection techniques identify measurable amounts of viral RNA copies in the plasma of most HIV-infected individuals.
- Viral load can provide significant information used to predict the course of disease progression, initiate ART, measure the degree of antiretroviral effect achieved, and note the failure of a drug regimen.
- Plasma levels of HIV RNA fall dramatically after effective ART.

- Detection of HIV RNA in plasma does not indicate whether any virus is present in lymphoid or other tissues.

Viral load and CD4⁺ cell counts are distinct markers that provide different information. Viral load can indicate disease progression and long-term clinical outcome; CD4⁺ cell measurements can indicate the damage sustained by the immune system (the loss of CD4⁺ or T cells) and the short-term risk for developing opportunistic infections. Each is an independent predictor of clinical outcome, and in combination they can give a more complete indication of clinical status, treatment response, and prognosis. Coffin (1996) used a metaphor to describe the infected patient without symptoms: as a train rushing along a track, heading for a bridge that has been destroyed. The time the crash will occur is determined by two variables: (1) where the train is at a particular instant (CD4+), and (2) how fast it is going (viral load).

A baseline determination of viral burden is recommended, with subsequent measurements every 3 to 4 months, in conjunction with CD4+ cell monitoring and clinical evaluations such as a history and physical examination. Guidelines continue to be revised as the implications of viral measurement evolve and its interpretation and use become better understood. In the future, opportunistic infection prophylaxis may be based on viral load, as well as on CD4+ cell counts.

RESISTANCE TESTING

Drug resistance to ART can make effective treatment of HIV challenging. In countries with high incomes, 10% to 17% of patients who have never taken HIV medications have mutations that indicate resistance to at least one ART medication (USDHHS, 2021). HIV mutates easily, which makes it hard to treat and contain. After multiple genetic mutations, the replication of HIV is chaotic and disorderly, which makes it more resistant to medication treatment and has prevented the development of an effective vaccine. ART resistance results from a patient's inability to adhere to ART protocols. Assay tests can detect HIV genetic mutations that result in ART resistance. Results of these tests are available in less than a month. A list of ART-resistant mutations has been developed by the International AIDS Society–USA. Phenotyping is available to help estimate how well the specific strain of virus will respond to treatment in people who have been receiving ART for a long time. To perform phenotyping, the patient must have a high viral load (USDHHS, 2021). Genotyping is less expensive to perform, and the results are often available faster than those of phenotyping. Genotyping is recommended for patients who have not received ART (USDHHS, 2021).

During the acute stage of HIV, resistance testing is important for administering appropriate ART to prevent extensive replication of HIV. Some health care providers identify baseline genetic mutations before starting ART. A patient-specific ART regimen can be created to avoid medications that would not work. Patients who are resistant to some ART medications may have cross-resistance issues with other ART medications. Resistant HIV strains are found in people who have undergone ART, as well as in other people who are newly infected and have not received treatment. Resistance to some ART drugs and the ability to transmit resistance to newly infected people are important issues for public health officials who are battling to control and prevent HIV infection.

OTHER LABORATORY PARAMETERS

Hematologic abnormalities are common in HIV infections and may be caused by the HIV, by opportunistic infections, or by drug or radiation therapy. The white blood cell count often is decreased, usually in conjunction with lymphopenia (decreased numbers of lymphocytes). Thrombocytopenia (decreased platelet count) may be caused by antiplatelet antibodies. Anemia is related to the chronic disease process and to HIV invasion of the bone marrow; it is a common adverse effect of antiretroviral agents.

Alterations in liver function tests are not uncommon. Abnormalities may be caused by viral hepatitis, alcohol abuse, opportunistic infections, neoplasms, or medications. Early identification of hepatitis B and hepatitis C viral infections is important, because these infections may follow a more serious course in patients with HIV disease. Patients who are HIV positive are often also seropositive for hepatitis B, both infections are bloodborne and sexually transmitted. In addition, about 25% of HIV-infected people in the United States are co-infected with hepatitis C, one of the most significant causes of chronic liver disease.

Syphilis testing is important because syphilis is more complicated and aggressive in HIV infected patients. It is also more difficult to treat with standard therapies and more likely to advance quickly to neurosyphilis. If a person with HIV infection is seropositive for syphilis, assessment and treatment must be performed immediately.

THERAPEUTIC MANAGEMENT

Therapeutic management of HIV-infected patients focuses on monitoring HIV disease progression and immune function, preventing the development of opportunistic diseases, initiating and monitoring ART, detecting and treating opportunistic diseases, managing symptoms, and preventing complications of treatment.

HIV-positive individuals must be linked to various resources, depending on their individual needs. Individuals often deny the infection, neglect their mental and physical health, and continue behaviors that put themselves and other people at risk. Interventions must be sustained and reinforced; the emotional effect of such devastating news ("You are HIV positive") can overshadow any initial information or education provided. Stress safer behaviors and the need for medical and emotional support, such as assistance in family planning, treatment for substance abuse, treatment for STIs, treatment for tuberculosis, and immunizations.

A transdisciplinary care approach is most appropriate for patients with HIV disease because of their complex medical and psychosocial needs. The HIV-infected patient should be the primary member of this team, working along with a physician who specializes in HIV, a social worker, a case manager, a dietitian, and a nurse. Other team members may include a dentist, a primary care provider (physician, osteopath, nurse practitioner, or physician assistant), a mental health worker, a substance abuse counselor, a nontraditional therapist (such as a massage therapist or acupuncturist), and the individual's family and significant other.

PHARMACOLOGIC MANAGEMENT

Opportunistic Diseases Associated With HIV

Probably the most difficult aspect of the medical management of HIV is dealing with the many opportunistic diseases that develop as the immune system degenerates. Although it is usually impossible to totally eradicate opportunistic diseases, the use of ART and prophylactic interventions can control their emergence or progression. However, these regimens must continue throughout the patient's life; otherwise, the disease will return. Advances in the diagnosis and treatment of opportunistic diseases have contributed significantly to increased life expectancy and decreased morbidity. Box 16.4 lists common opportunistic diseases associated with HIV disease.

Antiretroviral Therapy

Combination ART is an important component in the management of HIV infection (Table 16.4). In 1987, zidovudine was the only medication available to treat patients with HIV disease; since then, the FDA has approved more than 25 antiretroviral medications. Six different classes of ART are used to prevent the viral replication process: integrase strand transfer inhibitors, fusion inhibitors, CCR5 antagonists (also referred to as entry inhibitors), nucleoside reverse transcriptase inhibitors (NRTIs), nonnucleoside reverse transcriptase inhibitors (NNRTIs), and PI. Each class of medication interrupts HIV at different stages of the infectious process. Some ART medications are available as a combination of medications so that several medications are combined into one pill that is taken each day, which allows for better patient compliance (MedlinePlus, 2021). In ART, HIV is treated with three or more antiretroviral medications,

Scientists have found that the most effective medication regimen is the use of *cocktails* (generally three or more compounds given together). Medication combinations make it much more difficult for the virus to develop resistance to the drugs. Such intervention also may slow the progression from asymptomatic or mildly symptomatic HIV infection to a more advanced disease. Therapies that can reduce the quantity of circulating virus dramatically in the blood have been developed; in many cases, blood circulating levels become undetectable. It is still possible for one individual to infect another with the virus despite having undetectable viral levels. PIs directly reduce the ability of HIV to replicate, or make copies of itself, inside cells. As increasing numbers of therapeutic agents and clinical trial results become available, decisions about ART have become increasingly complex. For now, these combination therapies offer optimism for successful disease management and improvements in the quality and duration of life.

Considerations for ART include the following:
- Previous experience with ART may affect the efficacy of a proposed therapy, because the virus may have become resistant to medications taken by the patient in the past (e.g., zidovudine, lamivudine).
- Certain combinations of antiretroviral drugs may reverse the resistance to a single drug. Recycling drugs previously taken can sometimes improve viral suppression. Incorrect dosing (timing) or incorrect usage (missed doses) can cause drug resistance.

Box 16.4	Common Opportunistic Diseases Associated With HIV

- Candidiasis of bronchi, trachea, esophagus, or lungs
- Invasive cervical cancer
- Coccidioidomycosis
- Cryptococcosis
- Cryptosporidiosis, chronic intestinal (greater than 1 month's duration)
- Cytomegalovirus (CMV) disease (particularly CMV retinitis)
- Encephalopathy, HIV-related
- Herpes simplex: chronic ulcer(s) (greater than 1 month's duration); or bronchitis, pneumonitis, or esophagitis
- Histoplasmosis
- Isosporiasis, chronic intestinal (greater than 1 month's duration)
- Kaposi's sarcoma
- Lymphoma, multiple forms
- *Mycobacterium avium* complex
- Tuberculosis
- *Pneumocystis carinii* pneumonia
- Pneumonia, recurrent
- Progressive multifocal leukoencephalopathy
- Salmonella septicemia, recurrent
- Toxoplasmosis of brain
- Wasting syndrome resulting from HIV

HIV, Human immunodeficiency virus.HIV.gov: *What are opportunistic infections?*, 2019. Available at: https://www.hiv.gov/hiv-basics/staying-in-hiv-care/other-related-health-issues/opportunistic-infections.

Table 16.4	Pros and Cons of Highly Active Antiretroviral Therapy	
PROS		**CONS**
• Minimizes chance of emergence of resistant strain of virus • May play a role in the reduction of HIV transmission • Slows disease progression • Improves quality of life		• Can be toxic • Frequent side effects • Complexity of drug and dosing regimens • Difficulty with adherence to regimen (nonadherence can result in treatment failure) • High cost

HIV, Human immunodeficiency virus.

- Drug incompatibilities, similar side effect profiles, and toxic effects must be considered in the choice of a regimen.
- The patient's commitment to taking medication each day must be considered. Inadequate adherence can lead to drug resistance and, ultimately, to drug failure. This point must be stressed to the patient. Adherence is paramount for survival and success of treatment.

HIV-infected patients should begin taking HIV medications as soon as possible. A provider with expertise in HIV should supervise the care. Treatment should be offered to all patients with early HIV infection, who are pregnant, who have been diagnosed with AIDS or HIV-related coinfections or diseases (HIVinfo.nih.gov, 2020f).

Current HIV treatment is aimed at preventing the immune system damage that results from HIV replication. If HIV replication can be halted, then viral mutation can be prevented, and drug resistance issues can be decreased. ART is aimed at limiting viral loads to undetectable levels. With early ART, the patient's CD4+ cell counts will remain normal for a longer time.

Clinical trials being conducted by the AIDS Clinical Trials Group and the National Institutes of Health in conjunction with universities, pharmaceutical companies, and other agencies may be important considerations for people with HIV disease. Patients may be able to participate in clinical trials or may benefit from the results of such research studies. Benefits include (1) access to new and potentially effective treatments for HIV disease before they are released to the public, (2) the chance to have physician visits and laboratory work paid for by the research study, and (3) the opportunity to be cared for by a health care team with HIV experience (ACGT, n.d.).

Complementary and Alternative Therapies

People with HIV disease often use nontraditional or complementary therapies, such as massage, acupuncture or acupressure, and biofeedback. Some patients use nutritional supplements or herbal remedies with the hope of alleviating the side effects of the disease and the medications. Many patients prefer these therapies because of the limitations or side effects of approved drugs, mistrust of the health care system, easier access, lack of adequate insurance coverage, or the high cost of anti-HIV medications. These alternatives are best used in conjunction with approved therapeutic intervention.

Many patients may consider the use of complementary therapies. Alternative forms of therapy may be beneficial and always should be explored thoroughly. Patients should discuss their use with their health care team. It is important to educate the patient about selective review and use of complementary and alternative therapies. Their potential benefits and risks, along with the associated financial strain, should be evaluated carefully. Patients may need guidance to avoid expensive and particularly dangerous forms of alternative treatments. An open relationship and good communication with the patient build trust, creating a positive atmosphere for addressing difficult issues. They also reinforce the philosophy that the patient is an important participating member of the health care team.

Vaccine Development

Unfortunately, a vaccine for HIV is not yet available; however, clinical trials are under way. It has been difficult to develop a vaccine for HIV because the retrovirus easily mutates, many different viral strains exist, and poor adherence to ART has led to drug resistance issues. However, with greater understanding of the immune response to HIV and more effective ways to administer antigens, an aggressive push to create a vaccine continues. Since the mid-1980s, many initiatives and partnerships among organizations worldwide have attempted to develop a vaccine for HIV. Researchers continue to work to find an effective vaccine. The National Institutes of Health (NIH) is investing in multiple approaches to develop a vaccine. These research efforts include two late-stage, multinational vaccine clinical trials called Imbokodo and Mosaico(HIV.gov, 2021c).

NURSING INTERVENTIONS

Establish a comfort level in interacting with people with HIV disease. Patients must be treated in a nonjudgmental, empathetic, and caring manner regardless of their sexual practices or history of drug use. The nurse's attitudes, values, and beliefs should not interfere with the care of a patient with HIV disease. Patients are aware when their caregiver is not comfortable dealing with HIV disease. Knowledge of HIV transmission and competence in standard precautions and body substance isolation will minimize the fear of caring for HIV-infected patients. Boxes 16.5 and 16.6 and Table 16.5 list appropriate nursing assessments, activities, and interventions for HIV infection and disease.

Patient problems and interventions for the patient with HIV disease include but are not limited to the following:

PATIENT PROBLEM	NURSING INTERVENTIONS
Potential for Opportunistic Infection	Limit visitors Assess for early onset of infectious processes and unusual cancers Practice good hand hygiene
Insufficient Knowledge, related to • Health management • Disease process and progression • Prevention of complications • Medications	Provide patient and family teaching concerning diagnosis and health maintenance activities geared toward health promotion

PATIENT PROBLEM	NURSING INTERVENTIONS
Insufficient nutrition: Less than body requirements	Assess nutritional needs Provide between-meal snacks and supplements as indicated
Inability to Tolerate Activity	Encourage frequent rest periods Cluster care delivery to avoid tiring patient
Potential for Excessive Demand on Primary Caregiver, related to advancing disease in care recipient and inadequate caregiver coping patterns	Assess needs and capabilities of patient and caregiver Assess factors that contribute to caregiver strain Develop supportive and trusting relationship with caregiver Enlist the help of family members, significant others, and friends to assist caregiver Encourage interaction in support groups for caregivers Teach stress reduction techniques to caregiver Encourage caregiver to attend to own personal and health care needs
Frequent, Loose Stools, related to: • Gastrointestinal infections • Malabsorption • Medication side effects	Document quantity, quality, and frequency of stools Monitor intake and output, vital signs, and daily weight Assess for skin impairment Administer antidiarrheals on a routine schedule Encourage increased electrolyte-rich fluid intake (fruit juices, Gatorade, Pedialyte) Encourage high-protein, high-calorie, and low-residue diet

Health care needs can be unpredictable and assessment difficult because of the clinical diversity of HIV infection. HIV disease may necessitate alternating periods of long-term and acute care. The patient may fear isolation from the community or family and friends because of the social stigma associated with HIV disease.

The disease affects primarily young people who are at the most productive time in their lives, a time when they are expected to take control of their lives. For this reason, they often want an active role in the decision-making and planning stages of their care. Patients may experience bouts of serious, debilitating illness and then recover enough to function effectively for an unpredictable amount of time. People with HIV disease often prefer to stay at home as long as possible, and some prefer to die at home. Long-term care in an inpatient setting (e.g., long-term care facility) is not compatible with the social needs of young patients. Prolonged care is expensive. Patients who experience chronic diseases may find their insurance coverage is limited. In addition, the absence of insurance may affect availability and affordability of treatment options.

Health Promotion

Goals for the National HIV Strategy

1. Reduce the number of new HIV infections.
2. Increase access to care and improve health outcomes for people living with HIV.
3. Reduce HIV-related health disparities and health inequities.
4. Achieve a more coordinated national response to the HIV epidemic.

The following are indicators of the progress of this strategy:

- Increase the percentage of people living with HIV who know their serostatus to at least 95%.
- Reduce the number of new diagnoses of HIV by at least 75%.
- Reduce the percentage of young gay and bisexual men who have engaged in HIV-risk behaviors.
- Increase the percentage of newly diagnosed persons linked to HIV medical care within 1 month of their HIV diagnosis to at least 95%.
- Increase the percentage of persons with diagnosed HIV infection who are retained in HIV medical care.
- Increase the percentage of persons with diagnosed HIV infection who are virally suppressed to at least 95%.
- Reduce the percentage of persons in HIV medical care who are homeless by 50%.
- Reduce the death rate among persons with diagnosed HIV infection.
- Reduce disparities in the rate of new diagnoses in the following groups: gay and bisexual men, young black gay and bisexual men, black females, and persons living in the southern United States.

aFrom HIV.gov: What is the national HIV/AIDS strategy?, 2017. Available at https://www.aids.gov/federal-resources/national-hiv-aids-strategy/overview/.

Religious and community-based organization volunteers, such as AIDS project workers, provide support and care services for patients and families. Friends, family, and significant others are also important resources to be considered in the planning of care for the patient with HIV disease.

ADHERENCE

Adherence to a prescribed regimen (following a prescribed regimen of therapy or treatment for disease) is paramount to survival and the success of treatment. The nurse is in a unique position to help patients adapt and maintain vigilance in their treatment. Nurses must assist patients to understand that ART is a lifelong undertaking. The ability to incorporate anti-HIV treatment into a lifestyle is affected by multiple factors, including treatment knowledge or misinformation, underlying psychiatric or psychological pathologic conditions, physical status, family and caregiver support, socioeconomic status, culture, fear of side effects, denial, and skills (memory, impaired function) necessary to adhere to a medical regimen.

Box 16.5 Nursing Assessment of a Patient With HIV Infection

SUBJECTIVE DATA
Important Health Information
Past health history: Route of infection, risk factors, history of hepatitis or other sexually transmitted infections (STIs), frequent viral infections, parasitic infections, tuberculosis, alcohol and drug use, foreign travel
Medications: Use of immunosuppressive drugs
Functional Health Patterns
Health perception–health management: Chronic fatigue, malaise, weakness
Nutritional metabolic: Unexplained weight loss; low-grade fevers, night sweats; anorexia, nausea, vomiting; oral lesions, bleeding, ulcerations; abdominal cramping; lesions of lips, mouth, tongue, throat; sensitivity to acidic, salty, or spicy foods; problems with teeth or bleeding gums; difficulty swallowing; skin rashes or color changes, lesions (painful or nonpainful), blisters; nonhealing wounds, pruritus
Elimination: Persistent diarrhea, constipation, painful urination
Activity-exercise: Muscle weakness, difficulty with ambulation; cough, shortness of breath
Cognitive-perceptual: Headaches, stiff neck, chest pain, rectal pain, retrosternal pain; blurred vision, photophobia, loss of vision, diplopia; confusion, forgetfulness, attention deficit, changes in mental status, memory loss; hearing impairment, personality changes, paresthesias; hypersensitivity in feet
Sexuality-reproductive: Lesions on genitalia (internal or external), pruritus, or burning in vagina or on penis; painful sexual intercourse; changes in menstruation; vaginal or penile discharge

Objective Data
General: Vital signs, weight, general status, diaphoresis
Eyes: Exudate, retinal lesions or hemorrhage, papilledema, pupillary response, extraocular muscle movements
Oral: A variety of mouth lesions, including blisters (HSV type–1 lesions), white-gray patches (*Candida* organisms), painless white lesions on lateral aspects of tongue (oral hairy leukoplakia), discolorations (Kaposi's sarcoma), gingivitis, tooth decay or loosening
Neck: Enlarged lymph nodes, nuchal rigidity, enlarged thyroid
Throat: Redness or white patchy lesions
Integumentary: Skin integrity and skin turgor; general appearance; lesions, eruptions, discolorations; enlarged lymph nodes, bruises, cyanosis, dryness, delayed wound healing, alopecia
Respiratory: Crackles or rhonchi, dyspnea, cough (productive or nonproductive, color and amount of sputum), wheezing, tachypnea, intercostal retractions, use of accessory muscles
Lymphatic: Generalized lymphadenopathy
Abdominal: Tenderness, masses, enlarged liver or spleen, hyperactive bowel sounds
Genitourinary-rectal: Lesions or discharge, abdominal pain indicative of pelvic inflammatory disease, difficult or painful urination
Neuromuscular: Aphasia, ataxia, lack of coordination, sensory loss, tremors, slurred speech, memory loss, apathy, agitation, social withdrawal or isolation, pain, inappropriate behavior, changes in level of consciousness, depression, seizures, paralysis, coma

HIV, Human immunodeficiency virus.

Box 16.6 Nursing Interventions for the Patient With HIV Infection or HIV Disease

PREVENT INFECTION
- Wash hands frequently, and administer skin lubricants to patient and caregiver to prevent skin breakdown.
- Use a gentle liquid soap.
- Provide for daily showering or basin bath; do not give patient tub bath if rashes are present; avoid extremely hot temperatures.
- Use a separate washcloth for lesions.
- For oral hygiene, provide soft toothbrushes; nonabrasive toothpaste; and mouth rinses with sodium bicarbonate, saline, or lemon and hydrogen peroxide before and after meals and at bedtime.
- Use measures to prevent skin impairment, such as turning sheets, air mattresses.
- Elevate and support areas of edema.
- Observe biopsy sites and intravenous insertion sites daily for signs of infection.
- Change dressings at least every other day; avoid plastic occlusive dressings.
- Prevent exposure to sources of microbes, such as plants or uncooked fresh fruits and vegetables.
- Carry out measures to prevent spread of infection: Use gloves for contact with bodily secretions, double plastic

bags to dispose of bodily secretions, bleach and water (1:10) solution for cleaning contaminated areas.

MODIFY ALTERATIONS IN BODY TEMPERATURE
- Administer prescribed antibiotics, intravenous fluids, or antipyretics.
- Encourage fluid intake of more than 2500 mL/day.
- Maintain daily intake and output records.
- Weigh patient daily.
- Provide tepid sponge baths and linen changes as necessary.
- Instruct patient in deep-breathing and coughing exercises to prevent atelectasis and additional fever.

PROMOTE GOOD NUTRITION
- Provide instruction for high-calorie, high-protein, high-potassium, low-residue diet.
- Encourage high-calorie, high-potassium snacks.
- Suggest foods that are easy to swallow (gelatin, yogurt, puddings) when dysphagia is present.
- Advise patient to avoid foods that are spicy or acidic, rare meats, and raw fruits and vegetables.
- Provide oral care before and after meals patient eats.
- Encourage patient to get out of bed and sit up for meals, if possible.

Box 16.6   Nursing Interventions for the Patient With HIV Infection or HIV Disease—cont'd

- Avoid odors by aerating room.
- Refer patient and caregiver for appropriate dietary consultations.
- Educate patient and caregiver about food safety and food preparation.

PROMOTE SELF-CARE
- Assess realistic functional ability.
- Plan, supervise, and assist with activities of daily living as necessary.
- Encourage patient to be as active and independent as possible.
- Assist patient with range-of-motion exercise to prevent contractures.
- Provide equipment such as assistive eating devices, walkers, and commodes to promote patient independence.

- To prevent fatigue, pace activities and schedule rest periods.

PROVIDE COUNSELING
- Assess and support patient's coping mechanisms.
- Explore with patient and significant others normality of grief.
- Assist patient and significant others in acknowledging and planning for anticipated losses.
- Provide information as desired and necessary, depending on patient's ability to understand.
- Suggest appropriate religious support.
- Facilitate participation in support groups or individual counseling as appropriate.

HIV, Human immunodeficiency virus.

Table 16.5   Nursing Activities in HIV Disease

LEVELS OF CARE AND GOALS	ASSESSMENT	INTERVENTIONS
Health Care Promotion and Maintenance		
Prevention of HIV infection Early detection of HIV infection	Risk factors: What behavioral, social, physical, emotional, pathologic, and immune factors place patient at risk? Does patient need to be tested?	Educate patient, including knowledge, attitudes, and behaviors, with an emphasis on risk reduction: • Regarding general population (cover general information) • Regarding individual patient (specific to assessed need)Empower patient to take control of prevention measures. Provide HIV-antibody testing with pretest and post-test counseling.
Acute Intervention		
Promotion of health and limitation of disability Successful management of problems caused by HIV infection	Physical health: Is patient experiencing problems? Mental health status: How is the patient coping? Resources: Does the patient have family and social support? Is patient accessing community services? Are money and insurance a problem? Does patient have access to spiritual support?	Provide case management. Educate regarding HIV, the spectrum of infection, options for care, signs and symptoms to watch for. Educate regarding immune enhancement and harm reduction. Establish long-term, trusting relationship with patient, family, and significant others. Refer to needed resources. Provide emotional and spiritual support. Provide care during acute exacerbations: recognition of life-threatening developments, life support, rapid intervention with treatments and medications, patient and family emotional support during crisis, comfort, and hygiene needs. Develop resources for legal needs: discrimination prevention, wills and powers of attorney, child care wishes. Empower patient to identify needs, direct care, seek services.

Continued

Table 16.5	Nursing Activities in HIV Disease—cont'd	
LEVELS OF CARE AND GOALS	**ASSESSMENT**	**INTERVENTIONS**
Chronic and Home Management		
Maximizing quality of life Resolution of life and death issues	Physical health: Are new symptoms developing? Is patient experiencing drug side effects or interactions? Mental health status: How is patient coping? What adjustments have been made? Finances: Can patient maintain health care and basic standards of living? Family, social, and community supports: Are these supports available? Is patient using supports in an effective manner? Spirituality issues: Does patient desire support from an established religious organization? Are spirituality issues private and personal? What assistance does patient need?	Continue case management. Educate regarding treatment options. Empower patient to continue directing care and to make desires known to family members and significant others. Continue physical care for chronic disease process: treatments, medications, comfort and hygiene needs. Refer to resources that will assist in meeting identified needs. Promote health maintenance measures. Assist with end-of-life issues: resuscitation orders, funeral plans, estate planning, child care continuation.

HIV, Human immunodeficiency virus.

Patients with a higher level of motivation to take their medications as ordered can have much better outcomes than do patients who are less compliant. Drug resistance to ART can easily develop when even a few doses of medication are missed or taken incorrectly. Compliance rates increase when HIV-infected patients are prescribed one combination ART medication per day and receive positive reinforcement from their health care team members (HIVinfo.nih.gov, 2020b).

Strategies that can assist nurses in increasing patient adherence include determining their own level of comfort with regard to HIV, learning to listen, having knowledge about the disease, using therapeutic communication skills, giving the patient and caregivers permission to grieve and feel sad, acknowledging frustration and helplessness, providing a safe environment, and seeking expert assistance as needed. All of these can help patients incorporate this difficult treatment into their lifestyle (Box 16.7).

PALLIATIVE CARE

Palliative care helps patients and families deal with possibly fatal illnesses and quality-of-life issues. The focus of palliative care is on preventing and relieving suffering from pain and to address the stress that comes with a serious illness. The goal of palliative care is to improve and maintain quality of life as much as possible by focusing on all patient needs, including physical, spiritual, psychological, social needs. Palliative care can help coordinate care with the health care provider and provides support to loved ones (Center to Advance Palliative Care, 2021).

Palliative care is not seen as hastening the dying process or postponing death. Nurses realize that death is a natural process of life, but other people may believe that a patient's death signifies the failure of medicine and loss of hope. Palliative care often is delayed

Box 16.7	Barriers to Adherence

- Caregivers' incomplete knowledge of the demands of patients' lives
- Prejudice
- Insufficient appointment time
- Lack of resources for patients who have doubts or questions
- Negative stereotypes about doctors
- Insufficient multidisciplinary communication

From NAM Publications: *Common barriers to adherence,* 2013.

as a result of this false belief. Palliative care can be provided at any stage of a disease and can be provided even if a cure is being sought. This is why palliative care works well with HIV patients since many will live long, productive lives after diagnosis. Most hospice programs use a palliative care approach, with the understanding that impending death means a shift from curing to caring. Remember that the goal is to relieve suffering through management of pain and symptoms at *any* point in the patient's disease process.

For patients with HIV disease, it is important for palliative care to address not only the potential chronic debilitating conditions associated with HIV disease but also superimposed acute exacerbations of opportunistic infections and related symptoms. Intravenous therapy, blood transfusions, and antibiotic usage may be considered palliative in the end stage of HIV disease, because these interventions help keep the patient comfortable and help maintain quality of life. In AIDS care, short-term aggressive, curative therapy is often important in treating acute infections such as pneumonia, but the overall goal remains palliation.

The complex needs of patients with HIV disease necessitate the services of a multidisciplinary team of physicians, nurses, social workers, pharmacists, dietitians, physical therapists, and clergy. The nurse is the "voice" and advocate for the patient who may or may not be able to communicate his or her treatment desires. Because of this unique role, it is important to be comfortable discussing treatment issues and options with patients, as well as respecting their decisions. Become familiar with the causes and interventions necessary to alleviate the patient's symptoms. Remember that symptoms such as pain are a subjective experience and must be treated appropriately until the patient indicates the treatment has worked. Although this phase of life is difficult for the patient and nurse, many nurses express significant satisfaction with these interactions, relationships, and their outcomes.

As HIV numbers have changed over time as a result of the use of ART and aggressive approaches to treatment, fewer patients with HIV infection are requiring hospice or palliative care. In some patients, however, HIV is not diagnosed until they are in a later stage of the disease process. These patients may choose palliative or hospice care instead of treatment.

PSYCHOSOCIAL ISSUES

People who have received a diagnosis of HIV infection deal with a complex set of psychosocial issues. Often, they are uncertain, fearful, depressed, and isolated. HIV infection can be treated, but it is incurable and contagious. Many infected people feel isolated and abandoned by friends and family because of the stigma associated with HIV. Like the health care costs associated with many chronic diseases, the expenses involved in treating HIV infection are daunting for many patients.

Nurses and health care providers must be empathetic during contact with patients. Listening is an important skill to help convey compassion. Therapeutic communication skills should be used to enhance rapport with a patient. Help the patient plan and decide about health care options. The patient has the right to be supported even when the decision seems imprudent.

Assisting With Coping

Individuals who have been exposed to HIV infection but who are without any symptoms or complications live with uncertainty, anxiety, denial, and hopefulness (Box 16.8). The nurse's role in this stage of the disease process is to provide continued education about HIV disease and prevention and to assist in realistic goal setting. Make every effort to include the patient and the support system in planning care. Early in the care process, assess past coping styles and support systems and continually reevaluate these issues. Encourage healthy patterns of coping, such as talk therapy, relaxation, and meditation. Relationships with family, friends, and significant others should be maintained and in fact may become stronger during the HIV crisis. However, prior family conflicts may worsen as a result of the stress of the illness. Families with poor communication skills are at particular risk for this outcome.

Box 16.8	Psychological Crisis Intervals in the Course of HIV Disease

- Diagnosis of HIV infection
- Viral load testing
- Increases in viral load
- Initiation of antiretroviral therapy
- Signs of treatment failure
- Adding prophylaxis therapies (e.g., for *Pneumocystis jiroveci* pneumonia)
- Occurrence of opportunistic illnesses
- Change in antiretroviral treatment regimen
- Illness or death in support networks
- New treatment advances

HIV, Human immunodeficiency virus.

As HIV disease progresses through the clinical complications of infections and cancers, patients experience multiple losses, including the loss of energy; a self-care deficit that necessitates assistance with activities of daily living; and the loss of independence, employment, finances, and hope. The reality of death emerges. Nursing interventions should focus on a philosophy of facing life one day at a time and living each day to its fullest. This may be a time for strengthening personal and spiritual relationships and resolving any conflicts.

Anxiety and depression can become chronic, ultimately interfering with daily functioning, relationships, communication, and even the ability to make simple decisions. Although anxiety and depression are normal when a patient is dealing with a significant health care threat, refer patients to mental health professionals for possible pharmacologic or verbal counseling when these feelings affect daily functioning for more than 2 weeks. Patients with HIV disease and depression should be assessed regularly for suicidal ideation because this phenomenon occasionally occurs in terminally ill patients. Early recognition of depression and anxiety is critical because most cases respond to medications, psychotherapy, or a combination.

Severe anxiety can cause individuals to believe they have no control over the events in their lives. Helping the patient develop a schedule of activities may decrease anxiety and feelings of powerlessness. Explore opportunities for spiritual support and comfort. Community support groups for patients and significant others may contribute to healthy coping. Arrange to spend time with the patient and the support system, in hopes that this will decrease anxiety and promote better coping.

The use of therapeutic communication and helping patients find meaning in life are critical nursing interventions. Assisting families and significant others in providing support to the terminally ill patient despite their own anger and grief is a unique nursing challenge. Such care, although emotionally draining, can provide great satisfaction.

Minimizing Social Isolation

The psychosocial aspects of HIV infection can be devastating. Feelings may include denial, fear, depression, and anger. These are similar to those that may be seen in an individual who has been diagnosed with cancer. The first stressful issue faced by a patient with newly diagnosed HIV infection is disclosure of HIV status. A very real concern for HIV-positive patients is that family, significant others, and friends will be angry and may even reject or abandon the patients. Families and friends of a patient with newly diagnosed HIV infection may be misinformed about the disease. The patient and the family may benefit from sources of support such as a mental health provider with experience providing service to patients who are infected with HIV. Support groups for patients and significant others are often also available. HIV-infected individuals who have been exposed through contaminated blood or who contract HIV from their partner may experience feelings of anger and hostility. Showing support and providing education about the disease may help alleviate some of these feelings.

Assisting With Grieving

Many patients with HIV infection benefit simply from having another person listen and explore in detail the feelings, unfounded fears, and treatment options. However, many others need the more structured support found in therapeutic relationships or formal support groups. Significant others and family members also may need assistance to provide support to their loved one. Formal counseling can help a patient address issues such as continued employment, health insurance concerns, preparations for disability, and feelings related to death. Referral to medical or clinical social workers and appropriate community agencies is part of the nurse's responsibility in addressing psychosocial needs. For some patients, it is appropriate to refer them to clergy.

CONFIDENTIALITY

Respect for the patient's right to confidentiality is particularly important for a patient with HIV disease. The confidentiality of the diagnosis must be protected carefully and shared only with caregivers who need to know for the purpose of assessment and treatment.

Health care workers should use standard precautions with each patient to prevent exposure to the patient's blood or bodily fluids. Not every infected patient may know that he or she is seropositive for HIV. When this information is shared by the patient, the information should be shared with other health care workers who are managing this patient's care.

The patient should be in control of who is told of the diagnosis, but laws dictate the reporting of an HIV diagnosis to appropriate health agencies. As with any patient seeking health care services, guidelines of the Health Insurance Portability and Accountability Act (HIPAA) must be followed. Partner notification laws also must be considered when HIV infection is diagnosed. The health care provider must follow laws in his or her state regarding partner notification.

ACUTE INTERVENTION

Early intervention after detection of an HIV infection can promote health and limit or delay disability. Because the course of HIV infection is extremely variable, assessment is of primary importance. Nursing interventions are tailored to any patient needs noted during assessment. The nursing assessment of HIV disease should focus on the early detection of constitutional symptoms, opportunistic diseases, and psychosocial problems (Box 16.9).

HIV disease progression may be delayed by maintaining the health of the immune system. Useful interventions for an HIV-infected patient include (1) nutritional changes that maintain lean body mass, maintain weight in the range of ideal body weight, and ensure consumption of appropriate levels of vitamins and micronutrients; (2) elimination of smoking and drug use; (3) elimination or moderation of alcohol intake; (4) regular exercise; (5) stress reduction; (6) avoidance of exposure to new infectious agents; (7) mental health counseling; (8) involvement in support groups; and (9) safer sexual practices.

The patient should be taught to recognize clinical manifestations that may indicate progression of the disease; this will ensure that medical care is initiated promptly. Early manifestations that must be reported include unexplained weight loss, night sweats, diarrhea, persistent fever, swollen lymph nodes, oral hairy leukoplakia, oral candidiasis (thrush; Fig. 16.5), and persistent vaginal yeast infections. In addition, the patient should report unusual headaches, changes in vision, nausea and vomiting, and numbness or tingling in the extremities. Give the patient as much information as needed to make health care decisions. These decisions dictate the appropriate medical and nursing interventions.

Nursing interventions become more complicated as the patient's immune system deteriorates and new problems arise to compound existing difficulties. The nursing focus should be on quality-of-life issues and symptom management, rather than on issues regarding a cure.

When opportunistic diseases develop, provide symptom-based nursing interventions, education, and emotional support. For example, an acute case of *P. jiroveci* pneumonia necessitates intensive nursing interventions, including monitoring the respiratory status, administering medications and oxygen, positioning the patient to facilitate breathing, managing anxiety, promoting nutritional support, and helping the patient conserve energy to decrease oxygen demand. Because advanced HIV disease can lead to death, emotional support for the patient, caregiver, or significant other is particularly important (see Nursing Care Plan 16.1).

| Box 16.9 | Conducting a Risk Assessment |

Risk assessment specific to HIV and sexually transmitted infections (STIs), as well as bloodborne diseases, is crucial in health care delivery today. Perform regular risk assessments on all patients and when evaluating any new patient. Determine sexual and drug use risks, along with other risks, during routine history taking. Advise the patient, and provide education and resources regarding risky behavior.

KEY QUESTIONS TO ASK

Any "yes" responses necessitate further assessment and evaluation.

- "Have you ever had a blood transfusion? Have you ever received any other kind of blood product? Before 1985?"
- "Do you now or have you ever shared injection equipment?"
- "Are you now or have you ever been sexually active?"

KEY POINTS TO CONSIDER

- Begin by assuring confidentiality and telling the patient why asking these questions is important:
  - "I am going to ask some personal questions. I ask all of my patients these questions so I can provide better care. All of your responses will be kept confidential. Is it okay to proceed?"
- Ask direct questions about specific behaviors:
  - "When was the last time you ...?"
  - "How often do you ...?"
  - "Have you ever exchanged sex for money or drugs?"
- Exploratory questions may help (especially with adolescents and young adults):
  - "Do your friends use condoms?"
  - "What happens at parties?"
  - "How easy is it to get drugs?"
- Honest responses may be more forthcoming if the behaviors are described in a nonjudgmental manner:
  - "Some of my patients who use drugs inject them. Do you inject drugs or other substances?"
  - "Sometimes people have anal intercourse. Have you ever had anal intercourse?"

DRUG USE ASSESSMENT

- It is important to be nonjudgmental and nonmoralistic:
  - Injection drug use is illegal in the United States and many patients are afraid to be honest unless trust is established.
- Start with less-threatening questions:
  - "What over-the-counter or prescription medications are you taking?"
  - "How often do you use alcohol? Tobacco?"
  - "Have you ever used drugs from a nonmedical source?"
  - "Have you ever injected any kind of drug?"
- Do not assume anything.
- Drug use occurs in all socioeconomic strata. Do not forget that people inject substances such as insulin,

steroids, and vitamins. Any sharing, even one time, can result in HIV exposure.
- Look for other clues in the history and physical examination, including antisocial behavior, recurrent criminal arrests, and needle tracks.
- If the patient has a positive history of drug injection use, get more information:
  - "Do [did] you share needles or other equipment?"
  - "Is (was) the equipment you use (used) clean? How did you know it was clean?"
  - "What drugs did you inject?"

SEXUAL RISK ASSESSMENT

- Direct and nonjudgmental questions work best:
  - "Do you have sex with men, women, or both?"
  - "Do you have oral sex? Vaginal sex? Anal sex?"
  - "What do you know about the sexual activities of your partners?"
  - "What do you do to protect yourself during sex?"
  - "Do you use condoms? How often?"
  - "Have you ever had sex with someone you didn't know or just met?"
- Ask for an explanation of sexual practices:
  - "When you say you had sex, what exactly do you mean?"
  - "I don't know what you mean; could you explain ...?"
- Do not assume anything.
- Marriage does not always mean an individual is monogamous or heterosexual.
- People who identify as homosexual may also have heterosexual sex.
- Use specific terms:
  - Use "men who have sex with men" or "women who have sex with women" instead of "gay."
  - Some men who practice anal insertive intercourse do not consider themselves "gay," but their receptive partners are considered to be gay (can be culturally related).

CLINICAL RISK ASSESSMENT

- Assess the patient for constitutional signs, history of chronic infection and HIV, and associated problems:
  - Headaches
  - Diarrhea
  - Fatigue
  - Shingles
  - History of STI, hepatitis, or tuberculosis
  - Fever, chills, night sweats
  - Skin lesions
  - Weight loss
  - Oral thrush
  - Generalized lymphadenopathy

HIV, Human immunodeficiency virus.
Modified from Mountain Plains AIDS Education and Training Center: *HIV risk assessment: A quick reference guide,* Denver, 2009, Author.

Diarrhea is often a long-term problem for HIV-infected people. Damage to the intestinal villi, malabsorption, infections of the gastrointestinal tract, and the side effects of medications contribute to a large number of cases of diarrhea. Nursing interventions include recommending dietary interventions (Table 16.6), encouraging adequate fluid intake to prevent dehydration, instructing the patient about skin

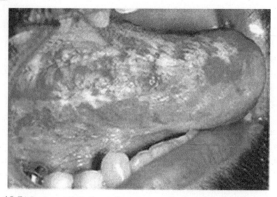

Fig. 16.5 Oral candidiasis, or thrush, manifests with a whitish, curdlike substance on the tongue or inside the mouth. (Courtesy Deborah Greenspan, DSC, BDS, University of California, San Francisco, and US Department of Veterans Affairs.)

care, and managing excoriation around the perianal area. In some cases, antidiarrheal agents may help control diarrhea and prevent further complications. Recommend the use of incontinence products to prevent soiling of the clothes and bed linens. In addition, assess for factors that may trigger the diarrhea, such as anxiety, medications, or lactose intolerance.

HIV wasting—the loss of lean body mass as a result of illness—has been a common clinical manifestation of HIV disease since early in the epidemic. Wasting is caused by disturbances in metabolism, which interfere with the effective use of nutrients, resulting in the loss of lean (muscle) body mass, often without reduction of body fat. This loss of lean body mass is a primary cause of functional decline in wasting, which results in increased risk of opportunistic infections, reduced quality of life, and reduced length of survival. A person with HIV is considered to have wasting syndrome when he or she has lost 10% of body weight and has had either diarrhea or weakness and fever for 30 days. The person infected with HIV who has wasting syndrome has a more advanced form of HIV or AIDS (US Department of Veterans Affairs [VA], 2019).

The causes of wasting are probably multifactorial. Food intake may be inadequate because of mechanical difficulties (e.g., thrush or esophageal ulcers), loss of appetite (e.g., side effect of medications, nausea, or neurologic disease), or psychological factors such as depression and anxiety. Absorption in the intestine may be decreased as a result of infections and a damaged mucosal barrier, which may lead to diarrhea. Some patients stop eating to decrease the number of bowel movements per day. An increased metabolic rate with muscle catabolism contributes to wasting syndrome.

Wasting disturbs self-concept and self-image and can be one of the most difficult consequences of HIV infection to accept. Useful interventions for these disturbances include creating an atmosphere of acceptance and reassurance, encouraging a focus on past accomplishments and personal strengths, and facilitating the use of positive affirmations.

Decreased levels of testosterone have been reported in HIV-infected men. Testosterone has two distinct biological properties: virilizing activity (androgenic effect) and protein building (anabolic effect). Because testosterone is an anabolic hormone, a deficiency may cause a loss of body cell mass, which contributes to HIV wasting. The role of gonadotropic hormones in women with wasting has not been studied sufficiently. Women with HIV wasting tend to lose a lot of body fat, but body cell mass is not significantly decreased. Conversely, men tend to lose a significant amount of lean body mass (e.g., exhibit skinny arms and legs), with preservation of fat, particularly in the truncal area.

With the advances in HIV treatment and opportunistic infection prophylaxis, serious malnutrition is less evident. However, nutrition does not return to normal after anti-HIV treatment begins. A syndrome of increased truncal obesity (visceral, abdominal), subcutaneous fat loss on the extremities and face (also called *lipoatrophy*), and metabolic abnormalities such as hyperlipidemia and insulin resistance have been reported in men and women.

The management of wasting and lipodystrophy is difficult and generally requires multiple nursing interventions. Diminished appetite and weight must be assessed and documented. Encourage nutritional supplementation (see Table 16.6) and increased protein intake, provide enteral supplements (through nasogastric or gastric tubes if necessary), and assist with total parenteral nutrition when it is needed. Medications to stimulate appetite, such as dronabinol (Marinol), can help; unfortunately, these medications tend to increase body fat and not lean muscle mass. Testosterone (anabolic steroid) can be administered by mouth, intramuscularly, or transdermally to increase lean body mass and weight. The effect of testosterone can be enhanced by a low-weight resistance-training program (e.g., weightlifting), which maintains muscle tone and improves appetite.

Nutrition counseling is vital to ensure that individuals with HIV disease maintain a well-balanced diet, including supplements if necessary. The dietitian can assist in counseling, provide the patient with high-protein and high-calorie diets, and suggest meal plans that fit the patient's lifestyle. Smaller, more frequent meals can be less overwhelming than larger meals. Teaching about food safety is of paramount concern because enteric infections (e.g., cryptosporidiosis, microsporidiosis, and amebas) in HIV disease are often not treatable or are relapsing. In some cases, enteral or parenteral feeding becomes necessary.

Management of elevated triglyceride and lipid (cholesterol) levels is common in HIV disease. The HIV infection and some types of HIV medications are responsible for the hyperlipidemia. As in other patient populations, these elevations can lead to cardiovascular disease and gallbladder disease, pancreatitis,

Nursing Care Plan 16.1   **The Patient Who Is HIV Positive**

Ms. J. is a 20-year-old who comes to the emergency department, accompanied by her mother, with complaints of severe vomiting and recent weight loss of 10 pounds. Ms. J. went to the 24-h clinic and learned that she is approximately 8 weeks pregnant and, because of risk factors for HIV exposure, gave informed consent for HIV antibody testing. The clinic determined that she is HIV positive according to ELISA and Western blot testing. Ms. J. is tearful and reluctant to answer questions about her recent HIV diagnosis and positive pregnancy test result. She states that she could not be HIV positive because she has had sexual intercourse only with her boyfriend of 5 years. In addition, Ms. J. is concerned about telling her mother about her HIV status and the pregnancy because she lives with her mother, who is also taking care of her sick elderly grandmother. Ms. J. does not have a job and depends on family members to help her meet financial obligations and needs. Ms. J. feels the added burden to her mother would "be too much" and is considering leaving home to live in a shelter.

PATIENT PROBLEM
Potential for Excessive Demand on Primary Caregiver, related to advancing disease in care receiver, inadequate caregiver coping pattern

Patient Goals and Expected Outcomes	Nursing Interventions	Evaluation
Caregiver will use available community and personal resources Caregiver will be able to complete necessary caregiving tasks Caregiver will receive effective support	Assess needs and capabilities of patient and caregiver. Assess factors that contribute to caregiver strain (unrealistic expectations, poor insight, inability to use resources, unsatisfactory relationship with care recipient, insufficient financial and psychosocial resources). Develop supportive and trusting relationship with caregiver. Enlist help of other family members or friends. Teach caregiver to perform care activities in a safe, efficient, and energy-conserving manner. Teach stress-reduction techniques. Encourage caregiver to attend to own personal and health needs.	The caregiver provides safe, supportive care to the HIV-infected patient. The caregiver acknowledges the need for personal support and accesses resources in family and community. The caregiver shares frustrations about difficulty of caring for a significant other. The caregiver receives assistance from family members and/or professional caregivers.

PATIENT PROBLEM
Insufficient Nutrition, related to chronic infections and/or malabsorption, nausea, vomiting, diarrhea, fatigue, or side effects of medications as evidenced by 10% or greater loss of ideal body mass.

Patient Goals and Expected Outcomes	Nursing Interventions	Evaluation
Patient's weight will remain stable Patient's nutritional intake will exceed metabolic needs Patient will regain lost weight	Assist with diagnosis of underlying opportunistic infections. Assess patient's knowledge of optimal nutritional intake. Increase protein, calorie, and fat intake. Offer nutritional supplements (e.g., Carnation Instant Breakfast, Boost, Sustacal). Schedule procedures that are painful, stressful, or nauseating so that they do not interfere with mealtimes. Provide the patient with several small meals throughout the day, as opposed to three large meals. Provide referrals to dietitians, social workers, and case managers. Weigh patient daily.	Patient's weight remains stable or increases. Patient reports increased energy level. Patient is able to complete activities of daily living. Patient experiences increase in lean muscle mass.

CRITICAL THINKING QUESTIONS
1. Ms. J. is tearful and asks the nurse if there is any treatment to prevent her baby from becoming HIV positive. What should be included in the nurse's information to Ms. J.?
2. Ms. J. asks the nurse whether she can legally require her boyfriend to be tested for HIV infection. What is the most appropriate response?
3. Ms. J. asks the nurse when she will develop AIDS now that she is HIV positive. What is the correct answer?

AIDS, Acquired immunodeficiency syndrome; *ELISA,* enzyme-linked immunosorbent assay; *HIV,* human immunodeficiency virus.

Table 16.6 Nutritional Management: HIV Infection

CONDITION	DIETARY RECOMMENDATION	INTERVENTION
Diarrhea	Lactose-free, low-fat, low-fiber, and high-potassium foods	Instruct patient to avoid dairy products, red meat, margarine, butter, eggs, dried beans, peas, and raw fruits and vegetables. Provide cooked or canned fruits and vegetables, which provide needed vitamins. Encourage patient to eat potassium-rich foods such as bananas and apricot nectar. Instruct patient to discontinue foods, nutritional supplements, and medications that may make diarrhea worse (Ensure, antacids, stool softeners). Advise patient to avoid gas-producing foods. Serve warm, not hot, foods. Plan small, frequent meals. Encourage patient to drink plenty of fluids between meals.
Constipation	High-fiber foods	Instruct patient to eat fruits and vegetables (beans, peas), cereal, and whole wheat breads. Gradually increase patient's fiber intake. Encourage patient to drink plenty of fluids and to exercise.
Nausea and vomiting	Low-fat foods	Advise patient to avoid dairy products and red meat. Plan small, frequent meals. Prepare nonodorous foods. Encourage patient to eat dry, salty foods. Serve food cold or at room temperature. Instruct patient to drink liquids between meals. Advise patient to avoid gas-producing, greasy, spicy foods. Encourage patient to eat slowly in a relaxed atmosphere. Enable patient to rest after meals, with head elevated. Administer antiemetics 30 min before meals.
Candidiasis	Soft or pureed foods	Serve moist foods. Encourage patient to drink plenty of fluids. Instruct patient to avoid acidic and spicy foods. Advise patient to use straw and tilt head back and forth when drinking. To decrease discomfort, encourage patient to eat soft foods, such as puddings and yogurt.
Fever	High-calorie, high-protein foods	Administer nutritional supplements. Increase patient's fluid intake.
Altered taste	Diet as tolerated	Encourage patient to try adding herbs and spices, as well as salt and sugar. Advise patient to marinate meat, poultry, and fish. Serve food cold or at room temperature. Encourage patient to drink plenty of fluids. Introduce alternative protein sources.
Anemia	High-iron foods	Encourage patient to eat organ meats and raisins. Advise patient to drink orange juice when taking iron supplements, to facilitate absorption.
Fatigue	High-calorie foods	Advise patient or caregiver to cook in large quantities and freeze meal-size portions in packets. Suggest the use of microwaveable and convenience foods. Encourage the use of easy-to-fix snack foods. Advise patient to use social support system to assist with meal planning and preparation. Help patient access in-home homemaker services and Meals-on-Wheels programs.

HIV, Human immunodeficiency virus.

and diabetes (HIVinfo.nih.gov, 2020a). Lipid-lowering agents such as the statins may be effective in treating this complication. However, because the liver metabolizes many of the antilipid agents, it is important to choose a drug that is safer than those that must pass through the liver to be activated; safer anticholesterol drugs include pravastatin, fluvastatin , and possibly atorvastatin . A program of diet, exercise, and medications can lower lipids safely and reduce the chances of a cardiovascular event.

Insulin resistance or diabetes sometimes responds to oral hypoglycemic agents (e.g., metformin or rosiglitazone). In some cases, the anti-HIV therapy must be changed. All medications belonging to the PI class increase lipid levels. Efavirenz (an NNRTI), abacavir, stavudine, zidovudine (NRTIs), and stibild (combination medication) have been linked to hyperlipidemia. Diet management, smoking cessation, weight loss, reduced alcoholic intake, and exercise can help control the elevations in blood glucose that can occur with the use of anti-HIV medications.

Unfortunately, as with any overwhelming viral infection, HIV infection increases the patient's metabolic needs. This hypermetabolism and consequent higher energy expenditure frequently exceed the number of calories taken in by the patient. Malnutrition, weight loss, and generalized wasting are common problems in patients with HIV disease (see Nursing Care Plan 16.1). Many patients with HIV disease experience wasting. Malnutrition contributes to wasting, and wasting hastens the negative immune consequences of HIV infection. HIV wasting contributes to slower recovery from infection, impaired wound healing, increased risk of secondary infection, and decreased cardiac and respiratory function. Wasting can lead to an earlier death. The weight loss associated with HIV disease is often severe and debilitating, producing a vicious cycle of anorexia, malnutrition, loss of tissue mass, muscle wasting, profound fatigue, and increased susceptibility to infections and drug interactions. Although typically seen in later stages of HIV disease, malnutrition and wasting can occur in the early stages of HIV infection.

NEUROLOGIC COMPLICATIONS

HIV-Associated Related Cognitive Issues

AIDS dementia complex (ADC), also known as HIV-associated dementia, is the term used to describe a common central nervous system complication of HIV disease. This condition is a complex combination of signs and symptoms, including dementia; impaired motor function; and, at times, characteristic behavioral changes that resemble those accompanying a stroke or head trauma. The disease generally does not cause alterations in the level of consciousness. It usually is described as a triad of cognitive, motor, and behavioral dysfunction that slowly progresses over a period of weeks to months. The cognitive changes involve primarily a mental slowing and inattention. Affected patients typically lose their train of thought and complain of slowed thinking. They may miss appointments and find themselves making lists of tasks and chores that need completing. The signs and symptoms of motor dysfunction ordinarily develop after those of cognitive impairment. They include poor balance and coordination (e.g., falling and tripping, dropping things); slower manual activities (e.g., writing, eating); and, ultimately, leg weakness that can limit ambulation. This type of dementia can be diagnosed through a simple physical examination, neurologic testing, magnetic resonance imaging and computed tomography, and cerebrospinal fluid analysis. Another less severe form of HIV-related cognitive issues is referred to as minor cognitive motor disorder. It manifests with forgetfulness, slowed movements, poor coordination, personality changes, and difficulty concentrating (Thomas, 2018).

Nursing interventions for neurocognitive dysfunction include administration of ART, antidepressants, psychostimulants, anticonvulsants, anti-dementia medications, benzodiazepines, and psychotherapy. Supervision of the patient, which includes a home safety assessment, is imperative. Ensure that orientation cues such as clocks and calendars are present, hallways and living areas are brightly lit, walkways are clear of electrical cords or throw rugs, and potentially dangerous objects (e.g., knives, poisons) are stored safely away from the patient.

Caring for patients with dementia is a collaborative effort between the health care provider and family. It is advisable to seek advice from a social worker, the home health care department, and a psychologist in developing a plan to care for an impaired individual.

Peripheral neuropathy. Neuropathies are diseases that affect the peripheral nervous system. They can affect sensory, motor, or autonomic nerves. The causes of neuropathies can be related to HIV disease or, more frequently, the side effects of many anti-HIV medications. Symptoms include numbness, localized tingling, hypesthesia (diminished sensitivity to stimulation) or anesthesia, loss of sense of vibration and position (proprioception), and decreased or increased sensitivity to pain. In most cases, patients complain of numbness in the fingers, the hands, and the feet and pain on walking. Patients also may experience autonomic neuropathy. Symptoms such as mild positional hypotension, cardiovascular collapse, and chronic diarrhea are suggestive of autonomic neuropathy.

Management of Opportunistic Infections

With the advent of effective ART and better understanding of opportunistic infection prophylaxis, the frequency of such infections has decreased dramatically. Opportunistic infections still occur in severely immunocompromised patients, so become familiar with the recognition, treatment, and prophylaxis of these diseases. Opportunistic infections typically are seen in individuals who are nonadherent to their antiretroviral regimen, nonadherent to prophylactic regimens against opportunistic infections, or at the end stage of HIV disease and in individuals who do not consistently access the health care system. (See Table 16.3 and Box 16.4 for common opportunistic infections, treatment, and prevention.)

Health Care Promotion

Because patients with HIV disease are living longer and more productive lives, attention to the promotion of health and healthy behaviors is important (see the Health Promotion box). Patients should be encouraged to eat well-balanced meals, stop smoking or at least reduce the number of cigarettes smoked, get adequate sleep and rest periods if possible, use stress-reduction modalities (e.g., biofeedback, referral for counseling), obtain dental care regularly, and keep scheduled appointments with all health care providers. Attention to comorbid conditions, such as hypertension and diabetes, helps minimize additional health problems. Encourage patients to get all immunizations and keep them up to date; female patients should regularly receive gynecologic examinations. If hospitalizations are necessary, encourage the patient and significant others to participate in treatment decision making, and arrange for home care follow-up if indicated.

 Health Promotion

The Patient Infected With HIV

- Remind patients that a positive diagnosis is not an immediate "death sentence." Patients are living increasingly longer, high-quality lives after diagnosis because of medications, more specialized care, and decreased morbidity and mortality related to opportunistic diseases.
- Stress the importance of health-promoting behaviors to reduce the risk of comorbidity.
- Encourage patients to maintain good nutritional status by eating regular, well-balanced meals that are high in protein and calories. Increased protein is necessary for cell and tissue repair, especially in patients who may be hypermetabolic.
- Encourage patients to limit their intake of alcoholic beverages and avoid the use of illicit or recreational drugs.
- Encourage patients to maintain an adequate sleep schedule.
- Encourage patients to use stress-reduction practices, such as biofeedback, massage, or progressive relaxation. They also should engage in relaxing or pleasurable activities.
- Advise patients to use safer sexual practices to avoid reinfection and exposure to other STIs.
- Encourage patients to establish an exercise regimen that includes aerobic activity and low-resistance weightlifting if possible.
- Of most importance, support patients in setting short- and long-term goals and assist them in achieving those goals.

Although some pets can pose risks for transmission of opportunistic infections, they are, overall, therapeutic and healing for the patient. Only minor modifications must be made for HIV-infected pet owners (e.g., birdcage and cat litter box cleaning). If possible, pet visits to the hospital or care facility should be arranged if a long separation is anticipated; the idea of benefit should not be dismissed just because this practice is not acceptable at the nurse's health care facility. Speak with managers and supervisors to obtain permission or help develop policies and procedures that allow the visitation of pets.

PREVENTION OF HIV INFECTION

HIV disease is *preventable*. However, prevention requires the cooperation and efforts of public health care providers, medical providers, nurses in all specialties, families, communities, churches, and schools (Box 16.10). Education on prevention is currently our best way to help reduce infection rates. Many patients admitted to acute care facilities have unrecognized HIV disease or are at risk for HIV infection. Assess each patient's risk, and counsel those at risk about HIV testing, the behaviors that put them at risk, and how to reduce or eliminate those risks. Today, every nurse is potentially an HIV nurse; that is, all nurses may find themselves responsible for teaching patients methods to reduce the risk of transmission. Nurses must be able to discuss, in a nonjudgmental way, behaviors related to sexual activity and substance use (e.g., condom application, using clean needles). Establish rapport with patients before asking sensitive, explicit questions related to behaviors typically not discussed.

Harm-reduction education is a fundamental element of HIV prevention methods. Harm reduction does not completely eliminate the risk of HIV transmission, but it minimizes the social harms and costs associated with certain behaviors. For example, attempts to quit smoking two packs of cigarettes per day all at once almost always result in failure. A harm-reduction approach may involve suggesting that the patient reduce the number of cigarettes smoked from 40 to 30 a day. Although the ultimate goal is for the patient to stop smoking altogether, the patient has at least reduced the risk of long-term effects by limiting the number of cigarettes smoked. The same is true for HIV prevention. Encouraging patients to use protective barriers such as male and female condoms helps reduce the risk of HIV transmission.

HIV TESTING AND COUNSELING

An important part of preventing HIV transmission is HIV screening tests and follow-up education and counseling (see Box 16.3). However, patients must not be coerced into having an HIV screening test. Nurses and health care providers should counsel their patients before and after HIV testing. HIV tests necessitate informed consent per state law before blood is collected. The informed consent always is accompanied by an explanation about the testing and implications of results. The limitations of the test also must be explained.

Performing HIV testing early in the course of the disease is important for increasing survival rates of HIV-infected patients and preventing the transmission to

Box 16.10   HIV Prevention Options

SEXUAL
No Risk
- Abstain from sexual contact that involves exchange of semen, vaginal secretions, or blood.
- Stay in a mutually monogamous relationship (the state of having one mate) in which neither partner is at risk of infection through injecting drug use and in which neither partner was previously exposed to HIV.

Reduced Risk
- Limit the number of partners, even though a potential risk exists if there was sexual contact with only one infected partner.
- Use protective measures through consistent and correct use of latex condoms with a spermicide in every act of sexual intercourse that would involve exchange of semen, vaginal secretions, or blood. The correct use of condoms is as follows:
  - Put on the condom as soon as erection occurs and before any sexual contact (anal, vaginal, oral).
  - Leave space at the tip of the condom.
  - Use only water-based lubricants.
  - Hold the condom firmly to keep it from slipping off; withdraw from partner immediately after ejaculation.

USE OF INJECTION DRUGS
No Risk
- Stop using injectable drugs; drug treatment opportunities should be provided.
- If drugs are going to be injected, use sterile needles and equipment.

Reduced Risk
- If needles and equipment are going to be shared, follow instructions on cleaning.
- Fill the syringe with sodium hypochlorite 5.25% (Clorox) bleach two times; empty two times. Fill the syringe with clean water two times; empty two times.

PERINATAL
No Risk
- Avoid pregnancy; this is the only certain way to prevent transmission of HIV to a fetus or infant.
- Women of childbearing age of unknown HIV status should be counseled about behaviors that would put them and their partners or spouses at risk for HIV infection. If risk factors are determined in either case, both individuals should be counseled about testing for HIV.

Reduced Risk
- Adhere to barrier birth control measures, including use of condoms, to avoid pregnancy.
- Use ART given during pregnancy and to infant for first 6 weeks of life.

HIV, Human immunodeficiency virus.

other people through high-risk behaviors. Guidelines from the CDC (2020a) mandated that all patients in health care agencies be informed about HIV screening and then be screened for HIV. However, these patients are allowed to refuse the test. HIV antibody testing should be offered to all patients, regardless of patient-specific risk factors. Also, test results should be made available rapidly to the patient so that education can be given to the patient, if needed. The CDC's recommendations state that informed consent is not needed. However, patients may opt out of testing if they wish. In rare emergency situations in which health care providers need to know a patient's HIV status to make a decision regarding health care and the patient is unable to speak, the patient may be tested without his or her consent.

Increasing numbers of people with HIV can be identified with the continued push for routine HIV screening. The antibody screening test (immunoassay) is the most common type of HIV test. It is used to test for the antibodies present when someone is infected with HIV. Blood or oral fluid may be tested. There are several blood tests available that can identity antigens and antibodies associated with HIV infection (HIV.gov, 2020). There is a rapid test available that can detect antibodies to HIV in 30 minutes or less. Oral fluids or blood may be used. Positive tests should be followed up with an antibody differentiation test to distinguish between HIV-1 and HIV-2 infections, an HIV-1 NAT to detect HIV which is used to identify antibodies. RNA tests can identify the virus directly. It can be used to detect the virus approximately 10 days after infection before the body's ability to develop antibodies. RNA tests are more expensive than antibody tests and typically are not used to screen. OraQuick and Home Access HIV-1 Test System are in-home, over-the-counter HIV tests approved by the FDA. OraQuick involves swabbing the mouth to collect oral fluid and can produce results in 20 minutes. This test is not as sensitive as other tests and can produce false-negative results if low levels of antibodies are present in the oral fluid (AIDS.gov, 2015).

HIV antibody testing may take place in a physician's office or at designated HIV counseling and testing sites. Many patients feel more comfortable being tested by someone who knows their medical and social history, but others prefer to be tested in a location where they are unknown. Be aware of the various options for HIV antibody testing in his or her state or community to advise patients appropriately.

HIV antibody testing can be done one of two ways: confidentially or anonymously. In *confidential testing,* patients provide identifying information, including a name; an address; and often demographic information such as age, sex, race, and occupation. Using this information, care providers can locate and provide information to an individual who does not return for the test results or counseling. All records are strictly confidential, and testing in physicians' offices, clinics, and hospitals is conducted in a confidential manner. Health care providers who share or use this information inappropriately can be sued for negligence and invasion of privacy, and they may be disciplined by licensing boards for unauthorized disclosure or breach of confidentiality. Patients should be informed that the results of their HIV antibody test will be linked to the patient's medical record.

In *anonymous testing*, individuals are not asked to provide identifying information. Records are kept through assigned numbers, and the patient must retain this number to receive test results. It is not possible to locate and provide information to an individual who does not return for test results and counseling. In either form of testing, the nurse can perform pretest and post-test counseling.

RISK ASSESSMENT AND RISK REDUCTION

Testing for HIV is an important part of the public health response to HIV disease. Risk assessment should be patient centered, a joint process between the nurse and patient. The patient should take "ownership" of the risk for HIV infection. The nursing assessment should include an evaluation of risky behaviors by the patient or a history of STIs. A patient will not get tested unless he or she perceives a need for testing and feels safe doing so. Help the patient assess the risks by asking some basic questions:

- Have you ever had a transfusion or used clotting factors? Was it before 1985?
- Have you ever shared needles, syringes, or other injecting equipment with anyone?
- Have you ever had a sexual experience in which your penis, vagina, rectum, or mouth came into contact with another person's penis, vagina, rectum, or mouth?

A positive response to any of these questions requires further exploration with the patient. Be prepared to refer the patient to centers that provide testing and counseling services. All testing should include pretest and posttest counseling (see Boxes 16.3 and 16.9).

BARRIERS TO PREVENTION

HIV prevention has numerous barriers, not the least of which is a denial of risk, an attitude that "it won't happen to me." Because the virus largely infects the MSM population in the United States, members of many other subpopulations have ignored their risks. Fear, misunderstanding, and the potential for social isolation and social stigma are significant barriers. Reinforcement is necessary for consistent, accurate information about the virus, the risks of transmission, and HIV disease.

Cultural and community attitudes, values, and norms can affect the success of prevention efforts. A community may be opposed to HIV education in the local school district because of the fear that certain values will be compromised. Those values may include views on sexuality, abstinence, the use of condoms, the use of drugs, and the provision of instructions about cleaning needles and syringes. Community organizations, churches, educators, and leaders can determine the community's expectations or norms. Cooperative efforts are essential for successful prevention of HIV transmission. The issues related to the HIV epidemic—sex, drug use, death, and homosexuality—are not easy issues for most cultures or communities.

Fear of alienation and discrimination are significant additional barriers to prevention. Some individuals are reluctant even to pick up a pamphlet about HIV because they fear that someone will believe they are gay or using illicit drugs. Some people will not go to a physician or to a testing and counseling site for HIV testing for fear of being seen there by people they know. This fear may be further compounded in smaller communities. Fear of discrimination includes fear of losing family, friends, prestige, job, housing, and insurance. Fortunately, many states have statutes to protect individuals with HIV disease from discrimination. Protection also is afforded by the Americans with Disabilities Act.

REDUCING RISKS RELATED TO SEXUAL TRANSMISSION

When patients have acute HIV disease and high viral loads, they are 10 times more likely to transmit HIV during sexual intercourse than during the chronic stage of HIV. Infection risk also is increased when sex is forceful or when mucosal membranes are disrupted (situations often associated with STIs). Most HIV infections are transmitted during the primary stage of the infection. This is when most people are unaware of their infection because they have no symptoms. Men are less likely to be infected with HIV during heterosexual intercourse than are women because women have more mucosal surface that can be exposed to infected body fluids in comparison to men. Male circumcision also can minimize a man's risk of becoming infected with HIV via heterosexual intercourse, according to the WHO (2020).

Safer sexual activities reduce the risk of exposure to HIV through semen, rectal secretions, and cervicovaginal secretions. Abstaining from all sexual activity is the most effective way to accomplish this goal. Limiting sexual behavior to activities in which the mouth, penis, vagina, or rectum do not come into contact with the partner's mouth, penis, vagina, or rectum is also safe because there is no contact with blood, semen, or cervicovaginal secretions. These activities may include massage and masturbation. Insertive sex is considered safe only in a mutually monogamous relationship with a partner who is not infected with, or at risk of becoming infected with, HIV. The problem with mutual monogamy is that both partners need to follow all of the rules all of the time. Unfortunately, cases of HIV

Box 16.11   Risk of HIV Transmission

HIV is spread primarily by the following:
- Not using a condom when having sex with a person who has HIV. All unprotected sex with someone who has HIV contains some risk. However:
  - Unprotected anal sex is riskier than unprotected vaginal sex.
  - Among men who have sex with other men, unprotected receptive anal sex is riskier than unprotected insertive anal sex.
  - Having multiple sex partners or the presence of other sexually transmitted diseases (STDs). Unprotected oral sex can also carry risk for HIV transmission, but it is a much lower risk than that with anal or vaginal sex.
- Sharing needles, syringes, rinse water, or other equipment used to prepare illicit drugs for injection.
- Being born to an infected mother: HIV can be passed from mother to child during pregnancy, birth, or breast-feeding.

Less common modes of transmission include the following:
- Being "stuck" with an HIV-contaminated needle or other sharp object. This risk pertains mainly to health care workers.
- Receiving blood transfusions, blood products, or organ/tissue transplants that are contaminated with HIV. This risk is extremely remote, however, as a result of the rigorous testing of the US blood supply and donated organs/tissue.
- Unsafe or unsanitary injections or other medical or dental practices. However, the risk is also remote with current safety standards in the United States.
- Eating food that has been prechewed by an HIV-infected person. The contamination occurs when infected blood from a caregiver's mouth mixes with food while chewing. This appears to be a rare occurrence and has been

documented among only infants whose caregiver gave them prechewed food.
- Being bitten by a person with HIV. Each of the very small number of cases has included severe trauma with extensive tissue damage and the presence of blood. There is no risk of transmission if the skin is not broken.
- Contact between broken skin, wounds, or mucous membranes and HIV-infected blood or blood-contaminated body fluids. Reports of these incidents also have been extremely rare.
- "French" or deep, open-mouth kissing with an HIV-infected person if the HIV-infected person's mouth or gums are bleeding. This chance, too, is extremely remote.
- Tattooing or body piercing. However, no cases of HIV transmission from these activities have been documented. Only sterile equipment should be used for tattooing or body piercing.
- Unsafe injections. There have been a few documented cases in Europe and North Africa in which infants have been infected by unsafe injections and then transmitted HIV to their mothers through breast-feeding. No cases of this mode of transmission have been documented in the United States.

HIV cannot reproduce outside the human body. It *is not* spread by any of the following:
- Air or water.
- Insects, including mosquitoes. Studies conducted by CDC researchers and others have shown no evidence of HIV transmission from insects.
- Saliva, tears, or sweat. No case of HIV being transmitted by spitting has been documented.
- Casual contact such as shaking hands or sharing dishes.
- Closed-mouth or "social" kissing.

All reported cases suggesting new or potentially unknown routes of transmission are thoroughly investigated by state and local health departments with assistance, guidance, and laboratory support from CDC.

HIV, Human immunodeficiency virus.
Modified from Centers for Disease Control and Prevention (CDC): HIV: HIV transmission, 2020. Retrieved from https://www.cdc.gov/hiv/basics/transmission.html.

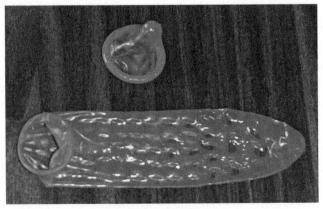

Fig. 16.6 Male condoms.

infection occur in individuals who are not aware that their partner has not remained monogamous. Serial monogamy (maintaining a monogamous relationship, often including unprotected intercourse, with one partner for a short time, followed by another relationship, and then another) also increases the risk of HIV exposure (Box 16.11).

ART can be provided to people who have been exposed to HIV through unwanted sexual intercourse (rape) or through injection drugs. The US Department of Health and Human Services (USDHHS) has developed some recommendations regarding these types of nonoccupational exposures. This is referred to as postexposure prophylaxis, or PEP. When a person has been exposed to body fluids from an HIV-infected person during high-risk activity less than 72 hours before seeking treatment, the exposed person should receive a 28-day supply of ART. This is recommended even if the HIV-infected source of the exposure has an undetectable viral load. However, if the activity is deemed to be low-risk exposure to body fluids, or if the exposed person seeks health care after the 72-hour window, ART is not recommended. Cases should be examined on an individual basis to determine the need for PEP, counseling, treatment, and education about preventing future exposures (CDC, 2021g).

The use of barriers (Fig. 16.6) reduces the risk of contact with HIV during sexual activity. Barriers should be used when a person engages in sexual activity with a partner whose HIV status is not definitely known or with a partner who is known to be infected with HIV. The most commonly used barrier is the male condom. Although not 100% effective, male condoms are very effective in the prevention of HIV transmission when used correctly and consistently. Other barriers include female condoms and latex dental dams. Female condoms consist of a vinyl sheath with two spring-form rings. The smaller ring is inserted into the vagina and holds the condom in place internally. The larger ring surrounds the opening to the condom. It keeps the condom in place externally while also protecting the external genitalia. The use of the female condom is complicated and cumbersome, and practice may be necessary to use this method effectively. Female condoms also can be used for anal sex, in men and women. Dental dams or microwave-safe plastic wrap can be used to cover the external genitalia or anus during oral sexual activity ("rimming"). Although the risk of HIV transmission is reduced significantly with the use of latex barriers, other STIs, such as human papillomavirus, warts, and HSV, can still be transmitted.

REDUCING RISKS RELATED TO DRUG ABUSE

The use of illicit or recreational drugs can cause immunosuppression, malnutrition, and emotional difficulties. Although using illicit drugs can increase a person's risk for acquiring HIV infection, drug use is not to blame. The major risks of HIV transmission are related to sharing injection equipment and having unsafe sexual experiences while under the influence of mood-altering chemicals. Essentially, people can reduce the risk of HIV infection by not using drugs. If drugs are injected, equipment should not be shared with other people. People should not engage in sexual activity while under the influence of any drug, including alcohol, that impairs decision making.

Abstaining from drugs is not always a viable option for a user who has no access to drug treatment services or who chooses not to quit. The risk of HIV for these individuals can be eliminated if they can find alternatives to injecting, such as smoking, snorting, or ingesting drugs. Risk also can be eliminated if the user does not share injection equipment, including needles, syringes, cookers, cotton, and rinse water. The safest tactic is for the user to have ready access to sterile equipment. Many states have laws that prohibit over-the-counter sale of needles and syringes, such as diabetic supplies. Some communities have needle exchange programs that supply sterile equipment to users to help reduce the risk of HIV transmission. The fear that needle exchange programs will result in increased illicit substance use has led to a lack of community support. However, studies have shown that in communities that have established exchange programs, drug use does not increase and rates of HIV infection are controlled (AVERT, 2019).

REDUCING RISKS RELATED TO OCCUPATIONAL EXPOSURE

As previously discussed, the risk of acquiring HIV through occupational exposure is low. The CDC and the Occupational Safety and Health Administration have instituted policies to protect employees from exposure to blood and other potentially infectious fluids (OSHA, n.d.). The use of standard precautions and body substance isolation has been shown to reduce the risk of bloodborne pathogens, the risk of transmission of other diseases between the patient and the health care worker, and the risk of transmission between patients. Hand hygiene in the form of handwashing still remains the most effective means of preventing the spread of infection.

Results of epidemiologic and laboratory studies suggest that several factors may affect the risk of HIV transmission after an occupational exposure. In a retrospective study of health care workers who had percutaneous exposure to HIV, the CDC (2001) found that the risk of HIV infection was increased with exposure to a larger quantity of blood from the source patient, as indicated by (1) a device visibly contaminated with the patient's blood, (2) a procedure that involved a needle being placed directly in a vein or artery, or (3) a deep injury. The risk also is increased for exposure to blood from a patient with terminal illness, which possibly reflects the higher viral load of the patient late in the course of HIV disease (CDC, 2001). Information about primary HIV infection (seroconversion) indicates that a systemic infection does not occur immediately. This leaves a brief window of opportunity during which initiation of antiretroviral PEP may prevent or inhibit systemic infection by limiting the proliferation of the virus in the initial target cells or lymph nodes.

For best prophylactic effect, PEP must be initiated within 72 hours but preferably as soon as possible after the exposure. PEP should include three or more ART medications (Familydoctor.org, 2019). In addition to possible exposure to an antiretroviral-resistant strain of HIV, other factors that may contribute to failures include a high titer or large volume of inoculum exposure, delayed initiation or short duration of PEP, and factors related to the exposed health care personnel (e.g., immune status).

Completion of a 4-week course of therapy after an occupational exposure is fundamental. The medications used have many side effects, and health care workers may stop PEP prematurely because of these. It is important to consult with experts in occupational exposure if side effects (headache, nausea, vomiting, and diarrhea) become unbearable. The use of PEP regimens has been associated with new-onset diabetes mellitus, hyperglycemia, hypertriglyceridemia, pancreatitis, elevated levels of lipids (cholesterol, low-density lipoproteins), liver dysfunction, and kidney stones. Despite these serious side effects, the exposed health care worker must continue therapy for 4 weeks or until it is determined that the source patient is not infected with HIV.

Hospitals or agencies should have policies that specifically address occupational HIV exposure, inasmuch as chemoprophylaxis must be undertaken immediately, even before testing of the source patient's and health care worker's blood for HIV or other blood-borne pathogens. Serial testing of the health care worker for HIV occurs immediately, 6 weeks, 3 months, and 6 months after the exposure.

Maintaining confidentiality for the exposed health care worker and the source patient is paramount. Many states and health care organizations have separate, distinct consent forms that are required before HIV antibody testing can be performed. Only in rare circumstances, such as the inability to give consent, can HIV antibody testing be completed without the patient's informed consent. Many ethical and legal issues surround HIV antibody testing; therefore nurses must be informed of the applicable laws in the state in which they practice. In many states, charges of assault and battery can be brought against health care workers who perform HIV testing against a patient's will. Appropriate counseling and referrals should be made for the health care worker and patient when HIV testing is indicated.

OTHER METHODS TO REDUCE RISK

HIV-infected people must be instructed not to give blood, donate organs, or donate semen for artificial insemination. They should not share razors, toothbrushes, or other household items that may contain blood or other body fluids. They also should avoid infecting sexual and needle-sharing partners, consider using birth control measures, and eliminate breast-feeding to avoid spreading the virus to infants.

OUTLOOK

During the HIV epidemic, much has been learned about transmission of the virus and ways to prevent infection. With no cure in sight, prevention of infection through education, prevention of mother-to-child transmission, and in some cases PEP or preexposure prophylaxis for people with a very high risk of becoming infected but are not currently infected can limit the effect of this disease on the human population.

The dynamics of the epidemic also have changed dramatically. In the United States, HIV disease has the characteristics of any other chronic illness, in that (1) it currently cannot be cured, (2) it continues throughout the patient's life, (3) it causes increasing physical disability and dysfunction if not treated, and (4) it ultimately results in significant morbidity and mortality. Chronic diseases are characterized by acute exacerbations of cyclic problems that compound each other. Despite a significant decrease in the number of opportunistic infections, new complications have emerged. Health care providers today must address body composition changes, cardiac disease, neuropathies, and the long-term effects of the very medications that have kept HIV at bay.

Since the discovery of HIV, knowledge about the viral cycle, resulting immune response, and disease progression of HIV has made significant advances. New medication treatments are very effective and can help the host manage the disease by limiting replication of the virus, which can allow the immune system to continue to function. Rates of survival among patients with late-stage HIV (and who have access to ART and are being cared for by health care providers with expertise in dealing with HIV) have increased dramatically. Patients who previously would have become disabled, quit jobs, and tended to end-of-life decisions are now reevaluating goals, returning to work, and rediscovering relative health. Now, couples with different HIV statuses have the option of having children with the use of sperm "washing" and in vitro fertilization.

For no other disease has there been such a rapid understanding and attempts at developing therapies as with HIV infection. The HIV research arena has provided insight into other diseases and scientific fields, including virology, immunology, and oncology. At this point, however, scientists' ability to develop new therapies depends on the patient's being nearly 100% adherent to regimens that are sometimes toxic. Adherence is poor even when therapy consists of only one pill per day. Even though treatment options for HIV have advanced, disease progression varies widely. Research is continuing into determining how psychological and social stressors alter immune system responses.

Minority MSM have become the fastest-growing segment of the population with HIV disease. Underdeveloped countries in Africa and Southeast Asia have been hardest hit; in fact, many villages have been destroyed because of HIV. The global threat of HIV is enormous, and nurses play a key role in the care and treatment of HIV-infected individuals. For the best possible outcomes, always seek guidance from HIV specialists when treating an individual with HIV disease because the care is very complex and multiple needs arise.

The field of HIV and AIDS nursing changes frequently, and nurses constantly must refresh their base of knowledge. Resources include local AIDS service organizations and state and regional AIDS education and training centers. As new therapies emerge, nurses are in a unique position to educate patients and the public about the virus and prevention of its transmission.

Get Ready for the NCLEX® Examination!

Key Points

- HIV, a retrovirus, is the agent that causes HIV disease and AIDS.
- Education on prevention is the best method for preventing HIV disease and AIDS.
- In the United States, HIV most commonly is spread by sexual activities and sharing injection equipment.
- AIDS is the third and final stage of HIV infection.
- When HIV enters the body, its primary target is the immune system.
- HIV is transmitted by three major routes: (1) anal and vaginal intercourse, (2) injecting drugs with contaminated needles or works, and (3) from infected mother to child.
- Blood, semen, vaginal secretions, rectal secretions, and breast milk are the body fluids that most readily transmit HIV.
- Each patient's risks for HIV infection must be assessed, and those at risk must be counseled about testing, behaviors that put them at risk, and how to eliminate or reduce those risks.
- A positive result of an HIV antibody test does not mean the patient has AIDS.
- A multidisciplinary care approach in which the patient is a primary member of the team is the most appropriate method of caring for patients with HIV disease because of their complex needs.
- As HIV infection progresses, the immune system loses its ability to fight infectious agents and cancer cells.
- Patients at risk for HIV infection should be encouraged to learn their HIV status.
- A person infected with HIV virus can transmit the virus, regardless of whether signs and symptoms are present.
- Barriers to HIV prevention include denial, fear, misinformation, and cultural and community norms.
- CD4$^+$ counts are important markers of disease progression and the status of the immune system.
- The stigma of HIV disease, because of its association with drug use, homosexuality, and sexual transmission, is a major concern.
- The 1993 expanded case definition of AIDS includes all HIV-infected people who have CD4$^+$ T lymphocyte counts of less than 200/mm^3; includes all people who have one or more of more than 20 opportunistic infections regardless of CD4 count.
- Measuring viral load in the blood helps assess effectiveness of therapy and possibly adherence.
- Adherence to medications is essential.

Additional Learning Resources

SG Go to your Study Guide for additional learning activities to help you master this chapter content.

Be sure to visit the Evolve site at http://evolve.elsevier.com/Cooper/adult for additional online resources.

Review Questions for the NCLEX® Examination

1. **What is responsible for causing the majority of HIV disease and AIDS?**
   1. Human immunodeficiency virus type 1
   2. Human immunodeficiency virus type 2
   3. African immunodeficiency virus type 1
   4. *Pneumocystis jiroveci* deficiency virus

2. **How does vertical transmission of HIV occur?** *(Select all that apply.)*
   1. Mother to fetus during breast-feeding
   2. Mother to fetus during pregnancy
   3. Mother to fetus during delivery
   4. Mother to fetus during the postpartum period
   5. Mother to fetus during the first year of the infant's life

3. **The nurse is assessing a patient who has requested HIV testing. What would be considered to be the most risky behavior?**
   1. Dry kissing a casual date
   2. Sharing a soda with an infected person
   3. Swimming with an infected person
   4. Having more than three sex partners in a year

4. **The student nurse is giving a presentation on the transmission of HIV to his class. The student is correct by sharing which information?** *(Select all that apply.)*
   1. Health care workers are at a high risk for contracting HIV.
   2. Risk for transmission of HIV is higher with anal intercourse than with other types of sexual intercourse.
   3. People who use injection drugs and share needles have an elevated risk for being infected with HIV.
   4. The leading mode of transmission of HIV worldwide is sexual intercourse, despite sexual preference.
   5. During sexual intercourse, the partner who is being penetrated is least likely to contract HIV.

5. **An 8-year-old boy receives a diagnosis of hemophilia. His mother is upset about his risk of acquiring HIV from blood products. What would be the nurse's best response?**
   1. "All blood and blood products are screened for bloodborne diseases, so it is impossible for your son to be infected."
   2. "Many blood products are treated with heat or chemicals to inactivate the HIV virus."
   3. "We can talk about this if your son requires transfusions or blood products."
   4. "All blood donors are asked about HIV status and risk factors before giving blood."

6. A 34-year-old patient comes to the clinic requesting HIV testing. He is a gay man with two significant others in his lifetime. His partner recently received a diagnosis of HIV infection. The patient asks the nurse how long it will take before the infection could show up in him. What would be the nurse's best response?

    1. "Antibodies may be detected in the blood within 1 to 12 weeks of exposure."
    2. "It takes at least a year to know if you will be infected with HIV."
    3. "You'll have to ask your doctor the next time you go in for an appointment."
    4. "We don't know how long it will take for a person to seroconvert to being HIV positive."

7. The patient is concerned that he may be infected with HIV. Which sign or symptom is most commonly associated with an HIV infection?

    1. Night sweats
    2. Rash on the legs only
    3. Constipation
    4. Pruritus

8. A patient receives a diagnosis of HIV disease. She visits the physician today for her prescriptions. What medication does the nurse expect the physician to order for the patient?

    1. Tenofovir and emtricitabine
    2. Efavirenz
    3. Lopinavir and ritonavir
    4. Combination of these drugs

9. What diet should the patient with HIV follow?

    1. High calorie, high fiber, low protein
    2. Low calorie, low fiber, high protein
    3. High calorie, high protein, low residue
    4. Low calorie, high fiber, high protein

10. What are the most common opportunistic infection and malignant neoplasm in the patient with advanced HIV disease (AIDS)?

    1. Streptococcal pneumonitis, myeloma
    2. *Pneumocystis jiroveci* pneumonia, Kaposi's sarcoma
    3. *Streptococcus pneumoniae,* malignant melanoma
    4. *Mycoplasma* pneumonitis, Kaposi's sarcoma

11. For most people who are HIV positive, marker antibodies are usually present 10 to 12 weeks after exposure. What is the development of these antibodies called?

    1. Immunocompetence
    2. Seroconversion
    3. Immunodeficiency
    4. Viral load

12. What is the expanded definition of AIDS?

    1. The patient has HIV infection.
    2. The patient has a dysfunction of the immune system and is HIV positive.
    3. The patient is HIV positive and has an opportunistic disease.
    4. The patient is HIV positive with a CD4+ lymphocyte count lower than 200/mm^3 or has an AIDS-related opportunistic infection.

13. What is the purpose of performing a viral load study once every 3 to 4 months in an HIV-positive person?

    1. To determine the CD4+ lymphocyte count
    2. To determine the progression of the disease
    3. To determine the effectiveness of the medication regimen
    4. To determine the results of the Western blot test

14. The health care provider asks the nurse to talk with a patient about how HIV is transmitted. Which routes of transmission are most important for the nurse to discuss with the patient?

    1. Receiving blood, donating blood
    2. Food, water, air
    3. Sexual intercourse, sharing needles, mother-to-child transmission
    4. Dirty toilets, swimming pools, mosquitoes

15. The patient asks the nurse, "How does HIV cause AIDS?" What is the nurse's best response?

    1. "HIV attacks the immune system, a system that protects the body from foreign invaders, and thus makes it unable to protect the body from organisms that cause diseases."
    2. "HIV breaks down the circulatory system, which makes the body unable to assimilate oxygen and nutrients."
    3. "HIV attacks the respiratory system, which makes the lungs more susceptible to organisms causing pneumonia."
    4. "HIV attacks the digestive system, which causes a decrease in the absorption of essential nutrients and results in weight loss and fatigue."

Objectives

1. Discuss the incidence rates of cancer in the United States.
2. Identify the three most common sites of cancer in men and women.
3. Discuss development, prevention, and detection of cancer.
4. List seven risk factors for cancer.
5. Discuss the American Cancer Society's recommendations for preventive behaviors and screening tests for men and women.
6. List seven warning signs of cancer.
7. Define the terminology used to describe cellular changes, characteristics of malignant cells, and types of malignancies.
8. Describe the pathophysiologic features of cancer, including the characteristics of malignant cells.
9. Describe the process of metastasis.
10. Define the systems of tumor classification: grading and staging.
11. List common diagnostic tests used to identify cancer.
12. Explain why biopsy is essential in confirming a diagnosis of cancer.
13. Describe nursing interventions for the individual undergoing surgery, radiation therapy, chemotherapy, bone marrow transplantation, or peripheral stem cell transplantation.
14. Describe the major categories of chemotherapeutic agents.
15. Explain the causes, pathophysiologic features, clinical manifestations, and medical management of tumor lysis syndrome. Then, describe the appropriate diagnostic tests, nursing interventions, and prognosis.
16. Discuss six general guidelines for pain relief in the patient with advanced cancer.

Key Terms

alopecia (ăl-ō-PĒ-shē-ă, p. 795)
autologous (ăw-TŎL-ŏ-gŭs, p. 799)
benign (bĕ-NĪN, p. 783)
biopsy (BĪ-ŏp-sē, p. 784)
cachexia (kă-KĔK-sē-ă, p. 800)
carcinogenesis (kăr-sĭn-ō-JĔN-ĕ-sĭs, p. 778)
carcinogens (kăr-SĬN-ō-jĕnz, p. 778)
carcinoma (kăr-sĭn-Ō-mă, p. 783)
chemo brain (Ke-mO Brain, p. 792)
differentiated (dĭf-ĕr-ĔN-shē-ā-tĕd, p. 783)
dysgeusia (dis-gyū-zē-ă, p. 801)
germline mutations (JĔRM-lĭn mū-TĀ-shănz, p. 779)
immunosurveillance (ĭm-yū-nō-sĕr-VĀ-lĕns, p. 783)

leukopenia (lū-kō-PĒ-nē-ă, p. 792)
malignant (mă-LĬG-nănt, p. 783)
metastasis (mĕ-TĂS-tă-sĭs, p. 783)
neoplasm (NĒ-ō-plăz-ĕm, p. 783)
oncology (ŏn-KŎL-ŏ-jē, p. 776)
palliative (PĂL-ē-ă-tĭv, p. 789)
Papanicolaou's [Pap] test or smear (pă-pĕ-NĬK-ō-lūz [PĂP] tĕst, smēr, p. 784)
sarcoma (săr-KŌ-mă, p. 783)
stomatitis (stō-mă-TĪ-tĭs, p. 795)
thrombocytopenia (thrŏm-bō-sīt-ō-PĒ-nē-ă, p. 794)
tumor lysis syndrome (TŪ-mŏr LĪ-sĭs SĬN-drŏm, p. 797)

ONCOLOGY

Oncology is the branch of medicine concerning the study of tumors. An oncology nurse is one with specialized training who cares for patients who have been diagnosed with cancer.

Until the appearance of human immunodeficiency virus (HIV), no other medical diagnosis produced as much fear as a diagnosis of cancer. The word *cancer* is thought by many people to be synonymous with death, pain, and disfigurement. However, advances in the treatment and control of cancer have outdistanced attitudes toward cancer. Education of health care professionals and the public is essential for promoting more positive and realistic attitudes about cancer and cancer treatment. The National Cancer Institute indicates that, in the United States, 38% of women and men living in the United States will be diagnosed with cancer at some point in their lifetime (NCI, 2018b.). The leading sites of primary cancer in men are the prostate, lungs, colon, and rectum (Centers for Disease Control and Prevention [CDC], 2021a). The leading sites of primary cancer in women are the breasts, lungs, and colorectal areas (ACS, 2019). Of every five deaths in the United States, one is

Leading New Cancer Cases and Deaths – 2018 Estimates

Estimated New Cases*		Estimated Deaths*	
Breast	268,670	Lung and bronchus	154,050
Lung and bronchus	234,030	Colorectum	50,630
Prostate	164,690	Pancreas	44,330
Colorectum	140,250	Breast	41,400
Melanoma of the skin	91,270	Liver and intrahepatic bile duct	30,200
Urinary bladder	81,190	Prostate	29,430
Non-Hodgkin lymphoma	74,680	Leukemia	24,370
Kidney and renal pelvis	65,340	Non-Hodgkin lymphoma	19,910
Uterine corpus	63,230	Urinary bladder	17,240
Leukemia	60,300	Brain and other nervous system	16,830
Pancreas	55,440	Esophagus	15,850
Thyroid	53,990	Kidney and renal pelvis	14,970
Oral cavity and pharynx	51,540	Ovary	14,070
Liver and intrahepatic bile duct	42,220	Myeloma	12,770
Myeloma	30,770	Uterine corpus	11,350
Stomach	26,240	Stomach	10,800
Brain and other nervous system	23,880	Oral cavity and pharynx	10,030
Ovary	22,240	Melanoma of the skin	9,320
Esophagus	17,290	Soft tissue (including heart)	5,150
Cervix	13,240	Cervix	4,170
Larynx	13,150	Gallbladder and other biliary	3,790
Soft tissue (including heart)	13,040	Larynx	3,710
Gallbladder and other biliary	12,190	Thyroid	2,060
Small intestine	10,470	Bones and joints	1,590
Testes	9,310	Small intestine	1,450
Anus, anal canal and anorectum	8,580	Vagina and other female genital	1,330
Hodgkin lymphoma	8,500	Vulva	1,200
Vulva	6,190	Anus, anal canal and anorectum	1,160
Vagina and other female genital	5,170	Hodgkin lymphoma	1,050
Ureter and other urinary organs	3,820	Ureter and other urinary organs	960
Eye and orbit	3,540	Testes	400
Bones and joints	3,450	Penis and other male genital	380
Penis and other male genital	2,320	Eye and orbit	350

Fig. 17.1 Cancer: 2018 estimates. (Data from American Cancer Society, Inc.)

from cancer, which makes cancer the second leading cause of death after heart disease (Fig. 17.1).

Cancer is any one of a group of diseases characterized by the uncontrolled growth and spread of abnormal cells in the body. Early detection and prompt treatment can cure some cancers and slow the progression of others. If not detected and controlled, cancer can result in death. Overall, it affects people of all ages, but most cases are diagnosed in people older than 55 (see the Lifespan Considerations box). Cancer incidence is higher among African American men than among members of any other race and African American women had the second highest rate of cancer. (CDC, 2020 see the Cultural Considerations box). In 2018, over 1.7 million new cancer diagnoses were anticipated, and 609,640 Americans were expected to die from cancer (NCI, 2018). Cancer death rates have decreased since 1991 in men and since 1992 in women. In comparison with the peak rates in 1990 for men and in 1991 for women, the cancer death rate for all sites combined in 2017 had dropped by 29% to 152 per 100,000 (ACS, 2020e). This is thought to be related to a reduction in smoking and better screening and treatment. Since the early 1960s, the 5-year survival rate has increased dramatically from 27% to 64% for Blacks and 39% to 70% for whites (ACS, 2020c).

 Lifespan Considerations

Older Adults

Cancer

- More cases of cancer occur among older adults than among people of any other age group.
- The incidence of cancer increases with aging, possibly as a result of decreased effectiveness of the immune system and changes in deoxyribonucleic acid (DNA).
- The most common types of cancers observed in older adults are prostate, lung, breast, and colorectal cancer. Cancers of the skin, urinary bladder, vagina, and vulva are seen primarily in older adults. Chronic lymphocytic leukemia and multiple myeloma are seen more frequently in older adults than in younger people.
- Many early signs and symptoms of cancer may be misdiagnosed as normal changes of aging. Stress the importance of routine medical screening and self-examination.
- Because of fear or experience, older adults may adopt a fatalistic frame of mind after hearing the diagnosis of cancer. Use of the terms *tumor* or *growth* may be more acceptable.
- The type of treatment for cancer should be based on the older person's wishes and overall state of health. Older individuals, their family members, and significant others should be presented with all options so that they can make informed decisions regarding treatment.

Cultural Considerations

Cancer in the United States

- The incidence of cancer is higher among African Americans than among white people.
- The death rate from the four most common cancers (lung, colorectal, breast, prostate) is higher among members of minority groups (except Asian Americans) than among white people.
- Of all ethnic groups, Asian Americans have the lowest rate of death from cancer.
- In comparison with white men, African American men have almost twice the rate of prostate cancer and are more than twice as likely to die from the disease.
- Hispanic women have the highest rate of invasive cervical cancer of any ethnic group other than Vietnamese, and the incidence rate is twice as high as that in non-Hispanic white women.
- Although African American women are less likely than white women to develop breast cancer, they are more likely to die from the disease if they develop it.
- Native Americans have a lower incidence of cancer than any other ethnic group in the United States but have the poorest survival rate when they do develop cancer.

Lung cancer is the leading cause of cancer-related death in men and women. Other cancers, such as breast and prostate, occur more often than lung cancer, but they have better cure and survival rates because of early detection and treatment.

DEVELOPMENT, PREVENTION, AND DETECTION OF CANCER

Carcinogenesis is the process by which normal cells are transformed into cancer cells. Cancer may be caused by external factors (infection, chemicals, radiation, and tobacco use) and internal factors (genetic mutations, immunologic conditions, and hormones).

Primary prevention of cancer consists of changes in lifestyle habits to eliminate or reduce exposure to **carcinogens**—substances known to increase the risk for developing cancer. Risk factors include the following:

- *Smoking:* According to the American Cancer Society, smoking is the most preventable cause of death from lung cancer. It is estimated that 80% of people who die from lung cancer are smokers. Other cancers associated with smoking are acute myeloid leukemia and cancers of the bladder, kidney, mouth, lip, stomach, colorectum, nasopharynx, larynx, paranasal sinuses, esophagus, pancreas, uterus, ovary, and cervix.
- *Dietary habits:* Nutrition is suspected to be a contributing factor to an estimated one-third of cancer deaths. Diets that are high in fat and low in fiber, as well as inadequate nutrient intake, are associated with cancer development. The National Cancer Institute (NCI, 2015b) estimates that dietary modifications could prevent as many as one-third of all cancer deaths in the United States. Excessive body weight and inactivity are also linked (NCI, 2015b); obesity is a risk factor for breast, endometrium, colon, rectum, esophagus, pancreas, kidney, and gallbladder cancer. Fruit and vegetable consumption may protect against cancers of the mouth and pharynx, esophagus, lung, stomach, and colon and rectum (see the Health Promotion box). Despite recommendations, just 10% of adults consume the recommended amount of fruits and vegetables per day (Lee-Kwan, 2017).
- *Ultraviolet radiation:* Excessive exposure to the sun's ultraviolet rays is a factor in the development of basal and squamous cell skin cancers and melanoma. Indoor tanning beds also emit ultraviolet rays and confer the same risks as does sunlight. (In addition, the effects of radiation commonly used for medical diagnosis and treatment are known to be carcinogenic. Exposure should be limited and monitored.)
- *Smoking tobacco:* Smoking tobacco is responsible for approximately 30% of all deaths attributed to cancer

🏃 Health Promotion

Foods to Reduce Cancer Risk

- Vegetables from the cabbage family, such as the following:
  - Broccoli
  - Cauliflower
  - Brussels sprouts
  - All types of cabbage and kale
- Vegetables and fruits high in beta-carotene, such as the following:
  - Carrots
  - Peaches
  - Apricots
  - Squash
  - Broccoli
- Rich sources of vitamin C, such as the following:
  - Grapefruit
  - Watermelon
  - Apricots
  - Oranges
  - Cantaloupe
  - Strawberries
  - Red and green peppers
  - Broccoli
  - Tomatoes

The American Cancer Society (2020d) has recommended including {1½–2} cups of fruit and {2½–3} cups of vegetables in the daily diet.

In addition are the following recommendations:

- Eat foods from protein sources such as legumes, fish, and skinned poultry.
- Choose monounsaturated and polyunsaturated fats instead of saturated or trans fats.
- Eat whole grains.
- Eat a variety of fruits, especially whole fruits with a variety of colors.
- Eat a variety of vegetables—dark green, red, and orange.
- Include fiber-rich peas and beans in the diet.
- Avoid salt-cured, smoked, or nitrite-cured foods.
- Avoid red or processed meat, highly processed grains, and sugar-sweetened drinks (Rock, 2020).
- Limit intake of added sugars.

in the US and 80% of those who have died due to lung cancer. In addition, smoking is linked to oral, esophagus, larynx, cervix, kidney, liver, pancreas, stomach, bladder, and colorectal cancers (ACS, 2020h).

Smokeless tobacco: Use of smokeless tobacco increases the risk of cancer of the mouth, larynx, pharynx, and esophagus. Long-term snuff users have an increased risk for cheek and gum cancers (ACS, 2020h).

Electronic cigarettes: Electronic or e-cigarettes contain nicotine, vegetable glycerin, and/or propylene glycol, which irritate respiratory airways. Also, e-cigarettes contain toxic volatile organic compounds, chemicals used for flavor, and formaldehyde, which is a known carcinogen (ACS, 2020j).

- *Environmental and chemical carcinogens:* Some of these include fumes from rubber and chlorine, as well as dust from cotton, coal, nickel, chromate, asbestos, and vinyl chloride. The incidence of bladder cancer is higher among people who live in urban areas and among those who work with dyes, rubber, or leather.
- *Frequent heavy consumption of alcohol:* Alcohol use is linked to cancers of the head and neck, esophageal, liver, breast, and colorectum (NCI, 2018a).

HEREDITARY CANCERS

About 5% to 10% of cancers are hereditary (ACS, 2020g). Hereditary cancers arise from germline mutations, which are changes in egg or sperm cells that are then incorporated into the DNA of each body cell of the children produced (NCI, 2017). Gene mutations occurring in specific genes are thought to be associated with more than 50 different hereditary cancer syndromes (NCI, 2017). Hereditary cancers usually are diagnosed 15 to 20 years earlier than cancers that are not inherited. Often, several relatives have the same or related cancers. In location, they are more likely to be bilateral, and the same person may have multiple cancers. These multiple cancers are often seen in unusual organ combinations, such as breast cancer and sarcoma, breast and thyroid cancers, and leukemia and brain tumors.

GENETIC SUSCEPTIBILITY

Scientific research has focused on genetic patterns in the most common cancer sites. The following patterns have emerged:

- *TP53* is the most commonly mutated gene found in all cancers. This gene is responsible for the synthesis of a protein that suppresses tumor growth. Germline mutations of this gene can produce Li-Fraumeni syndrome. This is an inherited and rare disorder that can lead to an elevated risk of developing specific cancers (NCI, 2017).
- The incidence of postmenopausal breast cancer is three times higher and the incidence of premenopausal breast cancer is five times higher in women with a family history of this disease. An estimated 13% of the general female population develops breast cancer during their lifetime. In comparison, women who have either of the genes *BRCA1* and *BRCA2* have a much greater chance of developing breast cancer. With the BRCA 1 gene the risk is 55%-72%, and with the BRCA 2 gene the risk is 45-69% breast cancer during their lifetime (NCI, 2020). These genes also increase a person's risk for developing pancreatic, prostate (men), and male breast cancer (NCI, 2017). Breast cancer is rare in Asian women and more common in white women.
- *PTEN* is a gene that assists with the production of another tumor growth suppressor. Mutations to *PTEN* can produce Cowden syndrome. This is an inherited disorder that can increase a patient's risk for developing endometrial, thyroid, and breast cancer (NCI, 2017).

- The incidence of lung cancer is greater among smokers with a family history of this disease than in smokers without a family history of the disease.
- The incidence of leukemia is higher in an identical twin of a person with the disease.
- The frequency of neuroblastoma is increased among siblings.
- Colon cancer is more likely to occur in women who have a history of breast cancer.

CANCER RISK ASSESSMENT AND GENETIC COUNSELING

When an individual or family has characteristics suggestive of a hereditary cancer (such as cancers that occur in several generations of a family, multiple primary cancers in one person, or rare cancers associated with birth defects), a cancer risk assessment is performed. The assessment begins with a comprehensive family history, including information on first-, second-, and third-degree relatives. Medical records, death certificates, and autopsy reports may be obtained to help confirm the cancer diagnoses previously identified in the family history.

Genetic counseling is an essential component of the genetic evaluation. The nurse who may be involved with the genetic counseling and genetic testing provides health care promotion education and support to individuals and families facing the uncertainty of hereditary cancer. Informed consent must be obtained before genetic testing.

CANCER PREVENTION AND EARLY DETECTION

The American Cancer Society (2020c) advises specific preventive behaviors and screening tests for men and women (Table 17.1). Education regarding early detection of cancer includes recognition of warning signs (Box 17.1). The nurse plays an important role in prevention and detection of cancer. Early detection and prompt treatment are directly responsible for increased

Table 17.1	Screening Guidelines for the Early Detection of Cancer in People With No Symptoms and Average Risk		
CANCER SITE	**POPULATION**	**TEST OR PROCEDURE**	**FREQUENCY**
Breast	Women, ages 20+	Breast self-examination (BSE)	Update: Research does not show a benefit of performing regular breast exams, by the patient herself or even by a health care provider. Most women find lumps when dressing or bathing. Lumps are also identified when women have mammograms (ACS, 2021a).
		Clinical breast examination (CBE)	For women of average breast cancer risk (no personal history or strong family history of breast cancer, no history of chest radiation therapy, no genetic mutation that increases risk), it is not recommended that CBE be part of a periodic health examination. No longer recommended.
Mammography			Women should begin receiving annual mammography (2D or 3D) from ages 45–54, with the option to begin at age 40. At age 55, women can receive a mammogram annually or every other year. Screening continues for as long as the woman is healthy and is expected to live for at least 10 more years. Recently, an advanced type of mammogram called digital breast tomosynthesis (three-dimensional [3D] mammography) has been developed and is becoming more commonly used. However, it is not available in all imaging centers. This type of mammography reduces the likelihood that the patient will be asked to return for follow-up diagnostic tests. It is a more sensitive test and may be helpful in finding more breast cancer sites and is also better suited for women with denser breasts. The 3D mammogram is more expensive and insurance companies do not cover all of the fees associated with this test (ACS, 2021a).
Cervix	Women, ages 21–65	Pap test and HPV DNA test	Regardless of HPV vaccination status, women should begin receiving cervical cancer screening beginning at age 21. Women who are 21–29 should receive a Pap test every 3 years. After an abnormal pap test, HPV testing should be used. At age 30, women should receive screening with a Pap test and an HPV test every 5 years unless the tests results are abnormal. This is referred to as co-testing and should continue until the age of 65. Another option for women aged 30–65 is to be screened every 3 years with only a Pap test.

Table 17.1	Screening Guidelines for the Early Detection of Cancer in People With No Symptoms and Average Risk—cont'd		
CANCER SITE	**POPULATION**	**TEST OR PROCEDURE**	**FREQUENCY**
Colorectal	Men and women, ages 45–75, if in good health and expected to live at least 10 more years, regular screening activities should continue until the age of 75. For those people between the ages of 76–85, screening activity decisions are based upon the person's preferences, overall health, life expectancy, and results from prior screening (ACS, 2020a).	Stool testing includes any of the following: Highly sensitive fecal immunochemical test (FIT) each year Highly sensitive (guaiac-based) fecal occult blood test (gFOBT) each year Multi-targeted stool DNA test (MT-sDNA) every 3 years for individuals at an average risk for colorectal cancer. It is not intended for high risk individuals.	Annual, starting at age 45. Testing at home with adherence to manufacturer's recommendation for collection techniques and number of samples is recommended. FOBT with the single stool sample collected on the clinician's fingertip during a DRE in the health care setting is not recommended. In comparison with guaiac-based tests for the detection of occult blood, immunochemical tests are more patient-friendly and are likely to be equal or better in sensitivity and specificity. There is no justification for repeating FOBT in response to an initial positive finding.
		Flexible sigmoidoscopy (FSIG), or	Flexible sigmoidoscopy (FSIG) every 5 years
		Colonoscopy	Every 10 years, starting at age 45
		CT Colonography	Every 5 years, starting at age 45
Endometrial	Women, at menopause		At the time of menopause, women at average risk should be informed about the risks and symptoms of endometrial cancer and strongly encouraged to report any unexpected bleeding or spotting to their physicians.
Lung	Patients with an elevated risk for developing lung cancer (within past 15 years), ages 55–74, who are in fairly good health with at least a 30 pack-year history and are receiving counseling to stop smoking (if they are current smokers) and have been informed by their health care providers regarding the potential benefits, limits, and harm associated with LDCT screening and have access to a facility with this type of screening available (ACS, 2021b).	Low-dose helical CT (LDCT)	Clinicians with access to high-volume, high-quality lung cancer screening and treatment centers should initiate a discussion about lung cancer screening with patients who have an elevated risk of developing lung cancer. A process of informed and shared decision making with a clinician related to the potential benefits, limitations, and harms associated with screening for lung cancer with LDCT should occur before any decision is made to initiate lung cancer screening. Smoking cessation counseling remains a high priority for clinical attention in discussions with current smokers, who should be informed of their continuing risk of lung cancer. Screening is not an alternative to smoking cessation.
Prostate	Men, ages 50+	Digital rectal examination (DRE) and prostate-specific antigen test (PSA)	Men who have at least a 10-year life expectancy should have an opportunity to make an informed decision with their health care provider about whether to be screened for prostate cancer, after receiving information about the potential benefits, risks, and uncertainties associated with prostate cancer screening. Prostate cancer screening should not occur without an informed decision-making process.
Cancer-related checkup	Men and women, ages 20+	On the occasion of a periodic health examination, the cancer-related checkup should include examination for cancers of the thyroid, testicles, ovaries, lymph nodes, oral cavity, and skin, as well as health counseling about tobacco, sun exposure, diet and nutrition, risk factors, sexual practices, and environmental and occupational exposures.	

CT, Computed tomography.
From American Cancer Society: Cancer prevention & early detection facts & figures, 2021-2022, 2021c. Retrieved from: *https://www.cancer.org/research/cancer-facts-statistics/cancer-prevention-early-detection.html*.

Box 17.1   Eight Warning Signs of Cancer

If you have a warning sign, see your health care provider.
1. Changes in bowel or bladder habits
2. Sores that don't heal
3. White patches inside the mouth or on the tongue
4. Unusual bleeding or discharge
5. Thickening or lump in breast or elsewhere
6. Indigestion or difficulty swallowing
7. Recent change in warts, moles, or skin
8. Nagging cough or hoarseness

Modified from American Cancer Society (ACS): Signs and symptoms of cancer, 2020. From *https://www.cancer.org/cancer/cancer-basics/signs-and-symptoms-of-cancer.html*.

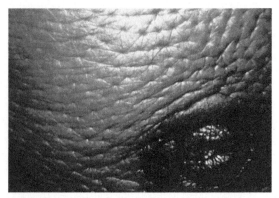

Fig. 17.2 Appearance of peau d'orange in the breast. (From Swartz MH: *Textbook of physical diagnosis*, ed 5, Philadelphia, 2006, Saunders.)

Health Promotion

Prevention and Detection of Cancer

- Reduce or avoid exposure to known or suspected carcinogens and cancer-promoting agents, including cigarette smoke and excessive sunlight.
- Eat a balanced diet that includes green, deep yellow, and orange vegetables; cruciferous vegetables (cabbage, broccoli, cauliflower, and Brussels sprouts); fresh fruits; allium vegetables (onion and garlic); nuts; legumes; soy products; whole grains; and adequate amounts of fiber. Reduce the amount of fat and preservatives, including smoked and salt-cured meats. Limit the consumption of processed foods and red meats.
- Exercise regularly. Adults should engage in 150–300 min of moderate-intensity or 75–150 min of vigorous-intensity physical activity per week; achieving or exceeding the upper limit of 300 min is optimal. The American Cancer Society recommends that adults engage in 150–300 min of moderate physical activity or 75–150 min of vigorous activity each week (ACS, 2020b).
- Obtain adequate, consistent periods of rest (at least 6–8 h per night).
- Schedule regular health examinations that include a health history, physical examination, and specific diagnostic tests for common cancers in accordance with the guidelines published by the American Cancer Society (see Table 17.1).
- Eliminate, reduce, or change the perceptions of stressors, and enhance the ability to cope effectively with stressors.
- Enjoy consistent periods of relaxation and leisure.
- Identify the eight warning signs of cancer (see Box 17.1).
- Seek immediate medical care if you notice a change in what is normal for you and if cancer is suspected. Early detection of cancer has a positive effect on prognosis.

rates of survival among patients with cancer (see the Health Promotion box).

A woman needs to become familiar with the appearance and feel of her breasts. This will help her identify any change in her breast tissue. Any abnormality—such as discharge from the nipples; puckering, dimpling, peau d'orange (skin appearance of an orange peel (Fig. 17.2), or scaling of the skin; and the palpation of a lump or thickness—is significant. Any delay is a waste of valuable time if cancer is present.

Teach boys, beginning at puberty, and men to check the scrotum for enlargement, thickening, and the presence of a lump in the testicles. This can be performed after a warm bath or shower. Emphasize that any changes from the normal, smooth consistency of the testes should be brought to the attention of a health care provider (see Chapter 12). Some clinical manifestations of testicular cancer include a lump in or enlargement of either testicle, a heavy feeling in the scrotum, dull aching in either the groin or the lower abdomen, fluid collection in the scrotum, and tenderness or enlargement of the breasts (this results from hormones produced by cancer cells) (ACS, 2018). The American Cancer Society currently has no recommendations for regular testicular self-exams because there are not enough studies about this topic to know whether they result in a reduction in the death rate.

Advise men older than 50 to discuss the prostate-specific antigen (PSA) test with their health care provider and whether they should undergo a rectal examination once a year. Populations at high risk for prostate cancer (African Americans and men who have positive family history for the disease) are urged to begin screening at ages 40 to 45 years. Blood in the urine, difficulty starting to urinate, a weak flow of urine, and other urination problems should be reported to the health care provider for evaluation.

PATHOPHYSIOLOGY OF CANCER

CELL MECHANISMS AND GROWTH

The basic unit of structure and function in all living things is the *cell*. The adult human body contains approximately 60,000 billion cells. Although there are many different types of cells, all of them have certain common characteristics. For example, all cells need nourishment to maintain life, and all cells use almost identical nutrients. All cells use oxygen, which combines with fat, protein, or carbohydrates to release the energy needed for cells to function. The mechanisms for changing nutrients into energy are generally the same in all cells, and all cells deliver their end product of chemical reactions into the nearby fluids.

Most cells are able to reproduce. When cells are destroyed, the remaining cells of the same type reproduce until the correct number has been replenished. This orderly replacement of cells is governed by a control mechanism that stops when the loss or damage has been corrected. Dynamic, active, and orderly, the healthy cell is a small powerhouse, laboratory, factory, and duplicating machine, copying itself over and over. The immune system aids in preventing the development of cancer by destroying the abnormal cells. On occasion, the immune system fails to recognize these abnormal cells, and cancer develops.

Cancer cells are not subject to the usual restrictions placed on cell proliferation by the host. When malignant cells change, they become unlike parent cells; they are not differentiated (recognizable as being the same in size or shape as normal cells). Cancer cells can divide and multiply, but not in a normal manner. Instead of limiting their growth to meet specific needs of the body, they continue to reproduce in a disorderly and unrestricted manner. The cellular features of cancer cells are a local increase in the number of cells, loss of normal cellular arrangement, variation in cell shape and size, increased nuclear size, increased miotic activity, and abnormal mitosis and chromosomes.

Proliferation is not always indicative of cancer, however. Abnormal cellular growth is classified as nonneoplastic growth and neoplastic growth. The four common nonneoplastic growth patterns are hypertrophy, hyperplasia, metaplasia, and dysplasia. Although not neoplastic conditions, these may precede the development of cancer. *Anaplasia* means "without form" and is an irreversible change in which the structures of adult cells regress to more primitive levels.

Neoplasm is a group of cells whose growth is uncontrolled or abnormal. Neoplasms may be benign (not recurrent or progressive; nonmalignant) or malignant (abnormal cell growths with a loss of normal role and function). Malignant neoplasms have the ability to spread to other body sites and resist treatment, as in cancerous growths (Table 17.2). Growths are also referred to as *tumors,* meaning "swelling" or "enlargement." Tumors may be localized or invasive. Benign tumors may become problematic because their increased size damages surrounding tissues, as in a benign brain tumor. Malignant neoplasms may progress and destroy surrounding tissues. They also may metastasize from the primary site of origin to distant sites.

Metastasis is the process by which tumor cells spread from the primary site to a secondary site. Once cancer cells have moved to another area of the body, secondary tumors may grow in that area. Metastasis can occur by (1) diffusion to other body cavities or (2) circulation via blood and lymphatic channels.

Table 17.2 General Characteristics of Neoplasms

BENIGN TUMORS	MALIGNANT TUMORS
Slow, steady growth	Rate of growth varies; usually rapid
Remains localized	Metastasizes
Usually contained within a capsule	Rarely contained within a capsule
Smooth, well defined; movable when palpated	Irregular; more immobile when palpated
Resembles parent tissue	Little resemblance to parent tissue
Crowds normal tissue	Invades normal tissue
Rarely recurs after removal	May recur after removal
Rarely fatal	Fatal without treatment

In addition to the identified carcinogenic factors that may cause malignant cellular changes, certain viruses have been suspected. Viruses linked to the development of cancers include human papillomavirus, Epstein-Barr virus (EBV), hepatitis B virus, hepatitis C virus, and HIV. There is also evidence to suggest that particular genetic factors result in a predisposition to the development of cancer (ACS, 2021d).

The body's immune system is responsible for recognizing and destroying malignant cells. The immune system may be weakened by cancer-producing substances, tumor cells, and the aging process. Some T cells are responsible for immunosurveillance (the immune system's recognition and destruction of newly developed abnormal cells). When a cell becomes malignant, its membranes carry a tumor-specific antigen that is recognized by the body as nonself and is destroyed. If T cell function is suppressed by age, drugs (e.g., corticosteroids), poor nutrition, alcohol, serious infections, or certain disease processes (e.g., neoplastic invasion of bone and lymph tissue), the risk of cancer increases. To suppress T cell rejection of a transplanted organ, steroids and other drugs are given. The resultant loss of immunosurveillance increases the risk of certain cancers.

DESCRIPTION, GRADING, AND STAGING OF TUMORS

Cancers are described according to the original site of the primary tumor. A carcinoma is a malignant tumor composed of epithelial cells, which tend to metastasize. Carcinomas originate from embryonal ectoderm (skin and glands) and endoderm (mucous membrane linings of the respiratory tract, gastrointestinal [GI] tract, and genitourinary tract). A sarcoma is a malignant tumor of connective tissues; sarcomas originate from embryonal mesoderm, such as muscle, bone, or fat, usually manifesting as a painless swelling. Sarcomas may affect bone, bladder, kidneys, liver, lungs, parotid glands, and the spleen. *Lymphomas* and *leukemias* originate from the hematopoietic system.

| Box 17.2 | TNM Cancer Staging Classification System |

T SUBCLASSES: PRIMARY TUMOR

T_x	Tumor cannot be adequately assessed
T_0	No evidence of primary tumor
T_{is}	Carcinoma in situ
T_1-T_4	Size and/or extent of the primary tumor

N SUBCLASSES: REGIONAL LYMPH NODES

N_x	Regional lymph nodes cannot be assessed
N_0	No regional lymph node metastasis
N_1–N_4	Degree of regional lymph node involvement (number and location of lymph nodes)

M SUBCLASSES: DISTANT METASTASIS

M_x	Distant metastasis cannot be evaluated
M_0	No distant metastasis
M_1-M_4	Distant metastasis present, specify site(s)

HISTOPATHOLOGY

G_x	Grade cannot be assessed (undetermined grade)
G_1	Well-differentiated grade (low grade)
G_2	Moderately differentiated (intermediate grade)
G_3	Poorly differentiated (high grade)
G_4	Undifferentiated (high grade)

From the National Cancer Institute. Cancer staging, 2015a. Retrieved from *https://www.cancer.gov/about-cancer/diagnosis-staging/staging*; and the National Cancer Institute. Tumor grade, 2013. Retrieved from *https://www.cancer.gov/about-cancer/diagnosis-staging/prognosis/tumor-grade-fact-sheet.*

A tumor may be named for its location, its cellular makeup, or the person by whom it was originally identified.

Grading of Tumors

Tumors are classified as grades 1 to 4 by the degree of malignancy. Grade 1 tumors are the most differentiated (most like the parent tissue) and the least malignant. Grade 4 tumors are the least differentiated (unlike parent tissue) tumor and the most malignant (Box 17.2).

Extent of Disease Classification

Classifying the extent and spread of disease is termed *staging.* This classification system is based on a description of the extent of the disease rather than on cell appearance. Although different types of cancer are staged similarly, there are many differences based on a thorough knowledge of the natural history of each specific type of cancer.

Clinical staging. The clinical staging classification system is used to determine the extent of the disease process of cancer by stages:

Stage 0: Cancer in situ

Stage I: Tumor limited to the tissue of origin; localized tumor growth
Stage II: Limited local spread
Stage III: Extensive local and regional spread
Stage IV: Metastasis

TNM classification system. The *TNM classification system* represents the standardization of the clinical staging of cancer. This classification system is used to determine the extent of the disease process of cancer according to three parameters: tumor size *(T),* degree of regional spread to the lymph nodes *(N),* and metastasis *(M)* (see Box 17.2). This system is used to direct treatment, predict prognosis, and contribute to cancer research by ensuring reliable comparison of different patients.

Bethesda system. Exfoliative (pertaining to the shedding of something) cytologic study (e.g., Papanicolaou's [Pap] test or smear) is a means of studying cells that the body has shed during the normal sequence of growth and replacement of body tissues. If cancer is present, cancer cells also are shed. The method is used most commonly to detect cancers of the cervix, but it may be used for tissue specimens from any organ.
- *Normal:* Inconclusive or ASC-US (atypical squamous cells of undetermined cause): Cells don't look normal.
- *Abnormal:* Cell changes most likely related to presence of human papilloma virus; may progress to cancer over a period of time; dysplasia
- *Low-grade squamous intraepithelial lesion (LSIL) or intraepithelial neoplasia (CIN):* Abnormal cells are found, but typically this issue resolves on its own.
- *High-grade squamous intraepithelial lesion (HSIL) or CIN2 or CIN3:* Moderately to severely abnormal cells; may indicate cancer is present (Johns Hopkins, n.d.)

DIAGNOSIS OF CANCER

BIOPSY

People who develop symptoms consistent with cancer should undergo diagnostic testing to confirm or rule out the diagnosis. The only definitive way to determine the presence of malignant cells is to perform a tissue biopsy (the removal of a small piece of living tissue from an organ or other part of the body for microscopic examination).

A biopsy is used to confirm or establish a diagnosis, establish prognosis, or follow the course of a disease. A variety of methods are used to perform a biopsy (Fig. 17.3). The *needle biopsy* is used to obtain fluid or to obtain tissue samples from the lesion. *Needle aspiration biopsy* is the aspiration of fluid or tissue by means of a needle (breast biopsy is performed with an aspiration needle). Transcutaneous needle aspiration biopsy has eliminated the need for most of the exploratory laparotomies for diagnosing metastatic cancer of the liver or for primary inoperable pancreatic cancer. Structures

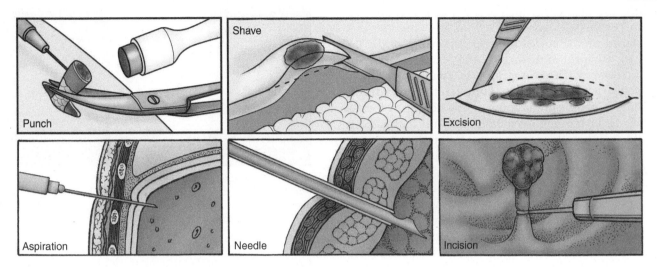

Fig. 17.3 Types of biopsy.

accessible to thin-needle biopsy under guidance of palpation include the breasts, skin, thyroid gland, prostate, palpable lymph nodes, and salivary glands. *Excisional biopsy* is the removal of the complete lesion, with little or no margin of surrounding normal tissue removed, as in polypectomy. Another example of excisional biopsy is the dissection of peripheral lymph nodes, such as those of the axilla for staging of breast cancer or those of the peritoneal region for staging of various abdominal cancers. *Incisional biopsy* is the removal of a portion of tissue for examination, such as the bite biopsy performed during endoscopy. *Skin biopsy* is used to assess suspect lesions of integument (e.g., shave biopsy, punch biopsy).

ENDOSCOPY

Cells or tissue also can be obtained by means of an *endoscope* to visualize an internal structure directly through a body cavity or a small incision. Endoscopes are rigid or flexible tubes containing a magnifying lens and a light. Endoscopes vary in diameter and length according to the structure being examined. The bronchoscope is used to visualize the tracheobronchial tree; upper GI endoscopy allows direct visualization of the upper GI tract (esophagus, stomach, duodenum); the colonoscope is used to visualize the entire colon; and the sigmoidoscope is used to examine the sigmoid colon, the rectum, and the anus.

DIAGNOSTIC IMAGING

Additional diagnostic studies may be used to determine the depth of the specific lesion and identify other structures that may have been invaded. These include radiography and scanning procedures. Commonly ordered radiographic studies are chest radiography, mammography, bone scanning, GI series, barium enema study, and intravenous pyelography.

Radioisotope Studies

Radioisotope studies require the injection or ingestion of a radioactive substance. A scanning device is then used to identify the distribution of the substance in different areas of the body. Concentration of the radioisotope in a specific organ, such as the thyroid gland or the brain, is indicative of a tumor in that location (it may be primary or metastatic).

Bone scanning is one type of radioisotope study. It involves several steps. Before the scan, a radioactive material is injected into a vein in the arm. The patient is encouraged to drink water over the next 1 to 3 hours to assist the kidneys in removing any radioisotope not picked up by the bone. Areas of concentrated uptake may represent a tumor or an abnormality. These areas of concentration can be detected days or weeks before an ordinary radiograph could reveal a lesion. Bone scanning is indicated to detect metastatic tumors that have spread into the bone. All malignancies capable of metastasis may reach the bone, especially malignancies of breasts, kidneys, lungs, prostate, thyroid gland, and urinary bladder.

Computed Tomography

In *computed tomography* (CT), radiographs and a computed scanning system are used to record images of specific structures at different angles. The entire body can be scanned to detect any abnormal lesion. CT is especially helpful in detecting small lesions that were missed on radiography or other types of diagnostic tests.

Ultrasonography

Ultrasonography is a noninvasive procedure in which high-frequency sound waves are used to examine internal structures. As a transducer is moved over the area being studied, an ultrasound beam is directed through the tissues and is then reflected back to the transducer. The sound waves are converted into electrical impulses, which produce an image on a display screen. Ultrasonography can show the size, consistency, and shape of the structure being studied. It is most helpful in distinguishing between cystic and solid tumors. Ultrasonography is not used to examine bones or air-filled organs. Although the procedure is painless, people undergoing ultrasonography feel the transducer moving over their skin and may need to hold their breath or remain still for brief periods.

Magnetic Resonance Imaging

Magnetic resonance imaging (MRI) is a painless diagnostic procedure that does not involve any exposure to radiation. The patient reclines on a narrow surface that moves into a cylindrical tunnel containing magnetic coils; radiofrequency energy waves produce signals that are processed by a computer and displayed as images on a video monitor. This test currently is used in the diagnosis of intracranial and spinal lesions and of cardiovascular and soft tissue abnormalities. The procedure also provides information about changes within the cells of soft tissues, arteries, veins, the brain, and the spinal column.

During the test, the patient must not have any metallic materials on the body, including jewelry. MRI cannot be performed on patients with metallic implants, such as a pacemaker, orthopedic nail, or aneurysm clip.

During the test, the patient can talk to the staff performing the test by means of a microphone placed inside the scanner tunnel. The patient will hear the sound waves thumping on the magnetic field and must lie still while the test is being done; it may take more than an hour to obtain the images needed.

Position Emission Tomography

Positron emission tomography (PET) is useful in many aspects of oncology. A radioactive chemical is given to the patient just before the procedure. PET can demonstrate glucose metabolism, oxygenation, blood flow, and tissue perfusion for any designated area. Alterations in the normal metabolic process in pathologic conditions are diagnosed during PET (Cancer.net, 2020c).

PET is useful for visualizing fast-growing tumors and specifying their anatomic location. PET also helps note tumor response to therapeutic intervention, helps identify a recurrence of a tumor after surgical intervention, and assists in differentiating a tumor from other abnormal conditions such as an infection. PET is extremely useful in visualizing regional and metastatic extension of a specific tumor. Oncologic staging is more accurate with PET than with CT. The CT scan is used to take detailed images of organs and tissues within the patient's body, whereas the PET scan can be used to identify abnormal activities. PET also is used to determine the specific site for performing a biopsy of a suspected tumor (Mayo Clinic, 2020b) (Fig. 17.4).

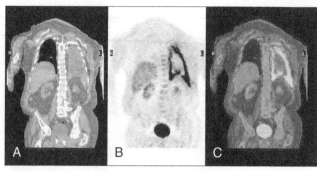

Fig. 17.4 Tomographic scans. (A) Computed tomography (CT). (B) Positron emission tomography (PET). (C) Combined CT and PET. (From Christian PE, Waterstram-Rich *KM: Nuclear medicine and PET/CT: Technology and techniques*, ed 7, St. Louis, 2012, Mosby.)

LABORATORY AND DIAGNOSTIC EXAMINATIONS

Measurement of Alkaline Phosphatase Blood Levels

The level of alkaline phosphatase is elevated in the presence of liver disease or metastasis to the bone or liver.

Serum Calcitonin Level

Calcitonin is a hormone secreted by the thyroid gland in response to a rise in serum calcium level. The level is increased in the blood of people who have cancer of the thyroid. It may be elevated with breast cancer and oat cell cancer of the lung. Calcitonin stimulation testing may be used in addition to the baseline level testing to confirm a diagnosis. Instruct the patient not to eat or drink anything the night before the test.

Carcinoembryonic Antigen Serum Level

Normally, production of carcinoembryonic antigen (CEA) stops before birth, but it may begin again if a neoplasm develops. Results of this test cannot be used as a general indicator of cancer because CEA level can be elevated for other reasons, such as smoking cigarettes or the presence of inflammation. CEA is found in increased amounts in the blood of people with colorectal cancer. The test may assist in the evaluation of cancer treatment, in which a rising CEA level may indicate tumor recurrence or metastatic disease. This test is used less frequently today because it is less accurate than was thought previously.

Tumor Markers

Several different tumor markers may be identified with laboratory studies of blood or urine to help with cancer screening and diagnosis. Tumor markers are substances that are present in the body when the patient has cancer. Three examples are the PSA for prostate cancer, CA-125 for ovarian cancer, and CA-19-9 for pancreatic or hepatobiliary cancer.

PSA is a biological marker, specific for cellular activity in the prostate gland. PSA is the only tumor marker for prostate cancer. The American Cancer Society suggests that men discuss this test with their physician.

Not all men should be screened routinely for this tumor marker. Men with a high risk of developing prostate cancer (family history, African American) should speak with their health care provider about this test beginning as early as the age of 40.

Although PSA levels usually are elevated when cancer is present, PSA level alone is not diagnostic of prostate cancer. Other common conditions, such as benign enlargement of the prostate, also can elevate PSA level. The finding of elevated PSA level necessitates further evaluation to determine the cause of increase. This may involve transrectal ultrasonography of the prostate gland.

The PSA assay requires a physician's interpretation. No specific level of PSA signals the presence or absence of prostate cancer. The PSA test is produced by different manufacturers, and the different products yield different results. In men with benign prostatic enlargement, levels defined as normal are different from those in men with normal prostate glands.

CA-125 is a cancer antigen detected in the blood and peritoneal ascites. The normal level is 35 units/mL. The CA-125 level may be elevated in patients with gynecologic cancers (including ovarian cancer) and cancer of the pancreas. A monoclonal antibody has been developed that reacts with this antigen, which gives physicians a method to measure the amount of CA-125 in blood samples. This test is used mainly to signal a recurrence of ovarian cancer. It is not a way to detect primary ovarian cancer, because other conditions (e.g., endometriosis, hepatitis, pelvic inflammatory diseases, or pregnancy) also may increase CA-125 levels in the blood.

CA-19-9 antigen, a tumor marker, is used in the diagnosis, monitoring, and surveillance of patients with pancreatic or hepatobiliary cancer. The CA-19-9 level is elevated in 70% of patients with pancreatic cancer and 65% of patients with hepatobiliary cancer. Measurement of CA-19-9 is not an effective screening tool for pancreatic or biliary tumors in the general population because of its lack of sensitivity and specificity (Pancreatic Cancer Action Network, n.d.). The following is a more comprehensive list of various tumor markers and how to interpret results of these tests (Vachani, 2020).

TUMOR MARKER	CANCERS ASSOCIATED WITH ELEVATED RESULTS	NONCANCEROUS REASONS FOR ELEVATED LEVELS	"NORMAL" RESULTS
Blood test (blood serum marker), except where noted	[a] indicates the most common association, if one exists		Different labs may have different high/low values
AFP Alpha-fetoprotein	Germ cell cancers of ovaries and testes[a] (nonseminomatous, particularly embryonal and yolk sac, testicular cancers) Some primary liver cancers (hepatocellular)	Pregnancy (clears after birth), liver disease (hepatitis, cirrhosis, toxic liver injury), inflammatory bowel disease	Low levels present in men and nonpregnant women (0–15 IU/mL); generally results >400 are caused by cancer (half-life 4–6 days)
Bence-Jones Proteins (urine test) or Monoclonal Immunoglobulins (blood test)	Multiple myeloma,[a] Waldenstrom macroglobulinemia, chronic lymphocytic leukemia	Amyloidosis	Generally, a value of 0.03–0.05 mg/mL is significant for early disease
B2M Beta-2-Microglobulin	Multiple myeloma,[a] chronic lymphocytic leukemia (CLL), and some lymphomas (including Waldenstrom macroglobulinemia)	Kidney disease, hepatitis	<2.5 mg/L
BTA Bladder tumor antigen (urine test)	Bladder cancer,[a] cancer of kidney or ureters	Invasive procedure or infection of bladder or urinary tract	None normally detected
CA 15-3 Cancer antigen 15-3 or carbohydrate antigen 15-3	Breast[a] (often not elevated in early stages of breast cancer), lung, ovarian, endometrial, bladder, gastrointestinal	Liver disease (cirrhosis, hepatitis), lupus, sarcoid, tuberculosis, noncancerous breast lesions	<31 U/mL (30% of patients have an elevated CA 15-3 for 30–90 days after treatment, so wait 2–3 months after starting new treatment to check)
CA 19-9 Cancer antigen 19-9 or carbohydrate antigen 19-9	Pancreas[a] and colorectal, liver, stomach and biliary tree cancers	Pancreatitis, ulcerative colitis, inflammatory bowel disease, inflammation or blockage of the bile duct, thyroid disease, rheumatic arthritis	<37 U/mL is normal >120 U/mL is generally caused by tumor

TUMOR MARKER	CANCERS ASSOCIATED WITH ELEVATED RESULTS	NONCANCEROUS REASONS FOR ELEVATED LEVELS	"NORMAL" RESULTS
CA 125 Cancer antigen 125 or carbohydrate antigen 125	Ovarian cancer,[a] breast, colorectal, uterine, cervical, pancreas, liver, lung	Pregnancy, menstruation, endometriosis, ovarian cysts, fibroids, pelvic inflammatory disease, pancreatitis, cirrhosis, hepatitis, peritonitis, pleural effusion, after surgery or paracentesis	0–35 U/mL
CA 27.29 Cancer antigen 27.29 or carbohydrate antigen 27.29	Breast[a] (best used to detect recurrence or metastasis) Colon, gastric, liver, lung, pancreatic, ovarian, prostate cancers	Ovarian cysts, liver and kidney disorders, noncancerous (benign) breast problems	<40 U/mL Generally, levels >100 U/mL signify cancer (30% of patients have elevated CA 27.29 for 30–90 days after treatment, so wait 2–3 months after starting new treatment to check)
Calcitonin	Medullary thyroid cancer[a]	Chronic renal insufficiency, chronic use of proton-pump inhibitors (medications given to reduce stomach acid)	<8.5 pg/mL for men <5.0 pg/mL for women
CEA Carcinoembryonic antigen	Colorectal cancers,[a] breast, lung, gastric, pancreatic, bladder, kidney, thyroid, head and neck, cervical, ovarian, liver, lymphoma, melanoma	Cigarette smoking, pancreatitis, hepatitis, inflammatory bowel disease, peptic ulcer disease, hypothyroidism, cirrhosis, COPD, biliary obstruction	<2.5 ng/mL in nonsmokers <5 ng/mL in smokers Generally, >100 signifies metastatic cancer
Chromogranin A	Neuroendocrine tumors,[a] carcinoid tumors, neuroblastoma, and small cell lung cancer	Proton-pump inhibitors (medications given to reduce stomach acid)	Normal varies on how tested, but typically <39 ng/L is normal
Cytokeratin fragment 21-1 (blood test)	Lung, urologic, gastrointestinal, and gynecologic cancers	Lung disease	0.05–2.90 ng/mL
HCG Human chorionic gonadotrophin or beta-HCG (B-HCG)	Germ cell, testicular cancers,[a] gestational trophoblastic neoplasia	Pregnancy, marijuana use, hypogonadism (testicular failure), cirrhosis, inflammatory bowel disease, duodenal ulcers	In men: <2.5 U/mL In nonpregnant women: <5.0 U/mL
5-HIAA 5-Hydroxy-indol acetic acid (24-h urine collection)	Carcinoid tumors	Celiac and tropical sprue, Whipple's disease, dietary: walnuts, pecans, bananas, avocados, eggplants, pineapples, plums, and tomatoes; medications: acetaminophen, aspirin, and guaifenesin	Normal 6–10 mg over 24 h
LDH Lactic dehydrogenase	Lymphoma, melanoma, acute leukemia, seminoma (germ cell tumors)	Hepatitis, MI (heart attack), stroke, anemia (pernicious and thalassemia), muscular dystrophy, certain medications (narcotics, aspirin, anesthetics, alcohol), muscle injury	Normal values are 100–333 U/L
NSE Neuron-specific enolase	Small cell lung cancer,[a] neuroblastoma	Proton-pump inhibitor treatment, hemolytic anemia, hepatic failure, end stage renal failure, brain injury, seizure, stroke	Normal <9 ug/L
NMP 22 (urine test)	Bladder cancer[a]	BPH (benign prostatic hypertrophy), prostatitis	Normal <10 U/mL
PAP Prostatic acid phosphatase	Metastatic prostate cancer[a] Myeloma, lung cancer, osteogenic sarcoma	Prostatitis, Gaucher's disease, osteoporosis, cirrhosis, hyperparathyroidism, prostatic hypertrophy	Normal: 0.5–1.9 U/L

TUMOR MARKER	CANCERS ASSOCIATED WITH ELEVATED RESULTS	NONCANCEROUS REASONS FOR ELEVATED LEVELS	"NORMAL" RESULTS
PSA Prostate-specific antigen	Prostate[a]	BPH (benign prostatic hypertrophy), nodular prostatic hyperplasia, prostatitis, prostate trauma/inflammation, ejaculation	Normal <4 ng/mL (half-life 2–3 days)
Tg Thyroglobulin	Thyroid cancer	Antithyroglobulin antibodies	<33 ng/mL; if entire thyroid removed <2 ng/mL
Urine catecholamines: **VMA** Vanillylmandelic acid (24-h collection of urine; it is a catecholamine metabolite)	Neuroblastoma,[a] pheochromocytoma, ganglioneuroma, rhabdomyosarcoma, PNET	Dietary intake (bananas, vanilla, tea, coffee, ice cream, chocolate), medications (tetracyclines, methyldopa, MAOIs)	8–35 mmols over 24 h
HVA Homovanillic acid (24-h collection of urine; it is a catecholamine metabolite)	Neuroblastoma[a]	Same as VMA, in addition: psychosis, major depression, dopamine (a medication)	Up to 40 mmols over 24 h

PNET, primitive neuroectodermal tumors.

Stool Examination for Occult Blood

The cause of blood in the stool must be identified to rule out the possibility of cancer. The *guaiac test* is used commonly to detect occult (hidden) blood in the stools. Other commonly used tests for occult blood in the stool are fecal occult blood test (FOBT), *fecal immunochemical test, hematest*, and *hemoccult test.* Early detection self-tests are available for home use. If blood is found, the person should seek immediate medical attention. Before these types of tests, it is essential that the person not ingest red meat, horseradish, uncooked broccoli, turnips, melons, aspirin, or vitamin C for 4 days before the test because this may result in a false-positive result. The test must be performed on three consecutive bowel movements. Urge patients to follow through with diagnostic tests recommended by their health care provider to screen for cancer.

CANCER THERAPIES

SURGERY

By the time it is decided that surgery is needed to remove a cancerous lesion, cancer cells already may have spread to other areas. The goal of surgery is to remove all malignant cells; this may include removal of the tumor, surrounding tissue, and regional lymph nodes. The combination of surgery with chemotherapy, radiation therapy, or both may destroy a higher number of cancer cells. The effects of cancer drugs and radiation treatments administered before, during, and after surgery are being investigated. A surgical cure may result from removal of an isolated lesion in the very early stages, as in cancer of the skin, testicle, breast, or cervix. Surgery may be performed for many reasons: preventive, diagnostic, curative, and palliative (designed to relieve uncomfortable symptoms but not to produce a cure).

Polyps in the colon may be removed during a colonoscopy before malignant changes occur. A prophylactic mastectomy may be performed to help prevent the development of breast cancer in patients identified to be at increased risk because of their family history or other factors. If a cancerous lesion has metastasized already, surgery may provide palliation by relieving some of the associated problems, such as obstruction, ulceration, hemorrhage, and pain. The pituitary, adrenal glands, ovaries, or testes may be removed surgically to help control the growth and spread of malignancies caused by hormonal stimulation.

A radical surgical approach to operable tumors is no longer routinely used because of more sensitive and accurate diagnosing methods, a greater variety of surgical procedures, more sophisticated staging techniques, and more available advanced treatment options. The more conservative surgical management of breast cancer (i.e., lumpectomy instead of total mastectomy) is one example of this trend.

Reconstructive surgery may be needed after some types of resection, such as modified radical mastectomy. Breast reconstruction is an option for women whose disease and treatment enable the surgeon to implant a prosthesis or to transplant tissue from other areas of the body to recreate a more natural-looking breast. In many cases, the oncology surgeon and the plastic surgeon work together. When this is anticipated, preoperative counseling by the surgeons and the nurse helps the patient consider the long-range outcome instead of the immediate surgical procedure.

Communication

Nurse-Patient Therapeutic Dialogue Before Modified Radical Mastectomy

Nurse: Good afternoon, Mrs. S. My name is J., and I will be your nurse this evening. How are you feeling? [Introduction and general lead]

Patient: I'm feeling all right now. It's tomorrow I'm dreading.

Nurse: You're dreading tomorrow? [Restatement]

Patient: Yes. My doctor told me he has to remove my entire breast. I hate thinking that I'll look so different.

Nurse: You're anxious about the fact that you won't look the same. [Reflection]

Patient: I'll be embarrassed to undress in front of my husband. He may think I'm no longer attractive.

Nurse: Have you had a chance to discuss your feelings with your husband? [Clarification]

Patient: No, he's out of town but will be back tonight. I guess I could talk to him then. Maybe he will accept it better than I think.

Nurse: We'll talk more after you've had a chance to talk to him about your feelings. Is there anything else on your mind that you'd like to talk about now? [Showing acceptance and general lead]

The use of laser beams as an alternative to some types of oncologic surgical procedures is increasing. The laser beam destroys tissue with little bleeding and low risk of infection. Laser surgery is used more commonly in the fields of ophthalmology, gynecology, urology, neurosurgery, and otolaryngology. The chief drawback with laser surgery is that the patient must lie very still while the laser is in use.

Nursing Interventions

If the LPN/ LVN is not present when the health care provider explains recommendations for care, then the nurse should ask the health care provider what he or she has told the patient and the family. This is essential to be able to reinforce the information given. Patients and families are usually anxious and may not remember everything that the health care provider has explained for them.

Patients should have confidence and trust in the health care professionals who are responsible for their care. Positive feelings and attitudes promote relaxation and help reduce anxiety and fear (see the Communication box). The patient should be encouraged to ask the health care provider any questions concerning potential risks of a given treatment. A patient needs to feel comfortable with the decision to follow through with the physician's recommendations.

The following are nursing guidelines to ensure that patients have the information needed to make an informed decision:

- Be present when the patient and health care provider are discussing treatment decisions.
- Assess the patient's progression in grieving for the loss of health and function related to the cancer diagnosis.

- If necessary, clarify explanations of treatments, including benefits and side effects, and help the patient formulate questions and voice concerns. Address patient or family concerns and questions concerning alternative treatments.
- Afterward, talk to the patient and the family about the information the health care provider presented; assess their understanding of the treatment and identify their goals and needs.
- Report any misunderstandings, unrealistic expectations, or other problems to the health care provider.
- Communicate with the patient to verify that his or her questions were answered.
- Accept and support the patient's choice, regardless of personal opinion.

Preparing the patient for a surgical procedure must include an explanation of what to expect postoperatively. Preoperative teaching is discussed in Chapter 2.

Regardless of the surgical procedure, assess the patient's nutritional status before and after surgery. Nutritional status has been found to be a significant factor in the amount of surgery that can be tolerated, the rate of recovery, the patient's role performance, and the adequacy of wound healing.

When surgery may produce a change in the patient's body image, as in mastectomy, laryngectomy, or the formation of an ostomy, the patient may benefit from talking with another person who has undergone the same type of surgery. The American Cancer Society sponsors support groups and prepares volunteers to visit patients who need these types of surgical procedures. Some of the special groups available in some communities are Reach to Recovery; the Lost Chord Club; I Can Cope; Look Good, Feel Good; and local chapters of the United Ostomy Associations of America.

RADIATION THERAPY

Radiation therapy can be used to cure or control cancer that has spread to local lymph nodes or to treat tumors that cannot be removed surgically. Radiation may be used preoperatively to reduce the size of a tumor. Postoperative radiation therapy may be indicated to destroy malignant cells not removed by surgery. Radiation also may be used to slow the growth of malignant tumors.

Radiation may be delivered externally or internally. External therapy may be directed toward superficial lesions or toward deeper structures within the body. Malignant cells lack the capacity for repair, so more cancer cells than normal cells are damaged by radiation and normal cells are able to recover more easily. However, normal cells can tolerate radiation only up to a certain amount before irreversible damage occurs. Treatment plans are designed to minimize the radiation dose to normal structures. Meticulous planning and recording of the doses are essential.

External Radiation Therapy

Radiation therapy is associated with skin damage and burning. Skin atrophy, changes in pigmentation, and chronic dermatitis may result. Frequent assessment and monitoring of the skin's condition are needed. When external radiation is planned, the specific area on the body is marked to indicate the port at which external radiation will be directed. These markings must not be washed off. Patients may be distressed about the presence of these markings. In a nonjudgmental manner, allow the patient the time to discuss these feelings. Management of the skin area marked for radiation should include the following:

- Keep the skin dry. If the area becomes wet during bathing, pat the skin dry with an absorbent towel.
- Do not apply lotions, ointments, creams, or powders in marked areas. Any lotions or creams designed specifically to manage drying skin must be prescribed by the physician.
- Protect the radiated area from direct sunlight.
- Avoid applications of heat or cold, because these would increase erythema, drying, and pruritus of the skin, which is common over an irradiated area.

Maintaining health during the treatment phase is important. Dietary interventions should focus on the ingestion of foods high in protein and calories. This helps promote healing and tissue regeneration. Fluid intake to maintain hydration is needed. The patient is encouraged to drink 2 to 3 L of fluid per day, unless this is contraindicated. In the event that the patient experiences severe anorexia or is unable to tolerate food and fluid intake, the health care provider should be notified to evaluate dietary needs and prescribe accordingly. Reassure the patient undergoing radiation therapy that lethargy and fatigue are common during treatment and that frequent rest periods are helpful.

Many people with cancer are treated with radiation therapy at some point. Sometimes, radiation therapy is the only therapy needed to destroy the cancer.

Internal Radiation Therapy

Treatment with a radioactive implant (brachytherapy) is the insertion of *sealed radioactive materials* temporarily or permanently into hollow cavities, within body tissues, or on the body's surface. The radioactive source delivers a specific radiation dose continuously over hours or days. A highly concentrated radiation dose is delivered into or near a tumor. This technique generally is combined with a course of external radiation therapy to increase the dosage to a specific site. Certain organs, such as the uterus and vagina, are natural receptacles for the placement of an applicator that can be loaded with radioactive material. Radioactive needles, wires, seeds, beads, or catheters may be inserted directly into tumor tissue.

Unsealed internal radiation is administered intravenously or orally so that it is distributed throughout the patient's body. Special precautions are needed to prevent exposure to the nurse of the sources of radiation during periods of patient care or disposal of care-related items (Box 17.3). Assemble materials needed to provide care. Provide several nursing interventions at the same time when entering the patient's room. Stand as far away as possible from the site where an internal radiation device is in the patient's body. In addition, limit the time needed for close contact near the irradiated site. If direct, prolonged care is needed, wear a lead apron.

Children younger than 18 years and pregnant women should not be allowed to visit implant recipients. Periods of visitation are limited to 10 minutes. Visitors are asked to stand as far away from the patient as possible.

When cancer of the cervix is treated with the use of an applicator containing a radioactive material, the applicator is placed in the vagina. The following special nursing measures are indicated:

1. Place "Radiation in Use" sign on the patient's door.
2. Prevent dislodgment. Keep the patient on strict bed rest. Instruct the patient not to turn from side to side or onto the abdomen. Do not raise the head of the bed more than 45 degrees.
3. Do not give a complete bed bath while the applicator is in place, and do not bathe the patient below the waist. Do not change bed linen unless it is necessary.
4. Encourage the patient to do active range-of-motion (ROM) exercises with both arms and mild foot and leg exercises to minimize the complications that can result from immobility. The patient also wears antiembolism stockings (thromboembolic disease hose) or pneumatic compression boots to prevent stasis of blood in the lower extremities.
5. Monitor vital signs every 4 hours, and be alert for elevations in temperature, pulse, and respirations. A temperature higher than 100°F (37.7°C) should be reported to the patient's health care provider.
6. Assess for and report any rash or skin eruption, excessive vaginal bleeding, or vaginal discharge.
7. Maintain an accurate intake and output record. Encourage the patient to consume at least 3 L of fluid intake daily. An indwelling urinary catheter is placed to reduce the size of the bladder and decrease the effects of radiation on the bladder. Monitor patency of catheter. Ensure that it continues to drain well.
8. Monitor the patient's dietary intake. Encourage low-residue selections to minimize peristalsis and bowel movement, which may lead to dislodgment of the applicator.
9. Check the position of the applicator every 4 hours.
10. Keep long-handled forceps and a special lead container in the patient's room for use by the radiologist, should the implant become dislodged. If an applicator or any other materials become dislodged or fall out of the patient, never touch them because the material may be radioactive. Any bed linens, dressings, or pads that have been changed for the patient must be checked with a radiation safety officer before they are removed from the patient's room.

11. After the applicator is removed, the indwelling catheter usually is removed, and a douche and enema commonly are prescribed.

12. Precautions are no longer needed after removal of the applicator. Encourage the patient to ambulate and gradually resume activities.

13. Sexual intercourse is usually delayed for 7 to 10 days.

14. Instruct the patient to notify the health care provider of nausea, vomiting, diarrhea, frequent or painful urination, or a temperature higher than 100°F (37.7°C).

Box 17.3	Instructions for Nursing Interventions for Patients Treated With Unsealed Internal Radiation for Thyroid Cancer

Spend as little time as possible for ordinary nursing care. The patient must be as self-sufficient as possible. The patient is radioactive and exposes the nurse to radiation while caring for the patient. The radioactive iodine-131 ($_{131}$I) leaves the patient through urine and perspiration. Therefore, the patient contaminates everything he or she touches and can spread contamination to the nurse in this way.

PRECAUTIONS TO REDUCE EXPOSURE TO MEMBERS OF THE HEALTH CARE TEAM

1. Assign patient to a private room.
2. Limit the time spent in the patient's room. Work quickly and enter only as necessary.
3. When in the room, maintain as much distance from the patient as possible. A few feet of distance makes a lot of difference in the amount of exposure to the nurse.
4. Wear personal protective equipment as indicated by the radiation safety officer (RSO).
5. Wear dosimeter when in patient room.
6. The patient is confined to the room.
7. Removal of trash, linen, and equipment from the room must be approved by the RSO.
8. Pregnant and breast-feeding personnel will not enter the area.
9. All clothes and bed linens used by the patient should be placed in the laundry bag provided and should be left in the patient's room.
10. No housekeeping staff is allowed until the room is officially released.
11. Food is delivered only by nursing staff. It is delivered to the door and picked up by the patient. Mail, flowers, and other items are delivered in the same way.
12. Whenever possible, only disposable items may be used in the care of these patients. These items should be placed in the designated waste container. Contact the RSO/designee for proper disposal of the contents of the designated waste container.
13. If a nurse, attendant, or anyone else knows or suspects that his or her skin or clothing (including shoes) is contaminated, that person should notify the RSO/designee immediately.

Policies may vary depending upon dosage and patient condition. Review individual facility policy and procedures for specifics concerning patient and environmental management.

CHEMOTHERAPY

Chemotherapy drugs are used to reduce the size or slow the growth of cancer. Most chemotherapeutic agents work by interfering with the cells' *replication* process (ability to multiply or reproduce). These drugs damage the cell and cause cellular death. Malignant and normal cells are affected by chemotherapy. Cells that multiply rapidly, such as cells of the *hematopoietic system, hair follicles,* and *GI system,* are affected the most. The majority of the side effects from chemotherapeutic agents result from the destruction of normal cells in these systems. Common manifestations include alopecia, nausea, and vomiting. The damage to tissue is not limited to the cancerous cells, and nephrotoxicity is a common adverse effect of the therapies.

Neurologic System

Chemo brain. Chemo brain is a mental fog or cloudiness that affects some patients in their cancer journey. It may occur during or after cancer treatment. It may be referred to as "cancer treatment-related cognitive impairment, cancer-related cognitive change, or post chemotherapy cognitive change" (ACS, 2020f). Some patients experience these mental changes for a short period of time and others experience this for years after treatment. Patients with chemo brain commonly have difficulty remembering things and experience poor concentration, slowed and disorganized thinking, and difficulty remembering common words. The condition can be worsened by the cancer itself, other types of medications used to treat the patient (such as antiemetics, steroids, and pain medications), depression, poor nutrition, hormone changes, anxiety, surgery, infections, stress, alcohol abuse, insomnia, advancing age, and anemia (ACS, 2020f).

Patients with chemo brain should be encouraged to use daily planners to help them remember appointments and schedules. When participating in care appointments, patients may require the attendance of a friend or family member to ensure that they have someone to help recall information afterward. Physical activity and mental puzzles can help. These patients should consume a nutritious diet, increase their intake of vegetables, try to get enough sleep, establish routines, and avoid attempting to multitask. Research studies are currently being performed to help prevent and protect the brain during chemotherapy (ACS, 2020f).

Hematopoietic System

Leukopenia. Leukopenia (reduction in the number of circulating white blood cells [WBCs] as a result of depression of the bone marrow) is a common problem for patients receiving chemotherapy. It can lead to life-threatening infections. The normal number of WBCs ranges from 5000/mm³ to 10,000/mm³. A patient with a total WBC count of less than 4000/mm³ is considered to be leukopenic. Lack of neutrophils, the type of WBC most often found to be suppressed in the differential WBC count, is called *neutropenia.* The normal number of neutrophils ranges from 60%

to 70%, or 3000/mm^3 to 7000/mm^3. When the neutrophil count is less than 1000/mm^3, neutropenia is considered to be present, and when the count is less than 500/mm^3, neutropenia is severe. A patient with neutropenia should be placed on neutropenic precautions, which sometimes is referred to as *protective precautions* or *reverse isolation*. Without enough neutrophils, the body's first line of defense collapses, paving the way for the development of pneumonia, septicemia, or other potentially overwhelming infections.

Protect the patient from pathogens, monitor the patient for signs of infection, and react quickly if an infection occurs. The patient's vital signs should be monitored every 4 hours. Notify the health care provider if the patient's temperature is elevated. A temperature of 100.4°F (38°C) or higher is considered a possible sign of infection (see the Safety Alert box).

Use the following systematic approach to assess the patient for infection.

Assessing the mouth. Stomatitis (inflammation of the oral mucosa) is one of the most common complications of chemotherapy and can lead to severe swallowing problems and systemic infections (Fig. 17.5). To assess for the presence of lesions, ulcers, or white plaque, a penlight and tongue blade may be used. Stomatitis may develop 5 to 14 days after chemotherapy and resolve after the end of treatments (Cancer.net, 2019).

Teaching the patient the importance of performing regular but gentle mouth care is important. Discuss the signs and symptoms of mouth infection, encourage the use of a soft toothbrush, and have the patient rinse the mouth with normal saline or sodium bicarbonate solution every 2 to 4 hours. A sponge-tipped applicator (Toothette) may help prevent the patient's gums from bleeding during or after mouth care.

To reduce the risk of an oral *Candida* infection, the health care provider may prescribe prophylactic antifungal medications such as an oral nystatin (Mycostatin) suspension, clotrimazole (Lotrimin) lozenges, or fluconazole (Diflucan). A bland soft or liquid diet also may be ordered.

Assessing the skin. A rash or eruption may indicate that the patient has an infection or is predisposed to one. Bacteria may flourish in skinfolds, such as those in the groin and axillae; ensure that these areas are cleaned twice a day with soap and water. Water-soluble moisturizers may be used to keep the patient's skin from drying. To prevent cuts, advise the patient to shave with an electric razor.

Vascular access sites are common portals of entry for infectious organisms. The sites of central and peripheral intravenous catheters must be monitored carefully. Check routinely for the presence of edema, drainage, erythema, or pain around catheter entry sites. Organisms also can grow along catheter tracts and infect the blood, resulting in septicemia. Signs and symptoms of a central line-associated infection in the

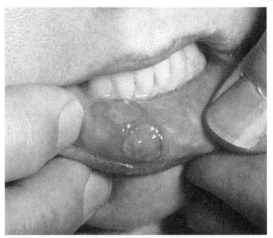

Fig. 17.5 Stomatitis. (Copyright Centers for Disease Control and Prevention/Robert E. Sumpter.)

⚠ Safety Alert

Neutropenic Precautions

- Monitor neutrophil count to identify signs of infection.
- Assess for presence of chills. Measure vital signs every 4 hours because fever may be the only indication of infection and septic shock.
- Report temperature elevations of more than 100.4°F (38°C) to the health care provider immediately so that antibiotic therapy can be initiated promptly to help avoid the rapidly lethal effects of infection.
- Ensure good hand hygiene techniques are used by all people in contact with patient, place patient in private room, and limit or screen visitors and hospital staff members with colds or potentially communicable illnesses to prevent transmission of pathogens to patient.
- Teach patient and family necessary personal hygiene techniques (e.g., hand hygiene, oral care, skin hygiene, pulmonary hygiene, and potential infection risks).
- Avoid invasive procedures (e.g., venipuncture, urinary catheter) as much as possible.
- Administer hematopoietic growth factors (e.g., granulocyte colony-stimulating factors such as filgrastim [Neupogen] or pegfilgrastim [Neulasta]) to increase patient's WBC count and reduce infection risk during periods of neutropenia. Provide neutropenic diet (avoid fresh fruits and vegetables because of presence of microscopic pathogens in uncooked produce). The patient's visitors should be discouraged from bringing fresh flowers or live plants to the patient's room. Mites, gnats, and other microscopic organisms could be a potential source of infection for the patient.

---

bloodstream include tenderness around the catheter site and pain.

Drugs should be administered orally whenever possible. Subcutaneous or intramuscular injections should be limited because they may cause abscesses in patients with neutropenia. These patients are also at risk for excessive bleeding because of the potential for an associated decrease in platelets and other formed elements in the blood.

Puncturing the skin is sometimes unavoidable, as when the patient needs a bone marrow biopsy. After a biopsy, carefully assess the site, clean the site with a facility-approved antiseptic, and apply a dressing over the site until the skin heals.

Assessing pulmonary function. Neutropenic patients with lung infections do not exhibit common clinical manifestations, such as sputum production or infiltrates demonstrable on chest radiographs. Assess the patient for other indications of a possible infection, such as changes in breath sounds, elevated respiratory rate and rhythm, and labored breathing. The patient also may complain of pain during inspiration or expiration.

To help prevent the patient from developing a lung infection, encourage the patient to perform deep-breathing and coughing exercises and to be as active as possible. Use of an incentive spirometer can help by maximizing ventilatory capacity.

Assessing urinary and bowel function. Changes in a neutropenic patient's urinary function are another indicator that the patient has developed an infection. Assess for decreased urinary output, changes in the odor or color of the urine, hematuria, or glycosuria. The patient also may complain of urinary frequency, urgency, or pain.

To reduce the risk of urinary tract infection, urinary catheterizations should be avoided in neutropenic patients. If catheterization is indicated absolutely, follow strict aseptic technique when inserting the catheter and must perform catheter care according to the facility's guidelines.

Assess the patient's bowel function. Chemotherapy can produce diarrhea or constipation. Characteristics of the stool include color, consistency, and the presence of blood. Dates of bowel movements should be recorded. The patient is instructed to report any changes in bowel habits.

If the patient needs to strain when defecating, the health care provider may prescribe a stool softener such as docusate (Colace). Straining can cause ulcerations or fissures in the rectum, which creates ports of entry for bacteria. Avoid the use of enemas, rectal medications, and rectal thermometers. They can abrade the mucosal lining, creating an entrance for pathogens. Neutropenia also predisposes patients to rectal abscesses. If the patient complains of perirectal pain, notify the health care provider immediately.

Medical management. Colony-stimulating factors (CSFs) have been very helpful when treating patients with neutropenia. CSFs are commercially made and are the only therapy that can prevent and manage neutropenia. CSFs are given subcutaneously or intravenously. Although CSFs are extremely expensive, they are administered prophylactically to patients at increased risk for neutropenia, such as those with a history of developing severe or prolonged neutropenia after chemotherapy.

Anemia. Anemia is a reduction in the number of circulating red blood cells (RBCs), hemoglobin, or hematocrit as a result of depression of the bone marrow. Normal values are as follows:

TYPE	MALE	FEMALE
Erythrocytes (RBCs)	4.7–6.1 million/mm^3	4.2–5.4 million/mm^3
Hemoglobin	14–18 g/dL	12–16 g/dL
Hematocrit	42%–52%	37%–47%

Hemoglobin levels of 10 to 14 g/dL indicate mild anemia, levels of 6 to 10 g/dL indicate moderate anemia, and levels lower than 6 g/dL indicate severe anemia. Patients with anemia often experience fatigue because of the decreased oxygenation to tissues. The plan of care should include a balance of activities to promote rest and prevent increased oxygen expenditure and hypoxemia. Such patients at home need to plan activities of daily living (ADLs) to allow for rest periods.

Recombinant human erythropoietin, or epoetin alfa (EPO; Epogen, Procrit), initially was approved by the US Food and Drug Administration (FDA) in 1987 for management of chronic anemia associated with end-stage renal disease. In 1993, the FDA approval was expanded to include management of chemotherapy-related anemia. EPO is administered subcutaneously or intravenously. Darbepoetin alfa (Aranesp) is a protein that stimulates erythropoiesis and is also identified as a synthetic form of erythropoietin.

Transfusion of packed RBCs is indicated if there is evidence of cardiac decompensation or if hemoglobin levels are low in combination with low platelet counts. The transfusion improves the patient's oxygen-carrying capacity, allows for a more efficient use of blood components, and lowers the risk of volume overload.

Thrombocytopenia. Thrombocytopenia is a reduction in the number of circulating platelets as a result of the bone marrow suppression. Normal platelet values are 150,000 to 400,000/mm^3. When the platelet count is less than 20,000/mm^3, spontaneous bleeding can occur. Platelet transfusions may be necessary. Patients with thrombocytopenia have an elevated risk of bleeding and may exhibit unexplained petechiae, ecchymoses, and bleeding (ACS, 2020i).

Patient teaching measures to prevent injury and hemorrhage caused by a decrease in platelets include (1) using a soft toothbrush or swab for mouth care; (2) keeping the mouth clean; (3) avoiding intrusions into rectum (such as rectally administered medications or enemas); (4) using an electric shaver; (5) applying direct pressure for 5 to 10 minutes if any bleeding occurs; (6) avoiding contact sports, elective surgery, and tooth extraction; (7) avoiding picking or blowing the nose forcefully; (8) avoiding trauma, falls, bumps, invasive procedures, and cuts; (9) avoiding the use of aspirin or aspirin preparations; and (10) using adequate lubrication and gentleness during sexual intercourse.

Integumentary System

Alopecia. Alopecia is loss of hair resulting from the destruction of hair follicles. It may occur by two mechanisms. If the hair roots are affected and have atrophied, alopecia occurs readily. The hair falls out either spontaneously or during hair combing, often in large clumps. If the hair shaft is affected, the hair breaks off very near the scalp. The root remains in the scalp, and a patchy, thinning pattern of hair loss occurs. Elsewhere on the body, other hair may be lost, such as eyebrows and eyelashes. Loss of leg, arm, pubic, axillary, and facial hair is less common.

The pattern and extent of hair loss is not predictable. When treatment involves a drug known to cause alopecia, education to the patient must include a frank discussion about the potential for hair loss that may begin within a few days or weeks of treatment and the fact that partial or complete baldness may occur rapidly. Drug-induced alopecia is temporary. The patient may note that the hair color or texture is different as the hair grows back. On occasion, hair growth may return while chemotherapy treatment continues. The loss of hair is a potential source of anxiety for the patient because it affects body image. Many patients tolerate this type of hair loss with minimal distress because the medication is necessary to control or cure the patient's cancer.

To meet the patient's needs, provide an education program that includes written materials and educational sessions with a hair stylist. The patient needs information about health care measures for scalp protection, such as using gentle shampoos; avoiding hair dryers, curling irons, permanents, and hair coloring; protecting the scalp; and wearing protective covering when outdoors (to reduce heat loss). A patient with long or thick hair may wish to trim or cut hair short before losing hair. There are organizations whose primary purpose is the provision of human replacement hair to patients in need. Express sincere concern and provide emotional support for the patient.

Gastrointestinal System

Stomatitis. Stomatitis is a condition that develops as a result of destruction of normal cells of the oral cavity, which results in the development of inflamed, sore, ulcerated areas within the patient's mouth. It may range from erythema of the oral mucosa to mild or severe ulceration. Methotrexate, 5-fluorouracil, doxorubicin, capecitabine, cisplatin, cytarabine, and etoposide are the chemotherapeutic drugs that are associated most frequently with the development of stomatitis (Mayo Clinic, 2020a). Patients also may develop a superimposed fungal infection of the mouth and esophagus, and oral nystatin or fluconazole usually is prescribed. Excellent oral hygiene is important. Frequent mouth rinsing is recommended.

Viscous lidocaine (Xylocaine) is used when stomatitis becomes intolerable. A light topical application can decrease pain so that the patient may eat and drink. Patients who suffer from stomatitis usually benefit from a soft or liquid diet. Small frequent meals and the avoidance of foods that are spicy or acidic is helpful.

Nausea, vomiting, and diarrhea

Risk of nausea and vomiting from chemotherapy and targeted therapy. Some drugs used for cancer treatment are more likely to cause nausea and vomiting than other drugs (Cancer.net, 2020a). The table below lists the likelihood that a certain cancer drug will cause nausea and vomiting.

NEARLY ALWAYS CAUSES NAUSEA AND VOMITING (HIGH RISK)	USUALLY CAUSES NAUSEA AND VOMITING (MODERATE RISK)	SOMETIMES CAUSES NAUSEA AND VOMITING (LOW RISK)	RARELY CAUSES NAUSEA AND VOMITING (MINIMAL RISK)
Carmustine (BiCNU)	Alemtuzumab (Campath)	Bortezomib (Velcade)	Bevacizumab (Avastin)
Cisplatin	Azacitadine (Vidaza)	Cabazitaxel (Jevtana)	Bleomycin (Blenoxane)
Cyclophosphamide at higher doses	Bendamustine (Treanda)		Busulfan (Busulfex, Myleran)
Dacarbazine	Carboplatin	Cytarabine at lower doses	Cetuximab (Erbitux)
Dactinomycin (Cosmegen)	Clofarabine (Clolar)	Docetaxel (Taxotere)	2-Chlorodeoxyadenosine
Daunorubicin (Cerubidine) when combined with cyclophosphamide	Cyclophosphamide at lower doses	Doxorubicin HCL liposome injection (Doxil)	Fludarabine
Doxorubicin (Adriamycin) when combined with cyclophosphamide	Cytarabine (Cytosar-U) at higher doses	(Etopophus, Toposar, VePesid)	Pralatrexate (Folotyn)
Epirubicin (Ellence) when combined with cyclophosphamide	Daunorubicin	Fluorouracil (5-FU, Adrucil)	Rituximab (Rituxan)

Continued

NEARLY ALWAYS CAUSES NAUSEA AND VOMITING (HIGH RISK)	USUALLY CAUSES NAUSEA AND VOMITING (MODERATE RISK)	SOMETIMES CAUSES NAUSEA AND VOMITING (LOW RISK)	RARELY CAUSES NAUSEA AND VOMITING (MINIMAL RISK)
Idarubicin *(Idamycin)* when combined with cyclophosphamide	Doxorubicin	Gemcitabine *(Gemzar)* Etoposide	Vinblastine
Mechlorethamine *(Mustargen, Valchlor)*	Epirubicin	Ixabepilone *(Ixempra)*	Vincristine
Streptozotocin *(Zanosar)*	Idarubicin	Methotrexate *(multiple brand names)* Fludarabine	Vinorelbine *(Navelbine)*
	Ifosfamide *(Ifex)* Irinotecan *(Camptosar)* Oxaliplatin *(Eloxatin)*	Mitomycin Mitoxantrone Paclitaxel *(Taxol, Abraxane)* Panitumumab *(Vectibix)* Pemetrexed *(Alimta)* Temsirolimus *(Torisel)* Topotecan *(Hycamtin)* Trastuzumab *(Herceptin)*	

Nausea, vomiting, and diarrhea are disorders of the GI tract that can be caused by the excessive breakdown of normal GI cells. There are several different types of nausea that can occur in the patient with cancer who is receiving chemotherapy. Nausea that occurs for this patient is referred to as chemotherapy-induced nausea and vomiting (CINV). Some patients experience breakthrough emesis, which can occur on any day of chemotherapy, even with appropriate medications used to prevent its occurrence. Others experience refractory emesis, which occurs with continued failure to prevent the nausea and vomiting using prophylactic techniques. Some patients develop anticipatory nausea and vomiting. This is triggered by negative experiences associated with chemotherapy and poor control of nausea and vomiting in the past. The prevention of nausea and vomiting during the early stages and cycles of chemotherapy is the best treatment. Nausea and vomiting are among the most uncomfortable and distressing side effects of chemotherapy. The onset and duration vary greatly among patients and with the drug given. For the ambulatory patient, nausea may interfere with the ability to continue working. Persistent vomiting may result in fluid and electrolyte imbalance, general weakness, and weight loss. Decline of nutritional status renders the patient more susceptible to infection and perhaps less able to tolerate therapy. Such physiologic symptoms can accompany or precipitate psychological responses such as depression and withdrawal. Use nursing interventions and ordered medications to help minimize CINV.

Antiemetics vary in success. There are several medication classes used to prevent and treat CINV. Serotonin receptor antagonists include ondansetron (Zofran) and granisetron. Neurokinin-1 receptor antagonists include aprepitant and fosaprepitant (Emend). Dopamine receptor antagonists (butyrophenones, phenothiazines, and metoclopramide) are also used. Common corticosteroids used to treat CINV are methylprednisolone and dexamethasone. Other medication classes that are used include benzodiazepines and cannabinoids. Cannabinoids are chemical compounds of cannabis, and they activate receptors in the body to reduce nausea and vomiting. Two of the commercially prepared cannabinoids are nabilone and dronabinol (NCI, 2021a). The patient may receive antiemetics orally, intramuscularly, rectally, or intravenously.

Changes in bowel habits commonly occur but usually do not necessitate intervention. If diarrhea becomes marked or persistent, an antidiarrheal medication such as diphenoxylate with atropine (Lomotil) may be prescribed.

Nursing interventions. Combinations of chemotherapy agents, as well as chemotherapy combined with other treatments, have increased the remissions and survival rates among patients with cancer. Some problems experienced by patients undergoing chemotherapy are similar to those that may result from radiation therapy (depending on the target site and amount of radiation). Help the patient realize that some of the problems are merely the result of the therapy and not a sign that the cancer is getting worse.

Patient problems and interventions for patients undergoing chemotherapy include but are not limited to the following:

PATIENT PROBLEM	NURSING INTERVENTIONS
Compromised Tissue Integrity: Oral Mucous Membrane, related to • Stomatitis (inflammation of the mouth) • Xerostomia (reduced salivation, "dry mouth")	Assist with frequent, careful oral hygiene and hydration; use very soft toothbrush. Provide meticulous mouth care. Administer prescribed antifungal medication such as fluconazole. Give soothing oral lozenges, ice chips, and frequent sips of ice water; do not give hot beverages; apply lip balm for lip dryness.

PATIENT PROBLEM	NURSING INTERVENTIONS
Insufficient Nutrition, related to • Anorexia (from changes in taste and smell) • Nausea and vomiting • Dysphagia (difficulty swallowing) • Aspiration • Diarrhea • Malabsorption • Cachexia	Provide adequate, easily digestible, soft, bland diet; avoid spicy foods. Keep room free of odors and clutter. Administer prescribed antiemetic medications. Provide small, frequent, highly nutritional meals to meet the extra demands placed on the body by rapidly dividing malignant cells. Provide pleasant surroundings in which to eat and allow plenty of time for meal.
Potential for Infection, related to • Weakened immune system • Leukopenia	Protect against infections. Limit visitors. Discourage visits by people who are ill or have been recently exposed to a communicable disease. Advise patient to avoid crowds. Discourage eating fresh fruit or placing fresh-cut flowers or live plants in room. Observe and promptly report any signs of inflammation at injection sites or insertion sites of any peripheral or central intravenous lines; report any temperature higher than 100°F (37.7°C). Use sterile technique whenever possible. Initiate reverse isolation as indicated. Monitor temperature and leukocyte count. Avoid areas with indwelling catheters, and avoid performing rectal procedures or examinations. Administer antibiotics as prescribed.

Tumor Lysis Syndrome

Tumor lysis syndrome (TLS) is an oncologic emergency with rapid lysis of malignant cells.

Etiology and pathophysiology. TLS may occur spontaneously in patients with inordinately heavy tumor cell burdens. However, it is usually a result of chemotherapy or, less commonly, radiation therapy. It may occur anywhere from 24 hours to 7 days after antineoplastic therapy is initiated. Patients most at risk are those who have heavy tumor cell burdens (e.g., high-grade lymphomas) or markedly elevated WBC level (acute leukemias). TLS also occurs in chronic lymphocytic leukemia and metastatic breast cancer.

The syndrome develops when chemotherapy or irradiation causes the destruction (or lysis) of a large number of rapidly dividing malignant cells. As malignant cells are lysed, intracellular contents are released quickly into the bloodstream. This results in high levels of potassium (hyperkalemia), phosphate (hyperphosphatemia), and uric acid (hyperuricemia). These conditions, plus secondary hypocalcemia, increase the risk for renal failure and alterations in cardiac function.

Clinical manifestations. Early clinical manifestations include nausea, vomiting, anorexia, diarrhea, muscle weakness, and cramping. Later signs and symptoms may include tetany, paresthesias, seizures, anuria, and cardiac arrest.

Diagnostic tests. TLS is diagnosed by assessment of the signs and symptoms and by confirmation of abnormal laboratory values. Early symptoms of TLS may not be readily apparent, and clinical manifestations may appear rapidly. The syndrome is detected most frequently from abnormalities in blood chemistry. Other important values include serum creatinine, blood urea nitrogen, and urine pH.

Medical management. The best way to prevent TLS is to recognize which patients are at risk and to initiate prophylactic measures before antineoplastic therapy begins. This includes pretreatment *hydration* to maintain a urinary output of 150 mL/h. Hydration should begin 24 to 48 hours before treatment and continue for at least 72 hours after treatment. *Diuretics* may be used to promote the excretion of phosphate and uric acid, to prevent volume overload, and to promote the excretion of potassium in the urine. *Allopurinol* prevents uric acid formation; administration is initiated a few days before treatment and should be continued for 3 to 5 days after treatment is completed. *Sodium bicarbonate* is used to maintain alkalinity of the urine (pH over 7), which prevents uric acid crystallization. Cation-exchange resins, such as sodium polystyrene, bind with potassium and so their administration enables excretion of potassium through the bowel. *Calcium gluconate* is administered intravenously to correct hypocalcemia. Cardiac monitoring is required. Phosphate-binding gels, such as aluminum hydroxide, form an insoluble complex that is excreted by the bowel. When these measures are not successful, renal failure may occur and renal dialysis is necessary.

Nursing interventions. Nursing interventions include identifying patients at risk for TLS and initiating hydration 24 to 48 hours before chemotherapy. Allopurinol is administered before and during chemotherapy to maintain alkalinity of the urine. Determine which medications contain phosphate or spare potassium and discuss discontinuation with the health care provider. Monitor potassium, phosphorus, calcium, and uric acid levels. Assess the patient for signs and symptoms of TLS, including the following:

- *Hyperkalemia:* electrocardiographic changes, muscle weakness, twitching, paresthesia, paralysis, muscle cramps, nausea, vomiting, lethargy, and syncope
- *Hyperphosphatemia:* azotemia, oliguria, hypertension, and renal failure
- *Hypocalcemia:* electrocardiographic changes (heart block, dysrhythmias, and cardiac arrest), tetany, confusion, and hallucinations
- *Hyperuricemia:* renal failure, nausea, vomiting, flank pain, gout, and pruritus

If hyperuricemia is detected, diuretics, sodium bicarbonate, cation-exchange resins, and phosphate-binding gels are administered as appropriate. Monitor intake and output and notify the health care provider if urinary output is less than 100 mL/h. Urine pH is monitored and maintained at higher than 7 with sodium bicarbonate. Prepare the patient and family for dialysis if other measures are not effective.

Prognosis. When treating TLS, health care providers must focus on preventing renal failure. TLS typically resolves within 7 days, once appropriate treatment is initiated.

Chemotherapy has proved to be an effective treatment for many patients with cancer. Chemotherapy can be used to cure the cancer, control the cancer, or help reduce cancer-related pain. Learn about each drug being administered, anticipate the side effects, and monitor the plan of care, making modifications as needed with condition changes.

Safety guidelines in accordance with facility policy must be followed when chemotherapeutic agents are prepared and administered. Because of their potential for absorption or inhalation, they are potentially dangerous for the people who administer the agents.

TARGETED CANCER THERAPY

Sometimes, in addition to standard chemotherapy, oncologists may prescribe targeted cancer therapy. They are medications that can interfere with specific molecules that allow for the cancer's growth and its ability to spread to other tissues. This medication is cytostatic, meaning that it blocks cancer cell proliferation. Targeted cancer therapy is also known as molecularly targeted therapies and precision medicines. Standard chemotherapy is used to kill cancer cells, but it also kills other types of rapidly dividing normal cells. Standard chemotherapy is cytotoxic. Research studies currently are being performed regarding precision medicine so that oncologists can one day use information on a patient's proteins and genetic makeup to treat cancer (NCI, 2021b).

There are some significant side effects that are experienced by patients using targeted cancer therapy. Patients may develop problems with diarrhea, as well as liver or skin changes (rash, dry skin, depigmentation of hair, and changes to their nails). Some have difficulty with wound healing, blood clotting, and hypertension (NCI, 2021b).

BIOTHERAPY

The observation of interactions between the immune system and malignant cells led to the development of therapies that could manipulate this natural process. Traditionally, this field has been known as *immunotherapy.* It has led to the modern era of biotherapy. Since the 1980s, biotherapy, or biological therapy, has emerged as an important fourth modality for treating cancer. *Biotherapy* may be defined as treatment with agents derived from biological sources or affecting biological responses.

Biological response modifiers (BRMs) work against the cancer in three different ways. One type of BRM increases, restores, or modifies the host defenses against the tumor (CSFs, filgrastim, erythropoietin, GM-CSFs). Other BRMs are directly toxic to tumors (interleukins, bacille Calmette-Guérin vaccine [BCG]) or modify biological features of the tumor (interferons alpha, beta, and gamma).

Most of these therapies are given via intramuscular or subcutaneous injection and must be administered to the patient over an extended time. While providing emotional support, help ensure that the patient remains compliant with treatment. Common side effects in patients receiving BRMs include fatigue, flulike symptoms, leukopenia, nausea, and vomiting.

Health care professionals must understand these therapies to help give the patient with cancer the best care available. These therapies and research are leading to the development of gene therapy today; this will improve outcomes for patients with cancer in the future.

BONE MARROW TRANSPLANTATION

Bone marrow transplantation (BMT) is the process of replacing diseased or damaged bone marrow with normally functioning bone marrow. BMT is used in the treatment of a variety of diseases and offers a chance for long-term survival.

Stem cell transplants are being used in some solid tumor cancers, such as high-risk breast cancer. Bone marrow harvests are becoming less frequent because many centers have turned to peripheral blood stem cells for hematopoietic support after high-dose chemotherapy.

Most bone marrow used for transplantation is obtained by multiple needle aspirations from the posterior iliac crest while the patient is under general or spinal anesthesia. The anterior iliac crest and sternum also may be used. The amount of marrow extracted ranges from 600 to 2500 mL for the average adult. After processing, the marrow is given to the patient intravenously through a transfusion bag, or it can be frozen (cryopreservation). Marrow may be kept for 3 years

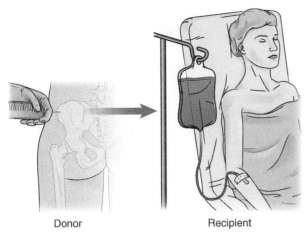

Donor   Recipient

Fig. 17.6 The process of bone marrow transplantation. (Copyright We Care Health Services. [n.d.]. *Bone marrow transplant in India.* Retrieved from *www.wecareindia.com/cancer-treatment/bone-marrow-transplant.html.*)

or more. When the bone marrow is infused, it is via a central line without a filter over 1 to 4 hours (Fig. 17.6).

Bone marrow may be removed from an individual for personal use (autologous, indicating something that originates within the patient, especially a factor present in tissues or fluids) at a later time. Alternatively, a patient may be given *allogenic* bone marrow (meaning the transplant came from someone else). Three types of allogenic bone marrow transplants are (1) *syngeneic* (donation from the patient's identical twin), (2) *related* (donation from a relative, usually a sibling), and (3) *unrelated* (donation from a nonrelative). The patient is at increased risk for developing infections during the process of transplantation because the immune defenses are weakened. Transplant recipients are cared for in special bone marrow units so that they can be monitored closely and carefully protected.

Interventions to prevent infections include protective isolation or laminar airflow rooms; prophylactic systemic antibiotics and antiviral agents (primarily acyclovir); and routine cultures of blood, urine, throat, and stool. Despite these and other interventions, the patient can become septic in hours, with multisystem failure.

Survival after BMT depends on the patient's age, remission, and clinical status at the time of transplantation.

PERIPHERAL BLOOD STEM CELL TRANSPLANTATION

An emerging and promising alternative to BMT is peripheral blood stem cell transplantation (PBSCT). This procedure is based on the fact that peripheral or circulating stem cells are capable of repopulating the bone marrow. PBSCT is a type of transplantation that differs from BMT primarily in the method of stem cell collection. Because there are fewer stem cells in the blood than in the bone marrow, mobilization of stem cells from the bone marrow into the peripheral blood can be done by means of chemotherapy or hematopoietic growth factors, such as GM-CSF and G-CSF.

Vascular access from the donor is initiated. Tubing from the donor enters a cell separator machine that is used to remove the peripheral stem cells. Then, the blood is returned to the donor. This procedure, called *leukapheresis,* usually takes 2 to 4 hours. In autologous transplantation, the stem cells are purged to kill any cancer cells and then frozen and stored until used for transplantation. Although many of the same steps (harvesting, intensive chemotherapy, reinfusion) of BMT are used in PBSCT, the hematologic recovery period in PBSCT is shorter and complications are less severe.

NURSING INTERVENTIONS

When discussing the expectations of specific treatments for the patient, communicate genuine concern. Encourage the patient to verbalize concerns and provide reinforced education as needed. Patients may become discouraged by toxic side effects and other problems they experience while undergoing conventional cancer treatment. Allow extra time to listen to patients with cancer express their feelings and encourage them to follow the guidelines of conventional medical practice that offer the most hope.

ADVANCED CANCER

PAIN MANAGEMENT

Patients with cancer may have pain at any point during the course of the disease and its treatment. There were approximately 15.5 million surviving cancer in 2016 and it is projected that by the year 2026 there will be almost 20 million cancer survivors. Pain is one of the most common symptoms of cancer (Gallaway et. al., 2020). Unfortunately, some patients seek care only after pain develops. Pain is usually a late symptom and indicates tumor obstruction, nerve damage, or invasion of bone.

It is estimated that in 85% of patients with cancer, pain can be managed effectively with appropriate therapy. The American Cancer Society, the American Pain Society, the World Health Organization, the Oncology Nursing Society, and other organizations consider pain control to be a significant issue for patients with cancer.

One of the many challenges in caring for the patient with pain is the assessment. The patient's communication of pain must be accepted. Remain nonjudgmental regarding the patient's complaints of pain and provide appropriate management interventions.

Cultural and religious practices in the patient's family play an important role in the perception of pain or expression of suffering. Some cultures tend to minimize pain, and patients with those cultural backgrounds may be less likely to express pain. Other cultures expect the expression of pain, and patients with such cultural backgrounds may exhibit a greater overt expression of pain.

Opioids used in the management of cancer pain include morphine, hydromorphone, fentanyl, and methadone. Sustained-release morphine in an oral form—such as MS Contin, Kadian, or morphine sulphate—is particularly effective in the management of the terminally ill person with pain. Administering opioids via transdermal method, inhalation, intravenous drips, intrathecally, and epidurally enhances the analgesic effect. The nurse can provide more consistent pain relief for the patient by administering bolus injections to the patient. Often, the most effective regimen involves round-the-clock dosage scheduling for effective pain control. Fixed dosage schedules of an adequate amount of pain medication provide more constant blood levels and predictable pain relief. Some patients have breakthrough pain that necessitates additional doses, but the fixed dosage schedule should be maintained. Monitor the patient for the development of any opioid-related side effects such as constipation, vomiting, and respiratory and central nervous system depression.

In addition to opioids, valuable nonopioid analgesics used in the treatment of certain levels of cancer pain are acetaminophen; aspirin; and nonsteroidal anti-inflammatory drugs (NSAIDs), such as ibuprofen, indomethacin, and naproxen.

The patient should be educated about nonpharmacologic pain management methods such as distraction and relaxation. Acupuncture, biofeedback, hypnosis, guided imagery, and massages also may be used to help manage the patient's pain. Many patients find that nonpharmacologic measures enhance the effectiveness of other prescribed pain interventions. The patient with cancer should receive enough sleep and rest. This can be challenging when the patient is admitted to an acute care setting. The patient with advanced cancer may experience cachexia, a profound state of ill health and malnutrition marked by weakness and emaciation (Fig. 17.7). Additional comfort measures include frequent position changes, meticulous skin care, nutritious foods and fluids, and the use of comfort measures to promote relaxation and reduce the perception of pain. The nurse's unique role in pain management for the patient with cancer involves acting as an advocate and a liaison between the patient and other members of the health care team. Spending time with the patient, assessing the patient's response to the pain, evaluating the effectiveness of the pain management plan of care, revising the plan of care as indicated, and educating the patient and the family are important for providing the patient with the best pain relief possible. Be able to monitor the patient's pain effectively and address patient and family concerns regarding the pain management strategies. Some patients and their families have opioid phobia, the irrational fear that even the appropriate use of opioids will result in addiction. This fear of addiction may contribute to undertreatment of pain. A goal for the patient and family includes the verbalization of understanding of the need for opioids in the care of ill patients. Appropriate use

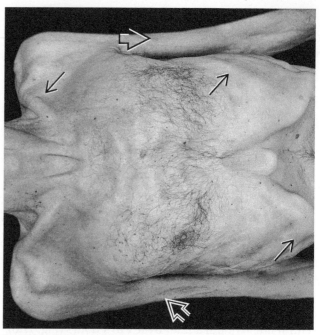

Fig. 17.7 Marked cachexia with severe loss of adipose tissue and muscle mass as noted here by prominent bony protrusions and marked muscular atrophy. (From Fyfe B, Miller D: *Diagnostic pathology*: Hospital autopsy. St. Louis, 2016, Elsevier.)

of pain management strategies enables patients and families to accept the therapeutic value of drugs such as opioids to ensure that patients do not suffer from potentially controllable pain.

Planning interventions to manage pain in the patient with cancer is challenging. Some general guidelines must be followed. The best management involves a variety of pain relief measures. These include medications and nursing interventions to promote comfort. Pain should be managed before it becomes unbearable. Assessing the patient's past history or pain management is vital. Be certain to determine what relief measures have been effective in the past. The best plan for pain management includes patient participation and engagement. Activities that the patient believes will be helpful should be incorporated. Debilitating pain can leave the patient feeling defeated. Encourage the patient to share concerns and make suggestions. Be aware of fears that the patient may have. Fear and anxiety may increase the perception of pain. Patients with cancer may feel that increased pain is a sign that their condition is worsening and death is imminent. The most effective pain relief is often a combination of pharmacologic and nonpharmacologic methods.

NUTRITIONAL THERAPY

Nutritional problems that most frequently occur in patients with cancer are malnutrition, anorexia, altered taste sensation, nausea, vomiting, diarrhea, stomatitis, and mucositis. These problems can be caused by a combination of factors, including drug toxicity, effects of radiation therapy, tumor involvement, side effects of medication, recent surgery, emotional distress, and difficulty with ingestion or digestion of food. If the patient is malnourished, the patient's normal cells cannot recover well from the effects of therapy, and the immune system may be compromised because of the depletion of protein stores.

Malnutrition

Patients with cancer are at increased risk for protein and calorie malnutrition, characterized by fat and muscle depletion. Encourage the patient to eat foods high in protein to facilitate repair and regeneration of cells, as well as high-calorie foods that provide energy and minimize weight loss.

The patient must be weighed daily. A 5% weight loss or other indications that the patient is at risk for developing malnutrition are signals for the nurse to confer with the health care provider concerning the patient's nutritional needs. Once a 10-pound (4.5-kg) weight loss occurs, it is difficult for the patient to maintain adequate nutritional status. A nutritional supplement may be necessary. The nursing assessment should include review of albumin and prealbumin levels. The patient may choose to use nutritional supplements in place of milk when cooking or baking. Nutritional supplements can be added easily to scrambled eggs, pudding, custard, mashed potatoes, cereal, and cream sauces. Packages of instant breakfast can be used as indicated or sprinkled on cereals, desserts, and casseroles. If the patient's malnutrition cannot be treated with dietary intake, it may be necessary to use enteral or parenteral nutrition as an adjunct nutritional measure.

Anorexia

Anorexia experienced by a patient with cancer can be a challenging problem. An intervention may be effective one day and ineffective the next. Continue to assess the patient and use interventions as necessary to help manage this problem. Nursing care should be geared to prevent or minimize anorexia. Evaluate the effectiveness of interventions and modify the plan of care as indicated to promote continuation of the interventions that are most successful. Megestrol (Megace) may be prescribed to manage anorexia and stimulate the appetite.

Altered Taste Sensation

Cancer treatments may cause the patient to experience an alteration in the sweet, sour, bitter, and salty taste sensations. This change in taste is known as dysgeusia. The patient needs information about this phenomenon. Discuss dietary selections that will incorporate foods preferred by the patient and help maintain caloric intake. The patient may feel compelled to eat certain foods because they are "healthy." Advise the patient to experiment with spices and other seasoning agents to mask the taste alterations. Lemon juice, onion, mint, basil, and fruit juice marinades may improve the taste of certain meats and fish. Bacon bits, onion, and pieces of ham may enhance the taste of vegetables.

COMMUNICATION AND PSYCHOLOGICAL SUPPORT

The patient and the family may become irritable and angry with caregivers when the patient is suffering and experiencing progressive problems. Remember that these feelings are not directed toward the caregivers personally but have developed as a result of the circumstances associated with the patient's disease. A display of anger toward the staff may be caused by deep-seated frustration or anxiety. Continue to use therapeutic communication techniques during these types of situations. The patient may not be able to accept or comprehend the explanations that are given when the patient's stress level has escalated. Administering kind, gentle nursing care may communicate more effectively than words. Touch also may be used to indicate awareness of the patient's emotional distress.

Nurses are able to help make the effects of cancer less psychologically traumatic through sensitivity and creativity. The health care system can foster dependency by stripping away the powers of decision making and the patient's personal identity. Care can be individualized by including the patient and family in the planning process. This also promotes compliance inasmuch as the patient feels more involved in the decision making. Offer as many areas of control in the decision-making process as possible. This fosters feelings of independence and increases self-esteem in the patient.

Psychological support of the patient is an important aspect of cancer care. Because of the effectiveness of cancer treatment, many cases of cancer are cured or controlled for long periods. Thus emphasis must be placed on maintaining an optimal quality of life after the diagnosis of cancer. If the patient, family, and caregivers have a positive attitude toward cancer and cancer treatment, then it may have a significant positive effect on the quality of life that the patient experiences. A positive attitude also may influence the patient's prognosis positively.

Most people view the diagnosis of cancer as a crisis. Cancer affects the quality of life of all affected patients in some way. Four quality-of-life factors affecting patients with cancer and their families are social, psychological, physical, and spiritual. The most common concerns voiced by the patient are (1) fear of recurrence, (2) chronic or acute pain, (3) sexual problems, (4) fatigue, (5) guilt for delaying screening or treatment, (6) behavior that may have increased the risk for cancer, (7) changes in physical appearance, (8) depression, (9) sleep problems, (10) change in role performance, and (11) being a financial burden on his or her loved ones.

Coping with these fears produces a range of emotions within the patient: denial, anger, bargaining, depression, and eventually acceptance. Some patients experience feelings of helplessness and hopelessness.

These feelings may occur at any time during the process of cancer. However, some patterns appear to occur more frequently or at a greater intensity at certain stages of the disease process. The following factors may determine how the patient will cope with the diagnosis of cancer:

* *Ability to cope with stressful events in the past* (e.g., loss of job, major disappointment): Assess the patient's past coping abilities. Review stressors in the patient's history and the coping skills demonstrated.
* *Availability of significant others:* Patients who have effective support systems tend to cope more effectively than do patients without such support systems.
* *Ability to express feelings and concerns:* Patients who are able to express their feelings and ask for help usually cope more effectively than do patients who internalize these types of feelings.
* *Age at the time of diagnosis:* Age determines the coping strategies to a great degree. For example, an adolescent and an elderly person may employ different coping strategies to psychologically manage the stress of the disease.
* *Extent of disease:* Cure or control of the disease process is usually easier to cope with than the reality of terminal illness.
* *Disruption of body image:* Disruption of the body image (e.g., radical neck dissection, alopecia, mastectomy) may intensify the psychological effect of cancer.
* *Presence of symptoms:* Symptoms such as fatigue, nausea, diarrhea, and pain may intensify the psychological effects of cancer.
* *Experience with cancer:* If the patient's previous experiences with cancer have been negative, the patient will probably view his or her current status as negative.
* *Attitude associated with cancer:* A patient who feels a sense of control and has a positive attitude regarding his or her health care and treatment is better able to cope with the diagnosis and treatment than one who feels hopeless, helpless, or out of control.

To facilitate the development of a hopeful attitude about cancer and to support the patient and the family during the various stages of the process of cancer, continue to be available, especially during difficult times. Exhibit a caring attitude and listen actively to fears and concerns. The nurse-patient relationship should be based on trust and confidence; be open, honest, and caring in the approach. Touch may be used to exhibit caring; touching the patient's hand may be more effective than words.

Essential information regarding cancer and cancer care should be provided. Provide relief from distressing symptoms. Assist the patient in setting realistic, reachable short- and long-term goals and in maintaining usual lifestyle patterns. Above all, maintain hope, which is the key to effective cancer care. The patient's perception of hope varies and is dependent on the patient's status. The patient may hope that the symptoms are not serious, hope that the treatment is curative, hope for independence, hope for relief of pain, hope for a longer life, or hope for a peaceful death. Recent research does not show a link between attitude and emotional states and the prevention of cancer growth.

TERMINAL PROGNOSIS

Coping with the multiple problems associated with advanced cancer can lead to a sense of helplessness and hopelessness, despite all efforts. The patient and the family may look forward to death as a relief from unrelenting suffering.

Many patients with advanced cancer know that they are dying. They may be able to recognize attempts to avoid the truth and may distrust and feel hostile toward people who make such attempts. Honesty and openness are the best approaches. Patients frequently express relief at a caregiver's willingness to discuss death. Remaining open and honest with patients as they near the end of life can be difficult for the nurse. It requires that the nurse be honest with his or her own personal feelings.

Spiritual activities may provide mental and emotional strength, despite physical deterioration. The patient may ask the nurse to read the Bible or to pray with him or her, or the patient may request that a minister, priest, imam, or rabbi visit. Spiritual strength may help the patient and family cope with the continuing problems encountered in the cancer experience.

If the patient wishes to die at home, the hospital social worker or discharge planner assists the patient and family in planning for home care. Arrangements for any special supplies and equipment are made before discharge. The nurse plays a major role in teaching the patient and at least one family member or significant other how to continue any special care needed at home, such as dressing changes, irrigations, the management of a feeding tube, or the care of a central venous line for administration of parenteral nutrition or medications.

Throughout the patient's hospital stay, take advantage of the time available to promote self-care to the greatest extent possible. Assess the patient's readiness to learn and ability to participate actively in self-care. If necessary, consult advanced clinical nursing specialists to provide individualized guidelines for teaching patients. Plans for patient education should be included in the nursing care plan. Evidence of the patient's ability to manage self-care should be documented, and any assistance needed from others should be planned. Continuity of care is the goal in discharge planning. Hospice services can be arranged in most communities for patients who have advanced cancer. There are freestanding hospices, hospices within a hospital or skilled nursing facility, or at-home arrangements. The primary focus of a hospice is enhancing the patient's quality of life, not prolonging it. Efforts are directed toward relief from pain and other problems. Skilled professional care and voluntary support services are provided to assist the patient and the family in living life to the fullest each day.

Get Ready for the NCLEX® Examination!

Key points

- Cancer is the second leading cause of death in the United States (after heart disease).
- There is strong evidence that what people eat or drink, as well as their lifestyle choices, may predispose them to the development of cancer.
- The American Cancer Society recommends specific preventive behaviors and screening tests for cancer prevention and early detection for men and women.
- People should report any changes that occur to their bodies to their health care provider immediately.
- It is important to have periodic physical examinations and to seek medical attention promptly if a person develops any warning signs of cancer.
- A common reason for a delay in diagnosing cancer is that early malignant changes are not accompanied by pain.
- Seeking medical attention when warning signs occur is also delayed frequently because people fear the possible diagnosis of cancer and hope that the signs and symptoms will just go away.
- The diagnosis of cancer has a profound effect on family members, as well as on the patient. They may experience denial, anger, fear, and depression.
- Most of the side effects from chemotherapeutic agents result from the destruction of normal cells of the hematopoietic system, hair follicles, and the GI system.
- TLS is an oncologic emergency that occurs in patients with cancer who have heavy tumor cell burdens after they receive chemotherapy or irradiation, which causes rapid lysis of malignant cells.
- The American Cancer Society sponsors organized support groups for individuals with the same types of cancer; some of these are Reach to Recovery; the Lost Chord Club; I Can Cope; Look Good, Feel Good; and the Ostomy Club. Prepared volunteers are available in most communities to visit a patient with newly diagnosed cancer.
- Spiritual strength assists the patient and the family in coping with the problems experienced as a result of cancer.
- The American Cancer Society, the American Pain Society, the World Health Organization, and the Oncology Nursing Society consider pain control a major issue in the management of a person with cancer.
- The concept of rehabilitation should be applied in the planning of care for the patient with cancer to promote the highest level of functioning possible.

Additional Learning Resources

SG Go to your Study Guide for additional learning activities to help you master this chapter content.

Be sure to visit the Evolve site at http://evolve.elsevier.com/Cooper/adult for additional online resources.

Review Questions for the NCLEX® Examination

1. A 58-year-old patient with colon cancer is receiving combined radiation therapy and chemotherapy. He has developed diarrhea. The patient asks the nurse why he is now having diarrhea. What nursing response is most accurate?
   1. "Your diagnosis of colon cancer has caused diarrhea."
   2. "Because you are unable to eat or drink much during treatment, you are having loose stools."
   3. "Radiation is very irritating to the lining of your GI tract, which may have caused diarrhea."
   4. "You most likely have an imbalance in your fluid and electrolyte levels."

2. Which is true regarding cancer prevention and health care promotion behaviors for patients with a diagnosis of cancer?
   1. They will not decrease the risk of developing a second malignancy.
   2. They will not be affected by personal choices related to diet and smoking.
   3. They are increasingly important with the growing population of cancer survivors.
   4. They would include only routine physical examinations.

3. A patient has received a diagnosis of stage I breast cancer. She is receiving adjuvant chemotherapy and radiation therapy after a lumpectomy. What teaching point should be included in this patient's plan of care? *(Select all that apply.)*
   1. Chemotherapy-related hair loss is usually temporary.
   2. All chemotherapeutic agents result in alopecia.
   3. Hair that grows back may have a different texture and color.
   4. Hair loss is most often related to radiation treatments.
   5. Avoid the use of lotions on the skin at and near the site of radiation treatment, unless prescribed.

4. A 61-year-old patient is receiving chemotherapy. The patient becomes anemic and has petechiae and ecchymoses. What side effect is the patient experiencing?
   1. Bone marrow suppression
   2. Cardiac suppression
   3. Liver toxicity
   4. Pulmonary toxicity

5. Before the insertion of a radioactive cervical implant, the nurse tells the patient what to expect while it is in place. Which statement is accurate? *(Select all that apply.)*
   1. "Nurses will always be available, but they will spend only a short time at your bedside."
   2. "Personal cleanliness is essential, so you will be given a complete bed bath each day."
   3. "We will be checking your vital signs at least every 4 hours."
   4. "Your bed linens will be completely changed each day to minimize radioactive contamination."
   5. "You should make diet choices that are low in fiber."

6. A 24-year-old patient has been receiving chemotherapy for acute lymphoblastic leukemia and has developed leukopenia. Which patient statement indicates that he understands discharge teaching concerning leukopenia? *(Select all that apply.)*

   1. "I am cured and have no limitations."
   2. "My family can catch leukopenia, so I need to be careful to not get too close to any of them."
   3. "I should avoid close contact with people who might give me an infection."
   4. "I need to be careful not to cut myself when shaving because I may not be able to stop the bleeding."
   5. "I should avoid being in large crowds until my white blood cell count rises to an acceptable level."

7. A 42-year-old patient has palpated a small lump in her left breast. She has scheduled an appointment with her health care provider. Which test will be used to make a definite diagnosis of a benign or malignant tumor of her breast?

   1. Biopsy
   2. Mammography
   3. Tomography
   4. Ultrasonography

8. The nurse educator is discussing the importance of the reduction of carcinogens in primary prevention of cancer. Which risk factor is considered significant in many types of cancer?

   1. Diet low in fat
   2. Occasional moderate use of alcohol
   3. High pollen count in the environment
   4. Smoking

9. The patient has been diagnosed with terminal cancer. Which of the following is the most therapeutic approach by the nurse?

   1. Anti-inflammatory agents are effective analgesics for severe pain.
   2. Opioids should be withheld because they are addictive.
   3. Pain is what the patient says it is.
   4. One can increase one's tolerance for pain.

10. A patient is receiving chemotherapy and has a low WBC count. What patient statement indicates the need for further teaching?

    1. "I check my mouth after each meal."
    2. "Fresh fruits and vegetables will help me get better."
    3. "My husband and I have been using a vaginal lubrication before intercourse."
    4. "My lips are dry and cracking. I need some lubricant."

11. The patient is receiving chemotherapy and has the patient problem of *insufficient nutrition.* What are likely reasons for this lack of nutrition related to side effects of this type of treatment? *(Select all that apply.)*

    1. The patient indicates that she doesn't feel hungry.
    2. The patient complains that she has developed small sores in her mouth.
    3. The patient has developed diarrhea.
    4. The patient complains that she has been nauseated.
    5. The patient has been having experiencing episodes of choking during meals.

12. A patient has a history of oat cell carcinoma of the lung and is being treated with chemotherapy. His WBC count is $2.5/mm^3$. What is the nurse's primary concern?

    1. Prevention of hemorrhage
    2. Prevention of infection
    3. Prevention of dehydration
    4. Prevention of electrolyte imbalance

13. A 63-year-old patient has a diagnosis of cancer of the prostate gland with metastasis and is experiencing cachexia. How is cachexia best described?

    1. Poor health, malnutrition, weakness, and emaciation
    2. Increased appetite and nervousness
    3. Irritability and anger
    4. Depression, fear, and anxiety

14. A woman, 58, is being treated for metastatic breast cancer with a heavy tumor cell burden. The first time she undergoes chemotherapy, she experiences nausea, vomiting, anorexia, and diarrhea—all of which are unusually severe, even for a very aggressive cancer. The nurse calls to check on her via telehealth and learns that the nausea and vomiting took a long time to subside. The patient reports that, when they finally did subside, she was left with abdominal cramping, leaving the patient anorexic. The nurse reports these effects to the oncologist, who calls the patient back and asks her to come in for lab tests, including a blood chemistry, serum creatinine, blood urea nitrogen, and urine pH. From these values, she is able to determine that the patient experienced tumor lysis syndrome (TLS), which results in high serum levels of potassium (hyperkalemia), phosphate (hyperphosphatemia), and uric acid (hyperuricemia). To prevent a recurrence, before the next treatment, the oncologist prescribes hydration to begin 36 hours before treatment and to continue 72 hours afterward. She also prescribes a diuretic, allopurinol, sodium bicarbonate, sodium polystyrene, calcium gluconate, and a phosphate-binding gel. Because of the number of preventive medications, she prescribes the lowest recommended dose of each. Afterward, in evaluating how treatment went this time, the nurse discovers that, although some of her previous negative reactions were prevented, the patient experienced a variety of new and disconcerting ones. The patient is kept in the hospital for evaluation and monitoring and the oncologist is called. It is determined that two preventive medications were prescribed at insufficient doses. The nurse tries to identify which reactions are due to which drug's underuse.

Use an X to indicate which post-treatment reaction is due to each drug's insufficient dosing. All should be used and can be used only once.

TLS REACTION	DUE TO INSUFFICIENT CATION-EXCHANGE RESINS	DUE TO INSUFFICIENT CALCIUM GLUCONATE
Muscle weakness		
Tetany		
Twitching		
Paresthesia		
Confusion		
Hallucination		
Syncope		

Abbreviations

http://evolve.elsevier.com/Cooper/adult/

Common Abbreviations

ABBREVIATION	MEANING	ABBREVIATION	MEANING
°C	degrees Centigrade	CPR	cardiopulmonary resuscitation
°F	degrees Fahrenheit	CT	computed tomography
@	at	dL	deciliter
≥	greater than	DNR	do not resuscitate
≤	less than	DTR	deep tendon reflex
↑	increase	Dx, dx	diagnosis
↓	decrease	ECG, EKG	electrocardiogram
1°	primary	EEG	electroencephalogram
2°	secondary	elix	elixir
Δ	change	ER/ED	emergency room/department
ABGs	arterial blood gases	ESR	erythrocyte sedimentation rate
ac	before meals	ETOH	ethyl alcohol
ADL	activities of daily living	FUO	fever of unknown origin
ad lib	freely as desired	Fx, fx	fracture
AED	automated external defibrillator	g/G	gram
AIDS	acquired immunodeficiency syndrome	GI	gastrointestinal
ama, AMA	against medical advice	gr	grain
BE	barium enema	gtt	drop; drops
bid, BID	two times a day	GTT	glucose tolerance test
BM	bowel movement	h, hr	hour
BMI	body mass index	H&P	history and physical examination
B/P, BP	blood pressure	HCT, Hct	hematocrit
BRP	bathroom privileges	Hgb	hemoglobin
BSA	body surface area	HIV	human immunodeficiency virus
BUN	blood urea nitrogen	hs	at bedtime, hour of sleep
C&S	culture and sensitivity	I&O	intake and output
$\bar{c}$	with	IM	intramuscular
cap	capsule	IV	intravenous
CBC	complete blood count	IVP	intravenous pyelogram
CDC	Centers for Disease Control and Prevention	K^+	potassium
		kg	kilogram
cm	centimeter	KUB	kidney, ureters, and bladder (radiograph)
c/o	complains of	KVO	keep vein open
CO	carbon monoxide	L	liter
CO_2	carbon dioxide	LLL	left lower lobe

Continued

Common Abbreviations—cont'd

ABBREVIATION	MEANING	ABBREVIATION	MEANING
LLQ	left lower quadrant	PO, po	orally, per os, by mouth
LMP	last menstrual period	prn	as often as necessary, when needed
LOC	level of consciousness	q	every
LUL	left upper lobe	qid, QID	four times a day
LUQ	left upper quadrant	RLL	right lower lobe
M	meter	RLQ	right lower quadrant
mcg	microgram	ROM	range of motion
mg	milligram	RUL	right upper lobe
mL	milliliter	RUQ	right upper quadrant
mm	millimeter	Rx	medication, prescription
mm Hg	millimeters of mercury	$\overline{s}$	without
MRI	magnetic resonance imaging	Sub-Q, subcut	subcutaneous
NG	nasogastric	$\overline{ss}$	half
NKA	no known allergies	SSE	soapsuds enema
NPO	nothing per os, nothing by mouth	stat	immediately
O_2	oxygen	tid, TID	three times a day
OD	optical density; overdose	TKO	to keep open
oz	ounce	TPN	total parenteral nutrition
pc	after meals	TPR	temperature, pulse, and respirations
PERRLA	pupils equal, round, and reactive to light and accommodation	TX, tx, Tx	treatment
pH	hydrogen ion concentration (acidity and alkalinity)	WBC	white blood cell

The Joint Commission "Do Not Use" Abbreviation List[a]

DO NOT USE	POTENTIAL PROBLEM	USE INSTEAD
U, u (unit)	Mistaken for "0" (zero), the number "4" (four), or "cc"	Write "unit"
IU (International Unit)	Mistaken for IV (intravenous) or the number 10 (ten)	Write "International Unit"
Q.D., QD, q.d., qd (daily)	Mistaken for each other	Write "daily"
Q.O.D., QOD, q.o.d., qod (every other day)	Period after the Q mistaken for "I" and the "O" mistaken for "I"	Write "every other day"
Trailing zero (X.0 mg)[b]	Decimal point is missed	Write X mg
Lack of leading zero (.X mg)	Decimal point is missed	Write 0.X mg
MS	Can mean morphine sulfate or magnesium sulfate	Write "morphine sulfate"
MSO_4 and $MgSO_4$	Confused for one another	Write "magnesium sulfate"

[a]Applies to all orders and all medication-related documentation that is handwritten (including free-text computer entry) or on preprinted forms.
[b]EXCEPTION: A "trailing zero" may be used only where required to demonstrate the level of precision of the value being reported, such as for laboratory results, imaging studies that report size of lesions, or catheter/tube sizes. It may not be used in medication orders or other medication-related documentation.
© The Joint Commission, Facts about the official "Do Not Use" list of abbreviations, 2019. Reprinted with permission.

Laboratory Reference Values

http://evolve.elsevier.com/Cooper/adult/

Reference Intervals for Hematology

TEST	CONVENTIONAL UNITS	SI UNITS
Acid hemolysis (Ham test)	No hemolysis	No hemolysis
Alkaline phosphatase, leukocyte	Total score, 14–100	Total score, 14–100
Cell counts		
Erythrocytes		
Males	4.6–6.2 million/mm³	4.6–6.2 × 10¹²/L
Females	4.2–5.4 million/mm³	4.2–5.4 × 10¹²/L
Children (varies with age)	4.5–5.1 million/mm³	4.5–5.1 × 10¹²/L
Leukocytes, total	5000–10,000/mm³	4.5–11.0 × 10⁹/L
Leukocytes, differential counts[a]		
Myelocytes	0%	0/L
Band neutrophils	3%–5%	150–400 × 10⁶/L
Segmented neutrophils	54%–62%	3000–5800 × 10⁶/L
Lymphocytes	20%–40%	1000–4000 × 10⁶/L
Monocytes	3%–6%	100–600 × 10⁶/L
Eosinophils	1%–4%	50–250 × 10⁶/L
Basophils	0.5%–1%	15–50 × 10⁶/L
Platelets	150,000–400,000/mm³	150–400 × 10⁹/L
Reticulocytes	25,000–75,000/mm³	25–75 × 10⁹/L
Coagulation tests	(0.5%–1.5% of erythrocytes)	
Bleeding time (template)	2.75–8.0 min	2.75–8.0 min
Coagulation time (glass tube)	5–15 min	5–15 min
D-Dimer	<0.5 mcg/mL	<0.5 mg/L
Factor VIII and other coagulation factors	50%–150% of normal	0.5–1.5 of normal
Fibrin split products (Thrombo-Welco test)	<10 mcg/mL	<10 mg/L
Fibrinogen	200–400 mg/dL	2.0–4.0 g/L
Partial thromboplastin time, activated (aPTT)	20–25 s	20–35 s
Prothrombin time (PT, Pro-time)	12.0–14.0 s	12.0–14.0 s
International normalized ratio (INR)	0.8–1.1	
Coombs' test		
Direct	Negative	Negative
Indirect	Negative	Negative
Corpuscular values of erythrocytes		
Mean corpuscular hemoglobin (MCH)	26–34 pg/cell	26–34 pg/cell
Mean corpuscular volume (MCV)	80–96 mm³	80–96 fL
Mean corpuscular hemoglobin concentration (MCHC)	32–36 g/dL	320–360 g/L
Haptoglobin	20–165 mg/dL	0.20–1.65 g/L
Hematocrit		

Reference Intervals for Hematology—cont'd

TEST	CONVENTIONAL UNITS	SI UNITS
Males	40–54 mL/dL	0.40–0.54
Females	35–47 mL/dL	0.37–0.47
Newborns	49–54 mL/dL	0.49–0.54
Children (varies with age)	35–49 mL/dL	0.35–0.49
Hemoglobin		
Males	13.0–18.0 g/dL	8.1–11.2 mmol/L
Females	12.0–16.0 g/dL	7.4–9.9 mmol/L
Newborns	16.5–19.5 g/dL	10.2–12.1 mmol/L
Children (varies with age)	11.2–16.5 g/dL	7.0–10.2 mmol/L
Hemoglobin, fetal	<1.0% of total	<0.01 of total
Hemoglobin A_{1C}	3%–5% of total	0.03–0.05 of total
Hemoglobin A_2	1.5%–3.0% of total	0.015–0.03 of total
Hemoglobin, plasma	0.0–5.0 mg/dL	0.0–3.2 µmol/L
Methemoglobin	30–130 mg/dL	19–80 µmol/L
Erythrocyte sedimentation rate (ESR)		
Wintrobe		
Males	0–5 mm/h	0–5 mm/h
Females	0–15 mm/h	0–15 mm/h
Westergren		
Males	0–15 mm/h	0–15 mm/h
Females	0–20 mm/h	0–20 mm/h

[a]Conventional units are percentages; SI units are absolute cell counts.
SI, International System of Units.

Reference Intervals[a] for Clinical Chemistry (Blood, Serum, and Plasma)

ANALYTE	CONVENTIONAL UNITS	SI UNITS
Acetoacetate plus acetone		
Qualitative	Negative	Negative
Quantitative	0.3–2.0 mg/dL	30–200 µmol/L
Acid phosphatase, serum (thymolphthalein monophosphate substrate)	0.1–0.6 units/L	0.1–0.6 units/L
Adrenocorticotropic hormone (ACTH), plasma, 8 AM	10–80 pg/mL	2–18 pmol/L
Alanine aminotransferase (ALT), Serum glutamic pyruvic transaminase (SGPT)	1–45 units/L	1–45 units/L
Albumin, serum	3.3–5.2 g/dL	33–52 g/L
Aldolase, serum	0.0–7.0 units/L	0.0–7.0 units/L
Aldosterone, plasma		
Standing	5–30 ng/dL	140–830 pmol/L
Recumbent	3–10 ng/dL	80–275 pmol/L
Alkaline, phosphatase (ALP), serum		
Adult	35–150 units/L	35–150 units/L
Adolescent	100–500 units/L	100–500 units/L
Child	100–350 units/L	100–350 units/L
Ammonia nitrogen, plasma	10–50 mmol/L	10–50 µmol/L
Amylase, serum	25–125 units/L	25–125 units/L
Anion gap, serum calculated	8–16 mEq/L	8–16 mmol/L
Ascorbic acid, blood	0.4–1.5 mg/dL	23–85 µmol/L
Aspartate aminotransferase (AST), Serum glutamic-oxaloacetic transaminase (SGOT)	1–36 units/L	1–36 units/L

Reference Intervals[a] for Clinical Chemistry (Blood, Serum, and Plasma)—cont'd

ANALYTE	CONVENTIONAL UNITS	SI UNITS
Base excess, arterial blood, calculated	0 ± 2 mEq/L	0 ± 2 mmol/L
Bicarbonate		
Venous plasma	23–29 mEq/L	23–29 mmol/L
Arterial blood	21–27 mEq/L	21–27 mmol/L
Bile acids, serum	0.3–3.0 mg/dL	0.8–7.6 µmol/L
Bilirubin, serum		
Conjugated	0.1–0.4 mg/dL	1.7–6.8 µmol/L
Total	0.3–1.1 mg/dL	5.1–19.0 µmol/L
Calcium, serum	8.4–10.6 mg/dL	2.10–2.65 mmol/L
Calcium, ionized, serum	4.25–5.25 mg/dL	1.05–1.30 mmol/L
Carbon dioxide, total, serum or plasma	24–31 mEq/L	24–31 mmol/L
Carbon dioxide tension (PCO_2), blood	35–45 mm Hg	35–45 mm Hg
β-Carotene, serum	60–260 mcg/dL	1.1–8.6 µmol/L
Ceruloplasmin, serum	23–44 mg/dL	230–440 mg/L
Chloride, serum or plasma	96–106 mEq/L	96–106 mmol/L
Cholesterol, serum or EDTA plasma		
Desirable range	<200 mg/dL	5.20 mmol/L
Low-density lipoprotein (LDL) cholesterol	60–180 mg/dL	1.55–4.65 mmol/L
High-density lipoprotein (HDL) cholesterol	30–80 mg/dL	0.80–2.05 mmol/L
Copper	70–140 mcg/dL	11–22 µmol/L
Cortisol, plasma		
8:00 AM	6–23 mcg/dL	170–630 nmol/L
4:00 PM	3–15 mcg/dL	80–410 nmol/L
10:00 PM	<50% of 8:00 AM value	<50% of 8:00 AM value
Creatine, serum		
Males	0.2–0.5 mg/dL	15–40 µmol/L
Females	0.3–0.9 mg/dL	25–70 µmol/L
Creatine kinase (CK), serum		
Males	55–170 units/L	55–170 units/L
Females	30–135 units/L	30–135 units/L
Creatinine kinase MB isoenzyme, serum	<5% of total CK activity	<5% of total CK activity
	<5% of ng/mL by immunoassay	<5% of ng/mL by immunoassay
Creatinine, serum	0.6–1.2 mg/dL	50–110 µmol/L
Erythrocytes	145–540 ng/mL	330–120 nmol/L
Estradiol-17β, adult		
Males	10–65 pg/mL	35–240 pmol/L
Females		
Follicular	30–100 pg/mL	110–370 pmol/L
Ovulatory	200–400 pg/mL	730–1470 pmol/L
Luteal	50–140 pg/mL	180–510 pmol/L
Ferritin, serum	20–200 ng/mL	20–200 mcg/L
Fibrinogen, plasma	200–400 mg/dL	2.0–4.0 g/L
Folate, serum	3–18 ng/mL	6.8–4.1 nmol/L
Follicle-stimulating hormone (FSH), plasma		
Males	4–25 mU/mL	4–25 units/L
Females, premenopausal	4–30 mU/mL	4–30 units/L
Females, postmenopausal	40–250 mU/mL	40–250 units/L
Gastrin, fasting, serum	0–100 pg/mL	0–100 mg/L

Continued

Reference Intervals[a] for Clinical Chemistry (Blood, Serum, and Plasma)—cont'd

ANALYTE	CONVENTIONAL UNITS	SI UNITS
Glucose, fasting, plasma or serum	70–115 mg/dL	3.9–6.4 nmol/L
γ-Glutamyltransferase (GGT), serum	5–40 units/L	5–40 units/L
Growth hormone (hGH), plasma, adult, fasting	0–6 ng/mL	0–6 mcg/L
Haptoglobin, serum	20–165 mg/dL	0.20–1.65 g/L
Immunoglobulins, serum (see table of Reference Intervals for Tests of Immunologic Function)		
Iron, serum	75–175 mcg/dL	13–31 mmol/L
Iron-binding capacity, serum		
Total	250–410 mcg/dL	45–73 mmol/L
Saturation	20%–55%	0.20–0.55
Lactate		
Venous whole blood	5.0–20.0 mg/dL	0.6–2.2 mmol/L
Arterial whole blood	5.0–15.0 mg/dL	0.6–1.7 mmol/L
Lactate dehydrogenase (LD), serum	110–220 units/L	110–220 units/L
Lipase, serum	10–140 units/L	10–140 units/L
Lutropin (LH), serum		
Males	1–9 units/L	1–9 units/L
Females		
Follicular phase	2–10 units/L	2–10 units/L
Midcycle peak	15–65 units/L	15–65 units/L
Luteal phase	1–12 units/L	1–12 units/L
Postmenopausal	12–65 units/L	12–65 units/L
Magnesium, serum	1.3–2.1 mg/dL	0.65–1.05 mmol/L
Osmolality	275–295 mOsm/kg water	275–295 mOsm/kg water
Oxygen, blood, arterial, room air		
Partial pressure (PaO_2)	80–100 mm Hg	80–100 mm Hg
Saturation (SaO_2)	95%–100%	95%–100%
pH, arterial blood	7.35–7.45	7.35–7.45
Phosphate, inorganic, serum		
Adult	3.0–4.5 mg/dL	1.0–1.5 mmol/L
Child	4.0–7.0 mg/dL	1.3–2.3 mmol/L
Potassium		
Serum	3.5–5.0 mEq/L	3.5–5.0 mmol/L
Plasma	3.5–4.5 mEq/L	3.5–4.5 mmol/L
Progesterone, serum, adult		
Males	0.0–0.4 ng/mL	0.0–1.3 mmol/L
Females		
Follicular phase	0.1–1.5 ng/mL	0.3–4.8 mmol/L
Luteal phase	2.5–28.0 ng/mL	8.0–89.0 mmol/L
Prolactin, serum		
Males	1.0–15.0 ng/mL	1.0–15.0 mcg/L
Females	1.0–20.0 ng/mL	1.0–20.0 mcg/L
Protein, serum, electrophoresis		
Total	6.0–8.0 g/dL	60–80 g/L
Albumin	3.5–5.5 g/dL	35–55 g/L
Globulins		
α_1	0.2–0.4 g/dL	2.0–4.0 g/L
α_2	0.5–0.9 g/dL	5.0–9.0 g/L

Reference Intervals[a] for Clinical Chemistry (Blood, Serum, and Plasma)—cont'd

ANALYTE	CONVENTIONAL UNITS	SI UNITS
β	0.6–1.1 g/dL	6.0–11.0 g/L
γ	0.7–1.7 g/dL	7.0–17.0 g/L
Pyruvate, blood	0.3–0.9 mg/dL	0.03–0.10 mmol/L
Rheumatoid factor	0.0–30.0 IU/mL	0.0–30.0 kIU/L
Sodium, serum or plasma	135–145 mEq/L	135–145 mmol/L
Testosterone, plasma		
Males, adult	300–1200 ng/dL	10.4–41.6 nmol/L
Females, adult	20–75 ng/dL	0.7–2.6 nmol/L
Pregnant females	40–200 ng/dL	1.4–6.9 nmol/L
Thyroglobulin	3–42 ng/mL	3–42 mcg/L
Thyrotropin (hTSH), serum	0.4–4.8 mIU/mL	0.4–4.8 mIU/L
Thyrotropin-releasing hormone (TRH)	5–60 pg/mL	5–60 ng/L
Thyroxine (FT_4), free, serum	0.9–2.1 ng/dL	12–27 pmol/L
Thyroxine (T_4), serum	4.5–12.0 mcg/mL	58–154 nmol/L
Thyroxine-binding globulin (TBG)	15.0–34.0 mcg/mL	15.0–34.0 mg/L
Transferrin	250–430 mg/dL	2.5–4.3 g/L
Triglycerides, serum, after 12-h fast	40–150 mg/dL	0.4–1.5 g/L
Triiodothyronine (T_3), serum	70–190 ng/dL	1.1–2.9 nmol/L
Triiodothyronine uptake, resin (T_3RU)	25%–38%	0.25–0.38
Troponin I	0.05–0.50 ng/mL	0.05–0.5 ng/mL
Urate		
Males	2.5–8.0 mg/dL	150–480 µmol/L
Females	2.2–7.0 mg/dL	130–420 µmol/L
Urea, serum or plasma	24–49 mg/dL	4.0–8.2 nmol/L
Urea, nitrogen, serum or plasma	11–23 mg/dL	8.0–16.4 nmol/L
Viscosity, serum	1.1–1.8 × water	1.1–1.8 × water
Vitamin A, serum	20–80 mcg/dL	0.70–2.80 mcmol/L
Vitamin B_{12}, serum	180–900 pg/mL	133–664 pmol/L

[a]Reference values may vary depending on the method and sample source used.
EDTA, Ethylenediaminetetraacetic acid; SI, International System of Units.

Reference Intervals for Therapeutic Drug Monitoring (Serum or Plasma)[a]

ANALYTE	THERAPEUTIC RANGE	TOXIC CONCENTRATIONS	PROPRIETARY NAME(S)
Analgesics			
acetaminophen	10–40 mcg/mL	>150 mcg/mL	Tylenol, Datril
salicylate	100–250 mcg/mL	>300 mcg/mL	Aspirin, Bufferin
Antibiotics			
amikacin	20–30 mcg/mL	Peak >35 mcg/mL Trough >10 mcg/mL	Amkin
gentamicin	5–10 mcg/mL	Peak >10 mcg/mL Trough >2 mcg/mL	Garamycin
tobramycin	5–10 mcg/mL	Peak >10 mcg/mL Trough >2 mcg/mL	Nebcin
vancomycin	5–35 mcg/mL	Peak >40 mcg/mL Trough >10 mcg/mL	Vancocin
Anticonvulsants			
carbamazepine	5–12 mcg/mL	>15 mcg/mL	Tegretol
ethosuximide	40–100 mcg/mL	>250 mcg/mL	Zarontin
phenobarbital	15–40 mcg/mL	40–100 ng/mL (varies widely)	Luminal

Continued

Reference Intervals for Therapeutic Drug Monitoring (Serum or Plasma)[a]—cont'd

ANALYTE	THERAPEUTIC RANGE	TOXIC CONCENTRATIONS	PROPRIETARY NAME(S)
phenytoin	10–20 mcg/mL	>20 mcg/mL	Dilantin
primidone	5–12 mcg/mL	>15 mcg/mL	Mysoline
valproic acid	50–100 mcg/mL	>100 mcg/mL	Depakene
Antineoplastics and Immunosuppressives			
cyclosporine A	150–350 ng/mL	>400 ng/mL	Sandimmune
methotrexate, high-dose, 48 h	Variable	>1 µmol/L, 48 h after dose	
sirolimus (within 1 h of 2-mg dose)	4.5–14 ng/mL	Variable	Rapamune
sirolimus (within 1 h of 5-mg dose)	10–28 ng/mL	Variable	Rapamune
tacrolimus (FK-506), whole blood	3–20 mcg/L	>15 mcg/L	Prograf
Bronchodilators and Respiratory Stimulants			
caffeine	3–15 ng/mL	>30 mcg/mL	Elixophyllin
theophylline (aminophylline)	10–20 mcg/mL	>30 mcg/mL	Quibron
Cardiovascular Drugs			
amiodarone (obtain specimen more than 8 h after last dose)	1.0–2.0 mcg/mL	>2.0 mcg/mL	Cordarone
digoxin (obtain specimen more than 6 h after last dose)	0.8–2.0 mcg/mL	>2.4 ng/mL	Lanoxin
disopyramide	2–5 mcg/mL	>7 mcg/mL	Norpace
flecainide	0.2–1.0 mcg/mL	>0.1 mcg/mL	Tambocor
lidocaine	1.5–5.0 mcg/mL	>6 mcg/mL	Xylocaine
mexiletine	0.7–2.0 mcg/mL	>2 mcg/mL	Mexitil
procainamide	4–10 mcg/mL	>12 mcg/mL	Pronestyl
procainamide plus NAPA (N-acetyl procainamide)	8–30 mcg/mL	>30 mcg/mL	
propranolol	50–100 ng/mL	Variable	Inderal
quinidine	2–5 mcg/mL	>6 mcg/mL	Cardioquin, Quinaglute
tocainide	4–10 ng/mL	>10 ng/mL	Tonocard
Psychopharmacological Drugs			
amitriptyline	120–150 ng/mL	>500 ng/mL	Elavil, Triavil
bupropion	25–100 ng/mL	Not applicable	Wellbutrin
desipramine	150–300 ng/mL	>500 ng/mL	Norpramin
imipramine	125–250 ng/mL	>400 ng/mL	Tofranil
lithium (obtain specimen 12 h after last dose)	0.6–1.5 mEq/L	>1.5 mEq/L	Lithobid
nortriptyline	50–150 ng/mL	>500 ng/mL	Aventyl, Pamelor

[a]Values may vary depending on the method and sample collection device used. Always consult the reference values provided by the laboratory performing the analysis.

Reference Intervals[a] for Clinical Chemistry (Urine)

ANALYTE	CONVENTIONAL UNITS	SI UNITS
Acetone and acetoacetate, qualitative	Negative	Negative
Albumin		
Qualitative	Negative	Negative
Quantitative	10–100 mg/24 h	0.15–1.5 µmol/day
Aldosterone	3–20 mcg/24 h	8.3–55 nmol/day

Reference Intervals^a for Clinical Chemistry (Urine)—cont'd

ANALYTE	CONVENTIONAL UNITS	SI UNITS
ᴅ-Aminolevulinic acid (d-ALA)	1.3–7.0 mg/24 h	10–53 µmol/day
Amylase	<17 units/h	<17 units/h
Amylase-to-creatinine clearance ratio	0.01–0.04	0.01–0.04
Bilirubin, qualitative	Negative	Negative
Calcium (regular diet)	<250 mg/24 h	<6.3 nmol/day
Catecholamines		
Epinephrine	<10 mcg/24 h	<55 nmol/day
Norepinephrine	<100 mcg/24 h	<590 nmol/day
Total free catecholamines	4–126 mcg/24 h	24–745 nmol/day
Total metanephrines	0.1–1.6 mg/24 h	0.5–8.1 µmol/day
Chloride (varies with intake)	110–250 mEq/24 h	110–250 mmol/day
Copper	0–50 mcg/24 h	0.0–0.80 µmol/day
Cortisol, free	10–100 mcg/24 h	27.6–276 nmol/day
Creatine		
Males	0–40 mg/24 h	0.0–0.30 mmol/day
Females	0–80 mg/24 h	0.0–0.60 mmol/day
Creatinine	15–25 mg/kg/24 h	0.13–0.22 mmol/kg/day
Creatinine clearance (endogenous)		
Males	110–150 mL/min/1.73 m²	110–150 mL/min/1.73 m²
Females	105–132 mL/min/1.73 m²	105–132 mL/min/1.73 m²
Cystine or cysteine	Negative	Negative
Dehydroepiandrosterone		
Males	0.2–2.0 mg/24 h	0.7–6.9 µmol/day
Females	0.2–1.8 mg/24 h	0.7–6.2 µmol/day
Estrogens, total		
Males	4–25 mcg/24 h	14–90 nmol/day
Females	5–100 mcg/24 h	18–360 nmol/day
Glucose (as reducing substance)	<250 mg/24 h	<250 mg/day
Hemoglobin and myoglobin, qualitative	Negative	Negative
Hemogentisic acid, qualitative	Negative	Negative
17-Hydroxycorticosteroids		
Males	3–9 mg/24 h	8.3–25 µmol/day
Females	2–8 mg/24 h	5.5–22 µmol/day
5-Hydroxyindoleacetic acid		
Qualitative	Negative	Negative
Quantitative	2–6 mg/24 h	10–31 µmol/day
17-Ketogenic steroids		
Males	5–23 mg/24 h	17–80 µmol/day
Females	3–15 mg/24 h	10–52 µmol/day
17-Ketosteroids		
Males	8–22 mg/24 h	28–76 µmol/day
Females	6–15 mg/24 h	21–52 µmol/day
Magnesium	6–10 mEq/24 h	3–5 mmol/day
Metanephrines	0.05–1.2 ng/mg creatinine	0.03–0.70 mmol/mmol creatinine
Osmolality	38–1400 mOsm/kg water	38–1400 mOsm/kg water
pH	4.6–8.0	4.6–8.0
Phenylpyruvic acid, qualitative	Negative	Negative

Continued

Reference Intervals[a] for Clinical Chemistry (Urine)—cont'd

ANALYTE	CONVENTIONAL UNITS	SI UNITS
Phosphate	0.4–1.3 g/24 h	13–42 mmol/day
Porphobilinogen		
Qualitative	Negative	Negative
Quantitative	<2 mg/24 h	<9 µmol/day
Porphyrins		
Coproporphyrin	50–250 mcg/24 h	77–380 nmol/day
Uroporphyrin	10–30 mcg/24 h	12–36 nmol/day
Potassium	25–125 mEq/24 h	25–125 mmol/day
Pregnanediol		
Males	0.0–1.9 mg/24 h	0.0–6.0 µmol/day
Females		
Proliferative phase	0.0–2.6 mg/24 h	0.0–8.0 µmol/day
Luteal phase	2.6–10.6 mg/24 h	8–33 µmol/day
Postmenopausal	0.2–1.0 mg/24 h	0.6–3.1 µmol/day
Pregnanetriol	0.0–2.5 mg/24 h	0.0–7.4 µmol/day
Protein, total		
Qualitative	Negative	Negative
Quantitative	10–150 mg/24 h	10–150 mg/day
Protein-to-creatinine ratio	<0.2	<0.2
Sodium (regular diet)	60–260 mEq/24 h	60–260 mmol/day
Specific gravity		
Random specimen	1.003–1.030	1.003–1.030
24-h collection	1.015–1.025	1.015–1.025
Urate (regular diet)	250–750 mg/24 h	1.5–4.4 mmol/day
Urobilinogen	0.5–4.0 mg/24 h	0.6–6.8 µmol/day
Vanillylmandelic acid (VMA)	1.0–8.0 mg/24 h	5–40 µmol/day

[a]Values may vary depending on the method used.
SI, International System of Units.

Reference Intervals for Toxic Substances

ANALYTE	CONVENTIONAL UNITS	SI UNITS
Arsenic, urine	<130 mcg/24 h	<1.7 µmol/day
Bromides, serum, inorganic	<100 mg/dL	<10 mmol/L
Toxic symptoms	140–1000 mg/dL	14–100 mmol/L
Carboxyhemoglobin, blood	Saturation, percent	
Urban environment	<5%	<0.05
Smokers	<12%	<0.12
Symptoms		
Headache	>15%	>0.15
Nausea and vomiting	>25%	>0.25
Potentially lethal	>50%	>0.50
Ethanol, blood	<0.05 mg/dL, 0.005%	<1.0 mmol/L
Intoxication	>100 mg/dL, 0.1%	>22 mmol/L
Marked intoxication	300–400 mg/dL, 0.3%–0.4%	65–87 mmol/L
Alcoholic stupor	400–500 mg/dL, 0.4%–0.5%	87–109 mmol/L
Coma	>500 mg/dL, 0.5%	>109 mmol/L
Lead, blood		
Adults	<20 mcg/dL	<1.0 µmol/L

Reference Intervals for Toxic Substances—cont'd

ANALYTE	CONVENTIONAL UNITS	SI UNITS
Children	<10 mcg/dL	<0.5 μmol/L
Lead, urine	<80 mcg/24 h	<0.4 μmol/day
Mercury, urine	<10 mcg/24 h	<150 nmol/day

SI, International System of Units.

Reference Intervals for Tests Performed on Cerebrospinal Fluid

TEST	CONVENTIONAL UNITS	SI UNITS
Cells	<5 mm³; all mononuclear	<5 × 10⁶/L; all mononuclear
Protein electrophoresis	Albumin predominant	Albumin predominant
Glucose	50–75 mg/dL (20 mg/dL less than in serum)	2.8–4.2 mmol/L (1.1 mmol/L less than in serum)
IgG		
Children, <14 years	<8% of total protein	<0.08 of total protein
Adults	<14% of total protein	<0.14 of total protein
IgG index	0.3–0.6	0.3–0.6
Oligoclonal banding on electrophoresis	Absent	Absent
Pressure, opening	70–180 mm H₂O	70–180 mm H₂O
Protein, total	<15–45 mg/dL	150–450 mg/L

SI, International System of Units.

Reference Intervals for Tests of Gastrointestinal Function

TEST	CONVENTIONAL UNITS
Bentiromide	6-h urinary arylamine excretion. 57% excludes pancreatic insufficiency
β-Carotene, serum	60–250 ng/dL
Fecal fat estimation	
Qualitative	No fat globules seen by high-power microscope
Quantitative	<6 g/24 h (>95% coefficient of fat absorption)
Gastric acid output	
Basal	
Males	0.0–10.5 mmol/h
Females	0.0–5.6 mmol/h
Maximum (after histamine or pentagastrin)	
Males	9.0–48.0 mmol/h
Females	6.0–31.0 mmol/h
Ratio: basal/maximum	
Males	0.0–0.31
Females	0.0–0.29
Secretion test, pancreatic fluid	
Volume	>1.8 mL/kg/h
Bicarbonate	>80 mEq/L
D-Xylose absorption test, urine	>20% of ingested dose excreted in 5 h

Reference Intervals for Tests of Immunologic Function

TEST	CONVENTIONAL UNITS	SI UNITS
Autoantibodies, Serum, Adult		
Anti-CCP antibody	0–19 units	
Anti-dsDNA antibody	0–40 IU	0–40 IU
Antinuclear antibody	<1:40	
Rheumatoid factor (total IgG, IgA, IgM)	0–30 mg/dL	
Complement, Serum		
C3	85–175 mg/dL	0.85–1.75 g/L
C4	15–45 mg/dL	150–450 mg/L
Total hemolytic (CH$_{50}$)	150–250 units/mL	150–250 units/mL
Immunoglobulins, Serum, Adult		
IgA	70–310 mg/dL	0.70–3.1 g/L
IgD	0.0–6.0 mg/dL	0.0–60 g/L
IgE	0.0–430 mg/dL	0.0–430 mg/L
IgG	640–1350 ng/dL	6.4–13.5 mcg/L
IgM	90–350 mg/dL	0.90–3.5 g/L

Anti-CCP, Anticyclic citrullinated peptide; *dsDNA,* double-stranded DNA; *Ig,* immunoglobulin; *SI,* International System of Units.

Reference Intervals for Lymphocytes Subsets, Whole Blood, Heparinized

ANTIGEN(S) EXPRESSED	CELL TYPE	PERCENTAGE	ABSOLUTE CELL COUNT
CD2	E rosette T cells	73–87	860–1880
CD3	Total T cells	56–77	140–370
CD3 and CD4	Helper-inducer cells	32–54	550–1190
CD3 and CD8	Suppressor-cytotoxic cells	24–37	430–1060
CD3 and DR	Activated T cells	5–14	70–310
CD16 and CD56	Natural killer (NK) cells	8–22	130–500
CD 19	Total B cells	7–17	140–370

Helper-to-suppressor ratio: 0.8–1.8.

Reference Values for Semen Analysis

TEST	CONVENTIONAL UNITS	SI UNITS
Volume	2–5 mL	2–5 mL
Liquefaction	Complete in 15 min	Complete in 15 min
pH	7.2–8.0	7.2–8.0
Leukocytes	Occasional or absent	Occasional or absent
Spermatozoa		
Count	60–150 × 10^6 mL	60–150 × 10^6 mL
Motility	>80% motile	>0.80 motile
Morphology	80%–90% normal forms	>0.80–0.90 normal
Fructose	>150 mg/dL	>8.33 mmol/L

SI, International System of Units.

References

CHAPTER 1

FamousScientists.org: Robert Hooke, 2014. Retrieved from: https://www.famousscientists.org/robert-hooke.

Lincoln D: Smaller than small: looking for something new with the LHC, 2014. Retrieved from: http://www.pbs.org/wgbh/nova/blogs/physics/2014/10/smaller-than-small/.

Moskowitz C: What is the smallest thing in the universe? LiveScience, 2012. Retrieved from: www.livescience.com/23232-smallest-ingredients-universe-physics.html.

Patton KT: Anatomy and physiology, ed 10, St. Louis, 2019, Mosby.

CHAPTER 2

American Society of Anesthesiologists (ASA): Practice guidelines for preoperative fasting and the use of pharmacologic agents to reduce the risk of pulmonary aspiration: Application to healthy patients undergoing elective procedures: An updated report by the American Society of Anesthesiologists Task Force on Preoperative Fasting and the Use of Pharmacologic Agents to Reduce the Risk of Pulmonary Aspiration. Anesthesiology 126:376-393, 2017. Retrieved from https://pubs.asahq.org/anesthesiology/article/126/3/376/19733/Practice-Guidelines-for-Preoperative-Fasting-and

Asthma and Allergy Foundation of America (AAFA): Types of latex reactions, n.d. Retrieved from: www.aafa.org/latex-allergy.aspx.

Blanchard JC, Denholm B: Association of operating room nurses, AORNJ 95(5):658–667, 2012.

Harris LJ, Moudgill N, Hager E, et al: Incidence of anastomotic leak in patients undergoing elective colon resection without mechanical bowel preparation: our updated experience and two-year review, American Surgeon 75(9):828–833, 2009.

The Joint Commission (TJC): The Universal Protocol for Preventing Wrong Site, Wrong Procedure, Wrong Person Surgery, n.d. Retrieved from: www.jointcommission.org/standards/universal-protocol/.

Kaiser Family Foundation (KFF): Prescription drugs and older adults. Retrieved from: https://www.kff.org/health-reform/issue-brief/data-note-prescription-drugs-and-older-adults/.

Kowalski TJ, Kothari SN, Mathiason M, et al: Impact of hair removal on surgical site infection rates: a prospective randomized noninferiority trial, Journal of the American College of Surgeons 223(5):P704-711, 2016. Retrieved from: http://www.journalacs.org/article/S1072-7515(16)30035-7/fulltext?rss=yes.

Mayo Clinic Staff: Latex allergy, n.d. Retrieved from: https://www.mayoclinic.org/diseases-conditions/latex-allergy/symptoms-causes/syc-20374287.

Mosby's 2021 Nursing Drug Reference. St. Louis, Elsevier, 2021.

National Council on Patient Information and Education (NCPIE): Medication management for older adults, 2018. Retrieved from: http://www.bemedwise.org/medication-safety/medication-therapy-management-for-seniors.

Nursing Interventions and Rationales: Latex allergy response, 2013. Retrieved from: http://nursinginterventionsrationales.blogspot.com/2013/07/latex-allergy-response.html.

Scabini S, Rimini E, Rairone E, et al: Colon and rectal surgery for cancer without mechanical bowel preparation: Onecenter randomized prospective trial, World J Surg Oncol 10:196, 2012.

CHAPTER 3

American Burn Association: Burn Injury Fact Sheet, 2018. Retrieved from: https://ameriburn.org/wp-content/uploads/2017/12/nbaw-factsheet_121417-1.pdf .

American Cancer Society: Survival rates for melanoma skin cancer 2020. Retrieved from: https://www.cancer.org/cancer/melanoma-skin-cancer/detection-diagnosis-staging/survival-rates-for-melanoma-skin-cancer-by-stage.html.

American Family Physician: STEPS New drug reviews: retapamulin (altabax) 1% topical ointment for the treatment of impetigo, 2007. Retrieved from: http://www.aafp.org/afp/2007/1115/p1537.html.

Carteret M: Traditional Asian health beliefs and healing practices. Dimensions of Culture, 2011. Retrieved from: http://www.dimensionsofculture.com/2010/10/traditional-asian-health-beliefs-healing-practices/.

Cancer.net: Melanoma: statistics, 2021. Retrieved from: https://www.cancer.net/cancer-types/melanoma/statistics.

Centers for Disease Control and Prevention (CDC): Skin cancer: what can I do to reduce my risk?, 2021. Retrieved from: https://www.cdc.gov/cancer/skin/basic_info/prevention.htm.

Centers for Disease Control and Prevention (CDC): Group A streptococcal (GAS) disease: impetigo, 2020. Retrieved from: https://www.cdc.gov/groupastrep/diseases-public/impetigo.html.

Centers for Disease Control and Prevention (CDC): Parasites—lice, 2019a. Retrieved from: https://www.cdc.gov/parasites/lice/index.html.

Centers for Disease Control and Prevention (CDC): Shingles (herpes zoster): about shingles, 2019b. Retrieved from: https://www.cdc.gov/shingles/about/overview.html.

Centers for Disease Control and Prevention (CDC): Shingles (herpes zoster): management of patients with herpes zoster, 2019c. Retrieved from: https://www.cdc.gov/shingles/hcp/hc-settings.html.

Centers for Disease Control and Prevention (CDC): Vaccines and preventable diseases: shingle vaccination, 2018. Retrieved from: https://www.cdc.gov/vaccines/vpd/shingles/public/shingrix/index.html.

Centers for Disease Control and Prevention (CDC): Genital Herpes, 2017. Retrieved from: https://www.cdc.gov/std/herpes/stdfact-herpes.htm.

Chrysopoulo, MT: Tissue flap classification. 2017. Retrieved from: https://emedicine.medscape.com/article/1284474-overview.

Daley BJ: Drugs, diseases, & procedures: Wound care treatment and management. Retrieved from: https://emedicine.medscape.com/article/194018-treatment.

Lewis LS, Steele RW: Medscape: Impetigo medication, 2019. Retrieved from: https://emedicine.medscape.com/article/965254-medication.

Lupus Foundation of America: Diagnosing lupus, 2018. Retrieved from: https://www.lupus.org/resources/diagnosing-lupus-guide.

Lupus Foundation of America: What is lupus? 2020. Retrieved from: http://www.lupus.org/answers/entry/what-is-lupus.

Mayo Clinic: Acne, 2020a. Retrieved from: https://www.mayoclinic.org/diseases-conditions/acne/symptoms-causes/syc-20368047.

Mayo Clinic: Genital herpes, 2020b. Retrieved from: https://www.mayoclinic.org/diseases-conditions/genital-herpes/diagnosis-treatment/drc-20356167

Mayo Clinic: Pityriasis rosea, 2020c. Retrieved from: https://www.mayoclinic.org/diseases-conditions/pityriasis-rosea/symptoms-causes/syc-20376405.

Mayo Clinic: Psoriasis, 2020d. Retrieved from: https://www.mayoclinic.org/diseases-conditions/psoriasis/diagnosis-treatment/drc-20355845.

Mayo Clinic: Self-injury/cutting, 2018. Retrieved from: http://www.mayoclinic.org/diseases-conditions/self-injury/symptoms-causes/dxc-20165427.

Mayo Clinic: Lupus, 2014. Retrieved from: http://www.mayoclinic.org/diseases-conditions/lupus/basics/tests-diagnosis/CON-20019676.

Melanoma Research Foundation: Facts and stats, 2017. Retrieved from: https://www.melanoma.org/.

National Library of Medicine (NLM): MedlinePlus.gov: Retapamulin, 2016. Retrieved from: https://medlineplus.gov/druginfo/meds/a607049.html.

National Library of Medicine (NLM): MedlinePlus.gov: Cellulitis, 2018. Retrieved from: https://medlineplus.gov/ency/article/000855.htm.

National Pressure Ulcer Advisory Panel (NPUAP): NPUAP Position Statement on Staging – 2017 Clarifications, 2017. Retrieved from https://cdn.ymaws.com/npiap.com/resource/resmgr/npuap-position-statement-on-.pdf

Sheehan MP, Rustin MH, Atherton DJ, et al: Efficacy of traditional Chinese herbal therapy in adult atopic dermatitis, Lancet 340:13–17, 1992

US Food & Drug Administration (FDA): Integra® dermal regeneration template, n.d. Retrieved from: www.accessdata.fda.gov/cdrh_docs/pdf/P900033S008d.pdf.

WebMD: Dermatitis medicamentosa, 2019. Retrieved from: https://www.webmd.com/skin-problems-and-treatments/picture-of-dermatitis-medicamentosa

WebMD: Skin condition and acne, 2020. Retrieved from: https://www.webmd.com/skin-problems-and-treatments/acne/default.htm.

CHAPTER 4

American Cancer Society (ACS): Osteosarcoma, n.d. Retrieved from: https://www.cancer.org/cancer/osteosarcoma.html.

Arthritis Foundation: Rheumatoid arthritis: causes, symptoms, treatment and more, n.d. Retrieved from: http://www.arthritis.org/about-arthritis/types/rheumatoid-arthritis/symptoms.php.

Centers for Disease Control and Prevention (CDC): Genomics & Precision Health: Osteoporosis, 2020. Retrieved from: https://www.cdc.gov/nchs/fastats/osteoporosis.htm.

Cleveland Clinic: Osteomyelitis, 2017. Retrieved from: https://my.clevelandclinic.org/health/diseases/9495-osteomyelitis.

Elam REW: Osteoporosis treatment & management, 2021a, Medscape. Retrieved from: https://emedicine.medscape.com/article/330598-treatment.

Elam, REW: What are the types of primary osteoporosis?, 2021b. Medscape. Retrieved from: https://www.medscape.com/answers/330598-82980/what%20-are-the-types-of-primary-osteoporosis.

Freeman J: RA facts: What are the latest statistics on rheumatoid arthritis?, 2018. Rheumatoid Arthritis Support Network (RASN). Retrieved from: https://www.rheumatoidarthritis.org/ra/facts-and-statistics/.

Gagel R: Preventing costly bone fractures – why don't we do what works?, 2019. American Journal of Managed Care.

Retrieved from: https://www.nof.org/news/preventing-costly-bone-fractures-why-dont-we-do-what-works/.

International Osteoporosis Foundation: Diagnosis, 2021. Retrieved from: https://www.osteoporosis.foundation/patients/diagnosis.

Kosova E, Bergmark B, Piazza G. Fat embolism syndrome. Circulation. 2015 Jan 20;131(3):317-20. https://doi.org/10.1161/CIRCULATIONAHA.114.010835. PMID: 25601951.

Lewis SL, Heitkemper MM, Dirksen SR, et al: Medical-surgical nursing: Assessment and management of clinical problems, ed 10, St. Louis, 2016, Mosby.

Mayo Clinic: Ankylosing spondylitis, 2019a. Retrieved from: https://www.mayoclinic.org/diseases-conditions/ankylosing-spondylitis/symptoms-causes/syc-20354808.

Mayo Clinic: Osteoporosis, 2019b. Retrieved from: https://www.mayoclinic.org/diseases-conditions/osteoporosis/symptoms-causes/syc-20351968.

Mayo Clinic: Carpal tunnel syndrome, 2021. Retrieved from: https://www.mayoclinic.org/diseases-conditions/carpal-tunnel-syndrome/diagnosis-treatment/drc-20355608.

National Institute of Arthritis and Musculoskeletal and Skin Diseases (NIAMS): Osteoarthritis, 2019. National Institutes of Health (NIH). Retrieved from: https://www.niams.nih.gov/health-topics/osteoarthritis.

National Institute of Arthritis and Musculoskeletal and Skin Diseases (NIAMS): Ankylosing spondylitis, 2020. National Institutes of Health (NIH). Retrieved from: https://www.niams.nih.gov/health-topics/ankylosing-spondylitis.

National Library of Medicine (NLM): Febuxostat, 2019. MedlinePlus. Retrieved from: https://medlineplus.gov/druginfo/meds/a609020.html.

National Library of Medicine (NLM): Glucosamine, 2021. MedlinePlus. Retrieved from: https://medlineplus.gov/druginfo/natural/807.html.

National Osteoporosis Foundation: Are you at risk?, n.d. Retrieved from: https://www.nof.org/preventing-fractures/general-facts/bone-basics/are-you-at-risk/.

NIH Osteoporosis and Related Bone Diseases National Resource Center: Bed rest and immobilization: Risk factors for bone loss, 2018. National Institutes of Health (NIH). Retrieved from: https://www.niams.nih.gov/Health_Info/Bone/Osteoporosis/Conditions_Behaviors/bed_rest.asp.

NIH Osteoporosis and Related Bone Diseases National Resource Center: Osteoporosis overview, 2019. National Institutes of Health (NIH). Retrieved from: https://www.bones.nih.gov/health-info/bone/osteoporosis/overview.

Pagana KD, Pagana TJ: Mosby's manual of diagnostic and laboratory tests, ed 5, St. Louis, 2014, Mosby.

Poindexter, KHC: Nursing Management of Fibromyalgia Syndrome. MEDSURG Nursing, 26(5), 349–351, 2017.

Rheumatoid Arthritis Support Network: RA Facts: What are the latest statistics on rheumatoid arthritis?, 2019. Retrieved from: https://www.rheumatoidarthritis.org/ra/facts-and-statistics/.

Skidmore-Roth L: Mosby's 2017 nursing drug reference, ed 30, St. Louis, 2016, Elsevier.

Spondylitis Association of America: Overview of psoriatic arthritis, 2019. Retrieved from: https://www.spondylitis.org/Psoriatic-Arthritis/.

US Food and Drug Administration (FDA): General information about hip implants, 2019. Retrieved from: https://www.fda.gov/medical-devices/metal-metal-hip-implants/general-information-about-hip-implants.

CHAPTER 5

Ackley BJ, Ladwig GB: Nursing diagnosis handbook: An evidence-based guide to planning care, ed 12, St. Louis, 2020, Mosby

American Academy of Family Physicians: Practice guidelines: IDSA updates guidelines for diagnosis and management. Am Fam Physician, 2018 May 15, 97(10):676-677.

American Cancer Society (ACS): Treatments and side effects, n.d. Retrieved from: https://www.cancer.org/treatment/treatments-and-side-effects.html.

American Cancer Society (ACS): Key statistics about Kaposi sarcoma, 2018. Retrieved from: https://www.cancer.org/cancer/kaposi-sarcoma/about/what-is-key-statistics.html.

American Cancer Society (ACS): American Cancer Society guideline for colorectal cancer screening, 2020. Retrieved from: https://www.cancer.org/cancer/colon-rectal-cancer/detection-diagnosis-staging/acs-recommendations.html.

American Cancer Society (ACS): Key statistics about stomach cancer, 2021a. Retrieved from: https://www.cancer.org/cancer/stomach-cancer/about/key-statistics.html.

American Cancer Society (ACS): Key statistics for colorectal cancer, 2021b. Retrieved from: https://www.cancer.org/cancer/colon-rectal-cancer/about/key-statistics.html.

American Cancer Society (ACS): Key statistics for oral cavity and oropharyngeal cancers, 2021c. Retrieved from: https://www.cancer.org/cancer/oral-cavity-and-oropharyngeal-cancer/about/key-statistics.html.

American Cancer Society (ACS): Risk factors of oral cavity and oropharyngeal cancers, 2021d. Retrieved from: https://www.cancer.org/cancer/oral-cavity-and-oropharyngeal-cancer/causes-risks-prevention/risk-factors.html.

American Cancer Society (ACS): Stomach cancer survival rates, 2021e. Retrieved from: https://www.cancer.org/cancer/stomach-cancer/detection-diagnosis-staging/survival-rates.html.

American Cancer Society (ACS): Survival rates for colorectal cancer, 2021f. Retrieved from: https://www.cancer.org/cancer/colon-rectal-cancer/detection-diagnosis-staging/survival-rates.html.

American Cancer Society (ACS): Survival rates for esophageal cancer, 2021g. Retrieved from: https://www.cancer.org/cancer/esophagus-cancer/detection-diagnosis-staging/survival-rates.html.

American Cancer Society (ACS): Survival rates for oral cavity and oropharyngeal cancer, 2021h. Retrieved from: https://www.cancer.org/cancer/oral-cavity-and-oropharyngeal-cancer/detection-diagnosis-staging/survival-rates.html.

Anand BS: Peptic ulcer disease, 2017. Retrieved from: http://emedicine.medscape.com/article/181753-overview.

Celiac Disease Foundation: What is celiac disease?, n.d. Retrieved from: https://celiac.org/about-celiac-disease/what-is-celiac-disease/.

Centers for Disease Control and Prevention (CDC): Healthcare-associated infections: Clostridioides difficile, 2019. Retrieved from: https://www.cdc.gov/HAI/organisms/cdiff/Cdiff_infect.html.

Centers for Disease Control and Prevention (CDC): C. diff (Clostridioides difficile): FAQs, 2020. Retrieved from: https://www.cdc.gov/cdiff/clinicians/faq.html.

Centers for Disease Control and Prevention (CDC): E. coli (Escherichia coli), 2021. Retrieved from: https://www.cdc.gov/ecoli/.

Cleveland Clinic: GERD (chronic acid reflux), 2019. Retrieved from: https://my.clevelandclinic.org/health/diseases/17019-gerd-or-acid-reflux-or-heartburn-overview.

Chahine A: Intussusception, 2018. Medscape. Retrieved from: https://emedicine.medscape.com/article/930708-overview.

Crohn's and Colitis Foundation: Crohn's diagnosis & testing, n.d.a. Retrieved from: http://emedicine.medscape.com/article/176319-overview.

Crohn's & Colitis Foundation: Overview of ulcerative colitis, n.d.b. Retrieved from: https://www.crohnscolitisfoundation.org/what-is-ulcerative-colitis/overview.

Daley BJ: Peritonitis and abdominal sepsis, 2019. Retrieved from: http://emedicine.medscape.com/article/180234-overview.

Drugs.com: Gastrografin, 2020. Retrieved from: https://www.drugs.com/pro/gastrografin.html.

Girard-Madoux MJH, Gomez de Agüero M, Ganal-Vonarburg SC, Mooser C, Belz GT, Macpherson AJ, Vivier E. The immunological functions of the Appendix: An example of redundancy? Semin Immunol. 2018 Apr;36:31-44. https://doi.org/10.1016/j.smim.2018.02.005. Epub 2018 Mar 2. PMID: 29503124.

Hidalgo JA: Candidiasis treatment & management, 2020. Retrieved from: http://emedicine.medscape.com/article/213853-treatment.

Johns Hopkins Medicine: Peptic ulcer disease, 2013. Retrieved from: www.hopkinsmedicine.org/gastroenterology_hepatology/_pdfs/esophagus_stomach/peptic_ulcer_disease.pdf.

Johns Hopkins Medicine: Barium swallow. n.d.a. Retrieved from: https://www.hopkinsmedicine.org/health/treatment-tests-and-therapies/barium-swallow.

Johns Hopkins Medicine: Peptic ulcer disease, n.d.b. Retrieved from: https://www.hopkinsmedicine.org/health/conditions-and-diseases/peptic-ulcer-disease.

Mayo Clinic: Inflammatory bowel disease, 2015b. Retrieved from: http://www.mayoclinic.org/diseases-conditions/inflammatory-bowel-disease/basics/treatment/con-20034908.

Mayo Clinic: Capsule endoscopy, 2019. Retrieved from: https://www.mayoclinic.org/tests-procedures/capsule-endoscopy/about/pac-20393366.

Mayo Clinic: Barrett's esophagus, 2020a. Retrieved from: https://www.mayoclinic.org/diseases-conditions/barretts-esophagus/diagnosis-treatment/drc-20352846.

Mayo Clinic: E. coli, 2020b. Retrieved from: https://www.mayoclinic.org/diseases-conditions/e-coli/symptoms-causes/syc-20372058.

Mayo Clinic: Esophageal cancer, 2020c. Retrieved from: https://www.mayoclinic.org/diseases-conditions/esophageal-cancer/diagnosis-treatment/drc-20356090.

Mayo Clinic: Gastroesophageal reflux disease (GERD), 2020d. Retrieved from: https://www.mayoclinic.org/diseases-conditions/gerd/symptoms-causes/syc-20361940.

Mayo Clinic: Stomach cancer, 2021. Retrieved from: https://www.mayoclinic.org/diseases-conditions/stomach-cancer/symptoms-causes/syc-20352438.

Mounsey A, Raleigh M, Wilson A: Management of constipation in older adults, Am Fam Physician 92(6):500–504, 2015.

National Cancer Institute: Head and neck cancer – Patient version. National Institutes of Health, n.d. Retrieved from: https://www.cancer.gov/types/head-and-neck.

National Institute of Diabetes and Digestive and Kidney Diseases (NIDDK): Virtual colonoscopy, 2016. National Institutes of Health (NIH). Retrieved from: https://www.niddk.nih.gov/health-information/diagnostic-tests/virtual-colonoscopy.

National Institute of Diabetes and Digestive and Kidney Diseases (NIDDK): Irritable bowel syndrome (IBS), 2017. National Institutes of Health (NIH). Retrieved from: https://www.niddk.nih.gov/health-information/digestive-diseases/irritable-bowel-syndrome.

National Library of Medicine (NLM): Misoprostol, 2017. MedlinePlus. Retrieved from: https://medlineplus.gov/druginfo/meds/a689009.html.

National Library of Medicine (NLM): Abdominal x-ray, 2019a. MedlinePlus. Retrieved from: https://medlineplus.gov/ency/article/003815.htm.

National Library of Medicine (NLM): Achalasia, 2019b. MedlinePlus. Retrieved from: https://medlineplus.gov/ency/article/000267.htm.

National Library of Medicine (NLM): Bernstein test, 2020a. MedlinePlus. Retrieved from: https://medlineplus.gov/ency/article/003897.htm.

National Library of Medicine (NLM): Gastroesophageal reflux disease, 2020b. MedlinePlus. Retrieved from: https://medlineplus.gov/ency/article/000265.htm.

National Library of Medicine (NLM): Hiatal hernia, 2021. MedlinePlus. Retrieved from: https://medlineplus.gov/hiatalhernia.html.

Nelson R: FDA approves Cologuard for colorectal cancer screening, 2014. Medscape. Retrieved from: https://www.medscape.com/viewarticle/829757.

Saltzman JR: Prevalence of H. pylori – Positive peptic ulcers is decreasing in the US, 2020. Retrieved from: https://www.jwatch.org/na50875/2020/02/24/prevalence-h-pylori-positive-peptic-ulcers-decreasing-us.

Skidmore-Roth L: Mosby's 2021 nursing drug reference, ed 34, St. Louis, 2020, Elsevier.

Skin Cancer Foundation: Ask the expert: What will help me less nervous about my lip cancer?, 2020. Retrieved from: https://www.skincancer.org/blog/ask-the-expert-what-will-help-me-feel-less-nervous-about-my-lip-cancer/.

The University of Texas of Southwestern Medical Center: Hereditary colon cancer: Guide for health pros, n.d. Retrieved from: https://utswmed.org/conditions-treatments/genetics-and-hereditary-cancers/guide-hereditary-cancer-health-pros/hereditary-colon-cancer-guide-health-pros/.

CHAPTER 6

American Cancer Society (ACS): About pancreatic cancer, n.d. Retrieved from: https://www.cancer.org/cancer/pancreatic-cancer/about.html.

American Cancer Society: Liver cancer, 2021a. Retrieved from: https://www.cancer.org/cancer/liver-cancer/.

American Cancer Society (ACS): Survival rates for pancreatic cancer, 2021b. Retrieved from: https://www.cancer.org/cancer/pancreatic-cancer/detection-diagnosis-staging/survival-rates.html

Centers for Disease Control and Prevention (CDC): Vaccine Information Statements: Hepatitis B VIS, 2019. Retrieved from: https://www.cdc.gov/vaccines/hcp/vis/vis-statements/hep-b.html.

Centers for Disease Control and Prevention (CDC): Vaccine Information Statements (VISs): Hepatitis A VIS, 2020a. Retrieved from: https://www.cdc.gov/vaccines/hcp/vis/vis-statements/hep-a.html.

Centers for Disease Control and Prevention (CDC): Viral Hepatitis: Hepatitis C questions and answers for the public, 2020b. Retrieved from https://www.cdc.gov/hepatitis/hcv/cfaq.htm.

Centers for Disease Control and Prevention (CDC): Hepatitis C questions and answers for health professionals, 2020c. Retrieved from: https://www.cdc.gov/hepatitis/hcv/hcvfaq.htm#section1.

Centers for Disease Control and Prevention (CDC): National Center for Health Statistics: Chronic liver disease and cirrhosis, 2021a. Retrieved from: https://www.cdc.gov/nchs/fastats/liver-disease.htm.

Centers for Disease Control and Prevention (CDC): Viral hepatitis: Viral hepatitis, 2021b. Retrieved from: https://www.cdc.gov/hepatitis/index.htm.

Centers for Disease Control and Prevention (CDC): Viral Hepatitis: Statistics & surveillance, 2021c. Retrieved from https://www.cdc.gov/hepatitis/statistics/index.htm.

Hepatitis B Foundation: Vaccine for hepatitis B, 2020. Retrieved from: https://www.hepb.org/prevention-and-diagnosis/vaccination/.

Hepatitis B Foundation: The 3-shot hepatitis B vaccine - Do I need to restart the series if I am off the recommended schedule?, 2017. Retrieved from: https://www.hepb.org/blog/the-3-shot-hbv-vaccine-do-i-need-to-restart-the-series-if-i-am-off-the-recommended-schedule/.

Mathew A: Pancreatic necrosis and pancreatic abscess, 2021. Retrieved from: http://emedicine.medscape.com/article/181264-overview.

May Clinic: Hepatitis B, n.d. Retrieved from: https://www.mayoclinic.org/diseases-conditions/hepatitis-b/diagnosis-treatment/drc-20366821.

Mayo Clinic: Liver transplant, 2021. Retrieved from: https://www.mayoclinic.org/tests-procedures/liver-transplant/about/pac-20384842.

Mayo Clinic: Esophageal varices, 2019. Retrieved from: https://www.mayoclinic.org/diseases-conditions/esophageal-varices/diagnosis-treatment/drc-20351544.

MedlinePlus: Alpha fetoprotein (AFP) tumor marker test, 2020. Retrieved from: https://medlineplus.gov/lab-tests/alpha-fetoprotein-afp-tumor-marker-test/.

National Institutes of Diabetes and Digestive and Kidney Diseases (NIDDK): Cirrhosis, n.d. National Institutes of Health. Retrieved from: https://www.niddk.nih.gov/health-information/liver-disease/cirrhosis.

Peralta R: Liver abscess, 2020. Retrieved from: https://emedicine.medscape.com/article/188802-overview#a4.

Wolf DC: Cirrhosis, 2020. Retrieved from: https://emedicine.medscape.com/article/185856-overview#a3.

World Health Organization (WHO): Hepatitis, n.d. Retrieved from: https://www.who.int/health-topics/hepatitis#tab=tab.

CHAPTER 7

Chaturvedi S, Arnold DM, McCrae KR: Splenectomy for immune thrombocytopenia: Down but not out, 2018. Retrieved from: https://www.ncbi.nlm.nih.gov/pmc/articles/PMC5855018/#:~:text=Efficacy%20of%20splenectomy%20for%20ITP,of%20patients%20achieve%20durable%20remission.

Joint United Kingdom (UK) Blood Transfusion and Tissue Transplantation Services Professional Advisory Committee (JPAC), 2020. Retrieved from: https://www.transfusionguidelines.org/transfusion-handbook/12-management-of-patients-who-do-not-accept-transfusion/12-2-jehovah-s-witnesses-and-blood-transfusion

Maakaron JE: Anemia workup, 2019. Retrieved from: https://emedicine.medscape.com/article/198475-workup#c9

Maerz LL: Transfusion and autotransfusion, 2019. Retrieved from: https://emedicine.medscape.com/article/434176-overview#a2

CHAPTER 8

American Heart Association: How to get your cholesterol tested, 2020. Retrieved from: https://www.heart.org/en/health-topics/cholesterol/how-to-get-your-cholesterol-tested#:~:text=The%20American%20Heart%20Association%20recommends,as%20their%20risk%20remains%20low.

American Heart Association: Risk for heart valve problems, 2020a. Retrieved from: https://www.heart.org/en/health-topics/heart-valve-problems-and-disease/heart-valve-disease-risks-signs-and-symptoms/risks-for-heart-valve-problems

Hinkle JL, Cheever, KH: Brunner & Suddarth's Textbook of Medical Surgical Nursing, Walters Kluwer, Philadelphia, 2018.

Bruss ZS, Raja A: Physiology, Stroke Volume. StatPearls Publishing, 2020. Retrieved from: https://www.ncbi.nlm.nih.gov/books/NBK547686/

Centers for Disease Control and Prevention (CDC): Rheumatic fever: All you need to know, 2018. Retrieved from: https://www.cdc.gov/groupastrep/diseases-public/rheumatic-fever.html

Centers for Disease Control and Prevention (CDC): Know your risk for heart disease, 2019. Retrieved from: https://www.cdc.gov/heartdisease/risk_factors.htm

Centers for Disease Control and Prevention (CDC): Health, United States Spotlight, Racial and ethnic disparities in heart disease, 2019a. Retrieved from: https://www.cdc.gov/nchs/hus/spotlight/HeartDiseaseSpotlight_2019_0404.pdf

Centers for Disease Control and Prevention (CDC): Preventing high cholesterol, 2020. Retrieved from: https://www.cdc.gov/cholesterol/prevention.htm

Center for Disease Control and Prevention (CDC): Facts about hypertension, 2020a. Retrieved from: https://www.cdc.gov/bloodpressure/facts.htm

Center for Disease Control and Prevention (CDC): Diabetes and your heart, 2020b. Retrieved from: https://www.cdc.gov/diabetes/library/features/diabetes-and-heart.html

Chen MA: Arterial embolism, 2018. Retrieved from: https://medlineplus.gov/ency/article/001102.htm

Cleveland Clinic: PAD: Atherectomy, 2019. Retrieved from: https://my.clevelandclinic.org/health/treatments/17310-pad-atherectomy#:~:text=An%20atherectomy%20is%20a%20procedure,is%20performed%20under%20local%20anesthesia.

Daskalov IR, Valova-Ilieva T: Management of acute pericarditis: treatment and follow up, European Society of Cardiology, e-Journal of Cardiology Practice 15(16), 2017. Retrieved from: https://www.escardio.org/Journals/E-Journal-of-Cardiology-Practice/Volume-15/Management-of-acute-pericarditis-treatment-and-follow-up#:~:text=Colchicine%20use%20is%20a%20first,they%20appear%20to%20encourage%20recurrences.

Dominguez JA, Rowe VL: Peripheral arterial occlusive disease, 2019. Retrieved from: https://emedicine.medscape.com/article/460178-overview

Foth C, Gangwani MK, Alvey H: Ventricular Tachycardia. StatPearls Publishing, 2020. Retrieved from: https://www.ncbi.nlm.nih.gov/books/NBK532954/

Harvard Health Publishing: More antidotes for newer blood thinners, 2018. Retrieved from: https://www.health.harvard.edu/diseases-and-conditions/more-antidotes-for-newer-blood-thinners

Health and Human Services (HHS): Heart disease and African Americans, 2020. Retrieved from: https://minorityhealth.hhs.gov/omh/browse.aspx?lvl=4&lvlid=19

Ludhwani D, Goyal A, Jagtap M: Ventricular Fibrillation. StatPearls, 2020. Retrieved from: https://www.ncbi.nlm.nih.gov/books/NBK537120/

Mayo Clinic: C-reactive protein test, 2017. Retrieved from: https://www.mayoclinic.org/tests-procedures/c-reactive-protein-test/about/pac-20385228

Mayo Clinic: Atrial Tachycardia, 2019. Retrieved from: https://www.mayoclinic.org/diseases-conditions/atrial-tachycardia/cdc-20355258

Mayo Clinic: Supraventricular tachycardia, 2019a. Retrieved from: https://www.mayoclinic.org/diseases-conditions/supraventricular-tachycardia/symptoms-causes/syc-20355243

Mayo Clinic: Buerger's Disease, 2019b. Retrieved from: https://www.mayoclinic.org/diseases-conditions/buergers-disease/diagnosis-treatment/drc-20350664

Mayo Clinic: Heart transplant, 2019c. Retrieved from: https://www.mayoclinic.org/tests-procedures/heart-transplant/about/pac-20384750#:~:text=Survival%20rates%20after%20heart%20transplantation,after%20five%20years%20for%20adults.

Mayo Clinic: Chest x-ray, 2020. Retrieved from: https://www.mayoclinic.org/tests-procedures/chest-x-rays/about/pac-20393494#:~:text=Because%20the%20outlines%20of%20the,your%20heart%20or%20blood%20vessels.

Mayo Clinic: Endocarditis, 2020a. Retrieved from: https://www.mayoclinic.org/diseases-conditions/endocarditis/symptoms-causes/syc-20352576

Mayo Clinic: Ankle brachial index, 2020b. Retrieved from: https://www.mayoclinic.org/tests-procedures/ankle-brachial-index/about/pac-20392934

MedlinePlus: Homocysteine test, 2018. Retrieved from: https://medlineplus.gov/lab-tests/homocysteine-test/

MedlinePlus: Pentoxifylline, 2017. Retrieved from: https://medlineplus.gov/druginfo/meds/a685027.html

Namana V, Gupta SS, Sabharwal N, et al: Clinical significance of atrial kick, QJM: An International Journal of Medicine 111(8):569–570, 2018. Retrieved from: https://doi.org/10.1093/qjmed/hcy088

Singh A, Saluja S, Kumar, A et al: Cardiovascular Complications of Marijuana and Related Substances: A Review. Cardiology and therapy 7(1):45–59, 2018. Retrieved from: https://doi.org/10.1007/s40119-017-0102-x

Sudheendra D: Ischemic ulcers – self care, 2020. Retrieved from: https://medlineplus.gov/ency/patientinstructions/000742.htm

Xie E, Yu R, Ambale-Venkatesh, B et al: Association of right atrial structure with incident atrial fibrillation: a longitudinal cohort cardiovascular magnetic resonance study from the Multi-Ethnic Study of Atheroslerosis (MESA). Journal of Cardiovascular Magnetic Resonance: Official Journal of the Society of Cardiovascular Magnetic Resonance, 22(1):36, 2020. Retrieved from: https://doi.org/10.1186/s12968-020-00631-1

Yallowitz AW, Decker LC: Infectious Endocarditis. StatPearls Publishing, 2020. Retrieved from: https://www.ncbi.nlm.nih.gov/books/NBK557641/

CHAPTER 9

American Cancer Society: Laryngeal and hypopharyngeal cancer, n.d. Retrieved from: https://www.cancer.org/cancer/laryngeal-and-hypopharyngeal-cancer.html.

American Cancer Society: Monoclonal antibodies and their side effects, 2019a. Retrieved from: https://www.cancer.org/treatment/treatments-and-side-effects/treatment-types/immunotherapy/monoclonal-antibodies.html.

American Cancer Society: What is lung cancer?, 2019b. Retrieved from: https://www.cancer.org/cancer/lung-cancer/about/what-is.html.

American Cancer Society: Key statistics for lung cancer, 2021a. Retrieved from: https://www.cancer.org/cancer/lung-cancer/about/key-statistics.html.

American Cancer Society: Tests for lung cancer, 2021b. Retrieved from: https://www.cancer.org/cancer/lung-cancer/detection-diagnosis-staging/how-diagnosed.html.

American Cancer Society: Treatment choices for small cell lung cancer, by stage, 2021c.

American Lung Association: Bronchiectasis, n.d.b. Retrieved from: www.lung.org/lung-disease/bronchiectasis.

American Lung Association: Antioxidants: lung cancer's friend or foe?, 2019. Retrieved from: https://www.lung.org/blog/antioxidants-lung-cancers.

American Lung Association: Lung cancer fact sheet, 2020a. Retrieved from: https://www.lung.org/lung-health-diseases/lung-disease-lookup/lung-cancer/resource-library/lung-cancer-fact-sheet.

American Lung Association: Treating and managing bronchiectasis, 2020b. Retrieved from: https://www.lung.org/lung-health-diseases/lung-disease-lookup/bronchiectasis/treating-and-managing

American Lung Association: COPD causes and risk factors, 2021. Retrieved from: https://www.lung.org/lung-health-diseases/lung-disease-lookup/copd/what-causes-copd.

Centers for Disease Control and Prevention (CDC): COVID data tracker: United States COVD-19 cases, deaths, and laboratory testing (NAATs) by state, territory, and jurisdiction, n.d. Retrieved from: https://covid.cdc.gov/covid-data-tracker/#cases_deathsper100k .

Centers for Disease Control and Prevention (CDC): Tuberculosis: drug-resistant TB, 2017. Retrieved from: https://www.cdc.gov/tb/topic/drtb/default.htm

Centers for Disease Control and Prevention (CDC): Vaccines and preventable diseases: Pneumococcal vaccination, 2017c. Retrieved from: https://www.cdc.gov/vaccines/vpd/pneumo/index.html.

Centers for Disease Control and Prevention: Asthma: Most recent asthma data. 2018. Retrieved from: https://www.cdc.gov/asthma/most_recent_data.htm.

Centers for Disease Control and Prevention (CDC): Leading causes of death – males – all races and origins – United States, 2017, 2019. Retrieved from: https://www.cdc.gov/healthequity/lcod/men/2017/all-races-origins/index.htm.

Centers for Disease Control and Prevention (CDC): Anthrax: Emergency use instructions for doxyclycline and ciproflaxin for post-exposure prophylaxis of anthrax. 2020a. Retrieved from: https://www.cdc.gov/anthrax/medical-care/cipro-eui-recipients.html.

Centers for Disease Control and Prevention (CDC): COVID-19: infection control, 2020b. Retrieved from: https://www.cdc.gov/coronavirus/2019-ncov/hcp/infection-control.html .

Centers for Disease Control and Prevention (CDC): Pneumonia: vaccines help prevent pneumonia, 2020c. Retrieved from: https://www.cdc.gov/pneumonia/prevention.html

Centers for Disease Control and Prevention (CDC): Tuberculosis: data and statistics, 2020d. Retrieved from: https://www.cdc.gov/tb/statistics/default.htm .

Centers for Disease Control and Prevention (CDC): Venous thromboembolism (blood clots): data & statistics, 2020e. Retrieved from: https://www.cdc.gov/ncbddd/dvt/data.html.

Centers for Disease Control and Prevention (CDC): Water, sanitation, & environmentally-related hygiene: coughing & sneezing, 2020f. Retrieved from: https://www.cdc.gov/healthywater/hygiene/etiquette/coughing_sneezing.html

Centers for Disease Control and Prevention (CDC): COVID-19: what to do if you are sick, 2021a. Retrieved from: https://www.cdc.gov/coronavirus/2019-ncov/if-you-are-sick/steps-when-sick.html.

Centers for Disease Control and Prevention (CDC): COVID-19: Symptoms, 2021b. Retrieved from: https://www.cdc.gov/coronavirus/2019-ncov/symptoms-testing/symptoms.html.

Centers for Disease Control and Prevention (CDC): COVID-19: Testing for COVID-19, 2021c. Retrieved from: https://www.cdc.gov/coronavirus/2019-ncov/symptoms-testing/testing.html .

Centers for Disease Control and Prevention (CDC): Legionella (legionnaires' disease and Pontiac fever), 2021d. Retrieved from: https://www.cdc.gov/legionella/index.html.

Centers for Disease Control and Prevention (CDC): Legionella (legionnaires' disease and Pontiac fever) fast facts, n.d. Retrieved from: https://www.cdc.gov/legionella/fastfacts.html.

Centers for Disease Control and Prevention (CDC), National Center for Health Statistics (NCHS): Chronic obstructive pulmonary disease, 2021. Retrieved from: https://www.cdc.gov/nchs/fastats/copd.htm.

Martines RB, Ritter JM, Matkovic E, et al. Pathology and Pathogenesis of SARS-CoV-2 Associated with Fatal Coronavirus Disease, United States. Emerging Infectious Diseases. 2020;26(9):2005-2015. Retrieved from: https://wwwnc.cdc.gov/eid/article/26/9/20-2095_article.

Mayo Clinic: ARDS, 2018. Retrieved from: https://www.mayoclinic.org/diseases-conditions/ards/symptoms-causes/syc-20355576.

Mayo Clinic: Anthrax, 2020a. Retrieved from: https://www.mayoclinic.org/diseases-conditions/anthrax/diagnosis-treatment/drc-20356209.

Mayo Clinic: Asthma, 2020b. Retrieved from: https://www.mayoclinic.org/diseases-conditions/asthma/symptoms-causes/syc-20369653.

Mayo Clinic: Pneumonia, 2020c. Retrieved from: https://www.mayoclinic.org/diseases-conditions/pneumonia/diagnosis-treatment/drc-20354210.

Mayo Clinic: Pulmonary edema, 2020d. Retrieved from: https://www.mayoclinic.org/diseases-conditions/pulmonary-edema/symptoms-causes/syc-20377009.

Mayo Clinic: Sleep apnea, 2020e. Retrieved from: https://www.mayoclinic.org/diseases-conditions/sleep-apnea/symptoms-causes/syc-20377631

Mayo Clinic: Asthma and acid reflux: are they linked?, 2021a. Retrieved from: https://www.mayoclinic.org/diseases-conditions/asthma/expert-answers/asthma-and-acid-reflux/faq-20057993.

Mayo Clinic: Tuberculosis, 2021b. Retrieved from: https://www.mayoclinic.org/diseases-conditions/tuberculosis/symptoms-causes/syc-20351250.

Medline Plus: Pulmonary ventilation/perfusion scan, 2020a. Retrieved from: www.nlm.nih.gov/medlineplus/ency/article/003828.htm.

Medline Plus: Allergy blood test, 2020b. Retrieved from: https://medlineplus.gov/lab-tests/allergy-blood-test/

National Cancer Institute: Laryngeal cancer treatment (adult) (PDQ®) – health professional version, 2021. Retrieved from: https://www.cancer.gov/types/head-and-neck/hp/adult/laryngeal-treatment-pdq.

Ortega VE, Genese F: Treatment of acute asthma exacerbations. Merck Manual: professional version, 2019. Retrieved from: https://www.merckmanuals.com/professional/pulmonary-disorders/asthma-and-related-disorders/treatment-of-acute-asthma-exacerbations.

Scholten, E. L., Beitler, J. R., Prisk, G. K., & Malhotra, A. Treatment of ARDS with prone positioning. Chest, 2017;151(1):215–224.

Sleepapnea.org: Sleep apnea information for clinicians, 2021. Retrieved from: https://www.sleepapnea.org/learn/sleep-apnea-information-clinicians/.

World Health Organization (WHO): Use of interferon-y release assays (Igras). In tuberculosis control in low- and middle-income settings, Geneva, Switzerland, 2011, Author.

World Health Organization (WHO): Tuberculosis, 2020. Retrieved from: https://www.who.int/news-room/fact-sheets/detail/tuberculosis.

CHAPTER 10

American Cancer Society: Radiation therapy for prostate cancer, 2019. Retrieved from: https://www.cancer.org/cancer/prostate-cancer/treating/radiation-therapy.html.

American Cancer Society: Risk factors for kidney cancer, 2020a. Retrieved from: https://www.cancer.org/cancer/kidney-cancer/causes-risks-prevention/risk-factors.html .

American Cancer Society: Survival rates for kidney cancer, 2020b. Retrieved from: https://www.cancer.org/cancer/kidney-cancer/detection-diagnosis-staging/survival-rates.html.

American Cancer Society: Hormone therapy for prostate cancer, 2021a. Retrieved from: https://www.cancer.org/cancer/prostate-cancer/treating/hormone-therapy.html.

American Cancer Society: Survival rates for bladder cancer, 2021b. Retrieved from: https://www.cancer.org/cancer/bladder-cancer/detection-diagnosis-staging/survival-rates.html.

BD: PureWick™ Female external catheter, n.d. Retrieved from: https://www.bd.com/en-us/offerings/capabilities/home-care/urinary-incontinence/external-catheters/purewick-female-external-catheter.

Centers for Disease Control and Prevention (CDC): Chronic kidney disease initiative: chronic kidney disease basics, 2020. Retrieved from: https://www.cdc.gov/kidneydisease/basics.html

Centers for Disease Control and Prevention (CDC): Chronic kidney disease initiative: chronic kidney disease in the United States, 2021, 2021. Retrieved from: https://www.cdc.gov/kidneydisease/publications-resources/ckd-national-facts.html.

Fung E: Autosomal dominant polycystic kidney disease (ADPKD). Merck Manual: professional version, 2021. Retrieved from: https://www.merckmanuals.com/professional/genitourinary-disorders/cystic-kidney-disease/autosomal-dominant-polycystic-kidney-diseaseadpkd.

Hinkle JL, Cheever K: Brunner & Suddarth's textbook of medical-surgical nursing, ed 14, Philadelphia, 2018, Lippincott, Williams & Wilkins.

Levy DA, Jones JS: Surveillance for recurrent bladder cancer. Medscape, 2019. Retrieved from: https://emedicine.medscape.com/article/458825-overview#a1 .

Mayo Clinic: Interstitial cystitis, 2019a. Retrieved from: https://www.mayoclinic.org/diseases-conditions/interstitial-cystitis/symptoms-causes/syc-20354357.

Mayo Clinic: Laser PVP surgery, 2019b. Retrieved from: https://www.mayoclinic.org/tests-procedures/laser-pvp-surgery/about/pac-20384877.

Mayo Clinic: Transurethral microwave therapy (TUMT), 2019c. Retrieved from: https://www.mayoclinic.org/tests-procedures/tumt/about/pac-20384886.

Mayo Clinic: Kidney cancer, 2020a. Retrieved from: https://www.mayoclinic.org/diseases-conditions/kidney-cancer/diagnosis-treatment/drc-20352669.

Mayo Clinic: Vesicoureteral reflux, 2020b. Retrieved from: https://www.mayoclinic.org/diseases-conditions/hydronephrosis/cdc-20397563.

Medline: Coude-Tip, 2017. Retrieved from: http://www.medline.com/product/Coude-100-Silicone-Foley-Catheters/Z05-PF02115.

Muruve NA: Transurethral needle ablation of the prostate (TUNA), 2017. Retrieved from: https://emedicine.medscape.com/article/449477-overview.

National Cancer Institute (NCI): Cancer stat facts: kidney and renal pelvis cancer, n.d. Retrieved from: https://seer.cancer.gov/statfacts/html/kidrp.html .

National Cancer Institute (NCI): Hormone therapy for prostate cancer, 2014. Retrieved from: https://www.cancer.gov/types/prostate/prostate-hormone-therapy-fact-sheet.

National Institute of Diabetes and Digestive and Kidney Diseases (NIDDK). Urinary retention, n.d. Retrieved from: https://www.niddk.nih.gov/health-information/urologic-diseases/urinary-retention#sec3

National Institute of Diabetes and Digestive and Kidney Diseases (NIDDK): Simple kidney cysts, 2019. Retrieved from: https://www.niddk.nih.gov/health-information/kidney-disease/simple-kidney-cysts.

National Institute of Diabetes and Digestive and Kidney Disease (NIDDK): Peritoneal dialysis, 2021. Retrieved from: https://www.niddk.nih.gov/health-information/kidney-disease/kidney-failure/peritoneal-dialysis.

National Kidney Foundation, 2017. Retrieved from https://www.kidney.org/atoz/content/kidneytests.

National Library of Medicine (NLM): Creatine blood test, 2021a. Retrieved from: https://medlineplus.gov/ency/article/003475.htm.

National Library of Medicine (NLM): Creatinine clearance test, 2021b. Retrieved from: https://medlineplus.gov/ency/article/003611.htm.

Prostate Cancer Treatment Guide: Prostate cancer treatment overview, n.d. Retrieved from: https://prostate-cancer.com/prostate-cancer-treatment-overview/prostate-cancer-treatment-overview.html.

Saginala K, Barsouk A, Aluru JS, Rawla P, Padala SA, Barsouk A: Epidemiology of bladder cancer. Med Sci (Basel, Switzerland) 8(1):15, 2020. https://doi.org/10.3390/medsci8010015

Urology Care Foundation: Neurogenic bladder, n.d.a. Retrieved from: https://www.urologyhealth.org/urology-a-z/n/neurogenic-bladder.

Urology Care Foundation: Prostatitis (infection of the prostate), n.d.b. Retrieved from: https://www.urologyhealth.org/urology-a-z/p/prostatitis-(infection-of-the-prostate).

Vasavada SP: Urinary incontinence, 2019. Medscape. Retrieved from: https://emedicine.medscape.com/article/452289-overview#a6.

WebMD: Blood urea nitrogen, 2010. Retrieved from: www.webmd.com/a-to-z-guides/blood-urea-nitrogen.

CHAPTER 11

Alkhalili E, Tasci Y, Aksoy E, et al: The utility of neck ultrasound and sestamibi scans in patients with secondary and tertiary hyperthyroidism, World J Surg 39(3):701–705, 2015.

American Addiction Centers: Alcohol & diabetes: can alcohol cause diabetes?, 2021. Retrieved from: https://americanaddictioncenters.org/alcoholism-treatment/alcohol-abuse-and-diabetes.

American Cancer Society (ACS): Thyroid cancer survival rates, by type and stage, 2021. Retrieved from: https://www.cancer.org/cancer/thyroid-cancer/detection-diagnosis-staging/survival-rates.html.

American Diabetes Association (ADA): Hypoglycemia (low blood sugar), n.d. Retrieved from: https://www.diabetes.org/healthy-living/medication-treatments/blood-glucose-testing-and-control/hypoglycemia.

American Diabetes Association (ADA): Statistics about diabetes. 2018. Retrieved from: https://www.diabetes.org/resources/statistics/statistics-about-diabetes.

American Diabetes Association (ADA): What is the Diabetes Plate Method?, 2020. Retrieved from: https://www.diabetesfoodhub.org/articles/what-is-the-diabetes-plate-method.html.

Buicko JL, Kichler KM, Amundson JR, et al.: The Sestamibi Paradox: Improving Intraoperative Localization of Parathyroid Adenomas. American Surgeon, 83(8), 832–835, 2017. https://doi.org/10.1177/000313481708300831.

Diabetes.co.uk: Diabetes and erectile dysfunction, 2019. Retrieved from: https://www.diabetes.co.uk/diabetes-erectile-dysfunction.html.

Funnel M, Barlage D: Managing diabetes wh "agent oral," Nursing 34(3):36, 2004.

Johns Hopkins Medicine: Hyperparathyroidism, n.d. Retrieved from: https://www.hopkinsmedicine.org/health/conditions-and-diseases/hyperparathyroidism.

Lewis SL, Heitkemper MM, Dirksen SR, et al: Medical-surgical nursing: Assessment and management of clinical problems, ed 8, St. Louis, 2011, Mosby.

Mayo Clinic: Dwarfism, 2018. Retrieved from: https://www.mayoclinic.org/diseases-conditions/dwarfism/symptoms-causes/syc-20371969.

Mayo Clinic: Addison's disease, 2020a. Retrieved from: https://www.mayoclinic.org/diseases-conditions/addisons-disease/symptoms-causes/syc-20350293.

Mayo Clinic: Gestational diabetes, 2020b. Retrieved from: https://www.mayoclinic.org/diseases-conditions/gestational-diabetes/symptoms-causes/syc-20355339.

Mayo Clinic: Hypothyroidism (underactive thyroid), 2020c. Retrieved from: https://www.mayoclinic.org/diseases-conditions/hypothyroidism/symptoms-causes/syc-20350284.

Mayo Clinic: Pheochromocytoma, 2020d. Retrieved from: https://www.mayoclinic.org/diseases-conditions/pheochromocytoma/symptoms-causes/syc-20355367.

Mayo Clinic: Acromegaly, 2021. Retrieved from: https://www.mayoclinic.org/diseases-conditions/acromegaly/diagnosis-treatment/drc-20351226.

National Institute for Diabetes and Digestive and Kidney Diseases (NIDDKD): Acromegaly, 2012. Retrieved from: https://www.niddk.nih.gov/health-information/endocrine-diseases/acromegaly.

National Institute of General Medical Sciences (NIGMS): Circadian rhythms, 2018. National Institutes of Health. Retrieved from: https://www.nigms.nih.gov/education/pages/Factsheet_CircadianRhythms.aspx.

National Library of Medicine (NLM): Growth hormone suppression test. 2019. MedlinePlus. Retrieved from: https://medlineplus.gov/ency/article/003376.htm.

National Library of Medicine (NLM): Congenital hypothyroidism, 2020. MedlinePlus. Retrieved from: https://medlineplus.gov/genetics/condition/congenital-hypothyroidism/#frequency.

National Library of Medicine (NLM): Simple goiter, 2021. MedlinePlus. Retrieved from: https://medlineplus.gov/ency/article/001178.htm.

Office of Dietary Supplements: Calcium: Fact sheet for health professionals, 2021a. National Institutes of Health. Retrieved from: https://ods.od.nih.gov/factsheets/Calcium-HealthProfessional/.

Office of Dietary Supplements: Iodine: Fact sheet for health professionals, 2021b. National Institutes of Health. Retrieved from: http://ods.od.nih.gov/factsheets/Iodine-HealthProfessional.

U.S. Department of Health and Human Services (DHHS) and U.S. Department of Agriculture (USDA): 2015-2020 Dietary Guidelines for Americans, ed 8, 2015. Retrieved from: https://health.gov/sites/default/files/2019-09/2015-2020_Dietary_Guidelines.pdf.

Walker RA: Identifying diseases that mimic strokes, J Emerg Med Serv 36(3):2011. Retrieved from: https://www.jems.com/patient-care/identifying-diseases-mimic-str/.

CHAPTER 12

American Cancer Society (ACS): American Cancer Society Recommendations for the Early Detection of Breast Cancer, November 17, 2020a. Retrieved from: https://www.cancer.org/cancer/breast-cancer/screening-tests-and-early-detection/american-cancer-society-recommendations-for-the-early-detection-of-breast-cancer.html.

American Cancer Society (ACS): American Cancer Society Guidelines for the Prevention and Early Detection of Cervical Cancer, November 17, 2020b. Retrieved from: https://www.cancer.org/cancer/cervical-cancer/detection-diagnosis-staging/cervical-cancer-screening-guidelines.html.

American Cancer Society (ACS): Breast cancer survival rates, 2021a. Retrieved from: https://www.cancer.org/cancer/breast-cancer/understanding-a-breast-cancer-diagnosis/breast-cancer-survival-rates.html.

American Cancer Society (ACS): Key Statistics for Endometrial Cancer, 2021b. Retrieved from: https://www.cancer.org/cancer/endometrial-cancer/about/key-statistics.html

American Cancer Society (ACS): Key Statistics for Ovarian Cancer, 2021c. https://www.cancer.org/cancer/ovarian-cancer/about/key-statistics.html.

American Cancer Society (ACS): Key Statistics for Testicular Cancer, 2021d. https://www.cancer.org/cancer/testicular-cancer/about/key-statistics.html.

American Cancer Society (ACS): Testicular survival rates, 2021e. Retrieved from: https://www.cancer.org/cancer/testicular-cancer/detection-diagnosis-staging/survival-rates.html.

American Cancer Society (ACS) Cancer Statistics Center: Ovary: at a glance, 2021. Retrieved from: https://cancerstatisticscenter.cancer.org/#!/cancer-site/Ovary.

Banks NK: Menopausal Hormone Replacement Therapy, 2021. Retrieved from: https://emedicine.medscape.com/article/276104-overview#a10.

Breastcancer.org: Halotestin, 2016. Retrieved from: https://www.breastcancer.org/treatment/druglist/halotestin.

Breastcancer.org: US Breast Cancer Statistics, June 25, 2020. Retrieved from: https://www.breastcancer.org/symptoms/understand_bc/statistics.

Brusch J, Cunha B: Which antibiotics are most effective in the treatment of prostatitis? January 2, 2020. Retrieved from: https://www.medscape.com/answers/231574-7871/which-antibiotics-are-most-effective-in-the-treatment-of-prostatitis.

Cedars Sinai: Stereotactic Breast Biopsy Procedure, 2021. Retrieved from: https://www.cedars-sinai.org/programs/imaging-center/exams/women/stereotactic-breast-biopsy/information.html

Centers for Disease Control and Prevention (CDC): Syphilis: a provider's guide to treatment and prevention, n.d. Retrieved from: https://www.cdc.gov/std/syphilis/Syphilis-Pocket-Guide-FINAL-508.pdf.

Centers for Disease Control and Prevention (CDC): Chlamydia - CDC Fact Sheet, 2014. Retrieved from: https://www.cdc.gov/std/chlamydia/stdfact-chlamydia.htm.

Centers for Disease Control and Prevention (CDC): Breast cancer: what are the risk factors, 2020. Retrieved from: https://www.cdc.gov/cancer/breast/basic_info/risk_factors.htm

Centers for Disease Control and Prevention (CDC): National overview of STDs, 2019, 2021a. Retrieved from: https://www.cdc.gov/std/statistics/2019/overview.htm

Centers for Disease Control and Prevention (CDC): Trichomoniasis: fact sheet, 2021b. Retrieved from: www.cdc.gov/std/trichomonas/STDFact-Trichomoniasis.htm

Cleveland Clinic, 2020. Dysmenorrhea. Retrieved from: https://my.clevelandclinic.org/health/diseases/4148-dysmenorrhea

Eunice Kennedy Shriver National Institute of Child Health and Human Development (NICHD): What are some possible causes of male infertility?, December 1, 2017. Retrieved from: https://www.nichd.nih.gov/health/topics/infertility/conditioninfo/causes/causes-male.

Gardasil 9: Complete the HPV vaccine schedule to help protect your child, n.d. Retrieved from: https://www.gardasil9.com/adolescent/hpv-vaccine-schedule/

Hofmeister S, Bodden S: Premenstrual Syndrome and Premenstrual Dysphoric Disorder. Am Fam Physician 94(3):236–240, 2016. Johns Hopkins: Breast biopsy, n.d.a. Retrieved from: http://www.hopkinsmedicine.org/healthlibrary/test_procedures/gynecology/breast_biopsy_92,P07763/.

Johns Hopkins Medicine: Toxic Shock Syndrome (TSS), n.d.b. https://www.hopkinsmedicine.org/health/conditions-and-diseases/toxic-shock-syndrome-tss

Komen.org: Breast cancer tumor characteristics, 2021a. Retrieved from: http://ww5.komen.org/BreastCancer/TumorCharacteristics.html.

Komen.org: Survival and Risk of Recurrence After Treatment, 2021b. Retrieved from: https://www.komen.org/breast-cancer/survivorship/health-concerns/survival-and-risk-of-recurrence/

Lewis SL, Dirksen SR, Heitkemper MM, et al: Medical-surgical nursing: assessment and management of clinical problems, ed 9, St. Louis, 2014, Mosby.

Mayo Clinic: Infertility, 2019a. Retrieved from: www.mayoclinic.com/health/infertility/DS00310

Mayo Clinic: Vaginal atrophy: diagnosis and treatment, 2019b. Retrieved from: https://www.mayoclinic.org/diseases-conditions/vaginal-atrophy/diagnosis-treatment/drc-20352294.

Mayo Clinic: Colposcopy, 2020a. Retrieved from: https://www.mayoclinic.org/tests-procedures/colposcopy/about/pac-20385036.

Mayo Clinic: Hot flashes: diagnosis and treatment, 2020b. Retrieved from: https://www.mayoclinic.org/diseases-conditions/hot-flashes/diagnosis-treatment/drc-20352795.

Mayo Clinic: Uterine prolapse, 2020c. Retrieved from: http://www.mayoclinic.org/diseases-conditions/uterine-prolapse/home/ovc-20343708.

Mayo Clinic: Erectile dysfunction, 2021. Retrieved from: http://www.mayoclinic.org/diseases-conditions/erectile-dysfunction/basics/treatment/con-20034244

National Cancer Institute (NCI): HPV and Pap Testing, 2019. https://www.cancer.gov/types/cervical/pap-hpv-testing-fact-sheet

National Cancer Institute (NCI): Endometrial cancer screening (PDQ)—health professional version, 2021. Retrieved from: https://www.cancer.gov/types/uterine/hp/endometrial-screening-pdq.

National Institute of Diabetes and Digestive and Kidney Diseases (NIDDK): Symptoms & Causes of Erectile Dysfunction, 2017. Retrieved from: https://www.niddk.nih.gov/health-information/urologic-diseases/erectile-dysfunction/symptoms-causes

National Library of Medicine (NLM): Endometrial cancer, Medline Plus, 2020. Retrieved from: www.nlm.nih.gov/medlineplus/ency/article/000910.htm.

Ollendorff AT: Cervicitis treatment & management, Medscape, 2017. Retrieved from: https://emedicine.medscape.com/article/253402-treatment#d9.

US Department of Health and Human Services (USDHHS) Office on Women's Health: Premenstrual dysphoric disorder (PMDD), 2018. Retrieved from: https://www.womenshealth.gov/menstrual-cycle/premenstrual-syndrome/premenstrual-dysphoric-disorder-pmdd.

US Food and Drug Administration (FDA): Cervarix, 2019. Retrieved from: http://www.fda.gov/BiologicsBloodVaccines/Vaccines/ApprovedProducts/ucm186957.htm.

US Preventive Services Task Force (USPSTF): Breast cancer: Screening, 2016. Retrieved from: https://www.uspreventiveservicestaskforce.org/uspstf/recommendation/breast-cancer-screening. Retrieved from: www.ahrq.gov/clinic/USpstf/uspsbrca.htm.

Webber J: Ayurvedic and Herbal Perspectives for Managing the Menopause. Positive Health Online. 260, 2020, N.PAG.

CHAPTER 13

American Foundation for the Blind, FamilyConnect: Functional visual assessment (FVA), n.d. Retrieved from: http://www.familyconnect.org/info/education/assessments/functional-vision-assessment-fva/135

American Macular Degeneration Foundation (AMDF): About macular degeneration - symptoms, risks, stargardt, anatomy, n.d. Retrieved from: https://www.macular.org/about-macular-degeneration

American Optometric Association (AOA): Dry eye, n.d. Retrieved from: https://www.aoa.org/healthy-eyes/eye-and-vision-conditions/dry-eye.

Centers for Disease Control and Prevention (CDC): Vision Health Initiative (VHI): fast facts about vision loss, 2020. Retrieved from: https://www.cdc.gov/visionhealth/basics/ced/fastfacts.htm

Glaucoma Research Foundation: Glaucoma facts and stats, 2017. Retrieved from: https://www.glaucoma.org/glaucoma/glaucoma-facts-and-stats.php.

Hakobyan L, Lumsden J, O'Sullivan D, Barlett H: Mobile assistive technologies for the visually impaired. Surv Ophthalmol. 58(6): 513–528, 2013.

InformedHealth.org [Internet]. Cologne, Germany: Institute for Quality and Efficiency in Health Care (IQWiG); 2006-. How does our sense of taste work? 2011 Dec 20 [Updated 2016 Aug 17]. Retrieved from: https://www.ncbi.nlm.nih.gov/books/NBK279408/

Li JC:. Meniere Disease (Idiopathic Endolymphatic Hydrops). Treatment & Management. 2020 May 7. Retrieved from: https://emedicine.medscape.com/article/1159069-treatment#d10

Mayo Clinic: Cataract surgery, 2019. Retrieved from: https://www.mayoclinic.org/tests-procedures/cataract-surgery/about/pac-20384765.

Mayo Clinic: Diabetic retinopathy, 2021. Retrieved from: https://www.mayoclinic.org/diseases-conditions/diabetic-retinopathy/diagnosis-treatment/drc-20371617

Mori Y, Miyata K, Ono T, Yagi Y, Kamiya K, Amano S: Comparison of laser in situ ketatomileusis and photorefractive keratectomy for myopia using a mixed-effects model. PLoS ONE. 12(3): 1–12, 2017. https://doi.org/10.1371/journal.pone.0174810

Munson, B: Now, listen up! Understanding hearing loss and deafness. Nursing Made Incredibly Easy 4 (2): 38, 2006.

National Library of Medicine (NLM): Visual Field. Medline Plus, 2019. Retrieved from: www.nlm.nih.gov/medlineplus/ency/article/003879.htm.

National Library of Medicine (NLM): Fluorescein angiography. Medline Plus, 2020a. Retrieved from: https://medlineplus.gov/ency/article/003846.htm.

National Library of Medicine (NLM): Tonometry. Medline Plus, 2020b. Retrieved from: https://medlineplus.gov/ency/article/003447.htm

Nikolatus L, Ring MH, Dirismar M, Mursch-Edlmayr AS, Kretzuer TC, Pretzl J, et al: Corneal epithelial remodeling induced by small incision lenticule extraction. Investigative Opthalmology & Visual Science. 57(6): 176–183, 2016.

Porter D: What is a slit lamp?, American Academy of Ophthalmology. 2018. Retrieved from: https://www.aao.org/eye-health/treatments/what-is-slit-lamp

Sjögren Foundation: Symptoms, n.d. Retrieved from: https://www.sjogrens.org/understanding-sjogrens/symptoms

CHAPTER 14

Alzheimer's Association: Stages of Alzheimer's, n.d. Retrieved from: https://www.alz.org/alzheimers-dementia/stages.

American Brain Tumor Association: Brain tumor education, n.d. Retrieved from: https://www.abta.org/about-brain-tumors/brain-tumor-education/.

American Stroke Association (ASA): Ischemic strokes (clots), n.d.a. American Heart Association (AHA). Retrieved from: https://www.stroke.org/en/about-stroke/types-of-stroke/ischemic-stroke-clots#.WJdf-DYiyM8.

American Stroke Association (ASA): Types of stroke and treatment, n.d.b. American Heart Association (AHA). Retrieved from: https://www.stroke.org/en/about-stroke/types-of-stroke.

American Speech-Language-Hearing Association: Swallowing disorders (dysphagia) in adults, n.d. Retrieved from: www.asha.org/public/speech/swallowing/Swallowing-Disorders-in-Adults/#tx.

Centers for Disease Control and Prevention (CDC): Vaccines and preventable diseases: Meningococcal, 2019. Retrieved from: https://www.cdc.gov/vaccines/vpd/mening/index.html.

Centers for Disease Control and Prevention (CDC): Alzheimer's disease and healthy aging: Alzheimer's disease and related dementia, 2020a. Retrieved from: https://www.cdc.gov/aging/aginginfo/alzheimers.htm .

Centers for Disease Control and Prevention (CDC): Epilepsy: Fast facts, 2020b. Retrieved from: https://www.cdc.gov/epilepsy/about/fast-facts.htm.

Centers for Disease Control and Prevention (CDC): Stroke: Stroke facts, 2021a. Retrieved from: https://www.cdc.gov/stroke/facts.htm.

Centers for Disease Control and Prevention (CDC): Traumatic brain injury & concussion: Get the facts, 2021b. Retrieved from: https://www.cdc.gov/traumaticbraininjury/get_the_facts.html.

Centers for Disease Control and Prevention (CDC): West nile virus: West nile virus, 2021b. Retrieved from: https://www.cdc.gov/westnile/index.html.

Cleveland Clinic: Alzheimer's Disease, 2019. Retrieved from: https://my.clevelandclinic.org/health/diseases/9164-alzheimers-diseases.

Cleveland Clinic: Huntington's disease, 2020. Retrieved from: https://my.clevelandclinic.org/health/diseases/14369-huntingtons-disease.

Cruz-Flores S, Chaisam T: Stroke anticoagulation and prophylaxis, 2018. Retrieved from: https://emedicine.medscape.com/article/1160021.

Foo CC, Loan JJM, Brennan PM: The relationship of the FOUR score to patient outcome: A systematic review. Journal of Neurotrauma, 36 (17), 20 Aug 2019. doi: https://doi.org/10.1089/neu.2018.6243

Glasgow Coma Scale: The Glasgow structured approach to the assessment of the Glasgow coma scale, n.d. Royal College of Physicians and Surgeons of Glasgow. Retrieved from: https://www.glasgowcomascale.org/.

Howes DS: What is the prognosis of encephalitis?, 2018. Medscape. Retrieved from: https://www.medscape.com/answers/791896-104293/what-is-the-prognosis-of-encephalitis.

Jalali R, Rezaei M: A comparison of the glasgow coma scale score with full outline of unresponsiveness scale to predict patients' traumatic brain injury outcomes in intensive care units, Crit Care Res Pract. Hindawi Publishing Corporation. 2014:2014;289803.

Ko DY: Epilepsy and seizures treatment & management. Medscape. Retrieved from: https://emedicine.medscape.com/article/1184846-treatment.

Kopstein M, Mohlman DJ. HIV-1 Encephalopathy And Aids Dementia Complex, 2021 In: StatPearls [Internet]. Treasure Island (FL): StatPearls Publishing; 2021 Jan-. Retrieved from: https://www.ncbi.nlm.nih.gov/books/NBK507700/.

Krel R, Thomas FP: Central nervous system complications in HIV, 2018. Medscape. Retrieved from: https://emedicine.medscape.com/article/1167008-overview.

Lewis SL, Heitkemper MM, Dirksen SR, et al: Medical-surgical nursing: assessment and management of clinical problems, ed 7, St. Louis, 2007, Mosby.

Mayo Clinic: Parkinson's disease, 2020. Retrieved from: https://www.mayoclinic.org/diseases-conditions/parkinsons-disease/symptoms-causes/syc-20376055.

Mayo Clinic: Epilepsy, 2021a. Retrieved from: https://www.mayoclinic.org/diseases-conditions/epilepsy/diagnosis-treatment/drc-20350098

Mayo Clinic: Migraine, 2021b. Retrieved from: https://www.mayoclinic.org/diseases-conditions/migraine-headache/symptoms-causes/syc-20360201.

Mayo Clinic: Stroke, 2021c. Retrieved from: https://www.mayoclinic.org/diseases-conditions/stroke/diagnosis-treatment/drc-20350119.

Medline Plus, 2021. Retrieved from: https://medlineplus.gov/hormonereplacementtherapy.html.

Mosby's dictionary of medicine, nursing & health professions, ed 10, St. Louis, 2017, Elsevier.

Myasthenia Gravis Foundation of America: MG quick facts, n.d. Retrieved from: https://myasthenia.org/What-is-MG/MG-Quick-Facts.

National Institute on Aging: Putting exercise to the test in people at risk for Alzheimer's, 2017. Retrieved from: https://www.nia.nih.gov/news/putting-exercise-test-people-risk-alzheimers.

National Institute on Aging: Alzheimer's disease fact sheet, 2021. National Institutes of Health. Retrieved from: https://www.nia.nih.gov/health/alzheimers-disease-fact-sheet.

National Institute of Neurological Disorders and Stroke (NINDS): Questions and answers about carotid endarterectomy, 2016. National Institutes of Health. Retrieved from: https://www.ninds.nih.gov/Disorders/Patient-Caregiver-Education/Hope-Through-Research/Stroke-Hope-Through-Research/Questions-Answers-Carotid-Endarterectomy.

National Institute of Neurological Disorders and Stroke (NINDS): Bell's palsy fact sheet, 2020a. National Institutes of Health. Retrieved from: https://www.ninds.nih.gov/Disorders/Patient-Caregiver-Education/Fact-Sheets/Bells-Palsy-Fact-Sheet.

National Institute of Neurological Disorders and Stroke (NINDS): Brain basics: Preventing stroke, 2020b. National Institutes of Health. Retrieved from: https://www.ninds.nih.gov/disorders/patient-caregiver-education/preventing-stroke.

National Institute of Neurological Disorders and Stroke (NINDS): Guillain-Barre syndrome fact sheet, 2020c. National Institutes of Health. Retrieved from: https://www.ninds.nih.gov/Disorders/Patient-Caregiver-Education/Fact-Sheets/Guillain-Barr%C3%A9-Syndrome-Fact-Sheet.

National Institute of Neurological Disorders and Stroke (NINDS): Myasthenia gravis fact sheet, 2020d. National Institutes of Health. Retrieved from: https://www.ninds.nih.gov/Disorders/Patient-Caregiver-Education/Fact-Sheets/Myasthenia-Gravis-Fact-Sheet

National Institute of Neurological Disorders and Stroke (NINDS): Amyotrophic lateral sclerosis (ALS) fact sheet, 2021. National Institutes of Health. Retrieved from: https://www.ninds.nih.gov/Disorders/Patient-Caregiver-Education/Fact-Sheets/Amyotrophic-Lateral-Sclerosis-ALS-Fact-Sheet.

National Institutes of Health (NIH): All about ALS: Understanding a devastating disorder, 2015. Retrieved from: https://newsinhealth.nih.gov/issue/aug2015/feature2.

National Library of Medicine (NLM): Cluster headache, 2019a. MedlinePlus. Retrieved from: https://medlineplus.gov/ency/article/000786.htm.

National Library of Medicine (NLM): Guillain-Barre syndrome, 2019b. MedlinePlus. Retrieved from: https://medlineplus.gov/ency/article/000684.htm.

National Library of Medicine (NLM): Basal ganglia dysfunction, 2020a. MedlinePlus. Retrieved from: https://medlineplus.gov/ency/article/001069.htm.

National Library of Medicine (NLM): CSF leak, 2020b. MedlinePlus. Retrieved from: https://medlineplus.gov/ency/article/001068.htm.

National Library of Medicine (NLM): Huntingdon disease, 2020c. MedlinePlus. Retrieved from: https://medlineplus.gov/genetics/condition/huntington-disease/.

Newsome Melton: Brain injury FAQs, n.d. Retrieved from: http://www.brainandspinalcord.org/brain-injury-faqs/.

Pappu S, Lerma J, Khraishi T: Brain CT to Assess Intracranial Pressure in Patients with Traumatic Brain Injury, J Neuroimag 26(1):37–40, 2016. https://doi.org/10.1111/jon.12289.

Parkinson's Foundation: Orthostatic hypertension, n.d.a. Retrieved from: http://www.parkinson.org/Understanding-Parkinsons/Non-Movement-Symptoms.

Parkinson's Foundation: Understanding Parkinson's, n.d.b. Retrieved from: https://www.parkinson.org/understanding-parkinsons.

United Spinal Association: Spinal cord injury facts and figures, 2020. Retrieved from: https://unitedspinal.org/spinal-cord-injury-facts-and-figures.

U.S. Environmental Protection Agency (EPA): DEET, 2021. Retrieved from: https://www.epa.gov/insect-repellents/deet.

CHAPTER 15

American College of Asthma, Allergy and Immunology: Latex allergy, 2014. Retrieved from: https://acaai.org/allergies/types/skin-allergies/latex-allergy.

Buelow B, Routes JM: Immediate hypersensitivity reactions, 2020. Retrieved from: https://emedicine.medscape.com/article/136217-overview.

Fernandez J: Overview of immunodeficiency disorders, 2021. Merck Manual. Retrieved from: https://www.merckmanuals.com/home/immune-disorders/immunodeficiency-disorders/overview-of-immunodeficiency-disorders.

Haroun, HSW: Aging of thymus gland and immune system. MOJ Anatomy & Physiology. 5, 2018. https://doi.org/10.15406/mojap.2018.05.00186.

Ignatavicius DD, Workman ML: Medical-surgical nursing: Patient-centered collaborative care, ed 8, St. Louis, 2017, Elsevier.

National Institute of Allergy and Infectious Diseases (NIAID): Immune cells, 2014. National Institutes of Health. Retrieved from: https://www.niaid.nih.gov/research/immune-cells.

National Institute for Occupational Safety and Health (NIOSH): Latex allergy: a prevention guide, 2014. Centers for Disease Control and Prevention (CDC). Retrieved from: https://www.cdc.gov/niosh/docs/98-113/.

National Library of Medicine (NLM): Aging change in immunity, 2020. Retrieved from: https://medlineplus.gov/ency/article/004008.htm.

US Department of Labor. Occupational Safety and Health Administration (OSHA). Latex allergy, n.d. Retrieved from: https://www.osha.gov/latex-allergy.

Wein H: Shaking out clues to autoimmune disease, 2013. National Institutes of Health: Research Matters. Retrieved from: www.nih.gov/researchmatters/march2013/03182013autoimmune.htm.

CHAPTER 16

AIDS Clinical Trials Groups (ACTG):About the clinical trials process, n.d. Retrieved from: https://actgnetwork.org/faq/.

AVERT: Needle and syringe programmes (NSPS) for HIV prevention, 2019. Retrieved from: https://www.avert.org/professionals/hiv-programming/prevention/needle-syringe-programmes.

AVERT: Global HIV and AIDS Statistics, 2021. Retrieved from: https://www.avert.org/global-hiv-and-aids-statistics.

AVERT: HIV and AIDS in the United States of America, 2021b. Retrieved from: http://www.avert.org/professionals/hiv-around-world/western-central-europe-north-america/usa.

Buonaguro L, Tornesello ML, Buonaguro FM: Human immunodeficiency virus type 1 subtype distribution in the worldwide epidemic: Pathogenetic and therapeutic implications, J Virol 81(19):10209–10219, 2007.

Centers for Disease Control and Prevention (CDC): MMWR: recommendations and reports, MMWR Morb Mortal Wkly Rep 30(RR–21):1–3, 1981.

Centers for Disease Control and Prevention (CDC): Updated U.S. Public Health Service guidelines for the management of occupational exposures to HBV, HCV, and HIV and recommendations for postexposure prophylaxis, MMWR Morb Mortal Wkly Rep 50(RR–11):1, 2001.

Centers for Disease Control and Prevention (CDC): Today's HIV/AIDS epidemic, 2016. Retrieved from: https://www.cdc.gov/nchhstp/newsroom/docs/factsheets/todaysepidemic-508.pdf.

Centers for Disease Control and Prevention (CDC): HIV in the United States: At a glance, 2018g. Retrieved from: http://www.cdc.gov/hiv/statistics/overview/ataglance.html.

Centers for Disease Control and Prevention (CDC): HIV: HIV testing, 2020a. Retrieved from: https://www.cdc.gov/hiv/guidelines/testing.html.

Centers for Disease Control and Prevention (CDC): HIV: people aged 50 and older, 2020b. Retrieved from: https://www.cdc.gov/hiv/group/age/olderamericans/.

Centers for Disease Control and Prevention: Diagnose and treat to save lives: decreasing deaths among people with HIV, 2020c. Retrieved from: https://www.cdc.gov/hiv/statistics/deaths/index.html.

Center for Disease Control and Prevention (CDC): HIV: African Americans, 2021a. Retrieved from: https://www.cdc.gov/hiv/group/racialethnic/africanamericans/.

Centers for Disease Control and Prevention (CDC): HIV: about HIV, 2021b. Retrieved from: https://www.cdc.gov/hiv/basics/whatishiv.html

Centers for Disease Control and Prevention (CDC): HIV: Hispanics/Latinos, 2021c. Retrieved from: http://www.cdc.gov/hiv/group/racialethnic/hispaniclatinos/.

Centers for Disease Control and Prevention (CDC): HIV: HIV and injection drug use, 2021d

Centers for Disease Control and Prevention (CDC): HIV: living with HIV, 2021e. Retrieved from: https://www.cdc.gov/hiv/basics/livingwithhiv/.

Centers for Disease Control and Prevention (CDC): HIV: people who inject drugs, 2021f. Retrieved from: https://www.cdc.gov/hiv/group/hiv-idu.html.

Centers for Disease Control and Prevention (CDC): HIV: PEP, 2021g. Retrieved from: https://www.cdc.gov/hiv/basics/pep.html.

Centers for Disease Control and Prevention (CDC): HIV: types of tests, 2021h. Retrieved from: https://www.cdc.gov/hiv/basics/hiv-testing/test-types.html.

Centers for Disease Control and Prevention (CDC): HIV: ways HIV can be transmitted, 2021i. Retrieved from: https://www.cdc.gov/hiv/basics/hiv-transmission/ways-people-get-hiv.html.

Centers for Disease Control and Prevention (CDC): HIV: women, 2021j. Retrieved from: https://www.cdc.gov/hiv/group/gender/women/index.html.

Centers for Disease Control and Prevention (CDC): Fungal diseases. Pneumocystis Pneumonia, 2021k. Retrieved from https://www.cdc.gov/fungal/diseases/pneumocystis-pneumonia/index.html.

Center to Advance Palliative Care: What is palliative care?, 2021. Retrieved from: https://getpalliativecare.org/whatis/.

Clinicalinfo.hiv.gov: HIV/AIDS glossary: antiretroviral pregnancy registry, n.d. Retrieved from: https://clinicalinfo.hiv.gov/en/glossary/antiretroviral-pregnancy-registry.

Coffin J: HIV pathogenesis. 11th International AIDS Conference, Vancouver, 1996, British Columbia.

Familydoctor.org: Occupational exposure to HIV: advice for health care workers, 2019. Retrieved from: https://familydoctor.org/occupational-exposure-to-hiv-advice-for-health-care-workers/.

Garry RF, Witte MH, Gottlieb AA, et al: Documentation of an AIDS virus infection in the United States in 1968, JAMA 260(14):2085–2087, 1988.

Henry J. Kaiser Family Foundation: The HIV/AIDS epidemic in the United States: The basics, 2021. Retrieved from: http://kff.org/hivaids/fact-sheet/the-hivaids-epidemic-in-the-united-states/.

HIV.gov: How is HIV transmitted?, 2019. Retrieved from: https://www.hiv.gov/hiv-basics/overview/about-hiv-and-aids/how-is-hiv-transmitted.

HIV.gov: Who should get tested?, 2020. Retrieved from: https://www.hiv.gov/hiv-basics/hiv-testing/learn-about-hiv-testing/who-should-get-tested.

HIV.gov: Preventing sexual transmission of HIV, 2021a. Retrieved from: https://www.hiv.gov/hiv-basics/hiv-prevention/reducing-sexual-risk/preventing-sexual-transmission-of-hiv

HIV.gov: U.S. Statistics, 2021b. Retrieved from: https://www.hiv.gov/hiv-basics/overview/data-and-trends/statistics.

HIV.gov: What are vaccines and what do they do?, 2021c Retrieved from: https://www.hiv.gov/hiv-basics/hiv-prevention/potential-future-options/hiv-vaccines.

HIVinfo.nih.gov: HIV medicines and side effects, 2020a. Retrieved from: https://hivinfo.nih.gov/understanding-hiv/fact-sheets/hiv-medicines-and-side-effects.

HIVinfo.nih.gov: HIV treatment adherence, 2020b. Retrieved from https://hivinfo.nih.gov/understanding-hiv/fact-sheets/hiv-treatment-adherence.

HIVinfo.nih.gov: Preventing mother-to-child transmission of HIV, 2020c. Retrieved from: https://hivinfo.nih.gov/understanding-hiv/fact-sheets/preventing-mother-child-transmission-hiv-0.

HIVinfo.nih.gov: The HIV life cycle, 2020d. Retrieved from: https://hivinfo.nih.gov/understanding-hiv/fact-sheets/hiv-life-cycle .

HIVinfo.nih.gov: The stages of HIV infection, 2020e. Retrieved from: https://hivinfo.nih.gov/understanding-hiv/fact-sheets/stages-hiv-infection.

HIVinfo.nih.gov: When to start HIV medicines, 2020f. Retrieved from: https://hivinfo.nih.gov/understanding-hiv/fact-sheets/when-start-hiv-medicines.

Holmberg SD: The estimated prevalence and incidence of HIV in 96 large US metropolitan areas, Am J Public Health 86(5):642–654, 2008, 1996.

Irshad U, Mahdy H, Tonismae T. HIV In Pregnancy. [Updated 2021 Apr 11]. In: StatPearls [Internet]. Treasure Island (FL): StatPearls Publishing; 2021 Jan-. Retrieved from: https://www.ncbi.nlm.nih.gov/books/NBK558972/.

MedlinePlus: HIV/AIDS medicines, 2021. Retrieved from: https://medlineplus.gov/hivaidsmedicines.html.

National Institute of Allergy and Infectious Diseases (NIAID): HIV replication cycle, 2018. Retrieved from: https://www.niaid.nih.gov/diseases-conditions/hiv-replication-cycle.

Nayamweya S, Hegedus A, Jaye A, et al: Comparing HIV-1 and HIV-2 infection: Lessons for viral immunopathogenesis, 2013. Retrieved from: http://onlinelibrary.wiley.com/doi/10.1002/rmv.1739/abstract;jsessionid=6A7F5352382E943A337A548E92EDDDD4.f01t04.

Peruski AH, Wesolowski LG, Delaney KP, et al. Trends in HIV-2 Diagnoses and Use of the HIV-1/HIV-2 Differentiation Test — United States, 2010–2017. MMWR Morb Mortal Wkly Rep 2020;69:63–66. DOI: https://doi.org/10.15585/mmwr.mm6903a2

SciDevNet: African HIV trials could create world's first vaccine, 2016. Retrieved from: http://www.scidev.net/sub-saharan-africa/hiv-aids/news/african-hiv-trials-could-create-world-s-first-vaccine.html.

Thomas, FP: Dementia due to HIV infection, 2018. Retrieved from: https://www.emedicinehealth.com/dementia_due_to_hiv_infection/article_em.htm#pictures_of_brains_with_aids_dementia_complex.

UNAIDS: Press release: UNAIDS report on the global AIDS epidemic shows that 2020 targets will not be met because of deeply unequal success; COVID-19 risks blowing HIV progress off course, 2020. Retrieved from: https://www.unaids.org/en/resources/presscentre/pressreleaseandstatementarchive/2020/july/20200706_global-aids-report

US Department of Health and Human Services (USDHHS): Guidelines for the Use of Antiretroviral Agents in Adults and Adolescents Living with HIV. Developed by the DHHS Panel on Antiretroviral Guidelines for Adults and Adolescents – A Working Group of the Office of AIDS Research Advisory Council (OARAC). 2021. Retrieved from: .https://clinicalinfo.hiv.gov/sites/default/files/guidelines/documents/AdultandAdolescentGL.pdf

US Department of Labor, Occupational Safety & Health Administration (OSHA): Bloodborne pathogens and needlestick prevention, n.d. Retrieved from: https://www.osha.gov/bloodborne-pathogens/general.

US Department of Veterans Affairs (VA): HIV wasting syndrome, 2019. Retrieved from: https://www.hiv.va.gov/patient/diagnosis/OI-wasting-syndrome.asp.

US Food and Drug Administration (FDA): Blood and blood products, 2021. Retrieved from: https://www.fda.gov/vaccines-blood-biologics/blood-blood-products.]

World Health Organization (WHO): Consolidated Guidelines on HIV Testing Services: 5Cs: Consent, Confidentiality, Counselling, Correct Results and Connection 2015, Geneva, 2015 Jul. 3, World Health Organization, PRE-TEST AND POST-TEST SERVICES. Available from: https://www.ncbi.nlm.nih.gov/books/.

World Health Organization (WHO): HIV/AIDS Key Facts, 2020. Retrieved from: http://www.who.int/en/news-room/fact-sheets/detail/hiv-aids.

World Health Organization (WHO): Zoonoses, 2020. Retrieved from: https://www.who.int/news-room/fact-sheets/detail/zoonoses.

CHAPTER 17

American Cancer Society (ACS): Signs and symptoms of testicular cancer, 2018. Retrieved from: https://www.cancer.org/cancer/testicular-cancer/detection-diagnosis-staging/signs-and-symptoms.html.

American Cancer Society (ACS): Breast cancer risk and prevention, 2019a. Retrieved from: https://www.cancer.org/cancer/breast-cancer/risk-and-prevention/breast-cancer-risk-factors-you-cannot-change.html.

American Cancer Society (ACS): Cancer facts and figures 2019, 2019b. Retrieved from: https://www.cancer.org/content/dam/cancer-org/research/cancer-facts-and-statistics/annual-cancer-facts-and-figures/2019/cancer-facts-and-figures-2019.pdf.

American Cancer Society (ACS): American Cancer Society guideline for colorectal cancer screening, 2020a. Retrieved from: https://www.cancer.org/cancer/colon-rectal-cancer/detection-diagnosis-staging/acs-recommendations.html.

American Cancer Society (ACS): American Cancer Society guidelines for diet and physical activity, 2020b. Retrieved from: https://www.cancer.org/healthy/eat-healthy-get-active/acs-guidelines-nutrition-physical-activity-cancer-prevention/guidelines.html.

American Cancer Society (ACS): American Cancer Society guidelines for the early detection of cancer, 2020c. Retrieved from: https://www.cancer.org/healthy/find-cancer-early/american-cancer-society-guidelines-for-the-early-detection-of-cancer.html.

American Cancer Society (ACS): American Cancer Society updates diet & physical activity guideline for cancer prevention, 2020d. Retrieved from: http://pressroom.cancer.org/DietPhysicalActivity2020.

American Cancer Society (ACS): Cancer Facts & Figures 2020, 2020e. Retrieved from: https://www.cancer.org/content/dam/cancer-org/research/cancer-facts-and-statistics/annual-cancer-facts-and-figures/2020/cancer-facts-and-figures-2020.pdf .

American Cancer society (ACS): Chemo brain, 2020f. Retrieved from: https://www.cancer.org/treatment/treatments-and-side-effects/physical-side-effects/changes-in-mood-or-thinking/chemo-brain.html,

American Cancer Society (ACS): Family cancer syndromes, 2020g. Retrieved from: https://www.cancer.org/cancer/cancer-causes/genetics/family-cancer-syndromes.html.

American Cancer Society (ACS): Health risks of smoking tobacco, 2020h. Retrieved from: https://www.cancer.org/healthy/stay-away-from-tobacco/health-risks-of-tobacco/health-risks-of-smoking-tobacco.html.

American Cancer Society: Low platelet count (bleeding), 2020i. Retrieved from: https://www.cancer.org/treatment/treatments-and-side-effects/physical-side-effects/low-blood-counts/bleeding.html.

American Cancer Society: What do we know about e-cigarettes?, 2020j. Retrieved from: https://www.cancer.org/healthy/stay-away-from-tobacco/e-cigarettes-vaping/what-do-we-know-about-e-cigarettes.html.

American Cancer Society: American Cancer Society recommendations for the early detection of breast cancer, 2021a. Retrieved from: https://www.cancer.org/cancer/breast-cancer/screening-tests-and-early-detection/american-cancer-society-recommendations-for-the-early-detection-of-breast-cancer.html.

American Cancer Society: Can lung cancer be found early?, 2021b. Retrieved from: https://www.cancer.org/cancer/lung-cancer/detection-diagnosis-staging/detection.html.

American Cancer Society: Cancer prevention & early detection facts & figures, 2021-2022, 2021c. Retrieved from: https://www.cancer.org/research/cancer-facts-statistics/cancer-prevention-early-detection.html.

American Cancer Society: Viruses that can lead to cancer, 2021d. Retrieved from https://www.cancer.org/cancer/cancer-causes/infectious-agents/infections-that-can-lead-to-cancer/viruses.html.

Cancer.net: Side effects of chemotherapy, 2019. Retrieved from: http://www.cancer.net/navigating-cancer-care/how-cancer-treated/chemotherapy/side-effects-chemotherapy.

Cancer.net: Nausea and vomiting, 2020a. Retrieved from: http://www.cancer.net/research-and-advocacy/asco-care-and-treatment-recommendations-patients/preventing-vomiting-caused-cancer-treatment.

Cancer.net: Positron emission tomography and computed tomography (PET-CT) scans, 2020b. Retrieved from: http://www.cancer.net/navigating-cancer-care/diagnosing-cancer/tests-and-procedures/positron-emission-tomography-and-computed-tomography-pet-ct-scans.

Centers for Disease Control and Prevention (CDC): Cancer incidence among African Americans, United States--2007-2016, 2020. Retrieved from: https://www.cdc.gov/cancer/uscs/about/data-briefs/no15-cancer-incidence-African-Americans-2007-2016.htm.

Centers for Disease Control and Prevention (CDC): Cancer: cancer and man, 2021a. Retrieved from: https://www.cdc.gov/cancer/dcpc/resources/features/cancerandmen/index.htm.

Gallaway MS, Townsend JS, Shelby D, Puckett MC: Pain among cancer survivors. Retrieved from: https://www.cdc.gov/pcd/issues/2020/19_0367.htm?s_cid=pcd17e54_x, 2020.

Johns Hopkins Medicine, n.d. Retrieved from: https://www.hopkinsmedicine.org/kimmel_cancer_center/cancers_we_treat/cervical_dysplasia/diagnosis_and_treatment/abnormal_pap_test.html.

Lee-Kwan SH, Moore LV, Blanck HM, Harris DM, Galuska D. Disparities in State-Specific Adult Fruit and Vegetable Consumption — United States, 2015. MMWR Morb Mortal Wkly Rep 2017;66:1241–1247. DOI: https://doi.org/10.15585/mmwr.mm6645a1

Mayo Clinic: Mouth sores caused by cancer treatment: how to cope, 2020a. Retrieved from: https://www.mayoclinic.org/diseases-conditions/cancer/in-depth/mouth-sores/art-20045486.

Mayo Clinic: Positron emission tomography scan, 2020b. Retrieved from: https://www.mayoclinic.org/tests-procedures/pet-scan/about/pac-20385078.

National Cancer Institute (NCI): Tumor grade, 2013. Retrieved from: https://www.cancer.gov/about-cancer/diagnosis-staging/prognosis/tumor-grade-fact-sheet

National Cancer Institute (NCI): Cancer staging, 2015a. Retrieved from: https://www.cancer.gov/about-cancer/diagnosis-staging/staging

National Cancer Institute (NCI): Obesity, 2015b. Retrieved from: https://www.cancer.gov/about-cancer/causes-prevention/risk/obesity.

National Cancer Institute (NCI): The genetics of cancer, 2017. Retrieved from: https://www.cancer.gov/about-cancer/causes-prevention/genetics.

National Cancer Institute (NCI): Alcohol and cancer risk, 2018a. Retrieved from: https://www.cancer.gov/about-cancer/causes-prevention/risk/alcohol/alcohol-fact-sheet.

National Cancer Institute (NCI): Cancer Statistics, 2018b. Retrieved from: https://www.cancer.gov/about-cancer/understanding/statistics.

National Cancer Institute (NCI), 2020. Retrieved from: https://www.cancer.gov/about-cancer/causes-prevention/genetics/brca-fact-sheet.

National Cancer Institute (NCI): Cannabis and cannabinoids (PDQ®)—health professionals version, 2021a. Retrieved from: https://www.cancer.gov/about-cancer/treatment/cam/hp/cannabis-pdq.

National Cancer Institute (NCI): Targeted cancer therapies, 2021b. Retrieved from: https://www.cancer.gov/about-cancer/treatment/types/targeted-therapies/targeted-therapies-fact-sheet.

Pancreatic Cancer Action Network: CA 19-9, n.d. Retrieved from: https://www.pancan.org/facing-pancreatic-cancer/diagnosis/ca19-9/.

Rock, C.L., Thomson, C., Gansler, T., Gapstur, S.M., McCullough, M.L., Patel, A.V., Andrews, K.S., Bandera, E.V., Spees, C.K., Robien, K., Hartman, S., Sullivan, K., Grant, B.L., Hamilton, K.K., Kushi, L.H., Caan, B.J., Kibbe, D., Black, J.D., Wiedt, T.L., McMahon, C., Sloan, K. and Doyle, C. American Cancer Society guideline for diet and physical activity for cancer prevention. CA A Cancer J Clin, 70: 245-271, 2020. https://doi.org/10.3322/caac.21591

Vachani C: Patient guide to tumor markers, 2020. Retrieved from: https://www.oncolink.org/cancer-treatment/procedures-diagnostic-tests/blood-tests-tumor-diagnostic-tests/patient--guide-to-tumor-markers.

Glossary

A

ablation Amputation or excision of any part of the body; removal of a growth or harmful substance.

ableism Discrimination and prejudice toward people with disabilities where the person is defined by their disabilities and preference is giving to people without disabilities.

achalasia Abnormal condition characterized by the inability of a muscle, particularly the cardiac sphincter of the stomach, to relax.

achlorhydria Abnormal condition characterized by the absence of hydrochloric acid in the gastric secretions.

acquired immunodeficiency syndrome (AIDS) Acquired condition that impairs the body's ability to fight infection; the end stage of the continuum of HIV infection, in which the infected person has a CD4+ (lymphocyte) count of 200 cells/mm^3 or fewer.

active transport The movement of materials across the membrane of a cell by means of chemical activity, which allows the cell to admit larger molecules than would otherwise be able to enter.

acute coryza Acute rhinitis, also known as the common cold; an inflammatory condition of the mucous membranes of the nose and accessory sinuses.

adaptive immunity Protection that provides a specific reaction to each invading antigen and has the unique ability to remember the antigen that caused the attack.

adherence Following a prescribed regimen of therapy or treatment for disease.

adventitious Abnormal sounds superimposed on breath sounds.

agnosia Total or partial loss of the ability to recognize familiar objects or people through sensory stimuli; results from organic brain damage.

air embolism An abnormal circulatory condition in which air travels through the bloodstream and becomes lodged in a blood vessel.

allergen A substance that can produce a hypersensitive reaction in the body but that is not necessarily inherently harmful.

alopecia Loss of hair resulting from destruction of hair follicles.

amenorrhea Absence of menstrual flow.

anaphylactic shock Severe, life-threatening hypersensitive reaction to a previously encountered antigen.

anasarca Severe, generalized edema.

anastomosis Surgical joining of two ducts or blood vessels to allow flow from one to the other.

anatomy The study, classification, and description of structures and organs of the body.

anemia Blood disorder characterized by red blood cell, hemoglobin, and hematocrit levels below normal range.

anesthesia Absence of sensation (*an-*, meaning "without," and *-esthesia*, meaning "awareness or feeling").

aneurysm A localized dilation of the wall of a blood vessel, usually caused by atherosclerosis, hypertension, and less commonly by a congenital weakness in a vessel wall.

angina pectoris Paroxysmal thoracic pain and choking feeling caused by decreased oxygen (anoxia) of the myocardium.

ankylosis Fixation of a joint, often in an abnormal position, usually resulting from destruction of articular cartilage and subchondral bone.

antigen A substance recognized by the body as foreign that can trigger an immune response.

anuria Urinary output of less than 100 to 250 mL in 24 hours.

aphasia Abnormal neurologic condition in which language function is defective or absent because of an injury to certain areas of the cerebral cortex.

aplasia In hematology, a failure of the normal process of cell generation and development.

apraxia Impairment of the ability to perform purposeful acts; inability to use objects properly.

arteriosclerosis Common arterial disorder characterized by thickening, loss of elasticity, and calcification of arterial walls, resulting in a decreased blood supply.

arthrocentesis Puncture of a joint with a needle to withdraw fluid; performed to obtain synovial fluid for diagnostic purposes.

arthrodesis Surgical fusion of a joint.

arthroplasty Surgical repair or refashioning of one of both sides, parts, or specific tissues within a joint.

ascites An accumulation of fluid and albumin in the peritoneal cavity.

asterixis Hand-flapping tremor usually induced by extending the arm and dorsiflexing the wrist; frequently seen in hepatic coma.

asthenia General feeling of tiredness and listlessness.

astigmatism Defect in the curvature of the eyeball surface.

ataxia Abnormal condition characterized by impaired ability to coordinate movement.

atelectasis Collapse of lung tissues, preventing the respiratory exchange of carbon dioxide and oxygen.

atherosclerosis A common arterial disorder characterized by yellowish plaques of cholesterol, lipids, and cellular debris in the inner layer of the walls of large and medium-sized arteries.

attenuation The process of weakening the degree of virulence of a disease organism.

audiometry Testing of hearing acuity.

aura Sensation, as of light or warmth, that may precede the onset of a migraine or an epileptic seizure. An epileptic aura may be psychic, or it may be sensory with olfactory, visual, auditory, or taste hallucinations.

autograft Surgical transplantation of any tissue from one part of the body to another location in the same individual.

autoimmune/autoimmunity Immune response (autoantibodies or cellular immune response) to one's own tissues.

autologous Something that has its origin within an individual, especially a factor present in tissues or fluids.

automated perimetry test Test places the patient in front of a computer-like device and asks patient to stare at a screen and to press a button when flashes of light enter the field of vision.

azotemia Retention of excessive amounts of nitrogenous compounds in the blood.

B

bacteriuria Presence of bacteria in the urine.

benign Not recurrent or progressive; opposite of malignant.

biliary atresia The absence of or underdevelopment of biliary structures that is congenital in nature.

biopsy The removal of a small piece of living tissue from an organ or another part of the body for microscopic examination to confirm or establish a diagnosis, estimate a prognosis, or follow the course of a disease.

bipolar hip replacement (hemiarthroplasty) Prosthetic implant used to replace the femoral head and neck in hip fractures when the vascular supply to the femoral head is or may become compromised.

blanching test A test of the rate of capillary refill; blanching means to cause to become pale by applying digital pressure.

bradycardia Slow rhythm characterized by a pulse rate of fewer than 60 beats per minute.

bradykinesia An abnormal condition characterized by slowness of voluntary movements and speech.

bronchoscopy Visual examination of the larynx, trachea, and bronchi using a standard rigid, tubular metal bronchoscope or a narrower, flexible fiberoptic bronchoscope.

B-type natriuretic peptide (BNP) A neurohormone secreted by the heart in response to ventricular expansion.

C

cachexia General ill health and malnutrition marked by weakness and emaciation; usually associated with a serious disease such as cancer.

callus Bony deposits formed between and around the broken ends of a fractured bone during healing.

candidiasis Mild fungal infection that appears in men and women; usually caused by *Candida albicans* and *C. tropicalis.*

carcinoembryonic antigen (CEA) Oncofetal glycoprotein antigen found in colonic adenocarcinoma and other cancers; also found in nonmalignant conditions.

carcinogen Substance known to increase the risk for the development of cancer.

carcinogenesis Various factors that are possible origins of cancer.

carcinoma Term used for a malignant tumor composed of epithelial cells; it displays a tendency to metastasize.

carcinoma in situ Preinvasive, asymptomatic carcinoma that can be diagnosed only by microscopic examination of cervical cells.

cardiac arrest Sudden cessation of functional circulation.

cardioversion Restoration of the heart's normal sinus rhythm by delivery of a synchronized electric shock through two metal paddles placed on the patient's chest.

catabolism Breakdown or destructive phase of metabolism. Catabolism occurs when complex body substances are broken down to simpler ones; opposite of anabolism.

cataract Opacity or clouding of the lens.

CD4⁺ lymphocyte A type of white blood cell; a protein on the surface of cells that normally helps the body's immune system combat disease.

cell The fundamental unit of all living tissue.

cellular immunity Acquired immunity characterized by the dominant role of small T lymphocytes; also called *cell-mediated immunity.*

Centers for Disease Control and Prevention (CDC) Federal agency that provides facilities and services for investigation, identification, prevention, and control of disease; headquartered in Atlanta, Georgia.

chancre Painless erosion of a papule that ulcerates superficially with a scooped-out appearance.

Chlamydia trachomatis A gram-negative intracellular bacterium that causes several common sexually transmitted diseases.

Chvostek sign Abnormal spasm of the facial muscles elicited by light taps on the facial nerve in patients who are hypocalcemic; seen in tetany.

circumcision Surgical procedure in which a part of the foreskin is removed, leaving the glans penis uncovered.

climacteric Phase of the aging process marking the transition from the reproductive phase to a nonreproductive stage of life.

Colles fracture A fracture of the distal portion of the radius within 1 inch of the joint of the wrist.

colporrhaphy Surgical correction of cystocele and rectocele by shortening the muscles that support the bladder and repairing the rectocele.

colposcopy Examination of the cervix and vagina using a colposcope.

compartment syndrome Pathologic condition caused by progressive development of arterial compression and reduced blood supply to an extremity. Increased pressure from external devices (casts, bulky dressings) causes decreased blood flow, resulting in ischemic tissue necrosis, most often occurs in the extremities.

conjunctivitis Inflammation of the conjunctiva.

conscious sedation Central nervous system depressant drugs and/or analgesia given to relieve anxiety and/or provide amnesia during surgical, diagnostic, or interventional procedures.

contracture Abnormal, usually permanent condition of a joint characterized by flexion and fixation and caused by atrophy and shortening of muscle fibers.

cor pulmonale Abnormal cardiac condition characterized by hypertrophy of the right ventricle of the heart as a result of hypertension of the pulmonary circulation.

coronary artery disease (CAD) Variety of conditions that obstruct blood flow in the coronary arteries.

coronary occlusion The partial or complete obstruction of a coronary artery.

coryza Acute inflammation of the mucous membranes of the nose and accessory sinuses, usually accompanied by edema of the mucosa and nasal discharge.

costovertebral angle Pertaining to a rib and a vertebra, one of two angles that outline a space over the kidneys.

crackle(s) Short, discrete, interrupted crackling or bubbling adventitious breath sounds heard on auscultation of the chest, most commonly upon inspiration. They are produced by passage of air through the bronchi that contain secretions of exudate or are constricted by spasms or thickening; usually heard during inspiration. Formerly called *rales.*

crepitus Sound that resembles the crackling noise heard when rubbing hair between the fingers or throwing salt on an open fire. It is associated with gas gangrene, the rubbing of bone fragments, or the crackles of a consolidated area of the lung in pneumonia.

cryosurgery Procedure to "freeze" the border of a retinal hole with a frozen-tipped probe.

cryotherapy A procedure in which a topical anesthetic is used so that a cryoprobe can be placed directly on the surface of the eye.

cryptorchidism Failure of testes to descend into the scrotum.

culdoscopy Diagnostic procedure that provides visualization of the uterus and adnexa (uterine appendages that include the ovaries and fallopian tubes).

cultural bias Thinking that the beliefs and practices of a particular culture are best.

curettage Scraping of material from the wall of a cavity or other surface, performed to remove tumors or other abnormal tissue for microscopic study.

Curling ulcer Duodenal ulcer that develops 8 to 14 days after severe burns on the surface of the body; the first sign is usually vomiting of bright red blood.

cyanosis Slightly bluish, gray, slatelike, or dark purple discoloration of the skin resulting from the presence of abnormally reduced amounts of oxygenated hemoglobin in the blood.

cytology/cytologic evaluation Study of cells and their formation, origin, structure, biochemical activities, and pathology.

cytoplasm "Living matter"; a substance that exists only in cells, composed largely of a gel-like substance that contains water, minerals, enzymes, and other specialized materials.

D

deaf culture A set of beliefs that are influenced by beliefs centered around an inability to hear.

débridement Removal of damaged cellular tissue from a wound or burn to prevent infection and promote healing.

deep brain stimulation (DBS) Involves placing an electrode in either the thalamus, globus pallidus, or subthalamic nucleus and connecting it to a generator placed in the upper chest (like a pacemaker).

defibrillation The termination of ventricular fibrillation by delivering a direct electrical countershock to the precordium.

dehiscence Partial or complete separation of a surgical incision or rupture of a wound closure.

dendrite Branching process that extends from the cell body of a neuron and receives impulses.

diabetes mellitus *See* type 1 diabetes mellitus, type 2 diabetes mellitus.

diabetic retinopathy Disorder of retinal blood vessels characterized by capillary microaneurysms, hemorrhage, exudates, and formation of new vessels and connective tissue.

dialysis Medical procedure for the removal of certain elements from the blood or lymph by virtue of the difference in their rates of diffusion through an external semipermeable membrane or, in the case of peritoneal dialysis, through the peritoneum.

differentiated Describes a tumor that is most like the parent tissue.

diffusion A process in which solid particles in a fluid move from an area of higher concentration to an area of lower concentration.

diplopia Double vision.

disseminated intravascular coagulation (DIC) Acquired hemorrhage syndrome of clotting, cascade overstimulation, and anticlotting processes.

diuresis Secretion and passage of large amounts of urine.

dorsal Toward the back.

drainage Free flow or withdrawal of fluids from a wound or cavity by a system (such as a urinary catheter or T-tube).

dumping syndrome A condition that results when food passes too rapidly from the stomach to the small intestine. It is often associated with high sugar-containing foods. It may be the result of gastrointestinal surgery, or it may be an independent condition.

dysarthria Difficult, poorly articulated speech resulting from interference in the control over the muscles of speech.

dysgeusia A distortion to the sense of taste.

dysmenorrhea Painful menstruation.

dyspepsia Vague feelings of epigastric discomfort.

dysphagia Difficulty swallowing.

dyspnea Shortness of breath or difficulty in breathing; may be caused by disturbances in the lungs, certain heart conditions, and hemoglobin deficiency.

dysrhythmia Any disturbance or abnormality in a normal rhythmic pattern, specifically irregularity in the normal rhythm of the heart. Also called *arrhythmia*.

dysuria Painful or difficult urination.

E

efficacy The effectiveness of the therapy to produce the intended effect.

embolism An abnormal circulatory condition in which an embolus (e.g., a foreign substance, blood clot, fat, air, or amniotic fluid) travels through the bloodstream and becomes lodged in a blood vessel.

embolus A foreign object, quantity of air or gas, bit of tissue or tumor, or a piece of thrombus that circulates in the bloodstream until it becomes lodged in a vessel.

empyema Accumulation of pus in a body cavity, especially the pleural space, as a result of infection.

endarterectomy Surgical removal of the intimal lining of an artery.

endocrinologist Physician who specializes in hormone imbalances and alterations in related body systems.

endometriosis Condition in which endometrial tissue appears outside the uterus.

enucleation Surgical removal of the eyeball.

enzyme-linked immunosorbent assay (ELISA) Antibody test that uses a rapid enzyme immunochemical assay method to detect HIV antibodies.

epididymitis Infection of the cordlike excretory duct of the testicles.

epistaxis Hemorrhage from the nose; nosebleed.

erythrocytosis Abnormal increase in the number of circulating red blood cells.

erythropoiesis The process of red blood cell production.

eschar Black, leathery crust; a slough that the body forms over burned tissue.

esophageal varices A complex of longitudinal, tortuous veins at the lower end of the esophagus.

evisceration Protrusion of an internal organ through a disrupted wound or surgical incision.

exacerbation An increase in the seriousness of a disease or disorder, marked by greater intensity in the signs or symptoms of the patient being treated.

excoriation Injury to the surface layer of skin caused by scratching or abrasion.

exophthalmos An abnormal condition characterized by a marked protrusion of the eyeballs.

extravasation The escape of fluids into surrounding tissue.

extrinsic Caused by external factors.

extubate To remove an endotracheal tube from an airway.

exudate Fluid, cells, or other substances that have been slowly exuded or discharged from body cells or blood vessels through small pores or breaks in cell membrane.

F

fibromyalgia A musculoskeletal chronic pain syndrome of unknown etiology that causes pain in muscles, bones, or joints.

filtration The transfer of water and dissolved substances from an area of higher pressure to an area of lower pressure.

fistula Abnormal opening between two organs.

flaccid Weak, soft, and flabby; lacking normal muscle tone.

flail chest Two or more ribs fractured in two or more places resulting in instability in part of the chest wall with associated hemothorax, pneumothorax, and pulmonary contusion.

flatulence Excessive formation of gases in the stomach or intestine.

folk medicine The traditional healing practices that are passed down within a culture.

G

germline mutations A variation in the composition of a germline cell.

Glasgow Coma Scale A quick, practical, standardized system for assessing the degree of conscious impairment in the critically ill; also used for predicting the duration and ultimate outcome of coma, primarily in patients with head injuries.

glaucoma An abnormal condition of elevated pressure within an eye because of obstruction of the outflow of aqueous humor.

global cognitive dysfunction Generalized impairment of intellect, awareness, and judgment.

gluten A protein primarily found in wheat, rye, and barley grains and products.

glycosuria Abnormal presence of sugar, especially glucose in the urine.

Goldmann tonometry A device used to assess ocular pressure.

Guillain-Barré syndrome (GBS) An immune disorder characterized by attacks on the peripheral nervous system. Symptoms may vary in intensity.

H

health disparities Preventable, negative health outcomes that disproportionately affect socially and economically disadvantaged populations.

heart failure (HF) Syndrome characterized by circulatory congestion due to the heart's inability to act as an effective pump; it should be viewed as a neurohormonal problem in which pathology progresses as a result of chronic release in the body of substances such as catecholamines (epinephrine and norepinephrine).

hemarthrosis Bleeding into a joint space, a hallmark of severe disease usually occurring in the knees, ankles, and elbow.

hematemesis Vomiting blood.

hematuria Blood in the urine.

hemianopia Defective vision or blindness in half of the visual field.

hemiplegia Paralysis of one side of the body.

hemophilia Hereditary coagulation disorder; caused by a lack of antihemophilic factor VIII, which is needed to convert prothrombin to thrombin through thromboplastin component.

hemoptysis Expectorating blood from the respiratory tract.

hepatic encephalopathy A type of brain damage caused by a liver disease and consequent ammonia intoxication.

hepatitis Inflammation of the liver resulting from several causes, including several types of viral agents or exposure to toxic substances.

heterograft (xenograft) Tissue from another species used as a temporary graft.

heterozygous Having two different genes.

hirsutism Excessive body hair in a masculine distribution.

HIV disease Symptomatic human immunodeficiency virus (HIV) infection that is not severe enough for a diagnosis of acquired immunodeficiency syndrome (AIDS); symptoms of HIV disease are persistent unexplained fever, night sweats, diarrhea, weight loss, and fatigue.

HIV infection The state in which HIV enters the body under favorable conditions and multiplies, producing injurious effects.

homeostasis A relative constancy in the internal environment of the body, naturally maintained by adaptive responses that promote healthy survival.

homograft (allograft) The transfer of tissue between two genetically dissimilar individuals of the same species, such as a skin transplant between two humans who are not identical twins.

homozygous Having two identical genes inherited from each parent for a given hereditary characteristic.

human immunodeficiency virus (HIV) An obligate virus; a retrovirus that causes AIDS.

humoral immunity One of the two forms of immunity that respond to antigens such as bacteria and foreign tissue. It is mediated by B cells.

hydronephrosis The dilation of the renal pelvis and calyces.

hypercapnia Greater than normal amounts of carbon dioxide in the blood.

hyperglycemia A greater than normal amount of glucose in the blood.

hyperopia Farsightedness; inability to see objects at close range.

hyperreflexia Neurologic condition characterized by increased reflex reactions.

hypersensitivity An abnormal condition characterized by an excessive reaction to a particular stimulus.

hypocalcemia A deficiency of calcium in serum.

hypoglycemia A lower than normal amount of glucose in the blood; usually caused by administration of too much insulin, excessive secretion of insulin by the islet cells of the pancreas, or dietary deficiency.

hypokalemia A condition in which an inadequate amount of potassium, the major intracellular cation, is found in the circulatory bloodstream.

hypoventilation An abnormal condition of the respiratory system that occurs when the volume of air is not adequate for the metabolic needs of the body.

hypoxemia An abnormal deficiency of oxygen in the arterial blood.

hypoxia An inadequate, reduced tension of cellular oxygen.

I

idiopathic Cause unknown.

idiopathic hyperplasia Increase, without any known cause, in the number of cells.

ileal conduit Ureters are implanted into a loop of the ileum that is isolated and brought to the surface of the abdominal wall.

immunity The quality of being unsusceptible to or unaffected by a particular disease condition.

immunization A process by which resistance to an infectious disease is induced or increased.

immunocompetence/immunocompetent The ability of an immune system to mobilize and deploy its antibodies and other responses to stimulation by an antigen.

immunodeficiency An abnormal condition of the immune system in which cellular or humoral immunity is inadequate and resistance to infection is increased.

immunogen Any agent or substance capable of provoking an immune response or producing immunity.

immunology Study of the immune system; the reaction of tissues of the immune system of the body of antigenic stimulation.

immunosuppression/immunosuppressive Administration of agents that significantly interfere with the ability of the immune system to respond to antigenic stimulation by inhibiting cellular and humoral immunity.

immunosurveillance The immune system's recognition and destruction of newly developed abnormal cells.

immunotherapy A special treatment of allergic responses; involves the administration of increasingly larger doses of the offending allergens to gradually develop immunity.

incentive spirometry A procedure in which a device (spirometer) is used at the bedside at regular intervals to encourage a patient to breathe deeply.

incision Surgical cut produced by a sharp instrument to create an opening into an organ or space in the body.

infarct Localized area of necrosis in tissue, a vessel, or an organ resulting from tissue anoxia; caused by an interruption in the blood supply to an area.

informed consent Permission obtained from the patient to perform a specific test or procedure.

innate immunity The body's first line of defense; provides physical and chemical barriers to invading pathogens and protects the body against the external environment.

integrative Care is the assimilation of complementary therapies into conventional medical care.

intermittent claudication A weakness of the legs accompanied by cramplike pains in the calves; caused by poor arterial circulation of the blood to the leg muscles.

intraoperative Pertaining to a period of time during a surgical procedure.

intrinsic Caused by internal factors.

introitus An entrance to a cavity (e.g., the vaginal introitus).

intussusception Infolding of one segment of the intestine into the lumen of another segment; occurs in children.

ischemia Decreased blood supply to a body organ or part, often marked by pain and organ dysfunction.

J

jaundice Yellowish discoloration of the skin, mucous membranes, and sclera of the eyes caused by greater than normal amounts of bilirubin in the blood.

K

Kaposi sarcoma (KS) Rare cancer of the skin or mucous membranes; characterized by blue, red, or purple raised lesions and seen mainly in middle-aged Mediterranean men and those with HIV disease.

Kegel exercises A series of contraction movements to the musculature of the perineum. The movements are intended to strengthen the pelvic floor.

keloids Overgrowths of collagenous scar tissue at the site of a skin wound.

keratitis An inflammation of the cornea.

keratoplasty Excision of the corneal tissue, followed by surgical implantation of a cornea from another human donor.

keratotomy A surgical procedure to correct myopia. The procedure involves making tiny incisions into the outer ring of the cornea.

ketoacidosis Acidosis accompanied by an accumulation of ketone in the blood resulting from faulty carbohydrate metabolism.

ketone bodies Normal metabolic products, beta-hydroxybutyric and aminoacetic acid, from which acetone may spontaneously arise.

kyphosis An abnormal condition of the vertebral column; characterized by increased convexity in the curvature of the thoracic spine.

L

labyrinthitis Inflammation of the labyrinthine canals of the inner ear.

laparoscopy The examination of the abdominal cavity with a laparoscope through a small incision beneath the umbilicus.

leukemia Malignant disorder of the hematopoietic system in which an excess of leukocytes accumulates in the bone marrow and lymph nodes.

leukopenia An abnormal decrease in the number of white blood cells to fewer than 5000 cells/mm^3 due to depression of the bone marrow.

leukoplakia A white patch in the mouth or on the tongue.

lipodystrophy Abnormality in the metabolism or deposition of fats. Insulin lipodystrophy is the loss of local fat deposits in diabetic patients as a complication of repeated insulin injections.

lipohypertrophy An abnormal mass under the subcutaneous tissue of the abdomen. It is associated with repeated insulin injections.

lordosis An increase in the curve at the lumbar space region that throws the shoulder back, making the appearance "lordly or kingly."

lumen Space within an artery, vein, intestine, or tube such as a needle or catheter.

lymphangitis Inflammation of one or more lymphatic vessels or channels; usually results from an acute streptococcal or staphylococcal infection in an extremity.

lymphedema Primary or secondary disorder characterized by the accumulation of lymph in soft tissue and edema.

lymphokine One of the chemical factors produced and released by T lymphocytes that attract macrophages to the site of infection or inflammation and prepare them for attack.

M

macules Small, flat, discolored blemishes; flush with the skin surface.

malignant Growing worse, resisting treatment; said of cancerous growths. Also tending or threatening to produce death; harmful.

mammography Radiography of the soft tissue of the breast to allow identification of various benign and neoplastic processes.

mastoiditis Infection of one of the mastoid bones.

melena Abnormal, black, tarry stool containing digested blood.

membrane Thin sheet of tissue that serves many functions in the body; it covers surfaces, lines and lubricates hollow organs, and protects and anchors organs and bones.

menorrhagia Excessive menstrual flow.

metastasis The process by which tumor cells are spread to distant parts of the body.

metrorrhagia Excessive spotting between cycles.

micturition Urination.

miotic Causing constriction of the pupil of the eye.

mitosis Type of cell division of somatic (i.e., nonreproductive) cells in which each daughter cell contains the same number of chromosomes as the parent cell.

MUGA scanning A nuclear medicine scan that is used to photograph the heart.

multiple myeloma A malignant neoplastic immunodeficiency disease of the bone marrow; the tumor is composed of plasma cells.

mydriatic Causing pupillary dilation.

myeloproliferative Excessive bone marrow production.

myocardial infarction An occlusion of a major coronary artery or one of its branches; it is caused by atherosclerosis or an embolus resulting in necrosis of a portion of cardiac muscle.

myopia Condition of nearsightedness; inability to see objects at a distance.

myringotomy A surgical incision of the tympanic membrane to relieve pressure and release purulent exudate from the middle ear.

N

neoplasm Uncontrolled or abnormal growth of cells.

nephrotoxin Substances with specific destructive properties for the kidneys, such as certain antibiotics, heavy metals, solvents, and chemicals.

neuropathy Any abnormal condition characterized by inflammation and degeneration of the peripheral nerves.

nevi Pigmented, congenital skin blemishes that are usually benign but may become cancerous.

nocturia Excessive urination at night.

nucleus Largest organelle within the cell; it is responsible for cell reproduction and control of the other organelles.

nystagmus Involuntary, rhythmic movement of the eyes. Oscillations may be horizontal, vertical, rotary, or mixed.

O

occlusion An obstruction or closing off in a canal, vessel, or passage of the body.

occult blood Blood that is hidden or obscured from view.

oliguria A diminished capacity to form and pass urine (less than 500 mL in 24 hours); result is that the end products of metabolism cannot be excreted efficiently.

oncology The sum of knowledge regarding tumors; the branch of medicine that deals with the study of tumors.

open reduction with internal fixation (ORIF) A surgical procedure allowing fracture alignment under direct visualization while using various internal fixation devices applied to the bone.

opportunistic Disease characteristic caused by a normally nonpathogenic organism in a host whose resistance has been decreased by a disorder such as AIDS.

organ A group of several different kinds of tissue arranged so that they can work together to perform a special function.

orthopnea An abnormal condition in which a person must sit or stand to breathe deeply or comfortably.

osmosis Passage of water across a selectively permeable membrane; the water moves from a less concentrated solution to a more concentrated solution.

oxygen saturation Measurement of how much oxygen has combined with hemoglobin in the red blood cell

P

palliative Designed to relieve pain and distress and to control the signs and symptoms of disease; not designed to produce a cure.

pancytopenia Deficient condition of all three major blood elements (red cells, white cells, and platelets); results from the bone marrow being reduced or absent.

panhysterosalpingo-oophorectomy Removal of the uterus, fallopian tubes, and ovaries. Also called *total abdominal hysterectomy with bilateral salpingo-oophorectomy.*

Papanicolaou test (Pap smear) A simple smear method of examining stained exfoliative cells; used most commonly to detect cancers of the cervix.

papules Palpable, circumscribed, red solid elevations in the skin; smaller than 0.5 cm.

paracentesis A procedure in which fluid is withdrawn from the abdominal cavity.

paralytic (adynamic) ileus Most common type of intestinal obstruction; a decrease in or absence of intestinal peristalsis and bowel sounds that may occur after abdominal surgery.

parenchyma Tissue of an organ as distinguished from supporting or connective tissue.

paresis A lesser degree of movement deficit from partial or incomplete paralysis.

paresthesia Any subjective sensation, such as a prickling "pins and needles" feeling or numbness.

passive transport The movement of small molecules across the membrane of a cell by diffusion; no cellular energy is required.

pathognomonic Sign or symptom specific to a disease condition.

pediculosis Lice infestation.

perimenopause The changes in the female body that lead the transition into menopause. Symptoms may include hot flashes, impaired sleep patterns, and weight gain.

perioperative Entire surgical inpatient period occurring immediately before, during, and immediately after surgery.

peripheral Pertaining to the outside, surface, or surrounding area of an organ, other structure, or field of vision.

pernicious Capable of causing great injury or destruction; deadly, fatal.

pessary A device that can be inserted into the vagina to support the bladder and reduce pressure on the bladder from the uterus in cases of prolapse.

phagocytic Refers to the ingestion and digestion of bacteria.

phagocytosis The process that permits a cell to surround or engulf any foreign material and digest it.

phimosis A condition in which the prepuce is too small to allow retraction of the foreskin over the glans penis.

photocoagulation Use of a laser beam to destroy new blood vessels, seal leaking vessels, and help prevent retinal edema.

physiology Explanation of the processes and functions of the various structures of the body and how they interrelate.

pinocytosis The process by which extracellular fluid is ingested by the cells.

plasmapheresis Removal of plasma that contains components causing or thought to cause disease. Also called *plasma exchange* because when the plasma is removed, it is replaced by substitution fluids such as saline or albumin.

pleural effusion An abnormal accumulation of fluid in the thoracic cavity between the visceral and parietal pleurae.

pleural friction rub Low-pitched, grating, or creaking lung sounds that occur when inflamed pleural surfaces rub together during respiration.

Pneumocystis jiroveci **(formerly** *carinii***) pneumonia (PCP)** An unusual pulmonary disease caused by a parasite that is primarily associated with people who have suppressed immune systems, especially in people with AIDS.

pneumothorax A collection of air or gas in the pleural space, causing the lung to collapse.

polycythemia Abnormal increase in the number of red blood cells in the blood.

polydipsia Excessive thirst.

polyphagia Eating to the point of gluttony.

polyuria Excretion of an abnormally large quantity of urine.

postictal period A rest period of variable length after a tonic-clonic seizure.

postoperative Pertaining to a period of time after surgery.

preoperative Pertaining to a period of time before surgery.

procidentia Protrusion of the entire uterus through the introitus.

proliferation Reproduction or multiplication of similar forms.

proning Turning the patient to a prone position for better posterior lung field ventilation and clearing of secretions

proprioception Sensation pertaining to stimuli originating from within the body regarding spatial position and muscular activity stimuli or to the sensory receptors that those stimuli activate. This sensation gives one the ability to know the position of the body without looking at it and the ability to "know the sense of touch objectively."

prostatodynia Pain in the prostate gland.

prosthesis Artificial replacement for a missing body part.

pruritus The symptoms of itching; an uncomfortable sensation leading to the urge to scratch; scratching often leads to secondary infection. Some causes of pruritus are allergy, infection, elevated serum urea, jaundice, and skin irritation.

pulmonary edema Accumulation of extravascular fluid in lung tissues and alveoli; caused most commonly by left-sided heart failure.

pulse oximeter Device used to measure the oxygen saturation

pustulant vesicles Small, circumscribed pus-containing elevations of the skin.

pyuria Pus in the urine.

Q

quarks The building blocks of protons and neutrons that comprise the atom.

R

radial keratotomy Microscopic incisions on the surface of the cornea outside the optical area. These eight spokelike incisions flatten the cornea to a more normal curvature, thus reducing or eliminating myopia.

Reed-Sternberg cells Atypical histocytes; large, abnormal, multinucleated cells in the lymphatic system, found in Hodgkin lymphoma.

refraction Light rays are bent as they pass through the colorless structures of the eye, enabling light from the environment to focus on the retina.

remission A decrease in the severity of a disease or any of its symptoms.

renal colic Abdominal pain that is associated with disorders of the kidney.

residual urine Urine remaining in the urinary tract after voiding.

retention The inability to void even in the presence of an urge to void.

retinal detachment Separation of the retina from the choroid in the posterior of the eye.

retrovirus Lentivirus that contains reverse transcriptase, which is essential for reverse transcription (the production of a deoxyribonucleic acid [DNA] molecule from a ribonucleic acid [RNA] model).

rule of nines Division of the body into multiples of nine; used to determine the total body surface area (BSA) involved in burn trauma.

S

saline infusion ultrasound Facilitates visualization of the uterus by infusing saline through a small catheter.

sarcoma Malignant tumor of connective tissues such as muscle or bone; usually presents as a painless swelling.

sclerotherapy Chemicals used to cause inflammation, followed by fibrosis and destruction of the vessels causing the bleeding.

scoliosisCurvature of the spine usually consisting of two curves: Curvature of the spine usually consisting of two curves:the original abnormal curve and a compensatory curve in the opposite direction.

sentinel lymph node mapping Diagnostic tool used before therapeutic surgery, which identifies the first lymph node most likely to drain cancerous cells; used in axillary lymph node biopsy, specifically in breast cancer staging.

sequestrum A fragment of necrotic bone that is partially or entirely detached from the surrounding or adjacent healthy bone.

seroconversion The development of detectable levels of antibodies; a change in serologic tests (e.g., ELISA and Western blot) from negative to positive as antibodies develop in reaction to an infection.

seronegative Negative result on serologic examination. The state of lacking HIV antibodies; confirmed by blood tests.

seroprevalence The overall frequency of findings of a disorder in a population as determined by blood testing.

sibilant wheeze Musical, high-pitched, squeaking, or whistlelike sound caused by the rapid movement of air through narrowed bronchioles.

singultus Hiccup.

Sjögren syndrome Dry eye syndrome; an immunologic disorder characterized by low fluid production by lacrimal (tear), salivary, and other glands, resulting in abnormal dryness of mouth, eyes, and other mucous membranes.

Snellen's test Eye chart test for visual acuity; letters, numbers, or symbols are arranged on the chart in decreasing size from top to bottom.

sonorous wheeze Low-pitched, loud, coarse, snoring sound.

spastic Involuntary, sudden movements or muscular contractions with increased reflexes.

spider telangiectases Dilated superficial arterioles.

stapedectomy The removal of the stapes of the middle ear and insertion of a graft and prosthesis.

steatorrhea Excessive fat in the feces.

stertorous Pertaining to a respiratory effort that is strenuous and struggling, which provokes a snoring sound.

stoma Combining form meaning a mouth or opening.

stomatitis Inflammation of the mouth due to destruction of normal cells of the oral cavity that may result from infection by bacteria, viruses, or fungi from exposure to certain chemicals or drugs, vitamin deficiency, or systemic inflammatory disease.

strabismus Condition in which the eyes are unable to focus in the same direction. Also called cross-eyed.

stroke An abnormal condition of the blood vessels of the brain characterized by hemorrhage into the brain; formation of an embolus or thrombus resulting in ischemia of the brain tissues normally perfused by the damaged vessels. The sequelae depend on the location and extent of ischemia.

subluxation Partial dislocation.

suppuration To produce purulent material.

surgery Branch of medicine concerned with diseases and trauma requiring operative procedures.

surgical asepsis A group of techniques that destroy all microorganisms and their spores (sterile technique).

system An organization of varying numbers and kinds of organs arranged so that they can work together to perform complex functions for the body.

T

tachycardia An abnormal condition in which the myocardium contracts regularly but at a rate greater than 100 beats per minute.

tachypnea An abnormally rapid rate of breathing.

tenesmus Persistent, ineffectual spasms of the rectum or bladder, accompanied by the desire to empty the bowel or bladder.

thoracentesis The surgical perforation of the chest wall and pleural space with a needle for the aspiration of fluid for diagnostic or therapeutic purposes.

thrombocytopenia An abnormal hematologic condition in which the number of platelets is reduced to fewer than $100,000/mm^3$.

thrombus Of or pertaining to a clot.

tinnitus A subjective noise sensation in one or both ears; ringing or tinkling sound in the ear.

tissue An organization of many similar cells that act together to perform a common function.

tophi Calculi containing sodium urate deposits that develop in periarticular fibrous tissue; typically found in patients with gout.

trichomoniasis A sexually transmitted disease caused by the protozoan Trichomonas vaginalis.

Trousseau sign A test for latent tetany in which carpal spasms are induced by inflating a sphygmomanometer cuff on the upper arm to a pressure exceeding systolic blood pressure for 3 minutes; used in hypocalcemia and hypomagnesemia.

tumor lysis syndrome Oncologic emergency that occurs with rapid lysis of malignant cells; most frequently associated with chemotherapy treatment. It is most commonly a result of treatment-related malignant cell death in patients with large tumor cell burdens.

turgor The normal resiliency of the skin caused by the outward pressure of the cells and interstitial fluid; may be assessed as increased or decreased skin turgor.

tympanoplasty One of several operative procedures on the eardrum or ossicles of the middle ear designed to restore or improve hearing in patients with conductive hearing loss.

type 1 diabetes mellitus Condition in which impaired glucose tolerance results because of destruction of beta cells in the pancreatic islets; results in deficient insulin production, but the patient retains normal sensitivity to insulin action. Also called insulin-dependent diabetes mellitus.

type 2 diabetes mellitus Condition in which impaired glucose tolerance results from an abnormal resistance to insulin action. Also called non–insulin-dependent diabetes mellitus.

U

unconscious bias An inherent decision-making shortcut that nearly all people possess as a part of brain efficiency.

unilateral neglect Condition in which an individual is perceptually unaware of and inattentive to one side of the body.

urinary retention The inability to empty the bladder completely.

urolithiasis Formation of urinary calculi.

urticaria Itching skin eruption characterized by welts of varying sizes with well-defined inflamed margins and pale centers. Also called *hives*.

V

vapotherm Noninvasive, mask-free high-flow oxygen delivery device delivering up to 40L/min

ventral Facing forward; the front of the body.

verruca Benign, viral, warty skin lesion with a rough, papillomatous (nipplelike) growth.

vertical transmission Transmission of HIV from a mother to a fetus; can occur during pregnancy, during delivery, or through postpartum breastfeeding.

vertigo The sensation that the outer world is revolving about oneself or that one is moving in space.

vesicle Circumscribed elevation of skin filled with serous fluid.

viral load Amount of measurable HIV virions.

virulent Having the power to produce disease; of or pertaining to a very pathogenic or rapidly progressive condition.

vitrectomy The removal of excess vitreous fluid caused by hemorrhage and replacement with normal saline.

Volkmann contracture A permanent contracture with clawhand, flexion of wrist and finger, and atrophy of the forearm; can occur as a result of compartment syndrome.

volvulus Twisting of the bowel on itself, causing intestinal obstruction.

W

wasting The loss of lean body mass as a result of illness.

Western blot A laboratory blood test to detect the presence of antibodies to a specific antigen; used in diagnosing HIV.

wheals Irregularly shaped, elevated areas, white in the center with a pale red periphery, with superficial localized edema; vary in size (hives, mosquito bite).

Index

O

Oat cell cancer, 416
Obesity
  breast cancer and, 577b
  cardiac disease and, 313
  and obstructive sleep apnea, 390
  peripheral vascular disorders and, 350
Obstruction
  ear, 646
  intestinal, 214–222, 214f, 218f
  urinary, 459
Obstruction series (flat plate of abdomen), 180
Obstructive sleep apnea (OSA), 389–390
Occlusion, 249
Occult blood, 179, 789
Occupational exposures
  to HIV, 744–745, 772–773
  recommendations for preventing allergic reactions to latex, 733
Occupational Safety and Health Administration (OSHA), 732
Occupational therapist, 678
Octreotide (Sandostatin), 493
Oculomotor nerve (cranial nerve III), 661f, 662t, 666, 673–674
Ofloxacin, 403, 458, 597–598
Oil (sebaceous glands), 57
Older adults
  blood disorders in, 294b
  cancer in, 778b
  cardiac disease in, 311b
  chronic constipation in, 220b
  diabetes mellitus in, 525b
  endocrine disorders in, 525b
  gallbladder, liver, biliary tract, or exocrine pancreas disorders in, 248b
  gastrointestinal disorders in, 213b
  HIV disease in, 741b
  immune disorders in, 728b
  integumentary system, 101b
  lymphatic disorders in, 294b
  musculoskeletal disorders in, 137b
  nervous system in, 663b
  obstructive sleep apnea in, 390
  reproductive disorders in, 543b
  respiratory disorders in, 408b
  surgical care for, 17b
  urinary disorders in, 440b
Olfactory nerve (cranial nerve I), 661f, 662t, 666
Oliguria, 465, 471
Olsalazine, 190t–191t
Omeprazole, 184, 190t–191t
Oncology, 776–778
Ondansetron (Zofran), 796
Ondansetron HCl (5-HT3 receptor antagonist), 34t
One-day (same-day) surgery, 16t, 17b
Open mitral commissurotomy, 344

Open reduction with internal fixation (ORIF), 141–142, 141b
Open surgical biopsy, 547
Open-lung biopsy, 383–384
Operating room, 40, 40f
  transport to, 40
Operative cholangiography, 227–228
Ophthalmologic examination, 631–632
Opioids, 799–800
Opportunistic infections, 741, 755, 755b, 767–768
Optic disc, 610, 610f
Optic disc cupping, 629, 629f
Optic nerve (cranial nerve II), 610, 661f, 662t, 666
Oral airway, 36, 36f
Oral cancer, 181–183, 183t
Oral candidiasis, 762, 764f, 766t
Oral contraceptives, 552, 553t–554t, 600t–602t
Oral corticosteroids, 397
Oral glucose tolerance test, 516b
Oral hypoglycemics, 531, 532t
Oral supplements, 99
OraQuick test, 769
Organ of Corti, 637
Organ systems, 11, 11t–12t
Organs, 4, 11, 11t–12t
Orientation assessment, 664
Oropharyngeal cancer, 181
Oropharynx, 376, 376f
Orthopedic assessment
  nursing process, 166–167
  rapid, 139–141
  seven Ps of, 139
Orthopnea, 336, 370, 380–381
OSA. See Obstructive sleep apnea
Osmolality, urine, 442
Osmosis, 8, 8t, 9f
Osmotic diuretics, 445
Osteoarthritis (OA, degenerative joint disease), 113–114, 116t, 122–124, 123b
  complementary and alternative therapies for, 124b
  joints most frequently involved in, 122, 123f
Osteochondroma, 163
Osteogenic sarcoma, 163
Osteogenic tumors, 163
Osteomyelitis, 129
Osteopenia, 127
Osteoporosis, 126–128, 126f, 127b
  cultural considerations, 127b
  diagnostic tests for, 126–127
  dietary needs in, 128b
  medications for, 127, 128t
  nursing interventions for, 128, 128t
  patient teaching for, 128, 128b
  surgical interventions for, 127
  type 1 (postmenopausal), 126
  type 2 (senile), 126

Otitis externa, 641–642
Otitis media
  acute, 642–645
  nursing interventions for, 643–645, 643t
  patient teaching for, 643–645, 645b
  purulent, 642
Otosclerosis, 646–647
Otoscopy, 638
Outpatient (ambulatory) surgery, 16t, 17b
Ovarian cancer, 573–574
  nursing interventions for, 574, 574t
Ovarian cysts, 570
Ovaries, 489f, 539, 540f
  ablation of, 582
  palpable, 574
Overactive bladder, 451
Overflow incontinence, 451
Over-the-counter decongestants, 397
Over-the-counter pain relievers, 397
Oviducts, 539
Ovulation, drugs to induce, 560–561
Oxaliplatin (Eloxatin), 795t–796t
Oxcarbazepine, 683t
Oxybutynin, 449–450, 452
Oxycodone-acetaminophen, 74
Oxygen
  arterial saturation (SaO_2), 384–385
  arterial tension (PaO_2), 384–385
Oxygen therapy
  for asthma, 429
  for bronchiectasis, 430
  home care considerations, 425b
  for increased ICP, 675
  for myocardial infarction, 329
  for pneumonia, 408
  for pulmonary edema, 342t
Oxymetazoline, 397, 403t–405t
Oxytocin, 489, 490f

P

P wave, 306, 307f
Pacemakers
  artificial, 314f–315f, 320
  sinoatrial node, 302f
Pacing, ventricular, 314f
Packed red blood cells, 268
Paclitaxel (Taxol, Abraxane), 186, 795t–796t
$PaCO_2$. See Partial pressure of carbon dioxide in blood
Pain
  angina pectoris, 322–323, 322f
  assessment of, 369
  back, 124f
  medications for, 670–671
  myocardial, 322–323, 322f, 327
  myofascial, 130
  neuropathic, 672–673, 673t
  phantom, 165
  postoperative, 33